DIFFICULT DIAGNOSIS

2

DIFFICULT DIAGNOSIS

2

ROBERT B. TAYLOR, M.D.

Professor and Chairman
Department of Family Medicine
The Oregon Health Sciences University
School of Medicine
Portland, Oregon

W.B. SAUNDERS COMPANY
Harcourt Brace Jovanovich, Inc.
PHILADELPHIA • LONDON • TORONTO • MONTREAL • SYDNEY • TOKYO

W. B. SAUNDERS COMPANY
Harcourt Brace Jovanovich, Inc.

The Curtis Center
Independence Square West
Philadelphia, Pennsylvania 19106

Library of Congress Cataloging-in-Publication Data

Difficult diagnosis 2 / [edited by] Robert B. Taylor.
      p.   cm.
    ISBN 0-7216-3481-8
    1. Diagnosis.   I. Taylor, Robert B.   II. Title: Difficult
diagnosis 2.
    [DNLM: 1. Diagnosis.   WB 141 D569]
RC71.D54   1992
616.07′5—dc20
DNLM/DLC   91-27416

Editor: John Dyson

DIFFICULT DIAGNOSIS   2   ISBN   0-7216-3481-8

Printed in Mexico

Last digit is the print number: 9   8   7   6   5   4   3   2   1

CONTRIBUTORS

JØRN AAGAARD, M.D.
Section of Urology, University of Wisconsin School of Medicine, Madison, Wisconsin.
Dysuria

TIMOTHY R. AKSAMIT, M.D.
Clinical Associate, Division of Pulmonary Diseases, Department of Medicine, University of Iowa; Staff, Division of Pulmonary and Critical Care Medicine, University of Iowa Hospitals and Clinics, Iowa City, Iowa.
Clubbing

CLARK W. ANTONSON, M.D.
Assistant Professor, Division of Gastroenterology, Department of Medicine, Kansas University Medical School, Kansas City, Kansas; Department of Gastroenterology, Kansas City Veterans Administration Medical Center, Kansas City, Missouri.
Hematochezia

STEPHEN M. AYRES, M.D.
Dean, School of Medicine, Professor, Department of Internal Medicine, Virginia Commonwealth University, Medical College of Virginia, Richmond, Virginia.
Tachypnea

TERESITA BACANI-OROPILLA, M.D.
Associate Professor, Department of Psychiatry and Behavioral Sciences, University of Louisville School of Medicine; Physician in Charge, Mental Health Clinic, Veterans Administration Medical Center, Louisville, Kentucky.
Hallucinations

SAMI L. BAHNA, M.D., Dr. P.H.
Chief of Pediatric Allergy, Immunology Division, Professor, Departments of Pediatrics and Medicine, East Tennessee State University College of Medicine, Johnson City, Tennessee.
Food Allergy and Intolerance

LAWRENCE D. BAILEY, JR., M.D.
Lee County Community Hospital, Pennington Gap, Virginia; Holston Valley Hospital, Kingsport, Tennessee.
Abdominal Pain, Chronic

GEORGE L. BAKRIS, M.D., F.A.C.P., F.C.P.
Assistant Professor, Division of Nephrology, Departments of Medicine and Pharmacology, University of Texas Health Sciences Center; University of Texas Medical Center; Audie Murphy Veterans Administration Hospital, San Antonio, Texas.
Secondary Hypertension

JEFFREY L. BARNETT, M.D.
Assistant Professor, Division of Gastroenterology, Department of Internal Medicine, University of Michigan; University Hospitals; Veterans Administration Hospital, Ann Arbor, Michigan.
Intestinal Bloating and Gas

MARY K. BEARD, M.D., F.A.C.O.G.
Assistant Clinical Professor, Department of Obstetrics and Gynecology, University of Utah School of Medicine, LDS Hospital, Salt Lake City, Utah.
Dyspareunia

SCOTT D. BENNION, M.S., M.D., F.A.C.P., F.A.A.D.
Immunodermatologist, Department of Dermatology, Fitzsimons Army Medical Center, Aurora; Assistant Clinical Professor, Dermatology Service, Department of Internal Medicine, University of Colorado School of Medicine, Denver, Colorado.
Vesiculobullous Disorders

PATRICIA BLUMENREICH, M.D.
Assistant Professor, Department of Psychiatry and Behavioral Sciences, University of Louisville School of Medicine; Staff Psychiatrist, Veterans Administration Medical Center, Louisville, Kentucky.
Hallucinations

KANCHANA BOONSANER, M.D.
Bhumipol Adulyadej Hospital; Chantrarubeksa Hospital, Thailand; Arthritis Immunology Center, Veterans Administration Medical Center, Philadelphia, Pennsylvania.
Hyperuricemia

LENORE J. BRANCATO, M.D.
Clinical Instructor, Division of Rheumatic Diseases, Department of Medicine, Mount Sinai School of Medicine; Director, Center for Lyme Disease; Rheumatory Associate, Division of Rheumatic Diseases, Hospital for Joint Diseases; Clinical Instructor, Department of Medicine, Beth Israel Medical Center, New York, New York.
Polyarticular Arthritis

JAMES K. BREDENKAMP, M.D.
Staff Physician, Saddleback Hospital, Laguna Hills; Staff Physician, Mission Hospital, Mission Viejo, California.
Hearing Loss, Sudden

ALEX H. BRUCKSTEIN, M.D.
Staff Physician, St. Vincent's Medical Center of Richmond, Staten Island; Clinical Associate Professor, Division of Gastroenterology, Department of Medicine, New York Medical College, Valhalla, New York.
Cholestasis; Diarrhea, Acute

STEPHEN A. BRUNTON, M.D.
Associate Clinical Professor, Department of Family Medicine, University of California School of Medicine—Irvine; Director, Department of Family Medicine, Medical Director, Department of Health Promotion, Long Beach Memorial Medical Center, Long Beach, California.
Weight Gain

JOEL N. BUXBAUM, M.D.
Professor, Section of Rheumatology, Department of Medicine, New York University School of Medicine; Chief of Rheumatology, New York Department of Veterans Administration Medical Center, New York, New York.
Polyarticular Arthritis

NANCY CARPENTER, R.D.
Department of Family Medicine, Long Beach Memorial Medical Center, Long Beach, California.
Weight Gain

BLANCHE M. CHAVERS, M.D.
Associate Professor, Nephrology Division, Department of Pediatrics, University of Minnesota School of Medicine, Minneapolis, Minnesota.
Proteinuria

ROLAND B. CHRISTIAN, M.D.
Assistant Professor, Division of Gastroenterology, Department of Medicine, Kansas University Medical School, Kansas City, Kansas; Westside Clinic, Department of Gastroenterology, Hospital Division, Green Bay, Wisconsin.
Hematochezia

JOHN P. CONOMY, M.D.
Chairman, Department of Neurology, The Cleveland Clinic Foundation, Cleveland, Ohio.
Amnesia

MARK J. COOK, M.B., B.S., F.R.A.C.P.
Clinical Research Fellow, The National Hospital for Nervous Diseases, London, United Kingdom.
Ataxia

ALBERT J. CZAJA, M.D.
Professor, Division of Gastroenterology, Department of Medicine, Mayo Medical School; Consultant, Department of Gastroenterology, Mayo Medical Clinic; Staff Consultant, Rochester Methodist Hospital; Staff Consultant, Saint Mary's Hospital, Rochester, Minnesota.
Hepatomegaly

MARILYN DOYLE, M.D.
Assistant Professor, Division of Infectious Diseases, Department of Pediatrics, University of Texas Medical School; Herman Hospital; M. D. Anderson Hospital and Tumor Institute; Lyndon Baines Johnson General Hospital, Houston, Texas.
Fever in Childhood

MITCHELL D. DRUCKER, M.D.
Assistant Professor, Departments of Ophthalmology and Neurology, University of Florida College of Medicine; Chief of Ophthalmology, Tampa Veterans Administration Hospital; Chief of Ophthalmology, Tampa General Hospital, Tampa, Florida.
Visual Loss, Unilateral

DANIEL A. DUMESIC, M.D.
Assistant Professor, Division of Reproductive Endocrinology, Department of Obstetrics and Gynecology, University of Wisconsin School of Medicine, Madison, Wisconsin.
Pelvic Mass in the Female Patient

EDWIN C. EVERTS, M.D.
Professor, Department of Otolaryngology/Head and Neck Surgery, Oregon Health Sciences University School of Medicine; Oregon Health Sciences University Hospitals; Oregon Veterans Administration Hospital, Portland, Oregon.
Hoarseness

LOUISE FERRAROTTO, B.S.C.
Research Associate, Division of Urology, Veterans Administration Medical Center, Northport, New York.
Scrotal Pain

ROBERT B. FICK, JR., M.D.
Associate Professor, Division of Pulmonary and Critical Care Medicine, Department of Internal Medicine, University of Iowa College of Medicine; University of Iowa Hospitals and Clinics, Iowa City, Iowa.
Clubbing

SCOTT A. FIELDS, M.D.
Assistant Professor, Department of Family Medicine, Oregon Health Sciences University School of Medicine; Oregon Health Sciences University Hospitals, Portland, Oregon.
Anorexia

JAMES E. FITZPATRICK, M.D.
Chief, Dermatology Service, Fitzsimons Army Medical Center, Aurora; Associate Clinical Professor, Department of Dermatology, University of Colorado Health Sciences Center School of Medicine, Denver, Colorado.
Vesiculobullous Disorders

FRANK J. FRASSICA, M.D.
Assistant Professor, Department of Orthopedics, Mayo Medical School; Department of Orthopedics, Mayo Clinic and Mayo Foundation, Rochester, Minnesota.
Bone Pain

STANLEY A. GALL, M.D.
The Donald E. Baxter Professor and Chairman, Department of Obstetrics and Gynecology, University of Louisville School of Medicine; Chairman, Department of Obstetrics and Gynecology, Humana Hospital—University of Louisville; Attending Physician, Norton Hospital, Louisville, Kentucky.
Pap Smear, Abnormal

MARK A. GETZ, M.D.

Rheumatology Section, Department of Internal Medicine, University of Wisconsin School of Medicine; University of Wisconsin Hospital and Clinics, Madison, Wisconsin.

Lymphadenopathy

A. JAMES GIANNINI, M.D.

Clinical Professor, Department of Psychiatry, Ohio State University School of Medicine, Columbus, Ohio; Corporate Medical Director, Chemical Abuse Centers, Incorporated, Youngstown, Ohio.

Fatigue, Chronic

ROBERT N. GOLDEN, M.D.

Associate Professor, Department of Psychiatry, University of North Carolina School of Medicine; Associate Director, University of North Carolina General Clinical Research Center; Attending Physician, University of North Carolina Neuropsychiatric Hospital, Chapel Hill, North Carolina.

Insomnia

NORA GOLDSCHLAGER, M.D.

Professor, Division of Cardiology, Department of Medicine, University of California School of Medicine; Director, Coronary Care Unit, San Francisco General Hospital, San Francisco, California.

Bradycardia

FRANK M. GRAZIANO, M.D., Ph.D.

Professor, Division of Rheumatology, Department of Medicine, University of Wisconsin Medical School; Chief, Rheumatology Section, University of Wisconsin Hospital and Clinics, Madison, Wisconsin.

Lymphadenopathy

FREDERICK L. GREENE, M.D.

Professor, Director of Surgical Oncology, Department of Surgery, University of South Carolina School of Medicine; Chief of Surgery, Richland Memorial Hospital, Columbia, South Carolina.

Breast Lump

TRACY D. GUNTER, M.D.

Department of Surgery, University of South Carolina School of Medicine, Columbia, South Carolina.

Breast Lump

JAMES M. HAGAR, M.D.

Clinical Instructor, Section of Cardiology, Department of Medicine, University of Southern California School of Medicine, Los Angeles, California.

Systolic Murmurs

RALPH R. HALL, M.D.

Senior Vice-President of Medical Affairs, Long Beach Memorial Medical Center, Long Beach, California.

Weight Gain

JOE G. HARDIN, JR., M.D.
Professor, Division of Rheumatology, Department of Medicine, University of South Alabama College of Medicine, Mobile, Alabama.
Antinuclear Antibody, Positive Titer

ROBERT I. HENKIN, M.D.
Taste and Smell Clinic, Washington, D.C.
Phantogeusia

GREGORY L. HOLMES, M.D.
Associate Professor, Department of Neurology, Harvard Medical School, Cambridge; Director, Clinical Neurophysiology Laboratory, Director, Epilepsy Program, Children's Hospital, Boston, Massachusetts.
Seizures in Childhood

LAURENE L. HOWELL, M.D.
Assistant Professor, Department of Otolaryngology/Head and Neck Surgery, Oregon Health Sciences University School of Medicine; Oregon Health Sciences University Hospitals; Oregon Veterans Administration Hospital, Portland, Oregon.
Hoarseness

ABDULMASSIH S. ISKANDRIAN, M.D.
Clinical Professor, Division of Cardiology, Department of Medicine, University of Pennsylvania; Co-director, Philadelphia Heart Institute, Presbyterian Medical Center, Philadelphia, Pennsylvania.
Chest Pain, Acute

THOMAS M. JULIAN, M.D.
Associate Professor and Director, Division of Gynecology, Department of Obstetrics and Gynecology, University of Wisconsin School of Medicine, Madison, Wisconsin.
Pelvic Mass in the Female Patient

D. M. KAJI, M.D.
Associate Professor, Renal Division, Department of Internal Medicine, Mount Sinai School of Medicine, New York; Staff Physician, Renal Section, Veterans Administration Medical Center, Bronx; Attending Physician, Mount Sinai Hospital, New York, New York.
Azotemia, Acute

JOYCE D. KALES, M.D.
Professor, Department of Psychiatry, Director, Sleep Research and Treatment Center, Pennsylvania State University College of Medicine, Hershey, Pennsylvania.
Sleepiness, Excessive

LEE D. KAUFMAN, M.D., F.A.C.P.
Assistant Professor, Division of Allergy, Rheumatology, and Clinical Immunology, Department of Medicine, State University of New York at Stony Brook School of Medicine; Attending Physician, University Hospital, Stony Brook; Attending Physician, Veterans Administration Medical Center, Northport, New York.
Polyarteritis

KENNETH M. KESSLER, M.D.

Professor, Department of Medicine, Associate Director, Division of Cardiology, University of Miami School of Medicine; Chief, Cardiology Section, Veterans Administration Medical Center, Miami, Florida.

Congestive Heart Failure

S. ALI KHAN, M.D., F.R.C.S. (C), F.A.C.S.

Associate Professor, Department of Urology, State University of New York at Stony Brook School of Medicine; Chief, Urology Service, Veterans Administration Medical Center, Northport; University Hospital, State University of New York at Stony Brook, Stony Brook, New York.

Scrotal Pain

ELLEN J. KILLEBREW, M.D.

Associate Clinical Professor, Division of Cardiology, Department of Medicine, University of California School of Medicine, San Francisco; Director, Coronary Care Unit, Kaiser-Permanente Medical Center, Oakland, California.

Bradycardia

ABBAS E. KITABCHI, M.D., Ph.D

Professor, Chief, Division of Endocrinology and Metabolism, Departments of Medicine and Biochemistry, Director, Clinical Research Center, University of Tennessee School of Medicine; Chief, Diabetes and Endocrine Services, Regional Medical Center; Consultant Endocrinologist, University of Tennessee Hospital; Baptist Memorial Hospital; St. Francis Hospital; LeBonhewr Children's Hospital; Veterans Administration Medical Center, Memphis, Tennessee.

Hypoglycemia

ROBERT A. KLONER, M.D., Ph.D.

Professor, Section of Cardiology, Department of Medicine, University of Southern California School of Medicine; Director, Research Department, Heart Institute, Hospital of the Good Samaritan, Los Angeles, California.

Systolic Murmurs

PHILLIP E. KORENBLAT, M.D.

Professor, Division of Allergy-Immunology, Department of Medicine, Washington University School of Medicine; Medical Director and Chief of Staff, Barnes West County Hospital; Attending Physician, Barnes Hospital; Attending Physician, The Jewish Hospital of St. Louis, St. Louis, Missouri.

Cough, Chronic

JOHN P. LAVERY, M.D.

Assistant Instructor, Division of Rheumatology, Department of Medicine, University of Texas Medical Branch, Galveston, Texas.

Raynaud's Phenomenon

GLEN A. LILLINGTON, M.D., F.R.C.P. (C), F.A.C.P.

Professor, Division of Pulmonary/Critical Care, Department of Medicine, University of California at Davis School of Medicine; Active Staff, University of California at Davis Medical Center, Sacramento, California.

Mediastinal Mass

STEVEN LIPPMANN, M.D.
Professor, Department of Psychiatry and Behavioral Sciences, University of Louisville School of Medicine; Medical Director, Psychiatric Services, Humana Hospital University of Louisville, Louisville, Kentucky.
Anxiety; Hallucinations

JEFFREY R. LISSE, M.D.
Associate Professor and Director, Division of Rheumatology, Department of Medicine, University of Texas Medical Branch, Galveston, Texas.
Raynaud's Phenomenon

WORAWIT LOUTHRENOO, M.D.
Assistant Professor, Department of Medicine, Chiang Mai University; Chief, Rheumatology Section, Department of Medicine, Chiang Mai University Hospital, Chiang Mai, Thailand.
Hyperuricemia

PAUL O. MADSEN, M.D.
Professor, Section of Urology, University of Wisconsin School of Medicine; Veterans Administration Hospital, Madison, Wisconsin.
Dysuria

MARY C. MAIER, M.D.
Staff Allergist/Immunologist, Central Hospital, Group Health Cooperative of Puget Sound, Seattle, Washington.
Food Allergy and Intolerance

ROCCO L. MANFREDI, M.D.
Assistant Professor, Department of Psychiatry, Director, Sleep Disorders Clinic, Pennsylvania State University College of Medicine, Hershey, Pennsylvania.
Sleepiness, Excessive

CURTIS E. MARGO, M.D.
Professor, Department of Ophthalmology, University of Florida College of Medicine, Gainesville, Florida.
Visual Loss, Unilateral

DAVID W. MARSLAND, M.D.
Professor and Chair, Department of Family Practice, Medical College of Virginia; Chief, Family Practice Service, Medical College of Virginia Hospital, Richmond, Virginia.
Tachypnea

E. WAYNE MASSEY, M.D., F.A.C.P.
Professor, Division of Neurology, Department of Medicine, Duke University School of Medicine; Duke University Medical Center, Durham, North Carolina.
Athetosis

PATRICK McBRIDE, M.D., M.P.H.
Assistant Professor, Departments of Medicine and Family Medicine and Practice, University of Wisconsin Medical School; Co-director, Preventive Cardiology Program, University Hospital and Clinics, University of Wisconsin, Madison, Wisconsin.
Hypercholesterolemia

RICHARD W. McCALLUM, M.D., F.A.C.P., F.R.A.C.P. (AUST), F.A.C.G.
Paul Jannsen Professor, Chief, Division of Gastroenterology, Department of Medicine, University of Virginia School of Medicine, Charlottesville; Director, Gastroenterology Training Programs, University of Virginia, Salem; Veterans Administration Medical Center, Salem; Roanoke Memorial Hospital, Roanoke, Virginia.
Abdominal Pain, Chronic

KAY F. McFARLAND, M.D.
Professor, Department of Medicine, University of South Carolina School of Medicine, Columbia, South Carolina.
Thyroid, Enlargement

DANIEL K. MILES, M.D.
Assistant Professor, Division of Neurology, Department of Pediatrics, Temple University School of Medicine, Philadelphia, Pennsylvania.
Seizures in Childhood

STEVEN A. MILES, M.D.
Assistant Professor, Division of Hematology/Oncology, Department of Medicine, University of California at Los Angeles School of Medicine, Los Angeles; University of California at Los Angeles AIDS Center, Los Angeles, California.
Human Immunodeficiency Virus Infection, Diagnosis, and Staging

J. DANIEL NELSON, M.D., F.A.C.S.
Associate Professor, Department of Ophthalmology, University of Minnesota Medical School; Chief, Department of Ophthalmology, St. Paul-Ramsey Medical Center; Staff Physician, University of Minnesota Hospitals, St. Paul, Minnesota.
Dry Eye

DAVID NEVIN, M.D.
Assistant Professor and Clinical Researcher, Department of Medicine, University of Wisconsin Medical School; University of Wisconsin Hospitals and Clinics, Madison, Wisconsin.
Hypercholesterolemia

J. ROBERT NEWLAND, D.D.S., M.S.
Associate Dean for Student Affairs, Professor, Department of Oral Diagnostic Sciences, University of Texas Health Science Center (Dental Branch), Houston, Texas.
Oral Ulcers

THACH N. NGUYEN, M.D.
Clinical Instructor, Section on Cardiology, Department of Medicine, University of Pennsylvania; Staff Cardiologist, Philadelphia Heart Institute, Presbyterian Medical Center, Philadelphia, Pennsylvania.
Chest Pain, Acute

PASCAL NICOD, M.D., F.A.C.C.

Professor, Department of Medicine, University of Lausanne School of Medicine; Director of Service B of Internal Medicine, Centre Hospitalier, Universitaire Vaudois, Lausanne, Switzerland.

Silent Myocardial Ischemia

PEADAR G. NOONE, M.B., M.R.C.P.I.

Pulmonary Division, Department of Medicine, Tufts University School of Medicine; New England Medical Center, Boston, Massachusetts.

Interstitial Pulmonary Disease

TIMOTHY T. NOSTRANT, M.D.

Associate Professor, Division of Gastroenterology, Department of Internal Medicine, University of Michigan School of Medicine; University Hospitals; Veterans Administration Hospital, Ann Arbor, Michigan.

Intestinal Bloating and Gas

SCOTT D. NYGAARD, M.D.

Division of Pulmonary and Critical Care Medicine, Department of Medicine, University of Iowa College of Medicine; University of Iowa Hospitals and Clinics, Iowa City, Iowa.

Clubbing

ANGELO S. PAOLA, M.D.

Department of Urology, West Virginia University Hospital, Morgantown, West Virginia.

Scrotal Pain

RAYMOND PARY, M.D.

Associate Professor, Department of Psychiatry and Behavioral Sciences, University of Louisville School of Medicine; Staff Psychiatrist, Veterans Administration Medical Center, Louisville, Kentucky.

Anxiety

RICHARD F. PEPPARD, M.B., B.S., F.R.A.C.P.

Clinical Instructor, St. Vincent's Hospital Clinical School, University of Melbourne; Neurologist, St. Vincent's Hospital, Melbourne, Australia.

Ataxia

DANA W. PETERSON, M.D.

Assistant Professor, Department of Family Medicine, Oregon Health Sciences University School of Medicine; Oregon Health Sciences University Hospitals, Portland, Oregon.

Anorexia

ANNE M. PITTMAN, M.D.

Instructor, Department of Medicine, Washington University School of Medicine; Attending Physician, Barnes Hospital, St. Louis, Missouri.

Cough, Chronic

STEVEN H. PURSELL, M.D.
Assistant Professor, Division of Gynecologic Oncology, Department of Obstetrics and Gynecology, University of Louisville School of Medicine; Humana Hospital—University of Louisville; Baptist East Hospital, Louisville, Kentucky.
Pap Smear, Abnormal

GEOFFREY P. REDMOND, M.D.
Head, Section of Pediatric and Adolescent Endocrinology, Department of Endocrinology, The Cleveland Clinic Foundation, Cleveland, Ohio.
Menstrual Dysfunction

JAMES B. RHODES, M.D.
Professor, Division of Gastroenterology, Department of Medicine, University of Kansas Medical School; University of Kansas Hospital, Kansas City, Kansas.
Hematochezia

FRANÇOIS RICOU, M.D.
Division of Cardiology, Department of Medicine, University of California School of Medicine, San Diego, California.
Silent Myocardial Ischemia

INGRAM M. ROBERTS, M.D.
Professor, Division of Gastroenterology, Department of Medicine, George Washington University School of Medicine; Attending Physician, Department of Internal Medicine and Gastroenterology, George Washington University Hospital, Washington, D.C.
Steatorrhea

GLENN S. RODRIGUEZ, M.D.
Assistant Professor, Department of Family Medicine, Oregon Health Sciences University School of Medicine; Oregon Health Sciences University Hospitals, Portland, Oregon.
Anorexia

PAUL C. ROUSSEAU, M.D.
Adjunct Professor, Department of Adult Development and Aging, Arizona State University, Tempe; Chief, Department of Geriatrics, Carl T. Haydin Veterans Administration Medical Center, Phoenix, Arizona.
Constipation, Chronic

MARK J. RUMBAK, M.D.
Assistant Professor, Division of Pulmonary and Critical Care Medicine, Department of Medicine, University of Tennessee School of Medicine; Consultant, University of Tennessee Hospital; Veterans Administration Medical Center; Regional Medical Center, Memphis, Tennessee.
Hypoglycemia

KENNETH W. RYDER, M.D., Ph.D.
Professor, Department of Pathology, Indiana University School of Medicine; Chief, Pathology Service, Wishard Memorial Hospital, Indianapolis, Indiana.
Hypomagnesemia

MARK H. SANDERS, M.D.

Associate Professor, Division of Pulmonary Medicine, Departments of Medicine and Anesthesiology, University of Pittsburgh School of Medicine; Director, Pulmonary Sleep Evaluation Center, Presbyterian University Hospital, University of Pittsburgh Medical Center; Assistant Chief, Pulmonary Service, Veterans Affairs Medical Center, Pittsburgh, Pennsylvania.

Stridor

CESAR C. SANTOS, M.D.

Department of Pediatric Neurology, Duke University School of Medicine; Department of Pediatric Neurology, Duke University Medical Center, Durham, North Carolina.

Athetosis

MARK V. SAUER, M.D.

Associate Professor, Department of Obstetrics and Gynecology, University of Southern California School of Medicine; Women's Hospital of Los Angeles County, University of Southern California Medical Center, Los Angeles, California.

Ectopic Pregnancy, Suspected

JOHN W. SAULTZ, M.D.

Associate Professor, Department of Family Medicine, Oregon Health Sciences University School of Medicine; Oregon Health Sciences University Hospitals, Portland, Oregon.

Anorexia

DAN SCHULLER, M.D.

Instructor, Division of Respiratory and Critical Care, Department of Medicine, Washington University School of Medicine; Attending Staff Physician, Barnes Hospital; Attending Staff Physician, The Jewish Hospital of St. Louis, St. Louis, Missouri.

Cough, Chronic

H. RALPH SCHUMACHER, JR., M.D.

Professor, Acting Chief, Rheumatology Section, Department of Medicine, University of Pennsylvania School of Medicine; Acting Chief, Rheumatology Section, University of Pennsylvania Hospital; Chief, Rheumatology Section, Director, Arthritis Immunology Center, Veterans Administration Medical Center, Philadelphia, Pennsylvania.

Hyperuricemia

GERALD M. SEGAL, M.D.

Assistant Professor, Department of Medicine, Division of Hematology and Medical Oncology, Oregon Health Sciences University School of Medicine; Medical Staff, Oregon Health Sciences University Hospitals, Portland, Oregon.

Polycythemia

ELLIOTT L. SEMBLE, M.D.

Associate Professor, Section on Rheumatology, Department of Medicine, Bowman Gray School of Medicine, Winston-Salem, North Carolina.

Myofascial Pain

PETER E. SHAPIRO, M.D.

Department of Otolaryngology, University of Missouri School of Medicine; University of Missouri Hospitals and Clinics, Columbia, Missouri.

Xerostomia

CLOUGH SHELTON, M.D.
Assistant Clinical Professor, Department of Otolaryngology, University of Southern California School of Medicine, Los Angeles; University of California at Irvine, California.
Hearing Loss, Sudden

LEONARD SICILIAN, M.D.
Associate Professor, Department of Medicine, Tufts University School of Medicine; Director, Medical Intensive Care Unit, New England Medical Center Hospital, Boston, Massachusetts.
Interstitial Pulmonary Disease

FRANK L. SILVER, M.D., F.R.C.P. (C)
Assistant Professor, Division of Neurology, Department of Medicine, University of Toronto; Toronto Hospital, Toronto Western Division; Riverdale Hospital, Toronto, Ontario, Canada.
Transient Ischemic Attacks

FRANKLIN H. SIM, M.D.
Professor, Department of Orthopedics, Mayo Medical School; Consultant, Department of Orthopedics, Mayo Clinic and Mayo Foundation, Rochester, Minnesota.
Bone Pain

RICHARD M. SLATAPER, M.D.
Department of Internal Medicine, Ochsner Foundation Hospital, New Orleans, Louisiana.
Secondary Hypertension

CHARLES H. SOWDER, M.D.
Assistant Professor, Department of Family Practice, Resident Director, Medical College of Virginia; Medical College of Virginia Hospitals, Richmond, Virginia.
Tachypnea

RONALD A. STILLER, M.D.
Assistant Professor, Departments of Medicine and Anesthesiology, University of Pittsburgh School of Medicine; Associate Director, Medical Intensive Care Unit, Presbyterian University Hospital, University of Pittsburgh Medical Center, Pittsburgh, Pennsylvania.
Stridor

RUEY J. SUNG, M.D.
Professor, Division of Cardiovascular Medicine, Department of Medicine, Stanford University School of Medicine; Director, Cardiac Electrophysiology and Arrhythmia Service, Stanford University Hospital, Stanford, California.
Tachyarrhythmias

ILONA S. SZER, M.D.
Associate Professor, Department of Pediatrics, University of Southern California School of Medicine; Associate Head, Division of Rheumatology, Children's Hospital, Los Angeles, California.
Limb Pain in Childhood

JERRY W. TEMPLER, M.D.
Professor, Division of Otolaryngology, Department of Surgery, University of Missouri School of Medicine; University of Missouri Hospital and Clinics; Harry S. Truman Veterans Administration Hospital, Columbia, Missouri.
Xerostomia

DANIEL J. TENNENHOUSE, M.D.
Lecturer, University of California at San Francisco School of Medicine, San Francisco; Lecturer, University of California at San Francisco School of Nursing, San Francisco; Staff Physician, University of California at San Francisco Hospital, San Francisco; Staff Physician, St. Lukes Hospital, San Francisco; Consultant, Risk Management Section, Kaiser-Permenante Regional Center, Oakland, California.
Bradycardia

R. STEVEN THARRATT, M.D.
Assistant Professor, Division of Pulmonary/Critical Care Medicine, Department of Medicine, University of California at Davis School of Medicine; Active Staff, University of California at Davis Medical Center, Sacramento, California.
Mediastinal Mass

CARMELITA R. TOBIAS, M.D.
Associate Professor, Department of Psychiatry and Behavioral Sciences, University of Louisville School of Medicine; Staff Psychiatrist, Veterans Administration Medical Center, Louisville, Kentucky.
Anxiety

WILLIAM L. TOFFLER, M.D.
Associate Professor, Department of Family Medicine, Oregon Health Sciences University School of Medicine; Oregon Health Sciences University Hospitals, Portland, Oregon.
Anorexia

TERESA A. TRAN, M.D.
Department of Neurology, The Cleveland Clinic Foundation, Cleveland, Ohio.
Amnesia

JAMES L. VACEK, M.D.
Clinical Professor, Division of Cardiology, Department of Medicine, University of Missouri School of Medicine at Kansas City; Consultant, Department of Cardiology, Mid-America Heart Institute, Kansas City, Missouri.
Pericarditis

ANNE D. WALLING, M.D.
Professor, Vice-Chairman, Department of Family and Community Medicine, University of Kansas School of Medicine, Wichita; Wesley Medical Center; St. Joseph's Medical Center; St. Francis Medical Center, Wichita, Kansas.
Hyperpigmentation, Generalized

WENG-LIH WANG, M.D.
Nephrologist, Gemet Valley Hospital District, California; Nephrologist, Menifee Valley Hospital, San Jacinto, California.
Azotemia, Acute

ROBERT WHANG, M.D.
Professor, Vice-Chairman, Department of Medicine, University of Oklahoma College of Medicine; Chief, Department of Medicine, Veterans Administration Medical Center, Oklahoma City, Oklahoma.
Hypomagnesemia

GARY L. WILSON, M.D.
Assistant Clinical Professor, Section on Infectious Diseases, Department of Medicine, St. Louis University School of Medicine; Vice-Chairman, Department of Critical Care Medicine, St. John's Mercy Medical Center, St. Louis, Missouri.
Intracranial Infection, Acute

PETER R. WILSON, M.D.
Associate Professor, Department of Anesthesiology, Mayo Medical School; Consultant, Department of Anesthesiology, Mayo Clinic and Mayo Foundation, Rochester, Minnesota.
Bone Pain

CHRISTOPHER WISE, M.D.
Associate Professor, Section on Rheumatology, Department of Medicine, Wake Forest University, Bowman Gray School of Medicine, Winston-Salem, North Carolina.
Myofascial Pain

PREFACE

Difficult Diagnosis 2, like the first volume in this series, presents a diagnostic approach to a selected group of challenging clinical problems. *The topics presented in this book are all new;* that is, none were covered in *Difficult Diagnosis 1,* which was published in 1985.[1]

The choice of problems is based on my clinical experience—which includes 14 years in private practice and 14 years as an academician. In my care of patients over the past 28 years, I have encountered each of the problems discussed in this book.

The topics discussed represent enigmatic clinical presentations; some are rare and some occur commonly. Some topics, like chronic fatigue, have become especially pertinent since the publication of the first volume. Many, such as hypomagnesemia and hepatomegaly, cross specialty lines. All present a circuitous path from earliest manifestation to the moment of diagnosis.

The approach is the one that I use in practice and in *Difficult Diagnosis 1:* an overview of the problem, a directed history with high pay-off questions, a focused physical examination, laboratory investigation, and a systematic analysis of data. Authors of the book's 71 chapters recognize the importance of the medical history and physical examination. As noted by Wilson, commenting on a report[2] of gynecomastia (a topic in *Difficult Diagnosis 1*) as a diagnostic dilemma: "In my experience the cause of gynecomastia is more commonly recognized by history and physical examination than by hormone assay."[3]

The emphasis in this book is on diagnosis, with information regarding therapy included only when pertinent to the diagnostic process, e.g., the significance of aspiration in the investigation of a breast lump. Because of the multidisciplinary nature of problems such as anorexia, cholestasis, lymphadenopathy, and chronic abdominal pain, chapters are arranged alphabetically, with a listing of synonyms and eponyms. Where appropriate, I have included cross-references to *Difficult Diagnosis 1* and *Difficult Medical Management* (1991).[4]

The authors who have contributed to this book are experts in their fields, chosen for both their clinical expertise and ability to communicate clearly. The intended readers are the primary care physician and the limited specialist who encounter patients with problems outside their field of expertise.

I am grateful for the work of Coelleda Koches-O'Neil and Sherri Johnson of Oregon Health Sciences University, Richard Bernard, M.D., John Dyson at W. B. Saunders Company, and Elise Oranges at Spectrum Publisher Services.

I invite readers to offer comments regarding the topics and methods presented in *Difficult Diagnosis 1* and *2,* and to offer suggestions for future volumes.

ROBERT B. TAYLOR, M.D.

REFERENCES

1. Taylor RB. *Difficult Diagnosis 1*. Philadelphia: W. B. Saunders Co. 1985.
2. Coen P, Kulin H, Ballantine T, et al. An aromatase-producing sex-cord tumor resulting in prepubertal gynecomastia. *N Engl J Med* 1991;324:317–22.
3. Wilson JD. Gynecomastia: a continuing diagnostic dilemma. *N Engl J Med* 1991;324:334–5.
4. Taylor RB. *Difficult Medical Management*. Philadelphia: W. B. Saunders Co. 1991.

CONTENTS

ABDOMINAL PAIN, CHRONIC 1
Lawrence D. Bailey, Jr., and Richard W. McCallum

AMNESIA...7
Teresa A. Tran and John P. Conomy

ANOREXIA 16
William L. Toffler, Scott A. Fields, Glenn S. Rodriguez, Dana W. Peterson, and
John W. Saultz

ANTINUCLEAR ANTIBODY, POSITIVE TITER 22
Joe G. Hardin, Jr.

ANXIETY 29
Raymond Pary, Carmelita R. Tobias, and Steven Lippmann

ATAXIA..36
Mark J. Cook and Richard F. Peppard

ATHETOSIS...41
Cesar C. Santos and E. Wayne Massey

AZOTEMIA, ACUTE 46
Weng-Lih Wang and D. M. Kaji

BONE PAIN 52
Frank J. Frassica, Franklin H. Sim, and Peter R. Wilson

BRADYCARDIA...60
Ellen J. Killebrew, Daniel J. Tennenhouse, and Nora Goldschlager

BREAST LUMP...67
Frederick L. Greene and Tracy D. Gunter

CHEST PAIN, ACUTE...73
Thach N. Nguyen and Abdulmassih S. Iskandrian

CHOLESTASIS 86
    Alex H. Bruckstein

CLUBBING...91
    Timothy R. Aksamit, Scott D. Nygaard, and Robert B. Fick, Jr.

CONGESTIVE HEART FAILURE 98
    Kenneth M. Kessler

CONSTIPATION, CHRONIC...105
    Paul C. Rousseau

COUGH, CHRONIC 110
    Anne M. Pittman, Dan Schuller, and Phillip E. Korenblat

DIARRHEA, ACUTE...117
    Alex H. Bruckstein

DRY EYE..122
    J. Daniel Nelson

DYSPAREUNIA..128
    Mary K. Beard

DYSURIA 135
    Jørn Aagaard and Paul O. Madsen

ECTOPIC PREGNANCY, SUSPECTED..142
    Mark V. Sauer

FATIGUE, CHRONIC..152
    A. James Giannini

FEVER IN CHILDHOOD 159
    Marilyn Doyle

FOOD ALLERGY AND INTOLERANCE...167
    Sami L. Bahna and Mary C. Maier

HALLUCINATIONS 172
    Patricia Blumenreich, Teresita Bacani-Oropilla, and Steven Lippmann

HEARING LOSS, SUDDEN...179
    James K. Bredenkamp and Clough Shelton

HEMATOCHEZIA..186
    James B. Rhodes, Clark W. Antonson, and Roland B. Christian

HEPATOMEGALY..195
    Albert J. Czaja

HOARSENESS..203
    Laurene L. Howell and Edwin C. Everts

HUMAN IMMUNODEFICIENCY VIRUS INFECTION, DIAGNOSIS, AND STAGING....215
    Steven A. Miles

HYPERCHOLESTEROLEMIA..223
    Patrick E. McBride and David Nevin

HYPERPIGMENTATION, GENERALIZED 233
    Anne D. Walling

HYPERURICEMIA...239
    Worawit Louthrenoo, Kanchana Boonsaner, and H. Ralph Schumacher, Jr.

HYPOGLYCEMIA..249
    Abbas E. Kitabchi and Mark J. Rumbak

HYPOMAGNESEMIA 258
    Robert Whang and Kenneth W. Ryder

INSOMNIA 263
    Robert N. Golden

INTERSTITIAL PULMONARY DISEASE 266
    Peadar G. Noone and Leonard Sicilian

INTESTINAL BLOATING AND GAS 274
    Timothy T. Nostrant and Jeffrey L. Barnett

INTRACRANIAL INFECTION, ACUTE...280
    Gary L. Wilson

LIMB PAIN IN CHILDHOOD 287
    Ilona S. Szer

LYMPHADENOPATHY...292
    Mark A. Getz and Frank M. Graziano

MEDIASTINAL MASS..300
Glen A. Lillington and R. Steven Tharratt

MENSTRUAL DYSFUNCTION..308
Geoffrey P. Redmond

MYOFASCIAL PAIN...315
Elliott L. Semble and Christopher M. Wise

ORAL ULCERS 321
J. Robert Newland

PAP SMEAR, ABNORMAL...328
Steven H. Pursell and Stanley A. Gall

PELVIC MASS IN THE FEMALE PATIENT 334
Thomas M. Julian and Daniel A. Dumesic

PERICARDITIS..341
James L. Vacek

PHANTOGEUSIA...348
Robert I. Henkin

POLYARTERITIS..357
Lee D. Kaufman

POLYARTICULAR ARTHRITIS..363
Lenore J. Brancato and Joel N. Buxbaum

POLYCYTHEMIA 372
Gerald M. Segal

PROTEINURIA 379
Blanche M. Chavers

RAYNAUD'S PHENOMENON 386
John P. Lavery and Jeffrey R. Lisse

SCROTAL PAIN...392
Angelo S. Paola, S. Ali Khan, and Louise Ferrarotto

SECONDARY HYPERTENSION...403
Richard M. Slataper and George L. Bakris

SEIZURES IN CHILDHOOD..411
  Daniel K. Miles and Gregory L. Holmes

SILENT MYOCARDIAL ISCHEMIA 419
  Pascal Nicod and François Ricou

SLEEPINESS, EXCESSIVE 425
  Rocco L. Manfredi and Joyce D. Kales

STEATORRHEA..432
  Ingram M. Roberts

STRIDOR..436
  Ronald A. Stiller and Mark H. Sanders

SYSTOLIC MURMURS 444
  James M. Hagar and Robert A. Kloner

TACHYARRHYTHMIAS 453
  Ruey J. Sung

TACHYPNEA..463
  Charles R. Sowder, David W. Marsland, and Stephen M. Ayres

THYROID ENLARGEMENT 470
  Kay F. McFarland

TRANSIENT ISCHEMIC ATTACKS..475
  Frank L. Silver

VESICULOBULLOUS DISORDERS...481
  James E. Fitzpatrick and Scott D. Bennion

VISUAL LOSS, UNILATERAL...492
  Mitchell D. Drucker and Curtis E. Margo

WEIGHT GAIN...499
  Stephen A. Brunton, Nancy S. Carpenter, and Ralph R. Hall

XEROSTOMIA..506
  Jerry W. Templer and Peter E. Shapiro

INDEX...517

ABDOMINAL PAIN, CHRONIC

LAWRENCE D. BAILEY, Jr., and RICHARD W. McCALLUM

SYNONYM: Abdominal Pain Syndrome

BACKGROUND

For the purposes of this chapter, *chronic abdominal pain* will be defined as continuous symptoms of greater than 9 months' duration or intermittent symptoms for 12 months or more. The diagnosis of abdominal pain is complicated by the fact that pain is a subjective sensation and is defined and perceived differently according to sex, culture, or ethnic group. Perception of pain is also markedly influenced by psychologic factors and stress. Chronic pain is both a common complaint to primary physicians and often the cause of referral to subspecialists. While there are numerous identifiable causes of chronic abdominal pain (see Table 1), many cases still remain idiopathic in nature.

Abdominal viscera do not respond to usual painful stimuli such as cutting, crushing, or contact. Distention or stretch is the most common stimulus for abdominal pain. Rapid stretching is associated with more severe pain than gradual changes. Inflammation is also a common cause for pain and may occur as a result of direct stimulation of nociceptors or making them more sensitive to other stimuli. Pain is also generated by ischemia and neoplastic involvement of nerves. Pain is detected by A-delta and C afferent fibers. The ends of these fibers function as nociceptors. A-delta fibers tend to transmit pain that is sharp and well localized and are found predominantly in muscle and skin. C fibers tend to carry dull, poorly localized sensation and are found mainly in viscera and parietal peritoneum. Sensations pass through the splanchnic ganglia, travel along the sympathetic chain, and enter the dorsal root. There, they synapse with the dorsal horn cell bodies that communicate with the brain via the lateral spinothalamic tract.[1]

Abdominal pain can be separated into visceral, parietal, and referred pain. Owing to the fewer nerve endings and the multisegmental innervation, visceral pain is usually dull and poorly localized and tends to occur near the midline. Noxious stimulation of the parietal peritoneum tends to lead to sharp, intense localized pain. Pain that is felt in areas distant from the stimulus is called referred pain. Referred pain is due to a common neurosegment and may occur at skin level or deeper. It is generally a response to more severe stimuli and may not begin immediately but develop after prolonged stimulation.[1]

HISTORY

Although the history will rarely establish an exact cause for chronic abdominal pain, an accurate history will permit a focused and directed workup that will be expedient and cost-effective. The history must serve to guide subsequent testing and therapy. Not only are superfluous tests expensive and potentially harmful to the patient, but they may cause the patient with functional or idiopathic pain to become more obsessed with the pain. Special attention should be paid to (1) timing (duration and frequency), (2) character, (3) location, (4) factors that improve or exacerbate the pain, and (5) symptoms in other organ systems.

Timing

Once an appropriate duration of symptoms is established to classify abdominal pain as chronic, then one must determine if symptoms have continued unchanged for more than two to three years. Symptoms of this duration make malignancy much less likely and allow for a more leisurely investigation. Daily symp-

1

TABLE 1.   Causes of Chronic Abdominal Pain

Gastric	Hepatoma
Ulcer disease	Adenoma
Gastritis	Simple cysts
Gastroparesis	Hepatitis
Lymphoma	Amyloid
Adenocarcinoma	Vascular insults
Duodenal	Portal vein thrombosis
Ulcer disease	Hepatic vein occlusion
Diverticula	Fatty liver
Congenital abnormalities	Primary biliary cirrhosis
Small intestinal	Sclerosing cholangitis
Partial obstruction	Sarcoidosis
Adhesions	Porphyria
Superior mesenteric artery syndrome	Pancreatic
Hernia	Tumor
Tumor	Chronic pancreatitis
Crohn's disease	Pseudocyst
Ischemia	Pancreas divisum
Meckel's diverticulum	Ischemia
Gallstone ileus	Biliary
Celiac disease	Cholecystolithiasis
Whipple's disease	Choledocholithiasis
Eosinophilic gastroenteritis	Dyskinesia
Giardiasis	Bile duct tumors
Colonic	Choledochocele
Irritable bowel syndrome	Choledochal cysts
Diverticular disease	Other
Constipation	Nephrolithiasis
Ulcerative colitis	Splenomegaly
Amebiasis	Ovarian
Appendicitis	Cysts
Endometriosis	Carcinoma
Ischemia	Torsion
Pseudo-obstruction	Uterine fibroids
Adenocarcinoma	Abdominal epilepsy
Hepatic	Abdominal wall pain
Metastatic tumor	

toms make inflammatory diseases more likely. Short, episodic patterns of pain are associated with intermittent obstructive phenomena such as small bowel obstruction or choledocholithiasis and spastic diseases such as irritable bowel syndrome. Dull, continuous pain is associated with enlargement of solid organs such as in hepatomegaly due to infiltrative diseases such as amyloid or sarcoid. Timing in relation to meals must be considered and will be discussed below. Relationship to menstrual cycle is important in endometriosis and uterine abdominal pain. Progesterone may also have effects on smooth muscle function, and increased symptom intensity in the second half of the menstrual cycle may be observed.

Character

As discussed above, perception and description of the character of pain vary greatly from patient to patient. It is often helpful to have the patient describe the pain in terms of more familiar types of pain such as a tooth-ache or a cut. Patients will often describe cramping pain associated with obstruction using squeezing motions of their hands. Dull, penetrating pain is often associated with inflammation in conditions such as chronic ulcer, inflammatory bowel disease, or pancreatitis.

Location

Although the location of abdominal pain is nonspecific, the areas where pain is localized and where it is referred are helpful in directing your investigation. Colonic pain tends to be diffuse and poorly localized in the lower midabdomen. Gastric and duodenal pain are usually perceived in the upper epigastric area. Liver, biliary, and pancreatic pain are often felt in the right upper quadrant and may radiate to the back. Small bowel pain is often localized to the midabdomen or in the umbilical area and also may radiate to the midback. It is often useful to make patients point to one spot where the pain is most intense, even though they may state that they hurt everywhere.

Factors That Alter Pain

The most useful diagnostic historical information is often determination of what precipitates, worsens, or improves pain. Almost no patient will present with chronic abdominal pain without having tried several remedies. Abdominal pain that is improved by antacids is more likely peptic. The relationship to eating and the types of food should be elicited. However, it must be remembered that the response to food is varied and occurs in several conditions. For example, pain that begins within a few minutes of eating is more likely a biliary or pancreatic than an obstructive problem where the pain will often start one to two hours after eating. The absence of change with food will make a solid organ or peritoneal problem more likely. The effect of fasting (often done in preparation for tests) is also very useful. Problems associated with obstruction such as adhesions, Crohn's disease, or gastroparesis will often improve with fasting.

Associated Symptoms

The most important concurrent symptoms are those in the gastrointestinal tract. Nausea and vomiting are most frequently observed in small bowel obstruction, pyloric channel ulcer, gastroparesis, pancreatitis, or biliary diseases. Diarrhea is most often found in small bowel or colonic diseases. Nocturnal diarrhea is almost never due to functional bowel syndromes, and a pathologic condition should be sought. The presence of rectal bleeding makes colonic neoplasia a more pressing concern. Dark-colored urine, acholic stools, or jaundice suggest hepatic disease, biliary tract disease, or rarely, porphyria. Weight loss is of great significance and makes functional problems less likely. Tumor and chronic obstruction are the biggest concerns, but severe gastroparesis or malabsorption must also be considered. Pain that is localized specifically and relieved by heat or nonsteroidal medications may be due to abdominal wall pain.

A careful history of extra bowel symptoms is also important. A thorough medication history should be obtained, including the use of alcohol and intravenous (IV) drugs. This is helpful in consideration of possible pancreatitis, gastritis, or hepatitis. Unexplained pruritus is a phenomenon of chronic biliary obstruction such as primary biliary cirrhosis or sclerosing cholangitis. Urinary symptoms may denote nephrolithiasis or bladder outlet dys-

function. Crohn's disease and ulcerative colitis may be associated with arthralgias, rash, or iritis. Raynaud's phenomenon or tight skin around the fingers may suggest previously undiagnosed scleroderma or CREST (calcinosis cutis, Raynaud's phenomenon, esophageal involvement, sclerodactyly, and telangiectasia) syndrome. Vaginal bleeding or irregular menses require careful gynecologic evaluation. A social and occupational history should be acquired in every patient. Not only will a majority of patients with chronic abdominal pain have no demonstrable physical problem, but patients with organic disease will be affected in how they function with their pain. Particular attention should be placed on stressors and their relationship to pain. This should include home and employment situations and any important events such as divorce or death of a parent.

PHYSICAL EXAMINATION

The physical examination, while rarely making a diagnosis, will serve to direct subsequent testing. It is important not to become overly centered on the pain location during the abdominal exam, as important information is often found in other organ systems. Careful examination of the sclera may reveal unnoticed jaundice or anemia. The skin is involved in numerous causes of chronic abdominal pain. Acanthosis nigricans is a manifestation of malignancy. Erythema nodosum and other rashes are seen in inflammatory bowel diseases. Subtle changes in skin on the fingers may suggest scleroderma. Telangiectasias, palmar erythema, and gynecomastia suggest chronic liver disease. Xanthomas are also seen in primary biliary cirrhosis. The presence of bruits makes ischemic disease of the bowel or pancreas or an abdominal aortic aneurysm more likely. Temporal wasting, edema, or dry skin may be signs of weight loss associated with malabsorption.

The abdominal exam should begin with visual inspection, with careful attention paid to any previously unmentioned surgical scars (patients often fail to mention simple operations such as an appendectomy). The abdomen should be auscultated for bruits and evidence of obstruction. Hyperactive bowel sounds associated with obstruction are not necessarily found in chronic partial obstructions and are also present in patients with irritable bowel syndrome. Palpation should attempt to establish tender areas. It is good to distract the patient or to use the stethoscope to press in order to determine if the pain is reproducible. One should attempt to determine if the pain is limited to the abdominal wall, especially in areas of surgical scars. A careful check for hernias is often productive. A rectal exam should always be performed to evaluate possible masses and heme test the stool. A careful pelvic exam is also necessary in females.

DIAGNOSTIC STUDIES

The clinician is presented with a vast array of diagnostic modalities for the evaluation of chronic abdominal pain. Although these choices allow for diagnostic accuracy, they must be strategically selected to maintain cost-effectiveness and also to prevent reinforcement of functional pain syndromes. Each test should always be ordered with the thought, "How will a positive or negative result affect my care of the patient?" One must take great care to avoid ordering tests that will not alter the patient's course. Such an approach should be applied sequentially to allow for accuracy and cost-effectiveness. A normal sequence of testing would be clinical laboratory studies followed by appropriate diagnostic radiology and endoscopic procedures. For episodic problems (e.g., pancreatitis, small bowel obstruction), it may be necessary to perform studies during the acute pain episodes. In these cases, the physician should carefully instruct the patient to come to the office or the emergency room immediately when the pain begins so that appropriate laboratory and radiologic studies can be performed.

Clinical Laboratory

Laboratory results will serve to further define the need for additional testing. Screening laboratories should usually include a complete blood count (CBC) and routine chemistries including liver enzymes, bilirubin, and amylase. A urinalysis is also helpful to look for red cells that may be due to nephrolithiasis or renal cell carcinoma. Sedimentation rates, while being nonspecific, are usually elevated in active inflammatory bowel disease.[2] Stool should be tested for occult blood, and in patients with diarrhea, it should also be examined for ova and parasites, white cells, and a stain for fat.

Anticentromere antibodies may help confirm a diagnosis of CREST syndrome. Hepatitis serologies for hepatitis B and C (previously called non-A, non-B) should be drawn if liver enzymes are elevated. Antimitochondrial antibodies, ceruloplasm, antinuclear antibodies, alpha-1-antitrypsin levels, and protein electrophoresis are also useful in pain associated with suspected liver disease. Rare tests that may be helpful include a serum gastrin screening for Zollinger-Ellison syndrome, urine 5-HIAA (5-hydroxyindoleacetic acid) levels in carcinoid, and a porphyrin screen.

Diagnostic Radiology

Plain films of the abdomen are of limited utility in chronic pain as compared with acute abdominal pain, but they may reveal the calcifications of chronic pancreatitis or gallstones, abnormal bowel gas patterns of obstruction, or large amounts of feces. Although barium x-rays of the upper tract have a lower yield than upper gastrointestinal (GI) endoscopy, they have the advantages of lower cost and the ability to visualize the distal small bowel.[3] In cases where subtle small bowel pathology is suspected, an enteroclysis may be performed. This involves the passage of a tube into the duodenum to administer the barium and allows for greater density of contrast and improved resolution. The barium enema has been supplanted by colonoscopy in many cases. However, because of its lower cost, some studies would suggest that an air contrast barium enema is more cost-effective in people under the age of 55.[4]

Abdominal ultrasound has become the study of choice to diagnose gallbladder disease, having largely supplanted oral cholecystography. Its excellent sensitivity and ease of performance make it an ideal test. There is also the added benefit of being able to examine other organs—in particular, the liver, bile ducts, kidneys, and ovaries. A recent development in ultrasonography is the ability to Doppler scan hepatic and splenic vessels to rule out thrombosis. Biliary scintigraphy (PRIDA, HIDA, or DOSIDA scans) is the test of choice in acute cholecystitis and is also helpful as a noninvasive test of partial common duct obstruction.[5]

Computerized tomography (CT) has revolutionized the diagnosis of chronic abdominal pain. Structures can be visualized that would have required laparotomy for diagnosis. The main limitations of CT are its relatively high cost, an inability to distinguish cystic from solid masses, and the radiation exposure. CT is especially effective in examining the pancreas and localizing other mass lesions. The pelvis is less well seen as compared with ultrasound. Because of the cost factor, patients should be carefully selected before undergoing CT scanning. Magnetic resonance imaging (MRI) shows promise in providing increased resolution of abdominal structures, but its importance in the diagnosis of abdominal pain remains to be established.

Interventional radiology may be useful in selected cases. Percutaneous transhepatic cholangiography (PTC) has largely been supplanted by endoscopic retrograde cholangiopancreatography (ERCP) but may be useful in patients where ERCP is technically impossible and in whom biliary obstruction is strongly suspected. The main disadvantages of PTC are patient discomfort, inability to visualize the pancreas, and decreased therapeutic options. Angiography is useful in suspected abdominal angina and in the demonstration of portal or splenic vein thrombosis. The use of angiography for the diagnosis of malignancy has become rare because of the availability of CT and ultrasound.

Endoscopic Diagnostic Procedures

Fiberoptic endoscopy provides the clinician with the ability to visualize the stomach, duodenum, bile ducts, pancreas, and colon. As with CT, patients should be selected judiciously to insure cost effectiveness. Upper endoscopy is more sensitive than barium studies,[6] especially in finding small lesions or gastritis. A recent development is the ability to diagnose *Helicobacter pylori* by biopsy and rapid urease test.[7] Unfortunately, the cost of endoscopy is two- to threefold that of a barium study. Colonoscopy, although the procedure of choice in the evaluation of colonic polyps and cancer, is usually not a first-line study in chronic abdominal pain unless there are specific symptoms of possible malignancy such as rectal bleeding, heme-positive stool, weight loss, or unexplained anemia.

Evaluation of the biliary tree and pancreas has been revolutionized by the advent of ERCP. This provides the physician not only with the ability to visualize the biliary tree and pancreas but also with the potential to intervene in many biliary diseases. There is also the ability to measure sphincter of Oddi pressures via manometry.[8] Obviously, this is not a first-line test and will almost always be performed after preliminary diagnostic workup. The disadvantages of ERCP are cost, radiation exposure, and risk of complications. However, these compare very favorably with PTC. More specific indications will be discussed below. Laparoscopy can also be a useful diagnostic tool. The most common indication in patients with chronic abdominal pain is in women with possible endometriosis or ovarian disease.

ASSESSMENT

In that chronic abdominal pain may present in numerous ways, it is impossible to give specific guidelines for assessment. However, this section will attempt to give a framework that will permit a rational and cost-effective diagnostic approach. We will concentrate on specific areas of pain as opposed to individual disease states.

Epigastric Pain

Pain in the epigastrium is the most common complaint of patients with abdominal pain. It is important to establish if the pain is peptic in nature. Previously mentioned historical points include relationship to meals and response to antacids. Because the incidence of gastric cancer is very low in this country, a diagnostic trial of an H_2 (histamine$_2$) blocker (cimetidine, ranitidine, nizatidine, or famotidine) is warranted in patients with pain consistent with peptic disease. If patients respond with pain relief, no further evaluation may be necessary. In patients who do not respond, upper endoscopy should be performed to allow an evaluation of possible *Helicobacter pylori* infection, unsuspected malignancy, unresponsive ulcer disease, or gastritis.

In patients who present with chronic epigastric pain associated with nausea or vomiting, the approach is different. The initial goal should be toward ruling out obstruction by endoscopy and a small bowel series, if necessary. If no obstruction is demonstrated, then one must consider pancreatobiliary causes and gastroparesis. Determination of predisposing conditions such as diabetes mellitus and laboratory examinations will help direct the evaluation. Especially helpful are liver enzymes and an amylase level. The workup for pancreatobiliary pain will be discussed below.

The diagnosis of gastroparesis is established by nuclear gastric emptying study.

Right Upper Quadrant (RUQ) Pain

One must guard against the impulse to identify all RUQ pain as being due to hepatobiliary or pancreatic causes. In fact, peptic ulcer disease often presents as RUQ pain. By carefully examining the character and timing of the pain in conjunction with laboratory tests, one may avoid a costly and time-consuming evaluation of biliary disease. If the pain does appear to be peptic in nature, the approach should be as above. If peptic disease is eliminated by endoscopy or felt unlikely, then an ultrasound is a reasonable first test after diagnostic laboratory. Findings that are most likely to be useful are gallstones, dilated bile ducts, pancreatic masses, or hepatic lesions (e.g., cysts, adenomas, metastases). Abdominal CT may be necessary to visualize the pancreas well. Even in the absence of ultrasound or CT findings, ERCP may be indicated. This is especially true if there are abnormal liver function tests or increased amylase values.

In the patient who has had a cholecystectomy, the approach is different in the patient with RUQ pain. The threshold for performing ERCP is much lower, especially if liver enzymes are elevated. Ultrasound is an insensitive test for common bile duct stones, and the common bile duct is dilated somewhat postcholecystectomy. In patients with a normal ERCP and chronic pain, some authors advocate measurement of sphincter of Oddi pressures to make the diagnosis of biliary dyskinesia or sphincter of Oddi dysfunction.[9]

Lower Abdominal Pain

The most common cause of lower abdominal pain is irritable bowel syndrome (IBS). Since there is no definitive diagnostic test for IBS, this is a diagnosis of exclusion. The clinician is faced with the dilemma of excluding treatable or serious illnesses yet accomplishing a cost-effective and safe evaluation. Lower abdominal pain is more difficult in females because uterine and ovarian causes must be considered. Therefore, in women a complete pelvic examination is mandatory. History is very important in lower abdominal pain. Relationship to meals, bowel movements, and menstrual cycle is very important. Also, signs and symptoms of rectal bleeding or heme-positive stool will directly alter the eval-

uation. The physical exam should also concentrate on possible hernias, as these may present only as nonspecific abdominal pain.

Diagnostic studies should focus on the colon and pelvic organs. In patients without diarrhea, constipation, rectal bleeding, or heme-positive stool, the yield of colonoscopy or barium enema is low. Alternatively, heme-positive stools or rectal bleeding makes colonic evaluation mandatory. In patients with abdominal pain alone, the need to examine the colon is determined by the patient's risk for colon cancer (age, family history) and the patient's desire to know definitively that there is no colonic pathology. The presence of diverticula on barium enema or colonoscopy is not sufficient for a diagnosis of diverticulitis. Diverticulitis is a clinical diagnosis based on symptoms and signs along with the presence of diverticula. The pelvic organs are best examined by ultrasound, as mentioned above. Endometriosis is a particularly difficult diagnosis to make and may require laparoscopy to confirm the diagnosis. (Also see Pelvic Pain in Women, *Difficult Diagnosis I*, 1985.)

Implications of Chronic Abdominal Pain

Although chronic abdominal pain may signify serious underlying disease such as malignancy or inflammatory bowel disease, the very fact that the pain is chronic makes a benign cause more likely. Even though conditions such as irritable bowel are benign, they may have profound effects on the life-styles of patients. Therefore, the physician must strive to reassure his or her patient, while economically minimizing the number of diagnostic evaluations necessary, keeping in mind the fact that a concrete diagnosis is not always possible. In the final analysis, patients will often benefit most from an effort by their physician for extensive discussion and time allocation to elaborate on the possible explanations and treatment decisions. Physician-patient rapport emphasizes that the art *and* the science of medicine are used to the maximum in managing chronic abdominal pain.

REFERENCES

1. Way LW. Abdominal pain. In: Sleisenger MH, Fordtran JS, eds. Gastrointestinal disease: pathophysiology, diagnosis, management. 4th ed. Philadelphia: WB Saunders, 1989:238–50.
2. Prantera C, Levenstein S, Capocaccia R, et al. Pre-

diction of surgery for obstruction in Crohn's ileitis. A study of 64 patients. Dig Dis Sci 1987;32:1963–9.

3. Mangan TF, Larson DE, Melton LJ III, et al. Use of gastroscopy in a community: a population-based study in Olmstead County, Minnesota. Mayo Clin Proc 1986;61:877–81.

4. Rex DK, Weddle RA, Lehman GA, et al. Flexible sigmoidoscopy plus air contrast barium enema versus colonoscopy for suspected lower gastrointestinal bleeding. Gastroenterology 1990;98:855–61.

5. Darweesh RM, Dodds WJ, Hogan WJ, et al. Efficacy of quantitative hepatobiliary scintigraphy and fatty-meal sonography for evaluating patients with suspected partial common duct obstruction. Gastroenterology 1988;94:779–86.

6. Martin TR, Vennes JA, Solves SE, Ansel HJ. A comparison of upper gastrointestinal endoscopy and radiography. J Clin Gastroenterol 1980;2:21–25.

7. Marshall BJ, Warren JR, Francis GJ, et al. Rapid urease test in the management of *Campylobacter pyloridis*–associated gastritis. Am J Gastroenterol 1987;82:200–10.

8. Touli J, Roberts-Thompson IC, Dent J, Lee J. Manometric disorders in patients with suspected sphincter of Oddi dysfunction. Gastroenterology 1985;88:1243–50.

9. Lebovics E, Heier SK, Rosenthal WS. Sphincter of Oddi motility: developments in physiology and clinical application. Am J Gastroenterol 1986;81:736–43.

AMNESIA

TERESA A. TRAN and JOHN P. CONOMY

SYNONYM: Memory Loss

BACKGROUND

Memory is the mental registration, retention, and recall of past experiences, knowledge, ideas, and thoughts. Memorization involves selection of material to be retained and selective destruction of material no longer needed. Memory is dependent on brain function perceiving a stimulus and recalling and reproducing the response. The perception itself is dependent on other factors including attention, emotional state, and content of the stimulus. *Recollection* signifies the patient's ability to bring the stimulus once removed into consciousness and the ability to express its representation. Memory is a constantly evolving process of higher cortical function consolidating new experiences into long-term store within brain cells. This requires integration of the human frontal, parietal, and temporal lobes with the older limbic portions of the brain: the hippocampus, mammillary bodies, and the thalamus.

HISTORY/PHYSICAL EXAMINATION/LABORATORY

Clinically, memory is differentiated into (1) remote memory, (2) recent memory, and (3) immediate registration, retention, and recall. In assessing memory function, one should obtain a history from either the patient or his or her family in regard to subtle mental changes such as forgetfulness, poor concentration, or difficulty with simple calculations. A differentiation should be made between the actual loss of memory (amnesia) and the more general failure of mental function, of which amnesia may be a prominent part (dementia).

One should determine the duration of memory deficit, noting whether it is of acute or insidious onset. In testing remote memory, one can elicit pertinent information by reviewing the verifiable portions of a patient's life. Useful questions include the patient's age, place and date of birth, dates and places of residence, education history, employment history with dates and wages, wedding date, and names and ages of children. The history obtained should be verified with a reliable family member. Remote memory can also be tested by asking the patient to name the presidents or to recall historical events such as wars. Recent memory can be tested by asking the patient about events that have transpired recently (last few hours, days). To test for registration, retention, and immediate recall, the examiner can instruct the patient to remember three objects, recalling them immediately; at one, three, and five minutes; and at one hour. The examiner can give a series of digits at one per second; then the patient is asked to repeat the series. A normal person should be able to recite seven to eight numbers forward and six numbers backward. He or she should also be able to repeat a sentence of 28 to 30 syllables without error. The Babcock sentence[1] is commonly used for this purpose: "One thing a nation must have to become rich and great is a large, secure supply of wood." Other means of testing immediate recall include asking the person to carry out a complex command or to summarize the salient features of a short story. One can also give him or her a series of paired words to learn. When given one of the words, the patient is to supply the other paired word. The patient may be shown a group of objects and later asked to recall as many objects as possible by memory.

Amnesia is, per se, an impairment of memory. It involves dysfunction in the learning of new material and in retention and retrieval of information from the recent or remote past. The clinical symptom of amnesia presents itself in many forms. Amnestic patients may present with global confusion or disorientation or have varying degrees of attention span deficits. Orientation of one's self to the surrounding environment requires consistent and reliable integration of attention, perception, and recall. Disorientation for place and person, particularly, is often the initial clue to a severe retention problem in an otherwise normal-appearing person. Orientation for time is man's most tenuous orientation—our need to be reminded of date and time reflected in a brisk business in calendar watches; normal men and women have little personal need for their own name tags. Disorientation is usually seen in diffuse central nervous system (CNS) dysfunction rather than in focal brain lesions. Difficulty with attention span forward is often seen in parietal lobe lesions rather than focal disturbances of other parts of the brain.

Temporal lobe diseases, on the other hand, affect selective attention capacity, whereby a person has difficulty concentrating on a single subject without interference from other ongoing distractions or activities. A defect in focus-ing attention or inability to concentrate when there are no competing external distractions may be a sign of temporal lobe dysfunction. The importance of the temporal lobes in human memory can be further defined according to the following observations: Verbal and nonverbal stimuli, for example, have different effects on the temporal lobes.[2] A left temporal lobe lesion will produce deficits in the acquisition, recall, or recognition of verbally received material, that is, word list retention or learning number series. If the hippocampal formation deep within the mesial temporal lobe is involved as well as the neocortical portion of the temporal lobe, the verbal memory loss is even more profound. A right temporal lobe lesion, on the other hand, produces difficulty in recall of geometric figures, topographic details, faces, and melodies.[2] Another form of functional memory loss can be expressed in the difficulty a person experiences in time-tagging an event. In this case, an amnestic person remembers the event that he or she experienced but cannot place it in time or in relation to other events. This is commonly seen in frontal lobe disorders.

At the clinical level, persons with memory impairment can be described to have elements of anterograde and retrograde amnesia. Anterograde amnesia is measured as that duration from the time of injury or disease into the future in which memory is impaired. Retrograde amnesia is measured by the time during which a person is unable to remember events prior to the onset of trauma or disease. The measurement of anterograde and retrograde amnesia is particularly important in head injury, where severity is indexed by the duration of anterograde amnesia.[3]

The factors causing amnesia are extensive and diverse. They vary from primary neurologic diseases to medical and psychiatric illnesses. The onset of symptoms in some amnestic syndromes may be sudden or insidious. The more treatable amnesias tend to be of the more acute type. Recognition of specific etiologies, therefore, becomes important in these cases, as it may afford immediate treatment for the patients.

ASSESSMENT

Transient Global Amnesia

In 1956, Bender described 12 cases in which generally elderly patients had sudden onset of gross memory impairment but otherwise had seemingly normal social behavior.[4] He referred to this amnestic syndrome as transient global amnesia (TGA). It was not until 1958 that Fisher and Adams[5] gave a more detailed clinical description of the syndrome. They described 17 patients between the ages of 55 and 80 years who suddenly developed amnesia. There were no associated neurologic deficits. The symptoms gradually improved over a few hours, leaving the patient only amnestic for the period of the event.

Today, over 400 cases of TGA have been reported, and the syndrome cannot be considered rare. TGA is a benign entity that occurs in middle-aged and elderly persons, usually over 50 years of age. Clinical features typify the syndrome. It is of acute onset. There is an inability to form new memories of any event occurring during the course of the episode. There is also temporary retrograde amnesia, which may extend from a few days to as far back as years. As the syndrome resolves, the retrograde amnesia shrinks in size also, with more remote memory returning first. The patient is left with a shorter and permanent retrograde amnesia lasting for the duration of the syndrome. Aside from the memory deficit, the patient remains fully alert during the episode, retaining spontaneity and continuing to perform complex behavior throughout the episode. The patient will be able, for instance, to drive a car or to play a musical instrument. Interestingly, a person with TGA is aware of sudden memory deficit and is disturbed by it. Such a person may not think or express himself or herself in a constant, predictable logical manner and may appear confused and anxious during the episode. The patient may ask the same question or make the same comments, such as, ''Where am I?'' or ''Who are you?'' or ''What are you doing here?'' TGA has sometimes been preceded by emotional experiences, coitus pain, or dizziness, but frequently no precipitating cause is found. The amnestic period can last anywhere from 30 minutes to 12 hours, although durations of 24 to 48 hours have been reported. The syndrome is usually a one-time occurrence. Recurrence is rare. According to one multicenter study,[6] TGA has an annual recurrence rate of 4.7 per cent. The rate increases with each successive year, so that at five years the recurrence rate is 21 per cent.

Despite its well-characterized clinical features, the etiology of TGA is not known. TGA has been implicated as a manifestation of several disease processes including cerebral ischemia, migraines, emotional stress, seizures, tumors, polycythemia, and drug intoxication such as digitalis, iodochlorhydroxyquin, and diazepam.[7] However, none of these inferences have been proved. The possible relationship between TGA and vascular diseases such as transient ischemic or embolic brain event remains a controversial topic.[8,9] The vascular territory involved in amnesia, in most cases, is in the distribution of the posterior cerebral arteries, which supply limbic-hippocampal structures and mesial temporal lobes.[10] A transient ischemic attack in this territory could account for the amnesic syndrome. However, there are several arguments against this theory.[6,11,12] Documented vertebrobasilar strokes in the distribution of these arteries are usually not preceded by amnesia. Furthermore, when amnesia is a presenting symptom in vertebrobasilar insufficiency, it is usually accompanied by other neurologic signs and symptoms, such as visual field defects, blindness, hemiparesis, and sensory abnormalities. Vertebrobasilar insufficiency is common. If TGA were a consequence of vertebrobasilar disease, one would expect to see an increased incidence of TGA. Miller et al.,[13] in their review of 277 patients with TGA, found the incidence of stroke among the TGA patients to be approximately equal to that expected for age-specific incidence rates in a number of normal populations. TGA has also been reported after cardiac catheterization or cerebral angiography[14,15] where it is thought to be due to cerebral emboli. The embolization here may involve both hippocampi, thereby producing amnesia. In this setting, amnesia is accompanied by focal neurologic deficits as well. Amnesia seen in the presence of cerebral ischemia, therefore, is not TGA in the pure, uncontaminated sense. In global cerebral ischemia, amnesia is associated with focal neurologic symptoms.

The relationship between TGA and migraine has been heavily emphasized.[7,16] Caplan et al. assert that migraine has many unexplained vascular disturbances with a predilection for the posterior circulation.[16] Fortification spectra and teichopsia, for example, are positive visual phenomena in classic migraine. These are thought by some to be localized to the occipital lobes, the vascular supply of which is in the distribution of the posterior cerebral arteries. These vessels also supply part of the thalami, hippocampi, and forniceal systems. The anterograde and retrograde amnesia; the repetitive, compulsive questioning; and the anxiety seen in TGA can be regarded as positive phenomena resulting from ischemia of the limbic system during a migrainous attack. Some precipitating factors for migraines and TGA are similar. These include sudden cold water immersion, hot showers, sexual intercourse, fatigue, and intravenous contrast dyes. Electroencephalogram (EEG) done during or soon after the onset of an episode of TGA may show bilateral temporal lobe slowing or temporal lobe seizure abnormalities or be normal.[17,18] These same EEG changes may occur in migraine. The pathophysiology for both syndromes is felt to be related to regional cerebral blood flow (rCBF) changes.[7] In migraine, there is an initial vasoconstriction resulting in decreased rCBF during the prodromal stage. This is then followed by vasodilation with hyperperfusion leading to the headache. It is postulated that transient global amnesia occurs in migraine because of an imbalance in perfusion pressure between the anterior and posterior circulation. There is more vasoconstriction in the posterior cerebral artery at the level of the arterioles during the prodromal stage. The subsequent vasodilatory phase is asynchronous with the middle cerebral artery territory being hyperperfused earlier, therefore causing more shunting from the posterior cerebral artery. This leads to a worsening of the already relative posterior cerebral artery insufficiency. The work of Matthew et al.[19] and Edmeads[20] in spatial and temporal irregularities in rCBF during migraine have lent some support to this hypothesis.

Fisher proposed that TGA may be a result of emotional stress.[21] In his review of 85 cases, 26 cases were related to one form of emotion or another. Emotion not only involves expression of joy and sorrow or sadness; emotion also involves fear, severe pain, and sexual pleasure. Fisher contends that the cortical expression of emotion runs parallel to the hippocampal-forniceal system. Therefore, the affection of one system may involve the other as well. Pathologic correlation to this hypothesis, however, has not been shown.

Other illnesses implicated in the cause of TGA have included seizures and CNS tumors, although these latter are exceedingly rare. Seizure presenting de novo as TGA has been reported.[22] However, amnesia as a sole symptom in seizure is rare. Seizures are usually associated with other symptoms such as auras, automatisms, or focal motor phenomenon. The ictus tends to recur without treatment. An EEG with the presence of focal spikes or sharp waves will be helpful in diagnosing seizure in such instances. Amnesia as a symptom of CNS tumor is always associated with focal neurologic deficits. Furthermore, the memory deficit persists and deteriorates with time in these cases.

The diagnosis of TGA is based largely on history. It has typical clinical features of variable retrograde and anterograde amnesia with intact cognition and normal social behavior. Persons with TGA have normal neurologic examinations, save for the abnormal mental status exam. That notwithstanding, initial presenting symptoms of other disease processes may appear at their onset to be no more than TGA. Therefore, patients with suspected TGA should undergo routine blood work, serum cholesterol, echocardiogram, and chest x-ray. Head computerized tomography (CT) with and without contrast or head magnetic resonance imaging (MRI) should be done. An EEG should be performed to rule out a seizure disorder. TGA requires no treatment and will resolve on its own. TGA is a benign syndrome with a very good prognosis and a very low recurrence rate.

Cerebral Concussion

Concussion refers to a transient period of altered consciousness following head injury. The victim can be dazed and confused or have a brief period of unconsciousness. Hemodynamic reflexes, sweating, and other autonomic functions are immediately altered. If examination is carried out at this point, a variety of abnormal reflexes may be elicited. The victim regains his or her senses within a few minutes to hours, then is initially confused and disoriented for a variable amount of time. Depending on the severity of injury, it may be moments to months later before the victim can form reasonable memories again. It is during this period of confusion that the characteristic amnesic syndrome emerges.

Russell,[3] Russell and Nathan,[23] and Symonds[24] studied amnesia extensively among head-injured military men in the British armed forces and among civilians. They described two components to the syndrome of trauma-related memory disturbance: a retrograde and an anterograde amnesia. The retrograde amnesia has a characteristic brief duration consisting of moments of amnesia prior to the sustained head injury. The victim usually recalls being struck by something or seeing someone coming but does not remember the events that follow. In more severe trauma, however, the initial duration of the retrograde amnesia may be much longer, extending as far back as several years. In these instances, victims may insist that they are several years younger than their stated age and behave according to memories and experiences prior to the period of memory loss. Recent memory is more affected than remote memory. The retrograde amnesia will shrink as confusion clears, with more remote memories returning before recent ones.

The duration of post-traumatic amnesia, measuring the ability to make memories timed from the onset of injury, has different clinical implications. It is an index of the duration of impaired consciousness, signifies the seriousness of concussion or lack thereof, and has prognostic implications. The more severe head injuries have been correlated with prolonged or permanent post-traumatic amnesia. The prognosis of recovery of normal memory function diminishes with lengthy post-traumatic amnesia. Some patients experience delayed post-traumatic amnesia. Such a head-injured person does not lose consciousness initially and remains quite lucid. It is not until a few hours later that the amnesia becomes evident. Persons so affected have frequently received aggressive external stimuli to maintain consciousness after a blow to the head. It is not until they drift into unconsciousness or sleep and upon awakening that the amnesia becomes obvious. Occasionally, delayed post-traumatic amnesia is seen in patients having initially undisclosed brain or skull trauma such as extradural, subdural, or subarachnoid hemorrhages and basilar skull fractures. In these late-onset cases, the patient frequently displays a deteriorating mental state, progressing to confusion, somnolence, stupor, and coma.

A person's behavior during post-traumatic amnesia is highly variable. Some patients are confused and disoriented. They may fail to recognize familiar persons and exhibit confusion. Others appear quite normal and may carry out routine activities without evident difficulty. When questioned, however, the head-injured person has no inkling of events that have passed. This observation has been well described in athletes, particularly in football players and boxers, who had suffered significant head injury.[25,26,27,28,29] The athlete may continue to perform impeccably well and go on to win the match, yet immediately afterward is unable to recall any of his or her performance. Language function during post-traumatic amnesia may be contaminated by varying degrees and types of aphasia and apraxia or be completely normal. Confabulation is sometimes seen and initially may not have any relation to the accident. However, as patients recognize the nature of the accident, they may draw patchy recollections from islands of returned memory or from visual hallucinations to construct their stories. The confabulation may sound quite rational and realistic. One should be careful in distinguishing between true and false statements, especially if the case has legal implications. Some patients experience an interesting visual hallucination after they have recovered full consciousness. These are transient, repetitive hallucinations based on experience just before the trauma.

The pathogenesis of amnesia is not well understood. The current theory centers around the shearing force exerted on the brain during an accident. As a consequence, nerve fibers are stretched, not torn, resulting in a reversible postconcussion amnesia.[30]

Memory impairment following cerebral concussion consists of retrograde and anterograde amnesia. The duration of the latter has prognostic significance and correlates directly with the severity of the head trauma. Head trauma victims should be evaluated for focal neurologic deficits and level of consciousness to exclude concomitant neurologic pathology. Of greater diagnostic concern is the development of extradural, subdural, subarachnoid, or intracerebral hemorrhages or basilar skull fractures. At-risk individuals should have an unenhanced head CT. Patients who were initially lucid and later demonstrate mental deterioration should have a repeat head CT scan to rule out a slowly expanding subdural or epidural hematoma. A neurosurgeon should be consulted for the management of acute head trauma.

Wernicke-Korsakoff Syndrome

Thiamine deficiency affects both the central and peripheral nervous systems. Centrally, it causes an acute clinical syndrome of depressed delerium, ophthalmoplegia, and gait ataxia called *Wernicke encephalopathy*. In the chronic stage, it causes a dense amnesic syndrome called Korsakoff psychosis. The two entities are closely related and represent a continuum of the same disease process, with the former progressing to the latter in 96 per cent of cases. Its clinical and pathologic manifestations were extensively studied by Victor et al.[31] in their series of 245 patients. Wernicke encephalopathy is reversible if treatment is instituted early. Once clearly established, Korsakoff's psychosis is unremediable, and response to treatment is poor. Early diagnosis of Wernicke encephalopathy is paramount if effective treatment is to be instituted—that consisting of parenteral administration of thiamine.

In 1881, Wernicke described the clinical and pathologic findings in three patients with a peculiar encephalopathy. One was a seamstress, and two were alcoholic men. The seamstress developed esophageal sclerosis after a suicide attempt by drinking sulfuric acid. She developed intractable vomiting. Shortly thereafter, she had mental confusion and drowsiness, gait ataxia, and poor visual acuity. She displayed strabismus due to bilateral abducens palsy and vertical nystagmus on upward gaze. Her symptoms progressively worsened until her death 12 days later. Wernicke's other patients had similar complaints of delerium, gait ataxia, and external ophthalmoplegia. Pathologically, all three cases had evidence of small punctate hemorrhages in the periventricular gray matter around the third and fourth ventricles.

In a series of papers from 1887 to 1891, Korsakoff described a specific amnestic dementia coexisting with peripheral neuropathy in alcoholics and other nutritional deprivation such as puerperal sepsis, typhoid fever, intestinal obstruction with intractable vomiting, and hyperemesis gravidarum. Korsakoff maintained that these were different manifestations of the same disease process and called the illness psychosis polyneuritica. In his later observations, Korsakoff asserted that the peripheral neuropathy was not essential to the syndrome and that often the severity of the psychosis was out of proportion to the mild neuropathy.

The relationship between the Wernicke and Korsakoff disease entities was not appreciated until 1896 by Gudden. He studied the brain pathology in five alcoholic patients with peripheral neuropathy and psychosis. He found pathologic changes in the mammillary bodies, walls of the third ventricle, and brainstem similar to Wernicke's findings. Bereberi demonstrated the pathologic cause of the Wernicke-Korsakoff syndrome to be due to thiamine deficiency.

Wernicke encephalopathy is characterized by the triad of ophthalmoplegia, gait ataxia, and mental confusion. The most common eye finding is nystagmus, seen in over 80 per cent of cases. This is followed by bilateral abducens palsy (54 per cent) and conjugate gaze palsy (44 per cent). The *ataxia* refers to gait instability and rarely involves ataxia of any other limb or speech. The early mental changes are quite pronounced and are referred to as *global confusional state* by Victor et al.[31] This state is characterized by a quiet, hypokinetic delerium. Patients appear lethargic and apathetic, with decreased responsiveness and awareness of surroundings. There is significant spatial and temporal disorientation. Patients often know who they are but have no idea of where they are or how they got there. Furthermore, they have no concept of time and often give the wrong date by one to two decades. When asked specific questions, they usually respond evasively. Early in the disease, this may be due to poor concentration. As patients are being treated and the delerium clears, the evasiveness reflects patients' realization of memory deficit and attempt to hide it. There is a pronounced impairment of perception as well, with patients failing to recognize and identify their surrounding environment and persons and to integrate that information into present situations. Consequently, patients misidentify position of body parts, old familiar friends and relatives, and places. It is during this stage that patients may confabulate as they construct answers to questions from misperception of their environment. There is usually a marked memory defect present as well that is not initially recognized by the examiner owing to the dense confusion and delerium. However, memory impairment becomes apparent as the delerium is treated. Global confusional state is responsive to thiamine therapy, and symptoms begin to subside within days to weeks. A small number of patients have complete resolution. Unfortunately, a number of patients have a residual memory deficit and go on to develop Korsakoff psychosis.

Korsakoff psychosis is a more chronic manifestation of thiamine deficiency. Eighty per cent of patients initially present with the global confusional state. Only 20 per cent of patients present de novo as Korsakoff psychosis. Patients with Korsakoff psychosis are mentally alert and responsive, with intact awareness of their surrounding environment, and maintain proper social graces. Their moods tend to be placid; their affect, bland or detached. Language comprehension and expression are not affected, and they can deduce appropriate answers on given premises. There is no apraxia or agnosia. Patients, however, demonstrate significant impairment of both anterograde and retrograde amnesia and have no insight of their memory deficit.

With respect to anterograde amnesia, patients have a very limited forward memory span and marked impairment of recent memory. Thus, they are unable to learn and form new memories and cannot register and retain three bits of information regardless of whether they are given in the form of persons, objects, or nonsensical syllables. This impairment is seen irrespective of the type of sensory stimulus employed— verbal, visual, or tactile. Interestingly, immediate recall is never affected, regardless of the severity of the learning disability, an example of which is seen in Victor's patient who displayed appropriate emotional response when told that his brother had died.[31] When asked about his brother a few hours later, he answered as if nothing had happened. Anterograde amnesia is not absolute. With time—usually weeks to months—there is some mild improvement in memory defect such that patients can learn simple tasks such as finding their way around the hospital to go to the bathroom or to the dining room. Recovery, however, is never complete and adequate enough to enable independent living again. Overall, the memory defect becomes a handicap, as patients are unable to acquire new information and integrate it with old experiences.

The retrograde amnesia is more variable in terms of degree of severity and time involved. It usually extends several years back without clear distinction as to when the amnestic period started. The memory impairment is never complete, and patients have islands of retained memory. These islands of retained memories are of varying degrees of accuracy and are not separated by proper temporal sequences. As a consequence, patients have a sense of telescoped time. An event that lasted over five years is retold by patients as only lasting over a few months. An experience that occurred 10 years ago is recalled by patients as occurring yesterday.

Confabulation has traditionally been described as a characteristic feature of Korsakoff psychosis. However, in Victor's series,[31] confabulation was not seen in many patients and was not a key feature for diagnosis. Part of the problem in evaluating confabulation deals with how one defines it. It has commonly been defined as "a fabrication of a ready answer to a question or a fluent recitation of fictitious experiences."[31] In the Wernicke-Korsakoff syndrome, there are two phases of the illness in which confabulation has been inferred. The first is during the global confusional state whereby patients give inappropriate answers owing to impaired perception of the environment. The second is during the convalescent period where patients relate fragments of past events and experiences without any regard to their proper temporal sequences. Thus, these inaccurate accounts of events are not, by definition, confabulation; rather, they are actually made up of real experiences related out of context with respect to time and perception.

The pathogenesis of amnesia in the Wernicke-Korsakoff syndrome is due to thiamine deficiency. There are no specific pathologic changes seen in the global confusional state. In Korsakoff psychosis, the dorsal median nucleus of the thalamus has consistently been found either to be necrotic or to have small punctate hemorrhages.[31] Similar lesions have sometimes been found in the mammillary bodies and medial part of the pulvinar. Treatment involves giving patients 100 mg of thiamine intravenously or intramuscularly at the time of diagnosis for three to five days. This is followed by daily multivitamin supplements and appropriate dietary intake. Early in the treatment, patients should not be given glucose supplement without initially receiving thiamine. Thiamine acts as a coenzyme at several steps in glucose metabolism, including the pentose phosphate pathway, conversion of pyruvate to acetyl-coA for utilization in the Krebs cycle, and the Krebs cycle itself. Adding glucose under such conditions would deplete the body further of whatever meager store of thiamine is left and can precipitate an acute Wernicke encephalopathy.

Diagnosis of the Wernicke-Korsakoff syndrome should be considered in patients who present with delerium and mental status changes and have a history suspicious for poor nutrition. Patients include chronic alcoholics as well as those who have chronic debilitations including dementia, end-stage malignancies, malabsorption syndromes, and chronic and recurrent emesis.

The prognosis for Wernicke encephalopathy varies depending on symptomatology and duration. With respect to ocular palsies, response to treatment is good, with onset of response seen within hours to days; most patients go on to have complete recovery. Gait ataxia, on the other hand, has a slower recovery time. Onset of recovery varies from days to weeks to months. In Victor's series, only 38 per cent of patients had complete recovery, 35 per cent had partial recovery, and 27 per cent showed no sign of improvement at all.[31] The global confusional state has the slowest rate of recovery, as alluded to earlier. Furthermore, as the confusional state subsides, the memory impairment of Korsakoff psychosis becomes apparent. Korsakoff psychosis, in itself, carries a poor prognosis, with only 20 per cent of patients showing partial, and rarely complete, recovery. Recovery takes months to years. As patients improve, there is less confabulation, and patients appear to have more insight into their deficits. Unfortunately, they never regain full competency to assume independence again.

Alcoholic Blackout

Goodwin et al.[32] described discrete episodes of memory loss for significant events in 64 per cent of alcoholics. These blackouts occurred during prolonged alcohol imbibition and severe intoxication. There are two types of alcoholic blackouts: fragmentary and en bloc. In the fragmentary type, alcoholics are not aware of deficits until told later. They have islets of preserved memory, and the amnesia tends to shrink with time. In the en bloc type, patients eventually become aware of their amnesia as if coming around from a sleep. They have "time lost" that cannot be accounted for. They appear to be in a fuguelike state where they can pay bills, travel, stay at a hotel, and yet have no recollection of it afterward. The amnesia may last for hours to a few days. Some 61 per cent of these patients experience a state-dependent phenomenon whereby they can only do certain things while intoxicated—for example, patients who hide money in a special place while intoxicated and cannot find it in their sober state; they can only find it when intoxicated again. Islets of preserved memory are rarely seen in this type of alcoholic blackout.

Electroconvulsive Therapy

The adverse effects of electroconvulsive therapy (ECT) in causing discrete memory loss is well known and was described as early as 1951.[33] Verbal memory seems to be consistently affected. Unilateral ECT to the non-dominant hemisphere appears to have little effect on memory loss, as opposed to bilateral ECT. Memory testing of these patients within

hours after ECT shows variable retrograde amnesia of one to three years and significant anterograde amnesia with poor ability to learn and retain new information. Examination of these patients at six to nine months after ECT shows that the amnesia has resolved except for that portion of memory within hours after ECT.

Cerebrovascular Disease

Amnesia can sometimes be a prominent feature in some stroke syndromes. Infarction of the anterior communicating arteries from an aneurysmal bleed can produce a disconnection syndrome involving the memory pathway. These patients have both defective anterograde and retrograde amnesia. However, given proper cuing, they can recall the specific details of an event. They can learn isolated modal stimuli; however, they lack temporal tagging and therefore cannot integrate the learned auditory-verbal and visual information. These patients also have a prominent propensity to confabulate wildly. The content of confabulation here is quite different from those of Korsakoff psychosis. It consists of interweaving a current event with imagined personal fantasies. Interestingly, the fabricated fantasy can sometimes be incorporated into that patient's memory and be perceived by the patient as reality. The main region involved in the infarction is the ventromedial sector of the frontal lobe. This area of the basal forebrain is interconnected with the hippocampus via the fornix. Both of these areas are involved in memory processing and store.

Infarction of the posterior cerebral arteries or its terminal thalamic branches can result in bilateral hippocampal and thalamic infarctions rendering an amnesic syndrome very similar to Korsakoff psychosis. An aneurysmal rupture at, or distal emboli to, the basilar artery tip will cause infarction of mesial temporal lobes as well as occipital lobes, rostral midbrain, and paramedian thalamic and subthalamic structures, rendering a very classic stroke syndrome.[34] These patients are found to have an agitated delerium with confusion and disorientation. They also have characteristic ocular movement disorders, skew deviations, visual field defects, and visual hallucinations.

Amnesia may also be a prominent symptom in watershed infarction, which occurs in cardiopulmonary arrest with severe hypotension and hypoperfusion and in severe hypoxia. The watershed zones are the borders between the posterior cerebral and middle cerebral arteries and between the middle and anterior cerebral arteries. Finally, multi-infarct dementia can initially present with mild amnesia. The symptoms occur in a stepwise progression and are associated with other cognitive impairments.

Infection

Amnesia is a common complication of some CNS infections, particularly herpes encephalitis and tuberculous meningitis. In herpes encephalitis, there is predilection for the temporal lobe. When both temporal lobes are affected, the resulting amnesic syndrome is very similar to Korsakoff psychosis. Patients are left with dense and prolonged, persistent retrograde amnesia and severe anterograde amnesia. Patients' insight into their illness, however, is good, and there is no impairment of perception. In tuberculous meningitis, there is meningeal infiltration of mycoplasma into the sellar and tentorial areas. Patients can be confused and have impairment of recent and remote memory. As the infection resolves, there is good recovery of recent memory. Recovery of the retrograde amnesia is variable and patchy.

Dementia

Amnesia can be seen as an early symptom in most dementing illnesses, particularly Alzheimer's disease. Early subtle symptoms such as poor concentration, forgetfulness, and disorientation can be early clues to dementia. It is not until later, as the disease progresses, that apathy and other cognitive dysfunctions such as aphasia and apraxia become apparent. Similar findings are seen in Creutzfeldt-Jakob disease, normopressure hydrocephalus, and multi-infarct dementia. Subarachnoid hemorrhages have also been known to cause forgetfulness.

Psychogenic Amnesia

Aside from organic causes of amnesia, there are some psychiatric circumstances in which amnesia has been known to occur: fugue states; situation-specific circumstances, especially in relation to unlawful offenses; and depression with pseudodementia.

The fugue state is characterized by the sudden loss of personal memory and of personal identity, associated with a period of wandering. The episode lasts for periods of hours to days. The patient is left afterward with a residual amnesic gap for that duration. Certain factors predispose to the fugue state. The most common one is stress, particularly those associated with wartime. Other stressors such as marital discord and financial problems may also precipitate a fugue. Depression occurring at the onset of a fugue state is common. The fugue may act as a flight from committing suicide. Stengel[35] maintains that suicide never occurs during a fugue. However, the period immediately following it is most dangerous, the time when the patient is most vulnerable to committing suicide. Fugues have also been seen in patients with a previous history of organic causes for amnesia, such as head injuries, alcoholic blackouts, and temporal lobe epilepsy. Feigning a fugue can also be seen in hysterical patients with a tendency to lie.

Situational-related amnesias are commonly seen in unlawful offenses, and 30 to 40 per cent of these are related to homicide. Taylor and Kopelman[36] found that this type of amnesia may occur under three circumstances:

1.   Homicide cases in which the victim was closely related to the offender; the crime was not premeditated and occurred under a state of high emotional arousal.

2.   Chronic alcohol abusers who commit a crime while severely intoxicated; the victim in this case can be anyone.

3.   The crime is committed by a schizophrenic who is floridly psychotic at the time of the crime.

Finally, in depression and pseudodementia, the patient may appear to be forgetful. The mechanism here is due to poor effort in remembering and is related to attention deficits and lack of motivation and drive.

REFERENCES

1.   DeJong RN. The neurologic examination. 3rd ed. New York: Harper and Row, 1950:44–6.
2.   McGlone J, Young B. Cerebral localization. In: Joynt RJ, ed. Clinical neurology. Philadelphia: JB Lippincott, 1988:(vol 1):30–4.
3.   Russell WR. Cerebral involvement in head injury; study based on examination of 200 cases. Brain 1932;55:549–603.
4.   Bender MB. Syndrome of isolated episodes of confusion with amnesia. J Hillside Hosp 1956;5:212–5.
5.   Fisher CM, Adams RD. Transient global amnesia. Trans Am Neurol Assoc 1958;83:143–6.

6. Hinge H, Jenson TS, Kjaer M, Marquardsen J, Olivarius B. The prognosis of transient global amnesia. Results of a multicenter study. Arch Neurol 1986;43:673–6.

7. Crowell GF, Stump DA, Biller J, McHenry LC, Toole JF. The transient global amnesia–migraine connection. Arch Neurol 1984;41:75–9.

8. Kushner MJ, Hauser WA. Transient global amnesia: a case-control study. Ann Neurol 1985;18:684–91.

9. Matias-Guiu J, Colimer R, Sigura A, et al. Cranial CT scan in transient global amnesia. Acta Neurol Scand 1986;78:298–301.

10. Benson DF, Marsden CD, Meadows JL. The amnestic syndrome of posterior cerebral artery occlusion. Acta Neurol Scand 1974;50:133–45.

11. Palmer EP. Transient global amnesia and the amnestic syndrome. Med Clin North Am 1986;70:1361–74.

12. Shuping LA. Transient global amnesia. Ann Neurol 1980;7:281–5.

13. Miller WM, Petersen RC, Metter EJ, Millikan CH, Yanagihara T. Transient global amnesia: clinical characteristics and prognosis. Neurology 1987;37:733–7.

14. Cochran JW, Morrell GF, Hickman MS, Cochran EJ. Transient global amnesia after cerebral angiography: report of seven cases. Arch Neurol 1982;89:593–4.

15. Shuttleworth E, Wise G. Transient global amnesia due to arterial embolism. Arch Neurol 1973;29:340–2.

16. Caplan LR, Chedru F, Lhermitte F, Mayman C. Transient global amnesia and migraine. Neurology 1981;31:1167–70.

17. Matthew NT, Meyer JS. Pathogenesis and natural history of transient global amnesia. Stroke 1974;5:303–11.

18. Tharp B. The electroencephalogram in transient global amnesia. Electroencephalogr Clin Neurophysiol 1969;26:96–9.

19. Matthew NT, Hrastnik F, Meyer JS. Regional cerebral blood flow in the diagnosis of vascular headache. Headache 1975;15:252–60.

20. Edmeads J. Cerebral blood flow in migraine. Headache 1977;17:148–52.

21. Fisher CM. Transient global amnesia. Precipitating activities and other observations. Arch Neurol 1982;89:605–8.

22. Croft PB, Heathfield KWG, Swash M. Differential diagnosis of transient global amnesia. Br Med J 1973;4:593–6.

23. Russell WR, Nathan PW. Traumatic amnesia. Brain 1946;68:280–300.

24. Symonds CP. Mental disorder following head injury. Proc R Soc Med 1937;30:1081–94.

25. Fisher CM. Concussion amnesia. Neurology 1966;16:826–30.

26. Burton HL. Discussion on minor head injuries. Proc R Soc Med 1981;24:27–34.

27. Quigley TB. Athletic injuries: some observations on their prevention and treatment. Nebr Med J 1957;42:435–40.

28. Blonstein JL, Clarke E. Further observations on the medical aspects of amateur boxing. Br Med J 1957;1:362–4.

29. Critchley M. Medical aspects of boxing, particularly from a neurology standpoint. Br Med J 1957;1:357–62.

30. Strich SJ. Diffuse degeneration of the cerebral white matter in severe dementia following head injury. J Neurol Neuropsychiatry 1956;19:163–85.

31. Victor M, Adams RD, Collins GH. The Wernicke-Korsakoff syndrome and related neurologic disorders due to alcoholism and malnutrition. 2nd ed. Philadelphia: FA Davis, 1989:1–135.

32. Goodwin DW, Crane JB, Guze SB. Alcoholic "blackouts": a review and clinical study of 100 alcoholics. Am J Psychiatry 1969;126:191–8.

33. Janis RL, Astrachan M. The effects of electroconvulsive treatments on efficiency. J Abnorm Soc Psychol 1951;46:501–11.

34. Caplan LR. Top of the basilar syndrome. Neurology 1980;30:71–9.

35. Stengel E. On the etiology of the fugue state. J Ment Sci 1941;87:572–99.

36. Taylor PJ, Kopelman MD. Amnesia for criminal offences. Psychol Med 1984;87:581–8.

ANOREXIA

WILLIAM L. TOFFLER, SCOTT A. FIELDS, GLENN S. RODRIGUEZ, DANA W. PETERSON, and JOHN W. SAULTZ

SYNONYMS: Appetite Loss, Dysgeusia, Hypogeusia

BACKGROUND

The intake of food plays a powerful social role in our society. Anorexia, or the loss of appetite for food, may be the expression of physiologic, psychologic, or social disruptions.

The physiologic mechanisms that control appetite are incompletely understood. The hypothalamus has a lateral "feeding center" and a ventromedial "satiety center." The feeding center is modulated by a variety of neurotransmitters. Norepinephrine and dynorphin (an endogenous opiate peptide) appear to be appetite stimulants. Corticotropin releasing factor is a potent centrally acting appetite depressant. The gastrointestinal system has important suppressive feedback via the vagus nerve to the ventromedial satiety center. A variety of gastrointestinal hormones have been demonstrated to decrease food intake, but the role of cholecystokinin has been the best studied.[1] Sensory (especially smell and taste), emotional, and social factors may alter hormonal effects.

Gastrointestinal causes of anorexia include ulcerative colitis, regional enteritis, celiac disease, parasitic infestation, esophageal dysmotility, and gastric outlet obstruction.[2,3] Individuals with chronic infectious diseases such as acquired immune deficiency syndrome or reactivation of tuberculosis may present with both anorexia and weight loss.[4] Endocrine disorders (such as Addison's disease, hyperthyroidism, and diabetes mellitus), autoimmune disorders (such as ankylosing spondylitis and systemic lupus erythematosus), and neoplastic processes must also be considered. Anorexia may be a manifestation of psychiatric illness including major depression, mania, schizophrenia, and eating disorders. Alcohol and drug abuse with barbiturates, benzodiazepines, or amphetamines are also common causes of anorexia and weight loss.

Anorexia associated with loss of body mass in patients with malignancies is defined as *cancer cachexia.* Physical features include skeletal muscle and visceral organ atrophy. Metabolic derangements include anemia, hypoalbuminemia, liver enzyme abnormalities, and glucose intolerance. Over 50 per cent of cancer patients note weight loss, and approximately 15 per cent had lost more than 10 per cent of their baseline weight.[5]

Etiologies of anorexia vary in prevalence, and can be grouped into age-specific categories (see Table 1). Feeding problems are common in infants between 3 and 12 months of age and commonly last approximately 4 months. Frequent complaints include refusal to eat, colic, and vomiting.[6] Evaluation must include a thorough history of the complaint and consideration of social and family factors.

Anorexia nervosa and bulimia are common and serious eating disorders that occur most often in adolescents. Anorexia nervosa is estimated to occur in up to 1 per cent of teenage girls (ages 12 to 18 years)—often in individuals with a positive family history. The ratio of females to males is approximately 20:1. Diagnostic criteria for anorexia nervosa include an intense fear of becoming obese, disturbance of

TABLE 1. Common Causes of Anorexia Related to Age Groups

Infants	Colic
	Milk intolerance
	Infection
Children	Emotional stress
	Depression
	Infection
	Parenting problems
Adolescents	Mental illness
	Anorexia nervosa
	Depression
	Schizophrenia
	Substance abuse
	Family dysfunction
	Infection
Adults	Gastrointestinal (GI) disorders
	Inflammatory bowel disease
	Peptic ulcer disease
	Irritable bowel syndrome
	Hepatitis
	Cholelithiasis
	Infection
	Depression
	Malignancy
Elderly	Physiologic aging
	Depression
	Medications
	Dementia
	Malignancy
	Infection

body image, weight loss, refusal to maintain body weight, and an absence of physical illness that would explain these symptoms. Bulimia, defined as binge eating often followed by self-induced vomiting, is common in college-age populations, involving 2 to 13 per cent of women and 1.4 to 6.1 per cent of males.[7]

Anorexia in the elderly may be due to decreased responsiveness of the norepinephrine system, decreased activity of the endorphin system, and increased corticotropin releasing factor levels. Other physiologic changes of aging such as decreased smell, taste, and vision may all decrease the attractiveness of food.

HISTORY

History of the Present Illness

The medical history will provide important clues in determining the etiology of anorexia. Basic information regarding duration and associated systemic symptoms (fever, night sweats, rash, arthritis, or arthralgias) should be elicited. A history of sitophobia (fear of eating due to subsequent or associated discomfort), persistent cough, visual field defects, or melena may provide useful information. The presence or absence of weight loss is one of the most important clues in distinguishing between organic and psychogenic causes.

Past Medical History

Anorexia is a common symptom of gastrointestinal diseases. A previous history of peptic ulcer disease may be present with esophageal or gastric outlet obstruction, or gastric carcinoma. Previous abdominal surgery may also be associated with an obstruction. A past history of ulcerative colitis or regional enteritis, exposure to individuals with hepatitis or tuberculosis, or a travel history may be important information. Pre-existing pulmonary disease or endocrine disorders may also play a role in anorexia. Congestive heart failure may be a cause of anorexia but may also be a complication of malnutrition. A history of mental illness, major affective disorder, schizophrenia, or paranoid ideation may be related to anorexia in a given patient.

Medication History

Seventeen of 50 medications (34 per cent) chosen at random from the *Physicians' Desk Reference* were found to have anorexia listed as a major side effect.[8] Drugs commonly associated with anorexia include methylxanthines, beta-sympathomimetics, cardiac glycosides, antiarrhythmics, antihypertensives, antituberculin, antifungal, and chemotherapeutic agents. Inappropriate use of amphetamines, diet pills, or laxatives may be seen in patients with anorexia nervosa.

Social History

Efforts should be made to quantify any use of tobacco products, alcohol, or street drugs. A history of intravenous drug use or homosexual or promiscuous heterosexual relationships may prompt evaluation for acquired immune deficiency syndrome. As many as 50 per cent of male patients with anorexia nervosa are homosexual.[9] Personality traits and family dynamics are important clues in evaluating eating disorders. Asking about changes in the patient's relationships with friends and family may add valuable diagnostic clues. Patients with anorexia nervosa are often described as coming from economically privileged families, seeking upward mobility, and possessing introverted, dependent, and perfectionistic traits.[9] Their families are characterized by conflict avoidance, parental dependency, and insecurity.[10]

Occupational History

Employment involving exposure to toxic substances may be associated with anorexia. Occupational stress may also be an important clue suggesting depression or anxiety disorders.

Family History

There may be a family history of alcoholism in alcoholic or drug-abusing patients. Studies of patients with anorexia nervosa have shown an increased incidence of affective disorders in first-degree relatives.[11]

Focused Queries

1. *Has there been associated weight loss?* A documented unintentional weight loss exceeding 5 per cent over a 6- to 12-month period is considered abnormal and warrants investigation.

2. *Have there been fevers or night sweats?* The presence of a fever is not typically associated with psychogenic causes of anorexia. A history of fevers should raise the possibility of an infectious process (reactivation tuberculosis), connective tissue disease (systemic lupus erythematosus, ankylosing spondylitis), malignancy (lymphoma), or inflammatory bowel disease.[12]

3. *What is the usual diet and exercise level over a 24-hour period?* Low caloric intake with high caloric exercise expenditure is often seen in patients with anorexia nervosa.

4. *What is the patient's perception of his or her physique, and what is perceived as an ideal body weight?* Intense fear of fatness, disturbed body image, and refusal to maintain a normal body weight are characteristic of anorexia nervosa.[12]

5. *What is the patient's menstrual history?* Virtually all young women with anorexia nervosa develop amenorrhea, and up to 25 per cent of these patients have cessation of menses prior to weight loss.[12]

6. *What stressors are present in the patient's life?* Such questioning may provide significant psychosocial information related to the symptoms, as well as insight into the impact of the illness on the patient's life.

PHYSICAL EXAMINATION

Because anorexia may be the presenting symptom of many organic diseases, a complete physical examination is warranted. Careful examination of the breasts and pulmonary, gastrointestinal, genital, urinary, and neurologic systems for occult malignancy should be performed. Areas deserving specific attention include the patient's vital signs and weight, general body habitus, and gastrointestinal and neurologic systems. Serial examination is important and may reveal significant changes over time that direct the course of further evaluation.

Vital Signs, Height, and Weight

Careful documentation of the patient's height and weight is important to determine deviation below ideal body weight and to establish weight loss over time. Patients with anorexia nervosa have significant changes in their vital signs.[7,12] Bradycardia with a heart rate as low as 34 beats per minute is occasionally observed.[7] In addition, blood pressure is often less than 100/50.[7] Body temperature can be decreased to 34 to 35° C (93 to 95° F).[12] If severe vomiting is present, respiration (minute ventilation) may decrease in compensation for the metabolic alkalosis associated with the loss of gastric acid.

General Appearance

Profound wasting of muscle mass and loss of subcutaneous and breast fat stores should be identified.

Head and Neck Examination

The oral cavity may reveal stomatitis and glossitis. Staining of dental enamel may occur in patients with repetitive self-induced vomiting. Elderly patients should be checked for poor dentition or ill-fitting dentures. The thyroid gland should be palpated for enlargement or nodules.

Pulmonary and Cardiovascular System

Findings consistent with chronic pulmonary disease may include barrel chest, wheezing, distant breath sounds, and poor air exchange. Patients should be examined for signs of congestive heart failure (pulmonary edema, S_3 gallop, jugular venous distension, hepatojugular reflux, and peripheral edema).

Gastrointestinal System

Significant findings may include jaundice, hepatic enlargement or tenderness, epigastric pain, and abdominal or rectal masses. Hemoccult testing should be performed to detect occult gastrointestinal blood loss.

Genitourinary System

Examination of the kidneys, testes and prostate, or uterus and ovaries may reveal an underlying neoplastic process.

Lymphatic System

Cervical, supraclavicular, axillary, epitrochlear, or inguinal adenopathy may be associated with an infection or a malignancy.

Skin, Hair, and Nails

The lack of vitamins and nutrients seen in malnourished patients may lead to the loss of scalp hair; lanugolike hair on the face and trunk; rough, scaly skin; brittle nails; petechia, or ecchymosis.[12] Scars on the knuckles may be present with self-induced vomiting.[11,12]

Neurologic System

Cranial nerves should be examined completely. Motor and sensory systems should be evaluated. Age-related changes in the sense of taste or smell (dysgeusia) may result in anorexia in the elderly.[13] Patients with anorexia nervosa may have mild signs of a peripheral neuropathy or mental status changes with acute dementia, delirium, impaired memory and judgment, and deterioration of mood.

Mental Status Exam

Careful mental status exam with attention to affect and thought processes will provide important evidence of underlying depression, psychosis, or dementory illness.

DIAGNOSTIC STUDIES

While careful attention to the history and physical examination will provide important etiologic clues in the majority of patients presenting with anorexia, laboratory studies provide objective measures of nutritional status and the function of particular organ systems.

The following laboratory tests may be indicated in the initial evaluation:

1. Complete blood count (CBC).
2. Sedimentation rate.
3. Chemistry panel (blood urea nitrogen [BUN], creatinine, total protein, albumin electrolytes, and hepatic enzymes).
4. Urinalysis.
5. Stool testing for occult blood.

Directed studies of value in certain groups are:

1. Chest x-ray (elderly).
2. Thyroid stimulating hormone (elderly).
3. Urine toxicology screen (suspicion of substance abuse).
4. Human immunodeficiency virus (HIV) antibody (high-risk groups).
5. Endoscopy (suspected gastrointestinal blood loss).

In a series of hospitalized patients with unintentional weight loss, the sedimentation rate, alkaline phosphatase, and serum albumin were most often abnormal in patients with physical causes for their weight loss. In a series of outpatients who were primarily older and male, the chest x-ray was the most useful examination, showing a pertinent abnormality in 40 per cent of patients.[14] Additional targeted laboratory and radiographic evaluation is indicated for patients with specific abnormalities on history and physical examination.

ASSESSMENT

The initial task is to identify the severity of anorexia and any associated findings. Clinically, objective weight loss or a clear history of weight loss corroborated by observers is the best indicator of food intake.

Infants and Children

The height, weight, and head circumference growth curves are the foundation of the evaluation of feeding problems in infants and children. Because they are dependent, children are at increased risk for weight loss due to dysfunctional social and family factors. In infants, congenital problems and primary feeding difficulties are common. In young children, emotional stress often presents as abdominal pain and anorexia. In older children, depression has been reported to have a prevalence of approximately 2 per cent.

Adolescents and Young Adults

This age group has the lowest prevalence of organic disorders causing anorexia and unintentional weight loss. However, they are at increased risk for psychosocial problems, especially substance abuse, depression, and eating disorders. Familial and personal beliefs related to increased risk for eating disorders include: idealization of a thin physique, pressure to perform and please others, family relationships that discourage autonomy, and the perception of being obese.[9] Bulimia differs from anorexia nervosa in that bulimics will tend to binge-eat, followed by episodes of self-induced vomiting. The typical presentation is of a young, white woman, ages 12 to 25, from an upper-middle-class family with a 1- to 2-year history of weight loss and dieting. Careful assessment of actual weight loss; social, family, and environmental influences; and nutritional status are important parameters in evaluation of this age group.

Middle-Aged and Elderly

With advancing age, there is increased risk for organic illnesses. There is also an increased incidence of interacting medical problems and adverse drug reactions. Older individuals are susceptible to the psychologic effects (depression and anxiety) of increasing social dependency. (Also see chapter on Anxiety.) Malnutrition itself may contribute to decreased appetite. While some weight loss may occur on a physiologic basis secondary to declining muscle mass and increased fat stores, weight loss exceeding 5 per cent over a six- to 12-month period suggests a significant abnormality. Although anorexia occurs commonly in the elderly, it is not always accompanied by weight loss. In one study of patients with substantiated weight loss, two thirds had an underlying organic cause, nearly 10 per cent had an underlying psychiatric cause, and more than 25 per cent had no identifiable causes.[13]

Fewer outpatients (52 per cent) were likely to have organic causes than inpatients (81 per cent). Possible etiologies for weight loss in the elderly include poor dentition, loss of taste and smell, dysphagia, underlying dementia, and drug intoxication.

Prognostic Implications of Anorexia

Anorexia is a serious complaint and may be caused by a variety of disorders. The subset of patients whose decreased appetite has led to weight loss or malnutrition has a one-year mortality rate of nearly 25 per cent.[14] The most common causes of anorexia in a primary-care practice are associated with little or no weight loss. These common causes include depression, occupational or family stress, medication side effects, and acute self-limited illness such as viral infections. Careful history and physical examination are the cornerstones of the diagnostic evaluation. For those patients in whom a self-limited diagnosis is suggested, reassurance, brief counseling, and close follow-up may be all that is required. A simple battery of laboratory tests will provide important diagnostic information for those patients with a more complex presentation. As with other nonspecific symptoms such as fever and fatigue, a discerning clinician, aware of physiologic, psychologic, and social factors, will be able to help the patient in the majority of cases.

REFERENCES

1. Morley JE, Silver AJ. Anorexia in the elderly. Neurobiol Aging 1988;9:9–16.
2. Stracher G, Kiss A, Wiesnagrotzki S, Bergmann H, Hobart J, Schneider C. Oesophageal and gastric motility disorders in patients categorized as having primary anorexia nervosa. Gut 1986;27:1120–6.
3. Lee S, Wing YK, Chow CC, Chung S, Yung C. Gastric outlet obstruction masquerading as anorexia nervosa. Clin Psychiatr 1989;50:184–95.
4. Crocker KS. Gastrointestinal manifestations of acquired immunodeficiency syndrome. Nurs Clin North Am 1989;24:395–406.
5. Kern KA, Norton JA. Cancer cachexia. J Par Ent Nutr 1989;12:286–98.
6. Dahl M, Sunderlin C. Early feeding problems in an affluent society. Acta Paediatr Scand 1986;75:370–9.
7. Casper RC. The pathophysiology of anorexia nervosa and bulimia nervosa. Annu Rev Nutr 1986;6:299–316.
8. Bruppacher R, Gyr N, Fisch T. Abdominal pain, indigestion, anorexia, nausea and vomiting. Bailliere's Clin Gastro 1988;2:275–92.
9. Garfinkel PE, Garner DM, Goldbloom DS. Eating disorders: implications for the 1990's. Can J Psychiatr 1987;32:624–31.
10. Shisslak KM, Crago M. Primary prevention of eating disorders. J Consult Clin Psychol 1987;55:600–67.
11. Halmi KA. Anorexia nervosa and bulimia. Am Rev Med 1987;38:373–80.
12. Long TJ. Anorexia nervosa. Adolesc Med 1987;14:177–201.
13. Robbins LJ. Evaluation of weight loss in the elderly. Geriatrics 1989;44:31–7.
14. Marton KI, Sox HC, Krupp JR. Involuntary weight loss: diagnostic and prognostic significance. Ann Int Med 1981;95:568–74.

ANTINUCLEAR ANTIBODY, POSITIVE TITER

JOE G. HARDIN, Jr.

SYNONYMS: Antinuclear Factor (Obsolete), ANA, Positive ANA, FANA (Fluorescent ANA)

BACKGROUND

Regarding a positive antinuclear antibody (ANA) as a "difficult diagnosis" is somewhat paradoxical, since the test should facilitate and not complicate the diagnostic process. If the test is used appropriately to help support a clinical impression, it will not itself become a diagnostic problem. In fact, a positive result is not itself a clinical problem, although it is widely perceived as being such. While the practice may not be appropriate, it is recognized, however, that the test is often used in a screening sense for a number of symptoms that may not be compatible with a specific rheumatic disease diagnosis or may not be compatible with a diagnosis that is ANA associated. When the clinician is surprised by a positive result, a new diagnostic problem is perceived, and that problem will be discussed in the following sections as if it were real.

Technique and Interpretation

It is generally accepted that the only satisfactory test for ANAs is the indirect immunofluorescent technique (FANA); other techniques cannot be regarded as reliable. For this test, nucleated cells are fixed to a glass slide, and that preparation is reacted with varying dilutions of the test serum, allowing antibodies in the serum to attach to their antigens in the cell nucleus. After washing, the slide is then treated with fluorescein-labeled antihuman immunoglobulin (usually IgG), which attaches to the antibody attached to its nuclear antigen. In effect, this serves as a developer, making the ANAs visible when the slide is examined under a fluorescent microscope. The greatest dilution of test serum permitting visible nuclear fluorescence is the ANA titer. Numerous commercial kits are available for this test, and some laboratories manufacture their own reagents. Unfortunately, this presents a problem with standardization, since sensitivity may vary from one kit to another or even from one batch of reagents to another.[1,2] As a general rule, kits that utilize human tissue culture lines are more sensitive than the others, but a number of other variables including the skill of the technician, influence results. It is essential that the clinician be familiar with trends in his or her laboratory(s); and it is preferable to have one technician use one type of kit in one laboratory in an effort to standardize results.

Most kits (or laboratories) begin with a 1 : 20 or 1 : 40 dilution to eliminate nonspecific background fluorescence. Consequently, a positive FANA in a titer of 1 : 20, 1 : 40, or even 1 : 80 may be of equivocal significance and might be interpretable as negative in some laboratories. Again, it is necessary to be familiar with the local experience. The best way to do this is to examine the log of the laboratory's recent ANA results. A large percentage of positives in the range of 1 : 80 to 1 : 160 suggests that 1 : 320 may be the first significant dilution. Conversely, if no titers greater than 1 : 160 are found, perhaps any positive result should be considered significant.

FANA Patterns

Patterns of nuclear fluorescence are reported by most laboratories, and these may contribute to the meaning of a positive FANA,[3] but patterns must be interpreted with caution since they may vary from one dilution to another and two or more patterns may coexist at one dilution. The smooth or homogenous pattern is highly nonspecific and correlates with antibodies to a deoxyribonucleic acid (DNA)–histone complex, which is the lupus erythematosus (LE) factor. A speckled pattern is also nonspecific and generally reflects antibodies to saline extractable nuclear antigens (ENAs). The halo (or rim or peripheral) pattern suggests antibodies to native DNA, but it is a very insensitive test for these antibodies. A nucleolar pattern reflects antibodies to one or more of three nucleolar antigens and is most often found in the scleroderma syndromes and polymyositis; it may be the most clinically useful of these four patterns. Finally, the only commercially available test for the centromere antibody is to perform a FANA test on mitotic cells and look for that pattern of nuclear fluorescence.

LE Cell Test

The LE cell test is of considerable historical interest since the discovery of the LE cell phenomenon led to everything we now know about the ANAs; however, it is now generally considered obsolete as a clinically useful diagnostic tool. The LE cell test is a crude assay for a highly nonspecific group of ANAs—those directed against a DNA–histone complex (DNP). It is a time-consuming test that is less sensitive and no more specific than the FANA test, and many, if not most, laboratories in this country have abandoned it. It cannot be recommended.

ANA Associations

As a diagnostic tool, the ANA is useful only in supporting the clinical impression of a connective tissue disease and in supporting the diagnosis of one subset of juvenile rheumatoid arthritis (JRA) (see Table 1). Therefore, seeking evidence for one of these disorders should be the first priority when one is faced with a

significantly positive test. An ANA may also *suggest* the possibility of other occult autoimmune disorders,[4] although it is not certain that these are sufficiently frequent or serious enough to justify routinely seeking evidence for them. ANAs are associated with certain nonrheumatic disorders such as chronic inflammatory liver and lung disease,[5,6] although these disorders are usually readily apparent clinically. Drugs that induce a syndrome similar to systemic lupus erythematosus (SLE) always induce ANAs before the syndrome becomes apparent, and the majority of individuals with drug-induced ANAs do not develop SLE.[7,8] First-degree relatives of patients with connective tissue diseases often have ANAs without clinical evidence of a disease.[9,10] Finally, significant titers of ANA are occasionally encountered in individuals, especially the elderly, who have none of these or any other reason to have them.

HISTORY

The importance of the history in establishing the significance of a positive ANA cannot be overemphasized. If the history does not at least suggest a reason for the test to be positive, it is relatively unlikely that any other maneuvers will be rewarding. All the items listed in the following paragraphs should be explored.

Symptoms

In seeking a history of symptoms suggestive of a connective tissue disease, especially SLE, the major ones to pursue are: arthritis (joint pain *and* swelling), arthralgias (pain alone), Raynaud's phenomenon (at least a two-phase color change on cold exposure), photosensitivity (rash in response to ultraviolet light exposure), facial rashes, pleurisy, unexplained fever, and pronounced malaise. Hair loss, oral lesions, other rashes, unexplained weight loss, and lesser degrees of malaise are less specific but worth asking about. With diseases other than SLE in mind, proximal girdle muscle weakness (polymyositis), dry irritated eyes and dry mouth (Sjögren's syndrome), and skin tightness (scleroderma syndromes) should be specifically addressed. While nonspecific, the presence and duration of morning stiffness also need to be addressed, since prolonged morning stiffness suggests rheumatoid arthritis (RA).

TABLE 1.   ANA–Rheumatic
Disease Associations

DISEASE	AVERAGE PERCENTAGE WITH POSITIVE FANA
Systemic lupus erythematosus	95
Cardiolipin antibody syndrome	50 (often weakly positive)
Mixed connective tissue disease	100 (by convention)
Drug-induced lupus	100
Primary Sjögren's syndrome	70
Scleroderma syndromes	60 (90 with diffuse)
Dermato/polymyositis	35
Adult rheumatoid arthritis	30
Juvenile rheumatoid arthritis	40 (75 in pauciarticular disease with iritis)

Arthritis, or at least arthralgia, is usually a prominent symptom of the connective tissue diseases, and its distribution should be established historically; the physical examination establishes the distribution at only one point in time. Symptoms in the wrists, metacarpophalangeal joints, proximal interphalangeal (PIP) joints, and metatarsophalangeal joints suggest RA, whereas joint symptoms in SLE often predominate in the PIPs and knees. In RA, symptoms tend to persist for long periods in any affected joints, whereas in the other connective tissue diseases, joint symptoms tend to be more fleeting or migratory. None of the connective tissue diseases affect the lower axial skeleton, so prominent back pain is an argument against any of these diagnoses. In young children (especially girls) with the JRA subset associated with ANAs, the arthritis is pauciarticular and often in the lower extremity.

Past History

The connective tissue diseases often evolve slowly, and seemingly remote events may represent their beginnings. Especially with SLE in mind would a prior history of pleuritis, pericarditis, unexplained renal disease, abnormal urinalysis, thrombocytopenia, or unexplained anemia be pertinent. Pulmonary symptoms sometimes antedate clinically apparent scleroderma syndromes or polymyositis. The recently described cardiolipin antibody syndrome[11,12] is often accompanied by positive ANAs; consequently, a prior history of deep venous thrombosis, stroke, recurrent miscarriage, and arterial thrombosis should be sought. While the event is rare, mothers of children with neonatal lupus or congenital heart block often develop SLE later in life, so that even the outcome of previous pregnancies could have a bearing on a positive ANA.[13] Thyroiditis is associated with all the connective tissue diseases and perhaps directly with a positive ANA[4]; therefore, a history of thyroiditis could be considered an explanation for a positive test or could be considered supporting evidence for a connective tissue disease diagnosis.

A number of clinically apparent chronic autoimmune, inflammatory, and infectious diseases not usually considered rheumatic in nature have been associated with a positive ANA test. A partial list is included in Table 2. A current or past history of one of these disor-

TABLE 2.   Partial List of Reported Nonrheumatic Disease–ANA Associations

Leprosy
Malaria
Tuberculosis
Pneumoconiosis
Interstitial lung disease
Sarcoidosis
Primary biliary cirrhosis
Chronic active hepatitis
Chronic hemodialysis for end-stage renal disease
Autoimmune thyroid disease
Other autoimmune endocrinopathies
Pemphigus
Discoid lupus erythematosus
Myasthenia gravis
Multiple sclerosis
Uveitis
Necrotizing vasculitis
Polychondritis
Normal aging

ders could be considered an explanation for a positive ANA.

Drug History

Numerous drugs have been reported to induce ANAs and, less often, an illness similar to SLE, and drug-induced ANAs may persist for years after the agent is discontinued. Consequently, current or prior use of one of these agents is one of the most common explanations for an ANA in an asymptomatic individual. As a general rule, a drug needs to be used regularly for at least several months in order to induce an ANA, and larger doses are more likely to do so than smaller doses. The more commonly used agents reported to induce ANAs are listed in Table 3. A history of the

TABLE 3.   Partial List of Drugs Reported to Induce ANAs (and SLE)

Atenolol	Methylthiouracil
Captopril	Methysergide
Carbamazepine	Minoxidil
Chlorpromazine*	Oral contraceptives
D-Penicillamine	Phenylbutazone
Ethosuximide	Phenytoin*
Griseofulvin	Primidone
Hydralazine*	Procainamide*
Hydrochlorothiazide	Propylthiouracil
Isoniazid*	Quinidine
L-Dopa	Sulfasalazine
Mephenytoin	Sulfonamides
Methimazole	Tetracyclines
Methyldopa	Trimethadione

* Most commonly reported or best studied.

regular use of any one or more of these could explain a positive ANA test even if no symptoms were experienced by the patient.

Family History

First-degree relatives of patients with connective tissue diseases, especially SLE, often have ANAs even though they are asymptomatic and remain so indefinitely.[9,10] Therefore, a detailed family history should be obtained. A positive family history is a common explanation for an ANA in an asymptomatic individual, although the family history (more so than the ANA) places that individual at increased risk for SLE or some other connective tissue disease in the future.

PHYSICAL EXAMINATION

The physical examination can be guided by the history, but it should be complete. It is relatively uncommon to uncover asymptomatic physical findings in patients with connective tissue diseases, but occasionally they occur. The emphasis should be on the skin, mucous membranes, and joints.

Skin

Common rashes of SLE include the malar rash; scarring discoid lupus; rather nonspecific rashes in light-exposed areas (photosensitive); widespread maculopapular lesions, which may be papulosquamous (subacute cutaneous lupus); and dependent palpable purpura (vasculitis). Common lesions of dermatomyositis include periungual capillary dilatation, bluish (heliotrope) discoloration of the eyelids, and red scaling papules over the metacarpophalangeal and other joints (Gottron's plaques or sign). Subcutaneous calcinosis may occur with dermatomyositis or with the scleroderma syndromes. Hidebound tight skin with loss of appendages is characteristic of the scleroderma syndromes and often predominates over the dorsum of the fingers (sclerodactyly). Raynaud's phenomenon may occur spontaneously or may be related to the patient's nervousness over a visit to the doctor. Finger pad atrophy and scarring are typical of severe Raynaud's phenomenon and the scleroderma syndromes.

Patchy loss of scalp hair is characteristic of active SLE and may be overlooked by the patient. Inflamed oral (buccal mucosa, palate, or tongue) or nasal lesions are often seen with active SLE and may also be asymptomatic; therefore, they should be looked for specifically. These lesions often have an intensely inflamed base with a raised gray center that may secondarily ulcerate.

Joints

All peripheral joints should be examined for signs of inflammation, although the yield will be low in patients with no joint complaints. Pain on motion or tenderness alone might suggest an arthritis, but some degree of joint swelling is required to confirm the diagnosis. Redness and warmth over the affected joints are less likely but helpful when found. Confirming the diagnosis of an inflammatory arthropathy in an adult with an ANA strongly suggests the likelihood of a connective tissue disease and may indicate further laboratory investigation, although the remainder of the clinical picture is usually more helpful diagnostically.

Other Aspects of the Physical Examination

In evaluating the significance of a positive ANA, primary Sjögren's syndrome should be addressed at least with a screening Schirmer test for abnormal tearing; the test strips are readily available, and ophthalmology referral is not necessary. (See chapter on Dry Eye.) In children with an ANA and arthritis, ophthalmology referral is recommended since they often have an associated iritis that may be difficult to diagnose. Additional physical findings that might suggest a connective tissue disease include lymphadenopathy, muscle weakness, signs of a sensory peripheral neuropathy, and evidence for pleuritis or pericarditis.

DIAGNOSTIC STUDIES

In the absence of direction provided by the history and physical examination, further laboratory evaluation of a positive ANA is unlikely to be rewarding. Even if the diagnosis is to be pursued in the laboratory, routine tests such as the complete blood count (CBC) and urinalysis may be more helpful than further serologic evaluation; however, the emphasis in this section will be on other commercially

TABLE 4. Available Serologic Tests Useful in Evaluating the Significance of a Positive ANA

TEST	USEFUL IN SUSPECTED
Antinative DNA	SLE
Anti-Smith (Sm)	SLE
Anti-RNP (U1-RNP) } Anti-ENAs	Mixed connective tissue disease
Antihistone	Drug-induced lupus
Anti-Scl₇₀	Diffuse scleroderma
Anticentromere	Limited scleroderma
Anti-SSA, -SSB (Ro-La)	SLE, Sjögren's syndrome
Anticardiolipin	SLE, cardiolipin antibody syndrome
Rheumatoid factor	Rheumatoid arthritis, Sjögren's syndrome

available serologic tests, most of which are aimed at detecting antibodies to *specific* nuclear antigens. It should be apparent that most of these tests cannot be positive if the FANA is truly negative since most of them represent ANAs of various specificities. These additional tests are listed in Table 4. Additional laboratory testing will be discussed below in terms of specific suspected disease entities; if none of these is suspected, additional testing is unnecessary and will be unrewarding.

SLE

There are two ANAs considered to be highly specific for SLE, and both should be ordered if this diagnosis is suspected and the FANA is positive. They are the antinative DNA antibody (positive in about 60 per cent of SLE patients)[14] and an antibody to one or more of five nuclear glycoproteins called Smith or Sm (positive in about 30 per cent of SLE patients).[15,16] Anti-Sm and antinative DNA tend to be somewhat mutually exclusive; therefore, one or both should be positive in 70 to 75 per cent of patients with the disease, permitting a reliable laboratory confirmation of the diagnosis in the majority. Antibodies to a nuclear riboprotein (U1-RNP or RNP) are usually done routinely when anti-Sm is requested since the two antibodies were initially described together as anti-ENA; in fact, a request for anti-ENA is generally regarded as a request for anti-Sm and anti-RNP, and it is a convenient way to order the test. Anti-RNP is nonspecific and is found in a number of

patients with SLE as well as in other connective tissue diseases (see Mixed Connective Tissue Disease below).

Additional less specific tests may help support an SLE diagnosis. Antibodies to SS-A and/or SS-B occur in 30 to 40 per cent of patients with SLE and may be more frequent in older patients with the disease.[17] These antibodies are not specific and occur in normal individuals and in patients with a number of other connective tissue diseases, especially Sjögren's syndrome (see below). SS-A and SS-B antigens are not present in some cells used for the FANA test and when present may predominate in the cytoplasm; hence, some subjects with these antibodies may be reported as FANA negative. Cardiolipin antibodies are found in a number of conditions in addition to the traditional connective tissue diseases (see Cardiolipin Antibody Syndrome below), but they are found in about 40 per cent of patients with SLE, in whom they may account for recurrent miscarriages or thrombotic events.[12] Hypocomplementemia (CH50, C4, and/or C3) is often encountered in active SLE and could be used to support both the basic diagnosis and the activity of the disease. Patients with SLE frequently have a positive Coomb's test, even when there is no evidence for ongoing hemolysis.

All patients suspected of having lupus should have a CBC looking for any cytopenia; a urinalysis looking for proteinuria and an active urine sediment should also be considered routine. An abnormal urinalysis is an indication for a careful measurement of renal function and quantitative protein excretion. Other studies, too numerous to mention here, might also be indicated if the clinical picture warrants; but these are usually used to confirm a pattern of organ-system involvement rather than the primary diagnosis.

Cardiolipin Antibody Syndrome

Clinical consequences of the cardiolipin antibody may be seen in patients with positive ANAs (often weakly positive) but without other clinical or laboratory features supporting a diagnosis of SLE. The syndrome usually consists of recurrent thromboses, recurrent miscarriages, the skin finding of livedo reticularis, and/or arthralgias.[11,12] These patients may also have false-positive serologic tests for syphilis and a lupus anticoagulant. The diagnosis is confirmed by a significantly positive test for cardiolipin antibody (usually defined by the reference laboratory performing the test).

Mixed Connective Tissue Disease

Mixed connective tissue disease (MCTD) is regarded by some authorities as a benign variant of SLE, whereas others consider its overlapping clinical features and serologic profile sufficiently distinctive to justify a separate designation. The serologic profile consists of anti-RNP (usually required for the diagnosis) in the absence of anti-Sm and antinative DNA.[18] The anti-RNP should give a speckled pattern on FANA testing. Consequently if this diagnosis is suspected in a patient with a positive FANA, anti-ENA and antinative DNA should be requested.

Drug-Induced Lupus

A large number of drugs induce ANAs, and most of these have also been reported to induce a lupus-like syndrome (see Table 3). This syndrome can be suspected in a patient taking one of these drugs who has a positive FANA (typically in high titer) and one or more clinical features suggestive of lupus. About 80 per cent of these patients have antibodies to one or more of several classes of histones (ordered as histone antibody) and typically lack antibodies to Sm or native DNA.[8,19] Consequently, in the right context, a positive histone antibody, in the absence of antibodies to Sm and native DNA, strongly supports the diagnosis of drug-induced lupus.

Primary Sjögren's Syndrome

Primary Sjögren's syndrome has recently been recognized as a common connective tissue disease especially in women.[20] It is suggested by a sicca syndrome (dry eyes and dry mouth) with arthralgias, cutaneous vasculitis, and perhaps other connective tissue disease manifestations. (See chapters on Dry Eye and Xerostomia.) Most have a positive FANA, and about 60 per cent have antibodies to SS-A and/or SS-B, and these help confirm the diagnosis; a positive rheumatoid factor test is also commonly found. However, a specific diagnosis may require salivary gland (usually minor) biopsy. Even with an exhaustive evaluation, it may be clinically and serologically difficult to distinguish primary Sjögren's syndrome from SLE with secondary Sjögren's.

Scleroderma Syndromes

The scleroderma syndromes are clinical diagnoses, but the majority are FANA positive, and specific ANAs may establish the prognosis (diffuse versus limited) in early cases. The centromere antibody argues for limited disease and is found in half or more of these cases[21]; it may be associated with a negative FANA if nonhuman cells are used for that test. An antibody to nuclear topoisomerase I called Scl_{70} is commercially available (as the scleroderma antibody or anti-Scl_{70}) and correlates strongly with diffuse scleroderma—although it is not very sensitive.[22] Consequently, in an early scleroderma syndrome, anticentromere antibody and anti-Scl_{70} might be ordered to help establish the future behavior of the disease.

Dermato/Polymyositis

The diagnosis of dermato/polymyositis is clinical (based on weakness, muscle enzyme tests, electromyogram [EMG], muscle biopsy, and typical skin changes), and a minority have a positive ANA. A nucleolar pattern may help suggest the diagnosis, and several specific ANAs are under investigation. Perhaps the most useful so far is an antibody to an antigen designated Jo_1; this antibody occurs in about 30 per cent of patients with polymyositis and suggests the likelihood of coexisting interstitial lung disease.[23] However, the final diagnosis of poly/dermatomyositis will not be a serologic one.

Rheumatoid Arthritis

About 25 to 30 per cent of patients with typical adult rheumatoid arthritis (RA) will have a positive ANA, usually in association with a positive test for rheumatoid factor.[24] Almost all patients with Felty's syndrome (RA, neutropenia, and splenomegaly) have a positive ANA. If the clinical impression is RA, a positive ANA need not be further investigated. However, it may weakly imply a relatively poor prognosis.

Juvenile Rheumatoid Arthritis

A subset of JRA that is pauciarticular and predominates in young girls is strongly associated with a positive ANA.[25] The ANA does not require further investigation unless SLE is in the differential diagnosis; but it increases the likelihood of an associated iritis and suggests even more careful ophthalmologic follow-up.

ASSESSMENT

In assessing the significance of a positive ANA, there are two important initial questions that should be asked: (1) Is the titer significant? and (2) Why was the test ordered in the first place? If the titer or degree of positivity is not significant for the laboratory in which the test was done, the result can be dismissed. If the test was ordered because a connective tissue disease or JRA was suspected clinically, then a significantly positive result supports the clinical impression, and it should be pursued in the manner outlined above. There are a number of inappropriate reasons for requesting an ANA; these include low back pain syndromes, chronic fatigue, unexplained weight loss, osteoarthritis syndromes, regional rheumatic complaints such as a local shoulder syndrome, and use as a routine screening test. If the test was requested for one of these inappropriate reasons or for unknown reasons, a significantly positive result could be perceived as a diagnostic problem.

The first step in pursuing a significantly positive ANA obtained for inappropriate or unknown reasons is to use the history and physical examination to be sure that evidence for a connective tissue disease (or JRA) is not coincidentally present. If any such evidence exists, the diagnosis should be pursued as outlined above. If no such evidence exists, a history of other chronic diseases associated with ANAs (Table 2) should be explored. If none of these diseases exists, a careful drug history (Table 3) is indicated. If this inquiry does not result in an explanation, then a family history is warranted. If the ANA remains unexplained after all these maneuvers, it will likely remain unexplained indefinitely.

It should be made perfectly clear to the patient that an unexplained ANA is not a disease, nor does it necessarily imply that there will be one. Whether or not this finding requires medical follow-up is a matter of opinion. It would be reasonable to acquaint the patient with the important connective tissue disease symptoms and have him or her report back if any of these develop. It would also be reasonable to repeat the test in a year on the chance that it has gone away. The implications of the chance finding of a positive ANA are unknown, but the test should not be allowed to create a problem when none exists. Probably the least done and said about it, the better.

REFERENCES

1. Feigenbaum PA, Medsger TA Jr, Kraines RG, Fries JF. The variability of immunologic laboratory tests. J Rheumatol 1982;9:408–14.
2. Chaiamnuay P, Johnston C, Maier J, Russell AS. Technique-related variation in results of FANA tests. Ann Rheum Dis 1984;43:755–7.
3. Gonzalez EN, Rothfield NF. Immunoglobulin class and pattern of nuclear fluorescence in systemic lupus erythematosus. N Engl J Med 1966;274:1333–8.
4. Shiel WC Jr, Jason M. The diagnostic associations of patients with antinuclear antibodies referred to a community rheumatologist. J Rheumatol 1989;16:782–5.
5. Conn HG, Maddrey WC, Soloway RD. Immunologic aspects of chronic active hepatitis. Hepatology 1983;3:724–8.
6. Nagaya H, Sieker HO. Pathogenic mechanisms of interstitial pulmonary fibrosis in patients with serum antinuclear factor. Am J Med 1972;52:51–62.
7. Lee SL, Chase PH. Drug-induced systemic lupus erythematosus: a critical review. Semin Arthritis Rheum 1975;5: 83–103.
8. Cush JJ, Goldings EA. Southwestern internal medicine conference: drug-induced lupus: clinical spectrum and pathogenesis. Am J Med Sci 1985;290:36–45.
9. Lowenstein MB, Rothfield NF. Family study of systemic lupus erythematosus. Arthritis Rheum 1977;20:1293–1303.
10. Maddison PJ, Skinner RP, Pereira RS, et al. Antinuclear antibodies in the relatives and spouses of patients with systemic sclerosis. Ann Rheum Dis 1986;45:793–9.
11. Asherson RA, Khamashta MA, Ordi-Ros J, et al. The "primary" antiphospholipid syndrome: major clinical and serologic features. Medicine 1989;68:366–74.
12. Mackworth-Young CG, Loizou S, Walport MJ. Antiphospholipid antibodies and disease. Q J Med 1989;72:767–77.
13. Scott JS, Maddison PJ, Taylor PV, Esscher E, Scott O, Skinner RP. Connective-tissue disease, antibodies to ribonucleoprotein, and congenital heart block. N Engl J Med 1983;309:209–12.
14. Chubick A, Sontheimer RD, Gilliam JN, Ziff M. An appraisal of tests for native DNA antibodies in connective tissue diseases. Ann Intern Med 1978;89:186–92.
15. Beaufils M, Kouki F, Camus JP, Morel-Maroger L, Richet G. Clinical significance of anti-Sm antibodies in systemic lupus erythematosus. Am J Med 1983;74:201–5.
16. Munves EF, Schur PH. Antibodies to Sm and RNP. Arthritis Rheum 1983;26:848–53.
17. Tsokos GC, Pillemer SR, Klippel JH. Rheumatic disease syndromes associated with antibodies to the Ro (SS-A) ribonuclear protein. Semin Arthritis Rheum 1987;16:237–44.
18. Sharp GC, Irvin WS, May CM, et al. Association of antibodies to ribonucleoprotein and Sm antigens

with mixed connective-tissue disease, systemic lupus erythematosus and other rheumatic diseases. N Engl J Med 1976;295:1149–54.

19. Fritzler MJ, Tan EM. Antibodies to histones in drug-induced and idiopathic lupus erythematosus. J Clin Invest 1978;62:560–7.

20. Drosos AA, Andonopoulos AP, Costopoulos JS, Papadimitriou CS, Moutsopoulos HM. Prevalence of primary Sjögren's syndrome in an elderly population. Br J Rheumatol 1988;27:123–7.

21. Chen Z, Silver RM, Ainsworth SK, Dobson RL, Rust P, Marico HR. Association between fluorescent antinuclear antibodies, capillary patterns, and clinical features in scleroderma spectrum disorders. Am J Med 1984;77:812–22.

22. Juarez C, Vila JL, Gelpi C, et al. Characterization of the antigen reactive with anti-Scl-70 antibodies and its application in an enzyme-linked immunosorbent assay. Arthritis Rheum 1988;31:108–115.

23. Fudman EJ, Schnitzer TJ. Clinical and biochemical characteristics of autoantibody systems in polymyositis and dermatomyositis. Semin Arthritis Rheum 1986;15:255–60.

24. Elling P. Antinuclear factors in rheumatoid arthritis. Ann Rheum Dis 1968;27:406–12.

25. Moore TL, Osborn TG, Weiss TD, et al. Autoantibodies in juvenile arthritis. Semin Arthritis Rheum 1984;13:329–36.

ANXIETY

RAYMOND PARY, CARMELITA R. TOBIAS, and STEVEN LIPPMANN

SYNONYMS: Nervous, Tense, Upset, Worried, Apprehensive, Afraid, "Keyed Up," "On Edge"
Related Phenomenon: Agitated

BACKGROUND

Definitions

Anxiety is an unpleasant emotional state related to anticipation of real or imaginary danger. Fear is its hallmark. Realistic threats are usually absent or, if present, are not proportionate to the high degree of evoked feeling. Somatic manifestations of anxiety include fidgeting, autonomic hyperactivity, and increased vigilance. Agitation is a form of anxiety accompanied by motor restlessness.

Fear is an emotion produced by an imminent danger. It has survival value in that it evokes avoidance of a threat. Fear and anxiety are subjectively experienced in the same way. They are differentiated from one another in that with fear, the danger is more realistic and the emotion is proportionate to the threat. In adults, examples include fear of heights or snakes. If the fears do not lead to major avoidances and do not handicap functioning in life, then no anxiety diagnosis is warranted and no treatment is required. Fears that interfere with daily living activity by causing significant avoidance behaviors are termed *phobias*.

Biological Theories

The role of norepinephrine in the subjective experience of anxiety is supported by experiments with the locus ceruleus using isoproterenol and yohimbine. The locus ceruleus, located in the pons, contains cell bodies for most of the noradrenergic neurons, which project into the rest of the central nervous system (CNS). Sensory information about pain or danger has input into the locus ceruleus. When monkeys receive electrical stimulation in this region, they react fearfully. Ablation decreases fear responses. A beta-adrenergic agonist, isoproterenol, when infused to susceptible persons experimentally, induces anxiety.[1] Yohimbine, a presynaptic alpha-2-adrenergic blocker, also precipitates anxiety in many subjects.[2]

The physiology of anxiety remains obscure, but experimentally it can be induced by lactate and carbon dioxide administrations or by hyperventilation. Sodium lactate intravenous infusions precipitate the emergence of symptoms in panic disorder patients.[3] Panic attacks have also been produced by the inhalation of 5 per cent carbon dioxide in those with panic disorder.[4] Breathing carbon dioxide creates an acidosis, whereas intravenous lactate produces metabolic alkalosis; therefore, the anxiety symptoms are not thought to be related to changes in acid-base balance. Hyperventilation also produces panic in those with agoraphobia, while causing a respiratory alkalosis.

Such diversity obscures understanding about the mechanism of anxiety.

An alternative focus to norepinephrine's role in anxiety has developed around studies of the gamma-aminobutyric acid (GABA) receptor complex. This complex contains the GABA receptor, a site that binds benzodiazepines, and the chloride channel. When the GABA receptor is stimulated, chloride ions flow into the neuron, causing neuronal hyperpolarization and a less excitable state. Subsequently, at this neuron's presynaptic terminal, there is a reduced release of norepinephrine, serotonin, dopamine, and other neurotransmitters, resulting in a lessening of anxiety.

Both the benzodiazepine and GABA receptors are distinctly involved in the manifestations of anxiety symptoms. Benzodiazepines are widely used compounds with well-recognized anxiolytic effects. They are thought to increase the affinity of GABA for its binding site, thus allowing more chloride to enter the neuron. This action reduces anxiety. There is, therefore, a clear implication of the GABA receptor complex having a central role in the pathophysiology of anxiety. Further supporting evidence comes from studies of the compound beta-carboline carboxylate ethylesther. This agent has an intrinsic pharmacologic profile opposite to the benzodiazepines. It induces intensive behavioral agitation in monkeys, manifested by struggling and distress vocalization.[5] These observations can be blocked by pretreatment with a benzodiazepine antagonist without an intrinsic antianxiety effect.

It is improbable that either the norepinephrine or the GABA receptor system is the entire physiologic substrate for anxiety. A more likely explanation involves the interaction of complex intercellular signals with these transmitters integrated by such second messengers as cyclic adenosine monophosphate and the calcium ion to induce changes in different parts of the brain and body.[6] The totality of these diverse effects would then presumably constitute the biologic mechanism of pathologic anxiety.

Psychologic Theories

In psychodynamic theory, anxiety serves as a signal of unacceptable sexual or aggressive drives seeking conscious expression. Repression is viewed as a counteracting unconscious defense mechanism. No anxiety is felt with complete repression. Other defense mechanisms are utilized when repression is only partially effective. If these also function inadequately, then anxiety emerges.

Psychoanalytically, anxiety can be classified into four types: *impulse, separation, castration,* and *superego* anxieties. Impulse anxiety is experienced when stimuli overwhelm the individual into a state of perceived helplessness. Separation anxiety refers to abandonment fears. Castration anxiety presents when there are fantasized fears of injury. Superego anxiety occurs when an individual behaves in opposition to a personal ethical code.

According to learning theory, anxiety is initially an unconditioned reaction to a perceived threat. Subsequently, it becomes conditioned to a more benign situation. Persons learn to reduce anxiety by avoiding circumstances that stir up discomfort. Eventually, through pairing of noxious with neutral events, the avoidance behavior extends beyond what was once regarded as dangerous.

Existential anxiety refers to the disquietude induced through an awareness of the possibility of nonbeing. It may be present through a failure to reach one's potential in life. A lack of personal development may result from choices that involve reduced responsibilities and a less meaningful life.

HISTORY

In evaluating patients with anxiety symptoms, the physician should obtain a comprehensive history of the clinical picture. Elicit historical data in routine manner, gaining a thorough knowledge of the medical and psychiatric background. Details about the past history, previous treatments, allergies, menstrual cycle, pharmaceuticals taken, and chemical dependencies must be included. A complete physical and mental status examination also is mandatory because anxiety can result from a wide variety of etiologies. For example, anxiety occurs in many medical diseases affecting the cardiovascular, respiratory, endocrine, gastrointestinal, neurologic, and genitourinary systems. Functional illness also often presents with anxiety.

The onset of symptoms, their duration, and pattern of occurrence must be explored. The social history can often be the most important part of the evaluation of anxious patients. Stressors, such as deaths, illness, marital or other interpersonal conflicts, and financial, social, family, or occupational problems may cause an anxiety response. Also elicit past historical data about serious threats to life or family, sudden loss of a home, the witnessing of a person being seriously injured, and so on.

The physician must always be aware of previous mental illnesses or emotional problems. Depression is a very prominent cause of anxious feelings. Because of the close relationship and confusion between anxiety and depression with anxiety, apply special attention to a review for a mood disorder. Psychoses can present with anxious complaints accompanied by bizarre ideation or behavior. Although anxiety is common in young adults, the initial onset may have been observed in childhood. Anxiety symptoms in children can encompass frequent nightmares, sleepwalking, bed-wetting, fear of injury, and the like. Investigate the possibility of depression by asking about mood, hopelessness, sleep, appetite, optimism, and suicidal thoughts. Ask also about panic or phobic symptoms.

A comprehensive review of systems and family history is essential in providing diagnostic tips and in focusing the direction of the workup on positive findings. In addition to the usual somatic assessment, psychiatric syndromes such as mood disorders, substance abuse, organic brain disease, psychosomatic illnesses, and schizophrenia should all be considered; nervousness may present as a part of any of these conditions. One must inquire about prescribed or over-the-counter medicines and other substances such as caffeine, nicotine, alcohol, stimulants, and other intoxicants. Drug abuse can result in toxic or withdrawal symptoms, manifested by anxiety. Even among the elderly, inquiry about chemical dependency is indicated. This includes prescription medicine misuses. Beyond the apprehensive emotional aspects of anxiety, there are also numerous physical symptoms reported by such people. Autonomic hyperactivity includes palpitations, dry mouth, flushing, and urinary frequency. Motor complaints include tremors and restlessness. Many organ systems exhibit typical anxiety manifestations—for example, shortness of breath, a "lump in the throat," heartburn, insomnia, or heightened vigilance with irritability and startle reactions.

PHYSICAL EXAMINATION

The physical examination is a requisite in the assessment procedure. The most common findings of a panic or anxiety attack are associated with motor, behavioral, and autonomic hyperarousal. Patients exhibit shakiness, tremulousness, and a nervous or tense outlook. Facial expression may reveal fear or inner turmoil. Anxious individuals are often observed to pace and to move their extremities restlessly. Patients can manifest profuse sweating; cold, clammy hands; facial flushing; and gooseflesh. A nervous person could have a mild, transitory elevation in blood pressure. The heartbeat is fast and forceful.

The physical assessment follows usual techniques. A complete examination is expected, yet some emphasis goes toward the cardiovascular, pulmonary, and neurologic systems. Always carefully review vital signs and thoroughly consider endocrine disorders, especially of the thyroid.

Hyperventilation, when it occurs, may lead to numbness or tingling sensations in the extremities and circumoral area. Chvostek's sign (spasm of the facial muscle while tapping the facial nerve) can sometimes be elicited during overbreathing. In very severe cases, tetanic contractions are experienced.

Mental Status Examination

Characteristic features of overt anxiety are hard to miss. Often, the anxious patient complains of nervousness or tension. Speech is pressured at times with occasional stuttering but without incoherence or irrelevance. Fears of dying, of going crazy, or of doing something uncontrolled are expressed. Increased vigilance is common. This is perceived as feeling "keyed up" or "on edge." Patients also manifest increased somatic preoccupations, irritability, insomnia, and exaggerated startle response. Some individuals may complain of confusion and impaired concentration; however, orientation, cognitive skills, and memory are usually intact.

Screening questions for anxiety, phobia, and panic symptoms would include asking about the situations that bring out these feelings. Questions for obsessive-compulsive disorders might be as follows: "Do you have troubling thoughts that you can't get rid of?" and "Do you have to do certain acts repetitively that seem unnecessary?" For people with post-traumatic stress disorder, inquire if their traumatic event is re-experienced in the form of unusual behavior, episodes of "flashbacks" and/or nightmares. If anxiety was a part of a mood disorder, there would probably be associated findings such as dysphoria or helplessness. When apprehension is a component of a psychotic process, symptoms such as hallucinations, delusions, or bizarre thoughts are to be anticipated.

DIAGNOSTIC STUDIES

A complete blood count (CBC), serum chemistry profile, thyroid function tests, serologic test for syphilis, urinalysis, chest x-ray, and electrocardiogram (ECG) would be the initial laboratory workup. Thyroid function is included because milder degrees of hyperthyroidism are not always otherwise detected. Review the assays of thyroxine (T_4), triiodothyronine resin uptake (RT_3U), and free thyroid index (T_7). Also request a true triiodothyronine (T_3), by radioimmunoassay, if hyperthyroidism is suspected. Toxicology screening should be ordered if clinically indicated to determine stimulants, intoxications, or even potential drug withdrawal syndromes, namely, from alcohol or other sedatives, and so on. The laboratory test results are aimed at specific diagnostic differentials to either confirm or rule out certain pathologies (see Table 1).

Comprehensive further assessments are obtained on an individualized basis as suggested by clinical and laboratory parameters. For example, a patient with abnormal cardiac findings on the history, physical, or ECG may warrant more extensive evaluation by Holter monitor, echocardiogram, and stress tests. An acutely anxious, dyspneic individual may

TABLE 1.   Laboratory Studies in Differential Diagnosis of Anxiety

Initial considerations
   Complete blood count
   Serum chemistry profile
   Thyroid function (RT_3U, T_4, T_7, T_3)
   Toxicology studies (e.g., stimulants and sedatives)
   Serologic test for syphilis
   Urinalysis
   Chest x-ray
   Electrocardiogram

Other studies are ordered on an individualized basis, in accordance with clinical and laboratory parameters; some examples follow
   Holter monitor
   Echocardiogram
   Stress tests
   Pulmonary function studies
   Catecholamine assays
   Radiographic studies of the adrenal gland

need a pulmonary review. Similarly, an anxious patient with paroxysmal hypertension should be checked for adrenal gland pathology. Pheochromocytoma is ruled out by various urinary catecholamine assays and radiographic studies. Any other tests are systematically ordered on specific indications and in accordance with findings thus far.

ASSESSMENT

A wide array of physical conditions present with anxiety. Endocrine disorders such as hyperthyroidism, hyperparathyroidism, adrenocortical hyperfunction, porphyria, hypoglycemia, and pheochromocytoma are particularly noteworthy for their association with anxiety. The same applies within the cardiovascular and respiratory systems, with angina pectoris, cardiac arrhythmias, mitral valve prolapse, and chronic obstructive pulmonary disease, and so on. Being tense or nervous is common to many different neoplastic or gastrointestinal disorders, too. Delirium, dementia, and partial complex seizures should be considered as well. Anxiety of recent onset, that is not related to environmental stress, should alert the clinician to the possibility of physical causes inducing the distress. A brief discussion about some of the somatic ailments associated with anxiety follows (see Table 2).

Hyperthyroidism is an anxiety-related endocrine condition characterized by an excess of thyroid hormone. Customary symptoms include nervousness, insomnia, weakness, increased activity and appetite, sweating, palpitations, heat intolerance, and weight loss. Typical signs of this disorder are tachycardia, fine tremor, thyroid enlargement, and exophthalmos. Atrial fibrillation also is a common presentation. Causes for the excessive thyroid activity can involve humoral thyroid stimulators from thyroid stimulating immunoglobulins (Graves' disease), various tumors, toxic goiter, thyroiditis, and exogenous thyroid intake. Elevation of serum T_4, RT_3U, T_7, and true T_3 are noted in hyperthyroidism and help differentiate this disorder from uncomplicated anxiety. Further laboratory evidence includes a low serum thyroid stimulating hormone (TSH) level and failure of TSH to increase after the administration of thyrotropin releasing hormone.

Mitral valve prolapse is an example of cardiac disease often associated with anxiety. Approximately 23 per cent of such patients

TABLE 2. Somatic Ailments Associated with Anxiety

Anxiety in medical disorders
  Endocrine
    Hyperthyroidism
    Hyperparathyroidism
    Adrenocortical hyperfunction
    Porphyria
    Hypoglycemia
    Pheochromocytoma
  Cardiovascular
    Angina pectoris
    Cardiac arrhythmias
    Mitral valve prolapse
  Respiratory
    Chronic obstructive pulmonary disease
    Pneumonia
    Pulmonary embolism
  Neurologic
    Delirium
    Dementia
    Partial seizures with complex symptomatology
  Infectious
    Acquired immunodeficiency syndrome
    Syphilis
    Tuberculosis
  Neoplastic
    Cancer
Anxiety in psychiatric conditions
  Depressive and psychotic conditions
  Somatoform disorders
  Chemical dependencies (e.g., sedative withdrawal, etc.)
  Drug intoxications (e.g., stimulant use, caffeine abuse, etc.)

have panic attacks, and 12 per cent of people with panic disorder are diagnosed with mitral valve prolapse.[7] The characteristic physical finding is a midsystolic click, which results from the tensing of the valve leaflet and its chorda tendinae as they reach full extension. If mitral regurgitation is present, a late systolic murmur follows the click. It is usually asymptomatic, but some individuals complain of dyspnea or fatigue. Although various hypotheses have been proposed, there is no accepted explanation for the increased occurrence of anxiety in this disorder. Hypoxia of any cardiopulmonary etiology induces nervousness, as well.

Another condition commonly occurring with anxiety is the acquired immune deficiency syndrome (AIDS) or the state of being human immunodeficiency virus (HIV) positive.[8] Individuals who have engaged in behaviors at risk for AIDS often worry about becoming infected with the virus. Some people, despite being informed of a negative HIV test result, will remain tense and/or preoccupied with health or become hypochondriacal. Persons who test positive for HIV antibodies have a combination of fear and anxiety. Realistic worries involve concern with the potential for a rapid decline in health, ending in early death. Anxieties occur with the development of new symptoms, which are often interpreted as indicating disease progression. A depressive syndrome, that includes anxiety, sadness, hopelessness, guilt feelings, and suicidal ideation, is also common.[8]

Neoplastic disease is another process frequently presenting with anxiety. When patients are told that they have cancer, a period of shock is followed by profound anxiety. Cancer is associated with pain, disfigurement, loss of normal functioning, death, and disruption of significant relationships. Sleep disturbances, anorexia, and weight loss follow and are common manifestations of anxiety or depression. Hormonal paraneoplastic phenomena, too, can play a role in producing anxiety, as in a hyponatremic syndrome. The diagnosis of anxiety or depression with anxiety in cancer patients must be based on prolonged nonsomatic psychologic manifestations, such as fearfulness, impaired concentration, and thoughts of suicide. With cancer, pain itself is also a primary cause of anxiety. Control of pain, then, becomes the first focus for the physician. Patients often interpret pain as an indication of disease progression, although this relationship is not clearly established.[9]

Once it has been determined that medical illnesses are not causing the anxiety, psychiatric syndromes other than the primary anxiety disorders should be ruled out. A search for psychotic or depressive symptoms thus is initiated. The presence of delusions or hallucinations suggests conditions such as schizophrenia, mania, or major depressive disorder with psychosis. A depressive disorder must also be excluded in patients presenting with nervousness. Most people suffering from depression have considerable accompanying anxiety, sometimes making the distinction difficult. Symptom profiles that suggest depression are anorexia, loss of weight, early morning awakening, lack of energy or pleasure, decreased sexual interest, and psychomotor retardation. Such individuals often blame themselves, acknowledge sadness, imply unworthiness, and express hopelessness. Thoughts of self-destruction are typical for those with a mood disorder and are unusual in individuals with uncomplicated anxiety. Complaints of poor concentration and memory, too, are more closely associated with depression than with anxiety. A family history of depressive ailments also favors a mood disorder.

The next category to be eliminated is the somatoform disorders, a group of illnesses whereby physical symptoms suggest a pathologic condition, but demonstrable organic findings are absent. The somatic complaints in such conditions resemble anxiety symptoms but are more diffuse and vague and may be associated with previous medical interventions. Hypochondriacal patients, if presenting with anxiety symptoms, also have the conviction that a dreaded disease must be present.

The physician should consider screening anxious persons for substance abuse because drug-induced dysfunctions, especially stimulant intoxications and sedative withdrawal syndromes, regularly produce much anxiety. Intoxication from caffeine, nicotine, or sympathomimetic compounds is also noteworthy in this regard. Dietary caffeine consumption in dosages of as little as 250 mg per day can sometimes induce restlessness, insomnia, and nervousness.[10] Coffee contains about 125 mg of caffeine per cup, with tea being half as strong and a glass of cola one third as potent. Thus, two to three cups of coffee per day can be a significant cause of anxiety; however, as a primary cause of anxiety, caffeine-related symptoms generally occur at higher dosages. The astute clinician inquires into the daily intake of caffeinated beverages and of over-the-counter caffeine pills consumed by tense individuals.

Sedative withdrawal is also a very prominent cause for agitation. Patients who are discontinued from as little as 15 mg of diazepam per day for several months or its equivalent in other drugs (e.g., barbiturates) can experience irritability, autonomic hyperactivity, insomnia, and tremor.[10] An essentially identical syndrome occurs in alcohol withdrawal. The onset of symptoms follows cessation of alcohol ingestion within hours or longer and from one to six days after termination of benzodiazepines, in a truly addicted person (see Table 2).

Specific Anxiety Syndromes

After having checked for medical, drug-induced, psychotic, and depressive reasons for anxiety, a consideration of specific anxiety disorders is then appropriate. These psychiatric syndromes are classified as generalized anxiety disorder, simple phobia, social phobia, agoraphobia, panic attacks, obsessive-compulsive disorder, post-traumatic stress disorder, and adjustment disorder with anxious mood (see Table 3).

TABLE 3.   Specific Anxiety Syndromes

Generalized anxiety disorder
Simple phobia
Social phobia
Agoraphobia
Panic attack
Obsessive-compulsive disorder
Post-traumatic stress disorder
Adjustment disorder with anxious mood

Generalized Anxiety Disorder

This condition is manifested in individuals by a persistent apprehensive expectation about possible misfortune. The worries should be either exaggerated or unrealistic and be present most of the time over a six-month period. Usually, this diagnosis is not confirmed when the anxiety is manifest with other anxiety-inducing disorders. Symptoms from the following three categories are also observed: (1) motor tension, including shakiness, restlessness, tension, fatigue, or muscle soreness; (2) autonomic hyperactivity, including sweating, palpitations, dry mouth, clammy hands, dizziness, nausea, and frequent urination; and (3) heightened vigilance, feeling on edge, with concentration difficulties, irritability, or insomnia.

Simple Phobia

The essential features of a simple phobia are persistent fears of a specific object or situation, which upon exposure produces an anxiety response. People with this disorder recognize that their fear is excessive or unreasonable, yet avoidance behavior occurs. A phobia is diagnosed only if it interferes significantly with the individual's usual functioning. Some common simple phobias include fears of animals, driving, closed spaces, air travel, and/or examinations.

Social Phobia

Patients who have a social phobia are fearful of embarrassment or humiliation when performing in public. They dread the exposure of themselves to the scrutiny of others. These individuals may have fears of public speaking or talking at a party, of choking on food in front of others, about being incapable of urinating in a public lavatory, and so on.

Agoraphobia

Among patients with a phobia, this is the most frequent one that requires treatment. Agoraphobia refers to a fear of being in places or situations from which escape might be difficult, embarrassing, and so forth. Representative fears for this syndrome include those of crowds, traveling away from home, or being on a bridge. This disorder is often associated with panic attacks; agoraphobia without panic is much less frequent. Individuals with panic attacks and agoraphobia become so apprehensive about having further episodes of anxiety that avoidance behavior develops.

Panic Attacks

People with panic attacks experience discrete periods of intense fear when confronting certain specific situations. Instances may also occur unpredictably. An acute sense of doom is often reported. These recurrent sensations may occur in panic or phobic disorders. The onset of the "attack" is sudden, lasting from several minutes to a few hours. Usually patients express both psychic symptoms, such as fear of dying, going crazy, or losing control, and somatic complaints like dyspnea, dizziness, palpitations, trembling, sweating, choking, nausea, numbness, flushing, or chest pains. They typically have one or more instances per week, with an accompanying persistent fear of having a recurrent attack. An estimate of the occurrence in the general population has been reported at 3 per cent, with a female preponderance of approximately 3 : 1.[11]

Obsessive-Compulsive Disorder

In such an anxiety syndrome, apprehension is not a defining feature. Patients with this condition experience obsessions that are intrusive, with recurrent thoughts, images, ideas, or impulses that are reprehensible to the person. There is an internal struggle within the person to ignore or suppress these unpleasant thoughts or impulses. The individual recognizes that these ideas are figments of the imagination, but they still invade consciousness. Examples of obsessions include maladaptive preoccupation with harm to self or others, developing an illness, sexual thoughts, potential embarrassment, and the need for order. Often such ruminations impair sleep and daily function.

Compulsions are performances of unreasonable behavior in a repetitive and stereotyped manner. Compulsions usually follow obsessions. The behavior is purposeful and intended to prevent some dreaded event. There is little realistic connection between the compulsive act and the anticipated discomfort. The individual realizes that the behavior is irrational but is unable to stop.

Examples of compulsions include rituals that involve washing, hoarding, counting, checking, questioning, apologizing, and avoiding. A classic example may be a person who repetitively checks throughout the night to confirm that the stove is off and the doors are locked. Excessive behaviors that are inherently gratifying such as the excitement resulting from gambling or sex or the satisfactions of eating or drinking can become, but are not necessarily considered, compulsive. Conversely, people who are orderly or perfectionistic but do not behave unreasonably do not meet criteria for this disorder.

Post-traumatic Stress Disorder

Individuals with such a condition experience considerable disruption in functioning. This is associated with re-experiencing a traumatic event in the form of recurrent memories, nightmares, or dissociative episodes. The latter phenomena are commonly referred to as flashbacks, whereby the patient feels as if actually reliving the suffering. The original trauma should be well outside the range of expectable human experience, an occurrence that would be distressing to anyone. Examples include natural catastrophies, violent crimes, terrorism, incest, and assault. Symptomatic periods induce an array of anxiety manifestations. When the trauma occurs within a family, concerns about family survival become evident.

Psychic trauma can affect others in a contagious manner.[12] Symptoms include diminished interest, avoidance of activities that symbolize the event, estrangement, reduced capacity for loving, and general numbing of responsiveness. Hyperarousal is expressed by insomnia, hypervigilance, outbursts of anger, exaggerated startle, and poor concentration. A diagnosis of post-traumatic stress disorder requires symptoms to be present for at least one month.

Adjustment Disorder with Anxious Mood

When nervousness, worry, or jitteriness become the predominant manifestation to a psychosocial stressor, an adjustment disorder with anxious mood may be the appropriate diagnosis. The maladaptive social or occupational reaction must occur within three months of the stressor, persist for no longer than six months, and not meet the criteria for any specific mental disorder.[10]

REFERENCES

1. Rainey JM Jr, Pohl RB, Williams M, Knitter E, Freedman RR, Ettedqui E. A comparison of lactate and isoproterenol anxiety states. Psychopathology 1984;17(Suppl):74–82.
2. Holmberg G, Gershon S, Beck LH. Yohimbine as an autonomic test drug. Nature 1962;193:1313–4.
3. Pitts FN Jr, McClune JN Jr. Lactate metabolism in anxiety neurosis. N Engl J Med 1967;277:1329–36.
4. Gorman JM, Askanazi J, Liebowitz MR, et al. Response to hyperventilation in a group of patients with panic disorder. Am J Psychiatry 1984;141:857–61.
5. Insel TR, Ninan PT, Aloi J, Jimerson DC, Skolnick P, Paul SM. A benzodiazepine receptor–mediated model of anxiety. Arch Gen Psychiatry 1984;41:741–50.
6. Dubovsky SL. Generalized anxiety disorder: new concepts and psychopharmacologic therapies. J Clin Psychiatry 1990;51 (Suppl 1):3–10.
7. Crowe RR. Mitral valve prolapse and panic disorder. Psychiatr Clin North Am 1985;8:63–9.
8. Fullilove MT. Anxiety and stigmatizing aspects of HIV infection. J Clin Psychiatry 1989;50 (Suppl 11):5–8.
9. Holland JC. Anxiety and cancer: the patient and the family. J Clin Psychiatry 1989;50 (Suppl 11):20–5.
10. American Psychiatric Association. Diagnostic and statistical manual of mental disorders. 3rd ed rev. Washington, DC: APA, 1987:138–331.
11. Cameron OG. The differential diagnosis of anxiety: psychiatric and medical disorders. Psychiatr Clin North Am 1985;8:3–18.
12. Terr LC. Family anxiety after traumatic events. J Clin Psychiatry 1989;50 (Suppl 11):15–9.

ATAXIA

MARK J. COOK and RICHARD F. PEPPARD

SYNONYMS: Unsteadiness, Clumsiness, Incoordination, Dyssynergia

BACKGROUND

The term *ataxia* refers to incoordination of movement. It is usually due to a disorder of central processing at the level of the cerebellum or its afferent or efferent connections. Lesions of the cerebellar inputs from higher centers or from the periphery may give rise to similar problems.

Primary motor system lesions may produce clumsiness, but this is referred to as ataxia only when the incoordination is out of proportion to the weakness. This may occur with upper motor neuron lesions at a variety of levels. Severe limb weakness produces clumsiness, but this is not generally regarded as being ataxia. Minimal weakness with marked incoordination is considered to be an ataxic syndrome, and this has implications for the site of the lesion. Such ataxic hemiparesis may be observed with lacunar infarction or hemorrhage involving the pons, midbrain, thalamus, and internal capsule. Crural, or sometimes upper limb, weakness is associated with hemiataxia.[1]

Internal capsule lesions may evoke ataxia by interfering with ascending proprioceptive pathways through the thalamic nuclei or their projections to the cortex or descending corticopontine fibers.[2]

Analysis of the type and distribution of the ataxia and of associated neurologic abnormalities allows estimation of the level of involvement in the nervous system. Regional organization of cerebellar function permits the distinction of midline and cerebellar hemisphere lesions.

Sensory ataxia is due to disordered afferent information reaching the cerebellum from the periphery. This may arise through peripheral nerve or axial (spinal cord or brainstem) disease.[3,4] Sensory ataxia is characterized by improvement in limb function with visual guidance.

Optic ataxia refers to incoordination that cannot be corrected with visual input. It depends on abnormalities of hemispheric mechanisms and may be regarded as a disconnection syndrome.[5,6] Hemispheric lesions, particularly involving the superior parietal lobule, may produce clumsiness of the contralateral upper limb.[7]

HISTORY

Temporal aspects, laterality, and associated neurologic symptoms must be determined. Family history is particularly important in chronic cases. Recent infections, drug ingestion, and alcohol abuse are pertinent.

The rate of onset of the ataxia should first be determined. Infarcts and hemorrhages usually begin abruptly but may progress in steady or stepwise fashion over 24 hours. Vertebral dissection should be considered if there is a history of acute neck pain or of cervical manipulation.

A gradual onset over a few days usually occurs with the demyelinating lesions of multiple sclerosis, with infections, and occasionally with neoplasms. Demyelination and neoplasia may produce ataxia developing over weeks to months. The insidious onset and slow progression of an ataxic syndrome suggests an hereditary degeneration or, less commonly, a structural abnormality such as platybasia (flattening of the base of the skull) or the Arnold-Chiari malformation (displacement of the cerebellar tonsils and the lower medulla through the foramen magnum).[8]

Infarcts, hemorrhages, and space-occupying lesions involving a cerebellar hemisphere produce ataxia of the ipsilateral limbs. Toxic, metabolic, and heredodegenerative ataxias are usually quite symmetric.

Associated symptoms may help with localization and give clues to etiology. Have there been previous resolving episodes of ataxia, limb weakness, loss of vision, dysarthria, or sphincteric disturbance (multiple sclerosis)? Was there recent cervical pain, manipulation, or trauma (vertebral artery dissection)? Has there been associated headache or vomiting (cerebrovascular accident or neoplasm)? Has the patient a known systemic malignancy (paraneoplastic syndrome, secondary tumor)? Is there a fever, ear infection, or risk factors for acquired immune deficiency syndrome (AIDS) (abscess)? Is there a recognized cardiac valvular lesion (embolus, bacterial endocarditis)?

Family history deserves special inquiry in the chronic ataxias; however, sporadic forms of degeneration of the cerebellum and its connections are seen, many of which may have recessive modes of inheritance. Generally, the early onset ataxias, under 20 years of age, have a recessive mode of inheritance. Associated clinical features (sensory, pyramidal signs, optic atrophy, retinitis pigmentosa, deafness) may permit recognition of a defined syndrome.[9] It should be remembered that other family members may have mild involvement that goes unnoticed. It is useful to communicate directly with immediate relatives regarding problems of similar type. Sometimes the patient with a hereditary ataxia is erroneously diagnosed as having multiple sclerosis.

Focused Queries

1. *Was the ataxia of abrupt onset?* If so, vascular lesions are more likely, but remember that demyelination and tumor can occasionally imitate stroke.

2. *Is there an associated headache?* Primary or secondary neoplasms and occasionally stroke affecting posterior fossa structures cause headache, often in association with hydrocephalus and other features of raised intracranial pressure.

3. *Have you had any prior episode of self-limiting neurologic dysfunction, particularly vertigo, unilateral visual loss, sensory symptoms in limbs, urinary urgency or incontinence, or previous episode of ataxia?* Such a history suggests multiple sclerosis.

4. *Are you a heavy drinker?* Alcoholic nutritional cerebellar degeneration affects mainly the vermis and produces an ataxia of gait.

5. *Are you on anticonvulsant medication?* Consider especially recent changes in therapy, infections, or concomitant alcohol use.

6. *Do you have a family history of similar disorder?* This inquiry may provide the clue to the presence of a heredodegenerative ataxia.

7. *Do you engage in practices that might put you at risk of contracting AIDS?* Cerebral lymphoma and abscess are common neurologic complications of AIDS.

PHYSICAL EXAMINATION

General Examination

General examination is directed toward the detection of etiologic factors such as chronic liver disease, pulmonary neoplasia, sepsis, and fever. Abscess is not always associated with fever and leukocytosis. Signs of chronic hypertension with retinal vascular changes, cardiomegaly, and renal impairment may suggest that acute ataxia is due to cerebellar hemorrhage, the fourth most common site of spontaneous intracerebral hemorrhage (after putamen, thalamus, and pons). Gingival hypertrophy, coarse facial features, and hypertrichosis suggest chronic phenytoin (Dilantin) use.

Other evidence of vascular disease, carotid or peripheral arterial bruits, absent pulses, or trophic changes point to a vascular cause. Diabetes and hypercholesterolemia should be sought with cerebellar infarction. Cardiomyopathy, pes cavus, and scoliosis may accompany Friedreich's or other heredodegenerative ataxias. Sinus disease and cutaneous and conjunctival telangiectasia are the hallmarks of ataxia-telangiectasia. Polycythemia can accompany cerebellar hemangioblastoma. (Also see chapter on Polycythemia.) Cachexia may be seen with systemic malignancies or with malabsorption. Generalized pustular or vesicular rash in the febrile, gravely ill patient suggests herpes zoster encephalitis, which typically has a cerebellar emphasis.

Neurologic Examination

Dementia may be a prominent clinical feature with multiple sclerosis, olivopontocerebellar atrophy (OPCA), hereditary ataxias, and Marinesco-Sjögren's syndrome.

Cranial nerve abnormalities may be present. A dysarthria with slow, scanning, or staccato character and loss of usual prosody is found. This implies bilateral cerebellar hemisphere disease. Dysarthria may, at times, be a manifestation of lower cranial nerve, rather than a cerebellar, disorder. Other features of lower cranial nerve dysfunction may result from vascular, neoplastic, demyelinating, and degenerative disorders, particularly of OPCA type. Acoustic and vestibular nerve involvement can accompany the familial ataxias and OPCA.[10]

Disorders of ocular motility due to cerebellar diseases include gaze-evoked nystagmus; fixation instability, which often takes the form of square wave jerks; ocular dysmetria and hypometric saccades with a fast eye movement that falls short of the target and is followed by a corrective movement; jerky, "cogwheel" or saccadic pursuit where in the face of a reduction in the velocity of smooth pursuit movement a series of fast, "catch-up" movements occur; and impaired suppression

of vestibulo-ocular responses.[11] Other ocular abnormalities such as retinitis pigmentosa (familial ataxias, Refsum's disease), optic atrophy (demyelination, familial ataxias), retinal vascular abnormalities (hypertension, diabetes, phakomatoses), and cataracts (Marinesco-Sjögren's syndrome) provide valuable diagnostic clues.

Limb ataxia is characterized by miscalculations of the force, velocity, direction, and distance of movements. Problems become evident in tasks requiring a large amplitude movement concurrently at several joints with acceleration/deceleration phases and with an accurate approach to a target as is required in finger-nose and heel-shin testing. Dysmetria, error of measurement of distance, is evident as the finger or heel at first partially arrests before, beyond, or to the side of the target and is followed by a series of corrective movements with reduction in error until the target is reached. If each corrective movement carries a similar error, an oscillation may occur—so-called intention tremor.

There is difficulty in performing rapid, repetitive movements that require alternating activity of agonist-antagonist muscle groups such as flexors and extensors or supinators and pronators of the forearm. This dysdiadochokinesis is demonstrated in tapping the palm with the fingers or the foot or, as a more demanding task, alternate tapping with the palmar and dorsal surface of the fingers.

This distribution of ataxia may indicate the site of the lesion. With midline lesions of the archi- and paleocerebellum (or spinocerebellum), gait and postural abnormalities are prominent. Hemispheric lesions of the neocerebellum (or cerebrocerebellum) result in peripheral, lateralized ataxia. Ischemic, demyelinating, and space-occupying lesions may involve both midline and lateral structures, producing mixed features of upper limb and gait ataxia.

Gait should be tested initially in walking a straight line. More subtle ataxia may only be evident on turning and when attempting to walk heel to toe. The ataxic gait has a wide base with variable step length and elevation of the feet. Truncal instability may be so severe as to prevent sitting or walking. The arms may be held out to the sides for balance. Standing with the feet together, there is excessive swaying, which, with disorders of proprioception, increases when the eyes are closed. With chronic ataxia, these nonspecific accommodations of slowing of gait, widening of base, shortening of step length, and holding the arms out may become more prominent.

Muscular atrophy is a feature of some of the hereditary ataxias and OPCA, as are parkinsonism and chorea.[12] Peripheral neuropathy may accompany hereditary ataxias and alcohol-nutritional lesions. The proprioceptive loss may contribute to the ataxia. Absent reflexes, impaired vibration and joint position sense, and adventitious movements of the outstretched hands suggest there may be a sensory component to the ataxia. Cortical sensory loss, corticospinal signs, cognitive disturbance, and hemianopia suggest a cerebral hemisphere lesion. Spinal cord abnormalities may cause ataxia, but weakness, sensory loss to a level, or sphincteric disturbance dominate the presentation. Brainstem signs with cranial nerve or long tract involvement indicate a posterior fossa lesion. Myoclonic jerks accompany the dementing process of Jakob-Creutzfeldt, which occasionally has a cerebellar emphasis (the Oppenheimer variant).[13] Autonomic involvement occurs in familial ataxia, OPCA, Shy-Drager syndrome of multiple system atrophy, and diabetes mellitus, as well as other generalized neuropathies.[14]

DIAGNOSTIC STUDIES

Imaging Studies

Imaging studies provide the most useful information. The urgency with which a computed tomography (CT) scan is sought and the ancillary investigations are guided by the clinical setting. Magnetic resonance imaging (MRI) and CT scanning have the highest yield. Plain skull x-ray is usually unhelpful but may show evidence of previous trauma or surgery, metastatic carcinoma, or structural posterior fossa lesions.

MRI is ideally employed in posterior fossa lesions, as it avoids the beam-hardening artifact that obscures the region of the pons in CT scans. Nevertheless, CT is able to provide diagnostic information in the majority of instances. Tumor, hematoma, and infarct, if sufficiently large, are all identified on CT scan. Plaques of demyelination and intrinsic brainstem lesions, especially ischemic, are better identified with MRI. Attention may be focused on a specific region such as the pons or cerebral hemisphere in a syndrome of hemiparesis and ataxia, the internal auditory meatus and cerebellopontine angle in a syndrome of deafness, tinnitus, and ataxia.

Angiography is indicated to assess the posterior circulation in certain cases of unexplained hemorrhage or infarction and vertebral artery dissection[15] and sometimes to evaluate tumor circulation. Chest x-ray is valuable in suspected paraneoplastic syndrome, as small cell carcinoma of the lung is a common cause.

Other Tests

Nerve conduction studies are appropriate if a sensory ataxia of peripheral origin is suspected or in familial ataxias. Brainstem, visual, or somatosensory evoked responses may provide evidence of the primary lesion, for example, abnormal somatosensory evoked responses with a spinal cord lesion. Evidence of asymptomatic lesions, such as abnormal brainstem or visual evoked responses in a patient with a cerebellar syndrome may suggest multifocal lesions of multiple sclerosis. Cerebellopontine angle tumors can cause lateralized disturbance of brainstem evoked responses. Electroencephalography usually provides little help.

Lumbar puncture is necessary in the setting of suspected infection or demyelination. The cerebrospinal fluid should be sent for cell count, glucose and protein estimation including albumin/globulin ratio, cytology where appropriate, and electrophoresis to detect oligoclonal bands.

Where an alcohol-nutritional etiology is suspected, liver function tests and red blood cell transketolase assay are ordered. Serum antibodies to Purkinje cells are associated with paraneoplastic cerebellar degeneration, and this assay is available at some centers. Leukocytosis and left shift on blood examination suggest an infection.

In the chronic ataxias, certain specific investigations are relevant, depending on the associated clinical abnormalities. Serum phytanic acid is elevated in Refsum's disease and should be determined when the triad of neuropathy, retinitis pigmentosa, and ataxia occurs. A similar syndrome with associated abetalipoproteinemia (on lipoprotein electrophoresis) and acanthocytosis (on wet blood smear) occurs with Bassen-Kornzweig syndrome.[16] Chromosomal fragility and low serum immunoglobulin A are found in ataxia-telangiectasia.[17] In Friedreich's ataxia, some experimental work has suggested abnormalities of pyruvate metabolism. In chronic vitamin E deficiency due to malabsorption, a syndrome of spinocerebellar degeneration and peripheral neuropathy occurs.[18]

Serum lactate may be elevated in the mitochondrial disorders that may feature ataxia; these syndromes may include progressive external ophthalmoplegia, generalized myopathy, peripheral neuropathy, cardiac conduction defects, strokelike episodes, myoclonus, and epilepsy.[19] If there is a strong suspicion of a mitochondrial disorder, a muscle biopsy may be performed to look for ragged red fibers. Fluctuating ataxia suggests an organic aciduria, and biochemical evaluation of amino acids in the urine should be performed.

ASSESSMENT

Midline Lesions

Midline lesions are characterized by gait ataxia and often sparse signs in the limbs. When due to hemorrhage or infarct with edema, hydrocephalus may rapidly develop with drowsiness, headache, and vomiting. The patient may present because of symptoms of raised intracranial pressure. Signs of brainstem compression, with bulbar palsy or long tract signs, may be present. The triad of headache, vomiting, and inability to walk should lead to urgent evaluation and CT scanning, as this situation may require life-saving surgical decompression. Neoplasms, especially secondaries, may give rise to an acute midline cerebellar syndrome.

Wernicke's encephalopathy, a medical emergency, is characterized by ataxia, nystagmus or ophthalmoplegia, and mental disturbance.[20] Incomplete forms of this triad have been described with pathologic lesions of Wernicke's.[21] If suspected, treatment should be immediately instituted with parenteral thiamine. Intravenous dextrose may precipitate the syndrome in patients with marginal thiamine stores. Alcohol intoxication rarely causes diagnostic difficulty, but it may be confirmed by serum ethanol estimation. In the setting of chronic alcohol abuse, a history of acute deterioration in gait is not always obtainable. Midline vermal lesions may persist from periods of thiamine deficiency.

Anticonvulsant toxicity may produce prominent gait ataxia. The diagnosis can usually be suspected from the clinical setting. Rare cases of surreptitious self-administration or deliberate overdose occur. Phenytoin and carbamazepine are most likely to cause ataxia, but other anticonvulsants have been implicated. Some patients develop toxicity even within the usual therapeutic range, particularly if there have been rapid changes in serum levels. Anticonvulsant use in the past may account for an enduring ataxic syndrome with midline or global cerebellar atrophy. Dilantin is usually cited as the cause, but the contribution of repeated major convulsions is uncertain.

Multiple sclerosis, trauma, and hereditary ataxias may be identified by the history and examination. Both primary and secondary neoplasms may give rise to chronic midline or hemispheric syndromes. Signs of raised intracranial pressure are present in most cases. There is often a known primary lesion (lung, breast, colon). Primary cerebellar tumors are rare in adults, but hemangioblastomas, medulloblastomas, and gliomas occur.

Hemispheric Lesions

Acute hemispheric lesions are usually vascular, demyelinating, or less frequently, neoplastic. Ipsilateral peripheral or limb ataxia is the consequence. Nystagmus is seen, but dysarthria is uncommon with unilateral lesions. Typically, the patient falls to the side of the lesion. Infarction of the inferior cerebellar peduncle occurs in the lateral medullary syndrome of Wallenberg and causes a recognizable constellation of findings. Hemorrhage less commonly produces a purely lateralized dysfunction as pressure distorts the whole cerebellum. Demyelination of the cerebellar white matter or its afferent or efferent connections is often asymmetric.

Chronic bilateral lesions may be toxic, residua of vascular events, demyelinative, or hereditary. They are separated on clinical grounds combined with imaging. The differentiation of progressive forms of multiple sclerosis and sporadic cerebellar degenerations may be difficult.

Importance of Early Diagnosis

Most causes of ataxia are not life-threatening, but in the case of hemorrhage or infarction, the risk of brainstem compression necessitates early diagnosis. Wernicke's encephalopathy is a fatal condition if untreated, and it requires urgent treatment. These conditions should always be considered in the acutely developing ataxias.

REFERENCES

1. Fisher CM. Homolateral ataxia and crural paresis: a vascular syndrome. J Neurol Neurosurg Psychiatry 1965;28:48–52.
2. Mori E, Yamadorii A, Kudo Y, Tabuchi M. Ataxi hemiparesis from small capsular haemorrhage: computed tomography and somatosensory evoked potentials. Arch Neurol 1984;41:1050–3.
3. Davidoff RA. The dorsal columns. Neurology 1989;39:1377–85.
4. Nathan PW, Smith CM, Cook AW. Sensory effects in man of lesions of the posterior columns and of some other afferent pathways. Brain 1987;109:1003–41.
5. Ferro JM, Bravo-Marques JM, Castro-Caldas A, Antunes L. Crossed optic ataxia: possible role of the dorsal splenium. J Neurol Neurosurg Psychiatry 1983;46:533–9.
6. Rondot P, De Rocondo J, Ribadeau Dumas JL. Visuomotor ataxia. Brain 1977;100:355–76.
7. Appenzeller O, Hanson JC. Parietal ataxia. Arch Neurol 1966;15:264–9.
8. Adams RD, Victor M. Principles of neurology. 3rd ed. New York: McGraw Hill, 1985.
9. Walton JN. Brain's diseases of the nervous system. The hereditary ataxias. Oxford: Oxford University Press, 1977: 669–82.
10. Duvoisin RC. The olivopontocerebellar atrophies. In: Marsden CD, Fahn S, eds. Movement disorders 2. London: Butterworths, 1987:249–71.
11. Spector RH, Troost BT. The ocular motor system. Ann Neurol 1981;9:517–25.
12. Duvoisin RC, Plaitakis A, eds. Olivopontocerebellar atrophy. In: Advances in Neurology, Vol 41. New York: Raven Press, 1984.
13. Oppenheimer DR. Diseases of the basal ganglia, cerebellum and motor neurons. In: Adams JH, Corsellis JAN, Duchen LW, eds. Greenfield's neuropathology. 4th ed. London: Edward Arnold, 1984:699–747.
14. Dyck PJ. Inherited neuronal degeneration and atrophy affecting peripheral motor, sensory, and autonomic neurons. In: Dyck PJ, Thomas PK, Lambert EH, Bunge R, eds. Peripheral neuropathy. Philadelphia: WB Saunders, 1984:1600–42.
15. Hart RG. Vertebral artery dissection. Neurology 1988;38:987–9.
16. Bassen FA, Kornzweig AL. Malformation of the erythrocytes in a case of atypical retinitis pigmentosa. Blood 1950;5:381–7.
17. Sedgwick RP. Ataxia-telangiectasia. In: Vinken PJ, Bruyn GW, eds. Handbook of Clinical Neurology, Vol 42 (Neurogenetic Directory, pt 1). Amsterdam:North Holland, 1981:119–21.
18. Muller DPR, Lloyd JK, Wolff OH. Vitamin E and neurological dysfunction. Lancet 1983;1:225–7.
19. Petty RKH, Harding AE, Morgan-Hughes JA. The clinical features of mitochondrial myopathy. Brain 1986;109:915–38.
20. Charness ME, Simon RP, Greenberg DA. Ethanol and the nervous system. New Engl J Med 1989;321:442–54.
21. Harper CG, Giles M, Finlay-Jones R. Clinical signs in the Wernicke-Korsakoff complex: a retrospective analysis of 131 cases diagnosed at necropsy. J Neurol Neurosurg Psychiatry 1986;49:341–5.

ATHETOSIS

CESAR C. SANTOS and E. WAYNE MASSEY

SYNONYMS: Hammond's Disease, Mobile Spasms

BACKGROUND

Definitions

Athetosis is one of several types of abnormal involuntary movement disorders that include tremor, myoclonus, chorea, tics and spasms, dystonia, and ballism. Among these, tremor is by far the most common.

Athetosis was first used by Hammond in 1871 in his book *Diseases of the Nervous System* to describe involuntary movements of the limbs appearing in previously normal adults.[1] The term is derived from the Greek word *athetos*, meaning "without position." It is a form of dyskinesia characterized by constant succession of slow, writhing, involuntary, and purposeless movements of flexion, extension, pronation, and supination of the fingers and hands and sometimes of the toes and feet. It usually occurs in concert with chorea—hence, the term *choreoathetosis* and seldom in its pure form. The two, however, are completely different (Table 1). Athetotic movements do not occur in limbs that are completely paralyzed, and in contrast to chorea, muscle tone is increased in an extremity with athetosis.[2] Like most involuntary movement disorders, athetosis worsens during stress and voluntary

TABLE 1.   Different Movement Disorders

	ATHETOSIS	BALLISM	CHOREA	DYSTONIA	MYOCLONUS	TICS OR SPASMS	TREMORS
Velocity	Slow	Fast	Fast	Very slow	Very fast	Fast	Variable
Rhythmicity	Nonrhythmic	Nonrhythmic	Nonrhythmic	Nonrhythmic	Nonrhythmic	Nonrhythmic	Rhythmic
Site	One or both sides of the body Distal segments of the limbs	Commonly one-sided More proximal segments of the limbs	May affect any part of the body (e.g., limbs, face, hands, tongue, or trunk)	May be focal (foot or hand), segmental (more commonly proximal segments), or generalized	May be focal, segmental, or multifocal, affecting single muscle or muscle groups; can be symmetric	May involve a muscle or functionally related muscles Usually affects the face	May involve a muscle or functionally related muscles Usually affects distal limbs
Characteristics	Continuous, slow, writhing movement of the limbs, trunk, head, face, and tongue	A form of chorea but larger in amplitude, producing a flinging movement of the affected limb	Brief, rapid, irregular, and unpredictable muscle contractions	Intense, irregular, and persistent spasm resulting in marked abnormality of body posture	Abrupt and irregular stimulussensitive movements	Patterned sequences of involuntary coordinated movements that appear suddenly and intermittently	Stereotyped to and fro movements resulting from alternating contractions of muscles or muscle groups

activity and may subside during rest or disappear with sleep.

Causes

In the pediatric population, athetotic movements are often generalized and usually begin during childhood as a result of birth injury, kernicterus, or genetic disorders. This is in contrast to adults, where such movements are more limited to specific muscle groups and are commonly caused by vascular lesions, neoplastic lesions, degenerative diseases, and drug toxicity.

Athetosis Due to Birth Trauma or Asphyxia

This is an important cause of athetosis of early onset. It may be caused by (1) direct mechanical trauma, that is, forceps extraction or breech delivery, or (2) birth asphyxia, which often impairs the basal ganglia selectively. Mixed forms of cerebral palsy that occur as a combination of spasticity and extrapyramidal signs are common and account for about 15 to 40 per cent of cerebral palsies.[3]

Double athetosis, which is also known as Vogt's disease, corpus striatum necrosis syndrome, congenital chorea, état marbre, or more commonly, status marmoratus, was described by Cecile and Oskar Vogt in 1919–20.

The clinical features include athetosis of the upper extremities, dysarthria, and later rigidity, sometimes accompanied by spasmodic laughing or crying. The pathology is characterized by an abnormal aggregation of myelinated nerve fibers, typically in the corpus striatum, producing a marbled appearance (hence, the name *status marmoratus*).

Athetosis Due to Neurometabolic Disorders

A number of neurometabolic disorders produce a combination of progressive dyskinetic and dystonic abnormalities. These include (1) amino acid disorders, that is, cystinuria, glutaric aciduria, glyceric acidemia, Hartnup's disease, homocystinuria, methylglutaconic aciduria, phenylketonuria, and propionic acidemia; (2) carbohydrate disorders, that is, galactosemia, keratin sulfaturia, lactosuric oligosaccharidosis, mucolipidosis I, and pyruvate dehydrogenase deficiency; and (3) lipid disorders, that is, ceroid lipofuschinosis, gangliosidosis (GM_1 and GM_2 variants), infantile Gauchers' disease, infantile globoid cell leukodystrophy, and metachromatic leukodystrophy.[4]

Other hereditary neurologic disorders that produce dyskinesias include Huntington's disease, Hallervorden-Spatz disease, Pelizaeus-

Merzbacher disease, and neuroacanthocytosis (choreoacanthocytosis).[5]

Athetosis Due to Drugs

Pharmacologically, athetosis and chorea are the antithesis of parkinsonism and are considered to be manifestations of dopaminergic overactivity in the basal ganglia. Drugs implicated as causes of athetosis include levodopa, amphetaminelike drugs,[6] anticonvulsants,[7,8,9,10] and lithium.[11] Of the anticonvulsant drugs, the most commonly implicated is phenytoin, which usually occurs in the setting of pre-existing cerebral disease and marked phenytoin toxicity. Transient choreoathetosis, however, has been reported in the absence of the above conditions following treatment with phenytoin for status epilepticus.[7] It has also resulted from therapeutic phenytoin levels probably secondary to high free fraction.[8] Other anticonvulsants that produce choreoathetoid movements include carbamazepine[9] and clonazepam.[10]

Athetosis Due to Other Generalized Metabolic Disorders

In mild hyperthyroidism, tremor is a common manifestation. In severe thyrotoxicosis, however, choreoathetosis can occur.[12,13] It may be due to the high dihydroxyphenylalanine level that occurs in this condition[12] or due to increased sensitivity of the striatal dopamine receptors associated with decreased cerebral dopamine turnover.[13] In Lesch-Nyhan syndrome, an inherited disorder of purine metabolism affecting males, choreoathetosis is a major manifestation. A new variant, without the accompanying mental retardation and self-mutilating behavior, also produces choreoathetosis.[14] Disorders of glucose metabolism, either hypoglycemia[15] or hyperglycemia,[16] can cause choreoathetosis.

Athetosis Due to Miscellaneous Disorders

Infectious or inflammatory disorders either concomitantly or as a sequela, brain tumors, toxins (i.e., drugs, carbon monoxide, and toluene[17]), head trauma, and focal cerebrovascular disease may produce athetosis.

Genetics of Paroxysmal Dyskinesias

Paroxysmal dyskinesias are classified into two types. The first and the more common is paroxysmal kinesigenic choreoathetosis (PKC), characterized by frequent brief dyskinesias (primarily chorea) precipitated by sudden movement, especially after a period of relaxation. Attacks are short (seconds to minutes) and occur up to 100 times daily. It usually begins in one arm or a leg, spreading to the entire side. It tends to recur on the same side. Age of onset is between 5 and 15 years. The prognosis is good. Attacks are often controlled by anticonvulsants. The majority of familial cases are inherited as an autosomal dominant trait with variable penetrance,[18] although autosomal recessive inheritance has also been reported.[19] Sporadic cases also occur as well as secondary cases, that is, following brain injury.[20]

Paroxysmal dystonic choreoathetosis (PDC) is the second form. It is a rare familial disorder of autosomal dominant inheritance with high penetrance characterized primarily by sustained attacks of dystonia with chorea and athetosis as variable features. The duration of each attack is brief, lasting between two minutes and four hours, with the frequency ranging from three per day to one per month. Age of onset of PDC is earlier (one to two years of age) compared with PKC, and PDC responds well to clonazepam.[18] Sporadic and secondary cases occur.[21] Some cases can occur in association with another inherited disorder such as familial periodic ataxia.[22]

HISTORY

Diagnosis of movement disorders relies primarily on direct patient observation. History and physical examination provide clues to etiologies.

Birth, Perinatal, and Neonatal History

This information should always be obtained, especially in patients with early onset. The majority of athetoid movements in childhood are due to birth asphyxia and trauma, which include the double athetosis and the hemiathetosis of mixed cerebral palsy. Immediate neonatal course is also of importance. Was hyperbilirubinemia present? How long was it present? What type of intervention was needed? What was it due to?

History of the Present Illness

Age at onset of the abnormal movement, initial part of the body involved, duration, and presence of aggravating or alleviating factors should be noted. Other pertinent questions include: Was there history of head trauma, prior brain surgery, or infection? History of peculiar habits, for example, glue sniffing? History of carbon monoxide exposure? Is the abnormal movement progressive? If yes, does it affect performance of activities of daily living (dressing, combing hair, brushing teeth, eating, or mobility)? Does anything make it less or completely go away?

A list of current and previous medications should be obtained, noting whether they increase or decrease the severity of the abnormal movement. For the same reason, a good psychiatric history with special emphasis on possible medications used should be obtained.

Family History

The mode of inheritance of paroxysmal dyskinesias is predominantly an autosomal dominant trait, but the degree of penetrance is variable, so it may skip generations. In addition to pertinent family history, it is important to examine immediate relatives. Positive family history lends information to hereditary metabolic diseases associated with athetosis.

Focused Queries

1. *Was there anything abnormal about the birth history?* A positive answer implies an associated static encephalopathy.

2. *Was the onset of dyskinesia generalized or limited to one extremity?* Athetosis in children is usually generalized and due most commonly to birth asphyxia/trauma or genetic disorders, whereas it is usually focal in adults and caused by vascular or neoplastic lesions, degenerative diseases, or drug toxicity.

3. *Was there any relative with the same problem?* A positive answer suggests hereditary disorders causing athetosis or one of the paroxysmal dyskinesias.

4. *Does the movement occur in paroxysms?* An affirmative answer suggests the possibility of paroxysmal dyskinesia.

5. *Did the abnormal movement occur in the presence of a previous fixed neurologic deficit?* Abnormal movements can be a long-term sequela of focal cerebrovascular accident, central nervous system tumor, or infection.

PHYSICAL EXAMINATION

As stated previously, direct patient observation to determine the presence or absence of abnormal movements is of primary importance. Its absence, especially after a brief encounter with a patient, does not rule it out. Ancillary information can be obtained through examination.

General Physical Examination

The presence of specific physical signs can lead to a diagnosis: examination of the eye for Kayser-Fleischer rings (Wilson's disease); examination of the retina to look for pigmentary changes (Tay-Sachs diseases and ceroid lipofuscinosis); examination for retinopathy (diabetes). Thyromegaly may suggest thyrotoxicosis. Skin changes over the extremities may give evidence of self-mutilating behavior. Joint deformities may occur secondary to long-standing severe dyskinesia.

Neurologic Examination

Neurologic examination identifies deficits associated with secondary athetosis, that is, hemiathetosis with hemiparesis. This may assist to differentiate one movement disorder from another—for example, muscle tone is increased in athetosis while the reverse is true in chorea; the muscle mass in a hemiparetic limb is usually decreased, but if it is complicated by an abnormal movement, muscle hypertrophy may be observed.

Evaluation of Involuntary Movements

Individuals should be observed for an extended period. This means observation during sleep, rest, and while performing physical activity (i.e., walking, eating, writing, combing hair, buttoning shirts, opening doors, or during playing). Efforts should also be made to expose patients to factors previously identified that alleviate or worsen the abnormal movement.

Observation should note onset, progression, pattern, and distribution. This will help to differentiate the types of dyskinesia. How severe is the movement disorder? Is it limiting the patient from performing daily activities? These are two important questions.

DIAGNOSTIC STUDIES

Few ancillary data are needed after a complete history and detailed examination. These are mainly performed to support the diagnosis of a primary disease entity producing the dyskinesia—for example, a glycosylated hemoglobin and fasting blood sugar for suspected diabetes mellitus; uric acid for disorders of purine metabolism; 24-hour urine copper excretion, serum copper, and ceruloplasmin for Wilson's disease; an organic and amino acid urine analysis, creatinine phosphokinase, nerve conduction studies, and fresh blood smear in choreoacanthocytosis.[23] Further tests are dictated by clinical clues.

Imaging and electrophysiologic studies may be helpful. Abnormal imaging[24] and electrophysiologic studies in paroxysmal dyskinesias are reported. In general, however, they are normal. Imaging studies can be used to identify focal structural lesions, for example, brain tumor, infarction, or degenerative diseases. Electroencephalogram can differentiate the paroxysmal dyskinesias from movement-induced reflex epilepsy (MIRE).[26]

ASSESSMENT

Emphasis is placed on history and patient observation with the purpose of identifying the presence or absence of a movement disorder and differentiating it from other dyskinesias (Table 1). Although they are quite different from each other, this is often easier said than done. They frequently occur in combination. The history should include present illness, birth history, growth and developmental history, past medical history, and family history. Only through repeated patient contact can the physician become familiar with the dyskinesias.

REFERENCES

1. Foley J. The athetoid syndrome. A review of a personal series. J Neurol Neurosurg Psychiatry 1983;46:289–98.
2. Barker LF. Diseases of the nervous system. In: Backer LF, ed. The clinical diagnosis of internal diseases. New York: D Appleton, 1916:232–4.
3. Molnar GE, Taft LT. Cerebral palsy. In: Wortis J, ed. Mental retardation and developmental disabilities, Vol 5. New York: Brunner/Mazel, 1973:85–112.
4. Hagberg E, Kyllerman M, Steen G. Dyskinesia and dystonia in neurometabolic disorders. Neuropaediatrie 1979;10:305–20.
5. Massey EW, Pericak-Vance MA, Payne CS, Vance JM, Honeycutt PJ, Bowman M. Choreoacanthocytosis. Neurology 1985; 35 (Suppl):175.
6. Rhee KJ, Albertson TE, Douglas JC. Choreoathetoid disorders associated with amphetamine-like drugs. Am J Emerg Med 1988;6:131–3.
7. Filloux F, Thompson JA. Transient chorea induced by phenytoin. J Pediatr 1987;110:639–41.
8. Tomson T. Choreoathetosis induced by ordinary phenytoin levels, explained by high free fraction?—a case report. Ther Drug Monit 1988;10:239–41.
9. Bimpong-Buta K, Froescher W. Carbamazepine-induced choreoathetoid dyskinesias [Letter]. J Neurol Neurosurg Psychiatry 1982;45:560.
10. O'Flaherty S, Evans M, Epps A, Buchanan N. Choreoathetosis and clonazepam [Letter]. Med J Aust 1985;142:453.
11. Walevski A, Radwan M. Choreoathetosis as toxic effect of lithium treatment. Eur Neurol 1986;25:412–5.
12. Marks P, Anderson J, Vincent R. Choreoathetosis with severe thyrotoxicosis. Postgrad Med J 1979;55:830–1.
13. Clements MR, Hamilton DV, Siklos P. Thyrotoxicosis with choreoathetosis and severe myopathy. J R Soc Med 1981;74:459–60.
14. Gottlieb RP, Koppel MM, Nyhan WL, et al. Hyperuricemia and choreoathetosis in a child without mental retardation or self-mutilation—new HPRT variant. J Inher Metab Dis 1982;5:183–6.
15. Newman RP, Kinkel WR. Paroxysmal choreoathetosis due to hypoglycemia. Arch Neurol 1984;41:341–2.
16. Rector WG, Herlong HF, Moses H. III. Nonketotic hyperglycemia appearing as choreoathetosis or ballism. Arch Intern Med 1982;142:154–5.
17. Bartolucci G, Pellettier JR. Glue sniffing and movement disorder [Letter]. J Neurol Neurosurg Psychiatry 1984;47:1259.
18. Harel S, Yurgenson U, Kutai M. Paroxysmal kinesigenic choreoathetosis. Childs Nerv Syst 1987;3:47–9.
19. Kertesz A. Paroxysmal kinesigenic choreoathetosis. Neurology 1967;17:680–90.
20. Richardson JC, Howes JL, Celinski MJ, Allman RG. Kinesigenic choreoathetosis due to brain injury. Can J Neurol Sci 1987;14:626–8.
21. Micheli F, Fernandez Pardal MM, Parera IC, Giannuala R. Sporadic paroxysmal dystonic choreoathetosis associated with basal ganglia calcifications. Ann Neurol 1986;20:750.
22. Mayeux R, Fahn S. Paroxysmal dystonic choreoathetosis in a patient with familial ataxia. Neurology (NY) 1982;32:1184–6.
23. Massey J, Bowman M, Massey EW. EMG changes in choreoacanthocytosis. Neurology 1986;36 (Supp 1):116.
24. Gilroy J. Abnormal computed tomograms in paroxysmal kinesigenic choreoathetosis. Arch Neurol 1982;39:779–80.
25. Busard HLSM, Renier WO, Gabreels FJM, Vos AJM, Declerck AC, Verhey FHM. Autosomal dominant paroxysmal kinesigenic choreoathetosis—an electrophysiologic study. Clin Neurol Neurosurg 1984;86:281–9.
26. Lishman WA, Symonds CP, Whitty CWM, Willison RG. Seizures induced by movement. Brain 1962;86:93–108.

AZOTEMIA, ACUTE

WENG-LIH WANG and D. M. KAJI

SYNONYM: Acute Renal Failure

BACKGROUND

Azotemia refers to the retention of nitrogenous wastes normally excreted by the kidney and is the result of a decrease in the glomerular filtration rate. Arbitrarily, *acute azotemia* is defined as an increase in blood urea nitrogen (BUN) or plasma creatinine (Pcr) above a normal or previously stable level over several days.

Most of the descriptions of acute azotemia are derived from World War II experience, when trauma accounted for most of the cases. In a more recent study, the incidence of acute azotemia was 5 per cent in over 200 medical and surgical admissions.[1] Approximately 50 per cent of cases of azotemia are related to surgery or trauma; 40 to 45 per cent occur in a medical setting, many of them related to nephrotoxic renal injury; and 2 to 5 per cent are related to pregnancy.

The causes of acute azotemia are divided into prerenal, renal, and postrenal causes (Table 1). Prerenal azotemia results from increased catabolism or decreased renal perfusion secondary to volume depletion or poor cardiac output and accounts for 30 to 40 per cent of patients with acute azotemia.[2,3] The kidney is intrinsically normal in prerenal azotemia and is only responding to a decrease in effective circulating volume. However, a prolonged period of renal hypoperfusion can eventually lead to intrinsic renal damage and acute tubular necrosis.

Postrenal azotemia is caused by urinary tract obstruction and accounts for 5 to 10 per cent of cases of acute azotemia.[1,2] It is most common in elderly men with prostatic enlargement. In women, it is relatively uncommon in the absence of pelvic surgery or malignancy. A single normally functioning kidney is sufficient to excrete nitrogenous wastes and keep Pcr within normal limits. Therefore, acute renal failure due to obstruction of the upper urinary tract is much less frequent in the absence of simultaneous obstruction of both ureters or unilateral ureteral obstruction with absence or severe disease in the contralateral kidney.

Renal azotemia refers to acute deterioration of renal function due to intrinsic renal disease. This is a syndrome representing a nonspecific renal injury in response to a variety of insults and exhibits a typical clinical course (see Assessment). Acute tubular necrosis (ATN) accounts for the vast majority of patients with hospital-acquired renal azotemia. Other intrinsic renal diseases, which include damage to the glomerulus, interstitium, or vasculature, account for only 5 to 10 per cent of cases with acute azotemia in adults but for 40 to 50 per cent of cases in children.[3]

HISTORY

Acute azotemia is a laboratory finding, not a symptom complex. Thus, history taking should be directed toward the detection of various causes.

Focused Queries

1. *Is the azotemia acute, chronic, or acute superimposed on chronic?* The physician should engage in an aggressive effort to determine the Pcr values drawn during previous admissions, in other hospitals or in the office or outpatient clinic in the past. A recent intravenous pyelogram (IVP), renal scan, or sonogram is also useful. A history of urolithiasis, repeated urinary tract infections, abnormal urinary findings (e.g., proteinuria, hematuria), family history of renal disease (i.e., polycystic kidney disease), and/or a history of systemic illness (diabetes mellitus, hypertension, systemic lupus erythematosus) suggests chronic renal insufficiency. Chronicity is also suggested by a history of occupational or accidental exposure to heavy metals (such as mercury, arsenic, or lead) or organic solvents (carbon tetrachloride).

2. *Is there evidence of body fluid losses (diarrhea, vomiting, poor intake, inadequate replacement during or after intraoperative loss of fluids, excessive diuresis and losses from drainage tubes, burns, or high fever)?*

3. *Are there medications that might impair renal function?* A list of potential nephrotoxic drugs is given in Table 1. A temporal

TABLE 1. Causes of Acute Azotemia

Prerenal causes
  Hypovolemia
    Gastrointestinal, renal, or skin loss; hemorrhage; sequestration in "third space" (peritonitis, pancreatitis); increased vascular capacity (sepsis, anaphylactic shock)
  Decreased cardiac output
    Heart failure, myocardial infarction, cardiac tamponade, pulmonary embolism
  Increased catabolism
    Burn, sepsis, GI bleeding
  Medications (tetracycline, steroids)
  Hepatorenal syndrome
Postrenal causes
  Urethral
    Stricture, valve
  Bladder neck
    Prostate hypertrophy or tumor, bladder tumor, atonic bladder, autonomic neuropathy, spinal cord lesions, ganglionic blocking agents
  Ureteral
    Intraureteral (stone, blood clots, sloughed papilla)
    Extraureteral (prostate, bladder, or cervical cancer; lymphoma; retroperitoneal fibrosis)
  Intrarenal
    Crystals (uric acid, methotrexate, oxalic acid)
Renal causes
  Acute tubular necrosis (ATN)
  Post-ischemic
    All conditions listed under hypovolemia and decreased cardiac output in prerenal causes
  Nephrotoxic
    Antibiotics (aminoglycoside), contrast media, anesthetic agents (methoxyflurane), heavy metal (mercury, lead), organic solvents, cisplatin
  Pigment-induced
    Hemoglobulinuria (transfusion reaction), myoglobulinuria (trauma, heat stroke, potassium or phosphate depletion)
  Specific renal diseases
    Glomerular
      Acute poststreptococcal glomerulonephritis, antiglomerular basement membrane disease, SLE, subacute bacterial endocarditis
    Interstitial
      Drugs (cephalosporins, anticonvulsants, diuretics, NSAIDs), hypercalcemia
    Vascular
      Vasculitides (polyarteritis nodosa, Wegener's granulomatosis, Henoch-Schönlein purpura), malignant hypertension, scleroderma, thrombotic thrombocytopenic purpura, hemolytic uremic syndrome, arterial thrombosis or embolism
      Renal vein thrombosis

association between the administration of the medications and the onset of azotemia suggests, but does not establish, a cause-and-effect relationship. A history of allergy is a tip-off to the presence of hypersensitivity vasculitis of the kidneys. History of chronic headache or backache should alert the clinician to ask for the use of aspirin and other nonsteroidal anti-inflammatory drugs (NSAIDs). A history of recent exposure to contrast media during diagnostic studies such as angiogram, cardiac catheterization, IVP, or computerized tomography (CT) suggests nephrotoxicity from radiocontrast media. The risk of nephrotoxicity is especially high in patients with diabetes, multiple myeloma, or chronic renal insufficiency and in patients with volume depletion.

4. *Is there a history of cardiac failure?* Ask for predisposing conditions (ischemic or valvular heart disease, cardiomyopathy, arrhythmia, or pericarditis), symptoms of congestive heart failure (shortness of breath on exertion, paroxysmal nocturnal dyspnea, orthopnea, edema), and medications with negative ionotropic effects (beta-blockers, some calcium channel blockers). (Also see chapter on Congestive Heart Failure.)

5. *Is there a systemic illness or recent trauma?* Arthralgias, fever, and malar rash may suggest systemic lupus erythematosus (SLE). History of pharyngitis or pyoderma often precedes acute poststreptococcal glomerulonephritis by two to three weeks. History of viral infection can lead to possible volume depletion or rhabdomyolysis. Fever, chill, and hypotension should alert the clinician to the presence of possible sepsis, which can cause either prerenal or renal azotemia. Trauma can cause azotemia by extensive muscle injury (rhabdomyolysis), internal bleeding (prerenal azotemia), or acute urinary retention (postrenal azotemia).

6. *Are urinary symptoms present?* Hematuria, frequency, hesitancy, poor urinary stream, and lower abdominal pain may suggest prostate hypertrophy or cancer.

PHYSICAL EXAMINATION

Acute azotemia can be associated with a constellation of signs caused by retention of toxic substances or electrolyte disturbances. Neurologic disturbances can range from shortened attention span, twitching, seizure, stupor, or coma. Mild hypertension is seen in 15 to 25 per cent of cases. Edema, weight gain, jugular vein distension, and pulmonary rales suggest water and salt retention. Hyperventilation is associated with metabolic acidosis or pulmonary congestion. Pericardial rub and diminished heart sound may occur with pericarditis. Flaccid paralysis can be seen with severe hyperkalemia.

Special attention should be directed toward the following:

Status of Extracellular Fluid (ECF)

Weight loss, postural change of pulse pressure more than 10 mm Hg or postural change of pulse rate more than 15 to 20 per minute, and loss of skin turgor (especially in sternum area and forehead) all suggest a reduction in ECF, which may cause prerenal azotemia.

Amount and Pattern of Daily Urine Output

Anuria (urine volume less than 100 ml per day) may be encountered in complete obstruction, diffuse cortical necrosis, and rapid progressive glomerulonephritis but is rare in ATN. Oliguria (less than 400 ml per day) is only seen in 50 to 70 per cent of the cases in acute azotemia.[4] The nonoliguric form is commonly seen following the administration of nephrotoxins (aminoglycosides) and in myoglobinuria. It is important to emphasize that the presence of normal urine output does not rule out urinary tract obstruction. In partial urinary obstruction, urine output can range from high (owing to concentrating defect) to low.

Signs of Obstruction

Enlarged prostate, suprapubic dullness, and postvoid residual volume of more than 200 to 300 ml suggest significant urinary retention. In women, bimanual pelvic examination is recommended to rule out obstruction by a pelvic mass. Signs suggestive of intra-abdominal lymphoma (lymphadenopathy and hepatosplenomegaly) or aortic aneurysm (abdominal bruit and pulsating mass) may also suggest obstruction.

Signs of Systemic Diseases

Atrial fibrillation and signs of peripheral vascular disease suggest that azotemia may have a renovascular cause. Focal neurologic signs, bleeding, and jaundice may suggest disseminated intravascular coagulation (DIC) or thrombotic thrombocytopenic purpura (TTP).

Skin Lesions

Patients with hypersensitivity vasculitis or allergic interstitial nephritis present with a diffuse rash, whereas those with scleroderma and SLE manifest characteristic skin lesions with Raynaud's phenomenon. Polyarteritis nodosa is associated with ischemic necrosis of skin and palpable purpura. Henoch-Schönlein disease is characterized by purpuric lesions on the extensor surfaces of the limbs and on the buttocks.

DIAGNOSTIC STUDIES

The magnitude of biochemical abnormalities depends on the catabolic state of the patient. Catabolic patients undergo massive tissue breakdown and have higher endogenous loads of metabolic wastes and electrolytes. Table 2 illustrates the expected biochemical changes in a patient with acute azotemia.

The following findings are associated with acute azotemia:

1. Hyperkalemia. Patients are generally without symptoms or electrocardiographic findings when serum potassium is below 6 mEq/l. Above this value, bradycardia, electrocardiographic (ECG) abnormalities (peaked T wave, prolonged QRS complex, prolonged PR interval, and absent P wave), and ultimately cardiac arrest can occur. It is worth emphasizing that the absence of ECG findings does not exclude hyperkalemia. Thus, patients with high serum potassium may still suffer from sudden cardiac arrest without interim ECG changes.

2. Mild hyponatremia between 125 and 135 mEq/l.

TABLE 2.   Biochemical Changes in Acute Renal Failure

DAILY CHANGE IN SERUM CONCENTRATION	NONCATABOLIC	CATABOLIC
BUN (mg/dl)	<20	>20
Creatinine (mg/dl)	<1.5	>2
Bicarbonate (mEq/l)	<1	>2
Potassium (mEq/l)	<0.5	>0.5
Uric acid (mg/dl)	<1.5	>2

3. Hypocalcemia, hyperphosphatemia, and high alkaline phosphatase. A calcium · inorganic phosphorus product (Ca in mg/dl, P in mg/dl) greater than 70 may be associated with metastatic calcification.

4. Metabolic acidosis with increased anion gap.

5. Normocytic normochromic anemia due to lack of erythropoietin and bone marrow suppression with a typical hematocrit between 25 and 30 per cent. Associated gastrointestinal bleeding from uremic gastritis may further worsen the degree of anemia.

6. Prolonged bleeding time.

7. Hyperuricemia.

8. Hypermagnesemia.

9. Mild elevation of serum amylase and creatine phosphokinase (CPK) concentration (twice or three times the normal level).

10. Glucose intolerance.

Prerenal azotemia and ATN, which together account for 70 per cent of all cases of azotemia, are distinguished by the urinary diagnostic indices given in Table 3. It is important to distinguish between these two conditions because the therapy for the two conditions is markedly different. The urine should be collected before the administration of diuretics because the latter may invalidate the interpretation of these indices for up to 24 hours. The findings on urinary sediment (Table 4) may provide clues to the presence of a specific disorder, but negative findings do not necessarily help to exclude these causes. Specific serologic tests (e.g., antistreptolysin O titer, complement level, antinuclear antibody, antiglomerular basement membrane antibody, and cryoglobulin) should be ordered when a glomerulopathy is suspected.

Diagnostic Imaging

A plain abdomen x-ray may be of help in estimating the kidney size and in detecting radio-opaque stones. The finding of subperiosteal bone resorption and other changes of secondary hyperparathyroidism suggests that the renal disease is chronic rather than acute. A chest x-ray may reveal large nodules or cavities associated with Wegener's granulomatosis or interstitial fibrosis and infiltration in SLE or scleroderma.

Increased recognition of the risk of nephrotoxicity has decreased the enthusiasm for IVP. A renal sonogram is the test of choice in assessing kidney size. Small kidneys (8 cm or less) suggest chronic rather than acute azotemia. The sonogram is also useful in detecting hydronephrosis. The sensitivity for detection of hydronephrosis 24 hours after obstruction was about 95 per cent in a recent study[5]. A renal sonogram may also detect stones in the pelvic-calyceal area that may lead to obstruction. CT (without contrast media to prevent nephrotoxicity) may help to localize the site of extraureteral obstruction.

Radionuclide studies with technetium diethylene triamine pentacetic acid (^{99}Tc^m-DTPA) and chromium ethylene diamine tetraacetic acid (^{51}Cr-EDTA) are useful for evaluating renal perfusion and glomerular filtration, respectively. A diminished blood flow in one area or one kidney may suggest renal artery stenosis or renal infarction, but a negative finding does not rule out these conditions. A radionuclide scan of the kidneys is also important in differentiating acute transplant rejection from ATN as the cause of acute azotemia in transplantation patients. An acute transplant rejection usually presents with a pattern of diminished perfusion, whereas in ATN renal perfusion is preserved.

Retrograde pyelography is a highly invasive procedure and is only indicated when obstruction is highly suspect and when a renal sonogram has failed to establish or rule out obstruction. Retrograde urethrogram and cystogram are most useful in children with acute

TABLE 4. Urine Sediment Findings and Related Disorders

FINDINGS	DISORDERS
Red blood cell (RBC) cast	Acute glomerulonephritis or vasculitis
Tubular cast	Acute tubular necrosis
Oxalate crystalluria	Ethylene glycol intoxication
Eosinophiluria (Wright's stain)	Interstitial nephritis
Strong heme-positive urine without RBC	Hemo- or myoglobulinuria
White blood cell (WBC) cast	Acute pyelonephritis

TABLE 3. Urine Diagnostic Indices

	PRERENAL	RENAL
Urine osmolarity	>500	<350
Urine sodium (Na)	<20	>40
U/P creatinine	>40	<20
Renal failure index: $\left(\dfrac{\text{Urine Na}}{\text{Urine/plasma creatinine}}\right)$	<1	>1
Fractional excretion of Na: $\left(\dfrac{\text{Urine/plasma Na}}{\text{Urine/plasma creatinine}}\right)$	<1	>1

DIAGNOSTIC ASSESSMENT OF ACUTE AZOTEMIA

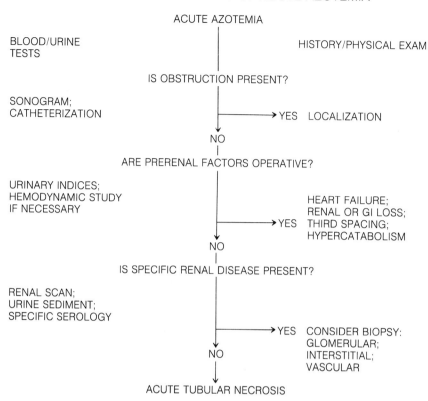

ACUTE AZOTEMIA

BLOOD/URINE
TESTS   HISTORY/PHYSICAL EXAM

IS OBSTRUCTION PRESENT?

SONOGRAM;
CATHETERIZATION   → YES   LOCALIZATION

NO

ARE PRERENAL FACTORS OPERATIVE?

URINARY INDICES;
HEMODYNAMIC STUDY
IF NECESSARY   HEART FAILURE;
                                                  RENAL OR GI LOSS;
                                          → YES   THIRD SPACING;
                                                  HYPERCATABOLISM
NO

IS SPECIFIC RENAL DISEASE PRESENT?

RENAL SCAN;
URINE SEDIMENT;
SPECIFIC SEROLOGY
                                          → YES   CONSIDER BIOPSY:
                                                  GLOMERULAR;
NO   INTERSTITIAL;
                                                  VASCULAR

ACUTE TUBULAR NECROSIS

azotemia to rule out the presence of urethral valves, strictures, or vesicoureteral reflux.

Renal venogram and arteriogram are highly invasive, associated with nephrotoxicity (worsening of azotemia) and should be considered in a patient with strong suspicion of renovascular disease.

Renal Biopsy

A renal biopsy is indicated when the cause of acute azotemia is unknown and a potential treatable renal parenchymal disease is likely. It should be considered in acutely azotemic patients with new onset of heavy proteinuria (urinary protein greater than 3 gm per 24 hours) and/or red blood cell casts (glomerulonephritis, vasculitis), or in such patients with aseptic pyuria, white blood cell casts, and/or eosinophiluria (acute interstitial nephritis). In two large series of patients with acute azotemia, 10 to 15 per cent of patients underwent a renal biopsy.[6,7] Of these patients, 30 to 50 per cent had glomerular disease, 10 to 15 per cent had interstitial disease, 20 to 30 per cent had vascular disease, and 15 to 25 per cent had ATN. Contraindications to percuta-

neous renal biopsy include a bleeding disorder, single functioning kidney, uncontrolled hypertension, and an uncooperative patient who cannot or will not hold the breath for the few seconds that a needle is in the kidney.

Other Studies

Assessment of central venous pressure (CVP) and pulmonary wedge pressure may be needed in patients who are in precarious cardiovascular balance and when routine clinical and laboratory tests cannot distinguish prerenal from renal causes.

ASSESSMENT

The algorithm provided suggests a pathway to determine the cause of acute azotemia. Acute tubular necrosis, once diagnosed, usually follows a relatively uniform course. The initial phase is the period between the precipitating event and the appearance of acute renal failure. The maintenance phase, characterized with oliguria in more than 50 per cent of cases, lasts between two and six weeks. This is followed by a recovery phase with diuresis and gradual improvement of renal function in four to six weeks. In nonoliguric ATN, the distinction between different phases is blurred because the urine volume is highly variable.

Implications of Acute Azotemia

Acute renal failure is associated with a mortality rate of 40 to 50 per cent.[8] The mortality rate has remained unchanged for the past four decades even after the introduction of hemodialysis and aggressive supportive care. Infection, gastrointestinal (GI) hemorrhage, complications resulting from fluid or electrolyte disturbances, and progression of the primary underlying disease are the major causes of mortality in acute renal failure.[9,10]

Factors that affect the prognosis of acute renal failure include the nature of underlying diseases, the amount of urine output, the age of the patient, and the number of clinical and biochemical complications.[11] Acute azotemia occurring with severe trauma or following operative complication is associated with a higher mortality (40 to 80 per cent) compared with azotemia from nephrotoxic or postpartum causes (10 to 30 per cent).[12,13] Nonoliguric patients generally show a lower mortality rate compared with oliguric patients (26 versus 50 per cent).[4,10,14] Bullock et al. reported the mortality rates in different age groups.[9] The mortality was 39 per cent between the ages of 10 and 29; 61 per cent between the ages of 30 and 59; 72 per cent between the ages of 60 and 79; and 79 per cent above the age of 80. The development of two or more complications or of specific types of complications such as peritonitis, congestive heart failure, severe GI bleeding, and jaundice is associated with a poor prognosis.[15]

Patients at high risk for developing acute azotemia include those with multiple trauma, burns, and rhabdomyolysis; those undergoing operative procedure; those receiving potential nephrotoxins; and those with underlying chronic renal insufficiency.[15] The recognition of such patients is important; while the incidence of acute azotemia can be reduced significantly with prophylactic treatment, the morbidity and mortality are high once acute azotemia is established.

REFERENCES

1. Hou SH, Bushinsky DA, Wish JB, et al. Hospital-acquired renal insufficiency. Am J Med 1983; 74:243–8.
2. Miller TR, Anderson RJ, Linas SL, et al. Urinary diagnostic indices in acute renal failure. A prospective study. Ann Int Med 1978;89:47–50.
3. Hodson EM, Kjellstrand CM, Mauer SM. Acute renal failure in infants and children. J Pediatr 1976;93:756–61.
4. Anderson RJ, Linas SL, Berns AS, et al. Nonoliguric acute renal failure. New Engl J Med 1977;296:1134–9.
5. Ellenbogen PH, Scheible FW, Talner LB, Leopold GR. Sensitivity of gray scale ultrasound in detecting urinary tract obstruction. AJR 1978;130:731–4.
6. Wilson DM, Turner DR, Cameron JS, Ogg CS, Brown CB, Chantler C. Value of renal biopsy in acute intrinsic renal failure. Br Med J 1976;2:459–62.
7. Sraer J-D. Renal biopsy in acute renal failure. Kidney Int 1975;8:60A.
8. Butkus DE. Persistent high mortality in acute renal failure. Are we asking the right question? Arch Int Med 1983;143:209–12.
9. Bullock ML, Umen AJ, Finkelstein M, Keane WF. The assessment of risk factors in 462 patients with acute renal failure. Am J Kidney Dis 1985;5:97–103.
10. Minuth AN, Terrell JB, Suki WN. Acute renal failure: a study of the course and prognosis of 104 patients and of the role of furosemide. Am J Med Sci 1976;271:317–24.
11. Scott RB, Cameron FS, Ogg CS, Bewick M. Why the persistently high mortality in acute renal failure? Lancet 1972;2:75–8.
12. Stone WJ, Knepshield JH. Post traumatic renal insufficiency in Vietnam. Clin Nephrol 1974;2:186–90.
13. Hall JW, Johnson WJ, Maher FT, Hunt JC. Immediate and long-term prognosis in acute renal failure. Ann Int Med 1970;73:515–21.
14. Meyer C, Roxe DM, Han JE. The clinical course of nonoliguric acute renal failure. Cardiovasc Med 1978;89:47–50.
15. McMurray SD, Luft FC, Maxwell DR, et al. Prevailing patterns and predictor variable in patient with ATN. Arch Int Med 1978;138:950–5.

BONE PAIN

FRANK J. FRASSICA, FRANKLIN H. SIM, and PETER R. WILSON

SYNONYMS: Musculoskeletal Pain, Bone Ache, Arthralgia, Rheumatism, "My Bones Hurt"

BACKGROUND

Musculoskeletal pain is a common presenting symptom. A wide range of physicians evaluate affected patients, including general practitioners, family physicians, internal medicine specialists, and orthopedic surgeons. It is impossible to cover the entire spectrum of causes of musculoskeletal pain in a single chapter. A simple classification of musculoskeletal pain might focus on pain secondary to bone lesions, intra-articular disorders, and disorders of muscles, tendons, and nerves. This chapter discusses the investigation of musculoskeletal pain secondary to bone lesions. Specifically, the goal of the chapter is to provide the clinician with useful clues and insights into the early identification of bone pain caused by destruction of bone by neoplastic processes. It is difficult to discuss evaluation of the patient with bone pain without mentioning intra-articular disorders and disorders of soft tissues. There is significant overlap in the pain patterns of intraosseous, intra-articular, and extra-articular soft tissue lesions. The overlap is explained by innervation of these structures from the same peripheral nerves.

Bone pain is not well understood at the physiologic level because of the difficulties in designing an appropriate experimental model. The periosteum is supplied by fine afferent fibers from nerves that act on the muscles around the bone.[1] Consequently, "dermatomal" patterns of innervation do not exist. For example, *Gray's Anatomy* simply states: "Nerves are most numerous in articular extremities of long bones, vertebrae and larger flat bones. They occur widely in periosteum, and fine myelinated and non-myelinate fibres accompany nutrient vessels into bone and even the perivascular spaces of Haversian canals."[2]

It must be assumed that some of these fine fibers are subserved by the usual nociceptors as mechanical pressure and deformation, and algogenic chemicals (released, for example, by infection or tumor)[3] produce particularly severe, deep-seated pain.[4] This pain has many of the characteristics of somatic (rather than visceral) pain: It is reasonably well localized, it is produced by the whole range of noxious stimuli, and it is relieved by measures that relieve somatic pain (such as anti-inflammatory agents and narcotics, which may be ineffective in visceral pain).

However, there may also be referral of bone pain, as with any other somatic pain. It may be a true referral (such as C-2 pain producing headache), stimulation of peripheral nerves by algogenic chemicals, or infection of the hip producing medial knee pain by stimulation of a sensory branch of the obturator nerve.

Muscle and muscle attachment pains are equally difficult to understand. Striated muscle contains nociceptors that appear to be high-threshold mechanoreceptors and polymodal nociceptors. Both might respond to chemicals released by tissue damage (and ischemia). Again, localization is not particularly accurate, and referral may occur.

Bone is a unique tissue with an immense capacity for self-repair. The functions of the skeleton include structural support, mineral metabolism, and hematopoiesis. The musculoskeletal system is complex, comprising many different structures with specific functions. As a tissue, bone fulfills different functions dependent on the organization of its two principal components: collagen and the hydroxyapatite crystal. Thick diaphyseal cortical bone serves as a structural member, whereas thin cortical bone and elaborate trabecular bone of the metaphysis serve to distribute forces about a joint. The clinical presentation of patients with bone pain is related to the underlying disease process and the particular anatomic area affected.

In the absence of a fracture, soft tissue trauma, or arthritis, bone pain implies the presence of bone destruction or resorption. In the normal turnover of skeletal tissue, bone is constantly undergoing resorption and formation. A pathologic process exists when resorption exceeds formation. Processes in which resorption and formation are not coupled include stress fractures, osteomalacia, and bone tumors. When a patient develops a stress fracture, the reparative process under the influence of repeated microtrauma favors resorption rather than bone formation. With activity, pain occurs at the site of microfracture.[5] Mineralization does not occur after the formation of osteoid in the patient with osteomalacia. The process affects all bones of the skeleton, and the patient will complain of diffuse pain.

Bone destruction and resorption by a tumor is painful. The pain may be caused by release of algogenic chemicals, such as prostaglandins, substance P, bradykinin, and others, from the tumor. A continuous level of pain will be present as the process continues. The pain will be worsened by activity when the pathologic process has progressed to the point that the remaining mineral and collagen have only enough strength to resist the forces of load application (such as walking or other daily activities). When there is insufficient strength to resist internal and external forces,

TABLE 1. Causes of Bone Pain in the Young Adult (20 to 40 Years Old)

Intra-articular lesions
  Avascular necrosis of femoral head
  Internal derangement of the knee
    Meniscus abnormality
    Anterior cruciate ligament insufficiency
    Osteochondritis dissecans
    Synovial proliferative disorders
      Pigmented villonodular synovitis
      Synovial chondromatosis
  Overuse syndromes
    Patellar tendon tendinitis
    Patellofemoral pain
    Popliteus tendon tendinitis
    Iliotibial band syndrome
Primary tumors of bone
  Malignant
    Osteosarcoma
    Chondrosarcoma
    Malignant fibrous histiocytoma
    Fibrosarcoma
    Adamantinoma
  Benign
    Giant cell tumor
    Osteoid osteoma/osteoblastoma
Stress fractures

TABLE 2. Causes of Bone Pain in the Older Adult (40 to 70 Years or Older)

Metastatic bone disease
Multiple myeloma
Primary bone tumors
  Chondrosarcoma
  Fibrosarcoma
  Malignant fibrous histiocytoma
  Lymphoma
Avascular necrosis
  Femoral head
  Medial femoral condyle
Osteoarthritis
  Hip
  Knee
  Spine
  Shoulder
Rotator cuff disease

a pathologic fracture occurs. The period of activity-related pain that occurs before fracture may be termed the *period of impending pathologic fracture*. The goal of the clinician is to detect and treat the pathologic process before fracture occurs.

Although it is sometimes difficult to determine the exact cause of musculoskeletal pain, the astute clinician can usually develop a differential diagnosis that will cover the most common causes on the basis of the history and physical examination. Blood tests and screening radiographs will further narrow the differential diagnoses. It is extremely important to identify pathologic neoplastic processes early in their course because early diagnosis may improve survival and will always improve the quality of remaining life in patients who have incurable disorders.

Many disorders will respond to nonoperative treatment. The key to successful treatment is an accurate diagnosis. Many of the common causes of bone pain in the young adult and older adult are shown in Tables 1 and 2, respectively. Patients with structural problems such as neoplasms, fractures, or arthritis should be referred to an orthopedic surgeon for evaluation and definitive care.

HISTORY

History of Present Illness

The medical history should include the nature, duration, and location of the pain.[6] One should ascertain whether the onset of pain was related to minor or major trauma. The nature of the pain is extremely important. Pain secondary to destruction of bone by neoplasms is intense, progressive, and unrelenting. Although the pain often begins insidiously, it invariably progresses. Most patients with primary malignancies of bone will have a 2- to 12-month history of pain before diagnosis. Many patients with nonmalignant conditions will have a history of pain for several years with multiple medical evaluations before a correct diagnosis is made. Pain secondary to bone destruction by tumors is often relieved significantly by nonsteroidal anti-inflammatory drugs (NSAIDs) early in the process or by oral narcotics. Discomfort at night is one of the characteristic symptoms of bone destruction caused by a tumor.

The medical history is of fundamental importance. In patients with a history of cancer, bony metastases should be suspected as a source of the bone pain until proved otherwise. Carcinomas of the breast, lung, prostate, thyroid, and kidney are the most common tumors that metastasize to bone and account for more than 80 per cent of bone metastases.[7,8,9] Among patients with visceral carcinomas, 60 to 70 per cent will develop bone metastases at some point. Jaffe[10] stated that with careful autopsy examination virtually all patients with breast, prostate, and lung cancers will be found to have bone metastases. Although bone metastases frequently occur within the first 5 years after the diagnosis of a visceral cancer, late bone metastases may occur up to 30 years after initial presentation. Therefore, the patient with a history of a visceral cancer and bone pain must always be suspected of having metastases to bone.

Patients with multiple myeloma will often present with bone pain.[11,12] The pain may be localized to the extremities or to the spine. These patients often develop vertebral compression fractures from tumor involvement or osteoporosis. In addition, patients with myeloma will often complain of weakness and easy fatigability secondary to anemia. Hypercalcemia may occur in patients with either multiple myeloma or bone metastases. Early symptoms include polyuria, polydipsia, anorexia, easy fatigability, and weakness. Late symptoms include apathy, irritability, profound muscle weakness, nausea or vomiting, pruritus, neurologic depression, and coma. The symptoms are related to both the increased serum calcium concentration and the rate of its elevation.

Pain secondary to metastases is uncommon in young patients. In this group, primary malignancies of bone are more common. Osteogenic sarcoma and Ewing's tumor are the most common neoplasms of the skeleton in children and young adults. However, bone pain in the young patient is most often secondary to overuse syndromes and acute injury. Stress fractures are common manifestations of overuse symptoms that cause bone pain. The young patient who is active in sports and has bone pain in the lower extremity should be questioned as to recent increases in training or competition.

The young patient with hip pain poses a special problem. When there is no history of trauma or concern for a stress fracture, it is necessary to exclude avascular necrosis of the femoral head and neoplasm. Risk factors for avascular necrosis include the use of oral or intravenous corticosteroids, sickle cell disease, excessive alcohol use, deep-sea diving, Gaucher's disease, rheumatologic disorders, and immunosuppression. In addition, some patients suffer from the idiopathic form of the disease.

The young adolescent with bone pain deserves a very careful evaluation. Young children seldom have significant bone pain without a pathologic process. Children usually enjoy sports and outside activities, so there is usually little to gain for them in feigning bone pain. The child with a painful scoliosis will almost always have a pathologic process. Although bone tumors and spinal cord tumors are rare, they must be considered in the differential diagnosis of the child with chronic back pain. Back pain, weakness, and a limp are characteristic findings in young adolescents with intraspinal lesions.[13] Spondylolysis of the posterior elements of the fifth lumbar vertebra is common and may be associated with low back pain in the young athlete (especially gymnasts and football players).

Focused Queries

1. *Is the pain related to activity?* This is an important question because it helps to differentiate pain that is caused by a neoplasm from the more common discomfort caused by arthritis, tendinitis, and bursitis. Bone destruction caused by neoplasm is usually not related to activity. In contrast, patients with arthritis often report that their pain occurs with activity and progressively increases as they be-

come more active. They usually feel better when resting. Patients with bursitis or tendinitis often describe certain motions or activities that exacerbate their symptoms. For example, patients with rotator cuff tendinitis may describe increased discomfort with overhead activities and pain when they sleep on the affected shoulder.

2. *Does the pain occur at night?* This is perhaps the most important question. Night pain is the hallmark of destruction of bone by tumors. Careful questioning will show that virtually all patients with primary malignant bone tumors and metastatic bone disease have night pain.

Although patients will note that their pain is constant, it is almost always worse at night. The increase in pain at night is not clearly understood. In the evening, the patient is often relieved of the distractions of daily routine (such as the stresses of the workplace or caring for children) and so can focus more on the pain. Pain from the common toothache or a simple fracture is also more prominent at night.

The patient should be questioned as to whether the pain awakens him or her from a sound sleep. If the patient awakens with severe, unrelenting pain in the back or an extremity, the physician must be very suspicious of bone pain caused by tumor destruction. Young children will often cry at night from the pain.

Another important clue concerning night pain is whether the patient needs to consume narcotics at night to relieve the pain and fall asleep. Pain requiring narcotics in the evening should prompt a search for malignancy. The patient should also be asked whether going back to sleep is a problem. If the patient notes only mild discomfort and is able to fall back to sleep with little effort, the discomfort is probably innocent in character.

Discomfort at night is also common in patients with arthritis of a major joint (such as the hip, knee, or shoulder) and in patients with chronic low back pain. In contrast to the patient with night pain caused by a tumor, such patients will often relate that their pain is positional in nature. The patient with osteoarthritis of the knee will often note that rolling over in bed causes enough discomfort to awaken him or her. The pain is probably related to motion of a joint during the rolling movement. Such patients can usually fall back to sleep with little effort. Patients with chronic low

back pain will often relate that they can sleep in only one position at night. They will often be disturbed in their sleep if they inadvertently change position.

3. *Is the pain relieved by nonsteroidal anti-inflammatory agents or aspirin?* The discomfort caused by arthritis, tendinitis, bursitis, or simple trauma is usually relieved partially or completely by nonsteroidal anti-inflammatory medications, including aspirin. In contrast, pain caused by tumor destruction may not always be relieved by NSAIDs.[14]

4. *Is the pain progressive?* Progressive and relentless pain is a key feature of bone pain caused by malignancies. In this regard, the physician should ask the patient whether the pain is worsening, staying the same, or subsiding. If the patient states that the pain is gradually resolving, it can be safely assumed that the source of the pain is not related to a malignancy. Pain that increases despite nonsteroidal anti-inflammatory medications, physical therapy, activity modification, and corticosteroid injections suggests that the differential diagnosis is incorrect and pain secondary to an occult malignancy should be considered.

A special category of progressive and relentless pain is pain caused by neural compression irritation. Affected patients will often have pain that is so severe that they cannot sit still and will often refuse to allow the physician to examine them. Nerve root or spinal cord irritation is very common in the patient with cancer (metastatic bone disease and multiple myeloma). Pathologic processes that compress the spinal cord or the sacral peripheral nerves (second, third, and fourth sacral nerve roots) may cause dysfunction of the bladder or rectum. In this regard, early diagnosis and prompt treatment are critical. The patient with low back pain should always be asked whether there has been a change in bowel, bladder, and sexual function. Incontinence of the bowel or bladder in the patient with low back pain implies the diagnosis of cauda equina syndrome. The cauda equina syndrome is a true emergency that requires emergency radiographic studies and surgical decompression or radiotherapy as appropriate. Nerve compression per se does not cause pain. Nerve irritation may be painful.

5. *Is the pain relieved by small doses of narcotics?* Bone pain caused by malignancies is often not relieved by small doses of oral narcotics (such as acetaminophen with co-

deine or propoxyphene). When patients relate that the pain is not relieved by two or three oral narcotic tablets, the physician should be very suspicious that the patient may have an occult malignancy, if narcotic dependence is eliminated.

PHYSICAL EXAMINATION

The physical examination is an integral part of the evaluation of the patient with musculoskeletal pain. Patients with malignancies of the musculoskeletal system may have only subtle physical findings, if any. Early in the course of the disease, there may be no physical findings. Subtle clues include small decreases in range of motion of a joint, synovitis, or muscle atrophy. Atrophy of the muscles about a joint usually occurs within one month of the onset of severe pain. When a malignancy has destroyed the cortex of a bone and spread into the soft tissues, one may palpate a soft tissue mass.

Stress fractures are often tender to palpation. Unfortunately, a stress fracture about the hip may yield no clues on physical examination because one cannot palpate the femoral neck.

A rectal examination is an important part of the examination of the patient with chronic low back or unexplained hip pain. Chordomas of the sacrum are often palpable on digital examination. Rectal cancers can also cause musculoskeletal pain by erosion of the anterior cortex of the sacrum.

For the patient with shoulder pain, the cervical spine and peripheral nerves should be examined carefully. Disorders of the cervical spine can present as shoulder pain. In addition, attention should be directed to the pulmonary system because tumors of the mediastinum and lesions in the upper lobe can present as shoulder pain. Diaphragmatic irritation can also present as shoulder pain.

Observation of the patient's gait is also important. A significant limp, an antalgic gait, and the inability to ambulate are usually good signs of a pathologic process.

DIAGNOSTIC STUDIES

The laboratory assessment of the patient with musculoskeletal pain is often complex and must be individualized. There are several principles in ordering blood tests, radio-graphs, radioactive bone scans (technetium, gallium, and gadolinium), and magnetic resonance imaging scans.

Initial blood tests for the patient with unexplained musculoskeletal pain should include complete blood count with differential leukocyte count, an erythrocyte sedimentation rate, and estimates of serum calcium and inorganic phosphate levels. Liver, parathyroid, and prostate hormone levels may need to be estimated. Significant anemia suggests metastatic bone disease with extensive marrow replacement or multiple myeloma. An elevation of the leukocyte count with a left shift suggests infection. The erythrocyte sedimentation rate is almost always elevated in patients with septic arthritis and multiple myeloma. Patients with acute osteomyelitis will often have an elevated erythrocyte sedimentation rate, but those with chronic osteomyelitis may have a normal rate. The calcium and phosphate levels may be abnormal in patients with metabolic bone diseases such as primary hyperparathyroidism and renal osteodystrophy or in patients with metastatic bone disease and multiple myeloma.

Radiographs in two planes (at 90 degrees to one another) should always be obtained in the patient with unexplained musculoskeletal pain. The clinician may feel that the radiographs are unnecessary in the patient with a known cause of pain, such as the patient with an acute back strain after lifting a heavy object. However, radiographs are necessary when the cause of the pain is unclear. When the pain is localized to a long bone, the joint above and below the area should be included in the radiographic examination. The choice of radiographic views must be individualized. Our initial choice of screening views is shown in Table 3.

When the radiographs are normal and do not shed light on an unexplained source of musculoskeletal pain, the clinician faces a difficult decision. Needless tests are expensive for the patient in terms of radiation exposure, time, and money. However, if the clinician halts the investigation after normal radiographs are obtained, certain patients with pathologic conditions will go undiagnosed. When the clinician believes that significant bone abnormality may exist and the radiographs are normal, the next diagnostic procedure should be a technetium bone scan. The technetium bone scan identifies areas of increased bone turnover. The active osteoblast takes up the radionucleotide. The technetium

TABLE 3. Radiographic Evolution of Musculoskeletal Pain

LOCATION OF PAIN	RADIOGRAPHIC VIEW
Shoulder	Anteroposterior view of shoulder
	Scapular axillary view
Arm	Anteroposterior view of humerus
	Lateral view of humerus
Elbow	Anteroposterior view of elbow
	Lateral view of elbow
Forearm	Anteroposterior view of the radius and ulna
	Lateral view of the radius and ulna
Wrist	Anteroposterior view of wrist
	Lateral view of wrist
	Oblique (scaphoid) view of wrist
Hand	Anteroposterior view of hand
	Lateral view of hand or digit involved
Hip	Anteroposterior view of the pelvis
	Anteroposterior view of the involved hip
Thigh	Anteroposterior view of the pelvis
	Anteroposterior view of the femur
	Lateral view of the femur
Knee	Anteroposterior view of the knee
	Lateral view of the knee
	Patellar view of the knee
Leg	Anteroposterior view of the tibia and fibula
	Lateral view of the tibia and fibula
Ankle	Anteroposterior view of the ankle
	Lateral view of the ankle
	Mortise view of the ankle
Foot	Anteroposterior view of the foot
	Lateral view of the foot
	Oblique view of the foot
Neck	Anteroposterior view of the cervical spine
	Lateral view of the cervical spine
	Oblique views of the cervical spine
	Odontoid view
Midback	Anteroposterior view of the thoracic spine
	Lateral view of the thoracic spine
Lowback	Anteroposterior view of the lumbosacral spine
	Lateral view of the lumbosacral spine
	Oblique views of the lumbosacral spine
	Anteroposterior view of the pelvis

scans are very sensitive in identifying bone tumors, stress fractures, and arthritis. There are two conditions in which the bone scan is not particularly helpful. The bone destruction caused by multiple myeloma does not incite increased activity in the osteoblast. In addition, patients with profound bone destruction secondary to metastatic bone disease may also have negative scans because there may be no osteoblasts left to take up the radionucleotide. When multiple myeloma or aggressive bone metastases are suspected, a skeletal survey is a superior diagnostic test to the technetium bone scan. The skeletal survey should include an anteroposterior view of the humerus, radius and ulna, pelvis, femur, and tibia and fibula bilaterally. The second situation in which the technetium scan may not be helpful is in the patient with avascular necrosis of the femoral head. The technetium scan may or may not show increased uptake, and when positive, the scan is not specific for avascular necrosis. Magnetic resonance imaging is the procedure of choice for the patient suspected of having avascular necrosis of the femoral head or knee because the scans are very sensitive and specific.

ASSESSMENT

The patient with unexplained bone pain presents a challenge to the clinician. The source of pain will often be apparent after the history, physical examination, and initial radiographs. When the patient has a history of significant trauma, physical examination and screening radiographs are usually all that are necessary to make a diagnosis. Patients with a fracture should be referred to an orthopedic surgeon. Although the nonorthopedist with experience can certainly manage minor nondisplaced fractures, there are many pitfalls in fracture management that may frustrate the inexperienced clinician, such as the development of reflex sympathetic dystrophy or pain dysfunction syndrome.

The patient with pain and no history of trauma presents the greatest diagnostic challenge. It must be ascertained whether the patient's pain is significant or a minor nuisance. Pain that is of only minor consequence, such as a long history of back strains that resolve with time, chronic anterior knee pain, or fleeting minor aches in the hip or knee, does not need expensive and time-consuming evaluations. In the patient with new onset of significant pain, a careful investigation is warranted. On the basis of the history, physical examination, laboratory tests, and screening radiographs, the clinician tries to classify the patient's disease into one of seven categories:

1. Congenital/developmental.
2. Metabolic.
3. Infectious.
4. Neoplastic.
5. Traumatic.
6. Vascular.
7. Arthritic.

TABLE 4.   Categories of Bone Disease

Congenital	Neoplastic
Multiple epiphyseal dysplasia	Benign primary bone tumor
Spondyloepiphyseal dysplasia	Malignant primary bone tumor
Dwarfism	Metastatic bone disease
Osteogenesis imperfecta	Multiple myeloma
Fibrous dysplasia	Arthritic
Osteofibrous dysplasia	Rheumatoid arthritis
Metabolic	Osteoarthritis
Primary hyperparathyroidism	Ankylosing spondylitis
Osteoporosis	Systemic lupus erythematosus
Osteomalacia	Psoriatic hip disease
Rickets	Reiter's syndrome
Renal osteodystrophy	Traumatic
Gaucher's disease	Acute injury
Vascular	Fracture
Avascular necrosis	Dislocation/subluxation
Femoral head	Contusion
Humeral head	Stress fracture
Medial femoral condyle	Heterotopic ossification
Sickle cell disease	
Infectious	
Septic arthritis	
Osteomyelitis	

Some of the more common entities in these seven categories are shown in Table 4. The formation of a logical differential diagnosis depends on the correct interpretation of the history, physical examination, and screening laboratory tests and radiographs.

In general, congenital and developmental problems are easy to recognize. Patients with bone dysplasia and dwarfism fit into this category. Most patients with these disorders develop pain as a result of arthritis of the large joints or a stress fracture through abnormal bone. Patients with dwarfism will often develop the symptoms of spinal stenosis secondary to deformities of the posterior elements of the spine. Radiographic studies in patients with congenital and developmental conditions will always show abnormal architecture of the bones. In addition, the changes are often bilateral and may or may not be symmetric.

Metabolic bone disease must always be considered in the differential diagnosis. Patients with osteomalacia may present with an insidious diffuse bone pain. Rarely will the patient with untreated primary hyperparathyroidism present with lower extremity pain and a large lytic lesion secondary to a brown tumor of hyperparathyroidism. Renal osteodystrophy results in osteomalacia and fractures. Patients with Gaucher's disease will often develop avascular necrosis of the femoral head.

Infections of the musculoskeletal system are common. The patient with bone and joint pain should always be questioned about recent fevers and respiratory and other bacterial infections. Exposure to tuberculosis and travel to areas endemic for coccidioidomycosis or other exotic diseases should also be ascertained. Patients with septic arthritis will resist passive range of motion of the joint because it causes intense pain. The erythrocyte sedimentation rate will always be elevated in septic arthritis. The physical findings may be very subtle in the immunocompromised patient, and joint aspiration may be the only definitive technique of excluding septic arthritis. Early diagnosis and prompt treatment are necessary to prevent destruction of the joint. Osteomyelitis poses greater diagnostic problems than septic arthritis. Infections in bone can mimic many other pathologic processes.[15] The leukocyte count, differential count, and sedimentation rate may be normal in the patient with chronic osteomyelitis. Often, open biopsy with cultures is required to establish the diagnosis.

The patient with acute trauma presents few problems in diagnosis. However, there are subsets of patients with acute trauma who are treated incorrectly because of failure to obtain appropriate radiographs. Patients with painful wrists secondary to scaphoid fractures and perilunate dislocations are often inappropriately treated because of incorrect interpretation of abnormal radiographic relationships of the carpal bones. Posterior dislocations of the shoulder (such as in patients who have had seizures or electrical injuries) are also often not recognized. Posterior dislocations of the shoulder joint may show only subtle changes if only an anteroposterior radiograph is obtained. One must therefore be aware that the patient may have more than a "simple sprain." Heterotopic ossification after trauma may result in pain and produce radiographs that appear ominous on initial inspection.[16] Ossification in the soft tissues may incorrectly lead to the diagnosis of osteosarcoma in this instance. The history of trauma and characteristic radiographic features allow a correct diagnosis without biopsy in most cases. Stress fractures may also be misinterpreted as neoplasms; however, if the right questions are asked, the diagnosis will be apparent.

Vascular insufficiency may lead to avascular necrosis of bone. The reparative process often leads to subchondral fracture and collapse, especially in the femoral head. Patients

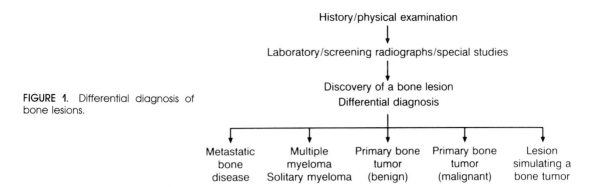

FIGURE 1. Differential diagnosis of bone lesions.

History/physical examination

↓

Laboratory/screening radiographs/special studies

↓

Discovery of a bone lesion
Differential diagnosis

↓

| Metastatic bone disease | Multiple myeloma Solitary myeloma | Primary bone tumor (benign) | Primary bone tumor (malignant) | Lesion simulating a bone tumor |

with avascular necrosis of the femoral head or medial femoral condyle will describe intense pain well localized to the hip or knee. When the joint surface has collapsed, the pattern of symptoms will change to activity-related pain with weight bearing and especially rotational motions of the joint.

Patients with arthritis will describe characteristic symptoms of morning stiffness and increased pain in the evening after a strenuous day.[2] They will often relate their symptoms to activity and will be able to describe how far they can walk before their pain forces them to stop. A rheumatologic disorder should be considered in the differential diagnosis of a patient with multiple joint complaints. (Also see chapter on Polyarticular Arthritis.) The young male with morning stiffness and low back pain may have the early symptoms of ankylosing spondylitis. Chronic effusions in a single joint should arouse the suspicion of Lyme disease if the patient has been exposed to the deer tick.

The careful clinician should be able to recognize when bone pain is being caused by the destruction of bone by a neoplastic process. Once this suspicion is aroused, attempts must be made to classify the pathologic process within the categories of metastatic bone disease, multiple or solitary myeloma, benign or malignant primary bone tumor, or a lesion that may simulate a bone tumor (Fig. 1). Once this further classification is made, the differential diagnosis can be further narrowed with special radiographic studies such as conventional tomography, computed tomography, and magnetic resonance imaging. The classification of the lesion aids in the choice of biopsy (e.g., incisional, excisional, or needle techniques). The classification system also allows the clinician to give the patient reasonable counseling as to the expected prognosis.

Many common conditions may mimic a primary bone tumor. An accurate diagnosis based on the history, physical examination, and radiographs can save the patient an expensive workup, needless anxiety, and even a surgical procedure for biopsy. Some of the most common lesions that may simulate primary bone tumor are listed in Table 5; an extensive review is beyond the scope of this chapter, but they are well summarized in several other sources.[17,18,19,20] Of particular importance is the recognition that many of the simulators of bone tumor such as fibrous cortical defects, avulsive cortical irregularities, bone infarcts, and bone islands require no treatment other than reassurance of the patient. However, pain from bone tumor might respond to appropriate therapy.[21]

In summary, assessment of the patient with bone pain requires a careful history and physical examination. All patients with unexplained bone pain need appropriate radiographic and

TABLE 5. Lesions That May Simulate Primary Bone Tumors

Paget's disease	Osteomyelitis
Fibrous dysplasia	Aneurysmal bone cyst
Osteofibrous dysplasia	Simple bone cyst
Avulsion fractures	Cysts associated with joint diseases
Stress fractures	
Histiocytosis X	Rheumatoid arthritis
Eosinophilic granuloma of bone	Osteoarthritis Gout
Hand-Schüller-Christian disease	Cyst of the calcaneus Ganglion cyst of bone
Letterer-Siwe disease	Epidermoid cyst
Pigmented villonodular synovitis	Hyperparathyroidism Exuberant callus
Synovial chondromatosis	Bone infarcts
Mastocytosis	Bone islands
Metaphyseal fibrous defect	
Avulsive cortical irregularity	

laboratory examinations. A diagnosis can be made in virtually all patients if the bone disease is classified into one of the five categories of bone disease and the differential diagnosis is narrowed with appropriate special radiographs and biopsy when needed. Successful treatment is contingent on an accurate and prompt diagnosis.

REFERENCES

1. Yates DAH, Smith MA. Orthopaedic pain after trauma. In: Wall PD, Melzach R, eds. Textbook of pain. 2nd ed. Edinburgh: Churchill Livingstone, 1989;327–34.
2. Williams PL, Warwick R, Dyson M, Bannister LH. Gray's anatomy. 37th ed. Edinburgh: Churchill Livingstone, 1989.
3. Payne R. Pathophysiology of cancer pain. Adv Pain Res Ther 1990;16:13–26.
4. Palmer E, Henrikson S, McKusick K, Strauss HW, Hochberg F. Pain as an indicator of bone metastasis. Acta Radiol 1988;29:445–9.
5. Devas M. Stress fractures. Edinburgh: Churchill Livingstone, 1975:190–211.
6. Agudelo C, Wise CM. Evaluation of the patient with symptoms of rheumatic disease. In: Schumacher HR Jr, ed. Primer on the rheumatic diseases. 9th ed. Atlanta: Arthritis Foundation, 1988:51–5.
7. Frassica FJ, Sim FH. Pathogenesis and prognosis. In: Sim FH, ed. Diagnosis and management of metastatic bone disease: a multidisciplinary approach. New York: Raven Press, 1988:1–6.
8. Sim FH, Frassica FJ, Edmonson JH. Clinical and laboratory findings. In: Sim FH, ed. Diagnosis and management of metastatic bone disease: a multidisciplinary approach. New York: Raven Press, 1988:25–30.
9. Sim FH, Frassica FJ. Metastatic bone disease. Contemp Issues Surg Pathol 1988;11:225–40.
10. Jaffe HL. Tumors and tumorous conditions of the bones and joints. Philadelphia: Lea & Febiger, 1958.
11. Sim FH, Frassica FJ. Metastatic bone disease and multiple myeloma. In: Evarts CM, ed. Surgery of the musculoskeletal system. 2nd ed., Vol. 5. New York: Churchill Livingstone, 1990:5019–53.
12. Frassica DA, Frassica FJ, Schray MF, Sim FH, Kyle RA. Solitary plasmacytoma of bone: Mayo Clinic experience. Int J Radiat Oncol Biol Phys 1989;16:43–8.
13. Tachdjian MO, Matson DD. Orthopaedic aspects of intraspinal tumors in infants and children. J Bone Joint Surg [Am] 1965;47:223–48.
14. Portenoy RK. Practical aspects of pain control in the patient with cancer. CA 1988;38:327–52.
15. Cabanela ME, Sim FH, Beabout JW, Dahlin DC. Osteomyelitis appearing as neoplasms: a diagnostic problem. Arch Surg 1974;109:68–72.
16. Ackerman LV. Extra-osseous localized non-neoplastic bone and cartilage formation (so-called myositis ossificans): clinical and pathologic confusion with malignant neoplasms. J Bone Joint Surg [Am] 1958;40:279–98.
17. Barnes GR Jr, Gwinn JL. Distal irregularities of the femur simulating malignancy. AJR 1974;122;180–5.
18. Kimmelstiel P, Rapp I. Cortical defect due to periosteal desmoids. Bull Hosp Joint Dis 1951;12:286–97.
19. Shives TC, Cooper KL, Wold LE. Lesions simulating tumors of bone. In: Sim FH, ed. Diagnosis and treatment of bone tumors: a team approach. Thorofare, New Jersey: Slack, 1983:155–89.
20. Dahlin DC, Unni KK. Conditions that commonly simulate primary neoplasms of bone. In: Bone tumors: general aspects and data on 8,542 cases. 4th ed. Springfield, Illinois: Charles C Thomas, 1986:406–81.
21. Robinson RG, Spicer JA, Preston DF, Wegst AV, Martin NL. Treatment of metastatic bone pain with strontium-89. Int J Rad Appl Instrum [B] 1987;14:219–22.

BRADYCARDIA

ELLEN J. KILLEBREW, DANIEL J. TENNENHOUSE, and NORA GOLDSCHLAGER

SYNONYMS: Slow Heart Rate. Underlying Rhythms: The following may be associated with slow heart rate: sinus bradycardia, sinus arrest, sinoatrial block, junctional rhythm, "idioventricular" rhythm, complete atrioventricular (AV) block, types I and II second-degree block, "slow" ventricular tachycardia, accelerated ventricular rhythm, ventricular escape rhythm

BACKGROUND

Bradycardia in the adult describes a heart rate of less than 60 beats per minute. In the neonate, 80 beats per minute or less constitutes bradycardia.

In the normal heart, the sinus node, located in the posterior right atrium, is responsible for

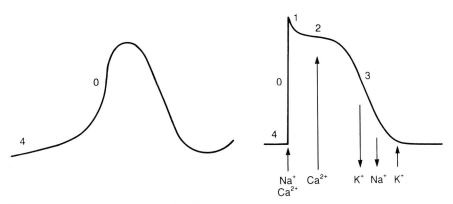

FIGURE 1. Schema of a pacemaker cell (*left*) showing phase 4 diastolic depolarization and a working myocardial cell (*right*). Ionic fluxes during the depolarization and repolarization phases are also depicted.

control of heart rate. The rate is, on average, between 60 and 100 beats per minute and is mediated by the input of the autonomic nervous system. Both vagal and sympathetic tones contribute to changes in heart rate in normal individuals. For example, pain can cause hypervagotonia, resulting in decreases in both heart rate and blood pressure, and even "vasovagal" syncope. Fear can initiate the so-called fight-or-flight phenomenon, causing the heart rate and blood pressure to rise owing to an increase in sympathetic output.

Impulse formation is a feature of the sinus node that allows it to generate electrical activity initiating each cardiac depolarization and resulting mechanical systole (heartbeat). Other lower pacemakers can initiate electrical activity if the sinus node either fails or conduction of its impulse to the lower pacemakers, discharging them, is delayed or blocked.

Certain characteristics are necessary for cardiac cells to act as pacemakers. Working myocardial cells utilize sodium channels (fast channels), whereas pacemaker cells are mediated by calcium channel activity (slow channels) rather than by the sodium channel activity (fast channels). Figure 1 depicts the action potential of a pacemaker cell. The action potential of pacemaker cells is characterized by a slow rate of rise of phase zero (depolarization) and a slowly rising phase 4 slope toward depolarization threshold that is mediated by potassium flux across the cell membrane. This slow ascent of phase 4 to threshold allows the cell to depolarize spontaneously and initiate a new contraction.[1,2]

If the sinus node fails, backup pacemaker cells exist in the AV junctional tissue and in the ventricular Purkinje system. These "fail-safe" pacemakers have a similar spontaneous phase 4 depolarization capability that allows initiation of electrical activity. The intrinsic rates of these backup pacemakers are slower than that of the sinus node and hence by definition are "bradycardic." The usual rate of a junctional rhythm is 50 to 60 beats per minute, and the usual Purkinje ventricular rate is 30 to 40 beats per minute. The junctional rate, unlike the ventricular rate, can be modified by autonomic tone.

In the case of AV block, depending on the site of the block, a backup pacemaker can usurp control of cardiac rhythm. The resulting rhythm is called an *escape rhythm*. If the block is at or above the bundle of His, the heart rate will be controlled by the AV junctional tissue at a rate of 50 to 60 per minute, and very often no hemodynamic compromise will occur. In these instances, the QRS complex is usually narrow and normal appearing (unless pre-existing bundle branch block is present).

If the site of block is below the bundle of His, the "escape" pacer will most likely be Purkinje-ventricular. The QRS complex should be wide (greater than 0.12 seconds) and the rate average 30 to 40 beats per minute. Often, the patient is hemodynamically compromised owing to the slow heart rate.

Causes of Bradycardia

Causes of slow heart rate are myriad and include drugs, ischemia, infarction, enhanced vagal tone, scarring due to trauma or degenerative disease, metabolic abnormalities, cerebrovascular abnormalities, and congenital cardiac disease (Table 1).[3,4,5,6,7,8,9,10,11,12,13,14,15,16,17,18]

TABLE 1.   Conditions Associated with Bradycardia

Drugs
  Analgesics
  Anesthetic agents
  Antiarrhythmics
  Beta blockers
  Calcium channel blockers (verapamil, diltiazem)
  Cholinergic agents
  Ionic contrast agents
  Digitalis (depending on prevailing vagal tone)
Metabolic
  Hyperkalemia
  Hypothermia
  Hypothyroidism
  Ischemia
  Jaundice
  Starvation
  Sudden infant death syndrome "near miss"
Physiologic
  Excessive vagotonia (Valsalva's maneuver, sleep, high
    degree of physical conditioning)
  Increased intracranial pressure
  Reflex (oculocardiac, diving)
Structural
  Calcific valvular disease (aortic and mitral)
  Congenital disorders
  Degenerative (Lenegre's diffuse conduction system dis-
    ease, "sick sinus" and bradycardia-tachycardia syn-
    dromes)
  Infarction
  Inflammation (viral hepatitis, infective endocarditis)
  Neurologic (Guillain-Barré syndrome)
  Trauma
  Tumor

Chronic heart block can be entirely or minimally symptomatic, particularly in the elderly and in patients with congenital heart block. In contrast, acute heart block often causes early symptoms.

Types of Bradycardia

Sinus Bradycardia

Impulse formation occurs normally in the sinus node, but the heart rate may be less than 60 per minute due to vagotonia, drugs, fibrosis, ischemia, or conditioning (Figs. 2A and 2B). The bradycardia may be transient. Unless the patient is hemodynamically compromised, sinus bradycardia requires no treatment. Sinus bradycardia is often seen in healthy athletes and normal young persons.

COMMON CAUSES OF SINUS BRADYCARDIA. Common causes of sinus bradycardia are: athletic conditioning; degenerative conduction system disease; effects of various drugs; ischemia and infarction, especially inferior infarction; and vasodepressor phenomena.

LESS COMMON CAUSES. Less common causes of sinus bradycardia are: hypothermia, increased intracranial pressure, jaundice, and metabolic abnormalities such as hypothyroidism.

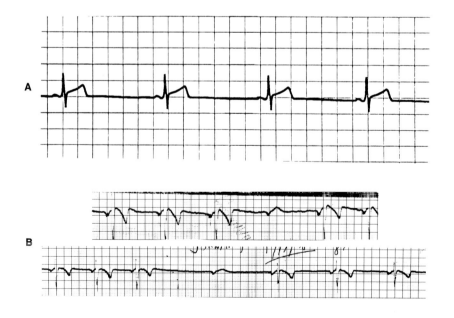

FIGURE 2.   (A) Sinus bradycardia. P waves are present and precede each QRS complex. The rate is just under 50 beats per minute. (B) Bradycardia due to increased vagal tone, resulting in a transient slowing of sinus rate and failure of conduction of a sinus impulse. Because this rhythm is "vagotonic," it is usually atropine responsive; since it is generally benign, treatment is not required.

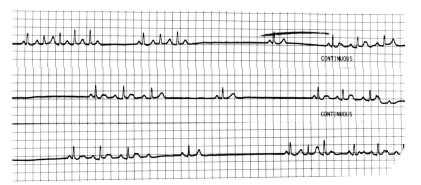

FIGURE 3. Pauses in sinus rhythm following, and possibly due to, bursts of nonsustained atrial tachycardia. This rhythm is known as the bradycardia-tachycardia syndrome; patients can complain of palpitations during the tachycardias and presyncope and syncope during the bradycardias.

Sinus Pause/Sinus Arrest

A failure in impulse formation in the sinus node results in a pause in, or slowing of, sinus rate (Figs. 3 and 4). Pauses in sinus rhythm can be distinguished from sinus arrhythmia, but the repetitive nature of the latter is helpful in the differentiation. The pause in rhythm is not a multiple of the basic PP interval. This rhythm is often seen as part of the bradycardia-tachycardia syndrome.[20,21,22]

COMMON CAUSES OF SINUS PAUSE/SINUS ARREST. Common causes of sinus pause/sinus arrest are: degenerative conduction system disease and effects of various drugs.

Sinoatrial Exit Block

Impulse formation does occur in the sinus node; however, owing to an infranodal or perinodal conduction disturbance, this impulse is not transmitted from the sinus node to the atria. Thus, no P wave is inscribed on the surface electrocardiogram (ECG). Because impulse formation continues undisturbed, the pause in P wave rate is equal to some multiple of the PP interval.

COMMON CAUSES OF SINOATRIAL EXIT BLOCK. Common causes of sinoatrial exit block are: degenerative conduction system disease and effects of various drugs.

Junctional Rhythm

Junctional bradycardia (Figs. 5, 6, and 7) is commonly an escape rhythm, arising by default when the sinus rate slows or if AV block is present. With junctional rhythm, there is either no visible P wave or an inverted P wave in leads 2, 3, and aVF. The PR (or RP) interval is short. The inverted P waves in leads 2, 3, and aVF indicate retrograde atrial depolarization. Usually, the QRS complex is narrow (unless pre-existing bundle branch block is present), and the rate is 50 to 60 beats per minute. Hemodynamic compromise does not usually occur, and the patient can be observed without treatment. Junctional rhythm can be seen in normal young persons or athletes but can also occur in the presence of myocardial ischemia or infarction and where hypervagotonia is present.

COMMON CAUSES OF JUNCTIONAL RHYTHM. Common causes of junctional rhythm are: athletic

FIGURE 4. Prolonged pause in sinus rhythm following an episode of probable atrial fibrillation. The pause is terminated by a ventricular escape complex, but sinus rhythm does not resume until an additional five seconds have elapsed.

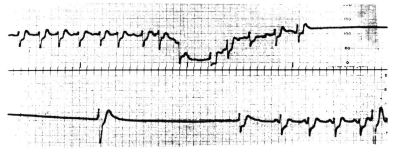

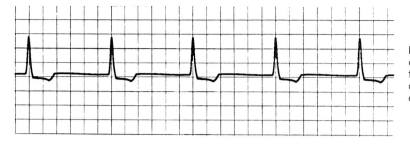

FIGURE 5. Junctional bradycardia. P waves are not seen, and the QRS duration and morphology are normal. The rate is just over 50 beats per minute.

FIGURE 6. Sinus bradycardia causes the emergence of a junctional escape complex (*E*), which begins a junctional escape rhythm. The earlier-than-expected QRS complexes (*arrows*) are capture beats by the preceding P wave.

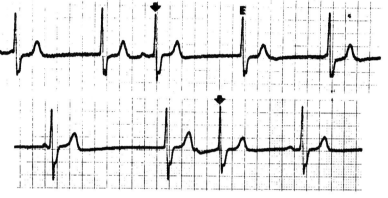

FIGURE 7. Junctional escape rhythm at a rate less than 30 per minute, resulting from complete AV block. This rhythm occurred in the setting of acute myocardial infarction. The slow rate of the rhythm suggests that the impulse-generating tissue within the junction is abnormal or that additional junctional block is present.

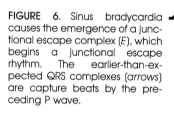

FIGURE 8. Continuous recording illustrating ventricular escape rhythm at about 35 beats per minute resulting from sinus bradycardia with further slowing of sinus rate. Resumption of sinus rhythm is hindered by retrograde atrial depolarization from the ventricular focus (*arrow*) but does occur at the end of the bottom strip.

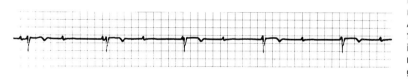

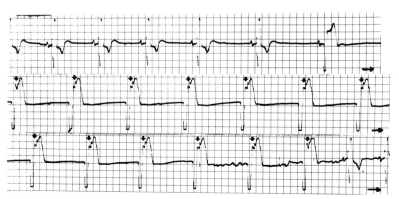

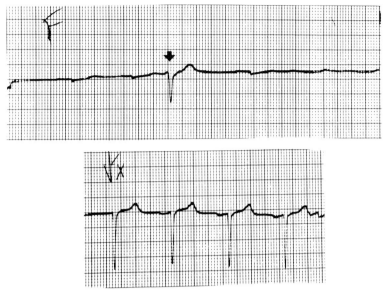

FIGURE 9. A type of "pseudobra-dycardia" due to low QRS signal magnitude in a properly standard-ized lead aVF. The clearly visible QRS complex (*arrow*) is in fact a premature ventricular complex. Normal sinus rhythm is demonstrated in aVL lead that had been simultaneously recorded.

conditioning; degenerative conduction system disease; effects of various drugs; ischemia and infarction, especially inferior infarction; and occasional normal finding.

Less Common Causes. Less common causes of junctional rhythm are: congenital (or familial) AV block,[19] hypothermia, and metabolic abnormalities such as hyperkalemia.

Ventricular Rhythm

Ventricular rhythms (Fig. 8) often occur in the presence of block below the bundle of His, owing to fibrosis or infarction (usually of the anterior wall). With ventricular rhythm, there is a wide QRS complex having a duration usually in excess of 0.12 seconds. The heart rate is between 30 and 40 beats per minute. The patient is often hemodynamically compromised and requires treatment.

Common Causes of Ventricular Rhythm. Common causes of ventricular rhythm are: degenerative conduction system disease and ischemia and infarction, especially anterior infarction.

Pseudobradycardia

The term *pseudobradycardia* refers to an apparent bradycardia found during physical examination but not by ECG. It is due to nonperfused beats causing a pulse deficit. Such nonperfusing beats may be atrial or ventricular extrasystoles, or pulsus alternans reflecting severe left ventricular dysfunction. The patient can be symptomatic, but the treatment should be addressed to the ectopy.

Common Causes of Pseudobradycardia. Common causes of pseudobradycardia are: ischemia and infarction, left ventricular dysfunction (such as cardiomyopathy), and nonpathologic.

Electronic (artifactual) pseudobradycardia has been described during ambulatory ECG monitoring and is usually due to electrode disconnection or transient acceleration in tape speed, but it can be patient induced. This has been called "electronic Munchausen's syndrome"[23] (Fig. 9).

Bradycardia-Induced Ectopy

At times, bradycardia can induce ventricular ectopy and nonsustained or sustained ventricular tachycardia, known as "bradycardia-dependent" or "pause-dependent" tachycardia.[24] The exact cause of the tachycardia is uncertain but involves fluxes in ion movement and dispersion of refractory periods. This ectopic activity can often be managed by treating the bradyarrhythmia.

HISTORY

The symptoms of bradycardia are those of cerebrovascular or, less commonly, cardiovascular, insufficiency. Common complaints are lightheadedness, confusion, presyncope or syncope, drop attacks (Stokes-Adams), and fatigue. Congestive heart failure symptoms and angina are relatively uncommon and suggest a concurrent disease process. Medications that can cause or contribute to bradycardia are listed in Table 1.

PHYSICAL EXAMINATION

In the bradycardic patient, the heart sounds, neck veins, and general mental state can point to the etiology of the bradycardia. In AV dissociation or complete heart block, the first heart sound will vary from beat to beat, reflecting the changes in position of the mitral valve relative to its fully closed position. In addition, "cannon waves" due to lack of AV synchrony may be seen in the neck.

Signs of congestive heart failure such as rales or an S_3 gallop should be investigated because cardiac output and ventricular filling may be adversely affected by slow heart rates. A new systolic heart murmur may be heard, generally at the left heart border, reflecting the larger stroke volume per beat. Mental status should also be carefully evaluated for evidence of decreased cerebral perfusion.

DIAGNOSTIC STUDIES

The 12-lead ECG should be the first examination. It has a high diagnostic yield in chronic bradyarrhythmias and in patients whose bradycardia is due to myocardial infarction. If the ECG does not provide a diagnosis and the patient presents with syncope, admission to a monitored hospital bed is the next appropriate step. If symptoms are subtle, the patient can then have a 24-hour ambulatory electrocardiographic examination performed to investigate paroxysmal heart block, tachyarrhythmias, or bradyarrhythmias. If symptoms are infrequent and unpredictable, ambulatory ECG monitoring is not useful. Instead, an event recorder may be carried by the patient, who must activate it to record his or her rhythm during symptoms. The ECG signals can then be transmitted by telephone to a nursing unit or other monitoring facility where a hard copy is obtained. Where the diagnosis of bradycardia is suspected but the physical examination does not suggest an etiology and the ECG is nondiagnostic, carotid sinus massage should be performed. Carotid sinus hypersensitivity is established if a three-second pause in QRS rhythm accompanies the carotid massage. The pause may be due either to sinus bradycardia/arrest or to high-grade or complete AV block. Although the demonstration of carotid sinus

hypersensitivity does not establish the *clinical* diagnosis of symptomatic bradycardia with certainty, it can be helpful in managing individual patients.

REFERENCES

1. Rosen MR. Electrophysiology of the cardiac specialized conduction system. In: Narula OS, ed. His bundle electrocardiography and clinical electrophysiology. Philadelphia: FA Davis, 1975:19–37.
2. Gadsby DC, Wit AL. Normal and abnormal electrical activity in cardiac cells. In: Mandel WJ, ed. Cardiac arrhythmias. Their mechanism, diagnosis, and management. Philadelphia: JB Lippincott, 1987:53–81.
3. Arnon R. Hepatitis, bradycardia, and the use of a cardiac pacemaker. JAMA 1974;228:1024–5.
4. Narayan D, Huang MTC, Mathew PK. Bradycardia and asystole requiring permanent pacemaker in Guillain-Barré syndrome. Am Heart J 1979;108:426–7.
5. Song E, Segal I, Hodkinson J, Kew MC. Sinus bradycardia in obstructive jaundice—correlation with total serum bile acid concentrations. S Afr Med J 1983;64:548–51.
6. Stober T, Sen S, Burger L. Bradycardia and second-degree AV block: an expression of the dominance of cholinergic activity in the rigid form of Huntington's disease. J Neurol 1983;229:129–32.
7. Montalescot G, Levy Y, Hatt PY. Serious sinus node dysfunction caused by therapeutic doses of lithium. Int J Cardiol 1984;5:94–6.
8. Nikolic G. Lidocaine bradycardia. Heart Lung 1984;13:290–1.
9. Dinai Y, Sharir M, Naveh N, Halkin H, Bradycardia induced by interaction between quinidine and ophthalmic timolol. Ann Intern Med 1985;103:890–1.
10. Margolis JR, Strauss HC, Miller HC, Gilbert M, Wallace AG. Digitalis and the sick sinus syndrome. Clinical and electrophysiologic documentation of severe toxic effect on sinus node function. Circulation 1975;52:162–9.
11. Arnon R, Ehrlich R. Hepatitis, bradycardia, and the use of a cardiac pacemaker. JAMA 1974;228:1024–5.
12. Ryden L, Cullhed I, Wasir H. Effect of lignocaine on heart rate in patients with sinus bradycardia associated with proven or suspected acute myocardial infarction. Cardiovasc Res 1972;6:664–70.
13. Sarachek NS, Leonard JL. Familial heart block and sinus bradycardia. Classification and natural history. Am J Cardiol 1972;29:451–8.
14. Burda CD. Cardiotoxic effects of Mellaril. Am Heart J 1970;80:147.
15. Abouganem D, Taylor AL, Donna B, Baum GL. Extreme bradycardia during sleep apnea caused by myxedema. Arch Intern Med 1987;147:1497–9.
16. Agruss NS, Rosin EY, Adolph RJ, Fowler NO. Significance of chronic sinus bradycardia in elderly people. Circulation 1972;46:924–30.
17. George M, Greenwood TW. Relation between bradycardia and the site of myocardial infarction. Lancet 1967;2:739–40.
18. Dreifus LS, Michelson EL, Kaplinsky E. Bradyarrhythmias: clinical significance and management. J Am Coll Cardiol 1973;1:327–38.

19. Swiryn S, McDonough T, Hueter DC. Sinus node function and dysfunction. Med Clin North Am 1984;68:935–54.
20. Scarpa WJ. The sick sinus syndrome. Am Heart J 1976;92:648–60.
21. Kaplan BM. The tachycardia-bradycardia syndrome. Med Clin North Am 1976;60:81–99.
22. Kaplan BM, Langendorf R, Lev M, Pick A. Tachycardia-bradycardia syndrome (so-called "sick sinus syndrome"). Pathology, mechanisms and treatment. Am J Cardiol 1973;31:497–508.
23. Mitchell CC, Frank MJ. Pseudobradycardia during Holter monitoring. The electronic Munchausen syndrome? JAMA 1982;248:469–70.
24. El-Sherif N, Bekheit SS, Henkin R. Quinidine-induced long QTU interval and torsade de pointes: role of bradycardia-dependent early after depolarizations. J Am Coll Cardiol 1989;14:252–7.

BREAST LUMP

FREDERICK L. GREENE and TRACY D. GUNTER

SYNONYM: Breast Mass

BACKGROUND

Anatomy and Physiology[1,2]

The breasts are the first of all ectodermal glands to appear in the embryo and are essentially modified sweat glands. In a six-week-old embryo, an ectodermal swelling known as the milk line is visible, but this will atrophy except for a small area in the pectoral region, which will become the mammary glands. If the milk line does not atrophy, one will see polythelia or polymastia. If the milk line is aberrant, this accessory breast tissue may be anywhere on the surface of the body. Another embryologic anomaly that may cause confusion is the congenitally inverted nipple. This is present, unilaterally or bilaterally, in many large-breasted women and may resolve spontaneously during pregnancy.

The breast lies between the second and sixth ribs anteriorly and between the sternal edge and midaxillary line. There is a projection of breast tissue into the axilla known as the axillary tail of Spence. About two thirds of the tissue lies laterally, superficial to the pectoralis major muscle. This upper outer area is the most common site of neoplasia. The remaining one third of the breast overlies the serratus anterior muscle. The nipple is located centrally and surrounded by the areola, which has small, rounded elevations representing modified sebaceous glands, which are called Montgomery glands. These glands may become infected and form abscesses that frequently present as subareolar masses.

Breast tissue has three major components. The first of these is glandular tissue. It is organized into 20 individual lobes that each terminate in a duct connecting the lobe to the nipple. The second major tissue type is the fibrous tissue that supports the glandular tissue. This category includes Cooper's ligaments connecting the breast to the overlying skin and underlying pectoralis major. And the third type of tissue is fat, which surrounds the breast and is particularly prominent superficially and peripherally. There are also lymph nodes and lymphatic vessels in the breast and tail of Spence, which may become palpable.

The arterial supply to the breast is provided by the internal mammary artery medially and the lateral thoracic artery laterally. The venous drainage follows the arterial supply. These vessels may become prominent during periods of rapid growth, especially during lactation and growth of a neoplasm.

The lymphatic drainage of the breast consists of three levels: cutaneous, areolar, and glandular. The cutaneous lymphatics terminate in the ipsilateral axillary nodes but may cross the midline to the contralateral axillary nodes when the medial aspect of the breast is involved. The areolar lymphatics drain into the anterior axillary nodes just lateral to the border of the pectoralis minor muscle. The glandular system may involve many sets of nodes including the infraclavicular, supraclavicular, axillary, and deep nodes of both the chest and abdomen.

The breast undergoes rapid development in the female at puberty but remains rudimentary in the male. Breast development occurs coincident with the appearance of pubic hair, between the ages of 8 and 13. It is essential to remember this fact when examining a pubescent female, as the most common cause of amazia (absence of breast with nipple present) is injudicious biopsy of a normal breast bud. Normal breast tissue may also be biopsied in cases of precocious puberty and premature thelarche.[3] Other causes of amazia include radiotherapy to the chest (especially in the treatment of breast hemangiomas) and accidental injury to the breast bud.

Statistics

As many as 50 per cent of premenopausal women have breast lumps noted on physical exam, and as many as 80 per cent of postmenopausal women have pathologic evidence of benign breast disease. In a large series of referrals to a surgical center for the evaluation of a breast lump, 30 per cent of women were found to have no disease, 40 per cent were found to have fibrocystic changes, 13 per cent were found to have other benign lesions, 7 per cent were found to have fibroadenoma, and 10 per cent were found to have cancer. The average age of the entire study was 40, with the youngest participant being 14 years of age. The average age of the patients with cancer was 56 years, and that for all benign disease was 37 years.[4]

Known risk factors for breast cancer include the female sex, increasing age, a history of previous breast cancer, and a family history of breast cancer in the first-degree female relatives of the patient. The younger the age of onset in those relatives, the higher the risk. Other risk factors include young age at onset of menses, nulliparity, late age at first-term pregnancy, late onset of menopause, obesity, and high-dose estrogen therapy. Previous primary malignancies involving the uterus, ovary, colon, and salivary gland have been implicated. Additionally, Hodgkin's lymphoma and malignant melanoma are associated with an increased risk of breast cancer. Hypothyroidism also places a woman at increased risk. Some softer associations include a high-fat diet, cigarette smoking, and alcohol consumption.[2,5]

Breast cancer is uncommon in males, occur-

ring less than 1 per cent as often in men as in women and comprising less than 1 per cent of all malignancies in men.[6] Because the disease is rare in males, the risk factors are not well defined. Some associations include increasing age, hyperestrogenism, radiation to the chest, and trauma.[6] Hyperestrogenism may be secondary to hypogonadism (Klinefelter's, XX male) or exogenous hormone administration. High-dose radiation is especially significant in those with a genetic predisposition. Trauma is an unclear association. It is likely that the traumatic event occurred by chance and merely called attention to a previously present breast mass.[2,6]

HISTORY

Focused Queries

When a woman presents with a breast lump, several questions are important in the evaluation of the lesion:

1. *How long has the mass been present?*
2. *Is the breast or mass painful?*
3. *Has the mass changed since it was first noticed?*
4. *Does it change cyclically?*
5. *Is it associated with a nipple discharge or changes in the nipples such as elevation, eczema, or retraction? How long have these changes been present (especially retraction)?*
6. *Is it associated with skin changes such as dimpling, ulceration, or erythema?*
7. *Has anything like this appeared before?*
8. *Have there been previous breast procedures? Diagnosis? Radiation?*
9. *Has there been trauma to either breast?*
10. *Has there been a change in bra size?*

A family history regarding breast disease and carcinoma is essential in evaluating a patient's risk of malignancy. An adequate past medical history should include a list of past and present medications, a reproductive history (including parity and menstrual history), and inquiry concerning previous neoplasms and thyroid disease.

PHYSICAL EXAMINATION

The physical exam should be conducted in a comfortable room with adequate lighting and warm hands. The examiner should begin by observing the breasts with the patient seated on the table and her arms at her sides. The physician should pay special attention to the gross configuration and symmetry of the breasts, including the nipples and the areolae. Next, have the patient raise her arms above her head, making the same observations. Then, have her press the palmar surfaces of her hands down on her iliac crests, and again observe. Ask the patient to lean forward and look for dimpling of the skin and asymmetry between the left and right sides.

With the patient leaning forward, palpate the breast tissue in an orderly fashion, using the flat surfaces of the second, third, and fourth fingers and employing a rotary motion. The breast may be divided into quadrants, strips, or spiraling circles for the purpose of thorough examination. The areolae should be palpated. An attempt should be made to express a discharge from each nipple. While still in the seated position, the axillary, supraclavicular, and infraclavicular regions should be evaluated.

The patient should then be instructed to assume a supine position, and a towel should be placed under the side to be examined. Examine each breast from the opposite side of the table, again in a systematic way. After both breasts have been palpated, move to the top of the table and examine the breasts for symmetry, with the patient in the supine position.

During or following the physical examination, the physician should instruct the patient in breast self-examination. It is best to guide her through the examination, giving instruction as she palpates her own breast. In this way, the physician may show the patient the texture of normal breast tissue and ensure that self-examination is being performed correctly. At this time, breast self-examination is the best screening test for breast cancer.

If a dominant mass is found, it should be mapped with any other breast findings. Consistency, tenderness, mobility, and margins (diffuse versus circumscribed) are qualities of the mass to be noted. Also note whether this is a diffuse or localized process confined to one breast or present in both breasts. Associated skin or nipple changes and adenopathy should also be mentioned.

The mass should be considered suspicious if it is singular, hard, poorly mobile, poorly defined, irregular, and asymmetric. Skin changes, nipple changes, and regional lymphadenopathy are almost diagnostic of breast cancer, especially in the appropriate age group.

DIAGNOSTIC STUDIES/ASSESSMENT

The early considerations in the differential diagnosis of a breast mass are age of the patient, whether or not the patient is pregnant, and whether the patient is pre- or postmenopausal.

Children[3,5,7]

As discussed previously, the most common breast masses of childhood involve an overgrowth of normal breast tissue. True neoplasms are quite uncommon in children, and carcinoma is a true medical curiosity. Inflammatory lesions such as staphylococcal mastitis and traumatic mastitis may occur at any age. Of the true neoplasms, fibroadenoma is the most common. If biopsy is decided on, the need to proceed with care cannot be overemphasized.

Nongravid Women

It is well known that fibroadenoma and fibrocystic changes constitute most masses in women less than 30.[4,8] Other less common benign lesions include tubular adenoma, intraductal papilloma, and fibromatosis.[9] Cancer is rare in this age group. Unless there is a significant family history of breast cancer occurring at a young age among the patient's first-degree female relatives, clinical suspicion must be very high to merit an open biopsy.

In women less than 35 years of age, one may aspirate a clearly cystic mass immediately following the physical examination and monitor the patient with a follow-up ultrasound or mammogram and physical exam. If the nature of the mass is solid or unknown after a careful physical examination, one should image the mass by ultrasound to determine whether it is cystic or solid. Aspiration of a cyst is performed with a 22- or 23-gauge needle and is said to be no more painful than venipuncture.[10] The procedure itself takes approximately five minutes to perform, and the results of fluid cytology are final in 24 to 48 hours. Although there is some discussion in the literature as to whether clear and cloudy fluid should be sent for cytology,[10,11,12,13] we feel that it is necessary to send all cystic fluid for cytology in order to be able to reassure the patient honestly. In the hands of an experienced cytologist, the false-negative rate of aspiration cytology is said to be similar to that of frozen section, and the false-positive rate approaches zero.[10] Suspicious cytology is an indication for open biopsy. If the cytology is benign, the mass disappears completely after aspiration, and the follow-up ultrasound or mammogram is not suspicious, then the patient should be followed every six months to one year with physical examination. Breast self-examination should be stressed.

If the dominant mass is solid or recurrent, an adequate imaging study should be obtained. This should be followed by open biopsy.[4,10]

Mammography in this population is not particularly useful at an early stage in the evaluation of a palpable mass because of the large amount of glandular tissue in the young breast. Imaging, however, has a place in the evaluation of a firm, persistent, or highly sus-

picious mass, with the understanding that a "normal" mammogram is never a reason to delay the timely biopsy of a highly suspicious mass in any age group.[14]

Other imaging techniques have been evaluated. Computerized tomography (CT) allows unacceptable radiation exposure and is too costly to be used routinely but may prove to be useful in those patients who have a known lesion that cannot be localized accurately by mammography and ultrasonography. Thermography has not been proved to be sensitive or specific enough to be useful. Diaphanography, breast imaging by transillumination utilizing visible light, gives information similar to that of mammography and ultrasound in the evaluation of a known breast mass greater than 1 cm.[15] Doppler flow studies are still in-

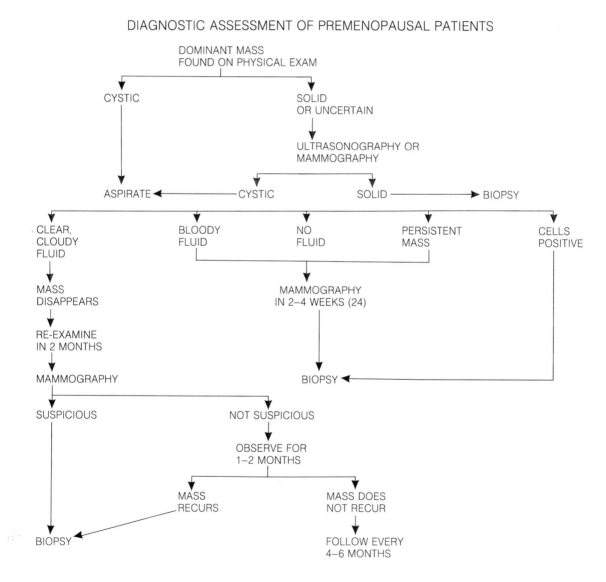

DIAGNOSTIC ASSESSMENT OF PREMENOPAUSAL PATIENTS

vestigational. Magnetic resonance imaging (MRI) is being investigated as a method of differentiating benign from malignant neoplasms. While the initial results are promising, MRI has an unacceptably high cost even when compared with open biopsy.[14,15,16,17]

In the 35 to 50 age group, the incidence of fibroadenoma decreases and that of fibrocystic changes, giant fibroadenoma, papilloma, granular cell tumors, and subareolar papillomatosis increases. Malignancy also increases with age in this group.[9,18] The algorithm (Diagnostic Assessment of Premenopausal Patients) presents the approach to a breast mass detected in the premenopausal patient.

In the age group between 40 and menopause, the degree of clinical suspicion and the risk factors of the patient determine whether the approach discussed previously should be used or whether the more aggressive approach, mentioned below for the postmenopausal woman, is more appropriate.

In the postmenopausal woman with a confirmed dominant mass, mammography and biopsy should be undertaken in that order[19] (see the algorithm Diagnostic Assessment of Perimenopausal, Postmenopausal, and Male Patients). Mammography has a sensitivity of approximately 80 per cent and a specificity of about 90 per cent.[8,16] Again, a ''normal'' mammogram is no reason to delay the biopsy of a clinically suspicious lesion.[10]

At any age, the differential diagnosis of a dominant mass must include fat necrosis, acute mastitis, granulomatous mastitis, chronic mastitis, breast abscess, and localized fibrosis.[2,9] Galactoceles and lactating adenomas must be considered, in addition to the above, in the postpartum breast.[9]

The indications for biopsy are a dominant solid mass, a cyst that cannot be aspirated, a cyst with bloody aspirate, a residual mass after aspiration, associated skin or nipple changes, a spontaneous nipple discharge, eczema of the nipple, and a suspicious mammo-

DIAGNOSTIC ASSESSMENT
OF PERIMENOPAUSAL,
POSTMENOPAUSAL,
AND MALE PATIENTS

DOMINANT
MASS PALPATED
↓
MAMMOGRAPHY
↓
BIOPSY

gram.[20] A mass is considered suspicious on mammogram if it contains multiple, small calcifications, is asymmetric, is stellate, or is vascular.[20] Mammography may also reveal previously unrecognized edema or nipple retraction.[5,20]

Once biopsy is decided on, three options are available: core biopsy, incisional biopsy, and excisional biopsy. Core biopsy may be attempted when the mass is large and the risk of cancer is high. A negative core biopsy is not sufficient to rule out carcinoma and does not preclude open biopsy. Although there is some controversy as to whether a core specimen is acceptable for receptor studies,[9,21] we feel that a larger specimen is necessary to overcome sampling error. This test is vitally important because it will be used in the selection of appropriate chemotherapy if the mass is malignant. Incisional biopsy is certainly adequate for receptor studies, but a tissue diagnosis of benign disease is not adequate to rule out cancer; consequently, the mass would have to be removed in its entirety.[19] Incisional biopsy is most useful for large, inoperable masses with a reasonable suspicion of malignancy.[5] Excisional biopsy is the most reliable means of determining the nature of the mass and may be curative.

Gravid Women[5,22,23]

The pregnant state is a neutral factor in the development of breast cancer. During pregnancy, there is increasing mass, firmness, and nodularity due to hypertrophy and hyperemia of the breast tissue. This makes clinical diagnosis and mammographic evaluation more difficult.

Nevertheless, a dominant mass discovered in the breast of a pregnant woman should be evaluated in the same manner as in the woman who is not pregnant. If ultrasonography is undertaken as an imaging modality, it is important to remember that there has been no standardization for the breast during pregnancy[23]; but it is still useful in discriminating cystic dominant masses from solid dominant masses. If a mammogram is deemed necessary, the abdomen should be appropriately shielded. If the mass is cystic, aspiration should be undertaken and the fluid sent for cytologic interpretation.[24] If the mass is solid, then open biopsy under local anesthesia is indicated. If open biopsy is undertaken in the postpartum period, the patient should be instructed to stop breastfeeding and take prophylactic antibiotics to decrease the risk of infection and fistula formation.

The differential diagnosis of a breast mass in the pregnant patient is essentially the same as that for other premenopausal women. Changes specific to pregnancy and lactation include hyperplasia, galactocele, lactational mastitis and abscess, and lactational adenoma. Breast infarcts are also more common in the pregnant breast.

Males[2,6,9]

When a male presents with a breast mass, the major differential diagnosis is between carcinoma and gynecomastia. As in the female, age is fundamental to the assessment of a mass in the male. Benign gynecomastia is an entity of adolescence. Breast cancer is a disease of elderly males. In middle-aged males, breast cancer is rare, but gynecomastia is most likely to be indicative of pathology. Gynecomastia is typically related to drug intake or an abnormal process involving estrogen production or metabolism, that is, hepatic cirrhosis, pituitary adenoma, hyperthyroidism, Cushing's syndrome, and testicular tumors.

A history of appropriate drug therapy (phenothiazines, digitalis, isoniazid, cimetidine, diazepam, estrogens) or excessive alcohol intake lends itself to a diagnosis of gynecomastia. There is no "typical" history for male breast cancer.

On physical exam, gynecomastia is suggested by unilateral or bilateral, tender, discrete breast masses. The findings of a serosanguinous nipple discharge, a unilateral periareolar mass, skin dimpling, skin ulceration, and a fixed firm mass strongly suggest carcinoma.

Evaluation of a dominant breast mass in a male is identical to that of a postmenopausal female: mammogram and biopsy.

REFERENCES

1. Osborne MP. Breast development and anatomy. In: Harris JR, Hellman S, Henderson IC, Kinne DW, eds. Breast diseases. Philadelphia: JB Lippincott, 1987:1–14.
2. Cotran RS, Kumar V, Robbins SL. The breast. In: Robbins SL, ed. Pathologic basis of disease. Philadelphia: WB Saunders, 1989:1181–1204.
3. Bower R, Bell MJ, Ternberg J. Management of breast lesions in children and adolescents. J Pediatr Surg 1976;11(3):337–46.
4. Ellis H, Cox PJ. Breast problems in 1000 consecutive referrals to surgical out-patients. Postgrad Med J 1984;60:653–6.
5. Leis HP Jr. Breast lesions: diagnosis and treatment. In: Barker HRK, ed. Gynecology. Practice of Surgery, Ltd: Woodbury, Connecticut, 1988:1–43.
6. Kinne DW. Male breast cancer. In: Harris JR, Hellman S, Henderson IC, Kinne DW, eds. Breast diseases. Philadelphia: JB Lippincott, 1987:577–80.
7. Farrow JH, Ashikari H. Breast lesions in young girls. Surg Clin North Am 1969;49(2):261–9.
8. Ferguson CM, Powell RW. Breast masses in young women. Arch Surg 1989;124:1338–41.
9. Kline TS, Kline IK. Breast. In: Kline TS, ed. Guides to clinical aspiration biopsy. New York: Igaku-Shoin, 1989.
10. Grady D, Hodgkins ML, Goodson WH. The lumpy breast. West J Med 1988;149(2):226–9.
11. Wile AG, Kollin M. Office management of the breast mass. Postgrad Med 1987;81(3):137–43.
12. Devitt JE, Barr JR. The clinical recognition of cystic carcinoma. Surg Gynecol Obstet 1984;159(2):130–2.
13. Bachman L. Breast problems. Office Gynecol Primary Care 1988;15(3):643–64.
14. Harris V, Jackson VP. Indications for breast imaging in women under age 35. Radiology 1989; 172(2):445–8.
15. Homer MJ. Breast imaging: pitfalls, controversies, and some practical thoughts. Radiol Clin North Am 1985;23(3):459–71.
16. Gisvold JJ. Imaging of the breast: techniques and results. Mayo Clin Proc 1990;65:56–66.
17. Greene F, Hicks C, Eddy V, Davis C. Mammography, sonomammography, and diaphanography (lightscanning): a prospective, comparative study with histologic correlation. Am Surg 1985;51(1):58–60.
18. Moskowitz MM. Benefit and risk. In: Bassett LW, Gold RH, eds. Breast cancer detection: mammography and other methods in breast imaging. Orlando, Florida: Grune and Stratton, 1987:132.
19. Kinne DW, Kopans DB. Physical examination and mammography in the diagnosis of breast disease. In: Harris JR, Hellman S, Henderson IC, Kinne DW, eds. Breast diseases. Philadelphia: JB Lippincott, 1987:77–80.
20. Cheek HJ. Experience with breast biopsies for mammographic findings. Breast 1978; 4(1):4–9.
21. Osborne K. Receptors. In: Harris JR, Hellman S, Henderson IC, Kinne DW, eds. Breast diseases. Philadelphia: JB Lippincott, 1987:210–32.
22. Greene F. Gestational breast cancer: a ten-year experience. South Med J 1988;81(12):1509–11.
23. Petrek JA. Breast cancer and pregnancy. In: Harris J, Hellman S, Henderson IC, Kinne DW, eds. Breast diseases. Philadelphia: JB Lippincott, 1987:600–5.
24. Sickles EA, Klein DL, Goodson WH, Hunt TK. Mammography after needle aspiration of palpable breast masses. Am J Surg 1983; 145(Mar):395–7.

CHEST PAIN, ACUTE

THACH N. NGUYEN and ABDULMASSIH S. ISKANDRIAN

SYNONYM: Substernal Pain

BACKGROUND

Chest pains are one of the most common symptoms encountered in clinical practice and often represent a major diagnostic challenge. Chest pain is an unpleasant sensation generally located in the thorax and upper epigastrium and may originate from various sources including the skin, musculoskeletal system, nerves, and deeper visceral structures. Occasionally, it may be of psychogenic origin.

Afferent sensory impulses enter the spinal cord through dorsal root ganglia and terminate on the posterior neurons. Both somatic and visceral pain fibers share common segmental neural distribution. Thus, visceral pain may be perceived in areas innervated by somatic nerve fibers. Examples are anginal pain referred to left chest, arm, neck, or jaw; or pain from diaphragmatic pleura referred to the shoulder. The precise localization of somatic pain differs from the wider distribution of visceral pain because, in general, visceral impulses are transmitted to several segmental levels, whereas somatic impulses are transmitted to a single segmental level.[1] An appreciation of the innervation pathways is important for the correct diagnosis and management of patients with chest pain.

Table 1 outlines the common causes of chest pain. One of the causes of acute chest pain is cardiac pain. Chest pain or angina due to myocardial ischemia occurs when the myocardial oxygen supply is inadequate to meet its oxygen demands. By far the most frequent cause of angina is atherosclerotic coronary artery disease. When the epicardial coronary atherosclerosis reaches a critical degree of narrowing, the intramyocardial arterioles dilate in an effort to maintain coronary blood flow at a marginally sufficient level to avert resting ischemia. Any condition associated with increased myocardial oxygen demand such as tachycardia, hypertension, and increased contractility will result in myocardial ischemia due to an imbalance between oxygen supply and demand.[2] In addition to a fixed coronary stenosis, there may be a dynamic component of decreased coronary blood flow secondary to spasm of the major epicardial vessels or to an intermittently occluding coronary thrombus at the site of the atherosclerotic plaque. When coronary thrombosis is complete, myocardial infarction usually ensues in the absence of adequate collateral supply. Myocardial ischemia or infarction can occur in patients with variant or Prinzmetal's angina due to coronary spasm. Such spasm usually involves atherosclerotic coronary arteries but may also be seen in coronary vessels free of significant atherosclerosis.[3] Typically, chest pain occurs at rest and has no relationship to physical exertion.

Another entity that has recently received attention is *syndrome X* or microvascular angina.[4] This term has been coined for patients with angiographically normal coronary arteries and no documented spasm of epicardial arteries or left ventricular hypertrophy. The intrinsic abnormalities of vasodilatory reserve of coronary microvasculature appear to be responsible for myocardial ischemia. Many patients with hypertrophic cardiomyopathy experience angina with angiographically normal coronary arteries. The mechanisms for angina in such cases are multifactorial and may be related to structurally abnormal small vessels with thickened media and narrowed lumen, decreased coronary flow as a result of diastolic dysfunction, smaller relative number of capillaries to muscle fibers, prolongation of systole and shortening of diastole, as well as increased demand because of hypertrophy. Increased myocardial mass and elevated left ventricular outflow tract gradient may increase oxygen demand and cause myocardial ischemia.[5] Hypertension with left ventricular hypertrophy alone can produce angina, although such patients may also have coexistent coronary artery disease. Myocardial ischemia usually results from increased oxygen demand and reduced coronary blood flow (abnormal vasodilatory reserve and inadequate capillary proliferation in left ventricular hypertrophy).[6]

Patients with significant pulmonary hypertension from both pressure and volume over-

TABLE 1. Causes of Acute Chest Pain

Cardiac
 Angina pectoris
 Variant angina (Prinzmetal)
 Microvascular angina (syndrome X)
 Myocardial infarction
 Coronary anomalies
 Coronary embolism
 Coronary arteritis
 Myocardial bridging
 Aortic stenosis/regurgitation
 Hypertrophic cardiomyopathy
 Pulmonary hypertension
 Pericarditis
 Mitral valve prolapse
 Cocaine use
Vascular
 Aortic dissection
 Aortic aneurysm
 Syphilitic aortitis
Pulmonary
 Pulmonary embolism
 Pneumothorax
 Pleurisy
 Pneumonia
 Neoplasm
 Mediastinitis
Gastrointestinal
 Esophageal spasm
 Reflux esophagitis
 Peptic ulcer disease
 Pancreatitis
 Cholecystitis
 Esophageal perforation/rupture
Musculoskeletal
 Costochondritis
 Rib fractures
 Thoracic outlet syndrome
 Cervical/thoracic spine diseases
 Herpes zoster
Psychogenic
 Neurocirculatory asthenia
 Hyperventilation syndrome

load such as chronic obstructive lung disease, restrictive lung diseases, left to right shunting, and mitral stenosis may have exertional chest pain due to increased right ventricular wall tension and distension of pulmonary arteries. Since right ventricular coronary flow occurs both during systole (the right ventricle exerts less compressive force from the left ventricle) and diastole, elevated right ventricular pressure may impede systolic coronary flow to the right ventricle.

Valvular aortic stenosis and insufficiency may be associated with angina. Although a large percentage of patients with calcific aortic stenosis have coexistent coronary artery disease, anginal discomfort can occur in the presence of normal coronary arteries as a result of increased oxygen demand and reduction in subendocardial oxygen supply.[7] Angina is less common in aortic insufficiency. Since coronary blood flow occurs primarily during diastole, low aortic diastolic pressure in chronic aortic insufficiency reduces coronary flow. Increased oxygen demand also contributes to myocardial ischemia. Other rare causes of angina include myocardial bridges, coronary anomalies, coronary arteritis, and embolism.

Myocardial bridging or milking of epicardial coronary arteries may be severe enough to constrict the vessel during systole and produce ischemia in some patients, especially during tachycardia. Bridging most commonly involves the proximal and middle third of the left anterior descending artery but may also be seen in the other epicardial vessels.[8]

Anomalous origin of the left main or left anterior descending artery from the right coronary sinus and its course between the aorta and pulmonary artery has been associated with myocardial ischemia and sudden death during strenuous activity.

A frequently encountered cause of recurrent chest pain is mitral valve prolapse (MVP). This syndrome is more common in women than in men. The leaflets and chordal structures are redundant owing to myxomatous degeneration and prolapse into the left atrium during systole, resulting in a sharp, high-pitched click and often a late systolic murmur as well.

Acute pericarditis most often presents with precordial pain.[9] The pericardium itself has relatively few pain fibers, and the pain of pericarditis is believed to be due to the inflammation of the adjacent parietal pleura. Acute pericarditis has various etiologies—most commonly viral infection—but can be secondary to noninfectious causes such as post-infarction Dressler's syndrome, uremia, myxedema, trauma, autoimmune disorders (lupus, rheumatoid arthritis, scleroderma), drugs (procainamide, hydralazine), postirradiation or postpericardiotomy, malignancy, and aortic dissection.

Acute aortic dissection or dissecting hematoma is a not-uncommon catastrophic illness that requires an aggressive diagnostic evaluation. Dissection of aorta is caused by degeneration of aortic media that results in blood entering the wall of the aorta through an intimal tear and separating its layers to form a false lumen. Hypertension is the major risk factor. Aortic dissection may be associated with Marfan's syndrome, a connective tissue disorder that is present in about 10 per cent of patients with dissection. Dissection may involve the arch, ascending or descending aorta, or both. Dissection can lead to acute aortic regurgitation, cardiac tamponade, acute myocardial infarction, transient ischemic attack, stroke, spinal cord infarction, ischemic limbs, acute renal failure, or mesenteric ischemia. Although most dissections are acute, this process can be subacute or chronic with gradual and insidious course.[10]

Syphilitic aortitis is a rare disorder that may cause myocardial ischemia through the involvement of coronary ostia.

One of the common and not infrequently misdiagnosed causes of chest pain is pulmonary thromboembolism.[11] The most common source of emboli is deep-vein thrombosis of lower extremities, but occasionally the thrombus may originate from right atrium, right ventricle, and tricuspid valve. Almost all pulmonary emboli consist of thrombotic materials (fibrin, platelets, red cells); rarely, nonthrombotic materials such as tumor, fat, bone marrow, amniotic fluid, and air may embolize to the lungs. Tricuspid valve infective vegetations can lead to septic embolism and pneumonia.

Pulmonary embolism results in arterial hypoxemia (due to ventilation-perfusion [V/Q] mismatch) and pulmonary hypertension. Less than 10 per cent of emboli lead to pulmonary infarction since the lungs also receive blood supply from the bronchial arteries. Infarction occurs infrequently and usually in the setting of left ventricular failure or severe mitral stenosis.

The visceral pleura and lung parenchyma are devoid of pain receptors, whereas the parietal pleura has rich sensory innervation. Therefore, a large pulmonary neoplasm may not cause many symptoms until it involves the parietal pleura or involves the chest wall. Pleuritic pain is highly characteristic of these disorders. Common causes of pleuritic chest pain are pneumothorax, viral pleurisy, bacterial pneumonia, pulmonary embolism/infarction, lung carcinoma, mesothelioma, and connective tissue diseases.

HISTORY

Despite the availability of a large number of diagnostic tests, the history and physical examination remain the initial and important methods of evaluating patients with acute chest pain. Incorrect diagnosis may lead to many unnecessary tests, and failure to recognize a serious illness may result in delay of appropriate therapy. The most important task of the clinician is to differentiate serious illnesses—such as acute myocardial infarction, aortic dissections, and pulmonary embolism—that require immediate intervention from less grave conditions. A thorough history and physical exam should provide significant clues that can be further confirmed with other diagnostic techniques.

Patients' descriptions of chest pain take on many different forms. Many times it is not possible to differentiate etiologies of chest pain on the basis of pain description; one has to rely on other factors such as location, duration, radiation of pain, accompanying symptoms, and provocative and relieving factors.[2,12]

Cardiac Causes of Chest Pain

Angina pectoris is the most common manifestation of myocardial ischemia. Angina pectoris can be classified as follows: (1) classic angina, a transient substernal discomfort precipitated by exertion and relieved with rest and nitrates; (2) atypical angina, similar symptoms, but the pain may not be consistently related to exertion or relieved with rest; and (3) anginal equivalent symptom such as indigestion, dyspnea, transient weakness, and toothache.

The term *angina* was originally described by Herberden in 1768 and connoted a sense of choking or strangling associated with anxiety. It is not actually pain. Indeed, many patients do not complain of pain but rather a discomfort, an unpleasant sensation that is sometimes difficult to describe. The discomfort may be a heaviness; tightness like a band across the chest; a weight on the chest, a fullness; pressure or constriction; or a choking, strangling, squeezing, or aching sensation. To complicate matters further, the discomfort may involve the epigastrium rather than midsternal area in the form of "nausea," a "burning feeling," or "indigestion." Angina may mean different things to different patients; a few may spontaneously clench a fist in the middle of the chest (positive Levine sign) when trying to describe the sensation. Sometimes dyspnea, fatigue, nausea, or indigestion may be the sole presensation of angina (angina equivalent), especially in elderly patients and diabetic patients. These patients may have a generalized reduced perception of painful stimuli related to autonomic dysfunction. Obviously in some patients, some or all episodes of ischemia may be painless and asymptomatic (silent ischemia). The quality of anginal pain is almost always dull and deep rather than sharp or superficial. The intensity of the discomfort varies widely from patient to patient, from day to day, or throughout the day in a given patient. There is a circadian rhythm, with more anginal events occurring between early and late morning. The variability of ischemic threshold is related to change in vasomotor tone at the site of coronary stenosis.[2,3]

Angina is typically located in the substernal, retrosternal, or left precordial area but may occur as isolated neck, shoulder, jaw, or left arm discomfort. (Also see Chest Pain, Atypical—in *Difficult Diagnosis I.*). The lower jaw or mandible is most often involved rather than the maxilla. Angina can sometimes be misdiagnosed as toothache. Chest pain may radiate up to the neck, jaw, left shoulder, and the ulnar aspect of the left arm along the hypothenar dominance, the fourth and fifth fingers. Right-sided chest pain is relatively uncommon. Not infrequently, angina limited to the subxiphoid or epigastrium can be confused with gastrointestinal disorders such as esophageal spasm and reflux esophagitis. However, cardiac ischemia may be suspected if symptoms are brought on by exertion and relieved with rest. Lower abdominal or back pain is unlikely to be angina. One important feature of angina and some other cardiac causes of chest pain is the diffuse, rather than localized, nature. If the patient can pinpoint the location of chest pain with one finger, the pain is usually not angina.

The duration of chest pain is also important in determining its etiology. Angina usually develops gradually and progresses in intensity over several minutes. The relief is also a gradual process. Angina is relatively short, lasting usually less than 10 to 20 minutes. A longer duration generally implies more severe or unstable angina or myocardial infarction. Chest pain lasting hours or days is unlikely to be angina. If pain is lancinating and brief and mounts rapidly in intensity, other conditions such as musculoskeletal pain or pericarditis should be considered.

Aggravating and relieving factors should be evaluated to determine the cause of chest pain. The main factors that provoke angina are physical exertion; exposure to cold, heat, emotion, or excitement; after a meal; or during sexual intercourse. Classic angina is characteristically induced by physical exertion. It may involve not only dynamic activity such as walking up the hall, hurrying to catch a bus, painting, or hammering but also isometric activity such as lifting and carrying a heavy object.

Exposure to cold may precipitate angina, usually in association with some exertion such as walking in a cold, windy weather or shoveling snow. Working in hot and humid weather can also induce angina. Angina usually develops after, rather than during, a heavy meal, especially when associated with some physical activity. Certain emotional reactions usually in the forms of excitement, anger, rage, or anxiety can precipitate angina. Emotionally induced angina tends to last longer than exertional angina, possibly because the sympathetic response does not terminate quickly. Sexual intercourse is associated with increased myocardial oxygen demand caused by both physical exertion and excitement and can induce angina and myocardial infarction.

Angina is commonly classified into different functional states according to New York Heart Association or Canadian Cardiovascular Society guidelines (Table 2). Angina usually subsides within a few minutes after cessation of physical activity or following sublingual nitroglycerin. Anginal relief does not occur instantaneously but usually within two to five minutes after sublingual nitrate. Severe angina may require two to three tablets for relief. Some patients only experience angina at the beginning of exertion but not during the continued activity (walk-through angina). The mechanism of this walk-through angina is not well understood.

The term *unstable angina* has been used quite frequently in clinical practice. The differentiation from stable or classic angina is very important because unstable angina carries an adverse prognosis, it may herald acute myocardial infarction, and it usually requires more intensive management.[13] The diagnosis

TABLE 2. **New York Heart Association Functional Classification of Angina Pectoris**

FUNCTIONAL CLASS	SYMPTOM OCCURRENCE
I	With unusual activity
II	With prolonged and slightly more than usual activity
III	With usual activity of daily living
IV	At rest

of unstable angina can be suspected when one or more of the following historical features are present:

1. Development of more severe, prolonged, and frequent angina superimposed on a chronic stable exertional pattern.
2. New onset angina (usually within one month and brought on by minimal exertion).
3. Angina occurring at rest or minimal exertion.
4. Recurrent angina following a recent myocardial infarction.

A history of a sudden change in the usual pattern of chest pain may be elicited in some patients with unstable angina, for example, chest pain awakening patient from sleep.

In contrast to exertional angina, some patients experience recurrent angina mostly during rest. This variant angina resembles classic angina in quality and location and its response to nitroglycerin, although the episodes are unusually severe and variable in duration. The pain may awaken patients at night or in the early morning hours. Some patients also report angina related to physical exertion and emotional stress. These episodes may occur after cessation of activity rather than during its peak. Palpitations are relatively common in variant angina. Most patients present between the ages of 35 and 50 years. There is a female predominance and a frequent history of smoking and migraine headaches. Some patients may also complain of Raynaud's phenomenon.

In most patients with acute myocardial infarction, the pain has similar quality to angina but tends to be deeper, more severe, and prolonged, lasting at least half an hour to several hours. Some patients may describe a crushing, oppressive sensation associated with severe dyspnea, nausea, vomiting, diaphoresis, cold sweat, lightheadedness, and profound weakness.[14] Occasionally the pain may be more of a dull aching sensation or an epigastric discomfort. In general, the pain of infarction does not subside with cessation of activity or sublingual nitrates. It is important to recognize that angina and infarction may be silent or asymptomatic, especially in elderly patients and patients with autonomic dysfunction (diabetes mellitus). These patients may have both symptomatic and asymptomatic episodes of angina during routine daily activities.

The evaluation of chest pain is incomplete without an adequate assessment of risk factors for coronary artery disease, namely, hypertension, diabetes, hypercholesterolemia, smoking, older age (males and females over age 55), obesity, type A personality, and positive family history of coronary artery disease. A history of drug use is very important. Chest pain occurs frequently following recreational use of cocaine and is probably related to a hyperadrenergic state.[15] Occasionally, acute myocardial infarction or ischemia may result from coronary vasospasm. Chest pain may start within minutes to hours after cocaine use and may last several hours. It is usually atypical, nonradiating, and nonexertion related. Relief with nitroglycerin is variable.

Angina due to isolated systemic hypertension, aortic stenosis, or hypertrophic obstructive cardiomyopathy may be indistinguishable from classic angina and may be associated with dyspnea and syncope.[5,6,7] Angina is less common in aortic regurgitation and often is somewhat atypical. The chest pain of chronic pulmonary hypertension due to chronic lung diseases, mitral stenosis, or left to right shunting resembles certain features of angina. It is usually brought on by exertion and varies widely in intensity and duration but rarely radiates to the neck or arms. Dyspnea is usually a more predominant symptom; response to nitroglycerin is variable.

The pain of acute pericarditis is often located in the left precordium and characteristically radiates to the left trapezius bridge.[9] Pericarditis can sometimes be misdiagnosed as myocardial infarction or postinfarction angina. However, there are certain features that allow pericarditis to be distinguished from angina or infarction. Pericardial pain has a pleuritic component, exacerbated by deep breathing, coughing, and recumbency and alleviated by sitting up and leaning forward. It tends to be more constant and unrelieved with nitroglycerin. Dyspnea, orthopnea, and fever may be the accompanying symptoms. Symptomatic response to salicylate and nonsteroidal anti-inflammatory agents may be a helpful clue.

The chest pain of mitral valve prolapse is rather atypical, usually not of the classic anginal type.[16] It is often sharp and has no relation to exertion. The pain may last for hours to days, is unrelieved with nitroglycerin, and may be localized anywhere in the precordium, but it rarely radiates to the neck or arms. Palpitation is a fairly common clinical finding.

Over 90 per cent of cases of acute aortic dissection present with acute chest pain.[10] The pain is usually of abrupt onset and extremely severe. It has a sharp, ripping, and tearing quality. The pain usually begins in the anterior chest, radiates to back, abdominal, or lumbar areas, and may involve the legs. In contrast to the crescendo nature of the pain of acute infarction, the pain of acute dissection is usually of maximal intensity at its inception. Aortic dissection can be misdiagnosed as acute myocardial infarction, although both may occur together as a result of dissection into the coronary artery. In general, symptoms depend on location and extent of dissection, and the pain may change location as the dissection is progressing. Sudden neurologic deficit, painful limb, paraparesis, or paraplegia may result from involvement of carotid artery, subclavian iliac arteries, or spinal cord artery. Syncope not associated with focal neurologic deficit is closely related to rupture into the pericardial sac with tamponade. Other manifestations include severe dyspnea due to aortic insufficiency, abdominal pain, hoarseness, and unexplained fever.

Pulmonary Causes of Chest Pain

Acute pulmonary embolism without pulmonary infarction usually does not cause chest discomfort. With massive thromboembolism, the chest pain may be severe and similar to myocardial infarction. When pulmonary infarction occurs, the pain is usually pleuritic.[11] In many patients, sudden onset of dyspnea is the most common and only presentation. A high index of clinical suspicion should be maintained in the appropriate settings such as prolonged immobility after surgery or low extremity/pelvic fractures, congestive heart failure, history of phlebitis, and hypercoagulable states (pregnancy, oral contraceptives, malignancy).

Other pulmonary causes of chest pain are bacterial pneumonia, viral pleurisy, and spontaneous pneumothorax. Chest pains are pleuritic and usually accompanied by dyspnea. Spontaneous pneumothorax is characterized by sudden onset of pain on either side of the chest and usually occurs in young patients, especially those with thin body habitus.

Neuromusculoskeletal Causes of Chest Pain

Chest wall pain is a common cause of chest discomfort and may be due to painful swelling of costochondral or chondrosternal joints (Tietze's syndrome). The pain may last for hours or days and is not consistently exertion related. Certain movements such as adduction, extension of the arms, rotation or twisting of the chest, deep breathing, or coughing tend to aggravate the pain. Patients usually can pinpoint the location of tenderness. Radiculopathic pain from cervical ribs or brachial plexus involvement tends to be constant stabbing with twinges of sharp, aching pain. The pain is accentuated by certain movements. Herpes zoster is another form of nerve root inflammation. The pain is usually intense, often burning or sharp, with paroxysms of greater severity. It usually precedes the appearance of a vesicular rash and persists after the rash has subsided. Patients with Hodgkin's lymphoma and those receiving immunosuppressive therapy are prone to develop herpes zoster.

Gastrointestinal Causes of Chest Pain

A variety of gastrointestinal disorders may cause precordial discomfort that mimics angina.[17] Patients with reflux esophagitis may complain of a dull squeezing or burning lower substernal or epigastric discomfort soon after recumbent position, especially following a heavy meal or certain foods/drinks (chocolate, coffee, tea). If pain occurs several hours or more after reclining, angina pectoris should be suspected. Nausea or heartburn may occur, and the pain may extend to the neck and arm. These symptoms are usually relieved with antacids or by raising the head of the bed up 30 degrees or more. This condition may or may not be associated with a hiatal hernia.

Esophageal motility disorders such as esophageal spasm also produce chest discomfort, particularly after meals, and dysphagia to both solid and liquid foods. It is important to note that both esophageal spasm and angina may coexist in approximately 25 per cent of patients. A confounding factor is that chest discomfort due to esophageal spasm may respond to nitroglycerin. Further testing may be necessary for diagnosis.

Peptic ulcer disease and gastritis can be distinguished from angina by the lack of relation to physical exertion and by their response to antacids. The discomfort typically is midepigastric burning and aching rather than substernal, is squeezing or heavy, and may radiate to the back.

Occasionally, cholecystitis may be difficult to differentiate from angina. The discomfort is usually located in the right upper quadrant but may radiate to the epigastrium and lower chest. Patients may move around to find a comfortable position and may have nausea, vomiting, and fever as accompanying symptoms.

Esophageal rupture or perforation is a catastrophic illness that can produce chest pain similar to angina. This condition may be preceded by a history of severe bouts of vomiting. Esophageal perforation may result from endoscopy and sclerotherapy.

Psychogenic chest pain is usually described as constant diffuse pain over the midsternum or left precordium without radiation, often associated with dyspnea, palpitation, and fatigue. Occasionally, patients may complain of circumoral numbness or tingling of the fingers due to hyperventilation. Patients with both coronary artery disease and psychologic problems can be very difficult to assess. They should be given a benefit of the doubt and treated for both problems. Further testings are usually needed to document objective evidence of myocardial ischemia.

PHYSICAL EXAMINATION

The general physical exam of patients with ischemic heart disease may be entirely normal. Certain clinical features may help identify patients with coronary artery disease (CAD) risk factors.[18] Xanthoma, xanthelasma, and arcus senilis in a white patient under the age of 50 years are suggestive of hypercholesterolemia. Arcus senilis in elderly and black patients is nonspecific. Examination of peripheral pulses may reveal decreased amplitude and bruits, which indicate the presence of diffuse atherosclerosis and increase the likelihood of concomitant coronary artery disease. Jugular venous pulses are usually normal but may be elevated in patients with chronic congestive heart failure or acute right ventricular infarction, especially in the presence of clear lung fields and hypotension. Palpitation of the left precordium may reveal a diffuse and large apical impulse indicative of left ventricular enlargement. A diffuse outward bulging during ventricular systole suggests apical aneurysm. The first heart sound, S_1, is usually normal. Occasionally, a soft S_1 and paradoxically split S_2 in the absence of left bundle branch block may be heard and generally reflects significant left ventricular dysfunction. An audible S_3 gallop also implies severe left ventricular failure

but can occur with significant aortic or mitral regurgitation. A new apical systolic murmur can be heard in some patients with ischemia or infarction due to papillary muscle dysfunction and secondary mitral regurgitation or ventricular septal defect. This murmur may sometimes be present only during episodes of chest pain and strongly suggests myocardial ischemia as the cause of chest pain.

The systolic murmur of acute severe mitral regurgitation (papillary muscle dysfunction) may not be holosystolic, as chronic mitral regurgitation, and may end before the A_2 component of S_2 owing to early aortic valve closure. The murmur is frequently loud and may be accompanied by a palpable thrill.

If a systolic murmur is heard along the right heart border and increases in intensity during inspiration, it is very likely due to tricuspid regurgitation in patients with acute right ventricular infarction or pulmonary hypertension. The P_2 component of S_2 may be accentuated. (Also see chapter on Systolic Murmurs.)

A harsh crescendo-decrescendo systolic murmur in right upper sternal border, especially if long and late peaking and in association with decreased A_2 and carotid upstroke/amplitude, suggests severe aortic stenosis (AS). Hypertrophic obstructive cardiomyopathy (HOCM) may be differentiated from AS by the nature of carotid pulses and the effect of Valsalva or amyl nitrate on the intensity of murmur. The systolic murmur of HOCM increases, whereas that of AS decreases during the straining phase of Valsalva and amyl nitrate. During handgrip systolic murmur decreases in both AS and HOCM but increases in mitral regurgitation.

Diastolic murmurs are uncommon in patients with coronary artery disease and suggest the presence of aortic or pulmonary insufficiency. A new early diastolic murmur in a patient with chest pain and hypertension should raise your index of suspicion of aortic dissection

Blood pressure should be checked in both arms, as there is often a significant difference. Blood pressure may be lower in one or both arms owing to compromise of blood flow through either or both subclavian arteries (pseudohypotension). Diminution or absence of peripheral pulses is an important clue to aortic dissection.[10] Neurologic exam may reveal Horner's syndrome, paraparesis or hemiparesis.

A mid- or late systolic click may be heard in patients with MVP.[16,18] It may or may not be associated with a late systolic murmur. The midsystolic click of MVP may sometimes be confused with ejection sound, but certain maneuvers can help confirm its presence. Clicks of MVP tend to occur earlier during the straining phase of Valsalva and later with squatting or handgrip. Clicks are best heard with the diaphragm of the stethoscope.

Rubs may be present in patients with pleuritis or pericarditis. They are usually of scratching, or grating, quality and are best detected with the diaphragm of the stethoscope. Pleural rubs are heard only during the inspiratory phase of respiration, whereas pericardial rubs are heard throughout the respiratory cycle. Pericardial rubs may have one, two, or three components (atrial systole, ventricular systole, and diastole). They may be evanescent.

Chest pain of musculoskeletal origins is often reproduced by palpation of chest wall or certain passive movements such as abduction, adduction, or extension of the arms. There may be some "trigger points" on the chest wall. Thoracic outlet syndrome may be detected by asking the patient to rotate the head toward the side of symptoms during deep inspiration with the neck extended. Chest pain is usually reproduced and radial pulse may be diminished owing to compression of the brachial artery. Pneumothorax may be diagnosed by unilateral decreased breath sound and increased resonance. The trachea may deviate to one side with tension pneumothorax.

Pleural rubs and egophony may suggest the presence of pneumonia. Lung exam is usually normal in pulmonary embolism, but pleural rubs may be present if there is pulmonary infarction.

Abdominal exam may be normal in patients with esophageal spasm/reflux or peptic ulcer disease. There is usually some tenderness in the right upper quadrant or epigastrium with deep inspiration in patients with cholecystitis (Murphy's sign).

DIAGNOSTIC STUDIES

Electrocardiography

The electrocardiogram (ECG) is a useful initial diagnostic test in patients with acute chest pain. The presence of pathologic Q wave in more than one lead usually indicates previous myocardial infarction. They are, however, nonspecific for CAD. "Pseudoinfarct" patterns (Q waves) may be seen in ventricular pre-exitation (Wolff-Parkinson-White syndrome) or HOCM. Q waves may also disappear after myocardial infarction. Rhythm disturbances such as atrioventricular block or ventricular tachyarrhythmia can sometimes occur during chest pain and may suggest an evolving myocardial infarction or severe unstable angina. ST-T wave abnormalities are often nonspecific and may be found with hyperventilation, mitral valve prolapse, ventricular hypertrophy, cardiomyopathy, drugs (digoxin), or electrolyte imbalance. However, new ST depression (horizontal or downsloping) or T wave inversion during chest pain is more suggestive of myocardial ischemia. ST elevation may be noted in variant angina or evolving myocardial infarction. However, diffuse ST elevation in multiple leads with PR segment depression is more likely due to early pericarditis. A random ECG is usually normal in patients with CAD. Ambulatory ECG (Holter) has recently been used to detect silent ischemia. However, routine use of ambulatory ECG is not recommended for the diagnosis of CAD because of high false-positive ST depression in patients without documented CAD.

Chest X-ray

Chest x-ray may provide useful information. It is often normal in patients with CAD. Cardiomegaly with or without vascular congestion, Kerley's B lines, may be seen in patients with left ventricular dysfunction and congestive heart failure. Widening of mediastinum with left pleural effusion and separation by more than 1 cm of calcium layers in aortic knob are highly suggestive of aortic dissection.[10] Pneumothorax, pneumonia, and neoplasm can be detected on chest x-ray. Chest radiography is usually normal in pulmonary embolism. Occasionally, elevated hemidiaphragm, atelectasis, pruning of pulmonary arteries, or wedge-shaped infiltrates may be seen.

Laboratory Tests

Laboratory tests are usually not useful except to detect acute myocardial infarction. An increase in creatine kinase (CK), lactate dehydrogenase (LDH), or aspartate aminotransferase (AST) is nonspecific and may be found in skeletal muscle trauma or intramuscular injection. However, elevation in isoenzymes CK-MB and the LDH_1/LDH_2 ratio is more specific for myocardial infarction. One single lab value neither confirms nor excludes myocardial infarction. These cardiac enzymes should be obtained serially over the first few days after onset of chest pain. CK is the earliest to appear (6 to 10 hours) and to peak (24 hours). LDH appears around 24 hours and peaks between 48 and 72 hours after acute myocardial infarction.[14]

Arterial blood gases can be useful in the differential diagnosis of chest pain. Hypoxemia associated with dyspnea, respiratory alkalosis, and normal chest x-ray in a patient with no known chronic lung disease strongly suggests pulmonary embolism in appropriate clinical settings (postoperative period, prolonged immobilization, etc.). A normal arterial oxygen pressure is rarely associated with significant pulmonary thromboembolism. Hypoxemia is a nonspecific finding and can be found in patients with pneumonia, pneumothorax, chronic obstructive or restrictive lung diseases, and congestive heart failure.

Exercise Testing

Exercise testing may be useful to establish the diagnosis of CAD.[19] Both treadmill and bicycle ergometer are available for exercise testing. Bruce protocol is the most popular for diagnostic purposes. Patients usually exercise until significant fatigue, dizziness, moderate angina, greater than 2 mm ST depression, arrhythmia, or hypotension develops. A stress test is considered positive or abnormal if the ST segment is depressed 1 mm or more horizontally or downsloping or 1.5 mm upsloping 0.05 seconds after the J point in three consecutive beats. Interpretation of test results is based on several parameters such as peak exercise heart rate, exercise blood pressure (BP) response, exercise tolerance, time of onset of ST segment changes, the duration and degree of ST segment abnormalities, and the number of leads showing ST segment changes. The pretest probability of CAD should be considered in the interpretation of test results. The extent of CAD can be determined on the basis of test results. An early appearance of horizontal or downsloping ST depression in the first 3 minutes of exercise at a heart rate of less than 120 beats per minute, persisting long into recovery period, is a good indication of extensive CAD such as left main or three-vessel disease. A blunted or hypotensive blood pressure response is also associated with severe coronary artery disease. The sensitivity of exercise testing is about 65 per cent and specific-ity about 80%. Exercise testing is contraindicated in patients with acute myocardial infarction, unstable angina, severe aortic stenosis, and HOCM.

Radionuclide Imaging

Perfusion Studies

The limitations of exercise testing are the high incidence of false-positive, false-negative, and nondiagnostic results due to inadequate exercise, beta blockers (less than 85 per cent predicted heart rate), and baseline ST-T abnormalities (left ventricular hypertrophy, digitalis, mitral valve prolapse, hyperventilation, ventricular preexcitation, pericarditis, bundle branch blocks). Exercise—perfusion imaging is more sensitive and specific than simple exercise testing for the detection of CAD.[19,20]

^{201}Thallium is injected intravenously about 1 minute before termination of exercise. Imaging usually begins within 10 minutes (initial images) and about 3 to 5 hours later (delayed images). After intravenous injection myocardial uptake of ^{201}thallium is dependent on regional blood flow. Myocardial thallium distribution is relatively homogenous in patients without significant coronary disease, except at the apex owing to normal apical thinning. In the presence of flow-limiting coronary stenosis, there is focal diminution in thallium uptake in the affected perfusion zones that correspond to one or more vascular supply territories.[20] Both ischemia and scar appear as focal areas with decreased thallium uptake on initial images. Comparison of the initial images to the delayed images is required to differentiate between ischemia and scar. Perfusion defects on initial images that show partial or complete "fill-in" (reversible) on delayed images are considered to represent ischemia. Perfusion abnormalities that remain unchanged or fixed on delayed images are usually considered to represent scar or infarction. However, recent studies suggested that delayed imaging at 24 hours or delayed imaging after reinjection of additional thallium is better at detecting viable ischemic myocardium. The lung thallium uptake and transient left ventricular cavity dilatation should be assessed along with perfusion pattern.

Imaging may be acquired using planar or tomographic techniques. Tomographic or single photon emission computed tomography (SPECT) imaging is superior to planar imaging because of three-dimensional view of the heart and lack of overlap of normal and abnormal myocardial segments in tomographic technique that allow better detection of smaller and more subtle abnormalities, especially in the left circumflex territory.

Thallium stress testing seems to be more useful than standard exercise ECG in women with suspected CAD and in patients who can achieve only moderate work load owing to poor conditioning or beta blockers. There are several limitations of thallium imaging. False-positive results may be due to breast attenuation of anterior wall or diaphragmatic attenuation of inferior wall. Most of these artifacts are fixed rather than reversible. Perfusion defects may also be seen in patients with aortic stenosis or hypertrophic cardiomyopathy in the absence of epicardial CAD. These defects, however, are not truly false positive but may be due to small vessel disease. False-negative results may occur if imaging begins late after thallium injection or if exercise level is submaximal (less than 85 per cent of predicted heart rate) or rarely in patients with severe three-vessel disease.

Alternate Tests

Some patients are unable to exercise owing to claudication, arthritis, neurologic deficits, or poor conditioning. Pharmacologic stress testing or atrial pacing tests in conjunction with thallium imaging are acceptable alternatives.

Dipyridamole and adenosine are potent coronary arteriolar vasodilators that create regional disparities in myocardial perfusion that can be detected by [201]thallium scintigraphy.[21] Dipyridamole and adenosine thallium imaging appear to have comparable sensitivity, specificity, and diagnostic accuracy to exercise–thallium imaging in the detection of CAD. Chest pain occurs commonly during dipyridamole and adenosine and is not specific for CAD. In patients with higher than first-degree atrioventricular (A-V) block, adenosine should be avoided because of risks of developing high-grade heart blocks; dipyridamole is the better option. Dipyridamole and adenosine are contraindicated in patients with significant bronchospastic diseases (asthma, chronic obstructive pulmonary disease [COPD]). An atrial pacing thallium test is a reasonable alternative in these patients. The atrial pacing test can be performed using an esophageal pacing lead or a transvenous pacemaker. [201]Thallium is injected at the peak pacing rate.

The sensitivity and specificity of the pacing thallium test are comparable with those of exercise-thallium test. The atrial pacing test cannot be done in patients with atrial flutter/fibrillation, or AV blocks due to intrinsic nodal disease or medications. Arm ergometry is less commonly used. Patients tend to become easily fatigued and do not usually achieve a reasonable rate-pressure product. The sensitivity of detecting CAD is lower with arm ergometry than with leg exercise.

Functional Studies

Global and regional left ventricular function may be evaluated by radionuclide ventriculography (first-pass or gated blood pool techniques).[19] The ejection fraction (EF) is a commonly used index of global left ventricular function. EF is normal (equal to or greater than 50 per cent) at rest and increases by more than 5 per cent during exercise in normal people. A failure to raise EF by greater than 5 per cent or a decrease in EF during exercise is an abnormal response but is not specific for CAD. This finding may be seen in patients with dilated cardiomyopathy or valvular heart disease. A new regional wall motion abnormality is more specific for coronary artery disease. Besides exercise, radionuclide ventriculography may be used in conjunction with cold pressor test, dobutamine, dipyridamole, or atrial pacing. However, the value of these tests is limited by low sensitivity of detecting CAD.

Infarct-Avid Imaging

The diagnosis of acute myocardial infarction is usually made on the basis of clinical evaluation, ECG, and cardiac enzymes. Scintigraphic techniques may be useful in cases of equivocal presentation or ECG or enzymatic changes.[14] $^{99}Tc^m$-pyrophosphate is taken up by infarcted myocardial tissues (hot spots). These scans tend to be positive between 2 and 5 days after acute infarction. $^{99}Tc^m$-pyrophosphate scan has a 90 per cent sensitivity for transmural infarction but only 70 per cent sensitivity for subendocardial infarction. The tracer is usually not taken up by old infarctions. Infarct-avid imaging is most useful in the setting of left bundle branch block (preventing diagnosis of myocardial infarction); ECG evidence of multiple previous infarctions, or delayed presentation to the hospital.

Echocardiography

Echocardiography is a very useful noninvasive imaging technique that provides both anatomic and physiologic information. The left ventricular wall normally thickens and the endocardial surfaces move concentrically toward the center of the left heart during systole. However, during myocardial ischemia or infarction, the systolic wall thickening decreases and is accompanied by a worsening segmental wall motion abnormality such as hypokinesis, akinesis, or sometimes dyskinesis. Wall motion abnormality usually precedes the development of ST depression or angina and is a more sensitive and specific finding for coronary artery disease. Two-dimensional echocardiograms obtained during chest pain may help differentiate ischemic from nonischemic etiologies.[19] However, a normal wall motion during pain-free episodes does not exclude CAD. Two-dimensional echo can be obtained during or immediately after treadmill or bicycle exercise or during dobutamine or dipyridamole infusion. New or worsening regional wall motion abnormality is highly suggestive of stress-induced myocardial ischemia and occurs more often with exercise and dobutamine than with dipyridamole. Exercise echo is limited by the difficulty in obtaining optimal images owing to motion and respiration.

Echocardiography is the diagnostic technique for MVP. Prolapse may occur in one or both leaflets in late systole or throughout systole. It may be associated with varying degrees of mitral regurgitation. Aortic dissection and aortic insufficiency can be detected by echocardiography, especially with transesophageal approach. Two-dimensional and Doppler echocardiography are very useful in evaluating the presence of the severity of aortic stenosis and hypertrophic cardiomyopathy.

Angiography

Coronary angiography provides important anatomic information about the presence, extent, and severity of CAD, coronary anomalies, and myocardial bridging.[19] Angiograms are usually obtained in multiple projections to better assess the degree of coronary stenosis because of the eccentric nature of many atherosclerotic plaques. The severity of stenosis is estimated visually in relation to the normal segment and reported as percent diameter stenosis. A 50 per cent or greater diameter stenosis is generally considered significant CAD. This visual assessment of coronary stenosis is fraught with significant subjective variability and does not consistently provide important physiologic information in terms of blood flow limitation, except in the presence of severe stenosis. Moreover, a normal cineangiogram does not exclude myocardial ischemia as cause of chest pain because some patients may have small vessel disease or coronary artery spasm. Coronary artery spasm can be detected with ergonovine challenge. Focal coronary spasm with reproducible chest pain or ST segment elevation is a specific finding for variant or Prinzmetal angina.

Although transesophageal echo, contrast computed axial tomography, and magnetic resonance imaging are useful for detecting aortic dissection, the gold standard remains aortography. Aortography outlines the site of dissection and the extent of involvement of major vascular structures.[10] These invasive techniques carry a small but definite risk of stroke, myocardial infarction, dye or atheroemboli-induced renal failure, bleeding and vascular compromise, or dye allergy.

Ventilation-Perfusion Imaging (V/Q Scan)

Ventilation-perfusion scans are important diagnostic tools in pulmonary embolism.[11] Perfusion scans are performed by intravenous injection of ^{99}Tc-labeled macroaggregates of albumin. A normal lung shows homogenous distribution of radioactivity. A normal perfusion lung scan essentially excludes pulmonary embolism. However, an abnormal perfusion scan is not specific for pulmonary embolism and can be seen in pneumonia, COPD, and neoplasm. In general, any condition that causes a radiographic infiltrate or causes regional obstruction to ventilation can cause a perfusion defect. Perfusion lung scans should always be evaluated in connection with a current chest film.

The number and size of perfusion defects are important in assessing the probability of pulmonary embolism. Single or multiple small subsegmental defects carry a low probability. Two or more segmental or lobar defects or one defect larger than a segment are associated with high probability. All these defects must be in an area of no radiographic abnormality or substantially larger than radiographic infiltrate.

Perfusion scans are often performed along with ventilation scans. Pulmonary embolism produces perfusion defects in areas with normal ventilation (V/Q mismatch), whereas pneumonia, congestive heart failure, and COPD diseases create both ventilation and perfusion abnormalities in the same area (V/Q match).

ASSESSMENT

The diagnosis of acute chest pain requires a thorough assessment of clinical history, cardiac risk factors, physical examination, and resting ECG. Which tests to order next depend on the clinical presentation and the pretest probability of disease.

Each patient must be evaluated individually. No single test provides 100 per cent diagnostic accuracy; each has its own merits and limitations. A clinician must decide whether a test is indicated and cost-effective. A list of diagnostic procedures for each condition is provided in Table 3. In patients with multiple cardiac risk factors and typical chest pain, a positive exercise ECG does not add significantly to the diagnosis of coronary artery disease, and a negative result is more likely false negative. However, exercise ECG may still be helpful in evaluating the extent and severity of CAD and in deciding whether a patient should have coronary arteriography. Early positive result (stage I, II) with or without hypotension suggests more extensive CAD and is an indication for coronary angiography.

At the other end of the spectrum, patients with no cardiac risk factors and atypical nonanginal chest pain may not need further testing. If there is still uncertainty, a negative exercise ECG may be useful for reassurance. A positive result is more likely false positive. The majority of patients have intermediate likelihood of coronary artery disease, for example, a young patient with typical angina or elderly men with atypical chest pain. Exercise ECG is most useful in this group. A positive result increases, and a negative result decreases, significantly the likelihood of CAD.

The decision to use radionuclide imaging with exercise ECG should be balanced by the benefit of additional information and relative costs of procedures. Table 4 outlines some indications for exercise–thallium imaging in patients with chest pain. Exercise ECG is associated with a high false-positive rate in women. Exercise–thallium imaging is more useful in

TABLE 3.   List of Diagnostic Studies

Angina
  Resting ECG
  Exercise ECG
    Thallium imaging
    Radionuclide angiography
    Echocardiography
  Pharmacologic stress
    Dipyridamole/adenosine thallium imaging
    Dipyridamole echocardiography
    Dobutamine radionuclide angiography
    Dobutamine echocardiography
  Atrial pacing ECG
    Thallium imaging
    Radionuclide angiography
  Coronary angiography
Myocardial infarction
  Resting ECG
  Cardiac enzymes
  Infarct-avid imaging (^{99}Tc-pyrophosphate)
Mitral valve prolapse
  Echocardiography
Aortic valve disease, hypertrophic cardiomyopathy
  Echocardiography
Pericarditis
  Resting ECG
  Echocardiography
Aortic dissection/aneurysm
  Chest radiograph
  Transesophageal echocardiography
  Contrast computerized tomography of chest
  Magnetic resonance imaging
  Aortography
Pulmonary embolism
  Arterial blood gases
  Chest radiograph
  Ventilation-perfusion scan
  Pulmonary angiography
Esophageal spasm/reflux
  Upper endoscopy
  Barium esophagogram
  Esophageal motility study
  24-hour Ph study
  Bernstein test

this group. Which radionuclide test to choose (thallium imaging versus radionuclide angiography) depends on the availability of the test, the expertise of nuclear laboratory, and individual clinical situation. Thallium imaging is

TABLE 4.   Indications for Exercise–Thallium Imaging for the Diagnosis of CAD in Patients with Chest Pain

- Baseline ECG abnormalities (digitalis, left ventricular hypertrophy, hyperventilation changes, left bundle branch blocks, mitral valve prolapse, ventricular pre-excitation)
- Nondiagnostic exercise ECG response (submaximal stress) with chest pain
- Positive exercise ECGs in patients with a low pretest probability of CAD
- Negative exercise ECGs in patients with a high pretest probability of CAD

more preferable in patients with atrial and ventricular arrhythmias or valvular heart disease. Radionuclide angiography may be more preferable if left ventricular (LV) function needs to be assessed for clinical purpose. If patients are unable to exercise adequately, pharmacologic stress tests or atrial pacing tests are acceptable alternatives.

Because of inherent risks and high costs, coronary angiography is usually not the first diagnostic test. If a patient has a high probability of CAD or has disabling symptoms or unstable angina, one may proceed directly to coronary angiography without initial noninvasive testing.

The diagnosis of acute myocardial infarction is usually made on the basis of history, physical exam, serial ECG, and cardiac enzymes. In the era of thrombolytic therapy for acute myocardial infarction, aortic dissection must be excluded because lytic therapy can lead to disastrous consequences. If clinical suspicion for aortic dissection is high (tearing chest/back pain, pulse deficit, blood pressure difference, diastolic murmur, widened mechastinum), one should proceed directly to aortography for definitive diagnosis and immediate therapy. If clinical presentation is not consistent and patient is stable, other noninvasive techniques can be used. Pericarditis can be very difficult to differentiate from unstable angina in patients with recent myocardial infarction. An audible rub and diffuse ST-T wave abnormalities are helpful clues. Coronary angiography is often indicated in equivocal cases.

The key to diagnosis of pulmonary embolism is a high index of suspicion. One must recognize the predisposing factors (immobility, thrombophlebitis, heart failure), especially when shortness of breath is the predominant symptom. Arterial blood gases and chest radiograph are useful initial screening tests, followed by perfusion scan. A normal perfusion scan is useful in excluding the diagnosis, and a high probability V/Q scan in patients with high pretest likelihood is helpful in confirming the diagnosis. If clinical suspicion is high but lung scans are of low or intermediate probability, pulmonary angiography should be considered. An abnormal venous Doppler, impedance plethysmogram, or venogram may provide useful information in patients with symptoms of pulmonary embolism but low or intermediate probability lung scan. Anticoagulation may be initiated for deep venous thrombosis without need for angiography.

REFERENCES

1. Adams R, Martin J. Pain. In: Petersdorf R., et al., eds. Harrison's principle of internal medicine. 10th ed. New York: McGraw Hill, 1983:7–12.
2. Karliner J. Stable angina pectoris. In: Parmley W, Chatterjee K, eds. Cardiology. Philadelphia: JB Lippincott, 1987:4:1–17.
3. Maseri A. Clinical syndrome of angina pectoris. Hosp Pract 1989; 24:65–80.
4. Kubler W, Opherk D, Tillmanns H. Syndrome X: diagnostic criteria and long-term prognosis. Can J Cardiol 1986;8 (Suppl-A):219–20A.
5. Wigle ED. Hypertrophic cardiomyopathy 1988. Mod Concepts Cardiovasc Dis 1988; 57:1–6.
6. Dunn FG, Pringle SD. Left ventricular hypertrophy and myocardial ischemia in systemic hypertension. Am J Cardiol 1987;60 (Suppl):19–22I.
7. Selzer A. Changing aspects of the natural history of valvular aortic stenosis. New Engl J Med 1987;317:91–8.
8. Faruqui AMA, Maaloy WC, Felner JM, et al. Symptomatic myocardial bridging of coronary artery. Am J Cardiol 1978;41:1305–10.
9. Spodick DH. The normal and diseased pericardium. J Am Coll Cardiol 1983;1:240–6.
10. DeSanctis RW, Doroghazi RM, Austin G, Buckley MJ. Aortic dissection. New Engl J Med 1987;317:1060–7.
11. Hirsh J, Hull R, Raskob G. Diagnosis of pulmonary embolism. J Am Coll Cardiol 1986;8:128–36B.
12. Braunwald E. The history. In: Braunwald E, ed. Heart disease. Philadelphia: WB Saunders, 1988:1–6.
13. VanDohlen TW, Rogers WB, Frank MJ. Pathophysiology and management of unstable angina. Clin Cardiol 1989;12:363–9.
14. Lavie CJ, Gersh BJ. Acute myocardial infarction: initial manifestations, management and prognosis. Mayo Clin Proc 1990;65:531–48.
15. Isner JM, Estes NAM, Thompson PO, et al. Acute cardiac events temporally related to cocaine abuse. N Engl J Med 1986;315:1438–43.
16. Shah P. Mitral valve prolapse syndrome. In: Parmley W, Chatterjee K, eds. Cardiology. Philadelphia: JB Lippincott, 1987:32:1–12.
17. Katz PO, Dalton CB, Richter JE, Wu WC, Castell DO. Esophageal testing of patients with non-cardiac-chest pain and dysphagia. Ann Intern Med 1987;106:593–7.
18. Chatterjee K. Bedside evaluation of the heart: physical exam. In: Parmley W, Chatterjee K, eds. Cardiology. Philadelphia: JB Lippincott, 1987: chap 31:1–55.
19. Dell'Halia LJ, O'Rourke RA. Evaluation of patients with signs and symptoms of ischemic heart disease. In: Parmley W, Chatterjee K, eds. Cardiology. Philadelphia: JB Lippincott, 1987: chap 3:1–19.
20. Iskandrian AS, Hakki A-H. Thallium-201 myocardial scintigraphy. Am Heart J 1985;109:113–29.
21. Iskandrian AS, Heo J, Askenase A, et al. Dipyridamole cardiac imaging. Am Heart J 1988;115:432–43.

CHOLESTASIS

ALEX H. BRUCKSTEIN

SYNONYMS: Impaired Bile Flow, Impaired Bile Formation, Excess of Biliary Substances in the Blood

BACKGROUND

Definition

The hallmark of cholestasis is impaired bile formation. A characteristic group of morphologic, physiologic, and clinical features have been described that represent various aspects of this primary underlying defect. Thus, morphologically, bile can be identified in the canalicular space of pericentral hepatocytes in liver biopsy specimens, and dilatation of the canaliculae and effacement of canalicular microvillae can be seen on ultrastructural examination. Pathophysiologically, reduction in excretion of organic and inorganic solutes and water can be measured. Clinically, cholestasis can be detected as the appearance in the blood of substances such as bile acids, bilirubin, and cholesterol, that should normally be excreted into the bile. Biochemically, cholestasis is described as an elevation in serum alkaline phosphatase activity, occasionally with an elevation of bilirubin, relative to serum aminotransferase elevations.

Biochemical Definition

Alkaline Phosphatase

The enzyme alkaline phosphatase is found primarily in liver and bone, with smaller amounts in kidney, placenta, intestine, and leukocytes. In healthy adults, the measured serum alkaline phosphatase is an approximately equal mixture of liver and bone isoenzyme. When skeletal alkaline phosphatase is elevated, it is related to osteoclastic activity, that is, new bone growth. Thus, it is commonly elevated in normal production of bone, that is, growing children, and in pathologic bone growth, for example, Paget's disease. On the other hand, skeletal alkaline phosphatase is generally not elevated in osteoclastic conditions, that is, lytic disease, such as multiple myeloma. In the later stages of pregnancy, the placental contribution may be substantial and serum alkaline phosphatase activity may be increased.

Biliary Substances

The substances usually excreted in the bile rise in the serum during cholestasis. Thus, bilirubin (mainly the conjugated form) and cholesterol rise, and their elevation can be measured in the routine lab. The bile acid level in the serum is raised, but this cannot be measured except in a few research labs.

Other Enzymes

In the setting of cholestasis, the activity of several serum enzymes, exemplified by alkaline phosphatase, is increased. This includes gamma-glutamyl transferase (GGT), leucine aminopeptidase, and 5′-nucleotidase, the activity of which is independent of bone production. (The latter two may increase during pregnancy.)

Is It Cholestasis or Jaundice?

Although physicians often use *cholestasis* and *jaundice* interchangeably, the terms refer to different aspects of pathophysiology. Thus, cholestasis indicates interference with the flow of bile into the duodenum, often associated with jaundice. Since the mechanism with which the liver metabolizes bile salts—conjugation with taurine and glycine—is different from the mechanism with which the liver metabolizes bilirubin—glucuronidation[1]—cholestasis can occur without jaundice and vice versa. As such, when the pathology involves only part of the liver (e.g., primary biliary cirrhosis in the early stage or hepatic metastases), cholestasis may be present (a high serum alkaline phosphatase) without jaundice. On the other hand, hyperbilirubinemia, clinically manifest as jaundice, without elevation of serum alkaline phosphatase, does not make a diagnosis of cholestasis. As such, the familiar defects of bilirubin transport (Gilbert's disease, Crigler-Najjar, Dubin-Johnson, and Rotor's syndromes) and the hemolytic diseases with jaundice are not cholestatic syndromes. (Also see chapter on Jaundice in *Difficult Diagnosis I*.)

Etiology

The impairment of bile flow may start at any point from the liver cell canaliculus to the ampulla of Vater. Thus, cholestasis can be characterized as either a functional defect in bile formation at the level of the hepatocyte (intrahepatic cholestasis) or an obstruction to bile flow within the biliary tract (extrahepatic cholestasis). The most common intrahepatic causes are viral or other forms of hepatitis, drugs, and alcoholic liver disease (see Table 1). Less common etiologies include primary biliary cirrhosis, cholestasis of pregnancy, metastatic carcinoma, pericholangitis secondary to ulcerative colitis, and numerous other disorders. Extrahepatic cholestasis is most often due to a common bile duct stone or to a pancreatic neoplasm. Less often, benign strictures of the common duct (usually related to prior surgery), ductal carcinoma, pancreatitis, or pancreatic pseudocyst are causes. The relevance of distinguishing between intrahepatic and extrahepatic etiologies of cholestasis is reflected in the differing diagnostic approach (as will be discussed) and management of patients with these different processes.

Pathophysiology

Cholestasis reflects bile secretory failure. The mechanisms of this are complex, even in the setting of extrahepatic mechanical obstruction. Contributing factors may include impaired activity of Na^+, K^+–ATPase (ATPase = adenosinetriphosphatase), which is necessary for canalicular bile flow; enhanced ductular reabsorption of bile constitu-

ents; interference with microsomal hydroxylating enzymes, which leads to the formation of poorly soluble bile salts; and interference with the function of microfilaments, thought to be important for canalicular function.

The pathophysiologic result of cholestasis reflects backup of bile constituents into the systemic circulation and their failure to enter the intestine for excretion. Bile salts, bilirubin, and lipids are the most important constituents affected. Since bile salts are needed for the absorption of vitamin K and fat, impairment in the excretion of bile salts can result in hypoprothrombinemia and steatorrhea. If the cholestasis persists, the concomitant malabsorption of calcium and vitamin D will eventually result in osteomalacia or osteoporosis. The retention of bilirubin results in hyperbilirubinemia with spillover of conjugated bilirubin into the urine; the stools will become pale because less bilirubin reaches the intestine. The retention of phospholipid and cholesterol produces hyperlipidemia.

HISTORY

Symptoms

Pruritus is the most frequent clinical manifestation of cholestasis. High levels of circulating bile salts are traditionally felt to be the etiology of the pruritus,[2] but the correlation with bile salt level is poor[3] and the pathogenesis of the pruritus remains unclear.[4,5]

In many patients, jaundice, dark urine, and pale stools are the other clinical hallmarks of cholestasis. However, as mentioned, patients can have cholestasis without jaundice, or they may have jaundice without cholestasis.

Many patients who present for evaluation of cholestasis will be asymptomatic, their cholestasis having been detected on a routine chemical analysis of the blood in which an isolated elevation of serum alkaline phosphatase was detected.

Focused Queries

The medical history should be focused on the following questions.

1. *Are you taking any drugs?* A wide variety of drugs have been reported to result in an elevation of serum alkaline phosphatase (Table 2). Obviously, only a small percentage of patients taking any of the drugs listed will

TABLE 1. Cholestatic Syndromes

INTRAHEPATIC	EXTRAHEPATIC
Acute hepatocellular injury	Pancreatic carcinoma
Viral hepatitis	Choledocholithiasis
Drug-induced	Bile duct stricture
Alcoholic hepatitis	Pancreatitis
Chronic hepatocellular injury	Periampullary carcinoma
Drug-induced	Biliary atresia
Chronic hepatitis	
Primary biliary cirrhosis	
Sclerosing cholangitis	
Postoperative state	
Parenteral hyperalimentation	

TABLE 2.   Drugs That Cause Elevated Alkaline Phosphatase Values

Chlorpromazine
Erythromycin
Phenytoin
Estrogens
Methyldopa
Oxacillin
Androgenic steroids

have an elevation of serum alkaline phosphatase. Additionally, some of the drugs may have a cholestatic as well as hepatotoxic effect, as indicated by elevation of aminotransferase levels.[6,7]

2. *Do you consume alcohol? If so, how much?* Patients who have stable, chronic liver disease may have no other biochemical abnormality except for an elevation of serum alkaline phosphatase activity.

3. *Have you traveled to areas of poor sanitation where infections such as amebiasis or hepatitis are prevalent?* Some forms of hepatitis may present with cholestasis without jaundice.

4. *Have you ever been diagnosed as having inflammatory bowel disease or malignancy? Other associated diseases?* Sclerosing cholangitis is a form of cholestasis that is associated with inflammatory bowel disease and that may present before the inflammatory bowel disease is apparent.[8]

5. *Have you ever received a blood transfusion or blood products? Have you been refused as a blood donor?*

PHYSICAL EXAMINATION

In the setting of an asymptomatic, isolated elevation of the alkaline phosphatase, the "routine" physical examination will generally be unable to help in determining the etiology of the cholestasis. However, when cholestasis has been present for an extended period of time, it may be associated with muddy skin pigmentation, a bleeding diathesis, bone pain, excoriations from pruritus, and cutaneous lipid deposits (xanthomas or xanthelasma). These physical findings are independent of the etiology of the cholestasis. Any systemic symptoms (e.g., fever, anorexia, vomiting), abdominal pain, or additional physical findings reflect the underlying etiology rather than the cholestasis itself and thus will provide a valuable etiologic clue.

DIAGNOSTIC STUDIES

Chemical Analysis (see Table 3)

Routine laboratory studies are of limited diagnostic value. The most common abnormality is a serum alkaline phosphatase level that is disproportionately elevated in relation to the serum aminotransferase activity. (Also see chapter on Alkaline Phosphatase Value, Elevated in *Difficult Diagnosis I.*) Most patients who have cholestasis will have elevation of serum bilirubin levels. An elevated serum bilirubin level reflects the severity but not the etiology of the cholestasis, and fractionation of the bilirubin will not assist in distinguishing intrahepatic from extrahepatic cholestasis. As mentioned, aminotransferase levels depend on the underlying etiology but are generally only modestly elevated. A significant elevation in serum aminotransferase level suggests a hepatocellular process but is occasionally seen in extrahepatic cholestasis, especially in the setting of acute obstruction due to choledocholithiasis. An elevated serum amylase level generally favors extrahepatic cholestasis. Following the administration of vitamin K, an improved prothrombin time favors an extrahepatic obstructive process, although occasionally hepatocellular disorders will respond to vitamin K therapy. The presence of an antimitochondrial antibody strongly favors primary biliary cirrhosis as the etiology of the cholestasis. This blood test must be ordered in

TABLE 3.   Differentiation of Extrahepatic from Hepatocellular Cholestasis

LABORATORY STUDY	EXTRAHEPATIC	HEPATOCELLULAR
Serum alkaline phosphatase	Significantly elevated	Mildly elevated
Serum aminotransferase	Mildly elevated	Significantly elevated
Serum cholesterol	Elevated	Decreased
Serum bile acids	Significantly elevated	Mildly elevated
Steatorrhea	Common	Rare
Response of prothrombin time to intramuscular vitamin K	Common	Rare

any middle-aged woman presenting with an asymptomatic elevation of alkaline phosphatase.[9]

Imaging Studies

There are noninvasive, as well as invasive, methods to image the biliary tract. At present, abdominal ultrasound and computerized tomography (CT) scanning have virtually done away with oral cholecystography in the evaluation of patients with cholestasis. The advantage of ultrasound is that it is cheaper, quicker, and more widely available than CT and is generally the first study for the evaluation of cholestasis. However, both ultrasound and CT are noninvasive and reliably demonstrate bile duct dilatation, which implies extrahepatic obstruction. However, the absence of this sign does not indicate intrahepatic cholestasis, especially in the setting of an acute process. The underlying etiology of the cholestasis may also be revealed; in general, gallstones are more reliably demonstrated with ultrasound analysis and pancreatic pathology more reliably demonstrated by CT.[10]

The more invasive procedures include percutaneous transhepatic cholangiography (PTC) and endoscopic retrograde cholangiopancreatography (ERCP). These procedures require specialized expertise and involve risk to the patient. These procedures are especially useful preoperatively to define extrahepatic obstruction.[9] Both have the advantage in that they can be used as part of the therapy of extrahepatic disease, such that a stent can be passed either transhepatically or via ERCP to aid in the drainage of an obstructed biliary system.

Liver biopsy is the invasive study that is useful in the diagnosis of intrahepatic cholestasis. It is safe in most conditions, but it should not be performed unless an ultrasound or CT scan shows that the bile ducts are not dilated, thus indicating that there is no evidence of increased intrahepatic pressure from extrahepatic obstruction.

ASSESSMENT

As in so many other medical conditions, cholestasis can be properly evaluated with a thorough history and physical examination and the judicious use of laboratory tests. The physician should avoid substituting an overreliance on laboratory data for inadequate clinical judgment.[11] In the setting of an isolated elevation of serum alkaline phosphatase, the first issue is to determine whether the source of the alkaline phosphatase is from a hepatobiliary process, reflecting cholestasis, or whether the source is bone. Table 4 outlines the approach. In a young patient, who is still growing, it is likely that it is skeletal alkaline phosphatase.

Determining the Site of Blockage

The first issue in most patients who have cholestasis will be to attempt to determine whether it is intrahepatic or extrahepatic (see Table 3).

Intrahepatic Cholestasis

Features in the history and physical examination that suggest this diagnosis include: (1) age younger than 40 (drug and viral hepatitis are most likely in this age group), (2) history of drug addiction or homosexuality (high risk for transmission of viral hepatitis B), (3) history of alcohol use or recent therapy with any of the medications outlined in Table 2 (recall that athletes may be receiving "steroids" but may not consider this as medicine), and (4) a physical finding of hepatomegaly (generally indicates a lesion within the liver; if tender, most likely is alcoholic hepatitis, whereas if nontender, most likely is malignancy).

Extrahepatic Cholestasis

Features in the history and physical examination that suggest this diagnosis include: (1) age above 40 (in males, the obstruction is most likely due to malignancy, whereas in females it is due to choledocholithiasis or malignancy), (2) a history of shaking chills and/or right up-

---

TABLE 4. Step Approach to the Asymptomatic Elevation of Alkaline Phosphatase

1. Is patient under 20?
   Yes. Skeletal growth is likely source of elevated alkaline phosphatase. Confirm with normal bilirubin, normal GGT, and elevation of skeletal fraction of alkaline phosphatase isoenzymes.
2. If no, is patient taking any medications? (See Table 2.)
   Yes. Discontinue all medications and repeat alkaline phosphatase determination after the drug-free trial period.
3. If no, is GGT elevated?
   Yes. Patient has cholestasis. Proceed to evaluate for etiology. (See algorithm.)
4. If no, obtain bone scan, skeletal survey, or parathyroid hormone assay.

DIAGNOSTIC ASSESSMENT OF THE PATIENT WITH CHOLESTASIS

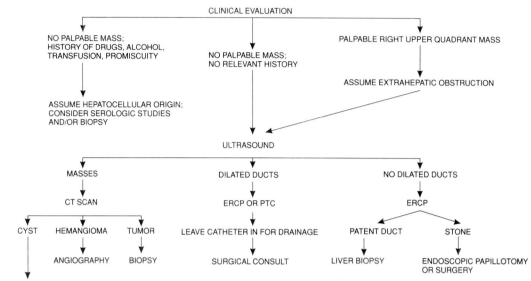

?NEEDLE ASPIRATION FOR DIAGNOSIS/THERAPY

per quadrant pain (suggests cholangitis or choledocholithiasis), (3) a history of acholic stools persisting for two weeks (indicates that bile is unable to enter the intestine), and (4) a palpable gallbladder (Courvoisier's law—almost pathognomonic of common bile duct obstruction, generally malignant).

Except for the patients who present with suppurative cholangitis, cholestasis is not an emergency. The approach to the diagnosis (see the algorithm) should be based on thorough clinical evaluation plus the judicious use of the locally available specialized studies. Thus, if the diagnosis is initially unclear, abdominal ultrasound should be the first study obtained.[12] If this shows dilated bile ducts, especially in a patient with progressive rise in serum alkaline phosphatase, mechanical obstruction is reasonably likely. Further delineation of the exact etiology of the extrahepatic mechanical obstruction can be done with direct cholangiography (ERCP or transhepatic).[13] If bile duct dilatation is not seen on ultrasound exam, an intrahepatic process is highly likely, and a liver biopsy should be the test to help make the diagnosis.

REFERENCES

1. Tiribelli C, Ostrow JD. New concepts in bilirubin chemistry, transport and metabolism: report of the International Bilirubin Workshop April 6–8, 1989, Trieste, Italy. Hepatology 1990;11:303–13.

2. Schonfeld LJ, Sjovall J, Perman E. Bile acids on the skin of patients with pruritic hepato-biliary disease. Nature 1976;213:93–4.

3. Freedman MR, Holzbach RT, Ferguson DR. Pruritus in cholestasis: no direct causative role for bile acid retention. Am J Med 1981;70:1011–6.

4. Gittlen SD, Schulman ES, Maddrey WC. Raised histamine concentrations in chronic cholestatic liver disease. Gut 1990;31:96–9.

5. Jones EA, Bergasa NV. Hypothesis. The pruritus of cholestasis: from bile acids to opiate antagonists. Hepatology 1990;11:884–7.

6. Kaplowitz N, Aw TY, Simon FR, Stolz A. Drug induced hepatotoxicity. Ann Intern Med 1986;104:826–39.

7. Bass NM, Ockner RK. Drug-induced liver disease. In: Zakim D, Boyer T, eds. Hepatology: a textbook of liver disease. 2nd ed. Philadelphia: WB Saunders, 1990:754–91.

8. Rabinovitz M, Gavaler JS, Schade RR, Dindzans VJ, Chien M, Van Thiel DH. Does primary sclerosing cholangitis occurring in association with inflammatory bowel disease differ from that occurring in the absence of inflammatory bowel disease? A study of sixty-six subjects. Hepatology 1990;11:7–11.

9. Chopra S, Griffin PH. Laboratory tests and diagnostic procedures in evaluation of liver disease. Am J Med 1985;79:221–9.

10. Balthazar E, Chako AC. Computed tomography of pancreatic masses. Am J Gastroenterol 1990;85:343–9.

11. Scharschmidt BF, Goldberg HI, Schmid R. Approach to the patient with cholestatic jaundice. N Engl J Med 1983;308:1515–9.

12. Olen R, Pickleman J, Freeark RJ. Less is better: the diagnostic workup of the patient with obstructive jaundice. Arch Surg 1989;124:791–4.

13. Richter JM, Silverstein MD, Schapiro R. Suspected obstructive jaundice: a decision analysis of diagnostic strategies. Ann Intern Med 1983;99:46–51.

CLUBBING

TIMOTHY R. AKSAMIT, SCOTT D. NYGAARD, and ROBERT B. FICK, JR.

SYNONYMS: Parrot Beak Nails, Hippocratic Fingers, Pachyonychia (literal *pachys* [thick], + *onych* [nail]), Acropachy (as with the entity thyroid acropachy), Acropathy

BACKGROUND

Clubbing refers to a bulbous, fusiform enlargement of the distal portion of the digits. It is a painless uniform swelling of the soft tissues of the terminal phalanx of a digit, most commonly identified clinically by disappearance of the hyponychial angle (see Physical Examination below and Fig. 1*A*). Another simple method measuring two circumferences (at the nailbed and digital interphalangeal joint) with creation of a ''digital index'' (Fig. 1*B*) also claims excellent reliability in distinguishing clubbed patients from normal controls with little interobserver variation.[1] Usually insidious in onset, clubbing has been documented to occur as rapidly as over a 10-day period of time.

Hereditary clubbing (autosomal dominant) or simple familial enlargement of the ends of fingers and toes occurs during childhood. In some individuals, hereditary clubbing may represent an incomplete expression of pachydermoperiostosis. Three additional distinct clinical categories of clubbing exist: *acquired secondary clubbing, clubbing with hypertrophic osteoarthropathy (HOA)*, and *pachydermoperiostosis*. Pulmonary HOA is a syndrome composed of clubbing, arthralgia, and periostitis of distal long bones. Periostitis is a well-known radiographic feature of HOA and is often associated with periarticular demineralization, as well as the classic irregular osseous proliferation. Periosteal spicules result from abnormal deposition of periosteal bone (''periostosis''). HOA is associated with a great number of diseases, including disorders of the respiratory, cardiovascular, and gastrointestinal systems (Table 1). Acquired secondary clubbing, with and without hypertrophic osteoarthropathy, is discussed in another section (see Assessment). Pachydermoperiostosis is a relatively rare disorder often clinically confused with acromegaly. The digital changes often begin around puberty in this insidiously progressive disease characterized by cylindric thickening of the legs and forearms (pachyderma), spadelike enlargement of digits (clubbing), and hyperkeratosis of the palms and soles. Seborrhea, bone periostosis, arthralgias, and acro-osteolysis also have a variable occurrence in this nondominant autosomal disease.[2]

Historical Background

Because of the poorly understood mechanism of clubbing and the association of this physical finding with many serious constitutional disorders (see Assessment), this disorder has intrigued physicians since the time of Hippocrates. Indeed, Hippocrates (460–375 B.C.) is credited with the first recorded description of these nail changes in a patient with empyema. During the second half of the nineteenth century, pachydermoperiostosis and HOA were described. In 1915, it was suggested[3] that HOA was invariably associated with clubbing and that clubbing was simply an early stage of HOA. Clubbing and HOA have many causes in common (Table 1), and this view found wide acceptance over the next 40 years. However, it has been recognized that HOA may rarely occur without clubbing.[4]

Etiology

It is remarkable that such a common physical sign that has attracted medical attention over a span of 2000 years should still be so poorly understood. Even though clubbing and HOA continue to arouse the curiosity of medical students, experienced clinicians, and investigators alike, the etiology and the pathogenesis of these familiar disorders remain elusive. It is clear that hypoxemia and hypercapnea do not provide an explanation. Several hypotheses are widely discussed and are re-

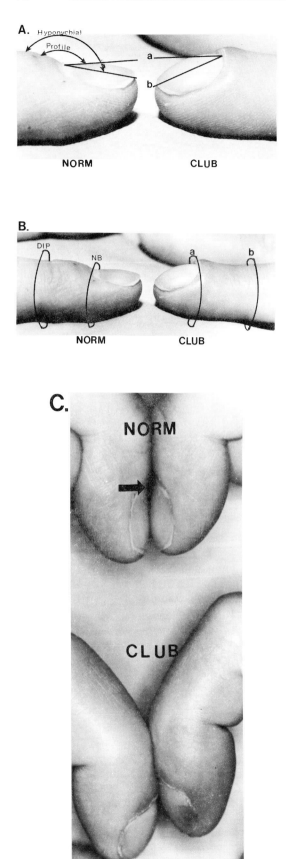

lated to vasodilators and local arterial pulse pressure, activation of nerve reflexes, and hormonal theories. Each in turn will be briefly reviewed below.

Vasodilation

It has been observed that there is an increase in the volume of the clubbed phalanx due to increased vascular flow and connective tissue proliferation. The occurrence of clubbing when an anatomic right to left shunt is the only lesion suggests that a vasodilator substance may bypass the lungs and reach the extremities unchanged. Additionally, the digital microvasculature appears to be uniquely sensitive to vasodilators. The fact that high levels of a vasodilatory prostenoid (PGE_2) have been described in conditions known to be associated with clubbing such as inflammatory bowel disease, lung malignancies, and cystic fibrosis[5] has provided indirect support for this theory. An additional example, ferritin, normally oxidized in healthy lungs, is known to inhibit the vasoconstrictor effect of catecholamines and may therefore act as a vasodilatory substance. Other pathogenic agents include the vasodilators bradykinin and adenine nucleotides, which are usually inactivated by passage through the lung.

Neural Mechanism

Regression of clubbing after vagotomy suggests a nerve reflex etiology to some clinical investigators. This is largely anecdotal, yet the theory holds that an impulse originating in the diseased organ moves by a vagal afferent and on an undetermined efferent route to cause reflex vasodilatation.[4] Appealing, yet unproved, intermediates include the neuropeptides substance P and vasoactive intestinal peptide. These substances have potent vaso-

FIGURE 1. Bulbous fusiform enlargement of the distal portion of the fingers referred to as clubbing. Three clinically useful methods of identification and measurement. In each panel, normal (*NORM*) is pictured on the *left* for comparison, and a clubbed phalanx (*CLUB*) is shown on the *right*. *A* provides measurements used in identifying loss of the hyponychial angle and the profile angle. A hyponychial angle greater than 195 degrees is compatible with a clubbed digit. The profile angle is drawn from the cuticle through the point where the lunula ends (nail plate begins). An angle greater than 160 degrees is compatible with a clubbed digit. *B* provides an example calculating the digital index, the sum of the 10 ratios of the circumferences at the nail bed (*NB*) and at the distal interphalangeal joint (*DIP*). In generalized clubbing, the sum of "a/b" will exceed 10. Panel *C* (*CLUB*) displays Schamroth's sign. The *arrow* indicates the diamond-shaped area that exists in normals.

TABLE 1.   Clubbing and Hypertrophic Osteoarthropathy

	REFERENCE
Primary—hereditary	
Clubbing	Medicine 1964;43:459
Hereditary, autosomal dominant	Chest 1985;88:627–8
Pachydermoperiostosis	Semin Arthritis Rheum 1988;17:156
Secondary	
Intrathoracic	
Non–small cell bronchogenic carcinoma	Semin Arthritis Rheum 1982;12:220
Pulmonary metastases from sarcomas; nasopharyngeal, uterine/cervical, esophageal, breast, stomach, kidney, prostate, and thyroid carcinomas	South Med J 1987;80:383
Pulmonary pseudotumor	Chest 1984;85:837
Lymphoma	JAMA 1977;238:1400
Benign (less commonly malignant) tumors of the pleura	Am J Surg Pathol 1989;13:620
Bronchiectasis	JAMA 1954;155:1459
Cystic fibrosis	Am J Med 1987;82:871
Tuberculosis	Thorax 1987;42:986
Emphysema	Surg Gynecol Obstet 1935;61:312
Sarcoidosis	JAMA 1981;246:1338
Asbestosis	Thorax 1987;42:117
Silicosis	S Afr Med J 1988;73:128
Interstitial pulmonary fibrosis	Chest 1985;88:84
Cardiovascular	
Arteriovenous malformation	Am Fam Physician 1988;38:187–91
Cyanotic congenital heart disease	Arthritis Rheum 1982;25:1186
Patent ductus arteriosus	Arch Intern Med 1963;111:346
Aortic aneurysm	Arch Intern Med 1965;98:700
Bacterial endocarditis	Ann Intern Med 1977;87:754
Infected vascular graft	Rev Infect Dis 1987;9:376
Takayasu's arteritis	Clin Exp Rheumatol 1988;6:329
Trauma	Br Med J 1988;297:1635
Gastrointestinal	
Inflammatory bowel disease	Br Med J 1979;2:825
Chronic active hepatitis	Am J Med 1979;67:88
Carcinoma of the colon	Medicine 1942;21:269
Achalasia	Am J Med 1986;81:355
Primary biliary cirrhosis	Gut 1967;22:2031
Biliary atresia	Pediatr Radiol 1983;13:44
Alcoholic liver disease	Arthritis Rheum 1969;12:261
Hepatocellular carcinoma	Gastroenterology 1972;63:340
Liver transplantation	Am J Med 1989;86:501
Laxative abuse	Br Med J 1981;282:1836
Other	
Laxative abuse	South Med J 1983;76:1071–2
Pregnancy	Ann Intern Med 1969;71:577
Nasopharyngeal carcinoma	Pediatr Radiol 1988;18:339
Heroin abuse	NEJM 1984;311:262
Hereditary hemorrhagic telangiectasia	Am J Med Sci 1988;295:545–7
Central nervous system tuberculoma	Indian J Pediatr 1988;55:304
Thyroid acropachy	Med Clin North Am 1968;52:393

dilatory, vasopermeable, and phlogogenic actions.[6]

Hormonal Theories

The final widely discussed postulated mechanism is that a hormonal substance(s) bypasses lung detoxification (as in the vasodilatory theory above) or gains direct access to systemic circulation. Early claims to the contrary, growth hormone has not been confirmed as an etiologic agent; however, gastrin and increased estradiol levels have been incriminated more recently. The most widely discussed theory is that of Dickinson and Martin,[7] which holds that finger clubbing in patients with respiratory disease may be initiated by platelet-derived growth factor (PDGF). It is theorized that PDGF may be released in digital arteries from megakaryocytes or platelet aggregates. PDGF has a growth promoting activity, increases vascular permeability, and has chemotactic effects. These authors argue that clubbing is an overgrowth of tissue and that a growth stimulating factor is more likely than is a vasodilator causing a simple increase in digital vascular volume.

HISTORY

The medical history may be helpful when attempting to ascertain the etiology of clubbing, although the majority of patients are asymptomatic with regard to the process of clubbing. The number of associated conditions is extensive (Tables 1 and 2), and it must be emphasized that clubbing may be the first early sign of a serious underlying disorder. It is helpful to think of clubbing as occurring in four distinct clinical categories[8]:

1. Acquired secondary clubbing.
2. Clubbing with HOA.
3. Pachydermoperiostosis.
4. Hereditary clubbing.

The importance of these distinctions is that the process of acquired clubbing with or without HOA is invariably associated with an underlying cardiac, pulmonary, gastrointestinal, or other condition (Table 1), which then may be identified early as a result of clubbing manifestation serving as a harbinger. The course of onset of clubbing without HOA is often gradual and painless. There is no family history, associated painful periostitis, or arthralgias. Clubbing associated with HOA[9] also occurs as the result of an underlying condition; however, there is an associated proliferative periostitis of the long bones and polyarticular arthritis (Table 1). This usually is symmetric and most commonly involves the ulna, radius, femur, tibia, fibula, metacarpals, and metatarsals. The joints most frequently involved are the knees, ankles, and wrists.

The third form of clubbing, pachydermoperiostosis, is a hereditary sex-linked condition that has a bimodal distribution with regard to time of onset. There is an initial peak in the first year of life, with a second peak occurring near puberty. This is a progressive disease with associated joint effusions and

skin abnormalities.[2,10] Lastly, hereditary clubbing, which affects both sexes equally, is inherited in an autosomal dominant pattern with variable penetrance. This form of clubbing is typically asymptomatic and symmetric (Table 1) and is associated with a normal life span.

Thus, the medical record should indicate reflection on the presence of these conditions associated with clubbing as noted above and in Tables 1 and 2. There should also be a thorough search for symptoms of long bone pain suggesting active periostitis.

Focused Queries

1. *Is there a history of primary lung cancer or other malignancy?*
2. *Are there any underlying pulmonary conditions such as cystic fibrosis, bronchiectasis, empyema, or tuberculosis?*
3. *Has there been exposure to silica or asbestos?*
4. *Is there a family history of clubbing?*

PHYSICAL EXAMINATION

The primary physical finding in clubbing is a swelling of the fingertips secondary to proliferation of soft tissue at the base of the nail. This proliferation of tissue secondarily causes obliteration of the normal angle between the nail base and the surface of the distal phalanx (Fig. 1A). In examining the nail and nail bed, the first step is to observe the skin surrounding the cuticle. Commonly, there are changes in color and texture of the skin at the base of the nail. The skin is usually shiny, flushed, and smooth, with less of the normal skin lines around the nail bed. The patient may describe this area as "itchy." There is also increased mobility of the nail plate on the nail bed, demonstrated by applying pressure to the proximal nail just beyond the cuticle and noting it is easily compressible on the underlying spongy tissues.

However, the objective finding of clubbing has been described as a change in the angle of the nail plate with regard to some other portion of the proximal fingertip. Lovibond's angle (profile angle), the angle between the nail plate and the proximal portion of the phalanx, is diagnostic of clubbing when greater than 160 degrees[11] (Fig. 1A). In a study by Regan et al.,[12] however, the hyponychial angle, the angle between the distal phalanx and a line drawn from the cuticle to the hyponychium,

TABLE 2.   Unilateral Clubbing

	REFERENCE
Pancoast's tumor nerve infiltration	Br J Dis Chest 1981;75:121
Vascular graft, infected	South Med J 1988;81:788–91
Trauma	ROEFO 1983;138:219–24
Aortoenteric fistula	Mo Med 1983;80:304–8. Rev Infect Dis 1987;9(2):376–81
Chronic venous stasis	Radiology 1960;74:279–88
Arteriovenous fistula	JAMA 1978;240:142–3
Subclavian stenosis	J R Army Med Corps 1973;119:81–5

was a better indicator of clubbing than the profile angle. A hyponychial angle greater than 195 degrees is defined as clubbing. This angle can most accurately be assessed from a shadowgram, made by projecting the lateral profile of a fingertip onto a screen and tracing the outline.[13]

Another method of assessing the presence of clubbing is the phalangeal depth ratio. This method determines a ratio of the distal phalangeal depth (DPD) to the interphalangeal depth (IPD)—DPD:IPD. This is the most objective criterion because it is independent of age, sex, and race.[14] In normal individuals, the DPD:IPD ratio averages 0.895 for the index finger, and thus the upper limit of normal has been set at 1.0, which is within 2.5 standard deviations of the average. Thus, a DPD:IPD ratio of greater than 1.0 is diagnostic of clubbing. However, this technique, as with the shadowgrams described above, is not particularly useful at the bedside.

The digital index, which is the sum of the 10 ratios of each finger's circumference at the nail bed (NB) and the sum of circumference at the distal interphalangeal (DIP) joint, NB:DIP, has been utilized to make the diagnosis of clubbing[1] (Fig. 1B). This is the easiest of all techniques to perform and utilize at the bedside. A digital index of 10 (10.2 to 11.32) is consistent with clubbing, whereas in normal individuals the index is 9 (8.51 to 9.99).

Lastly, diagnostically important increases in the soft tissues of the nail base can be detected by obliteration of the normally present clear space that appears as the dorsal surfaces of similar digits on right and left are opposed (see Fig. 1C). The loss of this wedge-shaped window is referred to as *Schamroth's sign*.

DIAGNOSTIC STUDIES

An important distinction to be made is between the true clubbing described above and pseudoclubbing (Table 3). Simple acro-osteolysis (not in association with pachydermoperiostosis) is a rare condition of bony destruction of the proximal phalanx that may be distinguished from true digital clubbing on the

basis of radiography. Acro-osteolysis will show characteristic signs of destructive changes in the terminal phalanges, whereas the osseous structures are normal in clubbed digits.[15]

Radiographs of the long bones may illustrate findings consistent with HOA. Periostitis generally appears as a thin sclerotic line or bony spicules separated from the cortical bone by an area of radiolucency. Most commonly affected are the ulna, radius, femur, and tibia.[16] Bone scans are more sensitive and may show evidence of periostitis in patients with HOA. Characteristically, there is increased osteoblastic activity in the pericortical and periarticular sites.[17]

ASSESSMENT

Once the findings of polyarthritis-periostitis and/or clubbing are established, the clinician *must* establish a list of differential diagnoses with the confidence that an explanation virtually always can be identified. The most direct approach begins with the determination of whether the underlying etiology is a primary or secondary process and, if secondary, what this associated disease is.

Hereditary Forms

One can usually differentiate the primary forms, hereditary clubbing and pachydermoperiostosis (the hereditary form of symptoms resembling HOA), from a secondary association given: (1) a complete family history, (2) age of onset of symptoms: and (3) lack of other organ system involvement. Symptoms of the hereditary forms are usually expressed by the time of puberty. The mode of inheritance remains uncertain but has been most consistent with an autosomal dominant pattern with variable penetrance. A male predominance has, however, been noted by others, suggesting an X-linked inheritance. The natural course of the primary forms tends to be insidious in onset, minimally progressive, and benign.

An interesting constellation of additional findings in pachydermoperiostosis includes hyperhydrosis of the hands and feet, prominent cylindric formation of the soft tissue of the lower legs and forearms, a peculiar thickening of the facial skin, and a similar scalp thickening known as cutis verticis gyrata. The dependent nature of the lower extremity pain associated with secondary hypertrophic osteoarthropathy is much less prominent with

TABLE 3. Pseudoclubbing	
CAUSE	REFERENCE
Sarcoidosis of bone	Arch Intern Med 1983;143:1017–9
Acromegaly	Chest 1985;88:627–8
Acro-osteolytis	AJR 1965;94:595–607

pachydermoperiostosis. Unilateral clubbing (Table 2) most often is associated with localized trauma or a vascular abnormality, although rarely this physical finding can be seen in an isolated form of hereditary clubbing.

Secondary Clubbing

The acquired secondary clubbing group (with and without HOA) accounts for an important group of associated diseases with clubbing often representing the only initial indicator for a significant underlying disease process. Characteristic features of the secondarily acquired forms not associated with congenital diseases are later age of onset of symptoms, relative acute onset, and progressive course of symptoms. Commonly associated diseases of the secondary group are listed in Tables 1 and 2. A more exhaustive list can be found in other reviews.[18] The consistent pattern of select associations with only clubbing can narrow such a broad differential diagnosis list. One must realize, however, that symptoms of clubbing, periostitis, and arthralgias may not occur simultaneously.

Pseudoclubbing

Forms of pseudoclubbing (Table 3) include acromegaly, acro-osteolysis (a rare resorptive bone disorder of the terminal phalanges), sarcoidosis of bone, and dystrophic nails. Growth hormone levels have been normal in patients with clubbing, and periostitis does not occur with acromegaly. Other disorders in which periostitis occurs include syphilis, scurvy, and poisoning with fluoride and strontium, as well as vitamin A and vitamin D.

Differential Diagnosis

Pulmonary Neoplasms

The most common association is with bronchogenic carcinoma. The onset of osteoarthropathy symptoms may precede the symptoms of intrathoracic disease by several months. Musculoskeletal symptoms are commonly misdiagnosed as rheumatoid arthritis or a carcinoma-associated inflammatory polyarthritis because of the similar distribution of joint involvement, similar response to nonsteroidal anti-inflammatory agents, and positive rheumatoid factor and antinuclear antibody titers. The latter findings are often present in the setting of a bronchogenic carcinoma. In the acquired secondary form of HOA, the synovial fluid is not inflammatory, the lower extremity pain is prominently increased with dependent positioning, and clubbing is nearly always present. The polyarthritis associated with carcinoma is similar to rheumatoid arthritis but usually not associated with periostitis or clubbing. Gynecomastia has been reported frequently in association with the HOA secondary to bronchogenic carcinoma but much less frequently in relation to other associated diseases. A high index of suspicion and complete physical examination are warranted for the clinician to establish a prompt diagnosis.

It is encouraging that the presence of HOA symptoms in association with neoplasms does not portend a negative prognosis in bronchogenic carcinoma. The most common cell types are of the non–small cell carcinoma type, with most reports noting similar distributions of squamous cell carcinoma, adenocarcinoma, and large cell carcinoma. In fact, small cell carcinoma has been associated only rarely with HOA. Interestingly, resection of the tumor results in nearly immediate and complete resolution of the symptoms of periostitis and arthralgias. The resolution of symptoms postthoracotomy may persist despite later recurrence of intra- and extrathoracic disease, supporting an etiology other than tumor burden alone. Because resolution of symptoms may occur with the interruption of vagal fibers without manipulation of the tumor, many authors postulate a role of vagal afferent nerve traffic as the important contribution to the development of symptoms (*vide supra*). In some patients, chemical vagotomy has been shown to improve symptoms.

Many different tumors metastatic to the lungs and mediastinum have been reported in association with HOA (Table 1), albeit infrequently. Primary tumors of the pleura have been noted distinctly in association with HOA, but these lesions more commonly present with isolated clubbing. However, there is a preponderance of benign tumors also found with HOA, most commonly benign pleural mesothelioma.

Respiratory Disorders

A number of other inflammatory and infectious intrathoracic processes are well known to be linked with clubbing and HOA. These include chronic idiopathic bronchiectasis, cystic fibrosis, pulmonary tuberculosis, empyema, and sarcoidosis. Clubbing without periostitis or polyarthritis is the general rule with the pneumoconioses and interstitial pulmonary fibrosis.

Cardiovascular Disorders

The interesting findings of clubbing with or without HOA are also found with various cardiovascular associations including cyanotic congenital heart disease, pulmonary arteriovenous fistulae, patent ductus arteriosus, aortic aneurysm, and bacterial endocarditis. Infected prosthetic vascular grafts and aortoenteric fistulae have been observed to be associated with unilateral (Table 2) and isolated lower extremity clubbing.

Gastrointestinal Disease

Other gastrointestinal neoplastic and inflammatory processes are well known to be associated with HOA. These include inflammatory bowel disease (much more common with regional enteritis than ulcerative colitis), colon carcinoma, chronic active hepatitis, primary biliary cirrhosis, ethanol-related liver disease, biliary atresia, liver transplantation, and hepatocellular carcinoma.

Other Associations

Miscellaneous but other noteworthy associations are laxative abuse, heroin abuse, and pregnancy. Thyroid acropachy is a special consideration in which the findings of digital clubbing and periosteal proliferation of the bones are associated with a prior history of Graves' disease and hyperthyroidism. Symptoms of clubbing and periostitis are often concurrent with those of exophthalmos and myxedema. The periosteal changes of thyroid acropachy, however, are characteristically different than HOA in that they are irregular and confined primarily to the hands and feet rather than the long bones of the extremities. Arthralgias are usually not present, and the treatment of Graves' disease has little impact on the course.

Diagnostic Decision Making

The findings of clubbing and HOA provide the clinician with a wide differential diagnosis. Nevertheless, frequently one experiences the satisfaction of making a specific diagnosis of an associated illness by pursuing a complete evaluation. This involves a thorough history with special emphasis on age of onset of symptoms, rate of progression of symptoms, and family history, followed by a careful examination of the heart, lungs, abdomen, and musculoskeletal system. In almost all instances, the secondary associated disease can be determined without difficulty. A chest roentgenograph, complete blood count with differential, general chemistry screen including liver enzymes, and occasional synovial aspirate will refine one's approach prior to the definitive microbiologic, cytologic, or histopathologic diagnosis.

REFERENCES

1. Vazquez-Abad D, Pineda C, Martinez-Lavin M. Digital clubbing: a numerical assessment of the deformity. J Rheumatol 1989;16:518–20.
2. Rimoin DL. Pachydermoperiostosis (idiopathic clubbing and periostosis). Genetic and physiologic considerations. N Engl J Med 1965;272:924–31.
3. Locke EA. Secondary hypertrophic osteoarthropathy and its relation to simple club fingers. Arch Intern Med 1915;15:659–64.
4. Shneerson JM. Digital clubbing and hypertrophic osteoarthropathy—the underlying mechanisms. Br J Dis Chest 1981;75:113–31.
5. Lemen RJ, Gates AJ, Mathe AA. Relationship among digital clubbing, disease severity and serum prostaglandins F2a and E concentrations in cystic fibrosis patients. Am Rev Respir Dis 1978;117:639–46.
6. Alberts WM. A clinician's guide to clubbing. J Respir Dis 1989;10:37–46.
7. Dickinson CJ, Martin JF. Megakaryocytes and platelet clumps as the cause of finger clubbing. Lancet 1987;ii:1434–5.
8. Kucirka S, Scher R. Heritable nail disorders. Dermatol Clin 1987;5(1):179–91.
9. Hansen-Flaschen J, Nordberg J. Clubbing and hypertrophic osteoarthropathy. Clin Chest Med 1987;8(2):287–98.
10. Martinez-Lavin M, Valdez T, Cajibas J, Weisman M, Gerber N, Steigler D. Primary hypertrophic osteoarthropathy. Semin Arthritis Rheum 1988;17(3):156–62.
11. Lovibond J. Diagnosis of clubbed fingers. Lancet 1938;1:363–4.
12. Regan G, Tagg B, Thompson M. Subjective assessment and objective measurement of finger clubbing. Lancet 1967;1:530–2.
13. Bently D, Moore A, Shwachman H. Finger clubbing: a quantitative survey by analysis of the shadowgraph. Lancet 1976; 2:164–7.
14. Sly M, Ghazanshahi S, Buran Akul B, et al. Objective assessment for digital clubbing in caucasian, negro and oriental subjects. Chest 1973;64:687–9.
15. Cheney W. Acroosteolysis. AJR 1965;94:595–607.
16. Greenfield G, Schorsch H, Shkolnik A. The various roentgen appearances of pulmonary hypertrophic osteoarthropathy. AJR 1967;101:927–31.
17. Lopez-Majano V, Sobti P. Early diagnosis of pulmonary osteoarthropathy in neoplastic disease. J Nucl Med Allied Sci 1984;28:69–76.
18. Altman RD, Tenenbaum J. Hypertrophic osteoarthropathy. In: Kelley WM, Harris ED, Ruddy S, Sledge CB, eds. Textbook of rheumatology. Philadelphia: WB Saunders, 1985:1594–1603.

CONGESTIVE HEART FAILURE

KENNETH M. KESSLER

SYNONYMS: Heart Failure, Circulatory Failure, Cardiac Failure

BACKGROUND

Definition of Terminology

Circulatory failure is a general term applied to the inability of the cardiovascular system to meet the metabolic demands of the cell. Circulatory failure may be related to cardiac or noncardiac abnormalities. *Heart failure* is circulatory failure due to a cardiac abnormality and may be defined as a condition wherein the heart (operating at normal filling pressures) cannot pump adequate blood to meet the metabolic requirements of the body. *Congestive heart failure* refers to a syndrome whereby heart failure has led to circulatory compensations resulting in systemic and pulmonary congestion. *Acute heart failure* implies heart failure of recent onset. *Intractable heart failure* refers to heart failure that fails to respond to aggressive treatment efforts.[1,2]

Approach to the Differential Diagnosis

Congestive heart failure is merely a syndrome that may result from a wide range of etiologies including rhythm abnormalities, myocardial abnormalities, mechanical abnormalities, high output states,[3] and diastolic dysfunction.[4] The evaluation of a patient with congestive heart failure is a three-step process (Table 1): (1) identifying the classic signs and symptoms of congestion, that is, systemic and pulmonary venous congestion (Table 2); (2) identifying the signs and symptoms of myocardial dysfunction per se, for example, third heart sound (Table 2); and (3) identifying the signs and symptoms of etiologic and precipi-

tating disorders, for example, valvular abnormalities, hypertension, thyrotoxicosis, alcohol abuse, coronary artery disease, anemia, and so on (Table 3).

Pathophysiology of Heart Failure

Myocardial Component

Congestive heart failure affects about 1 per cent of the population and once established significantly shortens longevity.[1,2] As such, it is a major cause of cardiovascular morbidity and mortality. When the myocardium is impaired, whether primarily, as in myocardial infarction or cardiomyopathy, or secondarily, as in volume or pressure overload, three basic pathophysiologic processes tend to interact. The overload state leads to cellular hypertrophy; there is primarily (as in myocardial infarction) or secondarily (as may accompany extreme left ventricular hypertrophy) cellular necrosis; and there is replacement fibrosis.[1,5] The common denominator in systolic heart failure is loss of contractile elements with a decreased ability to eject blood. The result may be reflected as a decrease in stroke volume, cardiac output, and/or ejection fraction. Myocardial failure leads to symptoms and signs of forward failure (due to an inadequate cardiac output) such as fatigue and signs of myocardial dysfunction such as displacement of the cardiac apex and gallop rhythms.

The congestive component of heart failure appears in response to inadequate blood supply at the tissue level. The decrease in flow activates the renin-angiotensin and sympathoadrenal systems. The result is salt and water retention, venous and arterial constriction, and an increase in heart rate. These compensatory mechanisms are directed to maintaining an adequate cardiac output, primarily, and an adequate blood pressure, secondarily. However, these compensatory mechanisms tend to overshoot, leading to circulatory con-

TABLE 1. Evaluation of Patients with Congestive Heart Failure

Three-step process
1. Identify the classic signs and symptoms of *congestion*
2. Identify the signs and symptoms of *myocardial dysfunction*
3. Identify the signs and symptoms of *etiologic and precipitating disorders*

gestion with signs and symptoms of backward heart failure, which is often divided into "right heart" and "left heart" components. The symptoms and signs of backward left heart failure include dyspnea on exertion and rales, whereas symptoms and signs of backward right heart failure include edema and jugular venous distension.

Systolic Versus Diastolic Dysfunction

Classically, heart failure related to myocardial dysfunction has been equated to a large poorly contracting left ventricle, that is, classic systolic left ventricular dysfunction. However, 40 per cent of patients with the classic signs and symptoms of congestive heart fail-

TABLE 2. Signs and Symptoms of Congestive Heart Failure*

Congestive component
  Forward failure
    Right heart
      Dyspnea
    Left heart
      Fatigue
      Weakness
      Cachexia
  Backward failure
    Right heart
      Jugular venous distension
      Edema (pedal, presacral, ascites, anasarca)
      Hepatomegaly
    Left heart
      Rales
      Dyspnea on exertion
      Orthopnea
      Paroxysmal nocturnal dyspnea
Myocardial component
  Left heart
    Displaced, diffuse PMI†
    S_3, S_4
  Right heart
    Heave
    S_3, S_4

* These signs and symptoms, although "classic," are nonspecific; furthermore, they cannot differentiate with certainty systolic from diastolic left ventricular dysfunction.
† PMI = point of maximal impulse.

TABLE 3. Classic Causes of Congestive Heart Failure

Abnormal ejection fraction
  Dilated congestive idiopathic cardiomyopathy
  Hypertensive myopathy (end-stage, dilated)
  Ischemic heart disease (chronic, acute myocardial infarction)
  Alcohol
  Valvular heart disease
  Peripartum cardiomyopathy
  Cor pulmonale
  Infection (viral, bacterial, protozoal, AIDS* related)
  Electrolyte abnormalities (calcium, magnesium, phosphate)
  Endocrine abnormalities (hypothyroidism, diabetes)
  Cardiotoxic agents (chemotherapeutics, cobalt)
  Collagen vascular diseases
  Neuromuscular diseases (muscular dystrophy, Friedreich's ataxia)
  Congenital heart disease
  Tumors (myxoma, metastatic tumors)
  Chronic tachy- or bradyarrhythmias
Normal ejection fraction
  Ischemic diastolic dysfunction
  Hypertensive diastolic dysfunction
  Hypertrophic cardiomyopathy
    Idiopathic hypertrophic subaortic stenosis
  High output states
    Hyperthyroidism
    Arteriovenous shunt
    Polycythemia vera
    Pulmonary disease
    Chronic anemia
    Renal insufficiency
    Nutritional (beri-beri)
  Pericardial disease
  Valvular heart disease
    Acute valvular insufficiency
    Mitral stenosis
  Restrictive/infiltrative myopathies
    Amyloidosis
    Hemochromatosis
    Radiation
    Sarcoid

* AIDS = acquired immune deficiency syndrome.

ure have a normal ejection fraction.[6] Heart failure in such individuals may be related to a variety of specific disorders, most notably diastolic left ventricular dysfunction. This is an important point in differential diagnosis and is discussed under Assessment.

HISTORY

Subjective Data

History of Present Illness

The classic historical data associated with congestive heart failure reflect: (1) the failure of the heart to provide an adequate cardiac output (forward failure) and (2) the symptoms of congestion (backward failure) (Table 2). Dyspnea is common and is related to the increased work of breathing. Dyspnea may become more pronounced or only be present on effort. Dyspnea on exertion has equivalents such as fatigue or an adaptive life-style in which the patient avoids dyspnea by restricting activities. Orthopnea refers to dyspnea that occurs when the patient becomes recumbent. When this occurs at night and awakens the patient from sleep, the term *paroxysmal nocturnal dyspnea* is used. The patient usually sits upright and seeks fresh air. A bronchospastic component of dyspnea may occur and is referred to as *cardiac asthma*.[2]

With extreme heart failure, pulmonary edema may occur. Additional findings are advanced breathlessness, blood-tinged sputum, and a graven appearance.[2]

Other symptoms of heart failure include: cough, insomnia, edema, weight gain, weakness, mental confusion, excessive abdominal fullness, right upper quadrant discomfort due to liver congestion, sweating, and at its extreme, weight loss and cardiac cachexia. Unfortunately, the symptoms of heart failure are nonspecific and may occur with lung disease, anemia, thyrotoxicosis, and the like. Symptoms also cannot differentiate heart failure primarily related to systolic versus diastolic left ventricular dysfunction.[4]

Family History

A family history of hypertension, coronary artery disease, early death, sudden death, hypertrophic cardiomyopathy, and congestive heart failure should be sought.

Social and Occupational History

A review of risk factors such as smoking, exercise habits, alcohol intake, and cholesterol level should be obtained.

Previous Medical History

Prior history of congestive heart failure is often present, and the duration and severity should be documented. Etiologies of heart failure may be suggested by a history of multiple myocardial infarctions (ischemic myopathy), recent viral symptoms (viral cardiomyopathy), trauma (arteriovenous fistula), a history of murmur (valvular or congenital heart disease), or hypertension (ischemic and/or hypertensive heart disease).

Focused Queries

1. *When did the symptoms occur or become dramatically worse?* Acute heart failure suggests acute myocardial infarction; acute viral myocarditis; acute valvular dysfunction, which may accompany bacterial endocarditis or acute myocardial infarction; or mitral chordal rupture.

2. *Have you changed your medications or salt intake?* Noncompliance with medications or diet is a common cause of the exacerbation of heart failure symptoms.

3. *Have you noted signs of infection such as fever or cough?* Pulmonary infection may precipitate congestive heart failure; conversely, a history of infection may be a clue to viral myocarditis or subacute bacterial endocarditis.

4. *Have you had any chest discomfort?* Angina may be a clue to myocardial infarction, ischemic myocardial dysfunction, or acute papillary muscle insufficiency. Chest discomfort occasionally occurs with cardiomyopathy without associated coronary artery disease. Pleuritic chest pain may be a clue to pulmonary embolism.

5. *Have you noticed any palpitations?* Arrhythmias can directly precipitate heart failure, may occur as heart failure worsens, or may exacerbate heart failure when accompanied by certain underlying diseases such as mitral stenosis or coronary artery disease.

6. *Have you ever had a heart murmur?* A history of murmur or rheumatic fever can point to significant valvular or congenital heart disease.

7. *Do you have high blood pressure?* Hypertension can be directly related to heart failure in hypertensive heart disease. Hypertension is a major risk factor for atherosclerotic coronary artery disease.

8. *Have you been pregnant recently?* Peripartum cardiomyopathy is an important, although fortunately rare, cause of heart failure in young women with specific implications for future pregnancies.

PHYSICAL EXAMINATION

Vital Signs

The blood pressure is usually low normal and equal in both arms. Inequalities in the blood pressure are suggestive of atherosclerotic disease, dissecting aortic aneurysm, or coarctation of the aorta. The blood pressure may be elevated in patients with systemic hypertension or may show a widened pulse pressure in patients with significant aortic insufficiency. The pulse rate is usually mildly increased. A markedly elevated pulse rate suggests marked cardiac decompensation, a cardiac tachyarrhythmia as the primary cause of the heart failure, or a dysrhythmia that has been caused by the hemodynamic abnormalities of heart failure. Inappropriate bradycardia may be seen with heart failure that has been precipitated by medications with combined negative inotropic and negative chronotropic activity. The respiratory rate is increased in depth and frequency. Marked breathlessness and ''air hunger'' are seen in acute heart failure and pulmonary edema. The oral temperature is unreliable in patients in heart failure who have been breathing through their mouths. The core temperature when more than minimally elevated is suggestive of an infective process, myocardial infarction, or pulmonary embolism.

Head and Neck Examination

Physical examination of the eyes may reveal jaundice related to chronic right heart failure with congestive hepatomegaly or pulmonary infarction.[2] Pale conjunctiva suggest anemia.

The neck veins are examined with the body elevated to 45 degrees. With severe congestion, an upright position may be needed. The right internal jugular vein is most reliable to examine. The upper limit of normal jugular venous pressure is 7 or 8 cm of water. Elevation of the mean systemic venous pressure is a sign of backward right heart failure. A prominent V wave suggests tricuspid regurgitation. When the venous pressure is near normal, pressing firmly on the abdomen (or right upper quadrant) will produce the so-called hepatojugular reflux, which is suggestive of an increase in venous volume and a heart that is unable to compensate for an abrupt increase in venous return.[2] The carotid impulses may be of normal contour but diminished in amplitude owing to the decrease in cardiac output. A delayed upstroke suggests significant aortic stenosis, whereas a bisferiens impulse suggests aortic regurgitation or idiopathic hypertrophic subaortic stenosis.

Cardiopulmonary Examination

Rales, suggesting pulmonary congestion, may be heard at the lung bases, or throughout the lung fields when heart failure is more pronounced. Wheezing may be a sign of bronchospasm and cardiac asthma. Evidence of pleural effusion on the right side or bilaterally may be found.

Findings of myocardial dysfunction include a diffuse and laterally displaced point of maximal impulse as well as a third heart sound originating from the left ventricle. In patients with diastolic dysfunction related to hypertension, a fourth heart sound and a nondisplaced but forceful apical impulse may be noted. However, the physical examination cannot be relied on to differentiate patients with systolic from diastolic heart failure. There may be signs of right ventricular failure with a right ventricular heave and a right ventricular third heart sound. When interpreting gallop rhythms, one should remember that a third heart sound is normal in adolescence, in some young adults, and during pregnancy,[7] and that a fourth heart sound is frequently heard in older patients.[8]

Other cardiac findings may reflect specific etiologies of the heart failure. Murmurs of hemodynamically significant mitral stenosis, mitral regurgitation, aortic stenosis, aortic regurgitation, tricuspid stenosis, tricuspid regurgitation, ventricular septal defect, and patent ductus arteriosus have characteristic findings.

Examination of the Abdomen and Extremities

Examination of the liver may reveal hepatomegaly resulting from chronic right heart failure, as well as the systolic pulsations of tricuspid insufficiency. Ascites may be present in patients with chronic cardiac dysfunction and right heart backward failure. The presence of an abdominal bruit is suggestive of underlying renovascular hypertension or diffuse atherosclerotic disease.

Examination of the periphery may reveal evidence of severely decreased cardiac output in the form of cool extremities or peripheral cyanosis. Edema is often present. The formation of edema is related to both total body salt and water content and local hydrostatic factors. Therefore, with minimal water accumulation in the upright position, edema fluid tends to accumulate in the ankles only. With greater degrees of fluid and more recumbency, presacral edema, ascites, or anasarca may be seen.

When the physical findings of heart failure are well defined but the etiology is not, additional findings should be sought. A warm, flushed skin suggests high output failure, thyromegaly suggests hyper- or hypothyroidism, and skin wounds suggest underlying arteriovenous malformations. Kussmaul's sign or paradoxical pulse suggests pericardial involvement, whereas bilateral arcus senilis and tendon xanthoma suggest underlying lipid abnormality and the presence of atherosclerotic disease (Table 3).

DIAGNOSTIC STUDIES

Chest X-ray

It has been taught that venous hypertension is associated with a wedge pressure of 14 mm Hg, whereas pulmonary edema will be noted with a wedge pressure of 25 to 30 mm Hg. Early findings of congestive heart failure are dilatation of the pulmonary veins as blood is shunted toward the upper lobe vessels and the lower lobe vessels become constricted. With increasing pulmonary venous, and subsequently arterial, pressure, there may be dilatation of the central right and left pulmonary arteries. Pulmonary interstitial edema may occur, which may range from mild haziness to the frank butterfly pattern of pulmonary edema. Thickening of pleural fissures may be seen as well as loculated subpulmonic or interlobar fluid. Correlation of Kerley lines with an 18-mm Hg wedge pressure has been noted in the past.[2]

Cardiac enlargement is defined when the transverse dimension of the cardiac silhouette is greater than 50 per cent of the transverse dimension of the thorax. This may be due to cardiac enlargement per se or to pericardial effusion. Specific etiologies of the heart failure syndrome may be suggested by pericardial calcification, valvular calcification, or a contour suggesting left ventricular aneurysm. It is important to note that despite classic teaching recent data indicate there is a poor correlation between clinical findings, roentgenographic findings, and the exact level of pulmonary capillary wedge pressure.[9] It is also impossible to differentiate with certainty the venous congestion and cardiomegaly associated with heart

failure due to systolic versus diastolic left ventricular dysfunction.[4,6]

Electrocardiogram

There are no specific electrocardiographic (ECG) findings of congestive heart failure. The ECG may show clues to the underlying heart disease such as an acute myocardial infarction pattern, diffuse ST-T abnormalities and arrhythmias associated with myocarditis, or left ventricular hypertrophy associated with aortic stenosis or hypertension. The ECG can help to evaluate arrhythmias that may be the cause of, or result from, heart failure.

Echocardiography

A powerful tool in the differential diagnosis of congestive heart failure is the echocardiogram.[4,6] Approximately 60 percent of the time, heart failure will be associated with a moderately to severely depressed ejection fraction (20 to 35 per cent). In such cases, there may be evidence of regional wall motion abnormality including frank left ventricular aneurysm in patients with coronary artery disease. However, the differential diagnosis of cardiomyopathy may be difficult. At its extreme, ischemic disease may be associated with left ventricular dilatation and global impairment of left ventricular function. Conversely, primary cardiomyopathies may, at times, show regional asynergy. Other etiologies of left ventricular systolic dysfunction should also be sought, such as evidence of aortic stenosis, aortic insufficiency, or mitral regurgitation. The severity of these valvular lesions can be further evaluated using Doppler echocardiography.

In approximately 40 per cent of individuals, a normal left ventricular ejection fraction will be noted. There are several cardiac and noncardiac causes for a patient with classic signs and symptoms of congestive heart failure to have a normal ejection fraction (see Assessment). Doppler echocardiography is used to assess left ventricular filling abnormalities associated with diastolic left ventricular dysfunction. Proper therapeutics depends on differentiating this subgroup of heart failure patients.

Swan-Ganz Catheterization

Swan-Ganz catheterization is rarely needed to define the congestive heart failure syndrome but may be helpful in patient management and the definition of the degree of filling pressure abnormality (particularly since physical findings and roentgenographic findings correlate poorly).[8,9]

Radionuclide Angiograms

Radionuclide angiograms are helpful in determining the ejection fraction and the degree of regional and global left ventricular wall motion abnormalities.[2]

ASSESSMENT

Signs, Symptoms, and Time Course of Onset

Chronic heart failure patients often present with a long-standing history of easy fatigability and dyspnea on exertion. At times, patients may be well compensated, with few or no symptoms, until a precipitating cause—such as pulmonary embolus, infection, dysrhythmia, or noncompliance with medication or diet—brings about rapid deterioration. With acute valvular abnormality or myocardial infarction, extreme degrees of heart failure may be seen with an acute onset. It is important to establish the time course of onset of the symptoms as a clue to the underlying disease process and/or precipitating factors. It is also important to realize that the signs and symptoms of congestive heart failure are not specific.[4,6] Dyspnea, orthopnea, and even paroxysmal nocturnal dyspnea may be seen in patients with pulmonary disease. The obese patient may complain of ankle edema and/or dyspnea and even have bibasilar "static" rales. Thus, it is extremely important to place the signs and symptoms of heart failure into the clinical context.

Underlying Etiologies

Acute myocardial infarction is a common etiology that needs aggressive management directed toward the ischemic process. Chest pain or a history of prior infarction is an obvious clue. But isolated heart failure may be the only clue to painless infarction. Cardiomyopathies are frequently noted and, while occasionally due to a discrete viral myocarditis, are often of a chronic, ill-defined etiology.

However, some patients have etiologies of myopathy of specific import.[10] These include chemotherapy-induced myopathy, hemochromatosis, and silent valvular abnormalities. Signs and symptoms of high output failure such as warm skin and persistent tachycardia suggest thyrotoxicosis, anemia, beri-beri, and the like. This subgroup is particularly important since heart failure may respond to therapy directed at the underlying disease process.[5]

Classic Congestive Heart Failure with a Normal Ejection Fraction

Over the last decade, it has become apparent that approximately 40 per cent of patients with congestive heart failure have a normal left ventricular ejection fraction.[4,6,11,12] There are several reasons for this apparent paradox. First, the signs and symptoms of congestive heart failure are nonspecific and are at times primarily related to obesity, pregnancy, pulmonary disease, or volume overload. At times, acute valvular abnormalities lead to congestive heart failure accompanied by a normal or even increased ejection fraction. Identification of these valvular abnormalities is paramount to appropriate therapy. Finally, there is the increasing recognition that a large number of patients present with a heart failure syndrome due to diastolic left ventricular dysfunction. The classic etiologies that lead to abnormal filling of the left ventricle, such as pericardial disease, mitral stenosis, and idiopathic hypertrophic subaortic stenosis,[10] are relatively rare when compared with the large number of patients who present with hypertensive heart disease,[12] ischemic heart disease, or undefined cardiac disease who have classic signs of a borderline low cardiac output and pulmonary and systemic venous congestion but who have a normal ejection fraction.[4,6,11,12]

Diastolic dysfunction forces the heart to operate at higher-than-normal filling pressures to eject a borderline to low cardiac output. These higher filling pressures can lead to all the same signs and symptoms of congestive heart failure as occur in patients who have systolic dysfunction. The differentiation of diastolic from systolic dysfunction is important because the prognosis and treatment differ.[4,6,14] Treatment for classic congestive heart failure includes digoxin, diuretics, and afterload reduction. The primary treatment for diastolic dysfunction is control of hypertension and ischemia, careful use of diuretics to avoid overdiuresis, and avoidance of digoxin and afterload reduction.[4] The use of beta-adrenergic blocking agents and calcium blocking agents is under investigation.

Clues to the Diagnosis of Diastolic Dysfunction

A high index of suspicion was always needed to diagnose the more classic causes of diastolic filling disorders such as pericardial disease, mitral stenosis, and idiopathic hypertrophic subaortic stenosis. However, in most patients the differentiation of systolic from diastolic dysfunction cannot be made on clinical grounds alone, and an objective measurement of ejection fraction is often needed. Worsening of low output symptoms using the classic treatment for congestive heart failure serves as a clue to the presence of diastolic rather than systolic dysfunction.[15] A history of episodic, reversible heart failure that is related to acute hypertension or ischemia, in a patient with residual signs and symptoms of congestive heart failure, suggests the clinical context in which diastolic dysfunction most often occurs. Patient management depends on the proper differentiation of congestive heart failure primarily related to diastolic versus systolic dysfunction. This may be done using clinical judgment combined with an objective measure of left ventricular function.

REFERENCES

1. Braunwald E. Pathophysiology of heart failure. In: Braunwald E, ed. Heart disease: a textbook of cardiovascular medicine. Philadelphia: WB Saunders, 1988:426–48.
2. Spann JF Jr, Hurst JW. The recognition and management of heart failure. In: Hurst JW, Schlant RC, Rackley CE, Sonnenblick EH, Wenger NK, eds. The heart. New York: McGraw Hill, 1990:418–41.
3. Fowler NO. High-cardiac-output states. In: Hurst JW, Schlant RC, Rackley CE, Sonnenblick EH, Wenger NK, eds. The heart. New York: McGraw Hill, 1990:462–72.
4. Kessler KM. Heart failure with normal systolic function [Editorial]. Arch Intern Med 1988;148:2109–11.
5. Schlant RC, Sonnenblick EH. Pathophysiology of heart failure. In: Hurst JW, Schlant RC, Rackley CE, Sonnenblick EH, Wenger NK, eds. The heart. New York: McGraw Hill, 1990:387–418.
6. Echeverria HH, Bilsker MS, Myerburg RJ, Kessler KM. Congestive heart failure: echocardiographic insights. Am J Med 1983;75:750–5.
7. Sloan AW, Campbell FW, Henderson AS. Incidence of the physioiogic third heart sound. Br Med J 1952;ii:853:5.
8. Spodick DH, Quary-Pigotti VM. Fourth heart sound as a normal finding in older persons. N Engl J Med 1973;288:140–1.
9. Chakko S, Woska D, Martinez H, et al. Clinical, radiographic, and hemodynamic correlations in chronic congestive heart failure: conflicting results may lead to inappropriate care. Am J Med 1991;90:353–9.
10. Wenger NK, Abelmann WH, Roberts WC. Cardiomyopathy and specific heart muscle disease. In: Hurst JW, Schlant RC, Rackley CE, Sonnenblick EH, Wenger NK, eds. The heart. New York: McGraw Hill, 1990:1278–1347.
11. Dougherty AH, Naccarelli GV, Gray EL, Hicks CH, Goldstein RA. Congestive heart failure with normal systolic function. Am J Med 1984;54:778–82.
12. Soufer R, Wohlgelernter D, Vita NA, et al. Intact systolic left ventricular function in clinical congestive heart failure. Am J Cardiol 1985;55:1032–6.
13. Topol EJ, Traill TA, Fortuin NJ. Hypertensive hypertrophic cardiomyopathy of the elderly. N Engl J Med 1984;312:277–83.
14. Cohn JN, Johnson G, Veterans Administration Cooperative Study Group. Heart failure with normal ejection fraction: the V-HeFT study. Circulation 1990;81(suppl III): III-48–53.
15. Kessler KM. Diastolic heart failure—diagnosis and management. Hosp Pract 1989;25(July):137–64.

CONSTIPATION, CHRONIC

PAUL C. ROUSSEAU

SYNONYMS: Obstipation, Costiveness

BACKGROUND

Constipation, derived from the Latin *constipare*, which means "to crowd together,"[1] is a common complaint among bowel conscious individuals. Although a precise definition is difficult, chronic constipation entails fewer than three bowel movements per week for a period longer than six weeks[2] and may be accompanied by prolonged or difficult evacuation,[3] expulsion of hard, painful stool,[4] or a feeling of incomplete emptying.[5] Lamentably, such a definition is clinically inadequate; therefore, a consummate description of constipation should include an inability to expel stool or a decline in the frequency of stool passage, even if in the "normal" range.[2]

Epidemiologically, the prevalence of constipation varies from 5 to 20 per cent,[5] with the ratio of males to females dependent on age. In younger age groups, boys are more often constipated than girls, whereas in the mid- to later years, females are more often constipated than males.[5] Older individuals reportedly suffer more episodes of constipation,[6] in part due to chronic laxative use fostered by the theory of autointoxication popular during the early part of this century.[3] This hypothesis suggested the absence of a daily bowel movement enhanced absorption of noxious substances, facilitating the onset of various diseases.[7] In an effort to preclude the development of bowel-associated maladies, laxative use was common, but after years of cathartic abuse, laxative-damaged bowel now contributes to chronic bowel dysfunction and constipation.

There are certain risks associated with chronic constipation, many with considerable morbidity. Urinary tract infection is related to the presence of constipation[5] and in children may precipitate enuresis and vesicoureteral reflux.[5,8] Chronic constipation may also increase the risk of colorectal cancer, particularly in women,[10] as well as stercoral ulceration, sigmoid volvulus, idiopathic megacolon, fecal impaction, urinary incontinence,[11] and unnecessary surgery.[5]

Constipation is, of course, a symptom, not a disease,[9] with known etiologies classified into five categories (listed in Table 1): environmental, pharmacologic, colorectal, metabolic, and neurologic. Many are encountered infrequently, although Hirschsprung's disease is the most common congenital disorder[5] and environmental precipitants the most common acquired maladies.

HISTORY

Subjective Data

History of Present Illness

The medical history should ascertain the onset of constipation and associated symptomatology. What is the patient's definition of constipation: infrequent bowel movements; hard, painful stools; or incomplete evacuation? What is the consistency of the stool? Has there been a recent change in bowel function, in spite of chronic "irregularity"? Has the patient experienced abdominal pain, nausea, vomiting, melena, or hematochezia? Has the patient noticed recent weight loss?

Other questions should disclose the use of drugs, both prescription and over-the-counter; dietary history; and extent of physical activity.

Past Medical History

Is there a history of colorectal or gynecologic surgical procedures? Is there evidence of trauma from accidents or obstetric injury?[12] Is there a history of psychiatric illness such as depression, bulimia, or anorexia nervosa?

105

TABLE 1. Classification of Constipation

Environmental
  Suppression of the defecation reflex
  Lack of adequate dietary fiber
  Limited physical activity/immobility
Pharmacologic
  Anticholinergics
  Narcotics
  Sympathomimetics
  Calcium channel blockers
  Aluminum
  Calcium
  Iron
  Nonsteroidal anti-inflammatory drugs
  Laxatives
Colorectal
  Anismus
  Descending perineum syndrome
  Tumors
  Ischemic colitis
  Anal fissure
  Chronic volvulus
  Hernias
  Anal stenosis
  Ulcerative proctitis
  Diverticulosis
Metabolic
  Diabetes mellitus
  Hypothyroidism
  Chronic renal failure
  Hypercalcemia
  Hypokalemia
  Porphyria
Neurologic
  Hirschsprung's disease
  von Recklinghausen's disease
  Cerebrovascular accidents
  Parkinson's disease
  Brain tumors
  Multiple sclerosis
  Trauma or tumor of the spinal cord
  Autonomic neuropathy

Focused Queries

1. *What is the frequency of bowel movements?* Since patients define constipation based on their concept of normal bowel function,[12] this question will help determine the presence of constipation and the need for further assessment. If the frequency of bowel evacuation falls within the province of normal, the individual should be questioned as to why he or she perceives the presence of constipation.[1] Concurrently, the patient should be queried about the use of laxatives and the frequency of colonic emptying, since cathartic use may contribute to the passage of stool on a regular basis.

2. *How long has the constipation been present?* The duration of constipation is inversely related to the presence of an organic disorder. Most individuals with factual chronic constipation suffer from a functional, or nonorganic malady (except persons with congenital disorders), whereas individuals with a recent or abrupt onset of constipation often harbor an organic etiology.[1] Moreover, ascertaining the duration of constipation will assist in categorizing the ailment into an acute or chronic disorder.

3. *Has there been a recent change in bowel function?* This is an important question, even in individuals with chronic constipation. If there has been a recent change in defecatory habits, such as a decline in frequency, suspect an intervening organic disorder.[1]

4. *Is there pain with passage of stool?* Chronic functional constipation is rarely associated with pain on defecation and, when present, suggests irritable bowel syndrome, bowel obstruction, anorectal mucosal injury (i.e., anal fissure/tear),[1] hemorrhoids, diverticular disease,[8] or herpetic proctitis.

5. *Is there blood with the passage of stool?* The presence of any amount of blood is incompatible with the diagnosis of functional constipation. The most common cause of blood-tinged stool is anal bleeding secondary to hemorrhoids, although an anal tear or fissure may also induce bleeding.[1]

6. *Is there lack of an urge to defecate or difficulty in expelling fecal matter?* If the patient relates an absence of a spontaneous urge to defecate, suspect long-term suppression of normal defecatory reflexes. On the other hand, difficulty expelling stool may indicate an underlying neuromuscular disorder or lack of dietary fiber.[1]

7. *What are the consistency and color of stool?* Most individuals describe a "normal" consistency of stool, but occasional patients complain of hard, rocklike feces, which may be associated with poor dietary habits or suppression of the defecatory reflex. Stools with a thin caliber may be seen with rectosigmoid carcinoma, although malignancy is unlikely in a patient with chronic constipation. Moreover, thin stools may also be observed with spastic colon.[13] Dark, tarry stools are significant, since occult gastrointestinal bleeding is the probable cause, necessitating further evaluation.

8. *What drugs are used, both prescription and over-the-counter?* Many drugs, particularly the concurrent use of multiple medications, are capable of inducing constipation.

TABLE 2.   Medications Capable of Causing Constipation

Anticholinergic agents
  Antidepressants
  Neuroleptics
  Antiparkinsonian drugs
  Antispasmodics
Narcotics
Sympathomimetic agents
  Ephedrine
  Isoproterenol
  Phenylephrine
  Phenylpropanolamine
  Pseudoephedrine
  Terbutaline
Calcium channel blockers
Aluminum
Calcium
Iron
Nonsteroidal anti-inflammatory drugs
Laxatives (primarily stimulant cathartics)

(From Rousseau PC. Managing constipation in the elderly patient. Fam Pract Recertification 1990;12:76–93. Used with permission.)

Culpable pharmaceuticals (listed in Table 2) include anticholinergic agents, narcotics, sympathomimetic agents, calcium channel blockers, aluminum, calcium, iron, nonsteroidal anti-inflammatory drugs, and laxatives.[11]

PHYSICAL EXAMINATION

The physical examination, which is often normal in patients with chronic constipation, should concentrate on the abdominal and perineal areas.

Examination of the abdomen includes assessment of bowel sounds, palpation of the liver and spleen to determine organ dimensions, and suprapubic palpation to appraise uterine and urinary bladder size. Noted abnormalities may include unusual tenderness,[1] abdominal or bladder distension, hepatosplenomegaly, uterine enlargement, or an occult mass.

Anorectal evaluation includes an inspection of the perineum for easily observable abnormalities. Perineal cutaneous sensation should be assessed, and a digital rectal inspection completed. With the examining finger in the rectum, sphincter tone may be estimated and pelvic muscular function assessed by asking the patient to bear down and strain. When this maneuver is performed, the puborectalis muscle should be felt to move anteriorly toward the pubic symphysis while the perineum descends.[12] If present, rectal prolapse may also be noted by straining maneuvers. Digital rectal examination may also reveal an obstructing lesion, while affording the opportunity to test any stool on the examining glove for occult blood.

DIAGNOSTIC STUDIES

Laboratory data are usually normal in chronic constipation, although occasional discovery of an underlying disorder mandates routine performance of a select group of pertinent tests.

Clinical Laboratory Tests

Recommended laboratory assessments include thyroid function studies, blood glucose, serum electrolytes, and serum calcium.[5,12,13] If physical examination suggests an underlying disorder, appropriate laboratory data should be requested (i.e., collagen vascular profile). When laxative abuse is suspected, a urine sample should be examined for evidence of cathartic residue or a stool sample stained with sodium hydroxide to detect the presence of phenophthalein (the active ingredient of Ex-Lax). If present, phenophthalein converts the stool to a pink-purple coloration.

Diagnostic Imaging

Routine radiographs of the abdomen may assist in the diagnosis of chronic constipation by disclosing gas patterns characteristic of Hirschsprung's disease or pseudoobstruction.[14]

Ingestion of 20 radiopaque markers each morning for three consecutive days will assist in the evaluation of colonic transit time by permitting radiographic determination of marker movement. Plain films of the abdomen obtained on days four and seven[14,15] will measure transit time of the entire colon, with normal passage averaging 11.5 hours for each segment.[14] Normally, the first markers should be excreted by the end of the third day, with 80 per cent eliminated by five days.[5] If the markers are widely distributed on radiographic visualization, motor dysfunction should be suspected, whereas accumulation of markers in the sigmoid area suggests an anorectal disorder.[12] Assessment of transit time not only permits appraisal of segmental transport but also detects patients who misrepresent their complaint of chronic constipation.[5] Radiopaque markers are available commercially or may be made by cutting 5-mm segments from a 16 French radiopaque Levin tube.[1]

Barium enema examination of the colon is suggested to determine whether bowel dysfunction is related to an underlying organic narrowing, particularly colorectal carcinoma.[5] In a chronically constipated individual, the size of the distal colon is usually larger than normal.[5] However, the largest normal diameter of the rectosigmoid area on lateral view is 6.5 cm[5,15]; a larger size suggests the possibility of Hirschsprung's disease[15] or megacolon.[5]

Defecography assesses defecation by infusing liquid or semisolid barium into the rectum and then videotaping the individual during active defecation.[12,14,15] This radiographic evaluation is particularly useful in detecting descending perineum syndrome, paradoxical contraction of the pelvic floor, posterior rectal hernia, rectal intussusception, and rectocele.[12,14] Although the test is fairly reliable, the great variation of normal defecation may make interpretation difficult.

Endoscopy

Endoscopy of the colon includes anoscopy, flexible sigmoidoscopy, and colonoscopy. Obviously, all three are not indicated for every episode of chronic constipation; rather, the clinician should determine which patients merit assessment based on history and physical examination. Anoscopy is useful for assessing abnormalities of the anal canal and distal rectal mucosa[12] and permits rectal biopsy of suspicious-looking lesions. Anoscopy is easily performed by all clinicians and is recommended for all patients with chronic constipation.

Sigmoidoscopy and colonoscopy are valuable in identifying obstructing lesions and strictures, as well as ulcerative colitis and melanosis coli.[15] Melanosis coli, a dark pigmentation of the colonic mucosa, occurs secondary to the chronic use of anthraquinone cathartics, which include cascara sagrada, senna, aloe, rhubarb, and danthron[4]; interestingly, the pigmentation spares any polyps that may be present.[15] Colonic biopsy is rarely useful in chronic constipation, although the histopathologic picture of ulcerative colitis or the aganglionosis of Hirschsprung's disease may be diagnosed by mucosal sampling.[15]

Manometry/Electromyography

When initial assessment reveals significant constipation or normal colonic transit, examination of the pelvic floor is appropriate.[14] Pelvic floor function is usually evaluated by anorectal manometry and/or electromyography (EMG) of the puborectalis muscle[14,15] and is contributory to the diagnosis of Hirschsprung's disease, anal fissure, megarectum,[14] paradoxic pelvic floor contraction,[12] and contributing neurologic disorders.

Other Tests

Rectal balloon expulsion is designed to assess pelvic floor function but is rarely utilized in the evaluation of chronic constipation. Urodynamics may also be considered to appraise sacral nerve root function but, like balloon expulsion, is seldom necessary.[12]

ASSESSMENT

Constellation of Findings

Environmental

This is indubitably the most common cause of chronic constipation. Lack of dietary fiber, little or no physical activity, and cortical suppression of the defecatory reflex are significant contributors to environmental constipation. Patients will frequently complain of a sensation of incomplete evacuation; sporadic bowel movements; and hard, pelletlike stools. Most diagnostic assessments are normal, although colonic transit studies may exhibit delayed transport, or radiopaque markers may accumulate in the rectosigmoid area with chronic suppression of the defecatory reflex. Anorectal manometry may also assist in confirming changes in the rectal vault secondary to suppression of the defecatory reflex.

Medications

The drug history will direct the practitioner to suspect medication use as the primary cause of chronic constipation, although bulimics, anorexics, and chronic laxative abusers will frequently test the diagnostic acumen of the most conscientious clinician. Most diagnostic studies are normal, although delayed colonic transit may be observed. If laxative abuse is suspected, urine screening for cathartic metabolites, or discovery of melanosis coli on colonoscopy, will facilitate diagnosis.

Colorectal

Most causes of colorectal constipation will be evident by radiographic studies or endoscopy. However, EMG and defecography may be necessary to diagnose two ailments of unknown etiology: anismus and descending perineum syndrome. Anismus occurs when the striated muscles of the pelvic floor fail to relax during straining, whereas descending perineum syndrome results when the pelvic floor dramatically descends during straining, bringing about a bulging of the perineum[14] with difficult evacuation.

Metabolic

Metabolic causes of chronic constipation are rare, although diabetes mellitus, hypothyroidism, and chronic renal insufficiency are three prominent causes. Autonomic neuropathic changes contribute to altered bowel function in diabetics, whereas hormonal deficiency induces constipation in hypothyroid individuals. Chronic renal insufficiency gives rise to constipation due to the underlying disease state and use of constipating medications.

Neurologic

Like metabolic etiologies, neurologic disorders are uncommon causes of chronic constipation. Hirschsprung's disease is one of the more common congenital disorders producing neurologic constipation and is easily diagnosed by barium enema, anorectal manometry, and full-thickness colonic biopsy. Constipation is also seen in patients with cerebrovascular ailments and Parkinson's disease, although the etiologic mechanism is unclear.

Implications of Chronic Constipation

While chronic constipation is often benign, it is important to exclude the presence of an underlying disorder. Most individuals experience bowel dysfunction secondary to poor dietary habits, suppression of the defecatory reflex, and limited physical activity—information readily secured by an assiduous history and physical examination. If the history and physical fail to identify the cause of constipation, consideration should be given to further diagnostic studies, including radiographic and endoscopic procedures.

REFERENCES

1. Haubrich WS. Constipation. In: Berk JE, ed. Gastroenterology. Philadelphia: WB Saunders, 1985:111–24.
2. Castle SC. Constipation: endemic in the elderly? Med Clin North Am 1989;73:1497–1509.
3. Jacknowitz AL. Gastrointestinal disorders. In: Covington TR, Walker JL, eds. Current geriatric therapy. Philadelphia: WB Saunders, 1984:178–238.
4. Rousseau PC. Treatment of constipation in the elderly. Postgrad Med 1988;83:339–49.
5. Devroede G. Constipation. In: Sleisenger MH, Fordtran JS, eds. Gastrointestinal disease: pathophysiology, diagnosis, management. 4th ed. Philadelphia: WB Saunders, 1989:331–68.
6. Thompson WG, Heaton KW. Functional bowel disorders in apparently healthy people. Gastroenterology 1980;79:283–8.
7. Brocklehurst JC. Colonic disease in the elderly. Clin Gastroenterol 1985;14:725–47.
8. O'Regan S, Yazbeck S. Constipation: a cause of enuresis, urinary tract infection and vesico-ureteral reflux in children. Med Hypotheses 1985;17:409–13.
9. Eastwood GL, Avunduk C, eds. Manual of gastroenterology. Boston: Little Brown, 1988:184–6.
10. Vobecky J, Caro J, Devroede G. A case-control study of risk factors for large bowel carcinoma. Cancer 1983;51:1958–63.
11. Rousseau PC. Managing constipation in the elderly patient. Fam Pract Recert 1990;12:76–93.
12. Miner PB. Constipation. Langhorne, Pennsylvania: Medicine Group, 1989:3–6.
13. Goldfinger SE. Constipation, diarrhea, and disturbances of anorectal function. In: Braunwald E, Isselbacher KJ, Petersdorf RG, Wilson JD, Martin JB, Fauci AS, eds. Harrison's principles of internal medicine. 11th ed. New York: McGraw Hill, 1987:177–80.
14. Pemberton J. Chronic constipation: matching type to treatment. Contemp Intern Med 1989;1(Sept):64–70.
15. Tremaine WJ. Chronic constipation: causes and management. Hosp Pract 1990;25(April):89–100.

COUGH, CHRONIC

ANNE M. PITTMAN, DAN SCHULLER, and PHILLIP E. KORENBLAT

SYNONYMS: A Sudden Noisy, Persistent Expulsion of Air from the Lungs

BACKGROUND

Cough is a normal reflex that protects the lung from injury by inhaled or aspirated foreign material. There are two specific mechanisms for clearing particles and secretions from the lung. The first is a thin layer of mucus propelled by continuous ciliary motion proximally from the terminal bronchi to the trachea. The second is cough. Cough can effectively remove secretions proximal to the segmental bronchi.[1]

Cough can also be a pathologic symptom elicited by stimulation at any point in the respiratory tract. A review of the afferent limb of the cough reflex and location of the cough receptors identifies many potential causes of cough. Cough receptors are found in the larynx, trachea, and major bronchi. They are located circumferentially in the airways; the number of receptors increases at points of airway bifurcations. Histologically, airway receptors have been shown to be myelinated nerve fibers located on the luminal side of the tracheobronchial basement membrane. A deeper site has also been postulated since removal of mucosa from the airways of experimental animals does not abolish their cough reflex.[2] Cough receptors can respond to either mechanical or chemical stimuli. Although functionally distinct, they are histologically indistinguishable. The mechanoreceptors are sensitive to pressure or changes in airway conformation and are found more frequently in large airways. Chemical, or irritant, receptors are found in greater number in small airways. In addition to the airways, it has been assumed that cough receptors exist in the nose, pharynx, paranasal sinuses, esophagus, tympanic membrane and ear canal, pleura, diaphragm, and pericardium.[3]

Afferent fibers from the cough receptors travel through the vagus, glossopharyngeal, tri-geminal, and phrenic nerves to the medulla. The efferent nerves travel back to the larynx, trachea, diaphragm, intercostal, and accessory muscles. The resulting muscular contractions are followed by sudden opening of the glottis and acceleration of intrathoracic gas.[3]

A chronic cough is one that has been persistent and bothersome for at least three weeks. Cough is very common in the general population, with up to 50 per cent reporting a cough of longer than three weeks' duration at some time. This chapter focuses on the diagnostic approach to chronic cough in the immunocompetent adult.

Clinical Spectrum of Chronic Cough

Many causes of chronic cough have been described (see Table 1). A minority of these account for the majority of cases. Cigarette smoking is associated with the highest prevalence of cough, followed by pipe and cigar smoking. In addition, estimates are that 8 to 14 per cent of nonsmoking adults report a chronic cough.[4]

Smoking Patients

There is a well-established relationship between cough and cigarette smoking. Among smokers of one pack of cigarettes per day, 25 per cent report a chronic cough. The prevalence increases with increasing number of cigarettes smoked. Smoker's cough usually responds to discontinuation of cigarette smoking. Wynder et al. found complete disappearance of cough in 77 per cent of patients after they had stopped smoking. In half, the cough resolved within one month.[5]

Although smoke-induced airway inflammation is the most common cause of chronic cough in smokers, other mechanisms appear to play a role. Direct stimulation of irritant receptors and increased risk of sensitization to certain inhaled antigens encountered in the workplace have been shown to be factors.[6] Cigarette smoke, by causing bronchial mu-

TABLE 1. Potential Causes of Chronic Cough by Receptor Location

Pulmonary
    Tobacco smoke
    Asthma
    Primary lung cancer
    Metastatic lung cancer
    Interstitial lung disease
    Hypersensitivity pneumonitis
    Postinfectious
    Occupational lung disease
    Sarcoidosis
    Cystic fibrosis/primary ciliary dyskinesia
    Endobronchial surgical sutures
Nose, pharynx, paranasal sinuses
    Postnasal drip
    Rhinosinusitis
Ear
    Cerumen impaction
    Cholesteatoma
    Auricular hair contact with tympanic membrane
Esophagus
    Gastroesophageal reflux
    Esophageal cyst
    Zenker's diverticulum
    Chronic aspiration
    Oculopharyngeal muscular dystrophy
Pleura
    Pleural effusion
    Pleural infiltration with tumor
    Mediastinal lymph nodes
    Mediastinal tumor
Pericardium
    Pericarditis
    Vagal nerve tumor
    Tumor infiltration
    Aortic aneurysm
    Enlarged left atrium
    Temporary pacemaker wires
Diaphragm
    Subphrenic abscess
    Hepatic abscess
Trachea, larynx
    Laryngeal disease
    Cervical vertebral osteophyte
    Thyroid mass lesion
    Aneurysm of ascending palatine artery

cous gland hyperplasia and impairment of ciliary function, leads to accumulation of mucous secretions in the airway, especially at night. This results in a morning cough that is frequently seen in patients with chronic bronchitis.

Nonsmoking Patients

In nonsmokers, Irwin et al.'s most recent prospective study of 102 consecutive patients found the most common etiology of chronic cough to be postnasal drip (41 per cent). This was due to sinusitis, allergic, nonallergic, or vasomotor rhinitis. Other causes included asthma (24 per cent), gastroesophageal reflux (21 per cent), and chronic bronchitis (5 per cent). It is important to note that rarely is cough found to be psychogenic.[7]

POSTNASAL DRIP.   Allergic, nonallergic, and infectious rhinitis are characterized by excessive mucous secretions. There can be profuse anterior rhinorrhea or posterior nasopharyngeal mucous drainage. Postnasal drip presumably causes cough by stimulation of cough receptors in the pharynx and larynx. This cough is frequently prominent at night and in the early morning.

SINUSITIS.   Sinusitis is inflammation of the mucosal membrane of one or more sinuses. Chronic sinusitis is defined by the presence of symptoms for more than four weeks. Cough is frequently one of the presenting symptoms in patients with acute or chronic sinusitis.

Obstruction of the sinus ostia is essential to the pathogenesis of sinusitis. Rhinitis, allergic and nonallergic, results in edematous obstruction of the ostia and decreased mucociliary function. Acute sinusitis also complicates 0.5 per cent of viral upper respiratory tract infections.[8] Ostia may be obstructed by polyps as well.

The anterior ethmoid sinuses are the most common site of chronic sinusitis. The maxillary and frontal sinuses drain near the ethmoid sinus and may be secondarily involved. Discomfort from sinusitis more typically arises from these secondarily involved sinuses. However, ethmoid sinusitis can be painless and frequently can be missed.

ASTHMA.   Isolated cough can be the sole presenting manifestation of bronchial asthma.[9] Cough in asthmatic patients was originally thought to be related to stimulation of airway mechanoreceptors secondary to large airway bronchoconstriction, where a large number of cough receptors are found. More recently, it has been recognized that cough and bronchoconstriction can be dissociated.[10] This cough may be especially bothersome at night.

GASTROESOPHAGEAL REFLUX.   Interestingly, chronic cough can also be the sole presenting manifestation of gastroesophageal reflux (GER). Irwin and coworkers found that up to 43 per cent of patients with GER documented by prolonged esophageal pH monitoring had no symptoms other than cough. This cough improved following specific antireflux therapy.[7] However, when cough was due to GER alone, it took more time to respond to specific therapy (mean 179 days) than when it was due to any other single condition.

HISTORY

History of the Present Illness

As is true for many other conditions, the diagnosis of chronic cough is facilitated by obtaining a detailed history. The characteristics of the cough can provide helpful clues. Attention should be given to onset, frequency, severity, and quality of symptoms. A dry, nonproductive cough can occur with pulmonary or extrapulmonary disease. With the exception of rhinosinusitis, a productive cough almost invariably implies pulmonary, as opposed to extrapulmonary, pathology. Sputum characteristics frequently narrow the spectrum of diagnostic possibilities. Large amounts of sputum (i.e., bronchorrhea) are seen in children with cystic fibrosis and patients with alveolar cell carcinoma, in whom up to 4 L of nonpurulent sputum per day have been described. More modest amounts of sputum are seen in patients with asthma, emphysema, and chronic bronchitis. The presence of large volumes of fetid sputum is associated with lung abscess and bronchiectasis. In pulmonary tuberculosis, cough is initially nonproductive, but as tissue necrosis ensues, sputum is usually produced and can be accompanied by hemoptysis.

The presence of associated symptoms may provide clues to the diagnosis. Postnasal drip may be described as a feeling of retropharyngeal phlegm or a need to clear the throat. These patients may also complain of sore throat or hoarseness. In addition, sneezing, nasal itch, profuse rhinorrhea, and ear popping of a seasonal or perennial nature suggest allergic or nonallergic rhinitis. The onset of either a pressurelike headache or dull pain and fullness of the upper teeth and zygomatic arch, in the setting of purulent postnasal drip, supports a diagnosis of sinusitis. Laryngeal pathology may be suggested by hoarseness and harsh cough.

Wheezing, dyspnea, and cough are cardinal symptoms of asthma. Cough, wheezing, and bronchial hyper-responsiveness are also common in patients with impaired left ventricular function—the so-called cardiac asthma.[11] A previous history of heart disease, orthopnea, paroxysmal nocturnal dyspnea, and pedal edema may support this diagnosis. Dysphagia, heartburn, and sour brash suggest GER. These symptoms of esophageal disease should be specifically looked for when assessing a patient with chronic cough. The association of cough with meals should alert the clinician to the possibility of a swallowing disorder. Halitosis should raise the possibility of a Zenker's diverticulum or an anaerobic lung abscess.

Medications

A detailed medication history (both prescription and nonprescription) should be obtained in every patient. A list of medications associated with cough is shown in Table 2. Angiotensin-converting enzyme (ACE) inhibitors such as captopril, enalapril, and cilazapril, increasingly used in the treatment of hypertension and congestive heart failure, are reported to cause cough. The overall incidence varies from 2 to 25 per cent, depending on the series. There is significant female predominance in some series. The cough may develop within days or after several months to a year of starting the medication and usually resolves within two weeks of discontinuation.[12]

Family History

Is there a family history of cystic fibrosis, asthma, pulmonary fibrosis, or hayfever? Are there any relatives who have been diagnosed with tuberculosis?

Social History

As previously stated, there is a well-established relationship between cough and tobacco smoking. There is also a significant incidence of chronic cough among those living in a house with smokers. Alcohol abuse has been associated with more frequent respiratory symptoms and slightly decreased respiratory function.[13] However, the data available are conflicting and confounded by other factors such as age, passive and active smoking, and occupational and socioeconomic status.

TABLE 2.   Drugs Associated
with Cough

Angiotensin-converting enzyme inhibitors
Beta-adrenergic blockers (oral or topical)
Aspirin
Nonsteroidal anti-inflammatory medications
Cholinesterase inhibitors
Tryptophan
Nitrofurantoin
Amiodarone
Neuromuscular blocking agents
Inhaled medications
Beclomethasone
Pentamidine
Sulfite sensitivity

Illicit drug use predisposes to conditions associated with chronic cough. Smoking freebase cocaine has been postulated to cause a variety of pulmonary complications that include barotrauma, pulmonary edema, pulmonary hemorrhage, hypersensitivity pneumonitis, and obliterative bronchiolitis.[14] The last two of these can be associated with chronic cough. Talc granulomatosis is seen in patients who crush tablets intended for oral use and inject them intravenously. Although dyspnea is the major symptom, cough occurs in some patients. Interestingly, talc granulomatosis can be associated with a normal chest roentgenogram in up to half of the patients with histologic evidence of disease.[15]

Patients should be questioned regarding intravenous drug use, sexual habits, and gender preference as risk factors for infection with human immunodeficiency virus (HIV). Acquired immune deficiency syndrome (AIDS) is associated with a variety of pulmonary problems, including chronic cough, the discussion of which is beyond the scope of this chapter.

Occupational History

A detailed occupational history is important. Many pneumoconioses are associated with chronic cough, pulmonary infiltrates, and fibrosis. Inquiry of specific work practices should include questions about specific contaminants (e.g., asbestos, cotton dust, or silica), the availability of respiratory protection devices, the ventilation in the workplace, and whether other coworkers have similar complaints. In addition, the occupational history should inquire about prior jobs and alternative sources for potentially toxic exposures, including hobbies or other environmental hazards at home or elsewhere.

Past Medical History

Is there a history of childhood asthma, hayfever, or recurrent sinus or ear problems? Is there a history of heart disease, malignancy, connective tissue disease, or neuromuscular disease that may predispose to chest pathology?

PHYSICAL EXAMINATION

In patients with chronic cough, the physical exam was found helpful 60 per cent of the time by Irwin and coworkers.[16] The general appearance of the patient may provide the first clue to the diagnosis. Weight loss and muscle wasting are seen in patients with AIDS, bronchogenic carcinoma, chronic infections such as tuberculosis, and severe emphysema. Malnutrition, nasal polyps, or poor growth or development in early age (rarely in late childhood or early adulthood) should raise the suspicion of cystic fibrosis.

The respiratory rate and pattern along with the examination of the accessory respiratory muscles provide an idea of the respiratory work required to compensate for the underlying respiratory or cardiac pathology.

Dermatologic Examination

Examination of the skin can reveal cyanosis, Kaposi's sarcoma, or erythema nodosum. The latter has been reported in association with sarcoidosis, tuberculosis, deep fungal infections, and psittacosis. (See *Difficult Diagnosis I*.)

Extremity Examination

Clubbing, either isolated or as part of hypertrophic osteoarthropathy, can occur in association with a variety of pulmonary problems including bronchogenic carcinoma, mesothelioma, bronchiectasis, lung abscess, empyema, cystic fibrosis, interstitial pulmonary fibrosis, asbestosis, and tuberculosis.

Head and Neck Examination

Periorbital puffiness, conjunctival injection, and infraorbital cyanosis ("allergic shiners") are seen in patients with allergic and nonallergic rhinitis. On examination of the ears, look specifically for fluid behind the tympanic membrane. Irritating hairs and impacted cerumen have been reported to induce cough by stimulating the auricular branch of the vagus nerve.[3]

Pale pink, boggy, enlarged inferior turbinates with visible mucus are characteristic of rhinitis. A granular "cobblestone" pharyngitis with erythematous lateral pharyngeal bands is evidence of postnasal drip. Mucopus in the nose, occasionally observed draining from sinus ostium, or streaming along the posterior pharynx, is suggestive of sinusitis. Tenderness to percussion over the maxillary or frontal sinus occurs too infrequently to be a reliable sign.

The neck exam may reveal lymphadenopathy, unsuspected masses, thyroid enlargement, or a trachea that is deviated or fixed.

Pulmonary Examination

The chest exam is of utmost importance. Attention should be paid to evidence of cardiac murmurs or gallops, pulmonary crackles or wheezes, pleural friction rubs, or physical findings consistent with pulmonary consolidation, atelectasis, hyperinflation, or pleural effusion.

DIAGNOSTIC STUDIES

History and physical examination constitute the basis upon which a diagnosis can be established in the majority of patients with chronic cough. Without any additional tests, a correct diagnosis was made in nearly three quarters of the patients.[7]

Clinical Laboratory Studies

Sputum examination, a complete blood cell count with differential, and nasal mucous examination are reasonable initial data to be collected in most patients with chronic cough. Occasionally, the sputum cytology can be positive for malignancy without abnormalities on the chest x-ray. This occurred in approximately 10 to 15 per cent of the asymptomatic patients who were "screened" for lung cancer with serial standard chest radiographs and sputum cytologic examination.[17]

Sputum cytologic examination should be considered in the early assessment of the patient with persistent cough and a normal chest roentgenogram. In smokers and those older than 50 years of age, it can be a cost-effective tool in determining whether bronchoscopy should be performed.[18]

A blood eosinophil count is of limited usefulness in the evaluation of chronic cough except in the case of allergic bronchopulmonary aspergillosis, eosinophilic pneumonia, or vasculitis. However, a clear distinction between patients with rhinitis is made by cytologic examination of nasal mucus for eosinophils. Nasal eosinophilia (greater than 10 per cent eosinophilia) is highly characteristic of allergic disease. It is also seen in the NARES syndrome (nonallergic rhinitis with eosinophilia) and occasionally in patients with nasal polyposis. Nasal neutrophilia is seen in infectious rhinosinusitis. Nasal smears are unsuitable for culture. Sinus aspiration is required to make a specific microbial diagnosis but is reserved for patients with severe illness, nosocomial infection, or immunodeficiency.

Diagnostic Imaging

Chest X-rays

A standard chest roentgenogram is an essential part of the evaluation. When the chest x-ray is normal, it is unlikely that the cause of the chronic cough is anything other than rhinosinusitis, asthma, GER, chronic bronchitis, or a combination of these possibilities. However, patients with various chest diseases may on occasion have a perfectly normal chest roentgenogram. As many as 14 per cent of patients with interstitial lung disease may have a normal chest film.[19] Endobronchial neoplasms, bronchiectasis, cystic fibrosis, endobronchial tuberculosis, bronchiolithiasis, and especially foreign bodies may also be radiologically undetectable.

Sinus X-rays

While maxillary or frontal sinusitis can often be diagnosed on clinical grounds, acute inflammatory sinus disease is best evaluated by x-rays of the paranasal sinuses. These may reveal an air fluid level or partial or complete opacification of the involved sinus.

Unfortunately, the anterior ethmoid sinus is most often involved in chronic inflammatory sinus disease and is not well visualized by plain films. Computerized tomography (CT) scan provides excellent definition of these sinuses.

Transillumination of the frontal or maxillary sinus may be a useful confirmatory test. However, transillumination cannot be relied on for definitive diagnosis. The technique is of limited usefulness when there is partial illumination or in patients with chronic sinus disease and ethmoid sinusitis.

Pulmonary Function Tests

Standard spirometry with measurement of the forced vital capacity (FVC) and the forced expiratory volume in the first second (FEV1) can be useful in revealing limitation of expiratory airflow consistent with asthma ("reversible") or chronic bronchitis/emphysema ("irreversible"). Decreased lung volume with a normal FEV1/FVC ratio is consistent with restrictive physiology and is seen in interstitial pulmonary fibrosis.

Bronchial inhalation challenge with methacholine or histamine is most useful for determining a diagnosis of asthma in patients with normal spirometry. The sensitivity of inhalation testing is very high, approaching 100 per cent at an agonist concentration of 8 mg/100 ml of methacholine.[20] Therefore, in the setting of chronic cough, the test is most useful in "ruling out" asthma. However, it should be noted that patients with seasonal allergic asthma tested out of the allergen season and patients with occupational asthma tested after a weekend away from work may have negative bronchoprovocation challenges.[20] A number of diseases other than asthma can be associated with bronchial hyperresponsiveness. These include chronic bronchitis, emphysema, bronchiolitis, viral upper respiratory infection, sarcoidosis, cystic fibrosis, hypersensitivity pneumonitis, and chemical irritant exposure.[20] Another interesting and common association with bronchial hyperresponsiveness occurs in patients with impaired left ventricular function.[11]

Gastrointestinal Evaluation

Since GER is a common entity, and some reflux episodes may be clinically silent, occasional patients will require specific evaluation. Barium swallow was positive in 44 per cent of Irwin's patients with GER (documented by a response to therapy) with a reported sensitivity of 48 per cent and specificity of 76 per cent. On the other hand, prolonged esophageal pH monitoring was abnormal and consistent with GER as the cause of cough in all patients tested, giving a sensitivity and specificity of 100 per cent in this series.[7]

Fiberoptic Bronchoscopy

The use of flexible fiberoptic bronchoscopy (FOB) in the evaluation of chronic cough has been controversial. Some find it useful in the early diagnosis of lung cancer. However, other authors have observed that although a chronic cough is commonly associated with bronchogenic carcinoma, it is almost never an isolated finding. In the presence of a negative chest x-ray, FOB is usually negative or nondiagnostic.[18]

Bronchoscopy is indicated when cough is accompanied by hemoptysis, when physical findings suggest an endobronchial lesion, or when sputum cytology is abnormal.

Rare situations other than tracheobronchial tumors that can be detected with FOB in patients with "occult cough" include foreign bodies, bronchioliths, and airway strictures.

ASSESSMENT

Since 1981, at least five published studies involving patients complaining of chronic cough have utilized an "anatomic-diagnostic" protocol. They have consistently found that the presumed cause can be determined in 88 to 99 per cent of the patients, leading to specific therapy that is successful at least 93 per cent of the time.[21] This approach is based on evaluating the locations of the afferent limbs of the cough reflex and encourages clinicians to consider extrapulmonary as well as pulmonary conditions in the differential diagnosis.

One must realize that an extensive evaluation is likely to uncover conditions common in the general population and commonly associated with cough. Finding them may not necessarily imply causation. In addition, some of the patients with chronic cough have more than one cause. Therefore, if there is lack of response to an initial therapeutic trial directed to a specific cause, other concomitant problems need to be excluded.

It seems reasonable to start with a thorough history and physical exam, accompanied by a posteroanterior and lateral chest x-ray. If the chest x-ray is normal, the patient is a nonsmoker, and a specific diagnosis cannot be established with the data available, then pulmonary function testing with or without bronchoprovocation should be obtained. If the results are consistent with asthma, the patient can be treated appropriately with bronchodilators, corticosteroids, or cromolyn as indicated. When the diagnosis is still in question, utilizing the clues provided in the history and physical exam, one can move to a more indepth ear, nose, and throat evaluation including sinus films or evaluate the possibility of GER with a 24-hour esophageal pH monitoring.

If the patient is a smoker and has a negative chest film, an aggressive strategy for smoking cessation should be instituted and the resolution of cough expected in four to six weeks.

Only rarely will FOB be helpful in the setting of a normal chest x-ray. It is most appropriate when the history, physical examination, pulmonary function testing, and perhaps esophageal pH monitoring are nondiagnostic. On the other hand, chronic cough, with an abnormal chest film suspicious for malignancy,

TABLE 3. Complications of Cough

Cardiovascular
  Syncope (cerebral hypoperfusion)
  Bradycardia, heart block
  Transient hypertension
  Hemorrhage (e.g., subarachnoid, epistaxis, subconjunctival, anal veins)
Pulmonary
  Barotrauma (pneumothorax, pneumomediastinum, subcutaneous emphysema)
  Bronchoconstriction
  Laryngeal injury
  Respiratory epithelial damage
Musculoskeletal
  Rib and vertebral fractures
  Rupture of rectus abdominis muscles
  Hernias
Miscellaneous
  Insomnia, depression, anorexia
  Vomiting
  Headache
  Urinary incontinence
  Vaginal prolapse
  Disruption of surgical wounds
  Displacement or occlusion of intravenous catheters

mandates the need for bronchoscopic evaluation.

Complications of Cough

Cough itself, in particular situations, can lead to a variety of complications that can be very disruptive to the patient. Most of these are the result of either a vagaly mediated reflex or high intrathoracic pressure with an associated decrease in venous return (Valsalva-like effect). In addition, pathology may arise as a result of violent muscular contractions and increased intra-abdominal pressure. Table 3 lists reported complications of cough.

REFERENCES

1. Pierce, JA. Cough. In: Blacklow R, ed. MacBryde's signs and symptoms. Philadelphia: Lippincott, 1985:317–29.
2. Sant' Ambriogio G, Remmers JE, DeGroot WJ, et al. Localization of rapidly adapting receptors in the trachea and main stem bronchus of the dog. Respir Physiol 1978;33:359.
3. Braman SS, Carrao WM. Cough: differential diagnosis and treatment. Clin Chest Med 1987;8:177–88.
4. Wynder EL, Lemon FR, Mantel N. Epidemiology of persistent cough. Am Rev Respir Dis 1965; 91:679–700.
5. Wynder EL, Kaufman PI, Lesser RL. A short term follow-up study of ex-cigarette smokers. Am Rev Respir Dis 1967;96:645–55.
6. O'Connor GT, Sparrow D, Weiss ST. The role of allergy and nonspecific airway hyperresponsiveness in the pathogenesis of chronic obstructive pulmonary disease. Am Rev Respir Dis 1989;140: 225–52.
7. Irwin RS, Curley FJ, French CL. Chronic cough. The spectrum and frequency of causes, key components of the diagnostic evaluation and outcome of specific therapy. Am Rev Respir Dis 1990;141:640–7.
8. Gwaltney JM Jr. Sinusitis. In: Mandell GL, Douglas RG Jr, Bennett JE, eds. Principles and practice of infectious disease. 2nd ed. New York: John Wiley, 1985:369–72.
9. Corrao WM, Braman SS, Irwin RS. Chronic cough as the sole presenting manifestation of bronchial asthma. N Engl J Med 1979;300:633–7.
10. Eschenbacher WL, Boushey HA, Sheppan D. Alteration in osmolarity of inhaled aerosols causes bronchoconstriction and cough but absence of a permeant anion causes cough alone. Am Rev Respir Dis 1984;129:211–5.
11. Cabanes LR, Weber SN, Matran R, et al. Bronchial hyperresponsiveness to methacholine in patients with impaired left ventricular function. N Engl J Med 1989;320:1317–22.
12. Meeker DP, Wiedeman HP. Drug induced bronchospasm. Clin Chest Med 1990;11:163–75.
13. Lebowitz MD. Respiratory symptoms and disease related to alcohol consumption. Am Rev Respir Dis 1981;123:16–9.
14. Ettinger NA, Albin RJ. A review of the respiratory effects of smoking cocaine. Am J Med 1989; 87:664–8.
15. Waller BF, Brownlee WJ, Robert WC. Self-induced pulmonary granulomatosis: a consequence of intravenous injection of drugs intended for oral use. Chest 1980;78:90–4.
16. Irwin RS, Corrao WM, Pratter MR. Chronic persistent cough in the adult; the spectrum and frequency of causes and successful outcome of specific therapy. Am Rev Respir Dis 1981;123:413–7.
17. Cohen MH. The natural history and clinical picture of carcinoma of the lung. In: Fishman AP, ed. Pulmonary diseases and disorders. 2nd ed. New York: McGraw Hill, 1988:1934.
18. Poe RH, Isreal RH, Utell, MJ, Hall WJ. Chronic cough; bronchoscopy or pulmonary funtion testing? Am Rev Respir Dis 1982;126:160–2.
19. Epler GR, McLoud TC, Gaensler EA, et al. Normal chest roentgenograms in diffuse infiltrative lung disease. N Engl J Med 1978;298:934–9.
20. Braman SS, Corrao W. Bronchoprovocation testing. Clin Chest Med 1989;10:165–6.
21. Poel RH, Harder RV, Isreal RH, Kallay MC. Chronic persistent cough. Experience in diagnosis and outcome using an anatomic diagnostic protocol. Chest 1989;95:723–8.

DIARRHEA, ACUTE

ALEX H. BRUCKSTEIN

SYNONYM: Acute Gastroenteritis

BACKGROUND

Definition

Clinically, healthy adults eating a regular diet have as many as three bowel movements per day or as few as three bowel movements per week.[1] The stool weight rarely exceeds 200 gm. The factors that account for variation in stool weight, percentage of water content, or frequency of bowel movements among various people without disease have not been fully clarified. A high-fiber diet will increase stool weight; an increase of stool weight often increases stool frequency without the patient necessarily complaining of diarrhea.[2] To the clinician, diarrhea is present when any of the following occur:

1. Abnormal increase in stool liquidity.
2. Abnormal increase in daily stool weight to an excess of 250 gm.
3. Abnormal increase in stool frequency.

Diarrhea is often accompanied by perianal discomfort, urgency, or rarely, incontinence. Acute diarrhea is defined as the persistence of these symptoms for less than three weeks in adults.

Diarrhea Versus Malabsorption

Diarrhea differs from malabsorption in that diarrhea means an excess of fecal water loss related to increased secretion of water or reduced absorption of water, whereas malabsorption implies an increase fecal loss of intestinal nutrients. Malabsorption is generally associated with diarrhea, whereas diarrhea frequently exists in the absence of fat or other nutrient malabsorption.

Physiology

For normal people eating three meals per day, approximately 9 L of fluid are handled by the gastrointestinal tract. Major components of this include: (1) dietary intake of 2 L, (2) salivary secretion of 1 L, (3) gastric secretion of 2 L, (4) biliary secretion of 1 L, (5) pancreatic secretion of 2 L, and (6) small intestinal secretion of 1 L. More than 98 per cent of this 9 L is reabsorbed daily. Only 0.1 to 0.2 L of fluid are excreted in the stool. Reabsorption of this fluid occurs such that in the upper small intestine 4 to 5 L of fluid are reabsorbed; the fluid is initially hyperosmolar, but as a result of rapid reabsorption of amino acids and sugars, it is iso-osmolar when it reaches the ileum. In the ileum, 3 to 4 L are reabsorbed; most of the nutrients have been reabsorbed before reaching this area, so the fluid is generally iso-osmotic. There is an efficient sodium pump, so ion exchange is rapid. In the colon, normal fluid reabsorption is about 0.5 to 1.5 L per day. However, the colon is very efficient at reabsorption; if necessary, the colon can reabsorb up to 7 L daily. Thus, unless it is damaged or its fluid reabsorptive capacity exceeded, the colon can often protect against diarrhea. In summary, the amount of fluid passing the duodenum is about 9 L; passing the ileocecal valve, 0.5 to 1.5 L; and passing the anal sphincter, 0.1 to 0.2 L. Stated differently, the small bowel absorbs about 8 L of fluid daily and empties 0.5 to 1.5 L into the colon, and the colon absorbs all but 0.1 to 0.2 L daily. Thus, considering the gastrointestinal tract as a single entity, more than 98 per cent of the volume that passes through it is absorbed daily.

Pathophysiology

Although diarrhea presents itself as an increase in fecal water loss, the clinician must consider that the transport of water in the gastrointestinal tract occurs as a result of solute movement, or as a result of hydrostatic and osmotic gradients. Therefore, abnormalities in either the absorption or secretion of water are the direct consequence of decreased absorption or increased secretion of osmotically active solutes, primarily electrolytes and carbohydrates. As such, it is useful to consider the major mechanisms that cause diarrhea as being altered osmotic load, active secretion with inhibition of normal active ion absorption, or abnormal intestinal motility. These mechanisms cause diarrhea with an excess of fecal water loss. In many clinical situations, however, the pathophysiologic process is often a combination of one or more of the above factors.

Osmotic Diarrhea

The pathophysiologic process in this situation is that a poorly absorbed solute accumulates in the intestinal lumen, with the result that sodium and water are drawn into the lumen, converting the intestinal luminal contents from hyperosmolar to iso-osmolar. The hallmark clinical feature of this diarrhea is that the diarrhea lessens and stops once the patient is fasted or placed on a clear liquid diet (see Table 1). The solute gap is greater than 40. (*Solute gap* is the stool osmolarity measured by the laboratory minus twice the concentration of fecal sodium and potassium.) When osmotic diarrhea is a result of carbohydrate malabsorption, the stool pH is low. The diseases that commonly cause osmotic diarrhea are either carbohydrate malabsorption, of which lactose intolerance is the most common, or surreptitious laxative abuse, especially true with laxatives containing polyvalent ions (e.g., magnesium, sulfate, or phosphate).

Another situation in which osmotic diarrhea occurs is in the patient who is given lactulose, an undigestible synthetic disaccharide, in an attempt to cause diarrhea as part of the therapy of hepatic encephalopathy. Additionally, sorbitol, a sweetener in diet drinks, diet chewing gum, or candy, is associated with an osmotic diarrhea. This is occasionally the mechanism of diarrhea in young patients who are diagnosed as having irritable bowel syndrome.

Secretory Diarrhea

The small intestine secretes and absorbs water and electrolytes. When the rate of secretion is less than the rate of absorption, the net effect on the small bowel transport process is absorption of fluid. The absorption of fluid occurs in the villus cells, and the secretion of fluid occurs in the crypt cells. Thus, the pathophysiology of secretory diarrhea can occur as a result of an inhibition of ion absorption or a stimulation of ion secretion. The two major causes of inhibition of ion absorption are related to alterations in cyclic adenosine monophosphate (AMP) levels and to congenital chloridorrhea. Active ion secretion is related to an increase of cyclic nucleotides as well. Some of the common intestinal secretagogues include bacterial enterotoxins (e.g., cholera, *Escherichia coli* enterotoxins), dihydroxy bile acids (ileal resection or disease), fatty acids (pancreatic insufficiency), laxatives (castor oil), and hormones (Zollinger-Ellison syndrome, carcinoid syndrome).

The clinical features are that the diarrhea is usually greater than 1 L per day, and the solute gap of the stool supernatant is less than 40, with a stool osmolality almost totally accounted for by $2(Na^+ + K^+)$ (see Table 1). The diarrhea will generally continue even after a 24- to 48-hour fast. Exceptions to this rule include secretory diarrhea resulting from malabsorption of fatty acids or bile salts, diarrhea as a result of laxative abuse when the laxatives are stopped, or situations where the colon compensates after the additional stimulus of the food is removed.

Abnormal Intestinal Motility

The pathophysiology here is most commonly secondary to some other underlying disease process. For example, there can be accelerated gastric emptying with resultant

TABLE 1. Clinical Features Distinguishing Osmotic from Secretory Diarrhea

CLINICAL FEATURE	OSMOTIC	SECRETORY
Daily stool volume	Less than 1 L	Greater than 1 L
Effect of 48-hour fast	Diarrhea stops	Diarrhea continues
Fecal fluid osmolality	400 mOsm/kg	290 mOsm/kg
$2(Na^+ + K^+)$	120 mEq/L	280 mEq/L
Solute gap	280	10

postgastrectomy diarrhea, or there can be delayed transit with secondary bacterial overgrowth as a result of scleroderma or diabetic diarrhea. There is no pathognomonic clinical finding; diagnosis is made after other causes of diarrhea have been excluded.[3]

HISTORY

The degree to which different aspects of the history are emphasized will vary depending on the duration of the diarrhea, the age of the patient, and the coexistence of evidence of systemic disease.

Focused Queries

The medical history should focus on the following questions:

1. *Has there been travel to areas where the drinking water is contaminated or where the fields are irrigated with suspensions of fecal matter?* The majority of these episodes would be related to enterotoxigenic *E. coli.* Additionally, *Salmonella, Shigella,* and *E. histolytica* infections must be considered because these may require specific treatment and may persist for a few days. Following an episode of "traveler's diarrhea" ("turista" or "Montezuma's revenge"), many patients are left with mild diarrhea, with or without other abdominal symptoms, for weeks to months, after which the initial agent can no longer be detected. These symptoms will occasionally resolve spontaneously. When questioning the patient about this issue, the patient should specifically be questioned about travel to the Soviet Union or China, where infection with *Giardia lamblia* may be acquired from the water supply. Additionally, travel to the Caribbean islands or South or Southeastern Asia can expose the patient to the risk of acquiring tropical sprue, especially if he or she does not remain in a Western-style environment.

2. *Are there synchronous cases in family members, coworkers, or participants at social gatherings?* This suggests an infectious or toxin-induced diarrhea. If the onset can be related to the intake of food or drink, the time between ingestion and onset of symptoms may be relevant. Early onset (within 14 hours) occurs with food poisoning, whereas a delayed onset suggests an infectious agent, which needs to proliferate in the intestine before producing symptoms.

3. *Has the patient been exposed to household pets or other animals? Salmonella, Yersinia,* and *Campylobacter jejuni* have been associated with this.

4. *Is the patient a homosexual?* Many unusual enteric and rectal infections have been observed in homosexual patients.[4]

5. *Is the patient immunosuppressed by disease or by taking corticosteroids,* or *could the patient have acquired immune deficiency syndrome (AIDS)?* These patients are at high risk for the development of opportunistic infections.[5,6]

6. *Does the diarrhea occur only with relation to specific foods?* The classic example here is the patient who has milk intolerance due to lactase deficiency; this patient will tell the clinician he or she dislikes dairy products but may not realize the reason for the dislike. In a new environment, such as in the hospital or while on a trip, this patient may consume extra amounts of dairy products and develop diarrhea.

7. *Is the patient eating many "low-calorie" foods?* Teenagers, patients trying to lose weight, and diabetics can develop diarrhea as a result of sorbitol.[7]

8. *Does the patient note that the diarrhea is related to alcohol?* Alcohol commonly causes a watery diarrhea as a result of a combination of mechanisms.[8]

9. *What medications does the patient take?* The patient must be questioned carefully as to the nature of any prescription or over-the-counter medications that he or she takes. Drugs that commonly cause osmotic diarrhea include antacids, especially those containing magnesium, and lactulose syrup. Any antibiotic, taken orally or even parenterally, can cause diarrhea that may persist for days or weeks after the antibiotic is discontinued. Most of these patients have a diarrhea that is perhaps related to an alteration in intestinal flora. Only the rare patient develops pseudomembranous enterocolitis due to *Clostridium difficile* toxin, but this is the most severe form of the complication. In the majority of patients who have antibiotic-associated diarrhea, the diarrhea is mild and nonbloody. Some of the other drugs that cause diarrhea are listed in Table 2.

10. *What is the patient's occupation or hobby?* Female patients in the health-related profession have the highest incidence of sur-

TABLE 2. Drugs That May Cause Diarrhea

Magnesium-containing antacids
Antibiotics
Antiarrhythmic drugs (e.g., digitalis, quinidine)
Gold compounds
Colchicine
Chenodiol
Surreptitious laxative abuse

reptitious laxative abuse.[9] Severe physical exertion, such as occurs in long-distance runners, may precipitate brief bouts of abdominal cramps and watery diarrhea.

11. *What is the nature of the diarrhea? Is there blood? Is there severe abdominal pain? Are there fever and associated weight loss?* An affirmative answer to any of these questions indicates that the diarrhea is organic as opposed to functional.

12. *Does the diarrhea awaken the patient at night?* Any serious cause of diarrhea will have associated nocturnal symptoms. Irritable bowel syndrome, on the other hand, is most common in the early part of the day.

13. *Where and when did the diarrhea develop? Specifically, if the patient is now hospitalized, was it the diarrhea that prompted the hospitalization, or was the patient hospitalized for another reason and then developed diarrhea in the hospital?* For community-acquired diarrhea, one should consider parasite infestation or bacterial infection with *Salmonella, Shigella, Campylobacter,* and other classic enteric pathogens in the spectrum of potentially responsible infectious agents. However, these organisms have rarely—if ever—been shown to cause nosocomial diarrhea, except in isolated outbreaks of food poisoning. For adult patients who develop infectious diarrhea while hospitalized, *Clostridium difficile* is the pathogen most often isolated.[10,11]

PHYSICAL EXAMINATION

In the setting of acute diarrhea, the physical examination rarely reveals diagnostic information. However, the physical examination is useful to assess the state of hydration, especially in the elderly, in the very young, or in patients with an ileostomy. Diminished skin turgor, hypotension, or orthostatic changes in pulse and blood pressure suggest significant dehydration. Hyperventilation suggests metabolic acidosis. Since one of the most common causes of acute diarrhea in elderly patients, especially those hospitalized or in those confined to nursing homes, is a fecal impaction, a careful rectal exam should be performed.

DIAGNOSTIC STUDIES

Routine Laboratory Tests

Laboratory Tests to Determine the Cause of Diarrhea

Since the most likely cause of acute diarrhea is either an infectious agent or some medication or food additive (see Table 3), the most useful laboratory study is a stool culture for ova and parasites and for enteric pathogens (see Table 4). Based on a recent study, this is the most cost-effective strategy for managing AIDS-related diarrhea.[12] It should be noted that the stool culture must be done on a fresh specimen of stool, promptly delivered to the laboratory. When parasitic infection is highly likely, three different stool specimens (one on each of three different days) should be examined before this diagnosis is reasonably excluded. Less useful tests of the stool include (1) a stool exam for fecal occult blood and (2) a Wright's stain of the stool to look for polymorphonuclear leukocytes, which would suggest bacterial infection or inflammatory disease. A complete blood count with differential may suggest a parasitic infection if there is an increased percentage of eosinophils.

A more invasive test would be a proctosigmoidoscopy. In the majority of cases of acute diarrhea, this will be unnecessary. It may, however, help make the diagnosis of a mucosal disease of the bowel.[13]

Laboratory Tests to Reflect the Severity of the Illness

Patients with diarrhea in whom the diagnosis is not obvious should have a complete blood count, chemical profile (including serum electrolytes, blood urea nitrogen, and creatinine), and urinalysis. This will help determine

TABLE 3. Most Likely Causes of Acute Diarrhea

Infections (viral, bacterial, parasitic, fungal)
Food poisoning
Medications (see Table 2)
Food additives (sorbitol)
Fecal impaction
Traveler's diarrhea

TABLE 4. Laboratory Studies in Acute Diarrhea*	
STOOL EXAMINATION	PROCTOSIGMOIDOSCOPY
Volume per 24 hours	Mucosal appearance
Frequency per 24 hours	Mucosal biopsy
Blood	Fecal aspirate for culture
Consistency	**PERIPHERAL BLOOD**
Wright's stain for white blood cells	Complete blood count
Sudan stain	Eosinophil count
Osmolality	Erythrocyte sedimentation rate
pH	Routine chemistry
Reducing substances	Ameba serology
Culture for enteric pathogens	
Culture for ova and parasites	
Clostridium difficile toxin	
Color change upon alkalinization	

* Diagnostic evaluation is determined by the nature of the problem. Selection and timing of individual investigations will vary.

the nutritional status of the patient and assess fluid and electrolyte status as well. Hypernatremic dehydration reflects a severe diarrhea and is occasionally found in children, nursing home patients, and those unable to have access to fluids.

Special Laboratory Tests

Stool Exam

A freshly passed stool should be inspected. If bright-red blood is seen, it favors active inflammation of the rectum or colon, rather than disease confined to the more proximal bowel. On the other hand, the absence of blood does not exclude proctocolitis. By the same token, the presence of blood does not indicate mucosal disease, since severe diarrhea may precipitate a minor degree of bleeding from pre-existent hemorrhoids or an anal fissure. If there is blood, pus, and mucous in the stool, but little solid matter, this suggests inflammatory bowel disease. Bulky, greasy stools suggest malabsorption. Oil in the toilet bowl suggests pancreatic insufficiency or points to the diagnosis of laxative abuse (when the patient is taking mineral oil).

In the majority of patients with acute diarrhea, it is rarely necessary to perform a quantitative stool collection. This is because the majority of cases subside spontaneously, and both the physician and patient are reluctant to perform this inconvenient test. In some instances, however, knowledge of quantitative stool volume is of direct aid in diagnosis and management. Very large volumes of stool will alert the physician to the potential need for vigorous fluid replacement.

Occasionally, the patient will complain of diarrhea, but when a quantitative stool test is performed in the hospital, he or she will have less than 200 gm of stool per day. This is useful, as it excludes the need for further studies. However, it does not imply that the patient has lied about the history; it may mean that he or she is passing stool that is abnormally frequent, abnormally urgent, or watery, all of which suggest either irritable bowel syndrome or anal sphincter dysfunction. On the other hand, the patient may have had true diarrhea that ceased in the hospital as a result of the fact that he or she was ingesting a food substance or drug (laxative) that is not available in the hospital or that in the hospital the patient is removed from a stressful home situation.

Osmotic Gap

As mentioned previously, the measurement of a fecal osmotic gap is a useful method to distinguish between secretory diarrhea and osmotic diarrhea. In the setting of osmotic diarrhea, the osmotic gap in the fecal fluid reflects the unabsorbed solute, whereas in secretory diarrhea the osmolarity of the fecal fluid is entirely a result of the fecal electrolytes.

ASSESSMENT

The initial encounter between the patient and the physician occurs under a wide range of circumstances, ranging from the apparently well patient who has two to three loose bowel movements per day to the acutely ill patient with fever and profuse diarrhea. The causes of acute and chronic diarrhea differ to a large extent. (Also see chapter on Diarrhea,

Chronic in *Difficult Diagnosis I*.) However, this distinction often cannot be made during the initial visit because chronic diarrhea may have an acute onset, and several diseases that are considered to be chronic—for example, idiopathic inflammatory bowel disease—may present acutely or may have an acute exacerbation intermittently. Thus, two decisions must be made by the physician before diagnostic studies are undertaken.

The first issue is whether the patient requires hospitalization. The indications for hospitalization include acute dehydration, manifesting clinically as orthostatic changes in pulse or blood pressure; poor skin turgor; active rectal bleeding; considerable weight loss; or fever with a tender abdominal mass. The second issue is whether there are indications of a common infectious source of the acute diarrhea, which will require notification of the local health authority. Once these issues have been addressed and a decision made, the physician is ready to evaluate the patient with acute diarrhea.

REFERENCES

1. Drossman DA, Sandler RS, McKee DC, Lovitz AJ. Bowel patterns among subjects not seeking health care. Gastroenterology 1982;83:529–34.
2. Tucker DM, Sandstead HH, Logan GM, et al. Dietary fiber and personality factors as determinants of stool output. Gastroenterology 1981;81:879–83.
3. Kirsch M. Bacterial overgrowth. Am J Gastroenterol 1990;85:231–7.
4. Phillips SC, Mildvan D, William DC, Gelb AM, White MC. Sexual transmission of enteric protozoa and helminths in a venereal disease clinic population. N Engl J Med 1981;305:603–6.
5. Antony MA, Brandt LJ, Klein RS, Bernstein LH. Infectious diarrhea in patients with AIDS. Dig Dis Sci 1988;33:1141–6.
6. Rolston KVI, Rodriguez S, Hernandez M, Bodey GP. Diarrhea in patients infected with the human immunodeficiency virus. Am J Med 1989;86:137–8.
7. Ravry MJR. Dietetic food diarrhea. JAMA 1980;244:270.
8. Burbige EJ, Lewis DR Jr, Halsted CK. Alcohol and the gastrointestinal tract. Med Clin North Am 1984;68:77–89.
9. Reich P, Gottfried LA. Factitious disorders in a teaching hospital. Ann Intern Med 1983;99:240–7.
10. Gilligan PH. Diarrheal disease in the hospitalized patient. Infect Control 1981;7:607–9.
11. Gilligan PH, McCarthy LR, Genta VM. Relative frequency of Clostridium difficile in patients with diarrheal disease. J Clin Microbiol 1981;14:26–31.
12. Johanson JF, Sonnenberg A. Efficient management of diarrhea in the acquired immunodeficiency syndrome (AIDS). A medical decision analysis. Ann Intern Med 1990;112:942–8.
13. Nostrant TT, Kumar NB, Appelman HD. Histopathology differentiates acute self-limited colitis from ulcerative colitis. Gastroenterology 1987;92:318–28.

DRY EYE

J. DANIEL NELSON

SYNONYMS: Keratoconjunctivitis Sicca, Sjögren's Syndrome

BACKGROUND

Dry eye refers to a group of diseases characterized by subjective complaints of burning, foreign body sensation, and grittiness. Symptoms arise from irritation of the sensory nerve endings in the surface of the cornea, conjunctiva, and eyelids. The ophthalmic division—and to a lesser extent, the maxillary division of the trigeminal nerve—carries sensory fibers from the eye and eyelids. The nasociliary nerve, a branch of the ophthalmic, carries sensory fibers from the cornea, medial eyelid, and conjunctiva. The frontal nerve carries the sensory fibers from the middle two thirds of the upper eyelid and the superior conjunctiva. The lacrimal nerve supplies sensory innervation to the lacrimal gland and the lateral portion of the upper eyelid and conjunctiva. The maxillary division of the trigeminal nerve carries sensory input from the lower eyelid and conjunctiva via the infraorbital nerve. It anastomoses with the infratrochlear nerve to provide sensory innervation to the medial corner of the eye. In general, most eye discomfort or pain is either surface irritation or deeper, "ache-like" pain. Symptoms of foreign body and burning sensations are quite specific for surface irritation. In eye conditions that involve the interior of the eye, such as iritis scleritis or glaucoma, the pain is more ache-like in nature.[1] Surface-type symptoms are caused by a variety of conditions that are termed *ocular surface diseases*. These diseases include keratoconjunctivitis sicca (KCS), blepharitis, ocular pemphigoid, Stevens-Johnson syndrome, allergic conjunctivitis, atopic eye disease, and toxic kerato-conjunctivitis (keratitis medicamentosa). Since the symptoms of these diseases are similar and as the treatment of these diseases varies, the correct diagnosis of the particular dry eye or ocular surface disorder is of great importance.

The ocular surface includes the precorneal tear film, eyelids, conjunctiva, and cornea. The precorneal tear film is the major refractive surface of the eye and has three layers. The meibomian glands, located along the posterior lid margin, secrete the superficial lipid or oily layer. This layer aids in preventing evaporation and provides stability to the tear film. The middle aqueous layer is secreted by the main and accessory lacrimal glands. This layer contains many substances that protect the ocular surface from microbial agents (IgA, lysozyme, lactoferrin, and various peroxidases) and provides for normal ocular surface homeostasis. Lack of the aqueous tears can result in an eye that is more vulnerable to microbial agents. Both sympathetic and parasympathetic nerve fibers innervate the lacrimal gland. The exact role of the sympathetic nerve fibers is not known. Control of reflex tear secretion is by the parasympathetic nerve fibers.[2] What controls emotional tearing is unknown, but it may be hormonal in nature.[3] Goblet cells, interspersed between the epithelial cells on the conjunctival surface, secrete the innermost mucin layer. Mucin interacts with a glycocalx secreted by the conjunctival and corneal epithelium. Mucin functions as a surfactant allowing hydrophilic tears to adhere to a hydrophobic corneal epithelium. The eyelids also contain cilia or lashes that function to protect the eye from airborne debris. The movement of eyelids spreads tears across the conjunctival and corneal surface, allowing renewing of the tear film. Lid closure also compresses the nasolacrimal sac, creating a negative pressure. Upon lid opening, tears and debris are literally sucked from the eye.

Classification

Dry eyes are usually classified into five broad categories (Table 1). The term KCS refers to aqueous tear deficiencies. KCS is most often associated with lacrimal gland atrophy due to aging changes, Sjögren's syndrome, scarring of the lacrimal gland excretory ducts (e.g., chemical burns, ocular pemphigoid), and contact lens wear.

Mucin layer deficiencies occur when goblet cells are reduced in numbers. Causes of mucin deficiency include: vitamin A deficiency, Stevens-Johnson syndrome, ocular cicatricial pemphigoid, chemical burns, long-term use of topical medications (epinephrine, pilocarpine), and environmental pollutants.

Lipid abnormalities are most common in patients with blepharitis, where inflammation of the meibomian glands alters the physical and biochemical properties of the lipid. Systemic agents containing retinoids, such as isotretinoin (Accutane), shrink the meibomian glands, leading to decreased lipid production.[4]

Keratinized conjunctival epithelium with loss of goblet cells (termed *squamous metaplasia*) results in a nonwettable ocular surface and a dry eye. Ocular cicatricial pemphigoid, Stevens-Johnson syndrome, vitamin A deficiency, and chemical burns are examples of ocular surface diseases that are associated with squamous metaplasia.

The eyelids are very important in maintaining a normal tear film. Malposition (ectropion or entropion), incomplete closure (lagophthalmos), and poor or incomplete blink (i.e., Bell's palsy) can cause a dry eye.

Epidemiology

There has never been a carefully conducted epidemiologic study to determine the incidence and prevalence of dry eye syndromes in the United States. However, a recent study from Sweden found a prevalence of 14.9 per cent for KCS in a randomly selected group of 705 subjects.[5] In a typical "dry eye" ophthalmology practice, where patients present with

TABLE 1. Classification of Dry Eye Syndrome

Aqueous tear deficiency (keratoconjunctivitis sicca)
Mucin deficiency
Lipid abnormality
Ocular surface pathology
Impaired lid function

symptoms of dry eyes, about one third of patients will have KCS; one third, blepharitis; and one third, keratoconjunctivitis medicamentosa due to topical drug toxicity. KCS is the most common ocular manifestation of rheumatoid arthritis and is present in 10 to 25 per cent of patients.[6] Sjögren's syndrome is the association of KCS and xerostomia (primary Sjögren's) or KCS and/or xerostomia and a connective tissue disease (secondary Sjögren's syndrome). About 25 per cent of patients with rheumatoid arthritis have Sjögren's syndrome. About 60 per cent of patients who present with dry eye and dry mouth have an associated connective tissue disease.[7] Sjögren's syndrome is more common in females as compared with males (range: 15:1 to 20:1). This chapter will deal specifically with the diagnosis of KCS and how to differentiate it from other dry eye conditions.

HISTORY

History of the Present Illness

The history should record the nature and timing of the symptoms, trying to be as specific as possible. Five important symptoms to look for are:

1. *Foreign body sensation.* The feeling of sand or gravel in the eye.
2. *Burning.* The feeling of soap or shampoo in the eye.
3. *Itching.* The sensation similar to a mosquito bite.
4. *Mattering or crusting on the eyelids.*
5. *Photophobia.* Discomfort with bright lights.

Each of these symptoms are graded as to mild, moderate, or severe; when they began; and when they are present. Are symptoms worse upon arising, gradually improving over the next few hours and then worsen later in the day (typical of blepharitis)? Are symptoms better upon arising and worsen as the day progresses (typical of KCS)? Are symptoms affected by changes in humidity, temperature, location, or work environment? Are the symptoms better/worse at work, at home, on weekdays or weekends? Are they increasing, decreasing, or variable? What makes them worse? What makes them less? Is matter or crusting present upon awakening? Does the patient use artificial tears or ointments, and do they help? What topical or systemic medications have been used, and what was their effect? Can the patient cry emotional and/or irritant (when peeling an onion) tears? If so, the lacrimal gland is still functional. When was the patient's last physical exam, and what were the results? Table 2 compares the historical findings in various dry eye disorders.

Review of Systems

Does the patient have systemic symptoms that may be associated with dry eye states? Is a dry mouth present? Does the patient have a sense of saliva in their mouth? Can they swallow meat or a cracker without water or fluids? Are vaginal secretions normal or decreased? Is the skin excessively dry? Does the patient have complaints of excessive fatigue or malaise? Are there problems with constipation? Are there frequent bladder infections? Is there any joint pain? Table 3 lists the various systemic diseases associated with decreased aqueous tear secretion (KCS).

TABLE 2.   Comparison of Historical Symptoms in Patients with Different Dry Eye Disorders

SYMPTOM	KCS	BLEPHARITIS	TOXIC KERATO-CONJUNCTIVITIS	ALLERGIC KERATO-CONJUNCTIVITIS
Foreign body sensation	+++	+	+++	+
Burning	+	+++	+++	+
Itching	−	−	−	+++
Photophobia	++	±	++	±
Symptoms worse	Afternoon, evening	Upon awakening, evening	When using eyedrops	Seasonal, environmental
Symptoms better	Upon awakening, morning	Mid-day	When not using eyedrops	Different environment
Crusting/mattering of lids	±	+++	±	−
Mucous discharge	++	−	±	+++

TABLE 3. Systemic Conditions Associated with KCS

Acquired immune deficiency syndrome (AIDS)
Allergy
Amyotrophic lateral sclerosis
Botulism
Chronic hepatobiliary disease
Deep anesthesia
Disseminated lupus erythematosus
Facial nerve lesion between nucleus and geniculate
   ganglion
Gougerot-Sjögren syndrome
Graft versus host disease
Hashimoto's thyroiditis
Lesions of the greater petrosal nerve, sphenopalatine
   ganglion, or lacrimal nerve
Lymphoma, leukemia
Mikulicz's syndrome (dacryoadenitis and parotitis)
Pheochromocytoma, medullary thyroid carcinoma, and
   multiple mucosal neuromas
Polyarteritis nodosa
Pulmonary fibrosis
Ramsay Hunt syndrome
Raynaud's phenomenon
Rheumatoid arthritis
Sarcoid
Scleroderma
Thrombocytopenic purpura
Typhus and cholera
Waldenström's hyperglobulinemia
Xerophthalmia

(From Roy FH. Ocular differential diagnosis. 4th ed. Philadelphia: Lea & Febiger, 1989:129–31.)

Family History

Family history is usually not helpful in the diagnosis of dry eye syndromes. There, however, may be a genetic predisposition to certain dry eye syndromes such as Sjögren's syndrome. One should, however, ask if any blood relatives have had Sjögren's syndrome, rheumatoid arthritis, systemic lupus, or other immunologic diseases.

Social and Occupational History

Home and work environments have a significant affect on dry eye syndromes, especially KCS. Is the atmosphere contaminated with cigarette smoke, chemicals, or pollutants? Is there new construction present at the job site or at home? Are there pets? What are the sleep habits, exercise, nutrition, and use of tobacco, alcohol, and caffeine of the patient? Does the patient wear makeup; and is it oil or water based, and is it hypoallergenic?

Past Medical History

Is there a previous history of collagen vascular type diseases, specifically rheumatoid arthritis or lupus? Have there been any laboratory tests done? Has the patient ever had any skin disorders, rashes, petechiae, or Raynaud's phenomenon? Is there a history of any previous eye diseases (specifically, any inflammatory eye diseases such as iritis or scleritis) or previous eye surgery?

Focused Queries

1. *Is the discomfort more foreign body (like sand or gravel in the eye), burning (like soap or shampoo in the eye), or itching (like a mosquito bite) in nature?* Patients with KCS usually complain more of foreign body discomfort. Patients with blepharitis or keratitis medicamentosa complain more of burning. Keep in mind, however, that patients with KCS can have blepharitis or keratitis medicamentosa and may complain of both foreign body and burning sensations. Itching (described as similar to a mosquito bite) is almost always due to an allergic problem—that is, hay fever, atopic disease, or vernal keratoconjunctivitis.

2. *Are the symptoms worse upon arising, toward midmorning, or later in the day?* Patients with KCS will have less symptoms upon arising and more symptoms as the day progresses, owing to the effects of evaporation and their environment. Cold days with low humidity, air from automobile heaters/air conditioners, and hot air from ovens make the symptoms of KCS worse. Patients with blepharitis will have more symptoms upon arising, improvement of their symptoms toward midmorning, and a worsening later in the day. Patients with keratitis medicamentosa will have worsening of their symptoms with instillation of their topical medication or artificial tear preparations.

3. *Is there mattering or crusting of the eyelids ("sleep") upon awakening?* Patients with blepharitis will have mattering or crusting upon awakening. This is due to the lack of blinking and close approximation of the eyelids while sleeping.

4. *Can the patient cry emotional and/or irritant tears?* Patients with KCS usually lose their ability to generate irritant tears, first followed by the inability to generate emotional tears.[8] If patients can generate tears by either

mechanism, it suggests that the lacrimal gland is still functional.

PHYSICAL EXAMINATION

The ocular examination by the nonophthalmologist will be limited by the lack of ophthalmic instruments and availability of diagnostic tests. Ideally, the minimum evaluation of a patient with a dry eye includes a history, a slit lamp exam with fluorescein staining, Schirmer test, and rose bengal staining. For the nonophthalmologist, a history, limited physical and ocular exam, fluorescein staining, and Schirmer test should be performed.

A limited physical exam to look for systemic diseases associated with KCS should be performed (Table 3). This includes examination for parotid gland swelling, lymphadenopathy, xerostomia (dry-fissured tongue), joint inflammation, rosacea, and skin rashes (petechiae). The eyelids are examined for incomplete lid closure, both with forced lid closure and with blinking. Incomplete lid closure (lagophthalmos) and blinking can lead to ocular surface irritation (exposure keratitis). Lid erythema, swelling, and crusting along the lid margins suggest blepharitis. Fluorescein, instilled using a moistened fluorescein paper strip, will identify corneal epithelial defects and filaments (mucus adherent to the cornea). Inferior staining is found in patients with blepharitis and lagophthalmos. Interpalpebral staining is found in KCS, whereas diffuse staining is seen in keratitis medicamentosa. If decreased visual acuity or redness of the conjunctiva or sclera is present, further evaluation by an ophthalmologist is needed.

Schirmer Test

Although the Schirmer test has high specificity (low degree of false negatives), it has low sensitivity (high degree of false positives). It is not used by itself to make the diagnosis of KCS.[9] However, if used along with a proper history, it is quite helpful. A test strip (Whatman No. 5 filter paper) is placed at the junction of the lateral and medial one third of the lower lid. The test may be done with or without anesthesia, with the amount of wetting (in millimeters) recorded after five minutes. Because of an initial reflexive tearing component (even when topical anesthesia is used), Schirmer test strips are left in place for a full five minutes. Removing the test strips at 2.5 min-

utes and doubling the result is not equivalent to a five-minute test.[10] In patients who have moderate to severe symptoms of a dry eye, a Schirmer test *without* anesthesia is most useful. Normal values are equal to or greater than 10 mm wetting per five minutes. In asymptomatic patients or those with mild symptoms, a Schirmer test *with* anesthesia is most helpful. Normal values with anesthesia are equal to or greater than 5 mm wetting per five minutes. Again, keep in mind that an abnormal Schirmer test does not make the diagnosis of KCS. Supportive history and other clinical and laboratory tests are also necessary.

Rose Bengal Staining

Rose bengal is a vital dye related to fluorescein. The dye comes in a 1 per cent solution and when instilled in the eye stains dead or dying epithelial cells. In KCS, the intrapalpebral conjunctiva is stained more than the cornea. In other dry eye states, the cornea stains more than the conjunctiva. The amount of staining can be graded.[11] Rose bengal will not stain the normal ocular surface. In KCS, increased staining correlates with disease severity.

DIAGNOSTIC STUDIES

Ophthalmologic Laboratory Tests

There are no convenient, easy-to-perform, practical laboratory tests for KCS that are readily available to the clinician. There are, however, several laboratory tests available for the diagnosis of KCS. These include tear film osmolality,[12] lysozyme,[13] and lactoferrin[14] and impression cytology.[15] Tear film osmolality is highly sensitive and specific in diagnosing KCS. However, it requires micropipette tear sampling and a nanoliter osmometer and is not practical in the everyday clinical setting. Commercially available test kits are available for tear lysozyme and lactoferrin determinations. Both tests are quite specific for KCS but suffer from decreased sensitivity. Impression cytology involves pressing cellulose acetate filter material onto the conjunctival ocular surface and then removing it. Surface epithelial and goblet cells adhere to the filter material and are stained with hematoxylin and periodic acid/Schiff's stain. The degree of squamous metaplasia is determined by microscopic evaluation. The technique has good specificity and sensitivity but requires an experienced technician to obtain and interpret the specimens.

Systemic Laboratory Tests

Blood studies reveal that about one third of patients with Sjögren's syndrome (SS) are anemic and one half have hypergammaglobulinemia; 20 per cent of SS patients have cryoglobulinemia. Primary SS and secondary SS, associated with systemic lupus erythematosus, commonly have SSA (anti-Ro) and SSB (anti-La) antibodies. Rheumatoid factor is found in 90 per cent, antinuclear antibodies in 70 per cent, and thyroglobulin antibody in 35 per cent of SS patients. One third of SS patients have decreased T lymphocytes.[16]

ASSESSMENT

Keratoconjunctivitis Sicca

Patients with KCS complain of foreign body sensation and photophobia. Symptoms are least upon awakening and worse as the day progresses. Low humidity, freezing temperatures, dry wind, airborne chemicals, and pollutants (especially cigarette smoke) make symptoms worse. In moderate to severe KCS, preservatives in topical artificial tears and medications worsen symptoms. KCS is much more common in women than men. Therefore, a man presenting with dry eye symptoms is unlikely to have KCS. If a dry mouth or a connective tissue disease is present, the patient may have SS. In moderate KCS, the patient cannot generate irritant tears. In severe KCS, the patient cannot generate irritant or emotional tears. On clinical exam, there is increased mucous production. With fluorescein and rose bengal, the conjunctiva stains more than the cornea in the intrapalpebral zone. The Schirmer test shows decreased tear production. If SS is present, laboratory workup may show the presence of anemia; rheumatoid factor; thyroglobulin, antinuclear, or SSA and SSB antibodies; or hypergammaglobulinemia.

Blepharitis

Patients with blepharitis complain of burning sensation. Symptoms are present upon awakening, improve toward midday, and worsen later in the day. Mattering or crusting along the eyelids is present upon awakening. Symptoms are worse in dry, windy environ-ments. Artificial tears and medications with preservatives worsen symptoms. Topical steroids improve symptoms. Blepharitis is common in women in their third through fifth decades and men after their third decade. Clinical evaluation shows lid erythema, swelling, and crusting. There is fluorescein and rose bengal staining of the inferior cornea and conjunctiva. Tear production as measured by a Schirmer test is usually normal. Examination of the facial skin may show evidence of rosacea, especially in younger women and older men. Laboratory workup is not usually helpful.

Allergic Conjunctivitis

Patients with allergic conjunctivitis complain of itching and excessive mucus. Symptoms vary considerably in intensity and duration, depending on the environment and season. They are consistently worse when in contact with the offending allergen and often seasonal in nature. Identifying the causative allergen is difficult and requires the patient to keep a careful diary as to when symptoms are better and worse. Although patients with allergic rhinitis often have allergic conjunctivitis, the reverse is not true. Clinical findings are variable. There may be a history of atopic dermatitis or hay fever. Fluorescein and rose bengal staining are usually not present. The Schirmer test is normal. Laboratory tests are noncontributory. Systemic workup for allergy is usually unproductive.

Keratoconjunctivitis Medicamentosa

Patients with KCS develop keratocojunctivitis medicamentosa due to a toxic reaction to the preservative in the topical artificial tears that they are using. In addition to having the symptoms of KCS, they experience burning with artificial tear instillation. A history of increasing use of artificial tear use is present. Patients present using preserved artificial tears every 5 to10 minutes without relief. Clinical exam shows those findings seen in KCS along with fluorescein and rose bengal staining of the entire cornea.

Ocular Cicatricial Pemphigoid and Stevens-Johnson Syndrome

These are rare diseases but common causes of dry eye syndrome. Acutely, patients present with an inflammatory conjunctivitis and increased mucous production. Chronically, patients have an intermittent, chronic conjunctivitis and complain of eye irritation. The cornea stains with fluorescein and rose bengal more than the conjunctiva. Trichiasis (aberrant lashes rubbing on the cornea), symblepharon (adhesion of the eyelid to the globe), subconjunctival scarring, and vascularization of the cornea are present in severe disease. If the excretory ducts of the lacrimal gland are scarred, tear secretion is decreased as measured by Schirmer testing.

Mild Chemical Burns

Patients who have sustained a mild chemical burn to the eye often complain of eye irritation, especially burning. Symptoms, although not often severe, are always present and quite bothersome. Dry, chemically laded environments are especially bothersome. Clinical exam shows minimal findings, often only a mild blepharitis.

REFERENCES

1. Burton H. Somatosensory features of the eye. In: Adler's physiology of the eye. Moses RA, Hart W, eds. St Louis: CV Mosby, 1987:60–3.
2. Midler, B. The lacrimal apparatus. In: Adler's physiology of the eye. Moses RA, Hart W, eds. St Louis: CV Mosby, 1987:24.
3. Frey WH II, Nelson JD, Frick ML, Elde RP. Prolactin immunoreactivity in human tears and lacrimal gland: possible implications for tear production. In: Holly FJ, ed. The precorneal tear film in health, disease, and contact lens wear. Lubbock: Dry Eye Institute, 1986:795–807.
4. Lambert RW, Smith RE. Pathogenesis of blepharoconjunctivitis complicating 13-*cis*-retinoic acid (isoretinoin) therapy in a laboratory model. Invest Ophthalmol Vis Sci 1988; 29:1559–64.
5. Jacobsson LTH, Axell TE, Hansen BU: Dry eyes or mouth—an epidemiological study in Swedish adults, with special reference to primary Sjögren's syndrome. In: Talal N, ed. Sjögren's syndrome: a model for understanding autoimmunity. San Diego: Academic Press, 1989:213–9.
6. Lamberts, DW. Dry eye and tear deficiency. Int Ophthalmol Clin 1983;23(1):123–30.
7. Sjögren, H, Bloch KJ. Keratoconjunctivitis sicca and Sjögren's syndrome. Surv Ophthalmol 1971;16:145–59.
8. Frey WH II. Crying the mystery of tears. Minneapolis: Winston Press, 1985:22.
9. Farris RL, Gilbard JP, Stuchell RN, et al. Diagnostic tests in keratoconjunctivitis sicca. CLAO J 1983;9:23–8.
10. Clinch TE, Benedetto DA, Felberg NT, Laibson PR. Schirmer's test: a closer look. Arch Ophthalmol 1983;101:1383–6.
11. Van Bijsterveld OP. Diagnostic tests in keratoconjunctivitis sicca syndrome. Arch Ophthalmol 1969;82:10–4.
12. Gilbard JP, Farris RL. Tear osmolality and ocular surface disease in keratoconjunctivitis sicca. Arch Ophthalmol 1979;97:1652–6.
13. Van Bijsterveld OP. Standardization of lysozyme test for a commercially available medium. Arch Ophthalmol 1974;91:432.
14. Boersma HGM, van Bijsterveld OP. Lactoferrin test for the diagnosis of keratoconjunctivitis sicca in clinical practice. Ann Ophthalmol 1987;19:152–4.
15. Nelson JD. Impression cytology. Cornea 1988;7:71–81.
16. Farris RL. Sjögren's syndrome. In: Gold DH, Weingeist TA, eds. The eye in systemic disease. Philadelphia: JB Lippincott, 1990:70–1.

DYSPAREUNIA

MARY K. BEARD

SYNONYMS: Painful Intercourse, Genital Pain During or Following Coitus

BACKGROUND

Dyspareunia is defined as pain or discomfort in the labial, vaginal, or pelvic area during or after sexual intercourse.[1] Other descriptions of the sensations experienced include irritation, rawness, pressure, aching, tearing, or burning, with a wide range of intensity and duration.[2] Dyspareunia is both a symptom as well as a cause of sexual difficulty.[3]

Types of Dyspareunia

1. *Primary* Pain present from initial intercourse.

2. *Secondary* Coital discomfort after initial pain-free intercourse.

3. *Complete* Pain that occurs during all episodes of coitus.

4. *Situational* Pain that occurs only during certain encounters or with certain partners.

5. *Positional* Pain only when female supine, on deep penetration or rear entry, and the like.

6. *Superficial* Pain at or near the introitus or vulva.

7. *Deep* Pain located deep in the vagina, at the cervix, pelvis, or lower abdominal area.

Dyspareunia is not a new problem, as descriptions date back to the ancient Egyptian Raesseum Papyri IV scrolls.[4] The Talmud mentioned dyspareunia as a cause for divorce.[1]

The true incidence of dyspareunia is unknown, as there is still a reluctance in our society to discuss sexual behavior, especially among older patients and physicians. Investigators over the last 60 years have reported that 4 to 40 per cent of women in various private practices or outpatient clinics identify recurrent coital pain as a major complaint.[1] In 1989, Bachmann et al. screened 887 women for sexual concerns and dysfunction in a gynecology outpatient clinic. The most common complaint was dyspareunia (48 per cent).[5] A recent collaborative study by Glatt et al. evaluated 313 questionnaires, and over 60 per cent of the participants had had dyspareunia at some point in their lives and one third still had discomfort.[1]

There has been a tendency by some authors to divide the subject of dyspareunia into physical and psychologic areas. This division may not necessarily be valid. A vicious cycle may arise in which any pain during intercourse will cause anxiety and inhibit arousal, resulting in a lack of lubrication, causing further pain. It is imperative that the physical or physiologic factors be ruled out before ascribing dyspareunia to the patient's mental state.[6]

In normal sexual response, arousal causes genital vasocongestion that results in vaginal lubrication. Sexual stimuli, as well as healthy vaginal tissue, are required for genital vasocongestion and vaginal lubrication. The second stage of sexual response is a series of involuntary contractions of the muscles of the pelvis under the control of the autonomic nervous system, resulting in a pleasurable sensory phenomenon known as orgasm.[7] It is also useful to keep in mind the normal patterns of vaginal lubrication, vaginal expansion, and uterine elevation that occur during sexual response and how these normal physiologic events may be altered by disease processes or postoperative changes. Masters and Johnson described an increase of approximately 35 to 40 per cent in the length and as much as 6 cm in the expansion of the width at the upper end of the vagina in response to sexual arousal.[8] Any organic or functional vulvar, vaginal, or pelvic disease that interferes with arousal or the orgasmic phase of sexual response will inhibit normal response because of dyspareunia.

Dyspareunia has been referred to as the most common female sexual dysfunction.[1,5,6] There is a high incidence of physical disease associated with dyspareunia compared with other sexual dysfunctions. On a continuum from primarily physical to primarily psychologic, many women fall in the middle when the etiology of dyspareunia is viewed.[2]

Causes of Dyspareunia

The causes of dyspareunia are listed in Table 1. Many of the possible etiologies are rare but must be kept in mind when a differential diagnosis is being considered for the patient presenting with dyspareunia either as a sole complaint or meshed with a variety of other complaints.

HISTORY

The history of a patient should record the chronology of the discomfort. Is the dyspareunia primary (onset with initial sexual experience), secondary (onset after a pain-free interval), or intermittent? Is it superficial with initial penetration, during all episodes of coitus, or only during thrusting, or does it occur only deep in the pelvis? Is it positional, or does it occur only in certain situations or with certain partners? How severe is it or how intense? Locate the site of origin if possible to the vulva, introitus, bladder, vagina, cervix, uterus, adnexa, pelvis, or lower abdomen. Review the menstrual cycle and see if there is a pattern to the occurrence of pain. Is there a discharge? If so, how much? What color is it, and is there an odor? Also inquire as to previous vaginal infections, treatment and results, hygiene practices, contraception, and sexual practices.

Assess the impact of the dyspareunia on the patient and on the couple's relationship. De-

TABLE 1. Causes of Dyspareunia

Infectious microorganisms causing vulvovaginitis	Vaginismus
Trichomonas vaginalis	Paraurethral vaginal leiomyoma
Candida	Reaction to Dacron buttress in urethropexy
Gardnerella vaginalis	Equestrian dyspareunia
Herpes progenitalis	Postoperative for genital descensus
Human papillomavirus	Urethral syndrome
Beta-hemolytic streptococci	Vaginal septum
Infectious microorganisms causing cervicitis and pelvic	Intrauterine devices
inflammatory disease	Adenomyosis
Neisseria gonorrhoeae	Pelvic inflammatory disease
Chlamydia trachomatis	Photocoagulation of the endometrium
Ureaplasma urealyticum	Pelvic adhesions
Mycobacterium species	Occult uterine prolapse syndrome
Angiokeratoma vulvae	Endometriosis
Bowenoid papulosis and neoplasia of vulva	Cervicitis
Skene's duct cyst	Uterine leiomyomata
Chemical allergens	Rotated hypoplastic hemipelvis
Vulvitis circumscripta plasma cellularis	Irritable bowel syndrome
Vestibulitis	Irradiated genital cancers
Focal vulvitis	Radical cystectomy
Postherpetic neuralgia	Bladder exstrophy
Vulvar dystrophies	Allen Masters syndrome (lacerations of the broad
Vulvodynia/"burning vulva syndrome"	ligament)
Colpoperineoplasty	Crohn's disease
Hymenal fissures	Laparoscopic sterilization
Introital adenosis associated with Stevens-Johnson	Surgery for rectal cancer
syndrome	Ovarian residual syndrome
Vestibular gland adenomas	Sjögren's syndrome
Glycerated impregnated chromic catgut	Pelvic congestion syndrome (pelvic varicosities)
Urethral diverticulum	Cement in pelvis from total hip replacement
Interstitial cystitis	Postabortal pelvic inflammatory disease
Postmenopausal vaginal atrophy	Pregnancy and postpartum
Glomus tumor	Penile curvature
Tight hymenal ring or stenosis	Overdeveloped perineal and levator muscles from
Premature ovarian failure	exercise
Postmenopausal use of Depo-Provera	True physical incompatibility
Urethral suspension procedures	Traumatic factors
Pudendal neuralgia	Postural lumbar backache
Vaginal cysts	Reflux dyspareunia in women with known gastroesopha-
Urinary tract infections	geal reflux

termine what prior experience the woman had had that may influence her development of dyspareunia. Are there social, cultural, or partnership relationships; traumatic sexual experiences in the past such as rape or incest; and/or lack of learning (sexual naïveté) factors that influence the perception of discomfort and sexual expectations?[8]

What evaluation and treatment have been done in the past, and what were the results? Do not expect information to be volunteered, as women raise sexual concerns only on direct inquiry.[5]

A thorough past history and review of systems are necessary to record medical illness, allergies, hospitalizations, medications, surgeries, and accidents or injuries. This information may provide clues as to the etiology of the dyspareunia.

PHYSICAL EXAMINATION

The focus of the exam will be the pelvic exam since dyspareunia is a symptom of pain with coitus. As the exam is carried out, it is important to keep in mind the normal patterns of vaginal lubrication, vaginal expansion, and uterine elevation that occur during sexual response,[8] especially in those patients who show signs of estrogen deprivation or who have had surgery or injury to the genital tract that could affect this area and result in dyspareunia.

The examination should begin with careful palpation of the abdomen, looking for masses (ovarian neoplasm, uterine leiomyomata), suprapubic tenderness (cystitis, uterine adenomyosis), and lower abdominal tenderness or guarding (bowel disease, pelvic inflammatory disease) as well as costovertebral angle (CVA) tenderness (urinary tract infection). The bowel should also be palpated and the bowel sounds noted for normal peristaltic sounds.

Gross examination of the external genitalia should be carried out under a bright light, evaluating the skin as to elasticity and turgor (poor, fair, excellent); pubic hair (normal, sparse); introitus (two finger breadths); vaginal mucosa (thin, friable, smooth, rugated); and the vaginal depth (shortened or normal). This will provide general information as to gross abnormalities, inflammation, scars, and lesions and a general hint as to estrogen status.

With magnification and a bright light, roll inward the hymenal ring with a cotton swab and expose the inner surfaces of the labia minora to look for focal inflammation, lesions, fissures, and hymenal crypts just lateral to the hymenal ring and urethral meatus. In focal vulvitis, vestibulitis, and Bartholin's gland inflammation, there will be exquisitely sensitive 3- to 10-mm areas of focal erythema. In most cases, there will not be swelling or ulcerations. "Touch test" of individual lesions with the tip of a cotton applicator is diagnostic.[9,10,11] Vulvar and vestibular papillomatosis are suggestive of human papillomavirus (HPV).[12] Any lesions suggestive of any infectious process should be cultured.

Proceeding through the introitus, the hymen should admit two fingers. If not, a tight hymen or hymenal stenosis may be the etiology of superficial dyspareunia. The vagina should be checked for scars from prior surgery, any distortion of the anatomic features of the vagina, tumors of the vaginal wall, tenderness of the levator muscles, vaginal septum, episiotomy scars, inflammation, loss of rugae, discharge, and lesions.

Inspect the cervix for color, smoothness, location of the transformation zone (junction between the squamous epithelium and the columnar epithelium), and evidence of discharge, irregularity, lesions, or growths. Feel the surface to see if it is smooth and firm but not rock hard or tender.

The bimanual examination is then done to feel the cervix as previously noted and to evaluate the uterus as to size (based on gestational weeks size), location (midlocated, deviated more to right or left), position (retroflexed, retroverted, or antiflexed), and shape. The adnexa are then palpated for size and location as well as to note if they are tender.

The rectal-vaginal exam is very important to evaluate for masses in the cul-de-sac, tenderness or nodularity of the uterosacral ligaments (endometriosis), and any irregularity and abnormalities on the posterior uterus (pedunculated myomas) and adnexa as well as any masses or abnormalities in the rectal vault.

It may be helpful to employ maneuvers to try to reproduce the same pain the patient felt during coitus. The exam may serve a useful function in reassuring the patient about anatomy and her ability to accommodate an intravaginal object.

DIAGNOSTIC STUDIES

In evaluating dyspareunia, laboratory testing will be confined to those tests pertaining to gynecologic problems, but a thorough workup is encouraged if the etiology appears to be gastrointestinal, urologic, or orthopedic, as suggested in the list of causes (see Table 1).

Cotton Swab Test

The cotton swab test is used to pinpoint areas of focal inflammation on the vulva, introitus, or opening of the Bartholin glands for women with vulvar vestibulitis, focal vulvitis, or bartholinitis. It is not particularly helpful in inflammatory processes such as *Candida* vulvovaginitis or generalized pain or burning from vulvar dystrophy. Ulcerations or lesions from herpes can also be exquisitely tender to touch.

Cultures

Cultures are done to identify aerobic, *Candida,* and *Chlamydia* organisms. Cultures are helpful in identifying infectious processes of the vulva, vagina, and cervix but usually cannot identify organisms causing pelvic inflammatory disease, as they are frequently polymicrobial.

Colposcopy

The colposcope may be used to look at suspected areas of vulvar dystrophy[13] or lesions suspected to be caused by the papillomavirus or to examine grossly normal appearing vulva, introitus, hymen, vagina, or cervix not responsive to routine treatments for infections, pain, burning, itching, and the like, associated with dyspareunia.

Biopsies

Biopsies help in diagnosing vulvar dystrophy, lesions suspicious for carcinoma, and any persistent, unidentifiable lesions of the vulva, introitus, vagina, or cervix. Biopsies have limitations in areas suspicious for focal vulvitis or vestibulitis, as the findings show only nonspecific inflammatory infiltrate.

Smears

Wet smears prepared with warm saline and examined under a microscope help differentiate between infections due to fungi, trichomonads, and bacteria. Adding a few drops of 10 per cent potassium hydroxide will aid in lysing all cells except those of *Candida* so as to identify *Candida* cells, buds, and pseudomycelia. Clue cells (stratified squamous cells with granular appearance due to a coating of organisms) are suggestive of *Gardnerella vaginalis*.

Complete Blood Count

The blood count is normal unless there is an infectious process as the etiology of the dyspareunia. However, even pelvic inflammatory disease may not show an elevation in the white count or shift in the differential.

Vaginal pH

This test uses pH tape that can be kept in the examining rooms. Normal range of the vaginal secretions are 3.5 to 4.5. A higher pH is suggestive of decreased glycogen production as the result of an infection.

Pelvic Ultrasound

Ultrasound is useful in defining irregularities of the uterus, pelvic masses, adnexal masses, ovarian cysts, or tubo-ovarian masses or abscesses. The ultrasound vaginal probe aids even further in defining pelvic pathology. The limitations are that ultrasound cannot be tissue specific and can only identify structures of differing densities.

Diagnostic Laparoscopy

Laparoscopy is used to diagnose endometriosis, adhesions, pelvic masses such as pedunculated myomas, pelvic inflammatory disease, uterine displacement, ectopic pregnancy, pelvic varicosities, adnexal cysts, neoplasms, normal pelvis, and any other pelvic pathology.

ASSESSMENT

The differential diagnosis of the etiology of dyspareunia can only be arrived at after a careful history and a physical exam that has included inspection and palpation of the external genitalia and internal pelvic organs. Dyspareunia is often associated with multiple symptoms such as vulvar burning and itching, dysmenorrhea, pelvic and abdominal pain, menstrual irregularities, problems with contraception, infertility, depression, and headaches. (Also see chapters on Menstrual Dysfunction and Pelvic Mass in the Female Patient.) For ease in categorizing dyspareunia, the lists of possible etiologies will be broken down into superficial and deep.

Superficial Dyspareunia

Superficial dyspareunia is the coital pain originating in the vulva, introitus, hymen, and lower vagina. The majority of causes are from infection, allergy, or trauma.[3] Possible causes are discussed in the following subsections.

Infectious Microorganisms

Although a variety of organisms can cause infections, those that typically cause vulvovaginitis that results in dyspareunia are the *Candida* species (most common), beta-hemolytic streptococci, herpes progenitalis (causes very tender vesicles that break and form painful ulcers), *Trichomonas,* and *Gardnerella vaginalis.* HPV causes condylomata acuminatum, which may form large, coalescing lesions that can become secondarily infected or which may be a cause of vestibulitis in which no gross lesions may be seen.[9,12]

Chemicals and Allergens

These are agents that contact the vulva and vagina and cause erythema, irritation, ulcerations, and discharge that can result in dyspareunia. These include soaps, douche materials, bubble bath, powder, cloth dyes, perfumed or colored toilet paper, feminine hygiene sprays, local medications, and contraceptive chemicals.

Inflammatory Diseases

These are inflammatory processes such as urethritis, trigonitis, interstitial cystitis, cystitis, vestibulitis, focal vulvitis, bartholinitis, or Bartholin abscesses that contribute to entrance dyspareunia. Minor vestibular gland syndrome (absence of active infection with a previous history of vaginal candidiasis) can also cause introital dyspareunia.

Surgical Procedures

Any surgical procedure involving the vulva, introitus, and vagina has the potential for leaving a tender or contracted scar such as perineoplasties, episiotomies, anterior and posterior colporrhaphy, and urethral suspensions. Reaction to materials used in the procedures such as Dacron buttress used in urethropexies and glycerol-impregnated chromic catgut sutures can also result in dyspareunia.

Atrophy

Atrophy will occur any time there is a loss of estrogen to the vagina, trigone of the bladder, and the urethra, such as in premature ovarian failure and menopause. The membranes become thin and with time atrophy, scar, and shrink. As a result, the membranes are easily traumatized, resulting in dyspareunia or even apareunia. Administration of medication such as the luteinizing hormone–releasing hormone (LHRH) analogue agonist for the treatment of endometriosis has superficial dyspareunia as a side effect owing to the low estrogen state.[14] Progestogens used in postmenopausal women will not restore the atrophic vagina. Thus, dyspareunia, if present, will continue or progress.

Developmental Anomalies

Müllerian anomalies such as a vaginal septum, transverse vaginal membrane, uterus didelphis, vaginal agenesis, or any of the other abnormalities that can occur during the embryo fusion process may be the etiology of dyspareunia. Congenital pelvic abnormalities—for example, a rotated hypoplastic hemipelvis with rotation of the pubic ramus into the vagina—can cause obstructive dyspareunia.

Traumatic Factors

Traumatic factors include error in sexual technique; absence of foreplay, leading to poor lubrication; overzealous clitoral stimulation; foreign bodies, including coital aids; coital injury; true physical incompatibility; and anal intercourse without sufficient lubrication.

Other Causes of Superficial Dyspareunia

Skene's duct cyst, glomus tumors, bowenoid papulosis and neoplasia of the vulva, urethral diverticulum, introital adenosis associated with Stevens-Johnson syndrome (adenosis with tubal glandular epithelium), paraurethral vaginal leiomyoma, adenomas in the minor vestibular glands, angiokeratoma vulvae (grayish-purple macular papular lesions on the labia majora), vulvitis circumscripta cellularis (also known as Zoon's vulvitis, is infiltration of the vulva by plasma cells), Sjögren's syndrome (progressive alteration of the exocrine glands with atrophy), pruritic vulvar squamous papillomatosis (progression of the development of squamous papillae possibly caused by HPV infection), and vaginal tumors (paraurethral, vaginal cysts, Gartner duct cyst, Bartholin duct cyst, endometriotic type, epidermal inclusion, mucus-secreting müllerian) may be etiologies for dyspareunia. Pudendal neuralgia can give pain without objective findings. Postherpetic neuralgia may also occur following an outbreak of herpes zoster or herpes simplex on the genitalia, causing unilateral pain and dyspareunia.

Deep Dyspareunia

Deep pelvic pain is often less obvious and more difficult to diagnose and is seldom due to or associated with psychologic problems.[15] The following are possible etiologies for deep dyspareunia.

Inflammatory Disease

Cervicitis, pelvic inflammatory disease, salpingitis, tubo-ovarian abscesses, and inflammatory bowel disease (Crohn's disease) can cause deep dyspareunia. Many organisms potentially involved in pelvic infections are polymicrobial, but *Neisseria gonorrhoeae, Chlamydia trachomatis, Ureaplasma urealyticum,* and *Mycobacterium* species are not only associated with pelvic infections that cause deep pelvic pain and dyspareunia but may have long-term sequelae if not properly eradicated. Induced first trimester abortions that result in postabortal pelvic inflammatory disease can also result in dyspareunia.

Pelvic Surgery

Any abdominal or pelvic surgery may cause scarring and/or adhesions to the pelvic organs or alter the axis of the vagina. Operative procedures that may result in dyspareunia are abdominal repair of vaginal prolapse (alters the axis of the vagina and can cause dyspareunia), laparoscopic tubal ligation by rings or electrocoagulation, photocoagulation of the endometrium, cement in the pelvis after a hip replacement, an ovary sutured to the vaginal cuff, and ovarian residual syndrome (pain and dyspareunia after a hysterectomy when one or both ovaries have been preserved). Dyspareunia may be even a more significant problem in women undergoing radical surgical procedures for carcinomas of the rectum, bladder, cervix, uterus, and ovaries (radical hysterectomy, cystectomy, proctocolectomy, low anterior resection for midrectal cancer, and abdominoperineal resection are examples) because of the marked disturbance in the anatomy and circulation, scarring, and adhesions that can occur.

Other Causes of Deep Dyspareunia

Occult prolapse of the uterus (very mobile uterus that descends easily down into the vagina), adenomyosis (enlarged, tender boggy uterus), uterine leiomyomas, endometriosis (may cause peritoneal inflammation, adhesions, scarring, and endometriotic adnexal masses resulting in pelvic pain and deep dyspareunia), irritable bowel (diffuse disorder of smooth muscle), equestrian dyspareunia (injury and inflammation of the levator muscles), intrauterine devices, overdeveloped perineal and levator muscles from exercise, vaginismus, bladder exstrophy, reflux dyspareunia (seen in women with known gastroesophageal reflux), and Allen Masters syndrome (lacerations of the broad ligament) can be etiologies for deep dyspareunia. Radiation therapy for pelvic carcinomas can result in deep dyspareunia that develops six months to one year later, probably secondary to pelvic fibrosis and/or vaginal stenosis. Diabetes is associated with inhibited sexual excitement and dyspareunia. Congenital penile curvature (ventral curvature) will cause dyspareunia in the partner. Intrauterine devices may cause a low-grade endometritis that results in a tender uterus, which can cause deep dyspareunia.

"Deep Thrust" Dyspareunia

A retroverted uterus, adnexa in the cul-de-sac, or ovaries adhered to the vaginal cuff as well as adhesions to the bladder, vaginal cuff, or cul-de-sac can result in deep thrust dyspareunia.

Ache After Intercourse

Pelvic congestion syndrome, which is felt to be due to pelvic varicosities or even broad ligament edema, can result in a deep pelvic ache that persists into the next day. Postural lumbar backache may be a cause of dyspareunia. The rhythmatic movement with the back flexed during intercourse can result in pain in the hypogastrium and result in a dull ache that persists into the next day.[16]

Pregnancy-Related Dyspareunia

Dyspareunia is seen more in primiparae and may be related to insufficient lubrication, fear of injury, and decreased sense of attractiveness. Three months after delivery, dyspareunia was a complaint after a mediolateral episiotomy (35 per cent), second-degree perineal laceration (29 per cent), delivery over intact perineum (9 per cent), and after cesarean delivery (16 per cent), evaluated by a retrospective questionnaire. By one year, the dyspareunia had diminished to prepregnancy rates except for the women who had had episiotomies, and 17 per cent still complained of dyspareunia.[17] With lactation, there is a diminished estrogen state that could contribute to dyspareunia.

Helping the Patient with Dyspareunia

Dyspareunia is a distressing symptom and a cause of sexual difficulty that can lead to serious conflicts in relationships.[3] Women do not readily volunteer information regarding their sexual practices and problems; therefore, a clinician must ask questions in a sensitive way in order to obtain this information. The etiology may be readily apparent or may be elusive, requiring extensive testing. It is imperative that physical and physiologic factors be ruled out before ascribing dyspareunia to the patient's mental state. The underlying cause must be elicited accurately if treatment is to be successful.[5]

REFERENCES

1. Glatt AE, Zinner SH, McCormack WM. The prevalence of dyspareunia. Obstet Gynecol 1990;75:433–6.
2. Sangberg G, Quevillon RP. Dyspareunia: an integrated approach to assessment and diagnosis. J Fam Pract 1987;24(1):66–9.
3. Riley AJ. Old and new causes of superficial dyspareunia. Br Med J 1987;295:513–4.
4. Fordney DS. Dyspareunia and vaginismus. Clin Obstet Gynaecol 1978;21:205–21.
5. Bachmann G, Leiblum S, Grill J. Brief sexual inquiry in gynecologic practice. Obstet Gynecol 1989;73:425–7.
6. Jarvis GJ. Dyspareunia. Br Med J 1984;288:1555–6.

7. Carr BR, Wilson JD. Disturbances of menstruation and sexual function in women. In: Braunwald E, Isselbacher KJ, Petersdorf RG, Wilson JD, Martin JB, Fauc AS, eds. Harrison's principles of internal medicine. 11th ed. St Louis: McGraw Hill, 1987: 214–6.

8. Steege JF. Dyspareunia and vaginismus. Clin Obstet Gynaecol 1984;27(3):750–9.

9. Michlewitz H, Kennison RD, Turksoy RN, Fertitta LC. Vulvar vestibulitis—subgroup with Bartholin gland duct inflammation. Obstet Gynecol 1989; 73:410–13.

10. Peckham BM, Maki DG, Patterson JJ, Hafez Gr. Focal vulvitis: a characteristic syndrome and cause of dyspareunia. Am J Obstet Gynecol 1986;154:855–64.

11. McKay M. Subsets of vulvodynia. J Reprod Med 1988;33(8):695–8.

12. Boden E, Eriksson A, Rylander E, Schoultz BV. Clinical characteristics of papillomavirus-vulvo-vaginitis. Acta Obstet Gynecol Scand 1988;67: 147–51.

13. Vulvar dystrophies. ACOG Technical Bulletin No. 139, January 1990:139.

14. Shaw RW. LHRH analogues in the treatment of endometriosis—comparative results with other treatments. Baillieres Clin Obstet Gynaecol 1988; 2(3):659–75.

15. Perimutter JF. Dyspareunia. In: Friedman EA, Borten MC, Japin DS, eds. Gynecological decision making. Toronto: Decker, 1988:46–7.

16. Rhodes P. Dyspareunia. Br Med J 1984;288:1916–7.

17. Bex PJ, Hofmeyr GJ. Perineal management during childbirth and subsequent dyspareunia. Clin Exp Obstet Gynecol 1987;14(2):97–100.

DYSURIA

JØRN AAGAARD and PAUL O. MADSEN

SYNONYM: Painful Micturition

BACKGROUND

Dysuria describes a sensation of pain or discomfort related to the micturition function. The pain may be slight discomfort on urination, or it may be excruciatingly painful, sharp, or burning. Dysuria can develop from disorders in the upper urinary tract (pyelonephritis) or from disorders in the lower urinary tract system or from organs closely related to the bladder and urethra, that is, prostate, seminal vesicles, epididymis, vulva, vagina, or cervix. Dysuria can have an acute onset (simple cystitis), or it can be chronic (interstitial cystitis, radiation cystitis, chronic bacterial prostatitis).

Dysuria can be localized either to the distal urinary tract (urethritis, balanitis, vaginitis), to the proximal part of the urethra (prostatitis), or to the suprapubic area (cystitis, pelvic inflammatory disease).

Dysuria is one of the most common clinical problems seen by clinicians, accounting for 3 million office visits per year in the United States.[1] Females have a much higher incidence of dysuria than males, and as many as a quarter of adult women may experience an episode of acute dysuria each year.[2] Dysuria can appear in both sexes from child to senescent patient and can be symptomatic of just natural aging or an indicator of serious disorders such as congenital anomalies or cancer.

Until recently, dysuria was believed most likely to indicate the presence of urinary infection, and subsequently, evaluation was often limited to detection of infection using the Kass definition: Quantitative urine cultures of more than 10^5 bacteria/ml indicate infection.[3] But many patients with symptoms of urinary infection failed to culture sufficient bacteria to meet this criterion of infection.[4] The condition of dysuria and frequent urination without appreciable bacteriuria has therefore been referred to as urethral syndrome in women and specific urethritis in men.

However, many patients with low-count bacteriuria have infection of the bladder. Komaroff[5] found positive urine culture collected by suprapubic aspiration among symptomatic patients. Furthermore, treatment of these patients resulted in prompt clinical and bacteriologic cure as compared with placebo therapy. This is in agreement with Stamm et al.,[6] who concluded the following:

1. The two most common infective agents associated with acute urinary symptoms in the women studied were *Escherichia coli* (*E. coli*) and *Chlamydia trachomatis*.

2. Bacteriuria of more than 10^5 organisms/ ml may be an insensitive diagnostic criterion when applied to symptomatic lower urinary tract infections.

3. *Chlamydia trachomatis* infection was implicated in most symptomatic women who had sterile bladder urine and pyuria.

We prefer the terminology *urethral syndrome* limited to the symptom complex dysuria, frequency, and urgency without documented bacteriuria and pyuria. The etiology of this disorder is not completely understood, but some studies seem to demonstrate, by using urodynamic tests, that these patients have dysfunctional voiding due to involuntary contractions of the external sphincter during micturition.[7]

Possible causes of dysuria other than infection vary from childhood to senescence. This chapter discusses etiology and diagnosis in childhood and adolescence, nonpregnant women, pregnant women, postmenopausal women, and younger and elderly men. Causes of dysuria are listed in Table 1. Many of the causes are encountered infrequently yet must be considered in the differential diagnosis of the patient presenting with dysuria.

HISTORY

History of Present Illness

The medical history should record onset and location as well as intensity of dysuria, the patient's age, and especially in the evaluation of adolescence, the stage of pubertal development and sexual activity. Furthermore, symptoms associated with dysuria such as hematuria, purulent urethral secretion, frequency, incontinence, and flank or back pain should be noted. Symptoms referrable to vaginitis such as abnormal vaginal discharge or itching, pain in the perineum or scrotum, history of associated systemic illness, upper respiratory tract infection, skin disorder, allergy, or diarrhea should be considered as well as use of any medications or irritants such as douches, feminine hygiene products, strong soap, bubble bath, contraceptive products, or deodorant sanitary pads and tampons.

Family History

Any family history of organic abnormalities (urethral valves, ureterovesical reflux, systemic diseases (e.g., diabetes mellitus, hypertension), or mental disorders should be recorded carefully.

Social and Occupational History

Consider the patient's job, emotional stress, allergy, social sanitary conditions, and use of tobacco or alcohol.

Past Medical History

Past medical history should include a history of sexually transmitted diseases and history of urinary tract infection. What is the patient's current contraceptive method? Has the patient had urogenital surgery? What kind of medicine is the patient taking (e.g., hypnotics, tranquilizers, antidepressants, diuretics, antihypertensives, alpha or beta blockers, narcotics, or antihistamines)?

PHYSICAL EXAMINATION

Full physical examination, including examination of the genital area, is essential in making the correct diagnosis. Complete physical examination includes evaluation of the upper respiratory system for signs of infection, examination for masses in the flank, examination of the abdomen for pain or tenderness, and examination of the skin for chronic or acute skin lesions that may also present on the perineum. The external genitalia should be examined to evaluate stage of pubertal development and to check for excoriations, dermatitis, balanitis, vulvitis, and vaginal discharge. The perineum should be examined for lesions.

DIAGNOSTIC STUDIES

Although history and physical examination should constitute the basis on which dysuria is assessed, laboratory tests are necessary in most patients. If a simple lower urinary tract disorder is present, a urinalysis is probably sufficient (see the algorithm). If symptoms suggest genital organ or upper urinary tract involvement, the procedure is much more complicated. Table 2 lists tests for specific mi-

TABLE 1.   Genitourinary System and Causes of Dysuria

LOWER URINARY TRACT

			→Benign prostatic hypertrophy
			→Ca prostate
			→Prostatitis
			→Stricture of urethra
			→Cystocele
	→Retention	→Descensus
	→Stone	→Prolapse
Bladder	Infection ———	→Tumor	→Neurogenic
	Carcinoma in situ	→Diverticulum	→Internal sphincter dyssynergia
	Interstitial cystitis	→Estrogen depletion
	Postradiation
Urethra	Infection
	Caruncles
	Condyloma
	Urethral prolapse
	Urethral diverticula	→Urethral stricture
	Structural anomalies ———
	Cancer	→Urethral valves
	Foreign bodies
Glans Penis	Infection
	Chemicals and irritants
Vulva	Infection (bacterial, virus)
	Chemicals and irritants
	Bartholin gland infections
	Tinea, molluscum, pinworms
	Scabies, folliculitis
	Dermatitis, excessive moisture
	Trauma, sexual abuse

UPPER URINARY TRACT

			→Vesicoureteral reflux
Kidney	Infection ———	→Acute pyelonephritis ———	→Ureteropelvic junction
		→Chronic pyelonephritis	→Stone
			→Stone
Pelvic	Infection ———	→Acute pyelonephritis ———	→Tumor
		→Chronic pyelonephritis	→Stone
			→Stone
Ureter	Obstruction	→Acute pyelonephritis ———	→Tumor
			→Megaureters (neurogenic)
			→Uterus, fibroma, pregnancy
			→Uterus, ovarian cancer
External			→Abdominal cancer
Compression	Obstruction	→Infection ———	→Retroperitoneal cancer
			→Cervical cancer
			→Bladder cancer
	Infection
Vagina	Chemicals and irritants
	Tampons
Cervix	Infection
	Carcinoma in situ
Adnexa Uteri	Infection	→Pyosalpinx
		→Acute bacterial prostatitis
Prostate	Infection ———	→Chronic bacterial prostatitis
		→Prostatodynia
		→Prostatosis
Vesicula	
Seminalis	Infection
Epididymis	Infection
Perineal Area	Chemicals and irritants

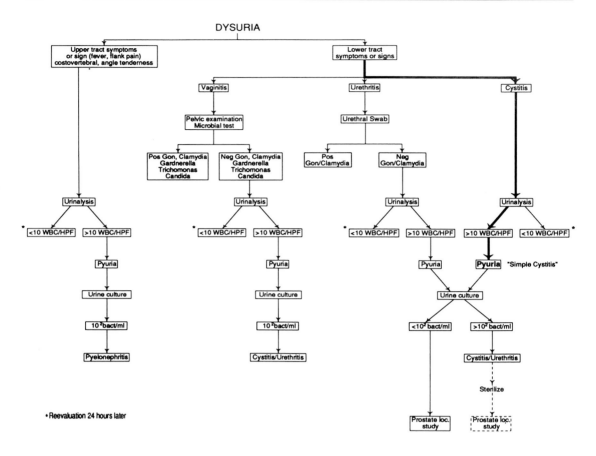

croorganisms involving related organs. Other tests utilized include cystoscopy, ultrasound, laparoscopy, colposcopy, and intravenous urography.

Cystoscopy

The presence of dysuria, frequency, and urgency without bacteriuria alerts one to the possibility of more serious disease, for example, carcinoma in situ of the bladder or interstitial cystitis. Cystoscopy can be performed safely and painlessly with the new flexible instruments and will often provide valuable information. Biopsy may be indicated.

Ultrasound

Noninvasive investigation has become more and more common and can provide important information about the urogenital organs—that is, ovarian cancer, cancer of the prostate, cancer of the bladder.

Laparoscopy

In the evaluation of women with pelvic inflammatory disease (PID), the laparoscopy procedure has been of help in classifying the infectious agents.

Colposcopy

Both inflammatory disease and carcinoma in situ of the cervix can be associated with disorders from the urinary tract, and colposcopy can be helpful.

Intravenous Urography (IVU)

IVU is still important in the evaluation of organ abnormalities in childhood and in the evaluation of organ damage after recurrent upper urinary tract infections, which can occur from systemic diseases such as diabetes mellitus or from stone formation in the pelvis or in the urethra/bladder.

TABLE 2.   Laboratory Tests for Infection of the Genitourinary Tract

URINALYSIS FOR PYURIA

The presence of more than 10 leukocytes per high power field of centrifuged urinary sediments indicates pyuria

URINE CULTURE

All organisms present with a concentration of more than 10^2 colony forming units (CFUs)/ml should be identified using standard laboratory techniques

NEISSERIA GONORRHOEAE

Urethral and cervical specimens should be gram-stained and examined for intracellular diplococci

CHLAMYDIA TRACHOMATIS

Urethral and cervical specimens should be cultured on irradiated McCoy cells pretreated with cycloheximide; inclusion bodies should be stained with iodine; serologic evidence for *Chlamydia* infection is a titer more than 1:64 using the *Chlamydia* IgG immunofluorescence technique

GARDNERELLA VAGINALIS

Urethral and vaginal specimens are suspended in saline, showing clue cells; vaginal specimens are cultured on human blood agar

MYCOPLASMA HOMINIS AND *UREAPLASMA UREALYTICUM*

Urethral swabs are placed in 1 ml of *Mycoplasma* and *Ureaplasma* phenol red broth

TRICHOMONAS VAGINALIS

Vaginal secretion specimens are suspended in 0.85 per cent sodium chloride to be examined at 400 magnification for characteristic motile forms

CANDIDA ALBICANS

A gram stain of the vaginal smear is examined for yeast cells and pseudohyphae; culture on Sabouraud's medium

HERPES SIMPLEX VIRUS

Specimens are obtained from blisters and ulcerative lesions; culture is performed on human embryonic lung cells

ANAEROBIC VAGINOSIS

Vaginal secretions with pH more than 5, potassium hydroxide test positive, and no evidence of *Gardnerella vaginalis, Trichomonas vaginalis,* or *Candida albicans* on microscopy or culture are diagnosed as anaerobic vaginosis

ASSESSMENT

Childhood and Adolescent Girls

The clinical conditions associated with dysuria in adolescents include (1) vulvitis and vaginitis and (2) urinary tract infection including upper urinary tract infection, trauma, and systemic disease or dermatitis.

Vulvovaginitis is an infection of the vulva and vagina that may cause an abnormal vaginal discharge that may be foul smelling or may produce itching or irritation. Vulvovaginitis has been well documented as the most common cause of dysuria in childhood and adolescent girls. Demetriou and colleagues[8] studied 53 adolescents (ages 12 to 21) with a chief complaint of dysuria. The patients underwent complete evaluation including (if indicated) an examination of the external genitalia and/or pelvic area. The results of this study indicate that 41 per cent had vulvovaginitis with the organism *Trichomonas vaginalis, Gardnerella vaginalis,* or *Candida albicans.*

However, many chemical agents such as those found in contraceptive foams, douche products, deodorant sanitary pads and tampons, and feminine hygiene products can also cause dysuria. In addition, other sexually transmitted organisms including *Neisseria gonorrhoeae, Chlamydia,* and herpes virus can cause inflammation of the urethra, cervix, and endometrium and may also result in abnormal vaginal discharge or dysuria. Organisms that are felt to be part of the normal vaginal flora can cause vulva vaginitis in adolescents, for example, *E. coli* or *Shigella.*

Organisms that commonly cause respiratory tract infections in children such as *Hemophilus influenzae* and group B streptococci are frequently found in cultures of vaginal secretions from young girls with concomitant abnormal vaginal discharge. The organism is most probably spread from mucosa to mucosa by a child's hands.

Childhood and Adolescent Boys

Dysuria in the childhood/adolescent boy is not very common, but after excluding infections from organisms like *E. coli* and sexually transmitted organisms such as *Neisseria gonorrhoeae, Chlamydia, Trichomonas,* and herpes simplex, often the following should be considered as potential causes for infection: various forms of trauma including excessive masturbation and sexual abuse, foreign bodies in the urethra, systemic diseases such as diabetes mellitus, and organ abnormalities (e.g., phimosis and secondary balanitis; anterior or posterior urethral valves).

Pregnant Women

Pregnancy does not appear to be associated with an increased susceptibility to urine infection. In different studies utilizing a variety of methods, the prevalence of bacteriuria among pregnant women ranges from 2.5 to 11 per cent; most investigators report a prevalence between 4 and 7 per cent.[9] This is similar to the prevalence of bacteriuria among other sexually active women of childbearing age. However, recurrent episodes of bacteriuria are common among pregnant women who have bacteriuria documented during their initial prenatal evaluation. (Studies show that there is a subset of women who are particularly prone to develop bacteriuria for biologic reasons that are independent of pregnancy per se.)

The complications of bacteriuria during pregnancy may be considered in terms of the mother and fetus. A variety of adverse effects on the mother have been described including development of acute and chronic pyelonephritis, persistent bacteriuria, and toxemia. The strongest association is between the presence of bacteriuria in the first trimester and the development of acute pyelonephritis, which usually occurs during the same period. A significantly increased rate of premature births occurs in women who have acute pyelonephritis during pregnancy.

Women of Childbearing Age

The majority of adult women with dysuria seen in general practice have urinary infection, and therefore evaluation of these patients is often still limited to obtaining urinalysis and cultures of urine. However, many of these women will have illnesses not detected by this limited evaluation. As for adolescent girls of childbearing age, dysuria and vaginal discharge are commonly associated. Therefore, sampling for *C. trachomatis* and *N. gonorrhoeae* from both the cervix and urethra is worthwhile (see the algorithm).

Studies have proved that between 30 and 40 per cent of women with dysuria and vaginal discharge have cultures positive for these organisms. The Western world is in the middle of an epidemic of sexually transmitted disease, and this has been associated with a secondary epidemic of acute pelvic inflammatory disease and ultimately infertility due to tubal occlusion and ectopic pregnancies.[10]

Postmenopausal Women

Lower urinary tract dysfunction is more common in women than in men at all ages.

The prevalence increases with age, and when looking at the etiology of dysfunction in elderly women, it is difficult to separate the influence of aging from that of menopause. However, the incidence of symptoms seems to aggravate in the middle-age woman. The symptoms include incontinence, urinary tract infections, and interstitial cystitis—all conditions that can be associated with dysuria.

It has been shown that the epithelium of the bladder and the vagina is estrogen dependent. In addition, it has also been demonstrated that lack of estrogen affects connective tissue, which can result in the lack of the usual support of the pelvic organs. These organs can therefore prolapse and interfere with the continence mechanism or inhibit complete bladder emptying.

Some women who do not have underlying urinary tract disorders are prone to recurrent urinary infection. Pathogenic mechanisms for recurrent infection are becoming clear, at least for coliform infection. Vaginal and periurethral colonization precedes infection. The uroepithelial cells of women who are prone to recurrent infection have an increased adherence for *E. coli* even when these patients are uninfected. This increased adherence may be due to a genetically determined increase in uroepithelial cell receptors.[11]

Certain behavioral factors also influence recurrence. After sexual intercourse, the concentration of bladder bacteria can transiently increase 10-fold.

The incidence of genitourinary cancer greatly increases with aging. It is therefore essential that the practitioner be sensitive to urinary tract symptoms and signs that herald malignancy in the older patient.

Younger and Elderly Men

Since both the vas deferens and the prostate are in continuity with the urethra, these accessory genital glands may be exposed to microorganisms that colonize and infect the urethra. Therefore, it is not surprising that infection of these organs may manifest as dysuria, suprapubic pain, perineal pain, testicular pain, and urethral discomfort. Except for cystitis, which is more common in elderly men primarily because of increased incidence of bladder outlet obstruction, epididymitis and prostatitis are not specifically age related. However, the etiology is different. In younger men under the age of 35, the infections are most commonly due to *N. gonorrhoeae* and *C. trachomatis*,

FIGURE 1. Bacteriologic localization in urethritis and bacterial prostatitis. For bacteriologic localization, the voided urine and expressed prostatic secretions are partitioned into segments: VB_1 = (voided bladder urine 1) is the first voided 5 to 10 ml of urine; VB_2 = (voided bladder urine 2) is the midstream aliquot; EPS = (expressed prostatic secretions) is the pure prostatic section expressed by prostatic massage; VB_3 = (voided bladder urine 3) is the first voided 5 to 10 ml immediately after prostatic massage. (From Meares EM Jr, Stamey TA. Bacteriological localization patterns in bacterial prostatitis and urethritis. Invest Urol 1968;5:492–518. Reprinted with permission.)

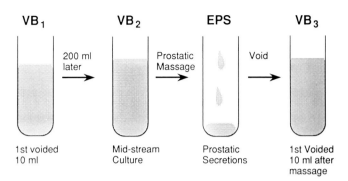

More than 10 WBC/HPF from EPS or VB 3, after 2 days without ejaculation, indicates prostatosis and possibly prostatitis

whereas the organisms found in elderly men are most often coliform bacteria.

Making the diagnosis of epididymitis is easy. However, the diagnosis of prostatitis is often made by the clinician to describe any condition associated with prostatic inflammation or prostatic symptoms but is rarely accompanied by objective evidence.

Some of the previous confusion over diagnosing and classifying has been dispelled by the introduction of uniform terminology by Drach et al.[12] based on objective evidence obtained by microscopic examination of the expressed prostatic secretion and differential quantitative bacteriologic localization status as evolved by Meares and Stamey[13] (Fig. 1). This classification divides the different entities into three main groups: bacterial prostatitis (acute and chronic), nonbacterial prostatitis, and prostatodynia.

The microscopic examination of the expressed prostatic secretion is, however, similar in acute and chronic bacterial prostatitis as well as in nonbacterial prostatitis, showing evidence of inflammation by the presence of more than 10 white blood cells (WBCs) per high power field. Acute and chronic bacterial prostatitis are definitely caused by bacterial infection of the prostate.

Patients with acute prostatitis present with perineal and suprapubic pain, dysuria, and fever. Rectal examination reveals a swollen and acute tender prostate. Chronic bacterial prostatitis is a much more common disease, even if it is difficult to diagnose. Complaints include genital discomfort, intermittent dysuria, frequency, micturition, and sometimes occasional urethral discharge or pain on ejaculation.

Chronic nonbacterial prostatitis is a poorly understood entity. It is undoubtedly over-

diagnosed, and many men given this diagnosis may be suffering from relapsing nongonorrheal urethritis or genital neurosis. However, there is leukocytosis in the prostatic fluid, but culture on conventional media is sterile. The etiology is unknown, but it is presumed to be infective, as there is some response to broad-spectrum antimicrobials. Because this population usually is sexually active, several sexually transmitted organisms that are responsible for a significant fraction of nongonococcal urethritis have been implicated as etiologic agents in nonbacterial prostatitis. These include *Chlamydia trachomatis* and *Trichomonas vaginalis*. However, contradictory results from studies concerning chronic nonbacterial prostatitis are numerous.

Managing Dysuria

Dysuria in its different variations is seldom a symptom of a life-threatening condition. It can be associated with high morbidity and even be a symptom of a serious condition. When a patient complains of dysuria, the correct diagnosis can be firmly established by evaluating symptoms and history carefully. However, the physical examination and, in most cases, various laboratory tests are necessary to confirm the diagnosis.

REFERENCES

1. Koch HK. The national ambulatory medical care survey, 1975 summer. Hyattsville, Maryland: U.S. Public Health Service, Department of Health, Education and Welfare, 1978:1–62.
2. Waters WE. Prevalence of symptoms of urinary tract infection in women. Br J Prev Soc Med 1969;23:263–6.
3. Kass EH. Chemotherapeutic and antibiotic drugs

and the management of infection of the urinary tract. Am J Med 1955;18:764–81.

4. Kass EH. Atraumatic infection of the urinary tract. Trans Assoc Am Physicians 1956;69:56–63.

5. Komaroff AL. Acute dysuria in women. N Engl J Med 1984;310:368–75.

6. Stamm WE, Runming K, McKevitt M, Counts GW, Tuick M, Holmes KK. Treatment of acute urethral syndrome. N Engl J Med 1981;304:956–8.

7. Barbalias GA, Meares EM Jr. Female urethral syndrome: clinical and urodynamic perspectives. Urology 1984;23(2):208–12.

8. Demetriou E, Emans SJ, Massland RP Jr. Dysuria in adolescent girls: urinary tract infection or vaginitis? Pediatrics 1982;70(2):299–301.

9. Sweet RL. Bacteriuria and pyelonephritis during pregnancy. Prenatal 1977;1:25–49.

10. Sweet RL. Pelvic inflammatory disease and infertility in women. Infect Dis Clin North Am 1987; 1(1):199.

11. Lomberg H, Hanson LA, Jacobson B, Jodal U, Leffler H, Eden SC. Correlation of P blood group vesicoureteral reflux and bacterial attachment in a patient with recurrent pyelonephritis. N Engl Med 1983;308:1189–92.

12. Drach TW, Meares EM Jr, Fair WR, Stamey TA. A classification of benign diseases associated with prostatic pain: prostatitis or prostatodynia? J Urol 1978;120:266.

13. Meares EM Jr, Stamey TA. Bacteriological localization patterns in bacterial prostatitis and urethritis. Invest Urol 1968;5:492–518.

ECTOPIC PREGNANCY, SUSPECTED

MARK V. SAUER

SYNONYMS: Tubal Pregnancy, Ectopic Gestation

BACKGROUND

Ectopic pregnancy results from the implantation and growth of an early conceptus outside the uterine cavity. Typically, ectopic gestations occur in the fallopian tube, but they may also be located in the ovary, cervix, or peritoneal cavity. Although rarely seen in animals, ectopic pregnancy is relatively common in humans. Rates vary slightly with locale, but in the United States, the incidence per live birth ranges from approximately 1 in 250 to 1 in 64.[1] Over the past 20 years, the number of ectopic pregnancies in the United States has steadily increased (Fig. 1). Consequently, annual hospitalizations for this condition have more than tripled since 1970, as reported by the Centers for Disease Control (CDC).[2] Suggested reasons for the increase include: (1) the higher prevalence of risk factors in the general population, particularly salpingitis; (2) improvements in the methods used for diagnos-

ing the condition; (3) the widespread use of the intrauterine contraceptive device (IUD); and (4) the postponement of childbearing until later reproductive life, when ectopic pregnancy rates are highest.

Despite the rising incidence, mortality rates remain low. The case-fatality rate is approximately 4.9 deaths per 10,000 ectopic pregnancies, demonstrating an 86 per cent decline from the 35.5 deaths per 10,000 ectopic pregnancies reported to the CDC in 1970.[2] This improvement is largely attributable to technologic advances in the diagnostic methods employed in managing these patients. Early diagnosis impacts on both morbidity and mortality rates. Although ectopic pregnancy accounts for but 1.4 per cent of all pregnancies, it is associated with over 13 per cent of all maternal deaths. Ectopic pregnancy remains the most common cause of maternal death in the first half of pregnancy and represents the most frequent cause of all maternal deaths experienced by black women (Fig. 2). Most deaths result from exsanguination following tubal rupture of a misdiagnosed ectopic pregnancy. A diagnostic delay estimated to be from 7 to 10 days was common in fatal cases. It was likely

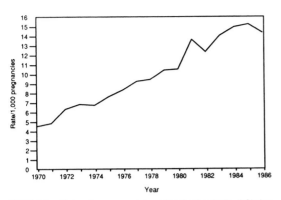

FIGURE 1. Ectopic pregnancy rates in the United States from 1970 through 1986. (From the Centers for Disease Control. MMWR 1990;45:335–47.)

that in the majority of cases maternal mortality was preventable. In reviewing these cases, the most common misdiagnoses were intestinal disorders, intrauterine pregnancy, and pelvic inflammatory disease.[3]

Ectopic pregnancy often occurs in women who have previously experienced one or more episodes of salpingitis. Nearly one half of all women operated on have clinical findings consistent with past tubal infection. Furthermore, women followed prospectively after experiencing an episode of acute salpingitis demonstrate an increased incidence of tubal pregnancies.[4] Other factors that contribute to tubal scarring, such as previous pelvic surgery, also increase the likelihood of tubal implantation.

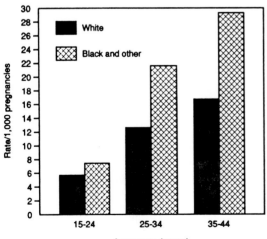

FIGURE 2. Ectopic pregnancy case-fatality rates by race and age group for women in the United States from 1970 through 1986. (From the Centers for Disease Control. MMWR 1990;45:335–47.)

Pregnancy following tubal ligation, especially if performed using electrocautery, is commonly ectopic in location.[5]

Most ectopic pregnancies occur in the fallopian tube. In the majority of cases, the pregnancy is located in the middle or distal third of the tube (Fig. 3).[6] Implantation occurs on the luminal surface. The villous trophoblast then invades the tubal mucosa to gain access to the blood supply located in the connective tissue space between serosa and endosalpinx. Subsequent growth may be intraluminal or extraluminal.[7,8] As the pregnancy grows, bleeding occurs and a hematoma forms. Eventually, rupture results from the stretching and overdistension of the tube.

Ovarian pregnancy represents 1 per cent of all ectopic gestations.[9] It is an infrequent finding, with an incidence of 1 in 7000 deliveries. Ovarian pregnancy is commonly misdiagnosed, even at laparoscopy. Usually, these pregnancies are mistaken for ovarian cysts. Even more rare are abdominal pregnancies, which are believed to result from the secondary implantation of an aborted tubal gestation.

Nearly 40 per cent of patients with ectopic pregnancies have no demonstrable pelvic pathology at the time of surgery. Presumably conditions creating a delay in embryo transit time may result in the blastocyst hatching and implanting in the tube instead of the uterus. Elevated levels of estradiol and progesterone are believed to slow embryo migration by interfering with normal cilial development and mesosalpingeal contractility.[10] This phenomenon may also explain why patients undergoing ovarian hyperstimulation with either clomiphene or human menopausal gonadotropin are predisposed to tubal gestations even in the absence of tubal pathology, as ovarian hyperstimulation leads to the endogenous production of supraphysiologic levels of sex steroid.[11] Similarly, contraceptive failures in women using progestin-only oral pills, high-dose postovulatory administered estrogen (morning-after pill), or a progesterone releasing IUD are likewise at an increased risk for tubal pregnancy.[5]

Although less common, other predisposing factors for ectopic pregnancy include chromosomal anomalies of the conceptus, a history of in utero exposure to diethylstilbestrol (DES) in the mother, and transmigration of the ova from the contralateral ovary to the site of the ectopic.[1,6] Also, women becoming pregnant following in vitro fertilization and embryo transfer may have a higher incidence of ec-

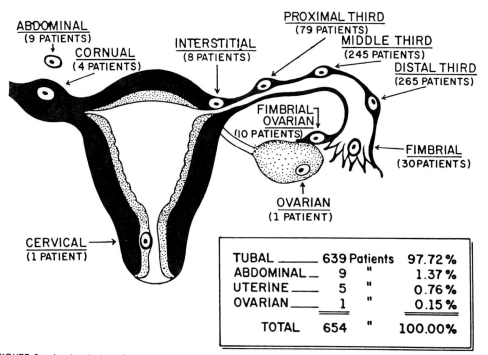

FIGURE 3. Anatomic locations of ectopic pregnancy. (From Breen JL. A 21-year survey of 654 ectopic pregnancies. Am J Obstet Gynecol 1970;106:1004–16. Reprinted with permission.)

topic pregnancy than generally seen in spontaneous conceptions.

Traditionally, serum measurements of the beta subunit of human chorionic gonadotropin (β-hCG) have been used to document and follow the normal progress of early pregnancy. Algorithms based on the mean doubling time of serum β-hCG in normal gestations have assisted in expediting the diagnosis of pathologic pregnancies.[12] Diagnostic accuracy can be further improved when combining serial quantitative measurements with ultrasound imaging.[13] Other hormones and serum markers have been utilized in pregnancy surveillance, including progesterone, estradiol, CA 125, human chorionic somatotropin, and pregnancy-associated plasma protein-A (PAPP-A).[1] However, with the exception of serum progesterone, most of these measures are either technically too difficult or lack the sensitivity and specificity to be practical for clinical use.

The ability to perform conservative fertility-preserving surgery depends on an early diagnosis. Significant delay decreases the likelihood that these measures can be implemented since trophoblastic growth and accompanying tissue damage increase with time. Because ectopic pregnancy occurs in younger reproductive age women, conservative measures are often desired and utilized. In addition, at least

one third to one half of all ectopic pregnancies are currently amenable to laparoscopic management, making this outpatient procedure both diagnostic and therapeutic.[14] By avoiding laparotomy, laparoscopy not only reduces the operative time but also significantly decreases the time spent recuperating postoperatively.

This chapter focuses on new approaches in establishing the diagnosis of ectopic pregnancy. Recognizing the patient at risk and obtaining timely serologic and ultrasonographic tests for evaluating the early pregnancy will facilitate the diagnosis and expedite the delivery of lifesaving and fertility-sparing care.

HISTORY

History of the Present Illness

Before recognizing an ectopic gestation, a diagnosis of pregnancy must first occur. Inquiry concerning the last normal menstrual period (LMP) is important in order to best date the pregnancy. Typically, menses are delayed from the expected time, but in many cases, spotting or light vaginal bleeding has been observed. Usually this happens between six and eight weeks gestation when the decidualized endometrium sloughs as a result of abnormal hormone support from the developing ectopic trophoblast. Other subjective complaints typical of pregnancy may be present but are only experienced by 10 to 25 per cent of patients.[15] Such complaints include breast tenderness, morning sickness, or fatigue. The triad of lower abdominal pain, amenorrhea, and vaginal bleeding has been reported in 80 to 100 per cent of patients presenting with tubal pregnancies. However, as diagnostic testing has improved, the discovery of a tubal pregnancy now often precedes the onset of signs or symptoms.

More specific complaints accompany the growth of the trophoblast within the fallopian tube. Abdominal pain is the most common symptom but initially may be vague and difficult to localize. Later, unilateral discomfort often develops. In the presence of intraperitoneal bleeding, shoulder pain may occur as a result of subdiaphragmatic irritation. As intra-abdominal bleeding increases, pain typically intensifies, and dizziness or syncope results.

Past Medical History

Risk factors for ectopic pregnancy should be established in obtaining both the past and present medical history (Table 1). Important to note are preceding events that directly violate the integrity of the fallopian tube and ovary. Not surprisingly, patients with previous ectopic pregnancies continue to have an increased risk for this condition in subsequent pregnancies.[6]

The gynecologic history should be thorough. A past history of salpingitis is a significant predisposing factor. The presence of tubal adhesions directly correlates with the number of episodes of clinical infections experienced by the patient.[4] Other conditions related to infertility or its treatment, such as

TABLE 1. Known Risk Factors for Ectopic Pregnancy

Previous salpingitis (pelvic inflammatory disease)
Low socioeconomic status
Previous tubal surgery (interruptive or reparative)
Previous ectopic pregnancy
Black and minority races
In utero exposure to DES
Progestin-only contraception, postcoital estrogen contraceptives
Progesterone-containing IUD
Advanced maternal age (> 35 years)
Ovarian hyperstimulation using clomiphene or human menopausal gonadotropin
In vitro fertilization and embryo transfer

endometriosis, a previous tuboplasty, or the reversal of tubal sterilization, predispose the patient to tubal disease and increase her risk of developing an ectopic pregnancy.

Although most ectopic pregnancies occur in sexually active women not using any form of contraception, certain medications and devices are believed to increase the likelihood for an ectopic implantation.[5] Progestin-only oral contraceptive pills and subdermal silastic implants containing progestins probably increase the risk. IUDs may increase the risk for an ectopic, especially if containing progesterone. This risk may be further compounded by extended use of the IUD for greater than two years. Combination estrogen/progestogen oral contraceptive pills carry no added risk. No matter which method of contraception is chosen, following its discontinuation the ectopic pregnancy rate is not appreciably increased. A history of abortion does not appear to increase the risk for an ectopic pregnancy, except for instances in which infection occurred postoperatively.[16]

Focused Queries

1. *Is abdominal or pelvic pain present?* Although often difficult to characterize, any pain complaint in a pregnant patient should heighten the suspicion for a tubal gestation. This is especially true for cases of unilateral lower quadrant complaints.

2. *Have you experienced a previous ectopic pregnancy?* Patients who have already experienced an ectopic pregnancy have a 10 to 30 per cent chance of another ectopic pregnancy in subsequent pregnancies.

3. *Have you ever been treated for a pelvic or tubal infection?* Clearly, the likelihood of developing tubal adhesions increases with the number of infectious episodes. Also, a history of pelvic infection raises the risk of developing an ectopic from approximately 5 per cent with one infection to 20 per cent following multiple episodes.

4. *Are you using contraception?* As previously stated, certain methods, particularly progestin-only pills, and IUDs are more likely to be associated with a tubal pregnancy. Furthermore, failed sterilization procedures increase the risk for an ectopic.

5. *Do you desire future fertility?* This is important to ascertain since it may dictate your approach to evaluating the patient. For instance, patients not interested in pregnancy may entertain a diagnostic uterine curettage in

order to discover the location of the pathologic pregnancy. Furthermore, patients later requiring surgery might be offered salpingectomy rather than salpingostomy if future fertility is not desired. These issues should be understood prior to placing the patient under anesthesia.

PHYSICAL EXAMINATION

Typically, patients with ectopic pregnancy have abdominal pain localized to the lower quadrant. Pain may be generalized to both sides of the pelvis but usually is more severe on one side than the other. Voluntary guarding is almost always present. Rebound tenderness is a frequent finding. A thorough pelvic examination should be performed including assessment of the vulva, vagina, cervix, uterus, and adnexa. On pelvic exam, the uterus may be slightly enlarged or normal in size. Tenderness may make it difficult to fully examine the adnexa, but in a third of patients, a distinct mass is appreciable. The patient is usually afebrile. Vital signs will vary according to the amount of anxiety and pain experienced by the patient. However, evidence of hemodynamic instability is usually associated with significant intraperitoneal bleeding. Less than 10 per cent of patients present in hemorrhagic shock. Significant findings on abdominopelvic examination include those shown in Table 2.

LABORATORY

Although the history and physical examination constitute the basis on which most ectopic pregnancies are initially assessed, when relying on these methods alone, a correct diagnosis is at best established in but 50 per cent of cases. Laboratory and ultrasonographic testing have become an integral part of the evaluation of early pregnancy states. Established algorithms utilizing serologic measurements of β-hCG and ultrasound provide well-defined growth parameters for identifying and tracking both normal and abnormal early gestations.[12,17] Following an algorithmic approach, many ectopics are diagnosed prior to tubal rupture and often are discovered prior to the manifestation of significant symptoms.

TABLE 2. Abdominopelvic Examination in Ectopic Pregnancy

PELVIC FINDING	POSSIBLE CAUSES
Adnexal tenderness	Majority of patients (75–90%) with ectopic pregnancy; also noted in salpingitis, adnexal torsion, endometriosis, hemorrhagic corpora lutea, appendicitis, enteritis
Adnexal mass	Seen in 30–50% of cases of ectopic pregnancy; also noted in corpora lutea, ovarian neoplasm, ovarian or periappendiceal abscess, or endometrioma
Vaginal bleeding	Evident in 50–80% of ectopic pregnancies; also noted in threatened abortion, spontaneous complete and incomplete abortion, dysfunctional uterine bleeding
Uterine enlargement	More commonly associated with an intrauterine gestation—only 20–30% of ectopics; also noted in leiomyomata, adenomyosis
Fever	Rare in patients with ectopic (5–10%); usually noted in salpingitis, appendicitis, enteritis, or colitis
Orthostatic change	Seen in 10–20% of ectopic pregnancies; massive intra-abdominal bleeding

Human Chorionic Gonadotropin

Measurement of β-hCG is an integral part of the evaluation of reproductive-age women with a history suggestive of pregnancy. Qualitative enzyme immunoassays (EIAs) that measure β-hCG in the urine are available in most offices and emergency rooms, with lower limit sensitivities of 50 mIU/ml. Thus, the diagnosis of pregnancy can be accomplished prior to the missed menstrual period. These assays are easy to perform, with results obtainable in less than 10 minutes. Although unlikely, a negative urine test does not absolutely rule out pregnancy. Rarely, ruptured ectopics have been reported in the presence of negative EIA and radioimmunoassay results.[18]

Levels of serum β-hCG rise exponentially in early pregnancy. Evaluation using serial estimations has been based on the linear regression of log-transformed values. However, changes in β-hCG levels change in a curvilinear manner as the pregnancy progresses, and a simple linear model is only applicable during the first six weeks of gestation. During this time period, β-hCG values normally increase by at least two thirds in two days and

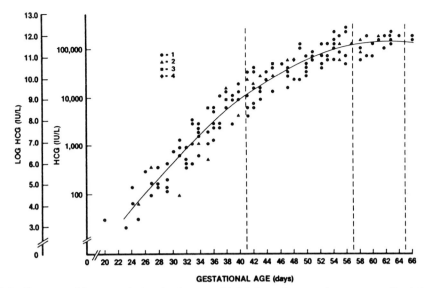

FIGURE 4. The normal increase in levels of serum β-hCG in early normal pregnancy. Depicted is a scattergram of log hCG plotted against gestational age, demonstrating that as gestational age advances hCG levels also increase until a plateau is reached at nine weeks of pregnancy. (From Daya S. Human chorionic gonadotropin increase in normal early pregnancy. Am J Obstet Gynecol 1987;156:286–90. Reprinted with permission.)

double every three days (Fig. 4).[12] Pregnancies demonstrating a slower rise, or a plateaued or decreasing slope, commonly are abnormal.[17] Thus, pathologic pregnancies, especially ectopic gestations, can be detected by defining an abnormal pattern of β-hCG secretion over time. However, beyond six weeks of gestation, the normal rate of increase for levels of β-hCG is slower, taking more than one week to double.[12] Thus, it is imperative to know the approximate gestational age of the patient when solely relying on β-hCG measurements. Since one third to one half of women presenting with ectopic pregnancy are uncertain of their last LMP, the clinical utility of a single value for β-hCG is limited.

Progesterone

Serum progesterone and its urinary metabolite pregnanediol glucuronide (PDG) are also known to be decreased in patients with pathologic pregnancies.[19] Direct radioimmunoassay of progesterone using nonextracted serum and a highly specific antibody provide reliable results in under four hours. It has been suggested that the EIA measurement of PDG has diagnostic advantage over serial samples of β-hCG. The PDG-EIA may be interpreted using a single sample, it is nonradioactive, and it

can be measured by office personnel in under 10 minutes. However, randomly collected urine specimens are only accurate if nondilute specimens (specific gravity greater than 1.015) are utilized, necessitating control over the patient's state of hydration at the time of specimen collection.

Approximately 50 to 75 per cent of patients with ectopic gestations will demonstrate a progesterone or PDG value below the 95 per cent confidence limit of normal for early pregnancy (Fig. 5). Progesterone and PDG levels remain relatively constant during the first eight weeks of pregnancy. Therefore, establishing a discriminatory zone for normal pregnancy using a single progesterone value would avoid the difficulties inherent in interpreting β-hCG values. Although most normal pregnancies will demonstrate progesterone levels above 15 ng/ml, occasional values as low as 6.0 ng/ml have been reported. Thus, overlap between normal and abnormal pregnancies does exist, making it difficult to recommend an absolute lower limit value that is 100 per cent inclusive of normal gestations. However, since approximately 25 per cent of ectopics are known to produce very low levels of progesterone (less than 3 ng/ml), rapid serum or urinary measurements may expedite the diagnosis and treatment of these patients, especially when used in conjunction with other diagnostic tests.

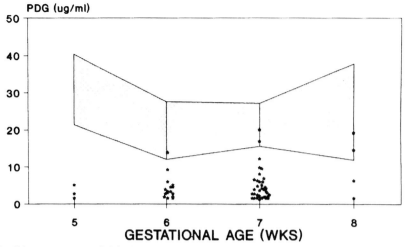

FIGURE 5.   Urinary pregnanediol-3-glucuronide (PDG) values measured in 60 patients with ectopic pregnancy in relation to the 95 per cent confidence limits of normal control subjects. (From Sauer MV, Vermesh M, Anderson RA, Vijod AG, Stanczyk FZ, Lobo RA. Rapid measurement of urinary pregnanediol glucuronide to diagnose ectopic pregnancy. Am J Obstet Gynecol 1988;159:1531–5.)

DIAGNOSTIC STUDIES

Ultrasound

Ultrasound imaging has been commonly used in conjunction with serum measurements of β-hCG to track the course of the developing early pregnancy. Traditionally, a discriminatory zone of 6500 mIU/ml (First International Reference Preparation [IRP] for hCG) defined the point at which a gestational sac should be visible using an abdominal transducer.[17] This usually occurred approximately six weeks from the date of the LMP. Those pregnancies not demonstrating a gestational sac at that time were usually pathologic. Thus, in cases where the quantitative value of β-hCG was known, abdominal sonography was helpful in discerning abnormal pregnancy states. However, patients with ectopic pregnancies often never reached the threshold value of 6500 mIU/ml, and technically transabdominal scanning was difficult to perform, thus restricting the application of this method.

The introduction of transvaginal ultrasound with its improved imaging capabilities and its relative ease of performance has circumvented many of the difficulties inherent to transabdominal scanning. Using a standard 5 mHz vaginal probe, visualization of the gestational sac becomes possible at the time of the missed menstrual period (2-mm size gestational sac).[20] The diameter of the sac normally continues to increase daily and by 40 days from the LMP approximates 10 mm. More importantly, a yolk sac normally becomes visible at five weeks of pregnancy within the developing gestational sac, confirming the presence of embryonic tissue within the uterine cavity. Thus, even prior to the appearance of embryonic heart activity, the intrauterine location of the pregnancy can be discerned with precision and accuracy.

Typically, pathologic pregnancies will deviate from this pattern of development, becoming identifiable on ultrasound even before abnormalities in the serum hormone values are detected. Other ultrasonographic signs suggestive of an ectopic gestation include a complex cystic adnexal mass and free fluid in the peritoneal cavity (Fig. 6). Earlier identification of the gestational sac has significantly lowered the discriminatory zone for normal pregnancy from 6500 mIU/ml to around 1500 mIU/ml (First IRP), shortening by approximately one week the time required to image an early normal pregnancy.

Culdocentesis

Culdocentesis has traditionally been considered an important test in the evaluation of ectopic pregnancy. The diagnosis of hemoperitoneum in a pregnant patient as ascertained by culdocentesis is highly predictive of an ectopic gestation.[15] Prior to the development of transvaginal ultrasound imaging, culdocentesis represented the only nonsurgical way to assess the intraperitoneal environment. When hemo-

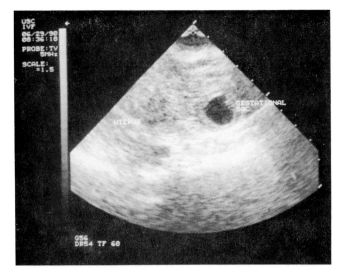

FIGURE 6. Right-sided unruptured ampullary ectopic visualized ultrasonographically in an asymptomatic patient 37 days following her LMP, using a 5-mHz vaginal transducer.

peritoneum was encountered, an exploratory laparotomy was usually performed.

However, beyond the diagnosis of hemoperitoneum, culdocentesis is of little value.[21] A negative or nondiagnostic tap does not exclude a tubal pregnancy and can also occur in the presence of a ruptured ectopic gestation. Furthermore, a positive tap does not correlate with tubal rupture and may be present in 1 to 2 per cent of women evaluated with intrauterine pregnancies. Therefore, proceeding directly to emergency exploratory laparotomy in hemodynamically stable patients with positive taps is unwarranted. The combination of data obtained from vaginal ultrasound and serum pregnancy tests is generally more helpful in making the diagnosis of ectopic pregnancy than the information obtained from culdocentesis alone.[13]

The advent of high-resolution ultrasound has in many ways superseded the need for performing a culdocentesis. Hemoperitoneum is quite apparent on imaging, and unlike culdocentesis, transvaginal scanning is neither painful nor invasive. Thus, culdocentesis should probably be utilized only if ultrasound is unavailable or in rare cases of dire emergency in order to best triage care.

Uterine Curettage

Uterine curettage should be performed in patients determined to have abnormal gestations based on the findings of the hormonal evaluations and ultrasound. The procurement of decidua without chorionic villi is highly suggestive of an ectopic gestation. Endometrial

curettage can easily be performed in the office or emergency room using a small caliber suction aspirator, with or without local anesthesia. When trophoblast is obtained, the procedure is both diagnostic and therapeutic.

Diagnostic Laparoscopy

Laparoscopy has the highest positive predictive value for diagnosing ectopic pregnancy as a single test and provides a correct diagnosis in more than 90 per cent of cases.[15] Direct visualization of the ectopic gestation is definitive. In many instances, the pregnancy may be treated using the operating laparoscope.[14] Thus, major surgery is avoided. If hemoperitoneum has been detected by culdocentesis prior to surgery in a stable patient, laparoscopy should still precede laparotomy since 50 per cent of such women will have an early unruptured gestation that is manageable using the laparoscope alone.

ASSESSMENT

Integration of hormone measurements, ultrasound imaging, and uterine curettage using diagnostic algorithms has promoted the early discovery of ectopic gestations. Improved detection expedites the delivery of care and allows a choice of treatment options, ranging from the traditional surgical approach to the more recent nonsurgical remedies.[22] Furthermore, early intervention significantly decreases morbidity and mortality rates.

DIAGNOSTIC ASSESSMENT OF SUSPECTED ECTOPIC PREGNANCY

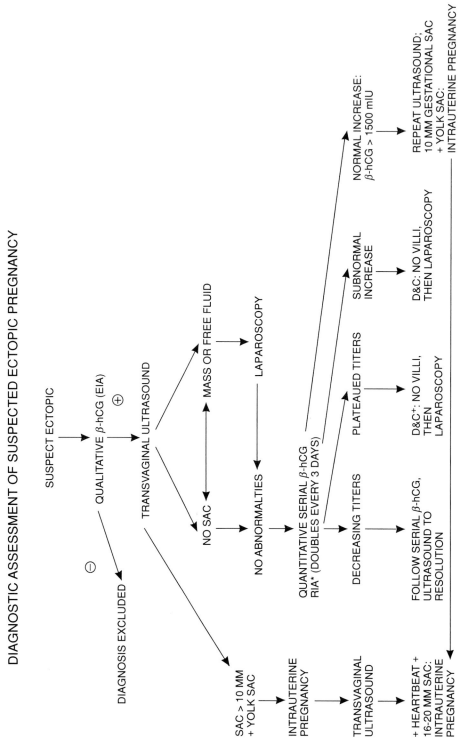

* RIA = RADIOIMMUNOASSAY.
+ D&C = DILATION AND CURETTAGE.

The algorithm presented here depicts the evaluation used in assessing a hemodynamically stable patient suspected of having an ectopic pregnancy. The algorithm works efficiently in practically all clinical settings, minimizing the need for patient follow-up and outside technical support. Implementation of diagnostic testing remains the key to successful management. Recognizing the pregnant patient is the initial, and perhaps most important step toward making the diagnosis. The combined use of ultrasound with serial β-hCG measurements should be considered in women known to be at risk for ectopic gestations, beginning at the time of the missed menses. Utilizing this approach, the majority of ectopic gestations will be successfully diagnosed prior to tubal rupture.

For symptomatic patients in need of acute emergency care, serial examinations may not be possible. In such instances, a rapid, qualitative urine pregnancy test combined with either transvaginal ultrasound or culdocentesis usually establishes the diagnosis. Diagnostic laparoscopy is definitive and should be used liberally.

Implications of Ectopic Pregnancy

The conception rate in women following an ectopic pregnancy is approximately 60 to 75 per cent.[15] It is estimated that one half of these pregnancies result in either another ectopic gestation or a spontaneous abortion. The rate of recurrence of ectopic implantation is in the range of 10 to 30 per cent. Thus, approximately one third to one half of women with an ectopic pregnancy ever experience a subsequent live birth. Age, parity, tubal status, and whether the ectopic pregnancy was ruptured or unruptured probably influence this prognosis. However, fertility outcomes following ectopic pregnancy are difficult to analyze since confounding variables exist within most studied populations that bias reported fertility rates.

The ability to diagnose and treat ectopic gestations early in their clinical course provides an opportunity to manage the majority of cases without laparotomy. Laparoscopic surgery has significantly reduced hospitalization and recuperation times, while maintaining treatment success rates. As imaging techniques and diagnostic assays continue to improve, ectopic pregnancy may someday be managed without surgery, reserving operative intervention for neglected or misdiagnosed cases.

REFERENCES

1. Stabile I, Grudzinskas JG, Ectopic pregnancy: a review of incidence, etiology, and diagnostic aspects. Obstet Gynecol Surv 1990;45:335–47.
2. Lawson HW, Atrash HK, Saftlas AF, Finch EL. Ectopic pregnancy in the United States, 1970–1986. MMWR 1990;38:1–10.
3. Dorfman SF, Grimes DA, Cates W, Binkin NJ, Kafrissen ME, O'Reilly KR. Ectopic pregnancy mortality, United States, 1979 to 1980: clinical aspects. Obstet Gynecol 1984; 64:386–90.
4. Westrom L, Bengtsson LPH, Mardh PA. Incidence, trends, and risks of ectopic pregnancy in a population of women. Br Med J 1981; 282:15–8.
5. Tatum HJ, Schmidt FH. Contraceptive and sterilization practices and extrauterine pregnancy: a realistic perspective. Fertil Steril 1977;28:407–21.
6. Breen JL. A 21-year survey of 654 ectopic pregnancies. Am J Obstet Gynecol 1970; 106:1004–16.
7. Pauerstein CJ, Croxatto HB, Eddy CA, Ramzy I, Walters MD. Anatomy and pathology of tubal pregnancy. Obstet Gynecol 1986;67:301–8.
8. Budowick M, Johnson TRB, Genadry R, Parmley T, Woodruff J. The histopathology of the developing tubal ectopic pregnancy. Fertil Steril 1980;34:169–71.
9. Vasilev SA, Sauer MV. Diagnosis and modern surgical management of ovarian pregnancy. Surg Gynecol Obstet 1990;170:395–8.
10. Jansen RPS. Endocrine response in the fallopian tube. Endocrine Rev 1984;525–51.
11. McBain JC. An unexpectedly high rate of ectopic pregnancy following the induction of ovulation with human pituitary and chorionic gonadotropin. Br J Obstet Gynecol 1980;87:5–9.
12. Daya S. Human chorionic gonadotropin increase in normal early pregnancy. Am J Obstet Gynecol 1987;156:286–90.
13. Weckstein LN, Boucher AR, Tucker H, Gibson D, Rettenmaier MA. Accurate diagnosis of early ectopic pregnancy. Obstet Gynecol 1985;65:393–7.
14. Silva PD. A laparoscopic approach can be applied to most cases of ectopic pregnancy. Obstet Gynecol 1988;72:944–7.
15. Weckstein LN. Current perspective on ectopic pregnancy. Obstet Gynecol Surv 1985; 40:259–72.
16. Levin AA, Schoenbaum SC, Stubblefield PG, Zimicki S, Monson RR, Ryan K. Ectopic pregnancy and prior induced abortion. Am J Public Health 1982;72:253–6.
17. Romero R, Kadar N, Jeanty P, et al. Diagnosis of ectopic pregnancy: value of the discriminatory human chorionic gonadotropin zone. Obstet Gynecol 1985;66:357–60.
18. Lonky N, Sauer MV. Ectopic pregnancy with shock and undetectable β-hCG. J Reprod Med 1987;32:559–60.
19. Sauer MV, Vermesh M, Anderson RA, Vijod AG, Stanczyk FZ, Lobo RA. Rapid measurement of urinary pregnanediol glucuronide to diagnose ectopic pregnancy. Am J Obstet Gynecol 1988;159:1531–5.

20. Fossum GT, Davajan V, Kletzky O. Early detection of pregnancy with transvaginal ultrasound. Fertil Steril 1988;49:788–91.
21. Vermesh M, Graczykowski JW, Sauer MV. Reevaluation of the role of culdocentesis in the manage-

ment of ectopic pregnancy. Am J Obstet Gynecol 1990;162:411–3.
22. Sauer MV, Gorrill MJ, Rodi IA, et al. Nonsurgical management of unruptured ectopic pregnancy: an extended clinical trial. Fertil Steril 1987;48:752–5.

FATIGUE, CHRONIC

A. JAMES GIANNINI

SYNONYMS: Burnout, Tiredness

BACKGROUND

Chronic fatigue syndrome (CFS) has traced its weary path through the entire history of Western civilization. It has struck at gods and heroes, kings and commoners. Both Odin and Zeus, retreating from the caves of heaven, and Sisyphus, pushing his stone in eternal toil, provide archetypes for this syndrome. The preclassical god-kings Akhenaton of Egypt and Gudea of Sumeria have left us documentation of their fatigue and irritability, headaches, and sour stomachs, to mark them as sufferers of the syndrome.

The Roman emperor Tiberius retreated to Capri when he was overcome with the effects of chronic fatigue. The Renaissance Italian merchant prince Lorenzo de Medici would regularly isolate himself in the cells of the abbey of San Marco. Following this example, Emperor Charles V, ruler of Spain, Austria, the Netherlands, and the New World, renouncing all for his spiritual and physical health, joined a monastery. Unlike the case of tired old King Arthur, there was no Holy Grail to cure them of their affliction. The medieval poet Dante Alighieri created chronic fatigue as fitting punishment for those strivers who found themselves in Hell. Ironically, he put them under the rule of Plutus, god of wealth.

Symptoms associated with CFS, as differentiated from simple physical fatigue, did not become common until after the Reformation. At this time, the Protestant ethic became one with the striving for efficiency and success. In John Bunyan's *Pilgrim's Progress*, his seventeenth-century hero is quite simply "burned out." His journey to salvation causes him to acquire many of the symptoms we commonly associate with chronic fatigue.

Today, chronic fatigue is recognized as a syndrome with worldwide distribution. In the West, it is seen as a compilation of symptoms that include fatigue, headache, gastrointestinal disturbances, tachycardia and palpitations, irritability, elevated blood pressure, insomnia, depression, and anxiety. It is not unique to a modern industrial society. Punjabi villagers, under stress of leadership and constant toil, complain of the *dil ghirda dai*—"the heart that falls in battle."[1] In the Andes, indigenous villagers note a similar complex that they label *pulsario*—"the sphere which vibrates under distress."[2] These syndromes, then, are not very different from "executive burnout" in New York, "drain" in Milan, or "college fatigue" in newly minted Tokyo University graduates.

ETIOLOGY

The syndrome of chronic fatigue actually refers to the similar effects of various different disease states, such as: anemia, depression, fibrositis, premenstrual syndrome, zinc deficiency, hypermagnesemia, and hypothyroidism). While these diseases are separate entities, they often have interactive effects (see Fig. 1).

Immune deficiencies often exacerbate the effects of viral and sometimes, bacterial infections, leading to chronicity.[3] This chronicity can be exacerbated by environmental stress or overwork.[4] It, in turn, can lead to opioid deficiencies, which may leave the woman patient more vulnerable to the effects of premenstrual syndrome (PMS, or late luteal phase dys-

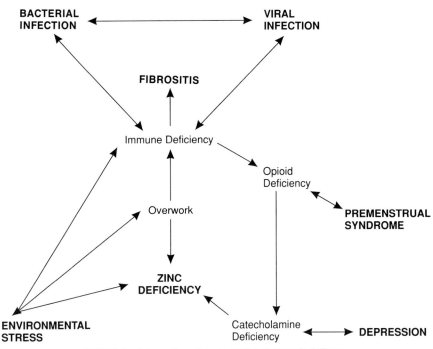

FIGURE 1. Interactive disease states of chronic fatigue.

phoric disorder).[5] The underlying PMS, the resultant opioid deficiency, or overwork itself can reduce central catecholamine levels, resulting in a tired depression. Stress, overwork, or reduced catecholamines can reduce zinc supplies, producing a rather anorectic fatigue.[6] These interactions produce many diagnostic difficulties. The clinician needs, then, to sort out many factors in the examination as well as the history.

Regardless of the etiology, there is a standard measure to diagnose "chronicity." The patient should have had a single episode of at least one year's duration or at least three separate episodes of at least three months' duration each. Episodes of shorter duration usually, while possibly of significance, do not meet criteria for chronic fatigue.

DEPRESSION

Depression is the most common cause of chronic fatigue. Major depression affects 7 per cent of the American population at some time, whereas dysthymia and manic depression account for another 10 to 15 per cent and 1 per cent, respectively. When patients complaining of chronic fatigue were examined at the National Institutes of Health, 55 per cent of all women and 25 per cent of all men studied met diagnostic criteria for major depression. Another 35 per cent of the women met criteria for dysthymia, although none of the men studied did.[7]

The average age of onset of major depression is in the midtwenties. Women account for 75 per cent of all episodes, although recent data indicate that the ratio is changing toward a 1:1 balance. The fatigue in this disease state is invariably most severe in the early morning. Anhedonia and depression are also most severe at this time. Other major symptoms include anorexia or hyperphagia with a weight loss or weight gain of at least 5 per cent of body weight per month. Sleep can be marked by hypersomnia or insomnia. Usually, the insomnia is characterized by nocturnal or early morning awakenings rather than difficulty falling asleep. Concentration and decisiveness are usually diminished. Hallmarks are feelings of worthlessness, guilt, and hopelessness. Usually, there is no identifiable environmental precipitant that would explain the amount of depression or fatigue. Severity is increased in autumn or spring. Symptoms may be either of several years' duration or intermittent.[8]

To assist the clinician in diagnosing depression, a number of laboratory tests have been developed. Depression is known to be due to decreased production of catecholamines, and most of these tests utilize this knowledge to make a diagnosis. 3-Methoxy-4-hydroxy phenethyleneglycol (MHPG) is a metabolite of norepinephrine. Approximately 50 per cent of all depressive tests show reduced levels of MHPG when 24-hour urines are assayed.[9]

The catecholamines also modulate endocrine secretion via the hypothalamic–pituitary–end organ axis. In assaying central modulation of thyroid function, the thyrotropin releasing hormone–thyroid stimulating hormone (TRH-TSH) stimulation test is used. If T_3, T_4, and TSH are within normal limits, the results can be read with confidence. For psychodiagnostic purposes, the baseline TSH level is subtracted from the highest level of TSH recorded during the test. If the difference is less than 5 mIU, a diagnosis of depression can be made with a high degree of confidence. If the difference is greater than 20 mIU, the diagnosis of manic-depressive illness can be made with a similar degree of confidence.[10]

In assessing the function of the hypothalamic-pituitary-adrenal axis, the dexamethasone suppression test (DST) may be used. In the absence of adrenal dysfunction, a failure to suppress adrenal function on two measures can be used to diagnose depression. This test can be employed assaying serum cortisol or salivary cortisol levels (Cortitest®, Princeton Diagnostic Laboratories, South Plainfield, New Jersey). When the DST is combined with the TRH-TSH test, 75 per cent of all depressions can be diagnosed with few false positives.[11]

Dysthymia presents with symptoms similar to major depression. The onset is usually in childhood or adolescence. Prevalence is about equal in males and females. Symptoms are similar though less severe than in major depression and last at least two years. There is usually a precipitant. Seasonal mood variation and diurnal mood variation are absent.

Manic-depression has all the symptoms of major depression except that at least one manic episode with unusually high energy levels, pressured speech, grandiosity, and racing thoughts has occurred. Cyclothymia incorporates all symptoms of dysthymia except there is a history of multiple mild manic episodes.

EPSTEIN-BARR VIRUS INFECTION

This herpes virus has received the major share of popular publicity as an etiologic agent for chronic fatigue. While 90 per cent of adults may be infected with the Epstein-Barr virus

(EBV), it usually is dormant.[12] Activation can be caused by an immunologic deficiency produced by stress, bacterial infection, or external toxin.[3] Chronic active EBV occurs via mechanisms similar to those of chronic mononucleosis and may coexist with chronic mononucleosis. Patients can present with recurring pneumonitis, chronic hepatitis, pancytopenia, or agranulocytosis.

The typical historical triad of the chronic EBV patient includes myalgia, depression, and low-grade fever of 99° to 100° F. The fever and depression are usually intermittent and present most frequently in the afternoon. Other common features include anxiety, arthralgia, confusion, insomnia (usually difficulty falling asleep), nausea, oral ulcerations, pharyngitis, photosensitivity, and tender adenopathy. Symptoms become progressively severe over several months. They then reach a plateau phase, which may continue for several years.[13]

Routine laboratory testing usually is nonspecific. Screening blood chemistry tests (SMAC) usually reveal elevated liver function, most often serum glutamic-oxaloacetic transaminase (SGOT) and serum glutamic-pyruvic transaminase (SGPT). The blood count is characterized by a low sedimentation rate, mild leukopenia (3000 to 5000 cu mm), and mild to moderate monocytosis (7 to 15 per cent).[14] Some authors have reported dimpled spherocytes, but others have challenged this observation.[15] Serum creatinine kinase can be elevated and is mildly correlated with persistent enterovirus ribonucleic acid (RNA) in muscle tissue. In assessing for immune deficiencies, one must ascertain the course of the disease for adequate interpretation. In the first two months of infection, there are elevated levels of IgG and IgM as the lysis of B cells expresses EB viruses. This is followed by production of antinuclear antibodies. Over a lifetime, IgE tends to be chronically elevated even in nonsymptomatic patients. IgM re-emerges intermittently. IgG is reduced in about 60 per cent of the chronic patients.[16] A naloxone challenge will cause a low lymphoproliferative response (17) because opioids help modulate immune functions. Bacterial infections can precipitate an immune reaction to an otherwise dormant EB virus. Bacterial infections, especially those of *Brucella* and *Borrelia burgdorferi*, can also mimic EBV infection. Routine blood counts, however, will generally differentiate between bacterial and viral infections.

FIBROSITIS

The symptoms associated with chronic fatigue in fibrositis are similar but not identical to those of EBV syndrome. They include arthralgia, nausea, myalgia, depression, anxiety, and insomnia. Fevers occur in only a fifth of these patients. In addition, fibrositis has many symptoms that set it apart from other diseases associated with CFS.[18]

In adults, there is low back pain, morning fatigue and stiffness, skinfold tenderness, head pain, migraine, hearing or vestibular abnormalities, localized numbness or parasthesias, chronic cough, carpal tunnel syndrome, Raynaud's phenomenon, and livedo reticularis. In children, there may be ankle pain and increased joint swelling but little low back pain or hand pain. In both adults and children, the "Symthe criteria" may be used to further establish a diagnosis. To do so, one should examine the patient for tenderness at "trigger points over the following 12 areas[19]:

1. Anterior cervical strap muscle.
2. Intertransverse ligament, C4–C6.
3. Epicondyle, lateral or medial.
4. Gluteal muscle, S1.
5. Heel pad.
6. Interspinous ligaments, C4–S1.
7. Medial foot pad at knee joint.
8. Occipital base.
9. Pectoral major over second rib.
10. Rhomboid, medial aspect.
11. Trapezius, upper border.
12. Trochanter, greater.

Tenderness over at least seven of these areas usually establishes a diagnosis of fibrositis. On the other hand, weight loss, fever, joint swelling, and vasculitic rash tend to exclude this diagnosis.

Routine laboratory testing is often noncontributory except as an exclusionary process. Electronystamography, however, will demonstrate positional and/or neck-torsion nystagmus. A sleeping electroencephalogram frequently will reveal a mixture of alpha and delta rhythms rather than normal pure delta, non–rapid eye movement (REM) sleep intervals. (This change, while suggestive of fibrositis, is not diagnostic. It also occurs with incubus, severe rheumatoid arthritis, pavor nocturnus, and sleep apnea.) Peripheral muscle stress testing usually shows abnormal xenon clearance. Skeletal muscle biopsy reveals scattered muscular degeneration of type I fibers and thin reticular banding between muscles.[19]

Primary fibrositis occurs in about 5 per cent of all adults and accounts for 15 to 25 per cent of all diagnoses in rheumatology practices. Cancer patients undergoing interleukin-2 therapy are at particular risk.

PREMENSTRUAL SYNDROME

Premenstrual syndrome (PMS) was first described by Frank in 1934, who also coined the term. Recently, the American Psychiatric Association has renamed this disorder "late luteal phase dysphoric disorder."[8] Both terms, however, are in common use.

This syndrome is usually associated with periods of fatigue associated with the menstrual cycle. However, the fatigue may be continuous, with monthly exacerbation. While the disease remits after menopause, it can occur posthysterectomy unless a bilateral ovariectomy is performed. It does not occur in the pregnant state.

Symptoms include affective lability; irritability; anxiety; depression; anhedonia; chronic fatigue associated with anergia or actual weakness; decreased concentration or memory; hyperphagia, cravings, or pica; hypersomnia or insomnia; tenderness or swelling of breasts; abdominal bloating; and arthralgia and myalgia. Physical examination usually confirms swelling and tenderness. Onset is usually after age 30 and independent of previous pregnancies.[20]

Some laboratory tests may be useful in confirming this diagnosis. Pseudocholinesterase levels tend to be elevated in this group as well as for patients with anxiety disorder.[21] The reason for this finding is unclear. Serial testing for beta-endorphin levels can also help resolve a diagnostic problem.[5] Serum levels of beta-endorphin are drawn every five to seven days for one menstrual cycle. While the specific time of the serum collection is unimportant, it should be consistent throughout the entire collection period. Women without PMS will have a decrease in their beta-endorphin level with a slope of less than 20 degrees, as measured from midcycle to onset of menses. PMS patients, on the other hand, will have a precipitous drop in their beta-endorphin level. It is hypothesized that fluctuating beta-endorphin levels are a primary cause of at least a large subgroup of PMS patients. Large monthly fluctuations in the level of the *opioid* beta-endorphin seem to bring about changes similar to those produced in addicts who abuse the *opiate* heroin. When levels of opioids or opiate suddenly drop, large amounts of the catecholamine norepinephrine are released from the locus ceruleus in the pons. This norepinephrine "flood" then accounts for the symptoms of PMS. Chronic fatigue is brought about by the low baseline levels of norepinephrine produced by the excessively large monthly depletions.

If beta-endorphin tests are not easily available or if serial testing is impractical, clonidine challenge testing may be used. Clonidine is an alpha-2 agonist that reduces the release of norepinephrine. It is given daily during the postluteal phase of one menstrual cycle. Dosage is 17 μg/k body weight divided on a q.i.d. (four times a day) basis. Symptoms will be reduced in about two thirds to three fourths of the patients. Theoretically, there should be no false positives except for placebo effects.[22]

STRESS

When confronted with a potentially dangerous stimulus, a mammalian system will go into selective overdrive. This overdrive is the "fight-or-flight" response. Adrenal production increases while catecholamines are released in accelerated fashion from both central and peripheral sources. This physiologic response then produces a predictable and logical behavioral response: The mammal uses the physiologic overdrive to either fight or run. Under these circumstances, strength and endurance are increased, whereas sensitivity to pain is decreased. In natural situations, this response is of great survival and evolutionary benefit.

Unfortunately, humans are mammals who live in a highly socialized and artificial environment. Under most circumstances, these fight-or-flight responses are not useful. When a perceived dangerous stimulus persists, however, the fight-or-flight reaction becomes a negative survival response. Continued production of hormones or catecholamines leads to depletion as well as aberrant physiologic and behavior responses. This, then, is the response to continued stress—the "burnout," the "overwork syndrome."

Generally, those people who do burn out tend to devote to their work hours far in excess to those given by their peers. In addition to the heavy work load, these people are driven more by extrinsic factors (e.g., recognition, status, money, promotion) than by intrinsic factors (e.g., personal satisfaction, creative expression). Their work tends to provide them with self-esteem, personal identity, and daily structure. It also excludes socialization, sexual expression, and creativity. These people generally become isolated, anxious, and/or depressed and irritable. Because of their fixation on work as an end, they tend to be perceived as controlling, selfish, and aloof.

Symptoms of chronic stress include difficulty falling asleep; anxiety; headaches, either of a frontotemporal or constricting band nature; stomach upsets; constipation; decreased libido, anorgasmia, dyspareunia, or impotence; tremors of an intermittent nature; intermittent micropsia; anhedonia; tachycardia or palpitations; fasciculations; epigastric "gnawing" pain, fatigue; amenorrhea or dysmenorrhea; emesis; decreased coordination; myalgia; dizziness; arthralgia; occasional confusion or memory gaps; and chest pain. Physical examination usually reveals a controlling or driven personality. The patient is usually tense or irritable. Speech is pressured, and hyperreflexia is often evident. Tachycardia with mild hypertension is also a common finding. Insight is poor.[23]

Laboratory testing shows mild to moderate decreases in serum testosterone, tyrosine, tryptophan, and cortisol levels. A blood count may reveal lymphocytosis without any other indication of infection. Zinc serum levels may also be low.[24]

ZINC DEFICIENCY

Zinc's function is an excitatory one. Neurons are stimulated by a group of amino acids that include glutamate and aspartate. These, in turn, activate NMDA (*N*-methyl-D-aspartate) receptors. These receptors then activate the neuron. Zinc acts to modulate activity of these receptors. The importance of zinc can be appreciated when it is understood that NMDA sites occur in the membrane surfaces of all neurons in the brain and spinal cord. The patient with a zinc deficiency gives a history of gradually accelerating fatigue. There is a history of acne, anxiety, confusion, constipation, emesis, hair loss, insomnia, joint pain, loss of senses of smell and taste, menstrual irregularities, poor healing of cuts, spasms, and striae. There may be a history of a diet deficient in sources of zinc such as peas, broccoli, spinach, shellfish, or red meat. Conversely, the diet may be high in grains that contain phytase, a protein that binds zinc. These include certain strains of wheat, corn, and millet. There may also be a history of diseases and conditions that decrease zinc levels. These include: alcoholic cirrhosis, cystic fibrosis, depression, diabetes mellitus, Down's syndrome, environmental stress, myocardial infarction, pica, pregnancy, schizophrenia, tuberculosis, and uremia. Penicillamine and oral contraceptives can also lower zinc levels, sometimes in dramatic fashion. Since copper can displace zinc, well water can be considered a possible etiologic agent for zinc deficiency.[24]

Physical examination generally reveals numerous white spots on the finger- and toenails. Occasionally, nails may be an opaque white. Hair is brittle and fair. There is an odd, sweetish breath. Moderately fine tremors are noted at rest. Tenderness is found in the upper left quadrant of the abdomen. Striae are seen across the abdomen, buttocks, or shoulders.[25]

Laboratory testing can detect hypoglycemia, hypoalbuminemia, or macrocytic anemia. Trace metals testing can reveal an absolute decrease in serum zinc levels. Alternatively, normal zinc levels may occur, but copper levels may be elevated. Since copper tends to antagonize zinc, both zinc and copper levels should be simultaneously drawn. The normal zinc : copper ratio ranges from 0.4 to 1.3.[24]

OTHER CAUSES

In addition to the previously cited causes of CFS, there are other pathologic states that may mimic this syndrome. Although they do not meet the criteria of the CFS-Surveillance Program at the Centers for Disease Control,[26] they are of diagnostic significance. They include anemia, hypermagnesemia, hypokalemia, and hypothyroid.

Anemia

The anemic state can be due to a variety of causes, which include nutritional deficiencies, neoplasms, parasitic infestations, metabolic disorders, autoimmune states, malabsorption syndromes, alcoholism poisoning, and kidney disorders. In addition to the fatigue, persons with anemia may give a history of cold insensitivity, palpitations, restlessness, irritability,

changes in menses and libido, constipation or diarrhea, emesis, abdominal cramping, or flatulence. Physical examination is noteworthy for pale nail beds, purpura, pale palms with red creases, slight tachycardia, and increased pulsation over the precordium as well as forceful carotid and femoral arteries. In severe anemia, systolic murmurs may be auscultated at the pulmonic area and a bruit (*bruit de diable*) over the carotids. Urinalysis may reveal a slight proteinuria or other signs of renal impairment.

Hypermagnesemia

Hypermagnesemia is usually an iatrogenically induced state. The clinician should be aware of a condition associated with *hypomagnesemia* that has been overtreated. Magnesium deficiency states include chronic alcohol abuse, aldosteronism, diabetic acidosis, prolonged dehydration, and postsurgical parathyroidectomy. These states are usually treated with intramuscular magnesium sulfate, followed by oral magnesium therapy. High magnesium levels associated with overtreatment produce depression, fatigue, confusion, weakness, slowing of movement and thought, and hyperphagia. Physical examination reveals hyporeflexia, lid lag, and diminished gag reflex. Laboratory testing shows high magnesium and phosphate levels but low calcium levels. The electrocardiogram (ECG) may demonstrate nonspecific conduction defects.

Hypokalemia

Hypokalemic fatigue is associated with anxiety, depression, confusion, myalgia, urinary frequency, polydipsia, and weakness. The history may give bulimia, metabolic acidosis, or treatment with potassium-wasting diuretics as the etiologic agent. The patient usually presents with hyporeflexia, decreased grip strength, respiratory depression, and diminished bowel sounds. The low potassium level is found on blood chemistry analysis. Usually, the bicarbonate level is high. A flat plate of the abdomen may reveal ileus. A variety of changes are seen on the ECG, including flattening of T waves, U waves, sagging ST segments, and prolonged QRS intervals.

Hypothyroidism

The sytmptoms associated with hypothyroidism are myriad. The patient may give a history of fatigue, angina, weakness, cold intolerance, constipation, hearing difficulties, depression, anxiety, menorrhagia, or visual hallucinations. The physical examination also reveals significant findings. The patient often moves slowly and may appear apathetic or depressed. The hair is typically coarse and the outer third of the eyebrows may be diminished or absent. The skin is pale and dry and has poor turgor, the nails are brittle, and there may be peripheral edema. Speech is slow, and the tongue appears thickened. Speech may be hoarse. Occasionally, carotenemia or ascites is present. The thyroid usually appears enlarged upon palpation.

Routine laboratory testing can demonstrate associated hypocholesterolemia, hyponatremia, and macrocytic anemia. Thyroid functions are decreased except in thyroiditis. TSH levels are elevated in primary hypothyroidism but decreased in secondary hypothyroidism. The 17-OH steroids may be decreased.

PERVASIVENESS OF CFS

Whatever the cause, chronic fatigue syndrome and diseases that mimic it can be debilitating and sometimes dangerous. The disease is not rare, only underdiagnosed. It affects people from all strata of society. The Centers for Disease Control describe receiving reports of 1000 new cases on a regular monthly basis. The first documented epidemic struck in Los Angeles 52 years ago and affected 3000 patients. In 1948, 1136 Icelanders were affected, and in 1984, 100,000 Americans reported onset of CFS. Clearly, this is not an isolated "Yuppie disease" but a true epidemic.[26]

REFERENCES

1. Krause IB. Sinking heart: a Punjabi communication of distress. Soc Sci Med 1989;4:563–75.
2. Finerman RB. The burden of responsibility: duty, depression and nervios in Andean Ecuador. Cult Med Psychiatry 1989;64:143–57.
3. Levine PH, Kreuger GRB, Strauss SE. The postviral chronic fatigue syndrome. J Infect Dis 1989;160:722–4.
4. Glaser R, Kiecult-Glaser JK, Speicher CE, Holliday JE. Marital stress carries immunoproliferative response. J Behav Med 1985;8:244–60.
5. Giannini AJ, Price WA, Loiselle RH. Beta-endorphin withdrawal as a possible cause for premenstrual syndrome. Int J Psychophysiol 1984;1:341–6.
6. Lockitch G, Halstead AC, Wadsworth L, Quigley C, Reston L, Jackson B. Age- and sex-specific reference intervals and correlations for zinc, copper, selenium, iron and related proteins. Clin Chem 1988;237:2616–20.
7. Krusei MJP, Dale J, Straus SE. Psychiatric diagnoses in patients who have chronic fatigue syndrome. J Clin Psychiatry 1989;5:53–6.
8. American Psychiatric Association. Diagnostic and statistical manual. 3rd ed, rev. Washington, DC: American Psychiatric Association Press, 1989.
9. Maas J. Biogenic amines and depression. Gen Psychiatry 1975;32:1357–61.
10. Extein I, Pottash ALC, Gold MS. Relationship of TRM test and dexamethasone suppression test in unipolar depression. Psychiatr Res 1981;4:49–53.
11. Greden JF, Albala AP, Hackett RF. Normalization of the dexamethasone suppression test. Biol Psychiatry 1980;15:449–57.
12. Icenhour ML, Calvert H. Managing the physiological and psychosocial implications of Epstein-Barr virus. J Psychosocial 1989;27:20–3.
13. Lloyd AR, Wakefield LJ, Boughten CR, Dwyer JM. Immunological abnormalities in chronic fatigue syndrome. Med J Aust 1989;151:122–4.
14. Tobi J, Doyle RW. Prolonged atypical illness associated with prolonged evidence of persistent EBV infection. Lancet 1982;61(1):62–7.
15. Lloyd A, Wakefield D, Smith L. Red blood cell morphology in chronic fatigue syndrome. Lancet 1989;75(2):85–6.
16. Jones JF, Ray GC, Minnich LL, Hicks MJ, Kibler R, Lucas DV. Evidence for active Epstein-Barr virus infection in patients with persistent unexplained illness. Ann Intern Med 1985;102–7.
17. Cliff LE, Treveri RW, Inboden JB. Medical and physiological effects of delayed convalescence. Arch Intern Med 1959;103:398–414.
18. Caro XJ. New concepts in primary fibrositis syndrome. Compr Ther 1989;15(5):14–22.
19. Wolfe F, Hawley DJ, Cathay MA. Fibrositis: symptom frequency and criteria for diagnosis. J Rheumatol 1985;12:1159–63.
20. Giannini AJ, Sorger LM, Martin DM, Bates L. Impaired reception of nonverbal cues in women with premenstrual syndrome. J Psychol 1988;122:591–9.
21. Giannini AJ, Price WA, Giannini MC, Loiselle RH. Pseudocholinesterase in premenstrual tension syndrome. J Clin Psychiatry 1985;139:45–9.
22. Giannini AJ, Sullivan BS, Loiselle RH, Sarachene JS. Clonidine in the treatment of a subgroup of premenstrual syndrome patients. J Clin Psychiatry 1988;49:62–7.
23. Rhoads JM. Overwork. JAMA 1977;237:2616–20.
24. Kiecolt-Glaser JK, Fisher LD, Ogrocki P, Stout JC, Speicher CE, Glaser R. Marital quality, marital disruption and immune function. Psychosom Med 1987;19:13–33.
25. Humphries L, Vivian B, Stuart M, McClain CJ. Zinc deficiency and eating disorders. J Clin Psychiatry 1989;50:456–9.
26. Williams L, Crooks C. Stalking a shadowy assailant: the government tries to find the cause of devastating fatigue. Time Oct 24, 1990:66.

FEVER IN CHILDHOOD

MARILYN DOYLE

SYNOMYMS: Pyrexia, Elevated Temperature

BACKGROUND

Fever in children is common. It is easily detected by parents and is generally recognized as a cardinal sign of disease. When presented with a febrile child, the physician's clinical acumen and judgment are sorely taxed. The fever may be the presenting symptom of a serious and life-threatening disease such as meningitis, or it may be the only manifestation of a trivial viral infection. Although the majority of fevers in childhood are the result of infectious causes, noninfectious etiologies must also be considered—such as the small infant swaddled in mounds of blankets and clothing; the child with an immunologic disorder, a malignancy, or autoimmune-mediated disease. In addition, the child is frequently accompanied by anxious parents who overestimate the danger represented by the fever. In two studies, 40 and 52 per cent of parents thought that fever within the range of physiologic tolerance would cause permanent harm, usually brain damage; 15 per cent of parents thought that an untreated fever could rise to 42° C (107.6° F) or higher.[1,2] Although normal body temperatures vary, rectal temperatures above 38.3° C (101° F) are generally considered abnormal.

Fever is the body's response to a host of infectious and noninfectious agents. The current concept of the pathogenesis of fever is that exogenous or foreign pyrogens such as bacteria or bacterial endotoxins induce the host's cells to produce endogenous pyrogens such as interleukin-1 (IL-1), tumor necrosis factor (TNF), interleukin-6 (IL-6), and interferons. These substances circulate to the hypothalamic thermoregulatory center and initiate fever by causing the release of arachidonic acid, which is metabolized to prostaglandins, largely prostaglandin E_2 (PGE_2). Prostaglandins increase the thermostatic set point in the anterior hypothalamus, which drives the mechanisms of heat conservation and heat production until the blood and body core temperature match the set point.[3]

It is hypothesized that the production of fever is a host defense mechanism. There are extensive in vitro data to support the hypothesis that certain host defense functions are enhanced by elevated temperatures. Microbial growth is suppressed, and lymphocyte activation and immunoglobulin synthesis are increased at elevated temperatures.[4,5] However, there is no convincing evidence that patients not taking antipyretics recover from their infections any more quickly than those who resort to aspirin or acetaminophen.[6]

The age and clinical status of the child as well as the duration of the febrile illness are important variables in evaluation. Fever in children may be grouped into three categories:

1. Acute fever, which is defined as fever of short duration with localizing signs in which the diagnosis can be established by history, physical examination, and laboratory tests; or fever present for less than one week where history, physical examination, and preliminary laboratory studies fail to detect a cause.

2. Fever of unknown origin, which, in pediatrics, is defined as fever persisting for more than eight days in a child in whom the initial evaluation fails to confirm a diagnosis.

3. Fever in an infant less than six weeks of age.

In most instances, the physician either identifies an agent or a local infection as the cause of the fever or the fever resolves in a short time. Although children in whom the diagnosis is not apparent from history, physical examination, and initial laboratory screening may not appear ill, the physician must be concerned about the possibility of occult bacteremia, generally due to *Streptococcus pneumoniae* or, less commonly, to *Hemophilus influenzae* or a variety of other organisms including *Neisseria meningitidis, Staphylococcus aureus,* and *Salmonella.*[7] The risk for occult bacteremia is age related, with most episodes occurring in children between 6 and 24 months of age (Table 1).

TABLE 1. Risk Factors for Occult Bacteremia

Age
 < 24 months
Temperature
 > 38.8° C (101.8° F) (especially if > 40° C [104° F])
Epidemiologic
 Exposure to *Neisseria meningitidis* or *Hemophilus
  influenzae*
 Underlying disease, for example, hemolytic anemia
  (including sickle cell disease)
 Immunodeficiency (including acquired immunodefi-
  ciency syndrome)
 Malnutrition
 Cancer
Clinical
 Appearance of illness, irritability, or lethargy
 Lack of appetite for food or water
Laboratory
 White blood cell count ≥ 15,000 cu mm
 Erythrocyte sedimentation rate ≥ 30 mm per hour

(From Doyle MG, Pickering LK. Is this child's fever a worry? Postgrad Med 1989;85:207–22. Reprinted with permission.)

In children with prolonged fevers, a bewildering array of diseases must be considered (Fig. 1). Obviously, not all possible causes can or should be pursued in a given patient. A systematic and individualized approach must be implemented. Several studies in patients with fever of unknown origin have demonstrated that an infectious cause is found in 40 to 50 per cent of cases, a connective tissue disease in 15 to 20 per cent, and a malignancy in 10 to 15 per cent. A diagnosis is not established in 10 to 15 per cent.[8,9]

The febrile infant less than six weeks of age presents a special situation. Fever in these infants is relatively rare. In one study, febrile children in this age group accounted for only 1.1 per cent of pediatric emergency room visits.[10] They are difficult to evaluate clinically, and infection is not easily localized to an organ system on the basis of history and physical examination.

HISTORY

Present Illness

The medical history should determine the duration of the fever, its diurnal variation, and the recorded height of the fever. Fever noted only after vigorous exercise or late in the afternoon is probably a normal physiologic variant. A high temperature for a prolonged period of time without other symptoms of illness suggests factitious fever. Fever that occurs only when a child is in a particular place,

such as a workshop, may represent a reaction to a toxin or chemical agent localized in that area. Any accompanying symptoms such as rhinorrhea, cough, diarrhea, rash, and joint swelling or tenderness must be noted. History concerning the general condition of the child is important. Has there been recent weight loss, decreased activity, or change in behavior? Any recent exposure to infection or illness in family members and/or school- or day-care center contacts is important. Has there been any travel, foreign or domestic, in the recent or distant past? Malaria, histoplasmosis, coccidiomycosis, blastomycosis, and other endemic infections may reappear years after exposure. Was the child born in the United States? Children born abroad are at higher risk for diseases such as tuberculosis and hepatitis B. Exposure to domestic or wild animals may result in unusual zoonoses. Tick bites have been implicated in a number of diseases such as Lyme disease and Rocky Mountain spotted fever. A history of ingestion of raw milk or wild game is also important to obtain. What is the water supply for the family? Pica by the child raises the possibility of visceral larva migrans or toxoplasmosis. An accurate history of exposure to drugs or medications must be elicited. Even antihistamines have been implicated in drug fever, and steroids are immunosuppressive.

Social History

High-risk sexual activity, intravenous drug use, or blood transfusions in either child or parents may be associated with infection by the human immunodeficiency virus (HIV). The parents' occupations may be important. Munchausen's syndrome by proxy generally occurs when a parent has a medical background.

Past Medical History

The past medical history of the child must include information regarding all past infections. A history of unusual infecting organisms or multiple serious infections may point to an underlying immunodeficiency. Does the child have any underlying disease such as cancer, diabetes, sickle cell anemia, or congenital or acquired immunodeficiency that makes him or her vulnerable to infection? Recently acquired immunizations may be the etiology of the fever. Children receiving the measles-mumps-

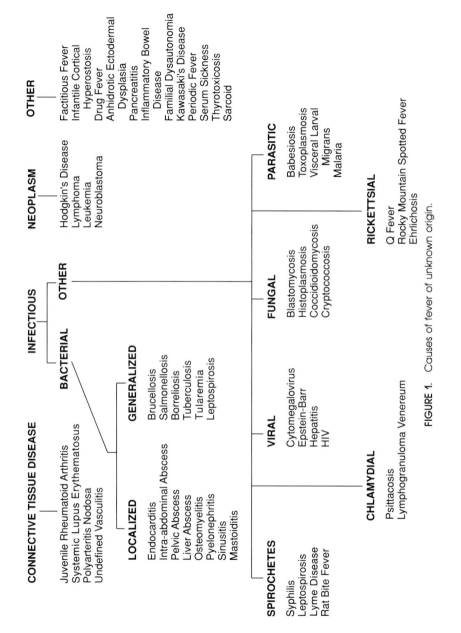

FIGURE 1. Causes of fever of unknown origin.

rubella (MMR) vaccine may develop fever and rash as long as 10 days postvaccination.

Family History

The child's ethnic background is important in that certain inherited illnesses are characteristic of distinct human populations. Familial Mediterranean fever is common among Arabs, Sephardic Jews, and Armenians, whereas familial dysautonomia is seen in the Jews of eastern Europe.

The history must be doggedly repeated. Parents and children will remember additional information with prodding and are more willing to share sensitive information after trust has been established with the physician.

Neonatal History

In evaluating a febrile infant less than six weeks of age, the history must include information concerning mother's pregnancy, birth, delivery, and any neonatal complications. Occasionally, infants present at this time with disease acquired from instrumentation—such as scalp electrodes—or from a procedure performed in the neonatal intensive care unit. A history of sexually transmitted disease such as herpes simplex or *chlamydia* in the mother must be sought. Respiratory and gastrointestinal tract viruses are the most common causes of fever in this age group and are usually acquired from ill family members. Genetically determined defects become symptomatic during this time. Some (such as galactosemia, which presents with gram-negative sepsis) may be heralded by fever. A family history of unusual illness, early deaths, or infections in young infants and children is an important clue to these problems.

Occasionally, the physician sees a young infant who has a history of fever at home but is afebrile in the office. These children rarely have significant illness, but their condition does merit a complete evaluation.[11]

PHYSICAL EXAMINATION

A thorough physical examination is imperative. The ability to identify the truly ill child from the majority with trivial illness is a skill obtained through training and experience. Assessment should be carried out in a setting where the child is allowed to relax and be comforted. Acutely febrile infants and chil-

dren should be given antipyretics and the fever controlled prior to evaluation. Quick, aggressive assessment and management are indicated in the toxic-appearing child. Children with signs referable to the central nervous system such as changes in sensorium and meningism deserve rapid evaluation for meningitis.

Acutely Febrile Children

In children with fever of less than a week's duration, who are acutely ill, the height of the fever is an important clinical sign. As the degree of fever increases, so does the risk for bacteremia. In one series of 264 children who had temperatures of 40.5° C (104.9° F) to 41° C (105.8° F), 13 per cent had bacteremia. The percentage increased to 23 per cent in children with temperatures higher than 41.1° C (106° F).[12] A fever of 41.1° C (106° F) is rare, occurring in only 1 child per 2100 patient visits in one study.[13] Special attention must be directed toward the areas where infection is occult in children such as the lungs, urinary tract, and central nervous system. It is important to realize that the classic stiff neck and other signs of meningitis are not always appreciated on physical examination in children under two years of age.

Signs of general illness such as irritability and lethargy and of focal disease such as lesions of the skin, soft tissues, and conjunctiva are identified by physical examination. Because almost 10 per cent of children have the first episode of otitis media by three months of age, the tympanic membrane must be visualized even in very young infants.

Fever of Unknown Origin

In the child with a more prolonged course of illness, the physical examination proceeds at a more deliberate pace. The child's fever should be documented with a health care worker in attendance to exclude factitious fever. The general condition of the child is assessed. The child's growth is charted, with special emphasis on weight.

The skin is examined for lesions, rashes, and petechiae. Careful examination of the eyes is important. Palpebral conjunctivitis suggests such conditions as measles, cat-scratch fever, tuberculosis, or infection with coxsackievirus or Epstein-Barr virus. Bulbar conjunctivitis indicates leptospirosis. Severe injection and tearing occur with collagen vascular diseases, most notably polyarteritis nododsa. Funduscopic examination can identify miliary tuberculosis, fungemia, endocarditis, leukemia, sarcoidosis, toxoplasmosis, and cytomegalovirus infection. Slit-lamp examination may demonstrate iritis associated with juvenile rheumatoid arthritis.

Tenderness over the sinuses and chronic purulent nasal discharge are signs of sinusitis. The presence of pharyngeal injection and/or exudate suggests infectious mononucleosis, tularemia, leptospirosis, or toxoplasmosis. Oral candidiasis is indicative of an immunodeficient state. The heart should be auscultated for murmurs associated with bacterial endocarditis.

A genital examination should be performed on all children. In sexually active girls, a pelvic examination should be done. Mild abdominal pain may be the only manifestation of intra-abdominal abscess or inflammatory bowel disease. Rectal examination may identify perirectal or deep pelvic abscesses.

Tenderness over the bone may indicate underlying osteomyelitis or invasion of the marrow by neoplastic disease. Generalized muscle tenderness occurs with arboviral infections, trichinosis, dermatomyositis, and polyarteritis. Palpation of the lymph nodes may reveal generalized lymphadenopathy, which occurs with herpesvirus, HIV infection, tuberculosis, toxoplasmosis, sarcoidosis, and brucellosis. Localized adenopathy is usually attributed to regional infection.

Neonatal Fever

Examination of the neonate is similar to the older child. However, physical signs of infection in this age group are poorly localized and often subtle. Careful attention must be paid to the overall appearance. Is the child lethargic or uncontrollably irritable? Is there any asymmetry of movement of the extremities or swelling of the joints? Are any lesions of the scalp or skin noted? Infections in this age group may represent an underlying defect or disability. For example, urinary tract infection with bacteremia is often the first indication of structural abnormality of the urinary tract.

DIAGNOSTIC STUDIES

Acutely Febrile Children

In the child between 6 months and 24 months of age who is at risk of occult bactere-

mia, the white blood cell (WBC) count is the laboratory test most studied when considering this diagnosis. It does not accurately predict bacteremia but helps divide the population into high- and low-risk categories. In one study, bacteremia was found to be five times as likely and pneumonia twice as likely if the WBC count was equal to or greater than 15,000/ cu mm.[14] The erythrocyte sedimentation rate (ESR), although a less convenient test, is also predictive of bacteremia when greater than 30 mm per hour (Wintrobe). In general, when a child presents with a temperature equal to or greater than 38.8° C (101.8° F) and an elevated WBC and/or ESR, a blood culture and a chest radiograph are usually warranted. Urinalysis and urine culture should also be run because urinary tract infection (UTI) is often accompanied by fever, irritability, and occasionally mild gastrointestinal tract symptoms. The decision to perform a lumbar puncture depends on the assessment of the child's clinical condition, taking into consideration that the risk of meningitis is increased when the temperature exceeds 41.1° C (106° F).[13] Rapid antigen detection tests, which are commercially available, are good tools for identification of invasive disease caused by *H. influenzae, N. meningitidis*, and *S. pneumoniae,* and should be performed on the urine and cerebrospinal fluid (CSF) in these patients.

Fever of Unknown Origin

In the child with prolonged fever or fever of unknown origin, laboratory and radiographic evaluation are directed by information obtained from the history and physical examination. The investigation proceeds in a stepwise fashion, from the least to the most invasive studies (Table 2). Before proceeding from one level to the next, the impact of fever on the child's health should be evaluated. Less vigorous evaluation is needed in the child who is only mildly ill, whereas aggressive study is indicated in children who are more seriously affected.

The WBC count is usually not helpful in assessing fever of unknown origin. However, an absolute neutrophil count below 5000/cu mm is evidence against a bacterial infection. Bacterial infection is more likely if the number of polymorphonuclear leukocytes is greater than 10,000/cu mm. An elevated ESR indicates inflammation and the need for further evaluation. Blood cultures for aerobic and anaerobic

**TABLE 2. Laboratory Evaluation
of Children with Fever
of Unknown Origin**

Level I
  CBC with differential and platelets
  Erythrocyte sedimentation rate
  Urinalysis/urine culture
  Rapid antigen detection of urine and serum
  Stool guaiac
  Chest radiographs
  Liver function tests
  Protein electrophoresis
  Three aerobic and anaerobic blood cultures
  Serology
    RPR* or VDRL†
    ANA‡
    Rheumatoid factor
    Serum complement
    HIV
  Skin tests
  PPD with tetanus, candida, mumps as controls
  One tube of serum for acute phase titers
  Lumbar puncture
Level II
  Bone marrow aspirate and biopsy
  Magnetic resonance imaging
  CT scan
  Intravenous pyelography
  Endoscopy or barium enema
  Radionucleotide scan
    Bone scan
    Liver/spleen scan
    Gallium scan
  Echocardiogram
  Ultrasonography
Level III
  Biopsy of suspicious lesions
  Exploratory laparotomy
  Arteriograms
  Lymphangiograms
  Empiric therapeutic trials

* RPR = Rapid plasma reagin.
† VDRL = Venereal Disease Research Laboratories.
‡ ANA = Antibodies to nuclear antigens.
(From Doyle MG, Pickering LK. Is this child's fever a worry? Postgrad Med 1989;85:207–22. Reprinted with permission.)

organisms need to be cultured, and urine culture is routine. A throat culture is easily obtained and should not be overlooked. Culture of pleural or peritoneal fluid, as well as biopsy and culture of any skin lesions or body organs, is performed as clinically indicated.

Tuberculin skin testing using purified protein derivative (PPD) is especially important in this era of increasing tuberculosis prevalence. Skin tests with tetanus, candidin, and mumps antigen should be done simultaneously to exclude anergy. Serologic testing may aid in the diagnosis of infectious mononucleosis, cytomegalovirus, toxoplasmosis, salmonellosis, tularemia, brucellosis, leptospirosis, HIV, and rickettsial diseases. More invasive testing includes bone marrow aspiration and biopsy for culture and histologic examination. Imaging techniques are also useful. Ultrasonography of the abdomen and pelvis is a good noninvasive screening examination to rule out abscess or masses; however, magnetic resonance imaging (MRI) and computed tomography (CT) are often more informative. Radionucleotide scans such as liver/spleen scan, bone scan, and gallium scan may help identify occult infections and abscesses. Radiographic imaging of the urinary tract may also be necessary. Echocardiography may indicate the presence of vegetation on the leaflets of heart valves. These procedures are generally safe for the patient, and consultation with radiologist or pathologist ensures that maximum information is obtained.

More complex tests such as surgical intervention, biopsy, and arteriogram are more invasive and represent increased risk of morbidity and mortality to the patient but may be necessary in seriously ill children.

Neonatal Fever

In the febrile neonate where history and physical examinations are not reliable indicators of disease, laboratory evaluation includes a complete blood count (CBC), blood cultures, urinalysis, and urine culture. The urine specimen should be obtained by suprapubic aspiration or catheterization since "bagged collections" are invariably contaminated with skin and gastrointestinal tract flora, leading to confusion and unnecessary treatment. Lumbar puncture is indicated in most circumstances. Rapid antigen detections should be performed on urine and CSF for previously mentioned bacteria as well as group B streptococcus, which is an important pathogen even at three months of age. Chest radiograph is indicated if tachypnea or signs of respiratory distress are evident. It is prudent to perform these studies even in the infant who is determined to be febrile at home but who is afebrile when seen in the physician's office.[15]

ASSESSMENT

Acutely Febrile Children

In most instances, the information gleaned from laboratory studies and cultures will direct appropriate therapy. The acutely ill child or infant who appears toxic should be hospitalized for evaluation and treatment. A mildly ill child with reliable caretaker can be managed as an outpatient. The mildly symptomatic child with laboratory studies placing him or her at risk for occult bacteremia may be started on an oral antibiotic such as amoxicillin (Amoxil, Larotid, Trimox), which is effective treatment for *S. pneumoniae* and *H. influenzae.* Close follow-up is imperative. If the parent or guardian cannot be contacted in 24 hours, the child should be admitted to the hospital, observed, and possibly treated. Children who are between six weeks and three months of age should be empirically treated with antimicrobials effective against group B streptococcus and *Listeria monocytogenes* as well as *H. influenzae, S. pneumoniae,* and *N. meningitidis* (Table 3).

A child with occult bacteremia at the initial visit has a 5 to 10 per cent chance of returning with meningitis regardless of antimicrobial treatment, a 10 per cent chance of developing a localized infection, and a 30 per cent chance of having persistent fever and bacteremia.[16,17] Patients treated with antibiotics improve more quickly than those not initially treated. However, careful follow-up and re-evaluation of the child's clinical condition are mandatory when the child is persistently febrile or unimproved in 24 hours.

If the child continues to appear significantly ill, the lumbar puncture may need to be repeated even if CSF findings were initially normal.

Children whose blood cultures are positive must be re-examined. If the organism isolated is *S. pneumoniae* and the child's clinical condition is improved, he or she may be treated as an outpatient. If the organism is *H. influenzae,* the child should be hospitalized, administered parenteral antibiotics, and observed closely, as this organism is invasive in 90 per cent of cases of bacteremia.[18]

Fever of Unknown Origin

In children with fever of unknown origin, at least 10 per cent of the time no etiology will be found despite extensive evaluation. Empirical therapy may be warranted in those children who are seriously ill.

Neonatal Fever

For infants less than six weeks of age, the recommendation remains that they should be hospitalized and treated empirically pending the outcome of cultures. Presently, several researchers are attempting to determine if febrile infants can be divided into low- and high-risk categories, as opposed to admitting all the children to the hospital. The results of these studies are inconclusive. At least 1 to 5 per cent of infants with serious infection will be missed on the basis of the recommended laboratory and clinical methods of evaluation.[19,20,21] To determine which infants are at risk is an important goal since in at least one study 19 per cent of infants admitted to the hospital experienced some complication related to the hospitalization.[22]

Appropriate antibiotic therapy for infants less than six weeks of age include ampicillin

TABLE 3.   Empirical Antibiotic Therapy for Common Organisms Causing Fever in Infants and Children

AGE	MOST COMMON ORGANISMS	ANTIBIOTIC
Less than six weeks	Group B streptococci *Listeria monocytogenes* Gram-negative enteric bacteria	Ampicillin and aminoglycoside *or* ampicillin and cefotaxime (Claforan)
Six weeks to three months	Group B streptococci *Hemophilus influenzae* *Streptococcus pneumoniae* *Neisseria meningitidis* *L. monocytogenes*	Ampicillin and cefotaxime *or* ampicillin and ceftriaxone (Rocephin)
Greater than three months	*S. pneumoniae* *H. influenzae* *N. meningitidis* *Staphylococcus aureus*	Ampicillin and chloramphenicol (Chloromycetin) *or* ampicillin and cefotaxime *or* ampicillin and ceftriaxone Penicillinase-resistant penicillin (Nafcil, Nalpen, Unipen) *or* oxacillin (Bactocill, Prostaphlin)
	S. aureus resistant to methicillin (Staphcillin)	Vancomycin (Vancocin, Vancoled)

(From Doyle MG, Pickering LK. Is this child's fever a worry? Postgrad Med 1989;85:207–22. Reprinted with permission.)

and an aminoglycoside. These antibiotics will treat group B streptococcus, gram-negative enteric organisms, and *L. monocytogenes,* the most prominent pathogens in this age group (Table 3).

REFERENCES

1. Schmitt BD. Fever phobia: misconceptions of parents about fevers. Am J Dis Child 1980;134:176–81.
2. Kramer MS, Naimark L, Leduc DG. Parental fever phobia and its correlates. Pediatrics 1985;75:1110–3.
3. Dinarello CA. The endogenous pyrogens in host-defense interactions. Hosp Pract 1989;24(Nov):111–28.
4. Duff GW, Durum SK. Fever and immunoregulation: hyperthermia, interleukin-1 and 2, and T cell proliferation. Yale J Biol Med 1982;55:437–42.
5. Hanson DF, Murphy PA, Silicano R, et al. The effect of temperature on the activation of thymocykes by interleukin-1 and interleukin-2. J Immunol 1983;130:216–21.
6. Dinarello CA, Wolff SM. Pathogenesis of fever. In: Mandell GL, Douglas RG, Bennett JE, eds. Principles and practice of infectious disease. New York: Churchill Livingstone Inc. 1990:462–4.
7. McLellan D, Giebink S. Perspectives on occult bacteremia in children. J Pediatr 1986;109:1–8.
8. Pizzo PA, Lovejoy FH, Smith DH. Prolonged fever in children: review of 100 cases. Pediatrics 1975;55:468–73.
9. McLung HJ. Prolonged fever of unknown origin in children. Am J Dis Child 1972;124:544–50.
10. McCarthy PL, Dolan TF. The serious implications of high fever in infants during their first three months. Clin Pediatr 1976;15:794–6.
11. Bonadio WA. Incidence of serious infections in afebrile neonates with history of fever. Pediatr Infect Dis J 1987; 6:911–4.
12. McCarthy PL, Jekel JF, Dolan TF. Temperature greater than or equal to 40° C in children less than 24 months of age: a prospective study. Pediatrics 1977;59:663–8.
13. McCarthy PL, Dolan TF. Hyperpyrexia in children. Am J Dis Child 1976;130:849–51.
14. Teele DW, Pleton SI, Myles MD, et al. Bacteremia in febrile children under 2 years of age: results of cultures of blood of 600 consecutive febrile children seen in a walk-in clinic. J Pediatr 1975;87:227–30.
15. Bonadio WA. Incidence of serious infections in afebrile neonates with a history of fever. Pediatr Infect Dis J 1987;6:911–4.
16. Bratton L, Teele DW, Klein JO. Outcome of unsuspected pneumococcemia in children not usually admitted to the hospital. J Pediatr 1977;90:703–6.
17. Feder HM. Occult pneumococcal bacteremia and the febrile infant and young child: a clinical review. Clin Pediatr 1980;19:457–62.
18. Marshall R, Teele DW, Klein JO. Unsuspected bacteremia due to *Haemophilus influenzae*: outcome in children not initially admitted to hospital. J Pediatr 1979;95:690–5.
19. Dagan R, Sofer S, Phillip M, Shachak E. Ambulatory care of febrile infants younger than 2 months of age classified as being at low risk for having serious bacterial infection. J Pediatr 1988;112:355–60.
20. Crain EF, Gershel JC. Which febrile infants younger than two weeks of age are likely to have sepsis? A pilot study. Pediatr Infect Dis J 1988;7:561–4.
21. Powell KR. Evaluation and management of infants younger than 60 days of age. Pediatr Infect Dis J 1990;9:153–7.
22. DeAngelis C, Joffe A, Wilson M, Willis E. Iatrogenic risks and financial costs of hospitalizing febrile infants. Am J Dis Child 1983;127:1146–9.

FOOD ALLERGY AND INTOLERANCE

SAMI L. BAHNA and MARY C. MAIER

SAMI L. BAHNA and MARY C. MAIER

SYNONYMS: Food Sensitivity, Food Hypersensitivity

BACKGROUND

Food intolerance is a general term that may encompass any type of adverse reaction to food. When the reaction is mediated by an immunologic mechanism, using the term *allergy, sensitivity,* or *hypersensitivity* would be more appropriate.

Adverse reactions to foods may result from any of several mechanisms: hypersensitivity, gastrointestinal irritation, toxicity, enzyme deficiency, psychologic, and other mechanisms that are not clear.[1] In evaluating a patient for possible food allergy, one should ascertain that the patient's illness seems to be allergic in nature and is related to food intake. The immunologic basis of the reaction may be clinically apparent by the nature of symptoms or by carrying out appropriate in vivo or in vitro tests. More than one mechanism may be involved in any single patient.[2]

Food allergy is more common in youngsters but may develop at any time during adulthood, and the offending food may have been previously tolerated for years. Clinical manifestations vary widely and may range from mild gastrointestinal, cutaneous, or respiratory symptoms to a life-threatening systemic reaction (Table 1). In some instances, the diagnosis of food allergy is so evident and may have been made, correctly, by the patient. More often than not, however, the diagnosis is a challenging task, even to the experienced physician.

To establish a clinical diagnosis of food allergy, information may be obtained through the medical history, physical examination, trials of elimination diets, food/symptom diary, allergy skin testing, and/or in vitro essays for food-specific IgE antibodies. Foods suspected by these procedures must then be verified by appropriate elimination-challenge testing, which is the definitive procedure in establishing a causal relationship between a certain food and a specific symptom. Challenge testing should be avoided, however, whenever systemic anaphylaxis or severe reactions are anticipated from exposure to a specific food. A stepwise approach to diagnosing food allergy is outlined in Table 2.

HISTORY

A detailed medical history is imperative and may provide information sufficient to establish the presence or absence of food allergy. Inquiry should be made about the nature of symptoms; age at onset; frequency of recurrences; duration, with or without intake of symptomatic medications; and relationship to food intake, regarding quantity and time interval. Other associated factors should also be explored, such as the appearance or exacerbation of symptoms to emotional stress, menstrual cycle, or physical exercise. Postprandial exercise–induced allergic reactions have been described and often are difficult to diagnose.[3]

Information learned from the medical history may be definitive enough to establish the diagnosis without any further testing. This is typically the case in a patient with well-defined allergy symptoms (e.g., anaphylaxis, urticaria, angioedema, or wheezing) that have occurred on multiple occasions shortly after ingestion of a specific food and where a psychologic component does not seem to be involved.

PHYSICAL EXAMINATION

A thorough physical examination should be performed, even in the absence of symptoms.

167

TABLE 1.   Common Manifestations of Food Allergy

Gastrointestinal	Abdominal pain
	Vomiting
	Diarrhea
	Bleeding
Dermatologic	Eczema
	Urticaria
	Angioedema
Respiratory	Rhinitis
	Cough
	Asthma
Other	Anaphylaxis
	Irritability in infants

All physical findings should be well documented, regarding their nature, severity, and extent, as baseline data. The findings might be compatible with a nonallergic disorder, which should be further explored with appropriate investigations. It should be noted also that no specific allergy signs are pathognomonic of food hypersensitivity.

DIAGNOSTIC STUDIES

The diagnosis of allergy per se is basically a clinical one, depending mostly on the medical

TABLE 2.   Stepwise Approach to Diagnosing Food Allergy

History and physical examination
   Nature of symptoms
   Age at onset
   Relation to meals or other factors
   Manifestations of nonallergic disease
Initial laboratory tests
   To support allergy diagnosis
      Total IgE level
      Eosinophilia
   To support or exclude nonallergic disease
      Complete blood count
      Urinalysis
      Stool analysis
      Microbiologic cultures
      Serology
      Radiology
      Immunologic screening
      Sweat chloride test
      Lactose tolerance or breath hydrogen test
Screening for food allergens
   Trials of elimination diets
   Food/symptom diary
   Allergy skin testing
   Serum IgE antibodies
Verification
   Elimination-challenge tests

(Data from Bahna SL. Food sensitivity: handling reactions to foods and food additives. Postgrad Med 1987;82:195–205.)

history and physical examination. Clinical or laboratory tests may be required to verify the diagnosis and to detect the causative allergens.

Basic Laboratory Tests

An elevated serum total IgE level and/or eosinophilia would support the diagnosis of allergy, although normal values do not exclude allergy. Depending on the patient's symptoms, other tests may be needed in pursuit of differential diagnosis. These tests may include complete blood count, urinalysis, stool analysis, microbiologic cultures, radiologic imaging, sweat chloride testing, immunologic screening, and selected serologic tests. When milk-induced gastrointestinal symptoms are suspected to be due to lactose intolerance rather than milk protein allergy, a lactose tolerance test—or more accurately, breath hydrogen test—is warranted.

Screening Tests for Food Allergens

Diagnostic Elimination Diets

Trials of elimination diets may be useful in those patients with frequent or persistent symptoms whose medical history is suggestive of food allergy without implicating any specific food.[4] These diets are designed to be free of certain groups of foods, such as Rowe elimination diets and their modifications.[5]

The use of an elimination diet is rather a random approach with unpredictable results and may be quite time-consuming. It is worth noting also that diet modification, in type or quantity, may improve the symptoms of certain nonallergic diseases, particularly of the gastrointestinal tract, for example, lactase deficiency, celiac disease, inflammatory bowel disease, and gastroenteritis from various causes. The selected diet may need to be individualized, especially for youngsters. If substantial clinical improvement is not noted within two weeks, another elimination diet may be tried. Once a certain diet becomes associated with significant clinical improvement, the eliminated foods are introduced singly at a few days' intervals. Those foods that the patient claims as offenders should be confirmed by blind oral challenges.

When a high degree of sensitivity to numerous foods is suspected, a strict, yet nutritionally adequate, diet may be attained by exclusive feeding of an elemental formula made of synthesized amino acids (e.g., Vivonex or Tolerex by Norwich Eaton Pharmaceuticals).

Food/Symptom Diary

The diary consists of daily recordings, in a chronologic time sequence, of foods eaten and the appearance or exacerbation of symptoms. The diary would be most informative by the inclusion of quantities and form of food as well as associated factors, such as physical exercise, emotional stress, menstrual period, and places visited. Such recordings should continue until symptoms have occurred several times, to allow for a high degree of suspicion of the offending food(s). The latter are then avoided until verified by challenge testing.

The diary is most helpful when the symptoms are well defined and occur shortly after eating. It is less informative when the symptoms are delayed in onset or caused by a food incorporated into food preparations that are eaten frequently. In fact, the patient may not be aware of such exposure, either because of incomplete food labeling or because of food listing under unfamiliar names such as whey, casein, ovalbumin, and ovomucin.

When symptoms are infrequent, the keeping of complete daily recordings is often impractical. In such cases, recording may be done only when symptoms occur and should cover the preceding 12- to 24-hour period.

Allergy Skin Testing

Skin testing is probably the most commonly used screening test for food allergy. It can be performed on patients of any age, and the results are known immediately. The test is supposed to be positive primarily in patients with the immediate type (IgE-mediated) allergic reactions. The reported reliability, however, varies widely. Several factors are responsible for such variation, including the testing technique, interpretation of the reaction, the shock organ, severity of symptoms, and type of food.[6]

Testing should be performed epicutaneously first (scratch, prick, or puncture) to minimize the risk of large local or systemic reactions that may result from intradermal injection of an allergen that the patient might be extremely sensitive to. The resulting wheal and flare should be compared with those produced by histamine (positive) and diluent (negative) controls.[2] Intradermal testing may be used for those allergens that were suspected by history but gave negative reactions by epicutaneous testing.

In a study of a series of patients with various allergy manifestations and clinical histories suggestive of food allergy, skin tests were positive in 58 per cent of those with positive double-blind oral food challenges and were negative in 65 per cent of those with negative challenges, with wide variations from one food to another. Skin testing showed an overall positive predictive accuracy of 48 per cent and an overall negative accuracy of 74 per cent.[7]

Purified or standardized food extracts are not commercially available and are not necessarily superior over crude extracts. In case of cow's milk, there was no advantage of testing with individual protein fractions over testing with whole milk.[8] Use of intradermal injection for provocation of symptoms has been advocated by some practitioners, but when this method was tested under double-blind conditions, the active and placebo injections were indistinguishable.[9]

Specific IgE Antibody Assays

The radioallergosorbent test (RAST) is the original assay for measuring allergen-specific IgE antibody levels in the serum. It was introduced more than two decades ago and is still widely used (Phadebas RAST by Pharmacia). Several analogues have been developed, either using radioisotopes (e.g., Allercoat RAST by Kallestad and VAST by Ventrex) or enzyme labels (e.g., Phadezym RAST by Pharmacia, IP-System by Ventrex, Allercoat EAST by Kallestad, IgE FAST by 3M Diagnostics, MAST-CLA by MAST Immunosystems, AlaSTAT by Diagnostic Products Corporation, and others).[10]

These assays may be considered the in vitro counterpart of skin testing; both detect specific IgE antibodies either in the circulation or on the mast cells of the skin. As in the case with skin testing, the reliability of these assays varied widely from one study to another.[10,11] Variations occur also in between the assays and from one laboratory to another. In 1983, the Centers for Disease Control reported the results of a proficiency survey[12] wherein positive and negative sera for wheat and cow's milk IgE antibodies were blindly tested by 33 laboratories. For the negative sera, a positive antibody result to milk was reported in 10 per cent and to wheat in 17 per cent. For the positive sera, a negative result for milk was reported in 7 per cent and to wheat in 0 per cent.

In a study[7] of allergic patients with clinical histories suggestive of food allergy, Phadebas

RAST results were compared with the outcome of double-blind oral food challenges. RAST was positive in 58 per cent of those with positive challenge and in 47 per cent of those with negative challenges, again with a wide variation from one food to another. The overall positive predictive accuracy was 44 per cent, and the negative predictive accuracy was 67 per cent.

Discordance between the results of skin testing or RAST (or its analogues) and the results of blind oral challenge testing may be due to several causes, such as poor technique, IgE antibodies mostly in the shock organ, non–IgE-mediated allergy, subclinical sensitization, and cross-reactivity between foods from the same botanical family or between foods and certain pollens.[2]

Less Commonly Used Tests

Several other tests have been attempted for food allergy diagnosis, including tests for plasma histamine level, leukocyte histamine release, specific antibodies of isotypes other than IgE, immune complexes, lymphocyte stimulation studies, neutrophil chemotaxis, and special intestinal biopsy studies. These tests are not routinely available in clinical practice either because of unestablished reliability, special expertise needed, or inconvenience for the patient.[10,13]

Testing the serum for precipitating antibodies to milk (mostly IgG and IgM) would be of value in evaluating infants suspected of having milk-induced chronic pulmonary disease (Heiner syndrome) or gastrointestinal bleeding.[14]

Controversial or Unproved Tests

Of great concern to the national societies of allergy and immunology has been the promotion by some practitioners or laboratories of certain tests without proof of reliability.[5,15] Among the most promoted of these controversial tests are the sublingual provocation, the intradermal or subcutaneous provocation, and the leukocyte cytotoxic test.

Verification by Oral Challenge

The only way of confirming a cause-and-effect relationship between a specific food and the patient's illness is through the documentation of improvement of the symptoms by dietary elimination and their recurrence by exposure to that food.

The oral challenge may be done openly or blindly, either single-blind or double-blind.[10,16,17] Open challenges may be acceptable in infants or young children whose allergy manifestations are objective and are unlikely to be emotional. Since negative challenges occur in more than two thirds of cases,[7] it might be reasonable, therefore, to use open challenge as a screening method in patients with mild symptoms, followed by blind challenges only for those foods that gave a positive open challenge.

Blind challenges are particularly recommended for older children and adults. Challenges with appropriate placebos should be randomly included in between the active challenges. The suspected food should be disguised regarding taste, odor, color, and texture, which can be a difficult task with certain foods particularly when large quantities need to be given. The most commonly used methods are providing freeze-dried foods in opaque capsules or hiding the suspected food in another appropriately chosen food or in an elemental formula (Vivonex). In clinical practice, single-blind challenges (the material is known to the observer but not to the patient) are usually satisfactory. For research studies and in certain clinical situations, it is more appropriate to conduct double-blind challenges where the active foods and placebo are prepared and coded by a third person. The code would be revealed after all planned challenges are completed.

Oral food challenges should be conducted when the patient is in a stable condition, with minimal symptoms, and is receiving no or minimal symptomatic medications. Only one substance is tested at a time, in a titrated fashion. All symptoms and signs should be accurately documented at the beginning of the challenge and before every challenge dose. The patient should be observed in a facility where equipment is easily available to manage possible severe reactions. Systemic anaphylaxis may occur in certain patients who had less severe reactions in the past. Challenge testing is not recommended in cases of anaphylaxis to a known food. However, if the patient had anaphylaxis linked to eating but the specific offending food is unknown, cautious challenges should be done in the hospital, preferably in the intensive care unit.

The initial challenge dose depends on the anticipated reaction and the usual quantity the patient used to consume of that food. Gradually increasing quantities are given at 20- to 30-

minute intervals as long as no definite symptoms appear. The total dose administered should be equivalent to the amount usually eaten by the patient. After a few hours of medical observation, the patient is sent home after being advised to report any symptoms that might develop later. If no symptoms occur within a couple of days, the food is probably a nonoffending one unless it requires the presence of other factors that were not duplicated during the challenges.

In addition to the recording by the observer of clinical symptoms and signs, certain laboratory measurements might be appropriate, for example, pulmonary function testing, rhinomanometry, eosinophilia in the circulation or in the secretion of the shock organ, and occult blood testing in stools. Whenever a challenge gives an equivocal result, a repeat challenge with larger doses is warranted. In some patients, particularly those with respiratory symptoms from occupational exposure, inhalation of food antigens may have a more important role than ingestion. In these instances, special inhalation challenges in certain centers would be indicated.

REFERENCES

1. Bahna SL. Food sensitivity: handling reactions to foods and food additives. Postgrad Med 1987;82:195–205.
2. Bahna SL. The dilemma of pathogenesis and diagnosis of food allergy. Immunol Allergy Clin North Am 1987;7:299–312.
3. Kidd JM III, Cohen SH, Sosman AJ, Fink JN. Food-dependent exercise-induced anaphylaxis. J Allergy Clin Immunol 1983;71:407–11.
4. Bahna SL. Critique of various dietary regimens in the management of food allergy. Ann Allergy 1986;57:48–52.
5. Anderson JA, Sogn DD, eds. Adverse reactions to foods. Bethesda, Maryland: American Academy of Allergy and Immunology Committee on Adverse Reactions to Foods, and National Institute of Allergy and Infectious Diseases, 1984; NIH publication no. 84–2442.
6. Bahna SL. In vivo diagnosis of food allergy. In: Hamburger RN, ed. Food intolerance in infancy: allergology, immunology, and gastroenterology. New York: Raven Press, 1989:75–81 (Carnation nutrition education series; vol 1).
7. Bahna SL, Gandhi MD. Reliability of skin testing and RAST in food allergy diagnosis. In: Chandra RK, ed. Food allergy. St. John's, Newfoundland: Nutrition Research Foundation, 1987:139–47.
8. Bahna SL. New aspects of diagnosis of milk allergy. Allergy Proc 1991 (in press).
9. Jewett DL, Fein G, Greenberg MH. A double-blind study of symptom provocation to determine food sensitivity. N Engl J Med 1990;323:429–33.
10. Bahna SL. Diagnostic tests for food allergy. Clin Rev Allergy 1988;6:259–84.
11. O'Connor RD. The use of the allergy immunology laboratory in food allergy. In: Hamburger RN, ed. Food intolerance in infancy: allergology, immunology, and gastroenterology. New York: Raven Press, 1989:83–92 (Carnation nutrition education series; vol 1).
12. Przybszewski VA, Taylor RN. Allergen-specific immunoglobulin E performance evaluation results. Atlanta, Georgia: USPHS Centers for Disease Control, 1983.
13. Bahna SL. The diagnostic dilemma of milk allergy. Ann Allergy 1989;63:475–6.
14. Bahna SL, Heiner DC. Allergies to milk. New York: Grune & Stratton, 1980.
15. Grieco MH. Controversial practices in allergy. JAMA 1982;247:3106–10.
16. Bock SA, Sampson HA, Atkins FJ, et al. Double-blind, placebo-controlled food challenge (DBPCFC) as an office procedure: a manual. J Allergy Clin Immunol 1988;82:986–97.
17. Bahna SL. Food challenge testing: practical considerations. Philadelphia: WB Saunders Co. Immunol Allergy Clin North Am. November 1991.

HALLUCINATIONS

PATRICIA BLUMENREICH, TERESITA BACANI-OROPILLA, and STEVEN LIPPMANN

SYNONYMS: Pychosis, Voices, "Hearing Things," Visions, "Seeing Things," Apparitions

Related Phenomena: Delusions, Illusions

BACKGROUND

Definition

Hallucinations are sensory perceptions experienced by a person without an external stimulus.[1] This term was introduced over 150 years ago, in an early effort to differentiate various psychotic symptoms.[2] Hallucinations were described as images internally derived but falsely judged to be of outside origin. Hallucinations can be auditory—"hearing" voices, music, or other noises when there is no sound; visual—"seeing" an object that is not there; gustatory—"tasting" a flavor when nothing has been ingested; olfactory—"smelling" an odor that is not present; or tactile—"feeling" a sensation without any skin contact. One must differentiate these phenomena from the fixed, false beliefs of a delusion and from the misperception of certain stimuli in an illusion (see Table 1).

Hallucinations are symptoms and are *not pathognomonic* of any specific disease. Without diagnostic implication, they occur in a broad range of medical, neurologic, and psychiatric conditions. All have in common their nonverifiable nature. Presence of such findings alerts the physician to the need for a diagnostic assessment to identify the causative pathology. Hallucinations have been described innumerable times throughout history in medicine and in literature. Identified as a hallmark of mental illness, they also can be present in normal individuals under certain circumstances, like sensory deprivation, or be caused by a variety of somatic ailments. There is no common etiologic factor, but they are a reflection of a nonspecific brain dysfunction. Multiple explanatory theories have been postulated from the biologic and psychologic points of view.

Biologic Theories

With the advent of sophisticated radiologic techniques, light is shed on the possible origin of hallucinations. The aim was to explain these changes in brain function regardless of the exact cause. Studies have documented decreased blood flow to postcentral cerebral regions during hallucinations.[3] Other researchers report increased temporoparietal flow.[3] Single photon emission computed tomography (SPECT) investigations in patients with auditory hallucinations has demonstrated relative frontal hypoactivity, with hyperactivity in basal ganglia and limbic structures.[4] In subjects with tactile hallucinations, there was a significant decrease in regional blood flow in the inferior temporal regions.[3] These results support earlier theories that postulated such perceptions occur mainly if higher cortical inhibitions are compromised in their control over basal ganglia and other deep structures.[3]

Radiologic findings appeared to be independent of antipsychotic drug treatment.[4] Positron emission tomography (PET) indicates that schizophrenic patients may have greater glucose uptake in auditory areas and the temporal lobe during hallucinations.[5] Research involving neurotransmitters suggests a defective serotonin state (low central levels) and involvement of the dopamine and cholinergic systems.[2] An investigation of brain stem responses found a significant relationship between auditory hallucinations and abnormal auditory brain stem response.[6] Disruption in the memory retrieval system and rapid eye movement (REM) sleep may be observed.[2] Skin conductance also can be affected by hallucinations.[2,7]

Psychologic Theories

Psychologic theories have assumed that hallucinations are the result of certain unconscious material being perceived as externally derived in response to personal needs. They may be similar to dreams, represent delusional ideas that are looking for other routes of ex-

TABLE 1. Types of Hallucinations

Auditory
Visual
Gustatory
Olfactory
Tactile

pression, or be a way to describe stressful internal experiences.[2]

Clinical Aspects

Hallucinations can be present in many different pathologic conditions and in nonmorbid states (see Table 2). They can be symptoms of various functional psychoses (e.g., schizophrenia), fever, drug intoxications (e.g., stimulant poisoning), withdrawal states (e.g., delirium tremens), certain other encephalopathies (e.g., hypoxia or hypoglycemia), and so on. The contents of the hallucinations may change to reflect historical events or the technology of the time.[8]

Hallucinations In Psychiatric Disorders

Hallucinations are frequent manifestations of mental illnesses such as schizophrenia or bipolar (manic-depressive) disorder. They are usually auditory, with "voices" making comments on the person, giving commands, or calling his or her name. The content may depend on the type of presentation. Depressed people may hear derogatory remarks, a manic one may hear something grandiose, and a schizophrenic individual perceives persecutory statements. Frequently, they are accompanied by other psychotic symptoms, like delusions, and significant mood changes. When visual hallucinations are present, they often do not change by closing or opening the eyes, as has been reported in certain drug-induced cases.[2] Other hallucinatory categories (e.g., gustatory) are described in schizophrenia, although they are more rare.

Neurologic Disorders

Many neurologic illnesses can create hallucinations as one of the symptoms. The olfactory sensations associated with complex partial seizures would be a classic example. During a migraine, visual hallucinations can appear in an aura just prior to the headache. Many encephalopathogens are among the most frequent sources of hallucinations. Indeed, this presentation is common to numerous delirium and/or dementia cases, regardless of their specific etiology. Cerebrovascular accidents in the occipital and temporoparietal lobes can cause such auditory and/or gustatory phenomena. Movement disorder patients with Parkinson's or Huntington's disease and Sydenham's chorea may hallucinate, too. People with head trauma, as in a concussion, or space occupying lesions can exhibit this symptom as well—e.g., auditory hallucinations with a sylvian lipoma[9] or visual ones with a pituitary adenoma.[10]

Sensory Diseases

Auditory hallucinations with hearing loss can exist in patients with brain stem lesions. They can also be present as a result of lesions along the auditory pathways. Visual hallucinations can be a consequence of damage to the optic tracts and may occur even when blindness has existed for years. Olfactory halluci-

TABLE 2. Causes for Hallucinations—Examples

	FUNCTIONAL	ORGANIC	NONMORBID
Auditory	Schizophrenia	High fever	Grief reaction
	Schizoaffective disorder	Delirium tremens	Sensory deprivation
	Mania with psychosis	Alcohol hallucinosis	
	Major depression with psychotic features	Sedative drug withdrawal	
		Stimulant abuse	
Visual	Schizophrenia (less common)	High fever	Grief reaction
	Post-traumatic stress disorder	Delirium tremens	Sensory deprivation
		Hallucinogens	Imaginary companions (childhood)
		Hallucinosis	Mirage
		Complex partial seizures	
		Atropine poisoning	
		Progressive loss of vision	
Olfactory	Schizophrenia (less common)	Temporal lobe lesions including complex partial seizures	
Tactile		Delirium tremens	
		Cocainism	
Gustatory		Temporal lobe lesions	

nations can be caused by pathology in olfactory pathways.

Drug-Induced Hallucinations

Hallucinations can be a result of drug intoxications. Substances with a wide variety of pharmacologic effects may precipitate hallucinations. Examples include phencyclidine (PCP), lysergic acid diethylamide (LSD), alcohol, cocaine, amphetamines and its derivatives, and the like. Drug-induced hallucinations are predominantly visual or tactile, but a substance can produce alternate types of hallucinations at different times, often depending on the dosage or the subject, his or her background, surroundings, and mood. Abrupt withdrawal from any sedative in a habituated person often produces hallucinations as a part of the abstinence syndrome. Alcohol withdrawal is the most well-known example and in its most overt form is called delirium tremens (DTs). All other sedatives such as barbiturates and benzodiazepines may precipitate such a presentation, when the addicted individual is experiencing an acute abstinence illness.

Hallucinations as a Medication Side Effect

Many medicines can cause hallucinations, even without the presence of toxicity or withdrawal. Among the group of psychotropics, several antidepressant pharmaceuticals such as amitriptyline, fluoxetine, phenelzine, trazodone, and doxepin are able to induce this symptom in susceptible individuals at routine doses or in toxic concentrations. Anticholinergic agents like diphenhydramine or benztropine may produce visual hallucinations, especially in older people. Hallucinations are reported in patients taking cimetidine, ranitidine,[11] bromocriptine, L-dopa, antihypertensives, anti-inflammatories, antineoplastics, antibiotics, corticosteroids, cough[12] or cold preparations,[13,14] muscle relaxants,[15] narcotics,[16] certain cardiovascular drugs (e.g, digoxin or beta blockers), and so forth. Pharmaceutical interactions in a person on several medications also can cause hallucinations.

Other Disorders

Metabolic abnormalities may precipitate hallucinations. This finding may occur quite prominently in association with fluid, glucose, or electrolyte imbalances; organ failures (e.g., uremia); vitamin deficiencies (e.g., Wernicke-Korsakoff); collagen diseases (e.g., lupus); and certain toxicities (e.g., poisonous mushrooms).

Nonmorbid States

During the grief process, many otherwise normal bereaved persons may "see" or "hear" the deceased. Imaginary companions are playmates to many children, without the presence of psychosis. Under conditions of prolonged isolation and/or sensory deprivation, emotionally healthy people also may hallucinate without other cause.[17] Likewise, hallucinations that appear on falling asleep (hypnagogic) or on awakening (hypnopompic) happen to some normal individuals. Sleep deprivation can induce visual and tactile hallucinations.[18] Members of certain societies or cults can hallucinate during religious activities; in such a case, they are usually the consequence of a culturally sanctioned emotional state.[19] Hallucinations can also present in a very high-stress hostage or similar situation as a result of isolation, sensory deprivation, physical restraint, or abuse and frightening threats.[17] Visual hallucinations can ensue in elderly patients with poor visual acuity and a clear sensorium as part of a condition called Charles-Bonnet syndrome.[20]

HISTORY

The diagnosis of hallucinations is clinical. Therefore, a detailed history is invaluable. Obtain such information according to usual procedure, just as applied to history taking in any other patient. Examples of good questions to get to the symptoms quickly are: Do you hear voices when there is nobody around? What about a vision or seeing things that other people do not see? Do you feel anything crawling on or under your skin?

It is important to investigate natural progression of the symptom. Assess the onset, type (auditory, visual, olfactory, gustatory, tactile), accompanying features (sadness, agitation, confusion, or paranoia), as well as the previous record of similar experiences and their treatment. Always explore the use of medications (including over-the-counter preparations) and abuse of drugs (by prescription or illegal). An alcohol intake history is essential. Get a thorough systems review and medical history, asking about head trauma, seizures, infectious processes, and family history of hallucinations or emotional illness. The social history with emphasis on recent losses and/or traumas (e.g., physical or sexual assault) can also yield significant data.

PHYSICAL EXAMINATION

A physical examination is a mandatory part of the assessment in all hallucinating patients. It is performed according to standard methodology. These patients, however, may be so agitated, scared, or even violent that the initial physical examination may not always be as easy to do or as thorough as it might otherwise be. If that is the case, a more definite evaluation will be completed at the earliest opportunity. In the meantime, a screening examination is *always* done. Even rudimentary observations must be recorded. Consistently include documentation of vital signs and autonomic functions. When hallucinations are purely the result of a functional illness, the examination may be normal. When they are a symptom of a medical condition, the findings will be those of the underlying ailment. The same applies to drug intoxication and withdrawal states. For example, a dry mouth and skin, with mydriasis, tachycardia, visual hallucinations, and confusion, is compatible with an anticholinergic delirium. Diaphoresis, tachycardia, tremor, agitation, illusions, and tactile or visual hallucinations are consistent with any hyperadrenergic state, which could point toward a diagnosis of alcohol or other sedative withdrawal or a stimulant drug toxicity.

MENTAL STATUS EXAMINATION

Utilize the mental status examination (MSE) to assess mental function. This evaluation augments the history and physical in making an accurate diagnosis. The assessment of a patient with hallucinations, as with all psychiatric presentations, always requires a thorough review of mental processes, but it need not take up much time. While cooperation greatly enhances the value of the data obtained, this procedure is a critical part of every evaluation and is done regardless of the level at which the subject can participate. The MSE is based on observation, listening, and response to questioning.

Observation

Look at the patient and make note of findings such as grooming, smell, hygiene, age and dress appropriateness, medical appliances (e.g., a bladder catheter, hearing aids, etc.), and general behavior. Also record information about facial expression, gestures, abnormal movements, and cooperation. Although these elements are themselves not diagnostic, the summation of them, together with the rest of the MSE, is of significant value. In patients with illnesses like schizophrenia or chemical dependencies, grooming and self-care may be poor or bizarre. They may not be fully cooperative with the interview because of an inability to concentrate, due to inner hallucinatory stimuli, agitation, or paranoid suspiciousness, for example. These people may look around, as if "hearing or seeing" something. They may be noted to be talking to themselves or screaming. Their arms may move as if fighting, and they can become combative or retreat into a corner to protect themselves from perceived danger. Picking at or brushing of the skin to "get rid of bugs" is common to many toxic or metabolic encephalopathy cases. Their level of distress will be affected by the nature and content of the hallucinations (e.g., menacing versus neutral comments, etc.) (see Table 3). Careful attention to such behavioral and other elements is of diagnostic value and provides clues about dangerousness and general health.

Listening

This segment of the MSE will examine speech, for its volume, rate, and coherence. Conversation can be clear or unintelligible. The volume can be loud or soft or have an unusual speed (e.g., as in mania or slow as in depression or myxedema). Some patients may be mute owing to functional or organic conditions or out of an oppositional nature. Always assess for memory, phasic, or paranoid disorders.

TABLE 3. Response to Hallucinatory Experience

HALLUCINATION	LEVEL OF DISTRESS
Acute	High
Chronic	Moderate to low
Content	
Nonthreatening or -commenting	Low
Menacing or demeaning	High

Active Questioning

During this stage of the MSE, the interviewer gathers data by making specific inquiries to evaluate thought content. The goal is to elicit information about the presence or absence of psychosis, mood changes, suicidal or homicidal ideation, and cognitive abnormalities. Much of this is very simply done while taking the routine history. Psychotic symptoms are explored by asking especially about hallucinations, illusions, and delusions. Command hallucinations—"voices" that give the patient some orders—can be dangerous because they may precede bizarre or dangerous episodes (i.e., self-mutilation, suicide, or homicide). Cognitive functions include orientation, short-term memory, intellectual function, and judgment. Disorientation and short-term memory impairment are common signs of an organic encephalopathy. Functional psychosis, as opposed to organic mental disorder, does not present with cognitive deficits. Thus, patients who hallucinate may or may not exhibit disorientation and memory deficits, for example, depending on the specific underlying etiology. Knowing their status by such testing quickly alerts the physician to the type of diagnostic workup required. If the patient is intact cognitively, first consider functional causes; if impaired, look toward an encephalopathic process.

DIAGNOSTIC STUDIES

Once the history, physical, and mental status examinations are completed, the physician may order certain laboratory tests and/or a psychologic evaluation to help clarify the diagnosis (see Table 4). These assessments are in-

TABLE 4. Laboratory Studies Indicated for Hallucinations

Complete blood count
Thyroid function tests
Serum chemistry profile
Urinalysis
Toxicology studies
FTA
Electrocardiogram
Chest x-ray
EEG
Head CT scan

dividualized and should confirm the original clinical impression into a more precise picture. The laboratory work will be directed first at *suspected* pathology. If no specific diagnosis is noted, a more generalized approach is ordered and would include a complete blood count (CBC); thyroid function tests; serum chemistry profile of electrolytes, glucose, renal and hepatic studies, and so on; urinalysis; a toxicology screen; fluorescent treponemal antibody (FTA) test; electrocardiogram; and a chest x-ray. The electroencephalogram (EEG) and head computerized tomography (CT) scan are useful when a neurologic disorder is considered. All other studies are obtained with specific conditions in mind, rather than in a "shotgun" approach (see Table 5). Systematically work up all appropriate differential diagnoses. Psychologic testing is a procedure, done by a clinical psychologist, that differentiates diagnostic categories (e.g., of psychotic or depressive disorders), personality styles (e.g., antisocial traits), and functional levels (e.g., retardation; deterioration due, for example, to substance abuse). It can be a valuable aid in diagnosis. Neuropsychologic evaluations are more detailed and focus

TABLE 5. Laboratory Results

	CBC	SERUM CHEMISTRY PROFILE	URIN- ALYSIS	TOXI- COLOGY SCREEN	EEG	HEAD CT SCAN
Schizophrenia	Normal	Normal	Normal	Normal	Normal	Enlarged or normal ventricles
Manic-depressive illness	Normal	Normal	Normal	Normal	Normal	Normal
Grief reaction	Normal	Normal	Normal	Normal	Normal	Normal
Alcohol withdrawal (possible)	Macrocytosis	Elevated liver function tests	Normal	Normal	Diffuse slowing	Normal or atrophic
Toxicity	Variable	Variable	Variable	Positive finding	Diffuse slowing	Normal
Complex partial seizures	Normal	Normal	Normal	Normal	Epileptiform discharges	Variable

particularly on detection and localization of brain diseases. Paper and pencil tests, an interview, and structured drawings are often requested in such an assessment.

ASSESSMENT

The most critical differential will be between the functional and organic syndromes (see Tables 6 and 7). This is of utmost importance for diagnostic and treatment purposes. Among the functional psychoses, schizophrenia and bipolar disorder are the main differentials. Expect cognitive functions to be normal and hallucinations to most often be auditory in such mental illnesses. Considering the organic disorders, alcohol and other drug-related states are frequent, and they must be ruled out immediately. Review all prescribed, over-the-counter, and illegal drugs. Hallucinations occur with certain intoxications (e.g., cocaine), withdrawal states (e.g., alcohol abstinence), metabolic abnormalities (as in uremia, hypoxia, hypoglycemia, and fluid or electrolyte imbalances), and certain neurologic disorders (e.g., partial complex seizures or brain tumor). In such encephalopathic cases, cognitive skills will most often be impaired and hallucinations will commonly be nonauditory.

Since hallucinations can be either acute or chronic, the person's reactions and adjustment to them will differ. Hallucinations can be very frightening and are at least disturbing; yet some patients with chronic conditions become used to their presence and may learn to ignore them. Other people are ashamed, afraid of "going out of their minds," and conceal these symptoms by denial. Regardless of the individual response, the doctor provides treatment as clinically indicated, after an evaluation reveals the etiology.

Specific Syndrome/Examples

Schizophrenia

A 20-year-old man over the last six months has become withdrawn, isolated, and disheveled. He believes there is a plot against him and does not eat out of fear of being poisoned. He "hears" voices telling him about those dangers, "hears" his own thoughts, and gets messages from the radio. He denies that there is anything wrong with him. The medical examination is unremarkable.

Psychotic Depression

A 50-year-old female is in the emergency room following an overdose with four ampicillin 250-mg capsules. She is, has been, and has a past history of being seriously depressed. Suicidal ideation is noted, and she volunteers concerns that she might kill herself since hearing her deceased husband calling her from heaven. A toxicology study reveals only caffeine. The physical and laboratory assessments were normal.

Grief Response

An elderly man whose wife just died three days ago is brought for evaluation by his children. For the past two nights he has barely slept and tearfully wanders about his children's home, convinced that his wife is calling him. The evaluation reveals occasional cardiac ectopy and no other abnormalities.

Alcohol Withdrawal

A 56-year-old professional male is admitted to the hospital for elective surgery. The day after admission, the patient becomes tremulous, agitated, and diaphoretic. His blood pressure, normal until then, increases, and he is also noted to be tachycardic. That evening, he screams that there are men in his room trying to attack him; is scared, flushed; and has a fever. He sees bugs on his bed and walls and tries to protect himself by throwing things. He does not know the time, where he is, or why he is in that setting.

Toxic Reaction

This teenage female is brought by police to the hospital hallucinating after being found down-

TABLE 6. Differential Diagnosis of Typical Functional Psychoses

	SCHIZOPHRENIA	MANIA	PSYCHOTIC DEPRESSION
Age of onset	Teenage or young adult	Young adult	Later in life
Sensorium	Clear	Clear	Clear
Expression	Flat, blunt, inappropriate	Labile	Sad, despondent
Speech	Bizarre	Pressured	Slow
Hallucinations	Religious, bizarre	Religious, grandiose	Religious, ominous
Delusions	Paranoid	Grandiose	Guilt-ridden
Orientation	Intact	Intact	Intact
Short-term memory	Unimpaired	Unimpaired	Unimpaired

TABLE 7. Differential Diagnosis and Typical Organic Mental Syndromes

	ALCOHOL WITHDRAWAL	TOXIC REACTION	PHARMACEUTICAL SIDE EFFECT
Sensorium	Hypervigilant, confused	Confused	Clear, confused, and/or obtunded
Expression	Agitated	Upset	Variable
Speech	Incoherent	Incoherent	Clear or incoherent
Hallucinations	Paranoid, visual, or tactile	Visual or tactile	Visual
Orientation	Disoriented	Disoriented	Disoriented
Short-term memory	Impaired	Impaired	Impaired

town wandering aimlessly and behaving in an upset, bizarre manner. She is agitated and admits taking "coke, speed, or something" obtained at a party. Tachycardia, mydriasis, diaphoresis, and skin excoriations are observed. Amphetamine and cocaine presence were reported on a drug screen, with all other studies being within normal limits.

Pharmaceutical Side Effect

An 85-year-old woman is delivered by ambulance after she called to say people were in her home. She has Parkinson's disease and takes L-dopa in an unknown quantity. Recently, she suffered worsening movement disturbance and increased the dose. For two days, she has experienced nightmares, dreams while awake, and sees people in her apartment. A comprehensive evaluation documents only symptoms and signs compatible with parkinsonism.

Over-the-Counter Drug Toxicity

A man, 64 years old, comes to the doctor because of confusion, blurry vision, visual hallucinations, and a dry mouth. Owing to nasal congestion, he has been taking allergy medicines for a week, in high doses. Because of insomnia, he recently added proprietary sleeping pills. There were a large number of diphenhydramine tablets in his pocket. The only other findings were mydriasis and a pulse of 100.

Complex Partial Seizures

A college student is referred for assessment of strange behavior spells. He has recently been observed periodically to pace about and mumble in a stereotypic manner. The history documents that he notices unusual "smells" and experiences strange feelings of unfamiliarity with his surroundings just prior to these instances. The evaluation was most remarkable for the EEG finding of bilateral epileptiform activity in the temporal regions, as recorded by the nasopharyngeal leads.

Clinical Comment

Hallucinations constitute a sensory experience without an external stimulus. Most often, they occur in major mental illnesses and in encephalopathies of toxic, metabolic, or certain other causation that induce brain dysfunc-

tion. They can present in nonmorbid conditions as well. The initial goal of the workup is to differentiate organic from functional processes. A complete history, physical, mental status, and laboratory assessment help to define an exact etiologic diagnosis. After the specific causative condition is identified, the physician can implement an appropriate, individualized therapeutic regimen.

REFERENCES

1. American Psychiatric Association. Diagnostic and statistical manual of mental disorders. rev. ed. Washington DC: APA, 1987 (DSMIII-R).
2. Asaad G, Shapiro B. Hallucinations: theoretical and clinical overview. Am J Psychiatry 1986;143(9): 1088–97.
3. Musalek M, Podreka I, Walter H, et al. Regional brain function in hallucinations: a study of regional cerebral blood flow with 99m-Tc-HMPAO-SPECT in patients with auditory hallucinations, tactile hallucinations, and normal controls. Compr Psychiatry 1989;30:99–108.
4. Musalek M, Podreka I, Walter H, et al. Neurophysiological aspects of auditory hallucinations. 99mTc-(HMPAO)-SPECT investigations in patients with auditory hallucinations and normal controls—a preliminary report. Psychopathology 1988;21:275–80.
5. Buchsbaum MS, Ingvar DH, Kessler R, et al. Cerebral glucography with positron tomography. Arch Gen Psychiatry 1982;39:251–9.
6. Lindstrom L, Klockhoff I, Svedberg A, Bergstrom K. Abnormal auditory brain-stem responses in hallucinating schizophrenic patients. Br J Psychiatry 1987;151:9–14.
7. Cooklin R, Sturgeon D, Leff J. The relationship between auditory hallucinations and spontaneous fluctuation of skin conductance in schizophrenia. Br J Psychiatry 1983;142:47–52.
8. Mitchell J, Vierkant AD. Delusions and hallucinations as a reflection of the subcultural milieu among psychotic patients of the 1930s and 1980s. J Psychol 1988;123(3):269–74.
9. Dyck P. Sylvian lipoma causing auditory hallucinations: case report. Neurosurgery 1985;16(1):64–7.
10. Ram Z, Findler G, Gutman I, Tadmor R, Sahar A. Visual hallucinations associated with pituitary adenoma. Neurosurgery 1987;20(2):292–6.
11. Price W, Coli L, Brandstetter RD, Gotz VP. Ranitidine associated hallucinations. Eur J Pharmacol 1985;29:375–6.

12. McEwen J, Meyboom RHB, Thijs I. Hallucinations in children caused by oxalamine citrate. Med J Aust 1989;150:449–52.
13. Ackland FM. Hallucinations in a child after drinking tripolidine/pseudoephedrine linctus [Letter]. Lancet 1984;1:1180.
14. Bain J, Drennan PC, Miller MG. Visual hallucinations in children receiving decongestants [Letter]. Br Med J 1984;288:1688.
15. Harrison SA, Wood CA Jr. Hallucinations after preoperative baclofen discontinuation in spinal cord injury patients. Drug Intelig Clin Psychiatry 1985;19:747–9.
16. Waller S, Bailey M. Hallucinations during morphine administration [Letter]. Lancet 1987;2:801.
17. Siegel RK. Hostage hallucinations visual imagery induced by isolation and life-threatening stress. J Nerv Ment Dis 1984;172(5):264–72.
18. Sing HC, Thorne DR, Genser SG, Hegge FW. Perceptual distortions and hallucinations reported during the course of sleep deprivation. Percept Mot Skills 1989;68:787–98.
19. Chittaranjan A, Srinath S, Andrade C. True hallucinations as a culturally sanctioned experience. Br J Psychiatry 1988;152:838–9.
20. Snyder BD. Case studies: atypical visual hallucinosis. Am J Prev Psychiatry Neurol 1990;2(2):29–30.

HEARING LOSS, SUDDEN

JAMES K. BREDENKAMP and CLOUGH SHELTON

SYNONYM: Sudden Deafness

BACKGROUND

Sudden hearing loss is commonly unilateral and may be mild or severe, temporary or permanent. Most otologists include in their definition of this disorder a hearing loss of greater than 30 decibels (dB) in three contiguous frequencies developing in three days or less.[1] Any interruption in the transmission of sound along the auditory pathway can lead to a sudden hearing loss. The site of lesion may be at the external, middle, or inner ear; internal auditory canal; cerebellopontine angle; or brain stem (Fig. 1). Depending on the location of the defect, the hearing loss can be sensorineural, conductive, or mixed.

This chapter focuses on sudden rather than chronic or congenital hearing loss. The majority of patients who experience a sudden hearing loss are young and healthy without previous otologic problems. They most often seek advice initially from their primary care physician or an emergency facility. The physician must recognize that sudden hearing loss is a symptom and not a diagnosis and that it may represent an important symptom of an underlying disease. Table 1 lists some of the many causes of sudden hearing loss.[1,2,3] Many of the problems outlined here are encountered infrequently and yet must be considered in the differential diagnosis. The majority of cases of sudden hearing loss are idiopathic. Clinically, this type of hearing loss is sudden, spontaneous, and sensorineural and occurs in a patient with no known previous otologic problems.[2,3] The annual incidence of idiopathic sudden hearing loss is 1 in 10,000. However, this estimate is probably low, since many people recover their hearing spontaneously before seeking medical attention.[4]

The patient with sudden hearing loss is usually anxious and concerned that the hearing loss will be permanent or that the hearing loss is a harbinger of more serious and life-threatening problems. Likewise, physicians quickly become exhausted considering the multitude of categories and causes of hearing loss. This chapter seeks to simplify the task of pinpointing a reason for sudden hearing loss by describing the most common causes and goes on to emphasize the important points in the history, physical examination, and radiologic and laboratory assessment of these patients.

HISTORY

Patients with sudden hearing loss should be questioned carefully about the details of the events leading up to the recognition of the hearing loss. It should be determined whether the hearing loss is fluctuating, progressive,

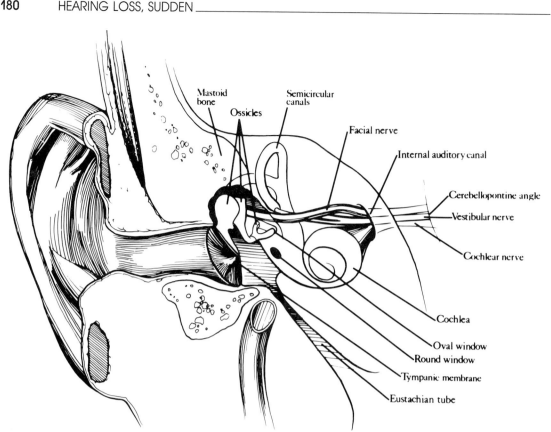

FIGURE 1. Anatomy of external, middle, and inner ear. Cochlear, vestibular, and facial nerves run from inner ear through internal auditory meatus and enter brain stem at cerebellopontine angle. (From Bredenkamp JK, Shelton C. Sudden hearing loss: determining the specific cause and the most appropriate treatment. Postgrad Med 1989;86:125–32. Reprinted with permission.)

partial, or complete, and if it is associated with vertigo, dizziness, or tinnitus. Any symptoms appearing around the time of the hearing loss as well as any previous ear problems or surgery, noise exposure, trauma, general medical problems, drug history (especially aminoglycoside and diuretics), and family history of hearing loss should be noted.

Patients who have a sudden hearing loss associated with a history of flying, diving, or straining should be suspected as having a perilymphatic fistula. They may note an audible pop followed by sudden hearing loss, vertigo, and tinnitus.[5]

Any patient who also complains of either decreased facial sensation, facial nerve paralysis, shoulder weakness, diplopia, tongue deviation, hoarse voice, or aspiration should be suspected of having an acoustic tumor or skull base tumor. Patients with a family history of von Recklinghausen's disease have a high likelihood of having an acoustic tumor.[6]

Patients with intolerance to loud noise and difficulty hearing speech in a crowded environment ("cocktail party") usually have a cochlear hearing loss. A retrocochlear loss is suggested by poor speech discrimination, including an inability to understand speech on the telephone. Patients who must stop chewing to hear better often have a conductive hearing loss. They may speak more softly because their own voice seems louder to them. Patients with sensorineural hearing loss speak more loudly because their own voice sounds softer.[5] Patients who are malingering may demonstrate poor eye contact with the examiner and a lack of attentiveness to visual speech clues (lip-reading).

Focused Queries

1. *What were the circumstances of the sudden hearing loss? Did it occur over minutes, days or hours? Was it associated with recent diving, flying, or straining?*

2. *Were there any associated symptoms of vertigo, dizziness, tinnitus, aural fullness, or an audible pop?*

TABLE 1.   Etiology of Sudden Hearing Loss

SITE OF ABNORMALITY	CAUSE	POSSIBLE UNDERLYING CONDITION
External ear	Foreign body or cerumen impaction	
	Otitis externa	Swimmer's ear
Middle ear	Trauma to temporal bone or skull base	
	Chronic otitis media with ossicular erosion	
	Acute otitis media	
	Postoperative complication	Previous stapedectomy
	Barotrauma	SCUBA diving
	Tumor	Glomus tumor
Inner ear	Infection	Viral cochleitis
		Viral or bacterial labyrinthitis
		Viral neuritis
		Bacterial meningitis
		Syphilis
	Vascular occlusion	Hyperviscosity syndromes
		Small vessel disease, sickle cell anemia
		Buerger's disease, hypercoagulability
		Vasospasm
		Inner ear hemorrhage
		Leukemia, anticoagulant therapy, and microembolic obstruction after bypass surgery
		Polyarteritis nodosa
		Cogan's syndrome
		Sarcoidosis
	Cochlear membrane rupture	Meniere's disease
		Round or oval window fistula
		Head trauma
		Barotrauma
	Drug toxicity	Treatment with ototoxic systemic agents
	Autoimmune	
	Idiopathic	
Internal auditory canal and cerebellopontine angle	Tumor	Acoustic tumor
		Meningioma
Brain stem	Vascular events	
	Tumor	
	Multiple sclerosis	
Psychogenic	Malingering	
	Conversion disorder	

(From Bredenkamp JK, Shelton C. Sudden hearing loss: determining the specific cause and the most appropriate treatment. Postgrad Med 1989;86:125–32. Reprinted with permission.)

3. *Is there a history of previous otologic problems or surgeries?*

PHYSICAL EXAMINATION

A general physical examination should be performed on all patients presenting with sudden hearing loss. Specific multisystem signs may be overlooked if one only examines the ear. A history and physical exam will usually reveal or suggest a diagnosis before tests are ordered.

The examination should include a careful neurotologic assessment that includes inspection of the ears and tuning fork tests. One should look for surgical scars, evidence of trauma, vesicles, and congenital defects. The external canal is examined for cerumen, foreign bodies, or infection. A cholesteatoma or mastoid cavity may be evident in the posterosuperior aspect of the canal.[5] All wax should be removed so that underlying areas can be visualized. If a tympanic membrane perforation is suspected, water irrigation should not be used to cleanse the ear.

The tympanic membrane's color and mobility should be assessed, and any scars, perforations, or tympanosclerosis should be noted. The posterosuperior area is carefully inspected for retraction pockets or attic cholesteatoma. Nystagmus or vertigo elicited by an increase in external auditory canal pressure ("fistula test") is suggestive of a perilymphatic fistula.[7]

The Weber test is performed with a 512-Hz tuning fork, which is placed on the center of the forehead. The patient will localize the sound to the ear with a conductive hearing loss or, in the case of sensorineural loss, to the better-hearing ear. The Rinne test compares the loudness of bone conduction to the loudness of air conduction. The 512-Hz tuning fork produces bone conduction greater than air conduction when the conductive hearing loss is greater than approximately 20 dB. Tuning forks provide an easy and inexpensive method to assess hearing loss at the bedside without the need for sophisticated equipment. They will also either confirm or refute the audiogram.[5]

Particular attention should be directed to the neurologic system, with emphasis on cranial nerve dysfunction. The facial nerve must be carefully assessed and its function documented. The eyes are observed for nystagmus, and the Romberg test and cerebellar tests are done to determine if a subtle balance disorder is present. Often a gradual unilateral vestibular loss, such as may occur with an acoustic neuroma, may not be associated with vertigo and is only suspected after careful vestibular testing.

DIAGNOSTIC STUDIES

Blood Tests

It is prudent to screen all sudden hearing loss patients with a complete blood cell count and an erythrocyte sedimentation rate. The possibility of syphilis should be evaluated with a fluorescent treponemal antibody (FTA) absorption test; RPR (rapid plasma reagin) and VDRL (Venereal Disease Research Laboratories) tests are generally negative in cases of inner ear syphilis. If the history and/or physical examination are suggestive of a systemic process, then specific tests are ordered to confirm the diagnosis.

Audiologic

All patients should undergo a complete audiologic workup early after presentation. The type of hearing loss suspected (sensorineural, conductive, or mixed) should be confirmed. The audiologist can also help identify those patients with unilateral hearing loss of psychogenic cause or who are malingering by performing a specific test called a Stenger. Those patients with bilateral fictitious hearing

loss often require more sophisticated audiologic testing. A standard audiologic test battery usually includes testing frequency-specific pure tones, speech discrimination, and middle ear impedance (tympanometry). Tympanometry helps to assess middle ear function and the status of the middle ear reflexes. The acoustic reflex is a tympanometric measure of the stapedial muscle's ability to maintain a contraction. Pathologic or absent acoustic reflex is 88 per cent sensitive in the detection of cerebellopontine angle tumors but has a 30 per cent false-positive rate.[8] A discrepancy between pure-tone hearing and speech discrimination is suggestive of a retrocochlear hearing loss. Further, special diagnostic tests can help to determine if the hearing loss is of possible retrocochlear etiology.[6,9] Auditory brain stem response (ABR) provides an objective test of the auditory signal from the cochlea to the brain stem. It is reported to be 96 per cent sensitive in the detection of retrocochlear tumors. Unfortunately, an ABR cannot be obtained if the hearing loss is greater than 70 dB. Approximately, 25 per cent of patients with an acoustic tumor will not have sufficient hearing to be eligible for an ABR[6,9] In these cases, radiologic studies will be required. The electronystagmogram is a relatively nonspecific test in patients with sudden hearing loss. However, acoustic tumors are unlikely in patients with bilateral symmetric caloric responses.

Radiologic

All patients with an asymmetric sensorineural hearing loss should be examined either audiometrically with an ABR or by imaging of the posterior fossa. Magnetic resonance imaging (MR) is more sensitive in this area than computerized tomography (CT) scanning. Gadolinium-DTPA (diethylenetriamine pentaacetic acid) enhanced MRI may be used to identify small tumors. Unlike MRI which allows superior soft tissue discrimination of the internal auditory canal, cerebellopontine angle, brain stem, and surrounding vascular structures, CT scanning is advantageous for its excellent visualization of the bony framework of the temporal bone. CT scanning is the procedure of choice in cases involving trauma, cholesteatoma, bony erosion, or inflammatory processes. Plain films of the skull base are generally insensitive because they will only show disease when it has caused bony erosion.

ASSESSMENT

Identifiable Causes

External Ear

Acute otitis externa or obstruction of the external auditory canal from either a cerumen impaction or a foreign body can cause sudden hearing loss. Patients may complain of otalgia and/or otorrhea and may give a history of trauma or water exposure. The hearing loss will be conductive and usually resolves following disimpaction or administration of drops and antibiotics.

Middle Ear

A conductive hearing loss usually accompanies acute otitis media. However, sudden sensorineural hearing loss associated with acute otitis media is suggestive of a toxic labyrinthitis. These patients will usually be vertiginous and have nystagmus. Sudden hearing loss associated with chronic otitis media with perforation usually implies disruption of the ossicular chain or erosion of the labyrinth by cholesteatoma. Patients with acute otitis media normally will have otalgia, but otalgia in patients with chronic otitis media may signify an impending intracranial complication.

Trauma to the temporal bone can cause either a sensorineural, conductive, or mixed hearing loss, depending on the line of fracture and on whether disruption of the ossicular chain has occurred. Temporal bone fractures should be suspected in any patient with signs of a skull base fracture (raccoon eyes, Battle's sign), cerebrospinal fluid otorrhea, or facial nerve paralysis. The external auditory canal may be lacerated or fractured, and often the posterior superior tympanic membrane is perforated. The patient may complain of vertigo or a sudden hearing loss and may have nystagmus. It is important to document facial nerve function carefully.

Sudden hearing loss also can result from movement of a previously placed middle ear ossicular prosthesis.

Inner Ear

A multitude of pathologic conditions can affect the inner ear: infectious, vascular, traumatic, autoimmune, and congenital. Infectious causes of inner ear sudden hearing loss include syphilis, viral cochleitis, labyrinthitis, neuritis, and bacterial meningitis. Any patient with an asymmetric, rapidly progressive sensorineural hearing loss and/or poor speech discrimination should be suspected as having inner ear syphilis. They may also have symptoms similar to Meniere's syndrome, with fluctuating hearing loss, vertigo, and tinnitus, or there may be a sensorineural hearing loss of any pattern. Patients may have a positive fistula test secondary to fibrous adhesions between the stapes footplate and membranous labyrinth (Hennebert's sign). It has been reported that as many as 6 to 7 per cent of adults with Meniere's-like syndrome or with a sensorineural hearing loss of unknown etiology may have inner ear syphilis. There may be a relationship between the human immunodeficiency virus (HIV) infection and otosyphilis.[10] Patients with a positive FTA absorption test should be treated for otosyphilis since deafness in the remaining ear may ensue if untreated. VDRL, RPR, and cerebrospinal fluid (CSF) tests may be negative.[11]

Sudden hearing loss can result from a viral cochleitis. Many viruses have been known to infect the inner ear and cause deafness. These include rubella, herpes, Epstein-Barr virus, mumps, and cytomegalovirus. Hearing loss occurs in about 5 of 10,000 cases of mumps, but may be as high as 4 to 5 per cent of adults following infection. In 80 per cent, the hearing loss is sudden and unilateral. A conductive sudden hearing loss occasionally occurs after chickenpox infection and is usually secondary to bacterial otitis media. Herpes zoster oticus (Ramsay Hunt syndrome) is a latent varicella zoster infection of the geniculate ganglion causing facial nerve paralysis and auricular vesicular eruption. In 6 per cent of cases, sudden sensorineural hearing loss may be present. Sudden hearing loss will often follow bacterial meningitis, and increasingly, sudden hearing loss has been associated with cryptococcal meningitis.

Rupture of the inner ear membrane and fistulae of either the round or the oval window has been hypothesized as a cause of sudden hearing loss.[7] Inner ear membrane rupture has been theorized to cause the hearing loss associated with endolymphatic hydrops (Meniere's disease). Round and oval window rupture are reported to occur when either CSF pressure or middle ear pressure suddenly increases and is subsequently transmitted to the inner ear, causing rupture of membranes. Any patient who notes onset of the hearing loss while flying, diving, or straining should be suspected as having a perilymphatic fistula. Exploration of the middle ear has revealed fistulae in some patients with sudden hearing loss that were thought to be associated with abrupt compression or decompression, head injuries, or heavy lifting.[2]

Sudden hearing loss can result from partial or complete occlusion of the cochlear vasculature. The hyperviscosity syndromes—Waldenström's macroglobulinemia and polycythemia vera—have caused sudden hearing loss secondary to vascular occlusion. (Also see chapter on Polycythemia.) Inner ear hemorrhage can occur as a complication of leukemia or heparin therapy, and small vessel destruction in polyarteritis nodosa can cause sudden hearing loss.[3] Microemboli during cardiopulmonary bypass cause immediate postoperative unilateral sudden hearing loss in about 0.1 per cent of patients; about 50 per cent of affected patients eventually recover hearing.[12]

Autoimmune-associated hearing loss has been demonstrated, and recently, a steroid responsive autoimmune hearing loss has been described in patients with no known systemic autoimmune disease. There is usually a bilateral progressive sensorineural hearing loss that may be sudden in onset and associated with complaints of pressure and tinnitus in the ear. There is an association with a positive lymphocyte inhibition test using inner ear antigen, and such patients will often have an elevated erythrocyte sedimentation rate (ESR). (Also see chapter on Erythrocyte Sedimentation Rate, Elevated in *Difficult Diagnosis I*.) Eventually, 20 per cent of patients with autoimmune hearing loss develop other systemic disease thought to be autoimmune in origin.[13].

Retrocochlear Area

An acoustic tumor in the internal auditory canal, at the cerebellopontine angle, or at the brain stem can cause sudden hearing loss. Seventy-five per cent of patients with proven acoustic tumors will have as their first symptom progressive sensorineural hearing loss. Although the loss is usually slow and progressive, 15 per cent patients will report that the hearing loss was sudden. Approximately 1 to 2 per cent of all patients with sudden hearing loss eventually are found to have an acoustic tumor.[6,14,15] Patients with sudden hearing loss who have spontaneous recovery may still harbor an acoustic neuroma. Unilateral tinnitus is the second most common symptom of an acoustic tumor. The ABR will show a retrocochlear pattern, and MRI will best demonstrate the tumor. Any patient with either a unilateral sensorineural hearing loss or unilateral tinnitus should be suspected of having retrocochlear pathology.[6,8,15]

Brainstem

Vascular events, tumors, or diffuse demyelinating disease, such as multiple sclerosis, may cause sudden hearing loss. Patients with brain stem stroke or tumors will usually have multiple cranial nerve deficits. Multiple sclerosis may present with isolated brainstem findings, like sudden hearing loss, or in combination with visual complaints, nystagmus, vertigo, clumsiness, or intention tremor.[3]

Idiopathic Cases

Sudden hearing loss is commonly idiopathic and is most frequent during the fourth decade. Sudden hearing loss has been reported in all ages and occurs in men and women equally. The hearing loss is almost always unilateral, and repeat episodes are unusual. About one third of patients awaken with the hearing loss, and about one half have an associated symptom of unsteadiness, dizziness, or vertigo. The severity of the disequilibrium often correlates with the severity of the hearing loss.[1] Identifiable causes of sudden hearing loss, as discussed previously, are always ruled out before this diagnosis is made.[3]

Mattox and Simmons observed a spontaneous recovery (either complete or good) in 65 per cent of patients.[4] They found that early presentation, low ESR, lack of vestibular symptoms, and an audiogram showing a mild midfrequency loss were good prognostic indicators. On the other hand, severe high-frequency hearing loss associated with vertigo and an ESR greater than 30 were poor prognostic indicators for return of function. They also found that patients who presented to physicians early after onset of their sudden hearing loss had a better prognosis. Therefore, these factors as well as the relative high spontaneous recovery rate must be taken into consideration when one examines any treatment program.[16]

Despite many reports on idiopathic sudden hearing loss, little is known about its pathophysiology. Possible causes include viral infection,[17] vascular occlusion,[1] and cochlear membrane rupture.[2,7] The evidence supporting any one of the above possibilities is not conclusive.

Viral cochleitis has been thought to be the leading cause of idiopathic sudden hearing loss.[1] Patients will often report coincidental viral infections or symptoms. However, 20 to 60 per cent of the general population will report recent symptoms, and idiopathic sudden hearing loss does not appear to be seasonal nor epidemic. Serologic data and temporal bone histology have been inconclusive. However, the mumps virus has been grown from the perilymph of a patient with idiopathic sudden hearing loss.[3,16] Similarly, temporal bone findings are not consistent with extensive destruction of the cochlea, as seen with experimentally induced vascular occlusion of the cochlear artery.[3]

Clinical Applications

Patients with sudden hearing loss should be approached systematically to exclude such obvious causes as external auditory canal obstruction or more subtle abnormalities such as an acoustic tumor. It is important to recognize treatable causes of sudden hearing loss, so that prompt treatment can be initiated. If the patient has given a history of sudden hearing loss associated with straining, lifting, flying, or diving, then this represents an otologic emergency, and immediate referral is necessary. When no discernible cause is found, then the hearing loss is considered idiopathic, and empirical treatment is indicated. Most patients with sudden hearing loss should be eventually referred to an otolaryngologist unless there is an obvious reversible cause of the sudden hearing loss. The otolaryngologist can initiate appropriate audiologic studies and do a more thorough otoscopic and head and neck examination.

REFERENCES

1. Wilson WR. Sudden sensorineural hearing loss. In: Cummings CW, Fredrickson JM, Harker LA, Krause CJ, Schuller DE, eds. Otolaryngology: head and neck surgery. St Louis: CV Mosby, 1986;4:3219–24.
2. Goodhill V, Harris I. Sudden hearing loss syndrome. In: Goodhill V, ed. Ear diseases, deafness, and dizziness. New York: Harper & Row, 1979:664–81.
3. Bredenkamp JK, Shelton C. Sudden hearing loss: determining the specific cause and the most appropriate treatment. Postgrad Med 1989;86:125–32.
4. Mattox DE, Simmons FB. Natural history of sudden sensorineural hearing loss. Ann Otol Rhinol Laryngol 1977;86:463–80.
5. House JW. Otologic and neurotologic history and physical examination. In: Cummings CW, Fredrickson JM, Harker LA, Krause CJ, Schuller DE, eds. Otolaryngology: head and neck surgery. St Louis: CV Mosby, 1986;4:2733–41.
6. Mattox DE. Vestibular schwannomas. Otolaryngol Clin North Am 1987;20:149–60.
7. Harris I. Sudden hearing loss: membrane rupture. Am J Otol 1984;5:484–7.
8. Hosford-Dunn H. Auditory function tests. In: Cummings CW, Fredrickson JM, Harker LA, Krause CJ, Schuller DE, eds. Otolaryngology: head and neck surgery. St Louis: CV Mosby, 1986;4:2779–2819.
9. Thomsen J, Tos M. Acoustic neuroma: clinical aspects, audiovestibular assessment, diagnostic delay, and growth rate. Am J Otol 1990;11:12–9.
10. Smith ME, Canalis RF. Otologic manifestations of AIDS: the otosyphilis connection. Laryngoscope 1989;99:365–72.
11. Dobbin JM, Perkins JH. Otosyphilis and hearing loss: response to penicillin and steroid therapy. Laryngoscope 1983;93:1540–3.
12. Plasse HM, Mittleman M, Frost JO. Unilateral sudden hearing loss after open heart surgery: a detailed study of seven cases. Laryngoscope 1981;91:101–9.
13. McCabe BF. Autoimmune sensorineural hearing loss. Ann Otol Rhinol Laryngol 1979;88:585–9.
14. Shaia FT, Sheehy JL. Sudden sensori-neural hearing impairment: a report of 1,220 cases. Laryngoscope 1986;76:389–98.
15. Pensak ML, Glasscock ME III, Josey AF, et al. Sudden hearing loss and cerebellopontine angle tumors. Laryngoscope 1985;95:1188–93.
16. Laird N, Wilson WR. Predicting recovery from idiopathic sudden hearing loss. Am J Otolaryngol 1983;4:161–4.
17. Wilson WR, Veltri RW, Laird N, et al. Viral and epidemiologic studies of idiopathic sudden hearing loss. Otolaryngol Head Neck Surg 1983;91:653–8.

HEMATOCHEZIA

JAMES B. RHODES, CLARK W. ANTONSON, and ROLAND B. CHRISTIAN

SYNONYMS: Bright Red Blood per Rectum, Gross Blood per Rectum, Rectal Bleeding, Maroon Stools

BACKGROUND

Hematochezia is the passage of bright red blood per rectum. In theory, hematochezia could result from gastrointestinal (GI) bleeding somewhere between the nasopharynx and the external anus. Hematochezia from an upper GI tract bleed is a dramatic, urgent event associated with moderate to severe shock and is life-threatening. Bleeding lesions in the distal small bowel, colon, and rectum may also present in a dramatic fashion with loose, bloody stools, and this is also an emergent event. These patients are likely to seek prompt help. The most common causes of emergent hematochezia are listed in Table 1.[1]

The great majority of patients with hematochezia pass smaller amounts of blood less frequently. The responsible lesions in the distal small bowel, colon, rectum, and anus are generally the same or similar lesions that account for emergent hematochezia. These patients usually present themselves to physicians in an outpatient facility. Some patients ooze smaller amounts of blood between the hematochezia episodes and have occult blood in their stools. The most common causes of non-emergent hematochezia are listed in Table 2. Hemorrhoids, polyps, and colorectal cancer account for about 85 per cent of the lesions judged to be the bleeding source.[2]

Hematochezia in children is quite different and usually of the nonemergent type. Table 3 summarizes the bleeding source of 52 children. Their mean age was 11 years (range: 1 month to 20 years). The most common lesion (50 per cent) was polyps, and of these, juvenile polyps are most common. Inflammatory bowel disease was the next leading cause (12 per cent). No bleeding site was detected in 13 per cent of the patients.[3] The colonic, rectal, and anal problems in children were recently reviewed.[4]

Several other causes have been reported to account infrequently for hematochezia. A partial list is provided in Table 4. These unusual causes are encountered in the United States but are more common in other countries. Some infectious causes may occur in sporadic epidemics.

The gross color of blood or blood products in the stool is dependent on the volume of blood lost per unit time, the transit time, the total amount of blood that is digested and absorbed, as well as the amount of bacterial degradation that occurs. A 50-ml bolus of blood in the upper GI tract can result in a black stool. A bolus of 100 to 200 ml of blood causes melena—a black, soft sticky stool. A 200-ml bolus of blood in the cecum is passed in less than a day as a soft maroon-colored stool that may disintegrate in the commode and release some red blood. A relatively large amount of blood in the GI tract has a laxative effect. A few milliliters of blood from the lower colon may appear as streaks on the periphery of a formed stool.[5] As little as 5 ml of bright red blood from the rectum or anus may turn the commode water red and be interpreted as an emergent event in the eyes of some patients.

TABLE 1. Emergent Hematochezia: Common Causes in 80 Patients

SOURCE	PERCENTAGE OF PATIENTS
Upper GI tract	11
Small bowel	9
No site found	6
Colon	74
AV* malformation	30
Diverticulosis	17
Polyp or cancer	11
Colitis or ulcer	9
Rectal lesion	4
Other	3

* AV = arteriovenous.
(Data from Jensen DM, Machicado GA. Diagnosis and treatment of severe hematochezia. The role of urgent colonoscopy after purge. Gastroenterology 1988;95:1569–74.)

TABLE 2.   Nonemergent Hematochezia:
Common Causes in 145 Patients

LESION	LESION SEEN	LESION BLED	
	Number of Patients*	Number of Patients*	Percentage of Patients*
Anal—74%			
Hemorrhoids	114	104	70
Fissure	8	6	4
Cancer	1	1	1
Other	5	4	3
Colorectal—26%			
Diverticulosis	38	5	3
Polyp(s)	25	11	7
Cancer	15	15	10
Proctitis	5	3	2
Prolapse	4	4	3
Other	5	2	1
No site found	3	—	2
Total	223	155	106

* Totals sum to more than 145, or 100 per cent, because many patients had more than one lesion. Patients with one lesion = 59 per cent; two lesions = 32 per cent; three or more = 9 per cent. Some 6 per cent of patients appeared to bleed from two lesions.
(Data from Goulston KJ, Cooke I, Dent OF. How important is rectal bleeding in the diagnosis of bowel cancer and polyps? Lancet 1986;2:261–4.)

The amount of blood lost in the GI tract can be quantitated. Normally, we lose up to 2 ml of blood per day from our GI tracts. The simplest and cheapest method of detection is the guaiac test for occult blood.[6] A peroxidaselike enzymatic activity in the red blood cells frees oxygen from hydrogen peroxide which combines with the colorless indicator to yield a blue color. This test can detect about 15 to 20 ml of blood in 100 gm of stool, which is about 7 to 10 times the normal amount of blood lost per day. In patients with more frequent hematochezia, or a slow leak, other tests may be helpful. The test that is quite sensitive is the radioactive chromium (^{51}Cr) isotope test. A sample of the patient's blood is incubated with ^{51}Cr and then reinjected intravenously. The ^{51}Cr released in the GI tract is not absorbed and is passed in the stool. The stools are quantitatively saved for several days, and the ^{51}Cr is measured and compared with the total counts injected. This sensitive method can measure normal blood loss.

The best test for hematochezia is probably the immunologic determination of the amount of hemoglobin contained in the feces. This test is specific for human hemoglobin and does not react with animal hemoglobin. This study is not commonly ordered.

Hemoglobin is further broken down by digestion and bacterial degradation to porphyrins, which do not react with the guaiac or hemoglobin tests. The porphyrins can be extracted from the stool and measured by fluorimetry. This sensitive test can measure normal blood loss and is probably most useful in upper tract oozing of an occult nature.[5,7] In clinical practice, the important point is how much blood remains in the body. This is estimated by hemoglobin, hematocrit, and iron studies. These tests are normal in most patients with hematochezia, who can make blood faster than they lose it.

Hematochezia appears to be a common event. A randomized population survey from Australia surveyed about 200 people over 30 years old. The authors found that 16 per cent

TABLE 3.   Hematochezia in Children:
Common Causes in 52 Patients

LESION	PERCENTAGE OF PATIENTS
Polyps	50
Inflammatory bowel disease	12
Vascular lesions	6
Nodular lymphoid hyperplasia	6
Meckel's diverticulum	6
Nonspecific colitis	4
Other	4
No site found	13

(Data from Hassall E, Barclay GN, Ament ME. Colonoscopy in childhood. Pediatrics 1984;73:594–9.)

TABLE 4.   Uncommon and Rare Causes of Hematochezia in the United States

INFECTIOUS	
Shigella	Sarcomas
Salmonella	Lymphomas
Escherichia coli	Leukemias
Campylobacter	Melanoma
Yersinia	Metastatic
Clostridium	Familial polyposis
Amebiasis	Peutz-Jeghers syndrome
Giardia	Gardner's syndrome
Cryptosporidia	Malacoplakia
Strongyloides	Hamartomas
Cytomegalovirus	
Herpes	**VASCULAR**
Antibiotic associated	Aneurysms
Staphylococcus	Aortic grafts
Tuberculosis	Arteritis
Syphilis	Arteriosclerotic
Gonorrhea	Clotting disorders
Chlamydia	Varices
Schistosoma	Thrombosis
Histoplasmosis	Venous lakes
Blastocystis	Hemangiomas
Coccidioidomycosis	Thrombocytopenias
Acquired immune deficiency syndrome	Blue rubber bleb
Isospora	Osler-Weber-Rendu disease
Aeromonas	Lymphangiectasias
Klebsiella	Chylous cysts
Plesiomonas	Purpuras
Vibrio	
Actinomycosis	**CONGENITAL**
Falciparum malaria	Pseudoxanthoma elastica
Oxyuris vermicularis	Ehlers-Danlos syndrome
Condyloma	Ectopic gastric mucosa
	Enteric duplication
INFLAMMATORY	
	MISCELLANEOUS
Sprue	Anastomosis
Whipple's disease	Episiotomy
Solitary ulcer	Endometriosis
Collagen diseases	Ectopic pregnancy
Lymphoid proctitis	Ovarian cyst
Eosinophilic enteritis	Ureterosigmoidostomy
Mucocutaneous syndromes	Stricture
Enteric fistulas	Intussusception
Necrotizing enterolitis	Foreign bodies
Epidemic jejunitis	Milk intolerance
Radiation	Running associated
	Amyloidosis
NEOPLASTIC	Factitious
	Trauma
Neuromas	Chemicals
Lipomas	Toxins
Leiomyomas	Drugs
Fibromas	Scurvy
Carcinoid	Uremia

of the people had noted hematochezia in the previous six months. This surprising percentage would underestimate the true incidence, because 43 per cent of the population rarely or never looked at their stools. Only 21 per cent always looked at their stools, whereas 32 per cent inspected the toilet paper. If these results are generally true in the United States, at least 16 per cent of the population over 30 experiences hematochezia every six months, a very common event. One could conclude that most people with hematochezia do not seek medical help. Perhaps one reason is that at least 43 per cent attributed their bleeding to hemorrhoids.[8]

HISTORY

The assessment of hematochezia begins with a thorough and targeted history. The history enables a more selected approach to the evaluation and generates a more specific differential diagnosis. Most important, a good history assists in distinguishing an urgent from an elective evaluation, acute from chronic disorders, and benign from potentially malignant disorders.[5,7]

Present Illness

An estimate of the quantity of blood lost is one of the first considerations. One is interested in the onset, duration, frequency, and volume of blood lost. The quantity of blood lost is estimated as a teaspoonful, a tablespoonful, a cup, or a pint. When did it start, and how long has it persisted? Has it been intermittent? Was the blood mixed in with the stool (suggesting a more proximal source)? Was blood coating a well-formed stool (suggesting a sigmoid, rectal, or anal source)? Was there associated dizziness or syncope (suggesting a large volume loss)? In general, the frequency and volume of hematochezia do not allow a more specific diagnosis.

A history of recent intermittent fevers, night sweats, and malaise suggests an acute or subacute inflammatory lesion. Weight loss, fatigue, and anorexia suggest a more chronic lesion such as chronic inflammation or a neoplasm.

If the patient has a recent change in bowel habit with abdominal pain or distress, one is interested in the onset, duration, location, and quality of these symptoms. The frequency of the complaints is of interest, as are any recognized associations, such as following meals. New-onset diarrhea with hematochezia suggests infectious colitis, inflammatory bowel disease, or ischemic colitis. New-onset constipation may suggest an obstruction from carcinoma or an inflammatory stricture. Passage of a hard stool may produce hematochezia due to painful anal fissures or hemorrhoids. The pain is frequent and associated with defecation of hard stools. Anorectal pain can often lead to a cycle of inhibited bowel movements, leading to harder stools and even more problems with pain and defecation. The quality of this pain is often described as burning, throbbing, or a tearing discomfort and at times can be quite severe.

Past Medical History

The past medical history may suggest an exacerbation of an old problem. A history of acid peptic distress or alcoholism suggests an upper GI tract lesion. The patient may have had previous x-rays, endoscopy, or operations that may be helpful.

Family History

A history of polyps in family members at a young age or colon cancer in relatives under 45 years of age raises the possibility of a familial cancer syndrome. A history of colon cancer in a parent increases the cancer possibility two- to four-fold. A significant number of patients with inflammatory bowel disease or polyps often have a positive family history. An older patient with a family history of vascular disease raises the possibility of an ischemic lesion.

Current Medications

The current use of heparin, warfarin, aspirin, and nonsteroidal anti-inflammatory agents has been associated with GI bleeding. Drugs such as antimetabolites for cancer chemotherapy and gold for arthritis have been associated with a drug colitis. Antibiotics commonly cause diarrhea, but hematochezia is uncommon. Hematochezia suggests pseudomembranous colitis.

Other sources of bleeding are occasionally mistaken for hematochezia. Bleeding from the vagina may be confused with hematochezia. A urinary source of blood may be rarely confused with hematochezia in males as well as females. In diarrhea, red food coloring (Jell-o) is sometimes mistaken for hematochezia. A black stool due to iron, bismuth (Pepto-Bismol), or green vegetables is occasionally mistaken for melena.

PHYSICAL EXAMINATION

Assessing the hemodynamic status, looking for evidence of systemic disease, and examining the anus are especially important. The patient's hemodynamic status includes looking for pallor, diaphoresis, and anxiety. A weak or rapid pulse suggests significant blood volume loss. A supine blood pressure of less than 100 mm Hg or a pulse greater than 100 usually represents a 25 per cent loss in the blood volume. Orthostatic changes are more sensitive. A pulse increase of 20 beats per minute and a systolic blood pressure drop of 20 mm Hg from the supine to the erect position suggest a blood volume loss of 1 L or more. Careful inspection of the skin, especially the lips, face, and chest, may show rare vascular lesions associated with GI lesions. About 25 to 50 per cent of the patients with an aortic heart murmur have colonic angiomata. Atrial fibrillation, especially if of recent onset, may be associated with arterial emboli and bowel ischemia or infarction.

Inspection of the abdomen may reveal hepatosplenomegaly, large masses, or prominent venous patterns on the abdomen consistent with portal hypertension. Auscultation may detect bruits, which may be significant for arterial lesions. Rapid bleeding causes rapid transit, and the bowel sounds are frequently increased. Tender masses may be consistent with inflammation. Hard, nodular, fixed, and tender masses may be associated with neoplasms. Firm, movable masses of constipated stool in the sigmoid colon may be accompanied by hemorrhoids and fissures.

The anus should be inspected for evidence of external hemorrhoids and fissures. Old hemorrhoidal tags suggest prior hemorrhoidal disease. Swollen, tender, thrombosed external hemorrhoids may be seen. Exophytic anal lesions suggest anal infections or neoplasms. A prolapsed mucosa is rarely seen. Perirectal inflammation may be associated with infectious or inflammatory diarrheas. Fecal soiling is consistent with diarrhea, rectal incontinence, or poor hygiene. Fistulous tracts are consistent with abscesses, inflammatory bowel disease, or neoplasms. Gentle palpation of the anus and rectum is helpful in most cases. Tenderness and palpable irregularities are sought. Mass lesions such as rectal cancer may be hard, firm, and nodular. Tender fissures may be felt in the anal canal. A palpable nodule in the rectum may represent a polyp, a neoplasm, or a prostatic nodule. Thrombosed internal hemorrhoids may be palpable. It is important during the examination to sweep the rectal ampulla a full 360 degrees to check both lateral and posterior rectal walls. Bright red blood on the examining finger is quite useful. Any stool in the rectum should be checked for blood by the occult blood test. Should the patient have to move their bowels during the examination, the stool should be inspected, which provides an amazing amount of information.

DIAGNOSTIC STUDIES

Laboratory

Laboratory assessment of GI bleeding allows an estimation of the amount and severity of bleeding. The more important laboratory studies include the hemoglobin, hematocrit, mean corpuscular volume (MCV), platelets, blood urea nitrogen (BUN), and prothrombin time.

The hemoglobin and hematocrit are usually accurate in assessing the overall amount of blood loss. In cases of severe GI bleeding, however, they may be misleading and lag behind other changes for 18 to 36 hours, depending on the rate and degree of volume re-expansion. The white blood cell count is often mildly elevated in severe GI bleeding, reticulocytes are usually increased, and the platelets may be mildly increased. The MCV may give a clue as to the chronicity of the problem if it is low (microcytosis), suggesting iron deficiency anemia. An elevated MCV (macrocytosis) may suggest significant alcohol consumption or a vitamin deficiency. A hemoglobin of 6 to 8 gm/100 ml suggests prior occult bleeding before the episode of hematochezia. A low serum iron with increased iron binding protein implies the rate of blood loss has exceeded the patient's ability to absorb iron and make hemoglobin. An occasional patient does not absorb iron well and can be identified by an iron absorption test. The BUN is helpful since blood in the GI tract is digested and absorbed, resulting in an elevated BUN with a normal or near normal creatinine. This is further reflected in the BUN/creatinine ratio which is generally greater than 20:1. A prothrombin time assesses coagulation parameters, which may be elevated owing to anticoagulants or decreased liver synthesis. None of the above tests are universally accurate and should be used in conjunction with a careful assessment of the patient.

Other laboratory data may be obtained in a case of GI bleeding when indicated. In a patient with diarrhea and hematochezia, an electrolyte panel would be useful. Serum transaminases and alkaline phosphatase are helpful in assessing possible metastatic disease or cirrhosis. Albumin, protein, and cholesterol reflect the nutritional status and may provide clues to systemic disease.

Endoscopy

A plastic disposable anoscope should be used after the digital rectal examination. Inflammation, hemorrhoids, tears, and fissures can be visualized. A 25-cm rigid proctoscope is available as a plastic disposable instrument. It can be advanced a mean distance of 18 cm if feces are not present. A hypertonic phosphate enema can be used to empty the lower colon. Rectal and rectosigmoid lesions such as inflammation and neoplasms may be seen. A 60-cm flexible fiberoptic sigmoidoscope can be passed a mean distance of 45 cm, which is somewhere in the sigmoid colon. In some cases, the splenic flexure can be reached. The distal colon is cleared of feces by a series of two hypertonic phosphate enemas immediately before the procedure. Diverticula, neoplasms, and mucosal abnormalities can be detected. The tip can be retroflexed in the rectum to visualize the anus from above.

Barium Enema

The first requirement for a barium enema is a clean colon. This is achieved by one to three days of a clear liquid diet with two courses of laxatives and a final large-volume enema. The barium enema may be a single column or preferably an air contrast examination. Barium enemas are better than colonoscopy in detecting diverticula and extraluminal masses. The liquid barium can pass through strictures that will not admit a colonoscope. The barium flows through loops of bowel fixed in position by adhesions or masses. The limitations of barium enemas include missing small polyps less than 5 mm in diameter and missing about 5 per cent of colon cancers, which tend to be in the cecum. Half of the cancer misses are due to technical problems, and half are due to observer distraction or oversight. Barium enemas may not detect superficial mucosal or submucosal lesions that do not alter the lumen. Examples are angiomata, superficial inflammation such as early ulcerative colitis, radiation colitis, or mild ischemic colitis. Complications are rare. About 10 to 25 per cent of the patients are referred for colonoscopy for biopsy or removal of a neoplasm or concern about a distorted segment with diverticula or a surgical anastomosis. Continued hematochezia after a normal flexible sigmoidoscopy and a normal air contrast barium enema is an indication for colonoscopy.

Colonoscopy

A clean colon is essential for colonoscopy, so that mucosal lesions such as angiomata will not be obscured by feces. A common preparation is an oral electrolyte solution that is not absorbed and cleans the colon from above. Approximately 4 to 6 L over two to four hours is usually sufficient. The patient usually receives an analgesic and a sedative medication for the examination. The advantages of colonoscopy are direct visualization of the mucosa with biopsy capability. Colonoscopy also has its limitations. Straightening out the sigmoid, transverse colon, and cecum on their mesenteries is an occasional problem. Long, redundant colons and severe diverticular disease can prolong the examination. Major problems are colonic loops fixed by adhesions or tumor extension and tight strictures, which may not permit passage of the colonoscope. In a survey of 674 colonoscopists doing prospective examinations in a total of 6614 patients, the cecum was reached in 75 per cent of the patients. The examination was limited in 18 per cent by patient discomfort or operator inability to advance the instrument. In 9 per cent of patients, the examination was limited by the colonoscopic findings.[9] Colonoscopy misses 6 to 8 per cent of all polyps, which tend to be at flexures and in the rectum.[10] The cancer miss rate is unknown, but we estimate about 0.2 to 1.0 per cent, and these tend to be in the cecum. Colonoscopy complications during diagnostic examination include a 0.15 per cent perforation rate and significant bleeding of 0.1 per cent. Other major complications such as cardiac arrhythmias, heart attacks, and medication reactions are 0.2 per cent.[11]

Nuclear Medicine

The radioactive technetium GI bleeding scan involves labeling the patient's red blood cells in a test tube and reinjecting the labeled cells. A gamma camera is used to detect abdominal pooling of the isotope in the GI tract. The tagged red cells and isotope can be measured for one to two days. The method detects GI bleeding at a rate of 0.1 to 0.5 ml per minute or about a unit of blood per day. Serial scans may detect subsequent bleeding if the bleeding temporarily stops or the bleeding rate slows. The method is useful in emergent bleeding and is more sensitive than current angiography. The method is not helpful in non-emergent hematochezia in small amounts.

Another radioisotope, pertechnetate, is avidly taken up by the gastric mucosa. Many Meckel's diverticula contain gastric mucosa and are detected on the abdominal scan. Some Meckel's diverticula bleed, whereas most do not. The pertechnetate scan does not differentiate bleeding from nonbleeding Meckel's diverticula.

Angiography

The abdominal arteries are serially injected, and radiopaque media pooling in the GI tract lumen is determined. This method detects rapid emergent bleeding at a rate of 0.6 to 1.0 ml per minute or about 3 units of blood per day. This method is especially useful in detecting arterial stenosis or occlusion, arteriovenous shunting in the intestine, and venous pooling. The lesions need to be larger than 0.5 to 1.0 cm in size. Newer contrast media are isotonic and should avoid some of the complications of the older hypertonic media. The disadvantage with bleeding lesions is that the bleeding must be at a rapid rate during the limited time of the examination. Many of the lesions associated with emergent hematochezia will not be detected by this test.

Exploratory Laparotomy

Ideally, the diagnostic role of laparotomy should be an early confirmatory test, should the patient experience a second or third emergent GI bleed. Mortality rates in the unstable elderly patient with multiple systemic diseases can be 20 to 40 per cent. However, the mortality rates in continued brisk bleeding may be higher. Laparotomy is more of a therapeutic option to treat specific lesions diagnosed with other studies.

ASSESSMENT

Most cases (80 to 90 per cent) of emergent GI bleeding are due to lesions in the upper GI tract. The frequent and loose stools are melenic or maroon in color, and hematochezia is associated with the most severe cases.[12] Emergent bleeding from the lower GI tract is less common (10 to 20 per cent) and associated with dark blood and more prominent hematochezia. Mortality rates from emergent GI

bleeding in the past have been 20 to 40 per cent. In the 1990s, mortality rates should be less than 10 per cent. The outcome is related to the rate of blood loss, blood replacement, and the severity of other diseases of the heart, blood vessels, and kidneys.[5,7] Viewed from the hematochezia reference point, emergent hematochezia accounts for less than 5 per cent of patients.

Emergent Hematochezia

Table 1 lists the bleeding sites in 80 patients with severe hematochezia prospectively evaluated at two hospitals. The mean age was 64 (range: 21 to 94), and the patients had unstable vital signs, received 6 units or more of blood in 24 hours, and required intensive care. Each patient had a negative anoscopy, sigmoidoscopy, and nasogastric tube aspiration. They were examined by upper GI endoscopy and emergent colonoscopy in the intensive care unit.[1] An upper GI source was documented by endoscopy in 11 per cent. Patients with bile but no blood in the nasogastric aspirate did not have an upper GI bleeding site, but bile is not routinely obtained in the nasogastric aspirate. In patients over 65, asymptomatic bleeding peptic ulcers are more common (9 versus 3 per cent). The elderly are more likely to have concomitant duodenal and gastric ulcers as well as duodenal ulcers greater than 2 cm.[13] The small bowel was the source in 9 per cent as blood or clots were seen coming through the ileocecal junction. No bleeding site was identified in 6 per cent of the patients.

Emergent lower GI bleeding classically presents suddenly, with little or no history and little or no clues obtained from the physical examination. Colonic lesions were the most common source (74 per cent). Angiomata (30 per cent) were the most common lesion. The usual lesion is a degenerative arteriovenous malformation in the mucosa. They are 5 mm in size, multiple, and commonly in the elderly right colon. These lesions can also ooze slowly and account for anemia with occult blood in the stool. They are best diagnosed with the colonoscope.

While 60 per cent of the patients had diverticulosis, a diverticulum accounted for only 17 per cent of the bleeding lesions. Bleeding, oozing, or a clot was seen in a diverticulum at colonoscopy. Diverticula are quite common in people from well-developed countries. A prospective dissection of 300 randomly selected autopsy colons found that diverticula were present in 10 per cent of the specimens from people less than 30 years of age. At age 50, diverticula were present in 28 per cent of the specimens and in 50 per cent of people 80 years or older.[14] A small (1-mm) artery in the dome of a diverticulum ruptures on the luminal side and bleeds through a normal mucosa. The bleeding stops in 75 to 95 per cent of the cases. Bleeding from active diverticulitis is usually of the nonemergent type.[15]

Polyps or cancer accounted for 12 per cent of the bleeding lesions. The incidence of polyps and cancers increases with increasing age. Colitis or colonic ulcers accounted for 9 per cent of the bleeding sites. Younger patients are more likely to bleed from inflammatory bowel disease. Rectal lesions accounted for 4 per cent of the bleeding sites, as seen by colonoscopy in the retroflexed position. The rectal lesions were missed at anoscopy or sigmoidoscopy or were obscured by blood in the rectum.[1] Bleeding from the anus or rectum is more likely to be suspected from the history of the present illness.

Nonemergent Hematochezia

Nonemergent hematochezia accounts for at least 90 per cent of all patients who seek medical help for hematochezia. Table 2 contains the results of a prospective study of 145 patients over 40 who had noticed hematochezia for less than six months. The mean age was 58 years (range: 40 to 95). They described their hematochezia as bright red (85 per cent), dark red blood (12 per cent), or maroon colored (3 per cent). In the preceding six months, only 39 per cent of the patients reported a change in bowel habits, and only 30 per cent noted abdominal pain or distress.[2]

Anal lesions were the most common, and hemorrhoids accounted for 70 per cent of the bleeding. Hemorrhoids come from the rich arteriovenous plexus of the anus. Small arterioles may leak a small amount of bright red blood. The external plexus, below the pectinate line, is covered with skin. Rapid subcutaneous bleeding results in a blue swollen external hemorrhoid that can be quite painful for a few days. These lesions can be surgically incised and drained. Internal hemorrhoids result from muscular and vascular breakdown with submucosal pools of blood that can thrombose. These larger lesions may prolapse with defecation and then retract. Even larger lesions may prolapse and not retract. They are

mucosa covered, and mucus may stain the underpants. Diverticulosis was common (26 per cent) but only accounted for 3 per cent of the bleeding sites. Diverticula probably account for more of the bleeding sites, but diverticula are rarely seen to be bleeding in nonemergent hematochezia when examined several days later.

Polyps were relatively common (17 per cent) and bleeding was attributed to 50 per cent of the polyps. Colorectal polyps are four to seven times more common than colorectal cancers and begin to occur about 10 years earlier than colorectal cancer. Small polyps (less than 5 mm) are benign (50 per cent) or neoplastic adenomas (50 per cent). The adenomas have a tubular histology (95 per cent) and show only mild dysplasia (97 per cent). These small adenomas rarely bleed. Infiltrating cancer in these small polyps is unusual (0.2 per cent). In contrast, larger polyps (greater than 1 cm) are largely (92 per cent) neoplastic with a villous histology (45 per cent), more severe dysplasia (17 per cent), and are more likely to have infiltrating cancer (7 per cent).[16] Larger polyps are more likely to bleed. Statistically significant risk factors for increasing grades of dysplasia include increasing polyp size, increasing villous histology, and increasing age of the patient. The sex of the patient and the location in the colon were not significant risk factors.[17] In the Rochester, Minnesota, population, 323 patients with polyps were identified and their outcome determined in retrospect. Follow-up was 80 per cent at 5 years and 65 per cent at 10 years. Twenty patients (6 per cent) developed colorectal cancer. Their risk of developing colorectal cancer was increased about threefold.[18] Another retrospective Mayo Clinic study identified 226 clinic patients in the six years before colonoscopy who had polyps greater than 1 cm in size that were demonstrated on x-ray. The patients elected to leave the polyp alone for one of several different reasons. While 37 per cent of the polyps enlarged with time on x-ray, only 21 patients (9 per cent) developed colorectal cancer in the polyp, and 11 patients (5 per cent) developed colorectal cancer at a site distant from the index polyp. The cumulative risk of developing cancer in the index polyp was 8 per cent at 10 years.[19] It seems clear that a small but significant number of polyps greater than 1 cm will become invasive cancer with time. Increasing size, villous histology, and increasing patient age fail to explain the development of colorectal cancer adequately. There are prob-

COLORECTAL CANCER WITH AGE

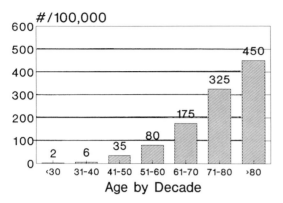

FIGURE 1.   The annual incidence of colorectal cancer in men, by age in decades. (Derived from Cutler SJ, Scotto J, Devesa SS, Connelly RR. Third national cancer survey—an overview of available information. J Natl Cancer Instit 1974;53:1565–75.)

ably more important factors that are yet to be described.

Cancer was present in 10 per cent of the patients, and all were considered a source of the hematochezia. Fissures, proctitis, rectal prolapse, and a number of other lesions were less common causes. A large percentage (40 per cent) of the patients had more than one lesion, and 60 per cent of the patients were judged to be bleeding from more than one site.[2] The documentation that hemorrhoidal bleeding is present does not exclude a neoplasm.

Occult Blood Positive

The cost-effectiveness of flexible sigmoidoscopy plus air contrast barium enema was compared with colonoscopy in 332 patients. All patients had hemoccult positive stools, and 35 to 40 per cent had noted hematochezia in the previous six months. They concluded that flexible sigmoidoscopy plus air contrast barium enema was more cost-effective for patients less than 55 years of age, whereas colonoscopy was more cost-effective in patients over 55. Colon cancer occurred in 1 per cent of the group less than 55 years and was 8 per cent in those over 55 years of age.[20] Angiomata, significant polyps, and cancer increase with age, accounting for the cost advantage of colonoscopy. It is our understanding that costs vary widely around the United States. Groups interested in cost-effectiveness should determine their local costs and options.

Colon Cancer

As depicted in Figure 1, colorectal cancer in men in the 41- to 50-age group begins to be a clinical problem with an incidence of 35 per 100,000 (0.04 per cent). The incidence increases with age to 450 per 100,000 (0.45 per cent) in those above 80 years of age.[21] Right-sided colon cancers are increasing, and more elderly women seem to be getting colon cancer. The symptoms of colon cancer, which include hematochezia, change in bowel habits, and abdominal pain or distress, occur late and are not very specific. Hematochezia is noted by only 50 per cent of the patients but is more common with distal cancers. The Dukes' stage of invasiveness is not related to the length of the history.[22] These problems have led to efforts to detect colon cancer earlier by occult blood screening in asymptomatic people. Interim reports of controlled clinical trials in people 50 to 74 years of age have shown that early Dukes A cancer, localized to the mucosa, is detected earlier (52 per cent of cancers) in screened groups compared with controls (11 per cent of cancers).[23] The question that remains is, Does earlier detection lead to increased survival? The answer to this question should be available in a few more years. Perhaps survival is more related to the genetic changes in the cells of the individual's colon, polyps, or cancer, rather than early detection.[24]

REFERENCES

1. Jensen DM, Machicado GA. Diagnosis and treatment of severe hematochezia. The role of urgent colonoscopy after purge. Gastroenterology 1988; 95:1569–74.
2. Goulston KJ, Cook I, Dent OF. How important is rectal bleeding in the diagnosis of bowel cancer and polyps? Lancet 1986;2:261–4.
3. Hassall E, Barclay GN, Ament ME. Colonoscopy in childhood. Pediatrics 1984;73:594–9.

4. Gryboski JD. Diseases of the colon, rectum and anus in children. In: Kirsner JB, Shorter RG, eds. Diseases of the colon, rectum and anal canal. Baltimore: Williams & Wilkins, 1988:595–686.

5. Bogoch H. Bleeding. In: Berk JE, ed. Bockus gastroenterology. Philadelphia: WB Saunders, 1985:65–110.

6. Knight KK, Fielding JE, Battista RN. Occult blood screening for colorectal cancer. JAMA 1989;261:587–93.

7. Peterson WL. Gastrointestinal bleeding. In: Sleisenger MH, Fordtran JS, eds. Gastrointestinal disease. Pathophysiology, diagnosis, management. Philadelphia: WB Saunders, 1989:397–427.

8. Dent OF, Goulston KJ, Kubrzycki J, Chapuis PH. Bowel symptoms in an apparently well population. Dis Colon Rectum 1986;29:243–7.

9. Gilbert DA, Shaneyfelt SL, Silverstein FE, Mahler AK, Hallstrom AP. The national ASGE colonoscopy survey. Analysis of colonoscopy practices and yield [Abstract]. Gastrointest Endosc 1984;30:143.

10. Laufer I, Smith NCW, Mullens JE. The radiological demonstration of colorectal polyps undetected by endoscopy. Gastroenterology 1976;70:167–70.

11. Gilbert DA, Hallstrom AP, Shaneyfelt SL, Mahler AK, Silverstein FE. The national ASGE colonoscopy survey—complications of colonoscopy [Abstract]. Gastrointest Endosc 1984;30:156.

12. Silverstein FE, Gilbert DA, Tedesco FJ, Buenger NK, Persing J. The national ASGE survey on upper gastrointestinal bleeding. II. Clinical prognostic factors. Gastrointest Endosc 1981;27:80–93.

13. Scapa A, Horowitz M, Waron M, Eshchar J. Duodenal ulcer in the elderly. J Clin Gastroenterol 1989;11:502–6.

14. Parks TG. Post-mortem studies on the colon with special reference to diverticular disease. Proc R Soc Med 1968; 61:932–4.

15. Almy TP, Howell DA. Diverticular disease of the colon. N Engl J Med 1980;302:324–31.

16. Gottleib LS, Winawer SJ, Sternberg S, et al. National polyp study (NPS): the diminutive colonic polyp [Abstract]. Gastrointest Endosc 1984;30:143.

17. O'Brien MJ, Winawer SJ, Zauber AG, et al. The national polyp study. Patient and polyp characteristics associated with high-grade dysplasia in colorectal adenomas. Gastroenterology 1990;98:371–9.

18. Lotfi AM, Spencer RJ, Ilstrup DM, Melton LJ III. Colorectal polyps and the risk of subsequent carcinoma. Mayo Clin Proc 1986;61:337–43.

19. Stryker SJ, Wolfea BG, Culp CE, Libbe SD, Ilstrup DM, MacCarty RL. Natural history of untreated colonic polyps. Gastroenterology 1987;93:1009–13.

20. Rex DK, Weddle RA, Lehman GA, et al. Flexible sigmoidoscopy plus air contrast barium enema versus colonoscopy for suspected lower gastrointestinal bleeding. Gastroenterology 1990;98:855–61.

21. Cutler SJ, Scotto J, Devesa SS, Connelly RR. Third national cancer survey—an overview of available information. J Natl Cancer Instit 1974;53:1565–75.

22. Payne JE. Symptoms and the diagnosis of bowel cancer: a critical review. Med J Aust 1988;148:505–7.

23. Hardcastle JD, Thomas WM, Chamberlain J, et al. Randomized, controlled trial of faecal occult blood screening for colorectal cancer. Results for first 107,349 subjects. Lancet 1989;1:1160–4.

24. Marx J. Many gene changes found in cancer. Science 1989 Dec 15: 1386–8.

HEPATOMEGALY

ALBERT J. CZAJA

SYNONYMS: Enlarged Liver, Hepatic Enlargement, Increased Liver Size

BACKGROUND

Hepatomegaly connotes abnormal enlargement of the liver, and its detection requires an appreciation of the variations of normal, the application of proper diagnostic techniques during physical examination, and recognition of the pitfalls in diagnosis.

Hepatic enlargement may be the first clinical indication of intrinsic liver disease or systemic illness, and its presence implies a pathologic disorder of an inflammatory, infiltrative, or congestive nature. An accurate assessment of liver size is essential to key the diagnostic workup, and reliable sequential assessments are necessary to monitor disease progression or resolution. Although most enlarged livers are palpable, palpable livers are not always enlarged, and estimates of hepatomegaly by palpation have not correlated with hepatic scintigraphy or necropsy findings.[1,2] Before embarking on an evaluation that may be costly, uncomfortable, anxiety provoking, and hazardous, the presence of hepatomegaly must be established with certainty.

The normal liver extends from the right fifth intercostal space in the midclavicular line to the right costal margin. With deep inspiration, its edge may descend 1 to 3 cm, and it can be palpated normally on physical examination.[3] Additionally, a normal-sized liver may be displaced inferiorly by disease processes, such as subdiaphragmatic abscess, chronic obstructive lung disease, or retroperitoneal mass, or its palpability may be enhanced by anatomic variations, such as pectus excavatum, flared costal margins, or Reidel's lobe.[3] The most objective assessment of hepatomegaly is by direct measurement at autopsy or at orthotopic liver transplantation. A liver weight that exceeds 1600 gm establishes the diagnosis of hepatomegaly but at a time when the information has little clinical advantage.

The most useful and practical method of estimating liver size is by percussion of the upper and lower borders of the liver in the right midclavicular and midsternal lines.[4] Scintiscans of the liver correlate well with measurements of liver size at autopsy, and percussion is better than palpation in correlating with scintigraphic findings.[1,2] Hard percussion of the liver borders is associated with a smaller estimate of liver span than soft percussion and it may improve the reproducibility of the findings between examiners.[4] Despite standardization of percussion technique, however, interexaminer variation in the estimate of liver dullness may be significant, and determination of liver size by percussion must be recognized as an imprecise but useful clinical assessment.[4]

Liver spans estimated by percussion have been shown to be reproducible by a given physician, larger for males than for females, and positively correlated with body height.[4] The expected liver dullness in the midclavicular line can be calculated from equations in men (span of dullness in centimeters = 0.032 × weight in pounds + 0.18 × height in inches − 7.86) and women (span of dullness in centimeters = 0.027 × weight in pounds + 0.22 × height in inches − 10.75) that predict the midclavicular line liver size for normal adults with a 95 per cent confidence limit of ±3 cm.[4] These analyses emphasize that the range of normal liver size varies according to sex, height, and weight and that such factors must be included in any clinical assessment of hepatomegaly. The normal liver dullness for an adult man weighing 200 lb and measuring 73 in is 11.7 ± 3 cm. The normal liver dullness for an adult woman weighing 120 lb and measuring 68 in is 7.4 ± 3 cm. Application of these principles in clinical practice should increase the sensitivity and specificity of the physical examination for the presence of hepatomegaly.

Hepatic scintigraphy is the most well studied and objective premortem method of assessing liver size, and its estimation of hepatomegaly has correlated well with necropsy findings.[1,2] Hepatic ultrasonography, computed tomography (CT), and magnetic resonance imaging (MRI) may also be used to evaluate liver enlargement. Fortunately, the clinical perception of hepatomegaly by percussion is sufficiently accurate to rarely require corroboration by one or more of these imaging techniques. Each, however, may be extremely useful later in the evaluation to clarify the causes of hepatomegaly.

HISTORY

History of the Present Illness

Symptoms should be accurately recorded, with emphasis on the rapidity and order of their development. A gradually evolving illness over a 6-month period or longer satisfies criteria for chronic liver disease and suggests the possibility of a chronic viral infection (hepatitis B or C infection), an autoimmune or idiopathic process (primary biliary cirrhosis, nonviral chronic active hepatitis, primary sclerosing cholangitis), metabolic disorder (hemochromatosis, alpha-1-antitrypsin deficiency, Wilson's disease, nonalcoholic steatohepatitis), infiltrative process (steatosis, amyloidosis), or chronic toxic exposure (alcohol, medication). Illness that evolves insidiously but over a period of less than six months' duration may be attributable to any of the above diseases, but other considerations should be malignancy (primary or metastatic), biliary obstruction, passive congestion (chronic heart failure, constrictive pericarditis, inferior vena caval obstruction, hepatic vein thrombosis, or veno-occlusive disease), and slowly resolving acute viral hepatitis or impaired regeneration syndrome. The abrupt onset of symptoms suggests an acute liver injury of an infectious (viral), toxic (medications, alcohol, organic solvents), congestive (acute heart failure), ischemic (hypotension), or hypoxic (respiratory failure) nature. Unfortunately, the assessment of duration of illness is mainly subjective, frequently inaccurate, and not disease specific. Up to 40 per cent of patients with chronic active hepatitis may present as an acute illness,[5] and patients with indolent chronic liver disease may have a superimposed disorder (viral infection, drug toxicity, or malignancy) that is expressed clinically as an acute decompensation.

The nature of the symptoms and the sequence of their evolution aid in the diagnosis of liver enlargement. Pruritus is a symptom of cholestasis, and if it is the main complaint, diseases of the interlobular bile ducts (primary biliary cirrhosis, small duct primary sclerosing cholangitis, ductopenic liver disease, cholestatic drug toxicity), intrahepatic bile ducts (primary sclerosing cholangitis, cholangiocarcinoma), and extrahepatic bile ducts (primary sclerosing cholangitis, ampullary cancer, cancer of the pancreatic head) must be excluded. Concomitant features of right upper quadrant abdominal pain and fever indicate cholangitis, and the entire symptom complex suggests mechanical obstruction of the biliary tract, typically of the extrahepatic system.

Jaundice, dark urine, and light stools also reflect cholestasis, but when they develop before pruritus or in its absence, an intrahepatic disorder should be considered such as acute viral or drug-induced hepatitis or advanced chronic liver disease.[3] Painless jaundice suggests a neoplasm obstructing the distal common bile duct, such as ampullary or pancreatic cancer, and the presence of a palpable gallbladder enhances the likelihood of this diagnosis. Silver-colored stools reflect the presence of blood in an acholic substrate, and they suggest bleeding from an obstructing biliary or ampullary malignancy. Intermittent jaundice and occult blood in the stool also suggest a neoplasm of the biliary tract. Lesions at the bifurcation of the common hepatic duct can slough, bleed, and unobstruct periodically.

Easy fatigability, diminished stamina, and malaise are common findings in acute and chronic liver disease.[6] The symptoms may be incapacitating, unassociated with other features, and out of proportion to other clinical, biochemical, or histologic findings. Malaise associated with acute viral hepatitis is commonly associated with other prodromal features that facilitate the diagnosis. Fever, headache, myalgias, and anorexia are compatible with acute hepatitis A infection. Serum sickness features such as urticaria and synovitis suggest acute hepatitis B infection, whereas pharyngitis, rash, and lymphadenopathy characterize infections with Epstein-Barr virus or cytomegalovirus.[7,8] Fever, nausea, and right upper quadrant pain may accompany the malaise and jaundice of acute alcoholic hepatitis, and increasing abdominal girth indicative of ascites may accompany the malaise of advanced chronic liver disease, hepatic malignancy, or hepatic vein outflow obstruction. Easy fatigability and malaise in the absence of other prodromal features suggest chronic liver disease or a malignant process.

Increasing abdominal girth connotes ascites formation, and it is a complaint that is typically associated with chronic liver disease, hepatic venous obstruction, and peritoneal inflammation or infiltration. Mental confusion, somnolence, and tremulousness are commonly features of hepatic encephalopathy. Hepatic encephalopathy that develops within eight weeks of an acute hepatitis connotes fulminant hepatic failure and a high mortality.

Anorexia is another common systemic manifestation of acute or chronic liver disease, and it has no disease specificity. Nausea and vomiting, however, suggest an acute severe hepatic insult of a viral, drug, or metabolic basis (Reye's syndrome). Significant weight loss is unusual except in malignant disorders, chronic cholestatic diseases associated with maldigestion or malabsorption (primary biliary cirrhosis), or advanced cirrhosis.

Hyperpigmentation is typically a feature of chronic cholestatic liver disease (primary biliary cirrhosis), but its recognition should also suggest the possibility of hemochromatosis. Hirsutism, acne, and cushingoid features are infrequent manifestations of autoimmune chronic active hepatitis, whereas hirsutism, photosensitive skin, and hyperpigmentation are typical features of porphyria cutanea tarda. Urticaria and petechiae are features of immune complex disease, and ecchymoses are most compatible with advanced chronic liver disease with hypersplenism and thrombocytopenia.

A thorough clinical history should permit classification of the hepatic disorder as acute or chronic, cholestatic or noncholestatic, and systemic or nonsystemic in nature. A review of epidemiologic factors, drug history, toxic exposures, and family history will clarify the basis of the disorder.

Family History

The family history should focus on the possibilities of an infectious or hereditary basis for the hepatomegaly. Secondary spread among family members of acute viral hepatitis should be considered in all patients with an acute hepatocellular inflammation. Hepatitis A virus is an enteric organism with a fecal-oral mode of transmission, and it can be spread by household contact or food contamination.[7] Hepatitis B virus is spread mainly by parenteral inoculation, and acute hepatitis B infection is uncommon in the household. Nevertheless, spouse or sexual contacts are at risk for developing type B infection, as are household contacts.[7] Secondary spread of hepatitis C infection within the family is rare.[8]

Perinatal transmission of hepatitis B virus from mother to infant is well documented.[7] and inquiry about the hepatitis status of the mother is warranted in all cases of type B infection in children, especially if the family has immigrated from areas of high endemicity for hepatitis B virus infection (Asia, Africa, Italy) or there is a familial background of illicit drug use.

Wilson's disease, hemochromatosis, and alpha-1-antitrypsin deficiency are chronic liver diseases with a familial basis, and a careful family history may suggest one of these diagnoses.[9] A family history of hepatocellular cancer may be an important clue to the presence of a familial basis for chronic liver disease such as hepatitis B virus infection, hemochromatosis, alpha-1-antitrypsin deficiency, or exposure to an environmental toxin (aflatoxin). Alcoholic liver disease may also have a familial association.

Social and Occupational History

Evidence of exposure to infectious or toxic agents must be sought, and a careful travel history should be obtained. Homosexual contact, promiscuous sexual activity, illicit drug use, receipt of blood transfusions, exposure to hepatotoxic medication or environmental toxins, and alcohol abuse must each be assessed by direct questioning. Health care providers and institutionalized or imprisoned patients are at risk for hepatitis infection. Vinyl chloride workers (angiosarcoma), asbestos workers (peritoneal meseothelioma), body builders using anabolic steroids (peliosis hepatis, hepatocellular cancer), and women on birth control pills (hepatic adenoma, cholestatic liver disease, hepatic vein thrombosis) are also at risk for hepatomegaly.

Past Medical History

A past medical history of diabetes or heart disease suggests the possibility of steatohepatitis, hemochromatosis, chronic passive congestion of the liver, or amyloidosis. Previous surgeries may have been associated with blood transfusions or exposures to anesthetic agents (halothane) or other potentially hepatotoxic medications, and a history of malignancy raises the specter of metastatic disease, especially if the primary lesion was of lung, colon, or breast origin. Any chronic disorder requiring regular medication on a long-term basis suggests the possibility of a drug-induced liver injury, and a history of ulcerative colitis suggests the diagnoses of primary sclerosing cholangitis, cholangiocarcinoma, amyloidosis, and chronic active hepatitis. Systemic sclerosis and Sjögren's syndrome may be associated with primary biliary cirrhosis, and thyroiditis, synovitis, nephritis, or iritis may be linked to autoimmune chronic active hepatitis. Systemic disorders such as sarcoidosis, polyarteritis, tuberculosis, lymphoma, myeloproliferative disorders, acquired immune deficiency syndrome, sepsis, and shock may all have hepatic manifestations. Pulmonary disease may be a result of the liver disease (intrapulmonary shunting) or a concomitant disorder (pulmonary hypertension, fibrosing alveolitis, alpha-1-antitrypsin deficiency). Recognition that intrinsic diseases of the liver frequently have extrahepatic manifestations or disease associations and that systemic disorders of an infectious, metabolic, immunologic, or malignant nature frequently have hepatic manifestations will facilitate the acquisition of a pertinent past medical history.

Focused Queries

1. *When was the first indication of liver disease?* Disease of six months or longer is chronic. Disease of 10 weeks or less is acute. Disease of 10 weeks' to 6 months' duration may be a slowly resolving acute process or early chronic disease. Such processes may be called subacute.

2. *What are the major symptoms?* Pruritus suggests cholestatic disease. Easy fatigability,

anorexia, and malaise are compatible with acute or chronic hepatocellular inflammation. Nausea and vomiting suggest acute hepatic necrosis, and weight loss is consistent with advanced cirrhosis and primary or metastatic malignancy. Fever may reflect systemic infection, acute viral hepatitis, severe chronic active hepatitis, hepatic abscess, or cholangitis. Jaundice in the absence of pruritus suggests viral infection, drug toxicity, decompensated chronic liver disease, or malignant obstruction of the biliary tract.

3. *Has there been an increase in abdominal girth, unexplained weight gain, or swelling of the ankles?* Ascites and fluid retention are most commonly manifestations of advanced chronic liver disease with cirrhosis, hypoalbuminemia, and functional renal insufficiency. The rapid accumulation of ascites suggests hepatic outflow obstruction or right-sided heart failure.

4. *Have there been any changes in sensorium?* Manifestations of hepatic encephalopathy indicate severe hepatic dysfunction. In association with acute liver disease, it signals fulminant hepatic failure (if present within 8 weeks of liver disease) or late onset hepatic failure (if present 8 to 24 weeks after liver disease). Cerebral edema may be a complicating factor that contributes to morbidity and mortality. In association with chronic liver disease, hepatic encephalopathy reflects progressive hepatic failure (endogenous encephalopathy) or portal systemic shunting and precipitating factors (exogenous encephalopathy). Chronic encephalopathy may be rapidly reversed if aggravating factors such as infection, drugs, electrolyte imbalance, gastrointestinal bleeding, excessive protein intake, and renal insufficiency are eliminated.

5. *Have there been black stools or vomiting of blood?* Features of gastrointestinal bleeding may be associated with portal hypertension, which is typically a manifestation of advanced chronic liver disease and cirrhosis. Bleeding may be from esophageal or gastric varices or a congestive gastropathy.

6. *Is there any history of previous jaundice, contact with individuals with liver disease, exposure to illicit drugs, homosexual contact, alcohol use, receipt of blood transfusion, or familial liver disease?* Once the acute or chronic nature of the disease has been established, cholestatic and hepatocellular manifestations detailed, and degree of liver decompensation assessed, the questioning can be directed toward etiologic considerations.

PHYSICAL EXAMINATION

Body Habitus

Facial rounding, dorsal hump formation, enhancement of supraclavicular fat pads, and truncal obesity are cushingoid features that suggest autoimmune chronic active hepatitis or corticosteroid-treated chronic liver disease. Cachexia and muscle atrophy indicate advanced cirrhosis or malignancy.

Skin Examination

Jaundice reflects hepatic excretory dysfunction of a hepatocellular or obstructive nature. Hemolysis or shortened red blood cell survival may be associated with acute viral hepatitis (glucose-6-phosphate dehydrogenase deficiency), Wilson's disease, hypersplenism, autoimmune chronic active hepatitis (Coombs' positive hemolysis), alcoholic hepatitis, and cirrhosis (disseminated intravascular coagulation, intravascular hemolysis), and it can accentuate the hyperbilirubinemia. Extreme jaundice usually signifies a combination of intrinsic liver disease and either shortened red blood cell survival or renal insufficiency or both.

Palmar and malar erythema, spider angiomata, Dupuytren's contractures, and striae are stigmata of chronic liver disease, and excoriations are hallmarks of severe pruritus. Hirsutism, acne, white finger-nails, and ecchymoses are features of chronic liver disease, especially chronic active hepatitis. Urticaria indicates immune complex disease, and photosensitivity suggests porphyria cutanea tarda. Hyperpigmentation is a clue to the diagnosis of chronic cholestatic disease (primary biliary cirrhosis) and hemochromatosis.

Head and Neck Examination

Icterus of the sclerae and buccal mucosa may be the only manifestations of jaundice. Kayser-Fleischer rings suggest the diagnosis of Wilson's disease. Nonwilsonian chronic cholestatic liver diseases may also be associated with Kayser-Fleischer rings, but these are detectable only by slit-lamp examination. Pharyngitis suggests Epstein-Barr virus infection, and dry eyes and dry mouth are commonly associated with primary biliary cirrhosis. Adenopathy may be associated with acute viral hepatitis, but it is always worrisome for a lymphoproliferative, granulomatous, or metastatic process. Thyromegaly suggests autoimmune chronic active hepatitis or Graves' disease, and distended neck veins infer congestive heart failure and hepatic congestion. Constrictive pericarditis may be suspected from the behavior of the neck vein pulsations. Fetor hepaticus reflects an impairment in hepatic detoxification.

Chest Examination

Gynecomastia connotes chronic liver disease and cirrhosis, whereas features of emphysema suggest alpha-1-antitrypsin deficiency. Wheezing may be a manifestation of congestive heart failure or carcinoid syndrome with metastases to the liver. Dyspnea suggests intrapulmonary shunting. It may improve in the supine position and be accompanied by clubbing of the fingernails. Diminished diaphragmatic excursion from ascites or the presence of pleural effusions in association with ascites may also cause dyspnea.

Cardiac Examination

Cardiomegaly suggests that congestive heart failure may be a cause of the hepatomegaly. Additionally, cardiomyopathies associated with hemochromatosis, alcoholism, and amyloidosis may be directly linked to the liver disease. Constrictive pericarditis and severe tricuspid insufficiency are treatable cardiac conditions that may cause hepatomegaly and ascites.

Abdominal Examination

The size (midclavicular and midsternal spans), shape (symmetric or asymmetric), consistency (soft, firm, stony-hard), surface texture (smooth, irregular, nodular), and edge (sharp, blunt) of the liver should be evaluated, and tenderness, rubs, and bruits should be sought.[10] Asymmetric enlargement suggests a space-occupying lesion (primary or metastatic tumor, bacterial or parasitic abscess, benign cyst). Lobar atrophy and compensatory hypertrophy may also produce asymmetric hepatomegaly, and it can result from proximal hepatic bile duct obstruction, nodular regeneration, hepatic ischemia, lobar infarction, or radiation injury. Firm hepatomegaly indicates an infiltrated, fibrotic, or congested state, as does a blunt or rounded liver edge. Rock-hard enlargement suggests malignancy and surface nodularity is compatible with cirrhosis and/or

hepatic neoplasm. Diffuse liver tenderness connotes generalized distension of the hepatic capsule, usually as a result of congestion or inflammation, and hepatic pulsation underscores the likelihood of passive congestion of a cardiac origin. Focal tenderness suggests an abscess, infected cyst, or hemorrhagic lesion (vascular tumor, hepatic adenoma, regenerative nodule). Rubs result from inflammation of the capsule, and they develop after capsular trauma (liver biopsy), infection (gonococcemia), or malignancy (surface implants). Hepatic bruits suggest a vascular tumor, arteriovenous fistula, or portal hypertension (venous hum).

Splenomegaly connotes viral infection, splenic or portal vein thrombosis, granulomatous disease, a lymphoproliferative disorder, or chronic liver disease with portal hypertension. Massive splenomegaly suggests a hematologic malignancy or storage disorder.

Ascites is usually a manifestation of chronic liver disease, hepatic vein outflow obstruction, or peritoneal inflammation or malignancy. A caput medusae signifies portal hypertension, whereas prominent superficial abdominal veins below the umbilicus that drain cephalad suggest an inferior vena caval obstruction.

Extremity Examination

The presence of pedal edema, clubbing of fingers and toes, cyanosis, and Dupuytren's contractures should be recorded.

Neurologic Examination

Disorientation may be an early sign of hepatic encephalopathy. Failure to complete simple calculations, connect numbers in sequence with facility, and write or draw without tremor is compatible with this diagnosis. A flapping tremor (asterixis) is a characteristic, but nonspecific, neurologic manifestation of this type of metabolic encephalopathy. Personality changes, slurred speech, hypertonicity, gross tremor, especially of a wing-beating type, suggest Wilson's disease.

DIAGNOSTIC STUDIES

Clinical Laboratory Tests

Laboratory tests permit classification of the liver disease into inflammatory, obstructive, or infiltrative categories. Biochemical profiles in which the predominant abnormalities are elevations of serum aspartate aminotransferase (AST) and alanine aminotransferase (ALT) levels indicate hepatocellular inflammation and necrosis. Extreme aminotransferase elevations (equal to or greater than 1000 U/L) connote acute viral, drug, toxic, or ischemic injury. Rarely, passage of a common duct stone will present in this fashion. Disproportionate elevation of the AST level above the ALT level suggests alcoholic liver disease.

Predominant elevation of the serum alkaline phosphatase level (hepatic isoenzyme) and/or gamma-glutamyl transferase concentration suggests an obstructive (cholestatic) or infiltrative disorder. Elevation of the total bilirubin level connotes a hepatic excretory defect, and it can occur with severe hepatocellular inflammation as well as biliary obstruction. A high alkaline phosphatase level in the absence of hyperbilirubinemia suggests infiltrative liver disease or partial extrahepatic biliary obstruction.

The synthetic functions of the liver can be assessed by determinations of the prothrombin time and serum albumin level. Correction of the prothrombin time by administration of vitamin K may distinguish extrahepatic obstruction from hepatocellular disease. An abnormal prothrombin time and normal albumin level indicate acute liver disease. The serum gamma globulin level as well as the albumin concentration can provide insight into the chronicity of the disorder. The more chronic the disease, the more likely that there will be derangements of these indices. Hypergammaglobulinemia may also reflect the severity of hepatocellular inflammation. The blood ammonia level is a reflection of the detoxification function of the liver and portal systemic shunting. Its elevation supports the diagnosis of hepatic encephalopathy.

Additional laboratory tests with etiologic implications for acute hepatomegaly include hepatitis A, B, C, and D serologic markers (IgM anti-HAV, HBsAg, anti-HBc, IgM anti-HBc, anti-HCV, anti-HDV), alcohol and drug screens, monospot test, and Epstein-Barr virus or cytomegalovirus serologic assays. Ferritin, ceruloplasmin, alpha-fetoprotein, carcinoembryonic antigen, immunoserologic markers (antimitochondrial, antinuclear, and smooth muscle antibodies), copper level, and alpha-1-antitrypsin phenotype should be determined as appropriate for the evaluation of chronic hepatomegaly.[9] Since decompensated chronic disease may present acutely, the laboratory assessment must be flexible and reflective of all diagnostic possibilities.

Diagnostic Imaging

Ultrasonography of the liver and upper abdomen is invaluable in the assessment of hepatomegaly. Focal defects (abscess, cyst, primary neoplasm, metastatic disease), dilated intrahepatic and extrahepatic bile ducts, gallbladder distension and stones, pancreatic enlargement, ascites, and patency of hepatic, portal, and splenic veins can be evaluated by this technique.[10] Hepatic scintigraphy can aid in the assessment of liver size, space-occupying lesions, hepatic vein occlusion (caudate lobe hypertrophy), and portal hypertension with shunting (increased uptake in spine and pelvis), but generally it is a nonspecific and insensitive technique that has been replaced by ultrasonography.

CAT scan of the liver and abdomen with contrast enhancement is an excellent method for evaluating hepatic masses, pancreatic lesions, retroperitoneal nodal metastases, ascites, and biliary tract dilatation.[10] CT can provide a confident diagnosis of cavernous hemangioma, suggest the possibility of hemochromatosis and Budd-Chiari syndrome, and assess the resectability of malignant lesions. MRI is ideally suited for the evaluation of vascular lesions, hepatic and portal vein patency, and tumor resectability.

Percutaneous transhepatic cholangiography (PTC) and endoscopic retrograde cholangiopancreatography (ERCP) are required for the assessment of the biliary tract.[10] PTC is used mainly to assess dilated bile ducts or the biliary tree that has been rendered inaccessible to ERCP by previous surgery. ERCP is useful in assessing nondilated ducts (primary sclerosing cholangitis), focal intrahepatic ductal disease, distal duct obstruction, and pancreatic masses. ERCP may permit sphincterotomy, stone extraction, brush cytology, and biliary stent placement. Biliary decompression, stenting, tissue sampling, and dilatation of strictures are also possible by PTC, and it is a preferred technique for proximal lesions.

Hepatic arteriography is used mainly to evaluate hepatic trauma, mass lesions, vascular fistulae, vascular anatomy before hepatic resection or portal vein surgery, and portal and splenic vein patency.[10] Hepatic venography is essential in the assessment of hepatic vein outflow obstruction. Right atrial, inferior vena caval, hepatic vein, and wedged hepatic vein pressures can also be determined to assess causes for portal hypertension and ascites formation.

Peritoneoscopy permits examination of the liver surface, gallbladder, spleen, and peritoneum. A visually directed biopsy from the most representative area of abnormality can be obtained.[10]

Tissue Examination

Liver biopsy examination is essential in the evaluation of chronic hepatomegaly if bleeding indices (prothrombin time, platelet count, bleeding time) are satisfactory or can be corrected. Tissue sampling may be necessary in the evaluation of acute hepatomegaly if there are questions of steatosis (Reye's syndrome), alcoholic liver disease, centrilobular congestion, or chronic liver disease. Transjugular liver biopsy can be performed in the presence of an uncorrectable bleeding disorder. Chronic inflammatory and diffusely infiltrative processes can be reliably sampled without direct visual guidance of the needle into the liver substance. Focal lesions, however, should be sampled under the guidance of ultrasonography, CT scan, or peritoneoscopy. Sampling error commonly prevents the diagnosis of cirrhosis, and this diagnosis may require peritoneoscopy for confirmation or exclusion.[11] Special stains (iron, periodic acid—Schiff's copper, acid-fast), fungal, viral, and mycobacterial cultures, and determinations of tissue concentrations of copper and iron enhance diagnostic accuracy.

ASSESSMENT

The causes of hepatomegaly are usually of an inflammatory, infiltrative, or congestive nature. The clinical history, physical findings, laboratory studies, imaging techniques, and tissue examination will usually establish the correct diagnosis.

Hepatic Inflammation

Hepatic inflammation is most commonly due to viral infection or drug toxicity. Hepatitis A, B, and C infections are responsible for most cases of acute hepatitis, and type B and C infections may produce chronic disease. Alcohol remains the major cause of acute and chronic liver disease, and it is associated with

TABLE 1. Causes of Hepatomegaly

INFLAMMATION
Hepatitis A, B, and C viruses
Alcohol, drugs, toxins
Chronic active hepatitis
Primary biliary cirrhosis
Primary sclerosing cholangitis
Wilson's disease
Sickle cell anemia
Polyarteritis
Infectious mononucleosis
Cytomegalovirus
Herpes simplex
Leptospirosis
Tuberculosis
Histoplasmosis
Actinomycosis
Brucellosis
Syphillis
Ascaris lumbricoides
Schistosoma mansoni
Echinococcus granulosus
Toxocara canis
Entamoeba histolytica
Opisthorchis sinensis
Leishmania donovani
Plasmodium falciparum and *vivax*

INFILTRATION AND STORAGE
Primary or metastatic cancer
Steatosis
Amyloidosis
Alpha-1-antitrypsin deficiency
Hemochromatosis
Sarcoidosis
von Gierke's disease
Niemann-Pick disease
Gaucher's disease
Lymphoma
Agnogenic myeloid metaplasia

VASCULAR AND BILIARY CONGESTION
Congestive heart failure
Cor pulmonale
Constrictive pericarditis
Hepatic vein occlusion
Inferior vena caval obstruction
Veno-occlusive disease
Common bile duct tumor
Biliary stricture
Choledocholithiasis
Pancreatic cancer
Ampullary cancer

the largest livers. Generalized viral and bacterial infections may be associated with hepatic inflammation, and various parasites have a predilection for the liver (Table 1).

Hepatic Infiltration

Infiltrative disorders include primary or metastatic malignancy, hematologic or reticuloendothelial (granulomatous) disorders, and metabolic or storage diseases (Table 1). The most common infiltrative disorder is fat accumulation from obesity, diabetes, protein-calorie malnutrition, hyperalimentation, or jejunoileal bypass (rare now).

Hepatic Congestion

Dilatation of the sinusoidal and vascular spaces of the liver produces hepatomegaly. The most common causes are congestive heart failure, cor pulmonale, and constrictive pericarditis (Table 1). Chronic large bile duct obstruction by strictures, stone, or tumor can also produce a "congestive" hepatomegaly.

REFERENCES

1. Naftalis J, Leevy CM. Clinical estimation of liver size. Am J Dig Dis 1963;8:236–43.
2. Peternel WW, Schaefer JW, Schiff L. Clinical evaluation of liver size and hepatic scintiscan. Am J Dig Dis 1966;11:346–50.
3. Czaja AJ. Axioms on hepatomegaly. Hosp Med 1980;16:43–57.
4. Castell DO, O'Brien KD, Muench H, Chalmers TC. Estimation of liver size by percussion in normal individuals. Ann Intern Med 1969;70:1183–9.
5. Davis GL, Czaja AJ, Baggenstoss AH, Taswell HF. Prognostic and therapeutic implications of extreme serum aminotransferase elevation in chronic active hepatitis. Mayo Clin Proc 1982; 57:303–9.
6. Czaja AJ. Clinical features of chronic active hepatitis. In: Gitnick G, ed. Modern concepts of acute and chronic hepatitis. New York: Plenum, 1989: 269–81.
7. Czaja AJ. Serologic markers of hepatitis A and B in acute and chronic liver disease. Mayo Clin Proc 1979;54:721–32.
8. Czaja AJ, Davis GL. Hepatitis non A, non B. Manifestations and implications of acute and chronic disease. Mayo Clin Proc 1982;57:639–52.
9. Czaja AJ. Diagnosis and treatment of chronic hepatitis. Compr Ther 1984;10:58–63.
10. Czaja AJ. Causes of liver enlargement. Hosp Med 1985;21:143–78.
11. Czaja AJ, Wolf AM, Baggenstoss AH. Clinical assessment of cirrhosis in severe chronic active liver disease. Mayo Clin Proc 1980;55:360–4.

HOARSENESS

LAURENE L. HOWELL and EDWIN C. EVERTS

SYNONYMS: Dysphonia, Laryngitis

BACKGROUND

Hoarseness is a general term used to describe an unnaturally rough, harsh, or deep voice. Patients may use the term to define any change in voice quality. The causes of hoarseness include a variety of functional and pathologic processes that affect the larynx. Voice quality can also be affected by problems separate from the larynx that interfere with normal resonance. The resonating chambers are located above the vocal cords and include the pharynx, oral cavity, sinuses, and nasal cavity (see Fig. 1). The sound produced by the larynx is amplified by these resonating cavities and can be modified by partial closure or changes in shape (i.e., uvula, soft palate, tongue position). The most easily identified resonance changes occur with total nasal obstruction (hyponasal sound) or a cleft palate defect (hypernasal sound). The following discussion is confined to alterations in voice resulting from laryngeal dysfunction.

Anatomy

A brief overview of anatomy is presented to aid in understanding voice production. The larynx serves several functions, one of which is phonation. Since the larynx is at the crossroads of the airway and foodway, it has life-dependent protective and respiratory functions.

The function of the larynx is dependent on an effective valvelike mechanism that has synchronized opening with diaphragmatic motion and respiration. The opening must be of a size to allow adequate air exchange. This valve must be very sensitive to ingress of any noxious fumes or foreign bodies, with a rapid reflex closure and cough response to remove the irritants.

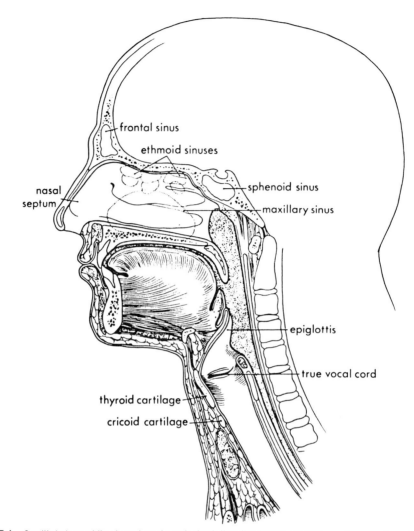

FIGURE 1. Sagittal view of the head and neck depicting the larynx, sinuses, and resonating chambers.

The larynx is housed by the thyroid cartilage. Each vocal cord consists of a vocal ligament and thyroarytenoid muscle. These structures are attached in the midline position anteriorly, and each muscle and ligament is attached to an arytenoid cartilage posteriorly (refer to Fig. 1 and Fig. 2).

The paired arytenoid cartilages sit on top of the cricoid cartilage in a posterior and lateral position. This important pair of joints (the cricoarytenoid joints) are synchronized to open the vocal cords during respiration and close the cords during phonation. If the cords are only partially closed during phonation, such as during whispering, a characteristic low-volume breathy voice is produced.

The intrinsic muscles of the larynx are used in the "fine-tuning" of phonation, with the thyroarytenoid muscles being the major adductors and the posterior cricoarytenoid muscles being the only abductors.

The larynx is lined by the same pink mucous membrane that covers the pharynx. Since the true vocal cords have a thin, delicate structure with few lymphatics or tissue bulk, they appear very white in contrast to the surrounding tissue (i.e., false vocal cords, aryepiglottic folds, arytenoids, and pyriform sinuses).

Voice Production

The voice is produced when the vocal folds are approximated and expiratory airflow escaping between the cords causes them to vibrate. Refinement of the voice is controlled by the tension of the vocal cords, thinness of the leading edges of the vocal cords, space between the vocal cords, and overall weight or

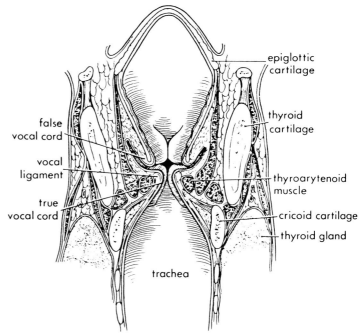

FIGURE 2. Coronal view of the larynx.

mass of the vocal cords, which all contribute to symmetry and frequency of vibration. With increased frequency of vibration, the voice has a higher pitch. Increased air velocity between the cords causes increased loudness of the sound.

Listening to the Voice

When listening to the voice, it is important to determine the source of the voice abnormality. Problems of resonance, articulation, and hoarseness should be distinguished. Resonance is affected by nasal obstruction, palatal incompetence, and sinus disease. Articulation problems and dysarthria result from oral muscular disorders. Hoarseness is an abnormal quality of the voice that originates with the larynx.

Evaluating the acoustic characteristics of the voice may be helpful when dealing with laryngeal problems. Acoustic evaluation includes such categories as range, loudness, pitch, register, and quality.

The patient's vocal range may be monotonal or excessively variable. Parkinson's disease has a characteristic monotonal voice. Voicing with lack of inflection may become a habit or reflect an underlining depression.

Generally, vocal loudness varies according to the surroundings. A patient who always uses a loud voice may have a sensorineural hearing loss. Excessive loudness may also indicate hyperfunction and be a contributing factor to vocal fatigue.

A soft voice may be characteristic of a patient's overall personality. Soft voicing can indicate neurologic disorders such as Parkinson's or bulbar palsy. The patient who is unable to speak in a loud voice may have vocal cord bowing, a laryngeal mass, or vocal cord paralysis.

The optimal vocal pitch requires the least physical effort and muscular energy. Forcing the voice above the usual high range results in a falsetto voice. The opposite of this is the very low pitched glottal fry. The usual speaking range is the modal register between these two extremes. A habitual low-pitched voice requires more effort to provide adequate volume. Very low pitched voices may slide into the glottal fry range and have a severe raspy sound. Men in particular may lower their vocal pitch intentionally, thinking it will enhance an authoritarian demeanor.

Pitch breaks are sudden changes in pitch during voicing. The most common example of this occurs in boys during puberty and is due to rapid growth changes in the larynx. Pitch breaks not associated with puberty usually occur with vocal hyperfunction and increased muscle tension. An abnormally low habitual pitch is much more common than an elevated pitch.

Phonation breaks are a temporary loss of voicing that may last for a single word or as long as a sentence. This sudden loss of voice is due to abductor spasm. It is associated with vocal hyperfunction and prolonged speaking. As vocal fatigue develops, many patients push harder, tightening muscles and increasing vocal tension.

If the voice quality is breathy, such as during whispering, this indicates a large air loss is occurring during phonation. Anything that prevents total vocal cord closure will result in a breathy voice. Vocal cord paresis or paralysis, vocal cord bowing, or atrophy will prevent total vocal cord adduction. A mass located on the leading edge of the vocal cord will also prevent total vocal cord closure.

HISTORY

History of the Present Illness

The information obtained about the onset, duration, and progression of symptoms will help guide any subsequent evaluation. Many forms of laryngitis look similar on initial examination but have very different causes. The best clues to the specific etiology for laryngitis are obtained through a very careful history. If the duration is less than two to three weeks, the laryngitis or hoarseness will be considered an acute problem, and the most likely etiology would be a viral upper respiratory infection. Symptoms that have extended beyond three weeks usually are due to a chronic laryngitis and are seldom due to an infectious etiology.

Additional questions about the initiating episode and mode of onset are helpful. If the patient noted persistent hoarseness after cheering vigorously at a sports event, the likely etiology is vocal abuse with physical findings, such as vocal cord edema, hemorrhage, vocal cord polyp formation, granulomas, or nodules. A history of easy onset vocal fatigue with pitch breaks is more likely due to vocal misuse and overuse resulting in intrinsic laryngeal muscle tension.

The history can become very detailed and extensive if the probable etiology is not apparent. Vocal abuse and misuse may take many forms and are frequently not acknowledged by the patient unless specific questions are asked. Does the patient talk frequently with hard-of-hearing friends, relatives, or coworkers? Are there small children in the house who prompt sudden, loud, verbal interactions for discipline or safety? Does the patient regularly talk from room to room or floor to floor in his or her home? Does the patient's work environment include noise, dust, fumes, or smoke? Does the patient have pollen allergies that have escalated this year? Is the patient a weight lifter who uses poor technique with a closed glottis? Does the patient travel frequently and talk during car and plane trips (when ambient noise levels are significant)?

Associated symptoms, such as frequent cough, shortness of breath, weight loss, symptoms of aspiration, odynophagia, dysphagia, ear pain, or throat pain, would raise a more urgent concern for neoplasm, systemic disease, or neurologic causes.

Additional information may be obtained from a list of the patient's current medications, including over-the-counter medications. Many drugs can and will affect the voice. A variety of medications cause drying and thickened secretions. The majority of these drugs also have a secondary effect of sedation. Drugs that affect proprioception and coordination may have a profound effect on the voice, especially during times of stress or performance. Medication containing androgens can permanently masculinize the female voice (see Table 1).

Focused Queries

1. *Is there a history of asthma?* Undiagnosed, poorly controlled asthma can result in a chronic cough with subsequent hoarseness. The reactive airway can include the trachea and larynx, with resulting mild edema and hoarseness.

2. *Are there symptoms of acid indigestion or heartburn?* Pharyngeal reflux may be relatively silent. The patient may complain of intermittent cough or chest discomfort. Reflux generally causes redness and edema of the posterior larynx, especially the arytenoid mucosa. In addition, the patient frequently develops a habit of throat clearing and has a sensation of a lump in the throat.

3. *Are there symptoms or a history of postnasal drainage or sinusitis?* Thick and/or purulent postnasal drainage often pool around the larynx, causing secondary edema, cough, and throat clearing. These all contribute to hoarseness.

4. *Does the patient have allergic symptoms such as rhinitis, nasal congestion, sneezing, or itchy, watery eyes?* Nasal congestion is generally associated with mouth breathing, es-

TABLE 1.   Drugs that Can Affect the Voice

DRYING AGENTS	COORDINATION AND PROPRIOCEPTION
Antihistamines (sedating)	Central nervous system depressants
Cold medication	Alcohol
Sinus medication	Barbiturates
Cough medication	Chloral hydrate
Sleep medication	Meprobamate (Equanil, Miltown)
Dizziness medication	Ethosuximide (Zarontin)
Seasickness medication	Benzodiazepines
Decongestants (thicken secretions, anxiety)	Diazepam (Valium)
Ephedrine	Chlordiazepoxide (Librium)
Pseudoephedrine (Sudafed)	Alprazolam (Xanax)
Phenylpropanolamine	Clorazepate (Tranxene)
Oxymetazoline (Afrin)	Flurazepam (Dalmane)
Naphazoline (Privine)	Oxazepam (Serax)
Antihypertensives (sedating)	Clonazepam (Klonopin)
Reserpine	Triazolam (Halcion)
Methyldopa (Aldomet)	Marijuana
Clonidine (Catapres)	Central nervous system stimulants
Prazosin (Minipress)	Caffeine (coffee, tea, colas, chocolate)
Captopril (Capoten)	Diet pills
Antidepressants (sedating)	Decongestants
Tranzodone (Desyrel)	Ephedrine
Doxepin (Sinequan)	Phenylpropanolamine
Maprotiline (Ludiomil)	Pseudoephedrine
Amitriptyline (Elavil)	Amphetamines (Benzadrine)
Desipramine (Norpramin)	Cocaine
Imipramine (Tofranil)	Topical anesthetics
Nortriptyline (Aventyl)	Alcohol
Amoxapine (Asendin)	Tetracaine (Cetacaine)
Major tranquilizers/antipsychotics (sedating)	Benzocaine (Hurricane, Chloraseptic
Chlorpromazine	spray/mouthwash/lozenges)
Fluphenazine	Extrapyramidal effects (muscle spasm/dystonia,
Haloperidol	dyskinesia, parkinsonian effects)
Thioridazine	Chlorpromazine (Thorazine)
Trifluoperazine	Fluphenazine (Prolixin)
Thiothixene	Haloperidol (Haldol)
Antispasmodics/antiemetics (sedating)	Thioridazine (Mellaril)
Atropine	Trifluoperazine (Stelazine)
Dicyclomine hydrochloride (Bentyl)	Thiothixene (Navane)
Scopolamine	Prochlorperazine (Compazine)
Phenobarbital	**HORMONES**
Promethazine hydrochloride (Phenergan)	Thyroid medication (if dose excessive)
Prochlorperazine (Compazine)	Androgens (can masculinize voice permanently)
Isopropamide	Danazol (Danocrine) prescribed for endometriosis,
Propantheline (Pro-Banthine)	fibrocystic breast disease
Diphenoxylate (Lomotil)	BCPs* with increased progesterone
Loperamide (Imodium)	Stanozolol (Winstrol)
Antidiarrheal (sedating)	Estrogens (can cause increased edema)
Diphenoxylate (Lomotil)	Corticosteroids
Loperamide (Imodium)	Anti-inflammatory effect early
Codeine	Edema late
Paregoric	
Vitamin C megadoses (acts like a mild antihistamine)	

* BCPs = Birth control pills

pecially at night, and promotes chronic pharynx and larynx dryness.

5. *What is the patient's stress level? Has it changed?* Increased stress generally causes increased muscle tension. The large muscles of the neck may become so tight that normal laryngeal function is hampered. The patient may also tense the intrinsic laryngeal muscles subconsciously. Increased tension during voice projection results in even more voice strain and fatigue, which perpetuates the problem.

6. *Is the patient able to produce a cough and laugh but cannot speak in a full voice?* This indicates that the vocal cords can be totally adducted, but the patient is consciously or subconsciously preventing their closure, making the problem a functional dysphonia.

7. *Is there any evidence of endocrine dysfunction? Has the patient noticed dry hair or dry skin, weight gain, fatigue, or a coarsening of features?* The mild vocal cord changes required to alter the voice may be the symptom that finally prompts a visit to the physician.

8. *Does the patient use alcohol?* Alcohol has an irritating and drying effect on the mucosa. Alcohol also interferes with normal coordination and proprioception and increases the risk of aspiration, cough, and vocal abuse.

9. *Does the patient smoke?* Smoking irritates all mucous membranes and immobilizes ciliary function with subsequent pooling of secretions around the larynx. In addition, it is a severe, direct irritant causing edema. It is the most significant risk factor for cancer of the larynx. Therefore, all smokers with hoarseness require a careful laryngeal examination to rule out this disease. If there is any question of cancer by examination, a biopsy must be recommended.

10. *Does the patient have a high caffeine intake?* Caffeine is a diuretic and often promotes relative dehydration. In addition, it is a stimulant and may create more irritability and tension in and around the neck and larynx. This will contribute to irritative habits, such as frequent throat clearing, especially if thick secretions do exist.

11. *What is the patient's usual daily fluid intake?* The hydration level of the patient is also a very important factor. Adults generally should drink the equivalent of 8 to 10 glasses of water a day. For adequate hydration, the fluid intake must be in addition to any alcoholic or caffeinated beverages.

12. *Has the patient undergone any surgery of the head and neck?* Prior history of intubation may have resulted in laryngeal trauma. If this has occurred in the last several months, it may be significant. Prior tonsillectomy may alter the voice if significant scarring occurs along the supraglottic tract, especially along the tonsil pillars and palate. Rhinoplasty surgery, in general, should not alter the voice unless the airway has been compromised, and this causes hyponasality. Prior neck surgery should be well documented. Carotid endarterectomies may cause injury to the vagus nerve. A thyroidectomy may cause injury to the superior, recurrent, or vagus nerve, with subsequent motion abnormalities. Any endolaryngeal surgery may create a scar, even if it is very subtle, and result in an abnormality of the voice. Abdominal and thoracic surgery may interfere with normal breath support. If the patient is a singer, he or she generally should not return to singing until able to do at least 10 situps.

PHYSICAL EXAMINATION

The initial examination includes an assessment of the patient's general physical condition. Evidence for rheumatoid arthritis will prompt concerns for possible cricoarytenoid joint inflammation or fixation. This usually results in a painful throat with swollen arytenoids and a poorly mobile or fixed vocal cord.

Muscular dystrophy or other myopathies may result in voice problems, especially a weak voice with poor projection, vocal fatigue, and possible vocal tremor or dysarthria.

Many neuropathies can affect the voice. Parkinson's generally causes a low-pitched, low-volume voice that lacks inflection and is quite monotonal in character. Amyotrophic lateral sclerosis patients may have a weak voice with associated progressive dysarthria and dysphagia. Palatal or laryngeal myoclonus often presents with "hiccup speech." Essential tremor of the larynx produces a rhythmic, quavering voice. The patient may also have an associated jaw, tongue, neck, or hand tremor. Many neurologic diseases cause microaspiration with chronic cough or throat clearing and resulting hoarseness.

Head and Neck Examination

A thorough examination of the head and neck is necessary. A neurologic examination of the cranial nerves, in addition to the tenth nerve, should be documented. If cranial nerves nine or eleven are involved, a subtle tenth nerve paresis should be carefully evaluated. This would increase the suspicion of a mass at the jugular foramen at the skull base.

Palpation of the neck should include the lymph node chains along the jugular vein, supraclavicular region, posterior neck triangle, submental, and submandibular regions. Enlarged lymph nodes in the deep cervical chain may indicate a hypopharyngeal or laryngeal cancer. Muscle tightness in the neck, as well as range of motion, should be assessed. Thyroid crepitus is evaluated by moving the thyroid cartilage across the cervical spine. Loss of crepitus raises concern for inflammation or tumor in the postcricoid region. The parotid gland is palpated for enlargement, masses, and decreased salivary flow, which could be associated with Sjögren's syndrome.

Thyroid gland palpation allows evaluation of size and nodularity. Since the recurrent laryngeal nerve travels in the tracheoesophageal groove immediately behind the gland, it is vulnerable to infiltration or compression from thyroid disease.

A general hearing screening by audiologic testing is recommended. A preliminary screening can be accomplished by voice testing. With one ear covered or distracted by rubbing the patient's hair between your fingers, it is possible to test the hearing level by voicing into the opposite ear. An audible whisper is equivalent to approximately 20 dB. Normal conversational speech is in the range of 50 dB. A patient with a neurosensory hearing loss may be using abnormal voice loudness or projection.

The nasal examination should include assessment for rhinitis, thick or purulent exudate, nasal polyps, postnasal drainage, excess swelling, chronic inflammation, or changes consistent with allergy. Septal perforations may suggest a granulomatous disease or recreational drug abuse.

The pharynx should be carefully examined for chronic pharyngitis, chronic tonsillitis, and evidence of hyperkeratosis or leukoplakia. In addition, aphthous ulcers in the pharynx may also affect the laryngeal region.

Oral cavity examination includes evaluation for unusual dryness, which would be consistent with Sjögren's syndrome. Muscle symmetry should be evaluated, especially in the tongue and palate region, since these are frequently associated with neurologic disease. If temporomandibular joint palpation confirms pain or crepitus changes, or the teeth have evidence of bruxism, the concern for muscle tension or stress is raised. If the patient wears dentures, these should be assessed for appropriate fit.

Laryngeal Examination

The traditional means of examining the larynx is with a light source and mirror looking indirectly at the hypopharynx and larynx through the oral cavity. Patient cooperation is mandatory. The patient is asked to extend the neck into a sniff position and open the mouth widely while protruding the tongue. A gauze is used to grasp the tongue, and the mirror is advanced above the tongue to contact the uvula and gently lift it while the patient continues to breathe through the mouth. The light must be focused on the mirror, and the mirror must be angled to visualize the larynx. The patient then phonates with a sustained "e" or "a" sound (see Fig. 3). The epiglottis may overhang the anterior cords and obscure their view.

Structures to be examined in the supraglottic larynx include the epiglottis (including its laryngeal surface), false vocal cords, and aryepiglottic folds, which extend from the epiglottis to each arytenoid cartilage (see Fig. 4, *inset*). The pyriform sinuses are collapsed spaces lying lateral and posterior in the hypopharynx. Pooling of secretions in this area or in the postcricoid region raises a concern for possible tumor. Arytenoid prominences should be examined for swelling or redness. If this is found, the possibility of pharyngeal reflux is high.

The true vocal cords are examined for any evidence of ulcer, polyp, nodule, mass, edema, or redness. Overall vocal cord motion is noted as well as subtle differences in symmetry of adduction and abduction. The leading edges of the vocal cords are examined for any irregularity, spasm, or tremor.

The mirror exam is limited by the physician's experience in the technique and the patient's ability to cooperate during the examination. The flexible fiberoptic laryngoscope has added significantly to our ability to examine the hypopharynx and larynx. This instrument is passed through the nose or oral cavity, is 3.2 mm in diameter, is flexible, and has a tip that allows anterior and posterior deflection for excellent visualization of the laryngeal sur-

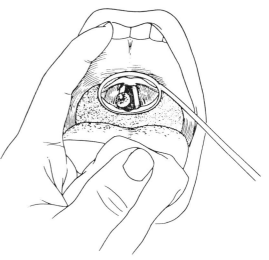

FIGURE 3. Mirror examination of the larynx. Image in mirror shows classic right vocal cord granuloma located over the vocal process.

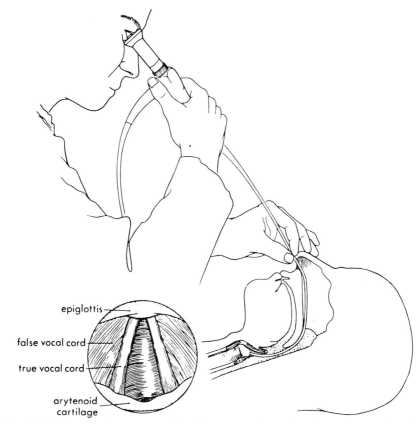

epiglottis

false vocal cord

true vocal cord

arytenoid
cartilage

FIGURE 4. Flexible fiberoptic laryngoscopy. *Inset* shows normal vocal cords and surrounding structures.

face of the epiglottis, the intrinsic larynx, and portions of the piriform sinus and hypopharynx. This is done as an office procedure and requires a special light source, and local anesthesia is applied to the nasal cavity and pharynx areas (see Fig. 4).

Real time and slow-motion videotape examination is available and allows a magnified view of the larynx during phonation. Certain laryngeal abnormalities can only be diagnosed with this specialized equipment. A stroboscopic examination is required to evaluate

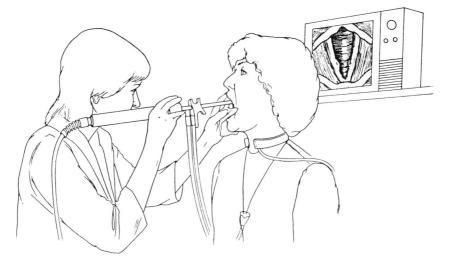

FIGURE 5. Videostroboscopy using a rigid right angle laryngoscope. Video monitor depicts bilateral vocal cord nodules.

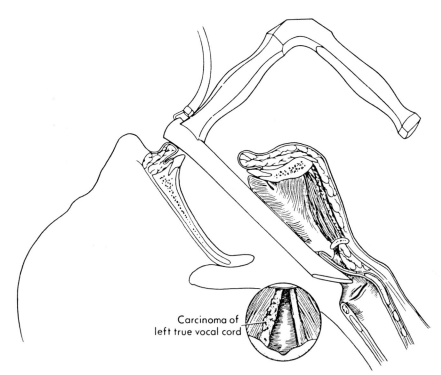

Carcinoma of
left true vocal cord

FIGURE 6.   Direct laryngoscopy. The tip of the laryngoscope can be moved from side to side to expose all areas including the piriform sinuses and postcricoid area. *Inset* illustrates left true vocal cord carcinoma.

phonation vibrations (see Fig. 5). Voice clinics exist in many areas of the country and are an excellent referral resource for community physicians.[1]

Direct laryngoscopy most commonly is done under general anesthesia. It allows the best means of inspecting the mucous membranes and anatomic structures of the hypopharynx and larynx (see Fig. 6). An operating microscope can be added to improve the detailed examination, and biopsy or definitive treatment is often performed utilizing this technique.

DIAGNOSTIC STUDIES

Laboratory Studies

Laboratory studies are generally ordered based on information obtained during the history and physical examination. Thyroid function tests are ordered if the thyroid is enlarged, if a thyroid nodule is present, if a family history of thyroid disease exists, or if the history and physical examination suggest hypofunction or hyperfunction.

Allergy, either seasonal or perennial, is often the source of laryngeal irritation, with chronic cough and throat clearing giving rise to edema of the vocal cords. Screening laboratory studies for elevated immunoglobins along with nasal smears for eosinophils may prompt the examiner to pursue further allergic workup. If chronic cough or other symptoms suggest reactive airway disease, pulmonary function tests should be ordered.

Diagnostic Imaging

Lateral soft tissue x-rays are often used in children and adults to evaluate hypopharyngeal structures for abnormalities in the region of the larynx or posterior pharyngeal wall.

When there is a suspicion of pharyngeal reflux, or aspiration, or there is evidence of pooling of secretions in the piriform sinuses or postcricoid region, a barium esophagogram with fluoroscopy is appropriate. Patients with allergic rhinitis or sinusitis should be evaluated with sinus x-rays. A limited sinus computed tomography (CT) scan is superior to plain x-rays. Many radiologists have created a protocol for a limited coronal CT scan in areas where the equipment is available.

If vocal cord paralysis is diagnosed, imaging studies to evaluate the entire course of the vagus nerve are indicated. A CT scan or magnetic resonance imaging (MRI) scan should be used to evaluate the nerve from the base of the skull through the neck and chest. In patients with cervical adenopathy in which the etiology is not apparent, MRI scanning beginning at the level of the nasopharynx and extending down through the neck is often helpful in defining a hidden primary tumor and allows better visualization of the parapharyngeal areas and neck structures.

ASSESSMENT

Hoarseness in Infants

Laryngomalacia

Lack of normal cartilage support allows the supraglottic laryngeal structures—that is, the epiglottis, aryepiglottic folds, and soft tissues around the arytenoids—to collapse into the airway with inspiration. Hoarseness and inspiratory stridor result. This occurs most commonly in the first 2 to 3 weeks of life and usually resolves as the infant matures between ages 6 and 18 months.

Vocal Cord Paralysis

Vocal cord paralysis is the second most common congenital anomaly of the larynx. If it is bilateral, the infants may have a normal cry but will have a very compromised airway with stridor. A unilateral paralysis will cause less airway compromise; the voice, however, is breathy. If the paralysis is due to birth trauma, return of vocal cord function may occur for a year or more after birth.

Laryngeal Webs

Mucosal webs, which alter the airflow through the larynx, commonly involve the vocal cords at the anterior commissure and produce an altered cry, hoarseness, and depending on the size, airway obstruction.

Subglottic Hemangiomas

The presenting symptom of subglottic hemangioma is progressive stridor or hoarseness often associated with progressive airway obstruction beginning at age two to three months. In about 50 per cent of cases, the infant will have a cutaneous hemangioma.[2] Diagnosis is made by direct laryngoscopy; more recently, MRI has been helpful in making this diagnosis.

Hoarseness in Children

Laryngeal Papillomas

Laryngeal papillomas are wartlike growths that occur in the larynx and trachea and are caused by a human papilloma virus. Papillomas can occur at any age but are more common in infants or children. Hoarseness associated with respiratory obstruction without systemic illness is characteristic of this disease process.

Vocal Nodules (Screamer's Nodules)

Vocal nodules are discrete swellings that occur at the junction of the anterior one third and posterior two thirds of the true vocal cords (see Fig. 5). Loud talking, yelling, and other vocal abuse behaviors are known to be causative for nodules in children. Hoarseness, breathiness, and voice breaks are common complaints.

Hoarseness in Adults

Acute Laryngitis

Acute laryngitis is the most common cause of short-duration hoarseness. A typical viral upper respiratory infection results in severe hoarseness and even short periods of aphonia. It is generally constant in nature, and the duration is most commonly three to five days. Examination shows edema and erythema of the true vocal cords. Sometimes these changes are quite subtle but still have a dramatic effect on the voice. Vocal cord mobility is entirely normal. Spontaneous improvement is expected. If hoarseness persists, this is no longer an appropriate diagnosis.

Chronic Laryngitis

Any factor that can incite chronic inflammation can result in chronic laryngitis. The examination shows some edematous changes of the true vocal cords with mild erythema. The voice may wax and wane and improve somewhat with voice rest. Inciting factors include vocal abuse and misuse, such as cheerleading, yelling, prolonged forced talking or singing, forced vocal projection, speaking over background noise, inhalation of irritants such as dust or chemicals, smoking, pharyngeal reflux, chronic cough, or throat clearing. Chronic laryngitis is seldom, if ever, caused by viral or bacterial infections. A rare exception would be granulomatous diseases, such as tuberculosis. Other causes of granulomatous disease or vasculitis are a rare cause (i.e., sarcoid, blastomycosis). The most common cause of chronic laryngitis is cigarette smoking. Polypoid corditis is a specific type of chronic laryngitis that results in a characteristic submucosal edema with a polypoid or scalloped appearance of the vocal cords.

Muscle Tension Dysphonia

Muscle tension dysphonia is an interesting cause of hoarseness that may be thought of as vocal strain/fatigue. It results from tension of the intrinsic and extrinsic laryngeal muscles. If the muscles of adduction and abduction are tensed at the same time, the vocal cords are unable to close completely.[3,4] A persistent posterior glottic chink remains during adduction. The voice is slightly breathy and raspy and fatigues easily. This causes the patient to push and work even harder when speaking and creates increased tension. It is not uncommon for the patient to wear his or her voice out with normal voice use. The neck and throat generally feel tight with voice use.

Vocal Cord Nodules

The most vibratory portion of the vocal cords is at the anterior middle one-third junction. This is actually the center of the membranous vocal cord since the posterior portion of the vocal cord attaches to a submucosal extension of the arytenoid cartilage. With excessive vibration, this area can develop a swelling or even tissue thickening. Nodules always occur at this characteristic location (see Fig. 5). There should be no pain or associated symptoms such as dysphagia or aspiration.

Vocal Cord Polyps

Vocal cord polyps have many sizes and shapes and usually occur on the superior or free margin of the true vocal cord, often starting as a subepithelial hemorrhage or localized edema. If vocal abuse persists, the polyp tends to increase in size, interfering with the apposition of the true vocal cords, giving rise to hoarseness. Bilateral polyps or diffuse polypoid corditis is often associated with a history of smoking, voice abuse, and gastric reflux.

Vocal Cord Granulomas (Contact Ulcers)

Vocal cord granulomas or contact ulcers are associated with vocal abuse and reflux pharyngitis. These are often seen in lawyers, teachers, preachers, and other professionals when voice use is excessive.

They occur at the vocal process of the arytenoid cartilage, may be unilateral or bilateral, and interfere with vocal cord apposition. Heartburn, nocturnal coughing, and localized pain in the laryngeal region are common associated complaints (see Fig. 3).

Intubation Granulomas

Occasionally, granulomas of the vocal cord can result from direct trauma to the vocal cord. During intubation, the most likely site for trauma is the vocal process, especially if an excessively large endotracheal tube is used during the surgical procedure. The resultant granuloma develops over a period of days to weeks, resulting in interference with vocal cord approximation and hoarseness. Partial airway obstruction can occur if an intense inflammatory reaction results in rapid enlargement of the granuloma.

Vocal Cord Paralysis

Vocal cord paralysis can be unilateral or bilateral. In the more common unilateral paralysis, the vocal cord is in the paramedian position (approximately 1.5 mm from the midline), and the voice is breathy, weak, and difficult to project. A chronic cough, especially when drinking liquids, is common. A careful search along the course of the vagus nerve and recurrent laryngeal nerve is necessary to determine the etiology of the paralysis. In approximately 20 per cent, no etiologic process is found.[5] In bilateral paralysis, the voice is often normal. The most characteristic symptom is expiratory and inspiratory stridor with shortness of breath, especially with any exertion. If the cords are paralyzed in a more lateral position, a breathy voice and aspiration may result.

Papillomas

Adult-onset laryngeal papillomas are much less common than childhood papillomas. The disease is usually not as aggressive in adulthood. Papillomas are often relentlessly recurrent. The voice is hoarse and may progress in severity with concern for possible airway obstruction symptoms.

Dysphonia Plica Ventricularis

Phonation with the false vocal cords is possible but results in a poor voice. The voice is unusually monotonous, and there is little ability to change the pitch. The resulting pitch is usually quite low, owing to the mass of the false vocal cords compared with the thin, delicate true vocal cords. Laryngeal examination will show false vocal cord closure during phonation, which completely obscures the true vocal cords from view. The cause may be true vocal cord pathology that prevents their adduction, such as in papillomas or polyps. It also may be due to hyperfunction or hypertrophy of the false vocal cords.

Vocal Cord Bowing

Atrophy or thinning of the thyroarytenoid muscle may result from normal aging. As the mass of the vocal cords decreases and their elasticity is lost, the cords may become somewhat flaccid, which results in a persistent gap during adduction. This bowing allows air loss and a breathy voice.

Amyloidosis of the Larynx and Trachea

Amyloidosis is a deposit of abnormal protein within the larynx usually seen on the vocal cords, epiglottis, and aryepiglottic fold. This protein deposit interferes with vocal cord motion and adduction, resulting in hoarseness. The disease process may be primarily in the larynx and trachea or may be secondary to severe, chronic, debilitating illness.

Sjögren's Syndrome

Sjögren's syndrome consists of a lymphocytic infiltrate of the major and minor salivary glands resulting in dryness of the oral cavity, hypopharynx, larynx, and eyes. (Also see chapter on Dry Eye.) The dryness is often associated with a chronic, irritating cough, and hoarseness is due to the edema caused by this cough. Patients will also have minor articulation problems.

Laryngocele

Dilatation of the laryngeal saccule occurs with increased laryngeal air pressure or air trapping. The resultant swelling of the saccule within the larynx causes hoarseness due to the edema and structural displacement. It is commonly seen in musicians who play wind instruments such as trumpets, and in glass blowers.

Rheumatoid Arthritis

Rheumatoid arthritis is an autoimmune process that involves the synovial membranes. The larynx is affected in approximately 20 per cent of the cases with ankylosis of the cricoarytenoid joint and swelling of the membranes surrounding the arytenoid cartilages. This results in impaired vocal cord mobility and hoarseness. Airway compromise is possible if both joints are involved. The diagnosis is made by direct laryngoscopy and palpation of the arytenoid cartilage.

Myasthenia Gravis

Myasthenia gravis is an autoimmune disease in which antibodies are directed against the specific acetylcholine receptors at the neuromuscular junction. Muscular weakness may affect the larynx, resulting in hoarseness and breathiness, which usually become more severe on prolonged conversation. Patients may have other symptoms such as dysphagia, diplopia, and nasal regurgitation.

Spastic Dysphonia

Spastic dysphonia is classically described as a strained, strangled voice. The patient appears to be speaking with great effort with a very tight or choked voice. Phonation breaks are frequent. The voice is usually worse in stressful situations. It is due most commonly to hyperfunction of the larynx with adductor spasm. A less frequent type with abductor spasm results in a strained but breathy voice. Recent information indicates that this is a dystonia much like blepharospasm; in fact, spastic dysphonia may be associated with blepharospasm and oromandibular dystonia in Meige's disease.[6]

Malignant Tumors of the Larynx

Hoarseness is the most common presenting symptom of a malignant laryngeal tumor. A history of smoking and alcohol abuse should alert the examining physician, and a complete visualization of the larynx is necessary in anyone who has progressive hoarseness or hoarseness persisting greater than three weeks. Squamous cell carcinoma is the most common malignant tumor and may occur anywhere within the hypopharynx or larynx. Hoarseness is the result of tumor mass interfering with vocal cord approximation or impairing vocal cord motion (see Fig. 6, *inset*).

REFERENCES

1. Rammage LA, Nichol H, Morrison MD. The voice clinic: an interdisciplinary approach. J Otolaryngol 1983;12(5):315–8.
2. Meyer CM, Cotton RT. Airway obstruction. In: Myer CM, Cotton RT, eds. A practical approach to pedi-

atric otolaryngology. Chicago: Yearbook Medical Publishers, 1988:199.

3. Belisle GL, Morrison MD. Anatomic correlation for muscle tension dysphonia. J Otolaryngol 1983; 12(5):319–21.

4. Morrison MD, Rammage LA, Belisle GM, et al. Muscle tension dysphonia. J Otolaryngol 1983;12(5):302–6.

5. Sobol SM, Alleva M. Hoarseness and voice change. In: Lucinte FH, Sobol SE, eds. Essentials of otolaryngology. 2nd ed. New York: Raven Press, 1988:273.

6. Blitzer A, Brin M, Fahn S, et al. Clinical and laboratory characteristics of focal laryngeal dystonia: a study of 110 cases. Laryngoscope 1988;98:636–40.

HUMAN IMMUNODEFICIENCY VIRUS INFECTION, DIAGNOSIS, AND STAGING

STEVEN A. MILES

SYNONYMS: HIV Infection, AIDS

BACKGROUND

The acquired immune deficiency syndrome (AIDS) was first identified in 1981 in the United States. At the time, it was primarily confined to the homosexual communities in New York, San Francisco, and Los Angeles.[1] As the prevalence of the human immunodeficiency virus (HIV) increased, cases of AIDS were diagnosed outside these cities. AIDS has now been diagnosed in every state in the United States and 137 countries worldwide. The Centers for Disease Control in Atlanta estimates that over 1.5 million persons in the United States are infected with HIV, the virus associated with AIDS. The World Health Organization estimates that an additional 5 to 10 million are infected with HIV worldwide.[2,3]

As the number of AIDS cases has risen, the demands placed on the health care system have risen. In some situations, the demands have exceeded the capacity of the governmental agencies to handle these patients. In addition, as our understanding of the clinical course of HIV infection has increased, we have recognized the importance of early diagnosis and treatment. As a result, in addition to providing care to patients with AIDS, we now offer a variety of experimental therapies to asymptomatic patients infected with HIV. We are rapidly approaching a time when all 1.5 million HIV-infected patients in the United States will be offered some form of therapy that will probably continue for the rest of their lives. In this sense, HIV infection has now become a chronic, treatable illness.

Clearly, the present system of caring for these patients will not keep pace with the growing demand for services. In the next several years, the responsibility for providing medical care to the majority of HIV-infected patients will fall on primary care physicians. Moreover, recent legal decisions have demonstrated that the failure of physicians to identify individuals as having HIV infection and to offer therapy carries significant liability risk. As a result of these events, it is important that these physicians learn about the diagnosis, staging, and treatment of patients with HIV infection.

HISTORY

Recognizing HIV infection in a young homosexual male with Kaposi's sarcoma is easy. In contrast, recognizing HIV infection in an elderly female with mild dementia and a history of blood transfusion is difficult. One must be cognizant of both the clinical spectrum of HIV disease and the risk of exposure to HIV. The important point is that in order to make a diagnosis of HIV infection, it must be considered. Next, the likelihood that the clinical symptoms are due to HIV infection must be ascertained. Finally, the clinical diagnosis must be confirmed with the most sensitive and specific laboratory test or biopsy available.

Determine the Risk of Exposure

Because the predictive value of the laboratory tests depends on the likelihood of infection (the posterior probability), it is important to determine this likelihood as accurately as possible. Unfortunately, owing to social stigmata associated with HIV high-risk behavior and the lack of training of physicians in taking an accurate sexual history, this risk is often underestimated. Specific questions about sexual practices that may be uncomfortable for the physician must be asked.

Focused Queries

1. *Has the patient had same-sex intercourse (if a male) or intercourse with men who have had same-sex intercourse (if a female)?* In particular, attention must be paid to the frequency of activity and the nature of the sexual acts performed. Specific questions must be asked about whether the patient has engaged in high-risk activities, which include the exchange of bodily fluids, rectal intercourse, unprotected vaginal intercourse, rimming, fisting, or "water sports."

2. *Has the patient ever used intravenous needles in his or her lifetime?* Because intravenous drug abuse can be episodic, it is important to ask about lifetime risk activities.

3. *Where did this activity occur?* Was the patient in San Francisco or Topeka? This is not meant to say that HIV infection has not

occurred in Topeka. Unfortunately, it has. However, the seroprevalence of HIV infection is several orders of magnitude higher in the homosexual communities in New York, Miami, Los Angeles, and San Francisco than many cities in more rural areas. As a result, given the same level of activity, the risk of disease acquisition is lower in some parts of the country than others.

4. *Has the patient had a lover or friend who has been diagnosed with HIV infection or AIDS?* The latter situation makes the risk of HIV-related illness substantially higher in the patient in the next year.

5. *Has the patient received blood or blood products including cryoprecipitate, clotting factor concentrates, fresh-frozen plasma, platelets, packed red blood cells, or whole blood since 1977?* All these products have been associated with the transmission of HIV infection. The highest risk is with the factor concentrates. The risk of transmission has decreased since March, 1985, when testing for HIV antibodies was mandated. Still, the risk of transmission of HIV is estimated at 1:50,000 per unit of blood product in high-risk cities to less than 1:200,000 in low-risk cities. To date, only three blood products have been shown to be free of the risk of transmission of HIV infection. These are immunoglobulin preparations, human serum albumin, and hepatitis B immunogens.

6. *Is the patient exposed to HIV in an occupational setting?* The risk is highest for laboratory personnel working with live virus concentrates and lowest for hospital personnel with a needle stick exposure. The risk for nee-

---

TABLE 1.   Relative Risk of HIV Infection*

High risk
  Unprotected anal intercourse
  Shared intravenous needles
  Child of HIV-infected mother
  Unprotected vaginal intercourse with intravenous drug
    abusers, bisexual men, or promiscuous partners
Moderate risk
  Multiple anonymous sexual partners
  Blood product recipient from 1981 to 1985 in Los
    Angeles, New York, or San Francisco
  Multiple sexually transmitted diseases
Low risk
  Blood product recipient from 1975 to 1981 and from
    1985 until now
  Needle stick exposure
  Protected intercourse with HIV-infected person
  Artificial insemination recipient

* All these activities have been documented to result in transmission even with only one exposure.

dle stick exposure is estimated at approximately 1:250.

Assuming an accurate and detailed history of exposure is obtained, patients can be classified into risk categories as in Table 1. The likelihood of infection with HIV can be further defined by examination of the patient for early signs of impaired cellular immunity.

PHYSICAL EXAMINATION

Early Manifestations of Impaired Cellular Immunity

The hallmark of infection with HIV is impaired cell-mediated immunity. Clinical signs and symptoms are widespread and varied in presentation. However, many of these findings are not unique to infection with HIV.

Two physical findings that are unique to HIV infection are hairy leukoplakia of the tongue and disseminated Kaposi's sarcoma. The former is a fine white growth usually on the lateral aspect of the tongue. Kaposi's sarcoma is a red to violaceous lesion, 1 to 4 cm in size, that can appear anywhere on the body. Frequent sites of involvement are the nose, mouth, chest, groin, and feet. In advanced stages, the tumor is associated with edema and lymphadenopathy, and the solitary lesions can coalesce, leaving large masses of tumor.

Cytomegalovirus (CMV) retinitis and recurrent oral candidiasis (thrush) in an adult not receiving antibiotics are also rarely seen outside the setting of HIV infection. The patient with CMV retinitis usually presents with low-grade fevers, "floaters" in the visual fields, and visual impairment. CMV lesions can be seen with ophthalmoscopy. These lesions occur anywhere in the fundus, are red and raised, and have a surrounding inflammatory exudate. In severe cases, the fundus can be obscured from retinal hemorrhage and scarring. Thrush (oral candidiasis) is seen as a white, cottage cheese–like exudate on the tongue and throat. Occasionally, the buccal mucosa can be involved. The exudate can be scraped free and examined with a potassium hydroxide preparation on a slide to confirm the presence of budding yeast forms.

Other physical findings suggestive of HIV infection include recurrent or refractory tineal infections, staphylococcal folliculitis, seborrheic dermatitis (especially involving the face), severe aphthous stomatitis, generalized extrainguinal lymphadenopathy, and refractory vaginal candidiasis.[4] Many physical findings will be brought to the attention of dermatologists, family practitioners, and internists. Without a high degree of suspicion, these problems would be treated and the patient dismissed without appropriate questioning and laboratory studies. Since the majority of patients with HIV infection are asymptomatic, the absence of physical findings in an at-risk individual unfortunately does not exclude HIV infection.

DIAGNOSTIC STUDIES

There are two types of commercially available serological tests for the confirmation of HIV infection. The enzyme-linked immunosorbent assay (ELISA) is inexpensive, has a high predictive value in high-prevalence populations, and is widely available.[5] Results are standardized and unambigous. Because of the gravity of the diagnosis of HIV infection, it has been recommended that the ELISA results be confirmed with an additional assay such as the immunoblot or immunofluorescence. The immunoblot or Western blot is more expensive and has a high predictive value but is available from only a few manufacturers as a federally licensed test. The immunoblot is widely available at commercial laboratories, but the reproducibility and reliability of this assay vary considerably.[6] Despite attempts to standardize these tests, diagnostic interpretation is not uniform, is often misleading, and can even be left to the physician ordering the assay. As a result, these tests should only be used to confirm a diagnosis.

In addition, there are several experimental assays available at National Institutes of Health (NIH) funded AIDS Clinical Trials Group (ACTG) centers. These include coculture assays of peripheral blood and plasma for HIV infection, ELISA assays for HIV p24 antigen and antibody in serum or plasma, and polymerase chain reaction (PCR) assays for the detection of HIV ribonucleic acid (RNA) and deoxyribonucleic acid (DNA) in peripheral blood or plasma.

HIV Enzyme-Linked Immunosorbent Assay

The ELISA, commonly referred to as the "AIDS antibody test" or the "AIDS test," was commercially licensed and has been available since March 1985.[5] Contrary to common belief, it is not a test for AIDS. It is a test for the presence of antibodies in the patient's serum against semipurified HIV viral antigens. Because the HIV antigen mixture is made from a cell culture supernatant, a variety of false-positive reactions can occur. These include clinical conditions where the patient may have antibodies to cellular antigens (such as systemic lupus erythematosus or pregnancy) or antibodies to immunoglobulins (such as rheumatoid factor or cryoglobulins).

Likewise, because the assay depends on the presence of antibodies to HIV antigens in the serum, a number of false-negative reactions can occur. These are seen in the early stages of infection (up to six months after exposure in rare cases) prior to the development of specific antibodies (the so-called window period).[7,8] False-negative reactions are also seen in the very late stages of AIDS when the immune system is so severely impaired that specific antibody production cannot be maintained.[9]

The vast majority of false-positive or -negative test results in the high seroprevalence group however, are due to laboratory errors. Given the inexpensive nature of the assay, most laboratories attempt to decrease this risk by repeating the test before releasing the results. Thus, a positive result is usually reported as "repeatedly positive." With the newer generation ELISAs, a positive test need not be repeated if the index of suspicion for HIV infection is high.

In contrast, the vast majority of positive tests in low seroprevalence groups are false-positive. Test results must always be considered in light of the patient's low risk for infection and confirmed using a different type of assay such as the immunoblot.

Because of the "window period" phenomenon when the suspicion for HIV infection is high, these tests should be repeated at six-month intervals for at least one year.

HIV Immunoblot (Western Blot)

The second most widely used test for the detection of antibodies to HIV antigens is the immunoblot or "Western blot." This assay is different from the ELISA and yields far more information. Unfortunately, it requires a higher level of technologic skill to perform and is therefore less reproducible. A survey by the U.S. Army suggests that fewer than 30 per cent of the laboratories around the country can reliably perform this assay.[6] With the ad-

vent of the first federally licensed kit and the widespread availability of viral lysate preparations, this may change.

In brief, the viral antigens are separated on a gel, transferred to a blotting strip, and exposed to the patient's serum. The patient's antibodies attach to these denatured HIV antigens, and after development (similar to the ELISA), bands corresponding to the major and minor HIV antigens are visualized. A patient is said to be "positive" based on criteria from the individual laboratory or manufacturer. Patients with some but not all the diagnostic bands are reported as "indeterminate." Those patients with no bands present are reported as "negative." As in the ELISA, indeterminate results in high-risk group members are almost always confirmed as "positive" on repeat testing or by clinical findings. In low-risk groups, these reactions usually remain isolated to a few indeterminate bands on repeat testing and do not represent HIV infection. Again, because of the window period phenomenon, when the suspicion for HIV infection is high, these tests should be repeated at six-month intervals for at least one year.

Experimental Assays for Detection of HIV Infection

Another reliable but difficult to perform serologic test for HIV infection is the radioimmunoprecipitation assay (RIPA). It is more specific than the immunoblot owing to the nondenaturing conditions of antigen recognition. It is equal to the immunoblot in its sensitivity for detecting HIV infection. This assay is useful in detecting seroconversion and in situations where there are cross-reacting antibodies present.

HIV core (p24) antigen can occasionally be detected for a brief time prior to the detection of antibodies to HIV antigens. The ELISA for HIV p24 antigen is widely available and, when used with the confirmatory serum neutralization assay, can be very specific for HIV infection. Its relative merit compared with other assays is unknown. As will be discussed later, the primary use for the HIV p24 antigen assay at the current time is in staging patients and evaluating response to antiviral therapy.[10]

Also available at participating institutions of the AIDS Clinical Trials Group are coculture assays for the detection of plasma HIV viremia and detection of HIV infection in the peripheral blood cells. These assays are expensive and often unreliable but when done properly can yield very useful quantitative data on patients infected with HIV.

Finally, a new assay technique called polymerase chain reaction (PCR) can be used to demonstrate the presence of integrated and transcribed HIV DNA and RNA in the plasma and peripheral blood cells of patients with HIV infection. The assay relies on the ability of a synthesized strand of DNA complementary to HIV proviral sequences to hybridize with HIV DNA or RNA.[7,8] Under high-stringency conditions and in the presence of the DNA polymerase enzyme Taq I, the duplex acts as a template for the extension and synthesis of new HIV DNA. This newly synthesized strand can then act as a template for further amplification after denaturation. The magnitude of amplification can be enormous, thus allowing for the detection of small amounts of HIV DNA or RNA.

The current limit of sensitivity of the assay is approximately 1 DNA copy in 1 million cells.[7] But, at the current time, false-positive reactions are quite common owing to "carryover" from a positive sample to a negative sample. Nonetheless, using this technique it has been possible to demonstrate the presence of HIV in peripheral blood cells in patients at risk for HIV infection up to 42 months prior to the detection of HIV antigen or antibodies.[8] It was also used to demonstrate HIV infection in two patients who transiently made antibodies to HIV.[9] While this test holds much promise for the future in diagnostics, it remains at present a research tool. It is available commercially in the United States from the developer of the assay, Cetus Inc., through an arrangement with Specialty Laboratories, Inc., Santa Monica, California.

Staging of the Patient with HIV Infection

Precise staging of patients with HIV infection is important for several reasons. First, it gives the patients some realistic assessment of life expectancy. Second, it can help guide physicians on how closely to follow patients for the development of complications. Third, it provides some data upon which to base therapeutic decisions and some parameters for measuring response to therapy. Finally, specific diagnoses may entitle patients to increased local and federal government assistance.

Examination of the patient with HIV infection should allow the physician to categorize the patient as asymptomatic or symptomatic. With the exception of a few specific disease states for which good survival data exist (i.e., first or second episode of *Pneumocystis carinii* pneumonia, disseminated *Mycobacterium avium,* or pulmonary Kaposi's sarcoma), clinical parameters alone are not very useful for determining prognosis.[11] Moreover, clinical parameters are only useful in assessing symptomatic patients, whereas the majority of patients are asymptomatic. For these latter patients, the evaluation by the physician of a relatively small number of laboratory parameters may be more useful in categorizing and following patients.[12] These tests include the absolute CD4 (helper) cell number, beta-2-microglobulin level, HIV p24 antigen level, and presence of HIV plasma viremia. The latter two tests are experimental, as are new tests for determining HIV p24 antibody levels (see Table 2).

Absolute CD4 (Helper) Cell Number in HIV Infection

The CD4 (helper) cell has a central role in HIV infection.[13] The HIV virus uses the CD4 receptor to gain entry to a number of cells.[14] The loss of CD4 cell number and functional activity gives rise to the immune deficiency seen in HIV infection.[15] Thus, it is not surprising that determination of CD4 cell number should be critical in staging patients.[11]

CD4 cell number remains normal (350 to 1200/cu mm) after infection until seroconversion. Coincident with seroconversion, the CD4 number declines (usually about 200 cells/cu mm) and then plateaus. During this long

TABLE 2.   Relative Risk of Progression to AIDS in Asymptomatic HIV-Positive Males over 18 Months

VARIABLE	LEVEL	%	RELATIVE RISK
HIV antigen	+	59	4.6*
	−	15	1.0
p24 Antibody	+	16	1.0
	−	43	3.2*
CD4 + lymphocytes	<200	87	13.4*
	201–400	46	3.6*
	>400	16	1.0
Beta-2-microglobulin	>5	69	16.9*
	3–5	33	4.5*
	≤3	12	1.0

* $p < 0.01$.
(Data from Moss AR, Seropositivity for HIV and the development of AIDS or AIDS related condition: three year follow up of the San Francisco General Hospital cohort. Br Med J 1988;296:745–50.)

plateau period, which may last for several years, patients are usually asymptomatic. This period roughly corresponds to the incubation period for AIDS and is attributed to low-level viral production termed *persistence*. Eventually, for as yet unclear reasons, viral replication increases and CD4 cell number declines. Coincident with the fall below 200 to 300/cu mm, the patient develops symptoms and may have his or her first opportunistic infection. Thus, patients with CD4 cell numbers greater than 500 cu mm have a low short-term risk for the development of AIDS, whereas those with CD4 cell numbers less than 200/cu mm have a high relative risk (see Table 2).

One note on the measurement of CD4 helper cell numbers: This value is a product of the white blood count (inaccurate), the per cent lymphocytes (inaccurate), the per cent T cells (accurate), and the per cent CD4-positive cells (accurate). As a result, the CD4 number often fluctuates by as much as 20 to 25 per cent, depending on the laboratory in which it is performed. It is important for patients and physicians not to place as much significance on the absolute number as on the trend.

Beta-2-Microglobulin Levels in HIV Infection

Beta-2-microglobulin is a small molecular weight protein that is synthesized and secreted from cells in concert with the expression of the major histocompatibility locus antigens (HLA class I). Beta-2-microglobulin expression on circulating cells is increased by interferons alpha and beta and by infections and other processes that are associated with increased levels of interferon production. Very early in the recognition of the clinical spectrum of AIDS, it was noted that patients frequently had high circulating levels of acid labile interferons (primarily alpha).[16] More recent work has extended this observation to show that patients with HIV infection who have high levels of beta-2-microglobulin have a greater relative risk for the development of AIDS than do patients with lower levels. Presumably, this elevated level reflects some ongoing immune stimulus that will ultimately manifest itself as disease.

This test is reliable and relatively inexpensive and may vary with specific forms of therapy (notably interferons). Still, of the markers studied, a level greater than 5 mg/L confers the single highest relative risk for the develop-

ment of AIDS (see Table 2). This assay is now being evaluated prospectively.

Experimental Assays Used to Stage HIV Infection

The most widely available and reproducible experimental assay used in the staging of HIV infection is an ELISA for the detection of HIV p24 core antigen. Although not federally licensed, this assay is available on an experimental basis at most centers where a large number of AIDS patients are treated. This assay uses two different antibodies to HIV p24 antigen to "capture" or "sandwich" the protein. This sandwich is developed in standard ELISA format. The assay can reproducibly detect as little as 2 to 30 pgm of HIV p24 antigen, depending on the manufacturer.[10]

Because patients in the latter stages of infection often produce HIV p24 antigen in excess of their ability to synthesize antibodies to HIV p24 antigen, we can readily detect free antigen in their serum or plasma.[17] Thus, this test is useful in detecting late-stage patients who are asymptomatic and who have a high relative short-term risk of developing AIDS. In addition, because antiviral agents suppress virus production, the amount of detectable HIV p24 antigen often falls with successful therapy.[18] As a result, the test is also used to follow late-stage patients on antiviral agents. In a small number of patients, HIV p24 antigen can be detected just prior to seroconversion.[19] When used with the HIV antigen neutralization serum, the HIV p24 antigen assay can be used to demonstrate HIV infection prior to the development of antibodies to HIV and seroconversion (the window period).

The plasma coculture assay for the detection of free HIV virus in the plasma is only available at selected centers in the United States. As reported recently by Coombs et al.,[20] this assay appears to be positive in a greater proportion of HIV-infected individuals than the HIV p24 antigen and may ultimately be more useful. It is also a marker of the later stages of disease. Whether it indicates the same relative risk for progression to AIDS as the HIV p24 antigen assay remains to be seen. It is used to follow antiviral therapy and can be diagnostic of HIV infection in newborns prior to antibody production against HIV antigens.

Finally, the PCR is the newest assay in the diagnostic arsenal. As mentioned previously, it is extremely sensitive and may eventually provide a means of following the success of antiviral therapy in early-stage patients where there is no free virus nor HIV p24 antigen detectable. Methods to quantify this assay remain experimental.

ASSESSMENT

Stages of HIV infection

Utilizing the presence of clinical manifestations, CD4 cell number, beta-2-microglobulin, and some experimental assays, we can classify patients into five categories (see Table 3). The first category is patients who were accidentally inoculated with HIV and those patients who were recently infected with HIV and had the HIV seroconversion syndrome. These patients may have no clinical or laboratory evidence of HIV infection. These individuals should be placed on one of the two available national experimental trials.

The second category includes patients who are positive on laboratory testing for HIV infection but have greater than 500/cu mm CD4 cells. These patients are nearly always asymptomatic and should be placed on zidovudine (azidothymidine [AZT], Retrovir), based on the results of the NIH AIDS Clinical Trials Group Study 019. This study showed decreased opportunistic infections in patients treated early in HIV infection with zidovudine. These patients can be seen every three to six months.

TABLE 3.   Stages of HIV Infection

Recent infection
    May have early HIV antibodies and p24 antigen
    May have acute seroconversion syndrome
    Normal T cells or elevated CD8
Asymptomatic, healthy
    No symptoms of HIV infection
    CD4 cell number greater than 500/cu mm
Asymptomatic but with poor prognosis
    No symptoms of HIV infection
    CD4 cell number less than 500/cu mm
    Detectable HIV plasma viremia
    Falling HIV p24 antibody or detectable p24 antigen
    Elevated beta-2-microglobulin
Impaired cellular immunity
    Tinea, thrush, or leukoplakia
    Laboratory markers of poor prognosis
Acquired immune deficiency syndrome
    Usually CD4 cell number less than 200/cu mm
    Elevated beta-2-microglobulin
    Detectable HIV p24 antigen

The third category includes patients who are positive for HIV infection and asymptomatic but also have poor prognostic indicators. These indicators include CD4 cell number less than 500/cu mm, HIV plasma viremia, falling HIV p24 antibody levels, and/or detectable HIV p24 antigen. These patients have increased viral expression and a high risk for the development of AIDS. They should be seen approximately every three months. Consideration should be given to prophylaxis against *Pneumocystis carinii* pneumonia (PCP) (see Table 4). A survival benefit associated with the use of zidovudine in these patients has been demonstrated. The use of zidovudine in

TABLE 4.   Prophylaxis for *Pneumocystis carinii*

AGENT	RECUR-RENCE (PRI-MARY)*	RECUR-RENCE (SECOND-ARY)†	DOSE	TOXICITY
Zidovudine	No experience	5.1	200 mg every four hours	Nausea, headaches, cytopenias
Trimethoprim-sulfamethoxazole	1.9	0	One double strength (d.s.) dose twice a day every Saturday and Sunday *or* one d.s. dose twice a week	Rash, fevers, cytopenias
Fansidar	3.8–6.67	0.26–0.76	One dose each week	Rash, cytopenias, Stevens-Johnson syndrome
Dapsone	0	0.11–0.14	25 mg twice a day or four times a day	Anemia, methemoglobinemia, rash
Intravenous Pentam	No experience	0.5	300 mg every three to four weeks	Diabetes, hepatic, leukopenia, renal
Aerosol Pentam	0.26–0.29	0.28–1.25	150 mg via hand held nebulizer (HHN) every two weeks	Cough, increased triglycerides, renal.

* Number of cases of first episode PCP per 100 patient months.
† Number of cases of second episode PCP per 100 patient months.

the patients must be discussed if not encouraged.

The fourth category includes those patients with clinical evidence of impaired cellular immunity such as tinea, thrush, or hairy leukoplakia. These patients may have some of the laboratory markers associated with a high risk of development of AIDS and should be treated with zidovudine. The current recommended dose is 100 mg five times a day. These patients should all receive PCP prophylaxis and should be seen at least every month.

Finally, the last category includes those patients who have AIDS. These patients should all be treated with zidovudine and given prophylaxis against PCP. Patients who are intolerant of zidovudine or who develop other complications that preclude its use should be referred to participating institutions of the NIH AIDS Clinical Trials Group for experimental therapy. A directory listing clinical trials of experimental therapy and location of research centers is available from the American Federation for AIDS Research (AmFAR) or from the National Institutes of Allergic and Infectious Diseases.

REFERENCES

1. Gottlieb MS, Schroft R, Schanker HM, et al. *Pneumocystic carinii* pneumonia and mucosal candidiasis in previously healthy homosexual men. N Engl J Med 1981;305:1425–9.
2. Centers for Disease Control. Human immunodeficiency virus infection in the United States. MMWR 1987;36:1–7.
3. World Health Organization. Acquired immune deficiency syndrome. 1987:362–9.
4. Hollander H. Work-up of the HIV infected patient: practical approach. In: Sande R, ed. The medical management of AIDS. Philadelphia: WB Saunders, 1988.
5. Centers for Disease Control. Classification system for human T-lymphotropic virus type III/lymphadenopathy-associated virus infections. MMWR 1986;35:334–8.
6. Burke DS. HIV screening by the US Army: two years of experience in quality control. Written testimony before the House Subcommittee on Regulation and Business Opportunities, House Small Business Opportunities, Oct 1987.
7. Rossi JJ, Murakana G, Arnold B, et al. Simultaneous amplification and direct deletion of HIV-1, T cell receptor and beta-actin in RNA sequences from peripheral blood samples [Abstract]. IV Int Conf AIDS, 1988:1612–9.
8. Wolinsky S, Rinaldo C, Farzedegan H, et al. Polymerase chain reaction (PCR) detection of HIV provirus before HIV seroconversion [Abstract]. IV Int Conf AIDS, 1988:1099–1104.
9. Farzedegan H, Polis MA, Wolinsky SM, et al. Loss of human immunodeficiency virus type I (HIV-1) antibodies with evidence of viral infection in asymptomatic homosexual men. Ann Intern Med 1988;108:785–7.
10. Wittek AE. Detection of human immunodeficiency virus core protein in plasma by enzyme immunoassay: association of antigenemia with symptomatic disease and T helper cell depletion. Ann Intern Med 1987;107:286–9.
11. Taylor J, Afrasiabi R, Fahey JL, et al. Prognostically significant classification of immune changes in AIDS with Kaposi's sarcoma. Blood 1986;67:666–70.
12. Moss AR. Seropositivity for HIV and the development of AIDS or AIDS related condition: three year follow up of the San Francisco General Hospital cohort. Br Med J 1988;296:745–50.
13. Fauci, AS. Immunopathogenesis of immunodeficiency virus infection. Science 1988;239:617–20.
14. Dagleish AG, Beverly PCL, Clapram PR, et al. The CD4(T4) antigen is an essential component of the receptor for the AIDS retrovirus. Nature 1984;312:763–70.
15. Hessol NA, Rutherford GW, O'Malley PM, et al. The natural history of human immunodeficiency virus infection in a cohort of homosexual and bisexual men: a 7 year prospective study [Abstract]. III Int Conf AIDS, 1987:1–5.
16. DeStefano E, Friedman-Kien RM, Friedman-Kien AE, et al. Acid-labile human leukocyte interferon in homosexual men with Kaposi's sarcoma and lymphadenopathy. J Infect Dis 1982;146:451–55.
17. Cao Y, Valentine F, Hojrat S, et al. Detection of HIV antigen and specific antibodies to HIV core and envelope proteins in sera of patients with HIV infection. Blood 1987;70:575–80.
18. Fischl MA, Richman DD, Grieco MH, et al. The efficacy of azidothymidine (AZT) in the treatment of patients with AIDS and AIDS related complex. A double blind, placebo controlled trial. N Engl J Med 1987;317:185–8.
19. Allain J-P, Laurian Y, Paul DA, et al. Serological markers of early stages of human immunodeficiency virus infection in hemophiliacs. Lancet 1986;2:1233–6.
20. Coombs RW, Collier AC, Allain JP, et al. Plasma viremia in human immunodeficiency virus infection. N Eng J Med 1989;321:1626–31–7.

HYPERCHOLESTEROLEMIA

PATRICK McBRIDE and DAVID NEVIN

SYNONYMS: High Blood Cholesterol, Hyperlipidemia, Dyslipidemia

BACKGROUND

Hypercholesterolemia is a major risk factor for coronary artery disease (CAD) and atherosclerosis, which are the leading causes of death and disability in the United States. CAD accounts for approximately 1.5 million myocardial infarctions and 520,000 deaths in the United States each year, resulting in health costs of $95 billion each year.[1] Over 300,000 people die from myocardial infarctions each year before reaching a hospital, and more than 45 per cent of all deaths from CAD occur in people under age 65.[1] However, there has been a 40 per cent decline in cardiovascular incidence and mortality in the United States in the past three decades, which has been attributed to modification of life-style, medical treatment, and surgery.[2] It is estimated that the national decline in average serum cholesterol levels of 7 to 12 mg/dl accounts for 30 per cent of the decline in CAD.[2]

Approximately 25 per cent of adults in the United States have serum cholesterol levels of 240 mg/dl or higher, and nearly half have a cholesterol exceeding 200 mg/dl.[3] A reduction in plasma cholesterol levels of 10 to 15 per cent can be expected in individuals consuming the average American diet when dietary saturated fatty acids are decreased to 10 per cent of total calories and dietary cholesterol to 300 mg per day.[4] Elevated low-density lipoprotein (LDL) and very low density lipoprotein (VLDL) and decreased high-density lipoprotein (HDL) are causally related to the development of atherosclerosis.[4,5] Evidence from epidemiologic, pathologic, genetic, animal, and metabolic studies has long supported the relationship between serum cholesterol and atherosclerosis.[6]

Treatment of hyperlipidemias has been demonstrated to be effective in reducing CAD morbidity and mortality in primary and secondary prevention clinical trials.[7,8,9,10] In the Lipids Research Clinics (LRC) Primary Prevention Trial,[7] men with LDL elevations treated with cholestyramine had a 19 per cent reduction in CAD death and nonfatal myocardial infarction compared with the placebo group and a greater than 20 per cent reduction in the incidence of positive exercise tests, angina, and bypass surgery. The Helsinki Heart Trial[8] used gemfibrozil treatment in middle-aged men with multiple types of lipoprotein disorders and found a 34 per cent reduction in the incidence of CAD. Neither study demonstrated a decrease in total mortality, but they were not designed to, owing to limitations in sample size and cost. The Coronary Drug Project[9] found that men treated with niacin for 5 years after myocardial infarction had an 11 per cent decrease in CAD and total mortality when evaluated 15 years after the trial. The Cholesterol Lowering Atherosclerosis Study[10] used coronary angiograms to evaluate the effect of aggressive lipid-lowering therapy (niacin and colestipol) to lower LDL to less than 110 mg/dl and found lack of progression and probable regression of coronary lesions with two years of treatment.

Given the high prevalence of hypercholesterolemia, the demonstration of effective therapies, and newly developed practical and accurate methods for testing blood cholesterol, it is timely to review the current diagnostic strategies for hypercholesterolemia. It is imperative that physicians detect and treat those individuals at risk to continue to reduce the burden of atherosclerosis and premature CAD.

It is currently recommended that all adults, and children from high-risk families, know their blood cholesterol.[4,11,12] Blood cholesterol measurement is an important component of periodic health maintenance and will identify a large number of individuals needing further diagnostic evaluation, management, and follow-up. Hypercholesterolemia can be detected easily, but in order to determine an appropriate diagnosis and plan for patients and families, an assessment of individual medical, social, and family histories; careful physical examination; and distributions of lipoproteins, are needed. Screening recommendations, special diagnostic tests, and clinical features of primary and secondary disorders will be discussed in this chapter to outline a useful diagnostic approach.

Lipoprotein Metabolism

Hypercholesterolemia includes common primary (genetically determined) disorders of lipoprotein metabolism and abnormal lipoprotein elevations induced by behavioral or secondary metabolic causes. A brief review of the structure and transport of lipoproteins, highlighting the mechanisms of genetic and acquired dyslipidemias, will set the stage for understanding key events in normal and abnormal cholesterol metabolism.

There are four major classes of lipoproteins, each with the same basic structure. Lipids (cholesterol, triglycerides, and phospholipids) are relatively insoluble in water but become miscible in water or plasma when combined with their specific proteins (apoproteins). Lipoprotein particles are arranged with hydrophobic cholesterol esters and triglycerides within the core and hydrophylic free cholesterol, phospholipids, and apoproteins on the particle surface.

It is useful to understand that VLDLs and chylomicrons are triglyceride-rich lipoproteins, and LDLs and HDLs are the principal cholesterol transport lipoproteins. Measurement of total cholesterol is the sum of the cholesterol contained in each type of lipoprotein. Normally, LDL and HDL are the principal carriers of cholesterol in the blood, with a small fraction being transported by VLDL.

Each of these lipoproteins can also be defined by its apoprotein constituents: chylomicrons (apo B-48, A-I, A-II), VLDL (apo B-100, E, C-II, C-III), LDL (apo B-100), and HDL (apo A-I, A-II, C-II, C-III). Apoproteins have multiple regulatory functions including lipoprotein assembly, enzyme activation, and recognition at the cellular receptors. The metabolism of lipoproteins is very complex in that, except for apo B-100, all the protein and lipid constituents can be exchanged among the different lipoproteins. Thus, an abnormality in one step of the transport path will often affect other lipoproteins and can lead to clinical disease.

The lipid transport system can be divided into the exogenous and endogenous pathways.

The exogenous pathway describes the movement of dietary fat to the liver. After ingestion of a fatty meal, triglycerides and cholesterol are packaged into chylomicrons, released into the mesenteric lymph, and reach the circulation. Lipoprotein lipase (LPL), an enzyme located in the capillary beds of adipose and muscle tissue, catalyzes the release of free fatty acids, resulting in the relatively cholesterol-enriched chylomicron remnant. Chylomicrons are cleared from the plasma within six to eight hours and are not normally found after an overnight fast. Mutations of apoprotein E, resulting in diminished binding to the remnant receptor, causes an accumulation of atherogenic remnant particles, termed beta-VLDL, seen in the disease dysbetalipoproteinemia.

The endogenous pathway has two paths: the VLDL-IDL-LDL pathway and the reverse cholesterol transport pathway mediated by HDL. Triglyceride and cholesterol are formed into VLDL. VLDL triglycerides are subsequently hydrolyzed by LPL, leading to a smaller intermediate particle that is enriched in cholesterol. Some of the VLDL is directly removed by the liver, whereas the rest follows a cascade through intermediate-density lipoprotein (IDL) to LDL through further hydrolysis.

LDL is the major lipoprotein that transports cholesterol to peripheral tissues (e.g., adrenal glands for steroid hormone biosynthesis) or back to the liver. LDL can be cleared from the plasma through the LDL receptor pathway or via non-LDL receptor pathways. Apo B-100 is the protein that mediates LDL uptake by the receptor. Patients with familial hypercholesterolemia (FH) lack, or have nonfunctional, LDL receptors and have markedly elevated plasma LDL levels. LDL is considered the major atherogenic lipoprotein, and prolonged residence in the plasma leads to deposition into the vascular wall and modification of LDL, which promotes macrophages to form foam cells, contributing to atherosclerotic plaque development. A mutation in apo B-100 has been found that causes this protein to be a poor ligand for the LDL receptor and may be a cause of premature atherosclerosis.

Reverse cholesterol transport, in which cholesterol in peripheral tissues is moved to the liver, is largely mediated by HDL. HDL is secreted by both the intestine and liver and acquires cholesterol, phospholipids, and other apoproteins from chylomicrons and VLDL undergoing lipolysis. Excess plasma membrane cholesterol from peripheral tissues can also be a cholesterol source for HDL. Nascent HDL (HDL-3) is a small, discoid form that increases in size during this cholesterol transfer process, becoming mature HDL (HDL-2). The enzyme lecithin acyltransferase (LCAT), with apo A-I as its cofactor, catalyzes the esterification of free cholesterol to cholesterol ester, which is trapped into the core of HDL. Cholesterol ester transfer protein (CETP) then facilitates exchange of cholesterol ester to VLDL or LDL for eventual return to the liver. Mutations in LCAT lead to very low levels of HDL, whereas mutations diminishing the function of CETP lead to elevations of HDL.

Lipoprotein(a) [Lp(a)] is a recently characterized lipoprotein that has been found to be a significant inherited risk factor for premature CAD. In a study of individuals with angiographically documented CAD, Lp(a) excess was noted in one third of patients and associated with a 2.7-fold increase in risk.[13] Lp(a) is similar in lipid composition to LDL and contains an apoprotein, apo(a), which is linked to this LDL molecule. Variation in plasma Lp(a) is largely genetically determined, with little apparent effect from diet. The normal function of Lp(a) is unknown but, owing to the striking structural similarity of apo(a) to plasminogen, is postulated to contribute to atherosclerosis by competing with plasminogen and diminishing fibrinolysis. Assays for Lp(a) are being tested and will be available in the near future.

HISTORY

The clinical evaluation includes a careful history, physical examination, and laboratory tests to accurately characterize overall risk, to rule out secondary causes, and to identify genetic and environmental influences on lipoproteins.

An assessment for the presence of underlying atherosclerosis and associated risk factors is the most important diagnostic goal for a patient with hypercholesterolemia. The presence of atherosclerosis, particularly documented CAD, requires a more aggressive approach to the patient and family, owing to well established risks and treatment benefits for those patients.[10,14]

Risk factor assessment is necessary because an elevated cholesterol has more influence on CAD risk when other risk factors are present.[15] The presence of multiple risk factors exponentially increases risk owing to their interactive nature in the atherosclerotic process.[15] The presence of multiple risk factors is more important, in many cases, than a single risk factor that is substantially elevated. For example, the presence of a cholesterol of 250 mg/dl approximately doubles the risk in a male without other risk factors, whereas the additional risk of a hypertensive, smoking male with high blood cholesterol is over 10 times that of a male with no other risk factors.[15] Therefore, every patient evaluation for CAD and atherosclerosis risk should be based on overall risk and likelihood of treatment benefit.

A risk assessment includes a personal health history (with an emphasis on cardiovascular review), family history, and life-style habits to guide diagnostic and management decisions. Major risk factors for CAD include: history of cerebrovascular or peripheral vascular disease, male sex, family history of premature coronary artery disease (one or more parents, grandparents, or siblings with CAD before age 55), hypercholesterolemia (LDL greater than 160 mg/dl), low HDL cholesterol (less than 35 mg/dl), high blood pressure (systolic greater than 150, diastolic greater than 95 mm Hg), cigarette smoking, obesity (greater than 130 per cent of ideal body weight), a sedentary life-style, and diabetes mellitus. An overall assessment of risk can be estimated using risk prediction equations which are particularly useful for the individual at substantial risk owing to multiple, marginal elevations of known risk factors.[15]

Focused Queries

1. *Do you, or anyone in your immediate family, have a history of heart disease, heart attack, angina, coronary bypass surgery, stroke, circulatory problems in your legs, or a past positive exercise tolerance test?*

2. *Do you have chest pain, shortness of breath, sweating, or other symptoms that occur at rest or during exertion?* Evaluate for dyspnea, orthopnea, lightheadedness, or syncope.

3. *Do you have any history of hypertension, current or past smoking, or obesity?*

4. *Is there a personal history of diabetes, kidney disease, hypothyroidism, and medication use?* Medications that may cause secondary elevations of cholesterol include beta blockers, thiazide diuretics, and steroid hormones.

5. *If immediate—that is, first-degree—family members (grandparents, father, mother, siblings, or children) have (had) cardiovascular disease, can you identify events, age at disease onset and death, whether autopsy was done, and known risk factors in other family members?*

6. *Can you provide lipoprotein levels for other first-degree family members?*

7. *Is there a history of abdominal pain, documented pancreatitis, alcohol intake, diabetes, or a family history of these problems?* This question is especially important if triglycerides are elevated. Individuals with pancreatitis should have a review of family histories of lipoprotein disorders and associated diseases.

Nutritional History and Assessment

A baseline nutritional assessment is needed prior to providing recommendations for behavior change in patients with hypercholesterolemia and to identify individuals with environmentally-induced dyslipidemias. A nutritional assessment can be performed efficiently in the office setting, using any of a variety of office instruments, by asking the patient to fill out the instrument while waiting or between visits.

Assessments can be made by using a history of the past 24 hour's food intake but are more specific for counseling when assessed by a three-day food diary or a food frequency instrument. A diary provides information on food eaten and can include times, locations, eating situations, feelings, and other information potentially useful for counseling strategies. A food frequency asks a patient to estimate food intake by categories as an "average" to attempt to provide an estimate of regular intakes instead of a single time period.

A dietary history will help identify those hypercholesterolemic patients with important environmental influences on their cholesterol level. Office staff can be trained to take very complete nutritional histories, to obtain information for referrals, and to provide initial nutritional recommendations for the patient. Referrals for detailed assessment can be made for patients requiring detailed histories and counseling, including patients with complicated nutritional needs, patients with adherence problems, or those who have not previously responded to initial recommendations. Nutritional assessment should be considered on a periodic basis to monitor adherence, as nutrition is the cornerstone of therapy for all patients with hypercholesterolemia.[4]

PHYSICAL EXAMINATION

The most important goals of the physical examination in the hypercholesterolemic patient are to assess for the presence of atherosclerosis and the manifestations of inherited dyslipidemias. Typically, a moderate cholesterol elevation is detectable only by laboratory testing and produces no physical findings. Table 1 lists skin signs that may be found in patients with unusual lipoprotein disorders. Xan-

TABLE 1.   Physical Examination Findings in Genetic Lipoprotein Disorders

PHYSICAL FINDING	LOCATION	LIPOPROTEIN DISORDER	SECONDARY DISORDER
Xanthomas			
Eruptive	Buttocks	Chylomicronemia (type I)	Pancreatitis
	Hands	Familial hypertriglyceridemias (type V)	Hepatosplenomegaly
	Abdomen		Diabetes
Tuboeruptive	Elbows	Familial dysbetalipoproteinemia (excess	Monoclonal gammopathies
	Knees	IDL—type III)	
Planar	Palms	Familial dysbetalipoproteinemia	Monoclonal gammopathies
	Diffuse	Apoprotein A-I deficiency	
Tendinous	Extensor tendons (hand, knees, Achilles)	Familial hypercholesterolemia	
Xanthelasma	Eyelids	Familial dysbetalipoproteinemia	Monoclonal gammopathies
		Familial hypercholesterolemia	
Corneal arcus	Cornea	Familial hypercholesterolemia	
Corneal opacities	Cornea	HDL deficiencies	Hepatosplenomegaly
			Lymphadenopathy
Tonsillar deposits	Tonsils	Apolipoprotein A-I abnormality (Tangier disease)	Hepatosplenomegaly
			Lymphadenopathy

thelasma and corneal arcus are more common in hyperlipidemic individuals but may occur in normolipidemic persons. If the other skin findings listed in Table 1 are found, they suggest a specific genetic disorder. Tendinous xanthoma, or deposits that produce irregular thickening of extensor tendons, can be a marker for familial hypercholesterolemia. Eruptive xanthoma, usually found on the hands or over extensor tendons of the extremities, is associated with severe hypertriglyceridemias (greater than 1000 mg/dl) and chylomicronemia. Chylomicronemia may be accompanied by lipemia retinalis, abdominal pain, pancreatitis, or memory loss. Tuberous, or tuboeruptive, xanthoma manifests as nodules over extensor tendons and is seen with familial dysbetalipoproteinemia (type III).

Genetic disorders producing HDL deficiencies may also have associated physical findings.[16] However, these disorders are very rare. Tangier's disease, a genetic disorder associated with hypercatabolism of HDL, and subsequent HDL deficiency, is identified by the presence of enlarged orange tonsils, hepatosplenomegaly, corneal opacification, lymphadenopathy, and premature CAD. Corneal opacification has also been noted in three other HDL-deficient familial disorders: fisheye disease (unknown cause), familial lecithin:cholesterol acyltransferase deficiency (associated with anemia and renal failure), and combined apolipoprotein A-I and C-III deficiency. Families with these disorders should usually be referred to a center specializing in lipoprotein disorders, owing to their rare occurrence and need for specialized studies and treatment.

The cardiovascular examination can identify patients with sequelae of CAD including enlargement or dysfunction of the left ventricle (sustained, displaced, or dyskinetic point of maximal impulse [PMI]), decreased compliance of the left ventricle (S_3,S_4), or other signs of myocardial/endocardial damage secondary to CAD (regurgitant murmurs due to papillary muscle dysfunction, ventricular aneurysm). Examination of the vasculature, including eye fundus, carotids, abdominal aorta, and peripheral arteries for evidence of atherosclerosis is essential to identify high-risk patients. Examination of the lower extremities may reveal evidence of peripheral vascular disease (decreased pulses, bruits, ischemic changes), signs of vascular congestion (edema), and tendinous signs of familial hypercholesterolemia (Achilles tendon xanthoma or thickening).

DIAGNOSTIC STUDIES

Testing for cholesterol is now more practical owing to the availability and reliability of office testing equipment and evidence that blood cholesterol is accurate in a nonfasting state.[4] Exceptions for the accuracy of cholesterol measurement in the nonfasting state include patients who are pregnant, acutely ill, or losing weight or the rare patient who is significantly hypertriglyceridemic (triglycerides greater than 500 mg/dl),[4] because cholesterol levels in such patients may not reflect their baseline levels.

Measurement of total cholesterol can be reliably obtained by either venipuncture or finger stick if the laboratory is participating in national standardization programs. Biologic variation and measurement error may produce measurements that do not necessarily reflect the true steady-state cholesterol, and therefore, a single test may not be representative. Blood should be drawn after the individual is seated for five minutes. Increasing lymphatic fluid in the specimen will inappropriately raise the serum cholesterol level, so the tourniquet should be applied just prior to drawing the blood, and finger stick measures should not be done after "milking" the finger to increase blood flow. Plasma cholesterols are approximately 5 per cent lower than serum samples. Serum cholesterol levels undergo physiologic fluctuations due to gender, stress, and season.[12] Owing to the possible variations in cholesterol measurement, the average of at least two tests should be used for any management decisions.

Adults with a total cholesterol averaging over 240 mg/dl on two separate occasions, with a family history of premature coronary disease or dyslipidemia, or more than one major risk factor when the average of at least two total cholesterols is 200 to 239 mg/dl should be considered for a fasting measurement of total cholesterol, triglycerides, HDL, and an estimated LDL (see Table 2). Determinations of risk based on all lipoproteins is an ideal, but owing to cost constraints, inconvenience, and other barriers, lipoprotein profiles cannot be considered for routine screening in all adults at this time.

Lipoprotein measurements are generally reported in milligrams per deciliter (mg/dl), but in the newer standard international units, these values are reported millimoles per liter (mmol/l). The conversion factor for total cholesterol, HDL, and LDL is used by multiply-

TABLE 2. Lipoprotein Testing for Adults Based on Screening Cholesterol Level*

CHOLESTEROL (mg/dl)	ATHEROSCLEROSIS,[†] FAMILY HISTORY,[‡] OR TWO RISK FACTORS[§]	RECOMMENDATION
<200	No	Total cholesterol level only; repeat in five years
<200	Yes	Lipoprotein profile
200–239	No	Total cholesterol level only; re-evaluate annually
200–239	Yes	Lipoprotein profile
>240	Yes/no	Lipoprotein profile

* Recommend average of two cholesterol values at minimum—nonfasting total levels.

† Known atherosclerosis (including coronary artery or peripheral vascular disease).

‡ Family history of sibling or parent with premature (less than age 55) atherosclerosis.

§ Male sex, smoking, hypertension, obesity, diabetes, low HDL (less than 35 mg/dl).

ing the mg/dl measurement by 0.026. The conversion factor for triglycerides is 0.0113.

The patient with premature atherosclerotic disease, that is, prior to age 55, represents a special situation.[14] This group includes men and women with premature myocardial infarction, coronary artery bypass grafting, angina pectoris, peripheral vascular disease, or cerebrovascular disease. Approximately two thirds of these patients will have an abnormal lipoprotein phenotype. The most common lipoprotein problems noted in those with premature CAD are those associated with low HDL cholesterol.[13] Testing family members will have a very high yield in finding individuals with dyslipidemias and other risk factors.[17] Following myocardial infarction, or any major systemic illness, lipoprotein levels may not return to baseline for a period of up to three to six months.[4]

Apoproteins (apo A-I and apo B-100) have been suggested by some as a potentially more accurate measure of risk than current lipid measures owing to their recognition at lipoprotein receptors, the potential for very accurate testing of proteins as compared with lipids, and case control studies that have shown greater specificity for CAD. However, despite the potential of the apoproteins, particularly Lp(a),[13] testing cannot currently be recommended unless performed at specialized centers because of lack of standardized measurements for these tests.

ASSESSMENT

Measurement of cholesterol is an important component of health maintenance for adults and should be incorporated into office practice routine. The National Cholesterol Education Program (NCEP) Expert Panel[4] has developed guidelines for office detection and management of the high-risk individual that can be adapted to each physician's practice style. Total cholesterol levels can be drawn nonfasting for routine testing but should be redrawn after a 12-h fast if confirmation of cholesterol or measurement of triglycerides and HDL are needed. A total cholesterol level greater than 240 mg/dl, if LDL is confirmed greater than 160 mg/dl, is clearly associated with increased risk of atherosclerosis and is considered high blood cholesterol. A total cholesterol level of 200 to 239 mg/dl, with LDL 130 to 159, is considered a borderline cholesterol level owing to the increasing risk of this range and the likelihood that a subsequent measure may be higher. A total cholesterol level of 200 mg/dl is greater than the 90th percentile for children aged 2 to 19 and, therefore a level ≥200 mg/dl is considered high in childhood.[18]

Lipoprotein levels help distinguish level of risk and likelihood of a genetic basis for the dyslipidemia. Lipoprotein phenotyping is most useful for distinguishing between disorders with very high triglyceride elevations—

that is, greater than 500 mg/dl—and generally not otherwise clinically useful.

Table 2 outlines the approach for measuring lipoprotein profiles (total cholesterol, triglyceride, HDL cholesterol, and calculated LDL cholesterol) in the office. This approach is based on the well-documented evidence that individuals with known atherosclerosis and CAD risk factors are more likely to be at risk with abnormal lipoprotein profiles.[6,13] A lipoprotein profile is used to guide risk assessment and decisions regarding therapy. A total cholesterol, triglyceride, and HDL can be drawn, and LDL calculated, if the specimen is drawn fasting and the triglyceride level is below 400 mg/dl. LDL is calculated using the formula:

$$LDL = Total\ cholesterol - HDL - \frac{Triglycerides}{5}$$

Lipoprotein phenotyping, or electrophoresis, is not recommended as a routine to evaluate patients. A lipoprotein profile will permit classification of common disorders, as outlined earlier. Lipoprotein phenotyping is useful to distinguish Fredrickson-Levy classifications of patients with triglycerides above 500 mg/dl not found related to secondary causes.

Secondary causes of hypercholesterolemias should be considered and ruled out prior to further testing and considering treatment. Secondary causes of altered lipoproteins include excess dietary fat, alcohol, or calories; obesity; diabetes; medications (steroids, beta blockers, thiazides); hypothyroidism; nephrosis; obstructive liver disease; and myeloma. In our experience, hypothyroidism is the most easily missed common cause of secondary hyperlipidemia and should be considered especially in older patients. Consideration of a secondary cause is also important when a sudden elevation of lipoproteins is noted in a patient who had previously normal levels. Treatment of secondary causes will often result in marked improvement, or normalization, of abnormal lipoprotein levels.

Patients with a total cholesterol greater than 240 mg/dl, and an LDL greater than 160 mg/dl, should have an evaluation for possible secondary causes of their apparent dyslipidemia. A directed history, a sensitive thyroid stimulating hormone (TSH) assay, and a fasting chemistry survey (including glucose, liver functions, proteins, and creatinine) will rule out major secondary causes of hypercholesterolemia.

Lipoprotein Classifications

Four classifications of lipoprotein disorders can simplify the basic approach to diagnosis and treatment (Table 3). These classifications provide a more practical office management by basing treatment initially on the triglyceride (TG), LDL, and HDL measurements and does not require phenotyping. This approach is currently recommended by the NCEP guidelines.[4] The Fredrickson-Levy classification remains important for more complicated dyslipidemias.[16]

Elevated LDL Cholesterol (LDL Greater than 160 mg/dl, TG Less than 200 mg/dl)

Elevation of LDL cholesterol, occurring without elevation of triglycerides, is considered either primary (i.e., without known cause) or familial. FH represents a fraction of individuals with hypercholesterolemia but has provided important insights into cholesterol metabolism. FH is caused by defects in the LDL receptor gene, which impair cellular uptake and clearance of LDL and result in lack

TABLE 3. Practical Approach to Classifying Lipoprotein Disorders

LIPID CLASSIFI-CATION DISORDER	FREDRICKSON-LEVY CLASS	GENETIC
LDL Elevated (normal HDL, TG)	II-A	Familial hypercholesterolemia Polygenic hypercholesterolemia
Triglycerides elevated (normal LDL, HDL)	I, V	LPL deficiency Apo C-II deficiency Familial hypertriglyceridemia
HDL decreased (normal LDL, TG)	—	Hypoalphalipoproteinemia
Combined hyperlipidemias (elevated LDL, TG; decreased HDL)	II-B, IV III	Familial combined hyperlipidemia Familial dysbetalipoproteinemia

of suppression of de novo cholesterol synthesis. Heterozygous FH (two to three times normal LDL cholesterol) affects 1 in 500 individuals in the general population[6] and approximately 5 per cent of the victims of premature myocardial infarction.[6,13] Homozygous FH is rare, affecting 1 in 1 million persons, and causes massively elevated LDL and total cholesterol levels (six to eight times normal LDL). Individuals with homozygous FH usually develop coronary artery disease in childhood and require special care. Distinguishing features of FH are the autosomal dominant pattern of expression, the selective elevation of plasma LDL (greater than 200 mg/dl), and the formation of xanthomas of the Achilles, patellar, or triceps tendons.

The vast majority of individuals with moderately elevated LDL (total cholesterol 240 to 300) do not have FH and are classified as primary, or polygenic, hypercholesterolemia. Multiple factors, including nutrition, obesity, and a number of genetic factors, contribute to this group. Recently, a mutation in apoprotein B-100 has been discovered in individuals with moderate or marked hypercholesterolemia and is termed familial defective apo B-100. Its clinical presentation may mimic FH.[19]

Hypertriglyceridemias (TG Greater than 500 mg/dl)

Clinically important hypertriglyceridemias are manifestations of either elevated VLDL and/or chylomicrons. Distinguishing between hypertriglyceridemias and hyperchylomicronemias is possible only by lipoprotein phenotyping, as these conditions both will produce elevated triglycerides on a routine evaluation. Hypertriglyceridemias are either genetically caused or due to the combination of genetic predisposition and secondary causes, including diabetes, obesity, or nephrosis. Patients presenting with fasting triglycerides greater than 1000 mg/dl usually have genetic forms, but secondary causes can exacerbate these conditions. Excessive use of alcohol and certain medications such as estrogens, progestins, beta blockers, or thiazide diuretics can also exacerbate hypertriglyceridemia.

Chylomicrons are normally absent after a 12–14-hour fast. Hypertriglyceridemia greater than 1000 mg/dl is associated with the appearance of chylomicrons, and levels above 2000 mg/dl have an increased risk of pancreatitis. This condition can be devastating, causing severe complications or death, emphasizing the importance of recognizing these patients. Familial lipoprotein lipase deficiency, familial apolipoprotein C-II deficiency, and familial inhibitor to lipoprotein lipase deficiency are rare genetic disorders causing chylomicronemia. These families can be identified by presentation in childhood, pancreatitis, and eruptive xanthomatosis. These diagnoses may be considered if triglycerides are greater than 1000 mg/dl and can be confirmed by lipoprotein lipase studies available in specialized laboratories.

Combined Hyperlipidemias (LDL Greater than 160 mg/dl and TG Greater than 200 mg/dl)

This very important category of lipoprotein disorders includes disorders with moderate to severe elevations of LDL and triglycerides and often a low HDL cholesterol. These disorders are either the type II-B or IV in the Fredrickson-Levy classification system but are very difficult to distinguish either clinically or in the laboratory; therefore, phenotyping is not generally clinically useful to distinguish between them. No specific physical examination findings are present in the combined hyperlipidemia disorders, although they are often noted in patients with obesity, particularly if the obesity is central (truncal).[20] Other secondary causes for combined hyperlipidemias include hypothyroidism, diabetes, nephrotic syndrome, and glucocorticoid use.

Familial combined hyperlipidemia (FCHL) is a very common lipoprotein disorder noted in 10 to 15 per cent of survivors of myocardial infarction[13] and a high percentage of patients who undergo coronary bypass surgery. Identification of FCHL relies on investigation of family members to make the diagnosis, as no specific test exists. This disorder usually does not manifest until young adulthood and is characterized by the presence of multiple combinations of abnormal lipoprotein phenotypes (II-A, II-B, IV, or V) in a family.[16] Approximately one third of family members with this syndrome have elevated VLDL-TG, one third have only elevated LDL, and in the rest, both are elevated. A useful diagnostic clue is elevation of VLDL-TG when drug therapy is directed at lowering LDL, or vice versa.

Hyperapobetalipoproteinemia is a subset of FCHL in which LDL particles are small and dense. These individuals have an increased risk for premature CAD with normal cholesterol levels and are distinguished by high levels of apoprotein B-100.[19]

Familial dysbetalipoproteinemia (type III) is an uncommon cause of combined hyperlipidemia, but should be noted because of its association with premature CAD and differences in treatment from other disorders with triglyceride elevations. This disorder should be suspected when both fasting cholesterol and triglyceride levels are greater than 300 to 400 mg/dl and when planar and tuboeruptive xanthomas are noted. The major genetic defect is delayed clearance of VLDL and chylomicron remnants associated with defects or absence of apoprotein E. This defect in apoprotein E is present in 1 per cent of the general population, but type III is present in only a fraction of these individuals, suggesting other factors must be implicated in its development. Remnant particles, which include cholesterol-enriched VLDL, can be detected on agarose electrophoresis. Indeed, individuals with familial dysbetalipoproteinemia may not present with xanthomas or CAD until middle age. This disorder requires specialized laboratory testing and may require evaluation at a specialized lipid program.

Low HDL Cholesterol (HDL Less than 35 mg/dl)

HDL cholesterol is inversely associated with atherosclerosis risk and is considered to be the most powerful predictor of premature CAD.[21] Whether low HDL is a manifestation of other metabolic or life-style factors rather than the source of CAD risk remains controversial, but studies to date have shown HDL to be an independent predictor of risk even when controlling for other risk factors.

Low HDL cholesterol is associated with genetic deficiencies, male sex, hypertriglyceridemias, obesity, smoking, and a sedentary life-style.[16] Familial hypoalphalipoproteinemia, a common low HDL cholesterol syndrome, is characterized by HDL levels below 35 mg/dl, normal triglyceride levels, and autosomal dominant inheritance.[16] This disorder is associated with premature CAD and is present in approximately 7 to 10 per cent of patients with CAD before age 60.[13] Low HDL cholesterol has also been noted in combined dyslipidemias (discussed earlier) and is also commonly associated with central obesity and the early onset of hypertension in families with a history of premature CAD.[20] Medications that lower HDL, and perhaps increase risk, include beta blockers (nonsympathomimetic), progestins, anabolic steroids, and possibly thiazide diuretics.[4] Other rare genetic forms of HDL deficiencies exist and are discussed in detail elsewhere.[16]

Assessment of Special Populations

Identification of secondary hyperlipidemias, such as hypothyroidism or diabetes mellitus, will aid the appropriate classification of patients and avoid unnecessary use of hypolipidemic drugs. Diabetes is particularly important to recognize owing to its major association with atherosclerosis and the additional risk of dyslipidemias in persons with diabetes. Careful control of blood glucose in type I diabetes will often correct associated lipoprotein abnormalities, but individuals with type II diabetes will often have residual dyslipidemias despite good control.[22] Individuals with type II diabetes typically have normal or moderately elevated LDL levels, moderate or markedly elevated triglycerides, and decreased HDL.[23]

Assessment of children for hypercholesterolemia remains controversial. Routine screening of all children as part of routine health maintenance has been advocated[18] but is not yet universally accepted. All children with parents, grandparents, or siblings with premature CAD should have lipoprotein profiles, at least once after age two, to identify genetic lipoprotein disorders. As the atherosclerosis process begins in childhood, identification and treatment of children with hypercholesterolemia will be an important strategy to reduce premature plaque development and atherosclerosis in high-risk children.

Increasing evidence indicates that an elevated LDL cholesterol remains an important risk factor beyond age 65.[23] Decisions to test older adults should be individualized and not based on age alone but based on an assessment of potential benefits and risks of possible testing or treatment. Evaluation of the older adult for dyslipidemias, especially when atherosclerotic complications or multiple risk factors are present, is recommended if the patient's long-term prognosis, motivation, and quality of life are reasonable.[4,24]

A decision to test for, or treat, hypercholesterolemia should be based on patient motivation and an appropriate cost-benefit balance for each individual. While benefit for adult males is well established, data on other population groups is less clear. Thus, women also represent a special population to consider in the evaluation of hypercholesterolemia. Nearly one fourth of premenopausal women with an elevated total cholesterol will have an LDL cholesterol considered low risk, and their cholesterol will be elevated owing to a high HDL cholesterol. These women have been shown to be at overall low risk if other risk factors are not present.[21] While clinical trials of cholesterol reduction are limited, epidemiologic evidence indicates that women with dyslipidemias are at risk equivalent to men with the same risk factors and should be evaluated for possible treatment.[4,5,15,21] Therefore, if any individual over age two has a high-risk profile—that is, with multiple risk factors—thorough evaluation is essential because of established risks independent of age or sex. Treatment guidelines for hypercholesterolemia are available for adults,[4] older adults,[24] and children.[18]

Managing Hypercholesterolemia

Targeted dietary recommendations are the first step in distinguishing between genetic and environmentally induced hypercholesterolemia. Nutritional recommendations to provide adequate calories, a variety of foods, and appropriate amounts of total fat, saturated fat, and cholesterol are available for all age groups.[4,18] Other nonpharmacologic strategies, such as weight loss, exercise, and smoking cessation, may improve blood cholesterol levels and eliminate the need for detailed diagnostic evaluations. LDL cholesterol levels should ideally be less than 130 mg/dl for reduction of risk but may need to be even lower in the individual with atherosclerosis to produce regression.[10,25]

A careful assessment of overall risk is the cornerstone of management of the high-risk individual and family. Lipoprotein measurements need to be included in the assessment of risk if the history, physical examination, or screening cholesterol levels indicate the presence of atherosclerosis, or significant risk, in the patient. Future clarifications of lipoprotein and apoprotein abnormalities and measurements will increase our abilities to predict risk and define treatment.

REFERENCES

1. American Heart Association. 1990 Heart facts. Dallas: American Heart Association, 1989.
2. Goldman L, Cook EF. The decline in ischemic heart disease mortality rates. Ann Intern Med 1984;101:825–36.
3. Sempos C, Fulwood R, Haines C, et al. The prevalence of high blood cholesterol levels among adults in the United States. JAMA 1989;262:45–52.
4. The Expert Panel. Report of the National Cholesterol Education Program Expert Panel on Detection, Evaluation, and Treatment of High Cholesterol in Adults. Arch Intern Med 1988;148:36–69.
5. Consensus Conference. Lowering blood cholesterol to prevent heart disease. JAMA 1985;253:2080–6.
6. Grundy SM. Cholesterol and coronary heart disease. A new era. JAMA 1986;256:2849–58.
7. Lipid Research Clinics Program. The Lipid Research Clinics Coronary Primary Prevention Trial results, I and II. JAMA 1984;251:351–74.
8. Frick MH, Elo O, Happa K, et al. Helsinki Heart Study. N Engl J Med 1987;317:1237–45.
9. Canner PL, Berge LG, Wenger NK, et al. Fifteen year mortality in Coronary Drug Project patients: long-term benefit with niacin. J Am Coll Cardiol 1986;8:1245–55.
10. Blankenhorn DH, Nessim SA, Johnson RL, et al. Beneficial effects of combined colestipol-niacin therapy on coronary atherosclerosis and coronary bypass grafts. JAMA 1987;257:3233–40.
11. Frame PS. A critical review of adult health maintenance, part 1: prevention of atherosclerotic diseases. J Fam Pract 1986;22:341–6.
12. US Preventive Services Task Force. Screening for high blood cholesterol. Am Fam Physician 1990;41:503–13.
13. Genest J, Martin-Munley S, McNamara JR, Salem DN, Schaefer EJ. Frequency of genetic dyslipidemias in patients with premature coronary artery disease. Arteriosclerosis 1989;9:701A.
14. Williams RR. Nature, nurture, and family predisposition. N Engl J Med 1988;318:769–71.
15. Kannel WB, Castelli WP, Gordon T. Cholesterol in the prediction of atherosclerotic disease: new perspectives based on the Framingham Study. Ann Intern Med 1979;90:85–91.
16. Schaefer EJ, Levy RI. Pathogenesis and management of lipoprotein disorders. N Engl J Med 1985;312:1300–10.
17. Becker DM, Levine DM. Risk perception, knowledge, and lifestyles in siblings of people with premature coronary disease. Am J Prev Med 1987;3:45–50.
18. Wynder EL, Berenson GS, Strong WB, et al. Coronary artery disease prevention: cholesterol, a pediatric perspective [Monograph]. Prev Med 1989;3:328–409.
19. Innerarity TL, Weisberger KH, Arnold KS, et al. Familial defective apolipoprotein B-100: low density lipoproteins with abnormal receptor binding. Proc Natl Acad Sci USA 1987;84:6919–23.
20. Williams RR, Hunt SC, Hopkins PN, et al. Familial dyslipidemic hypertension. Evidence from 58 Utah families for a syndrome present in approximately 12% of patients with essential hypertension. JAMA 1988;259:3579–86.
21. Castelli WP, Garrison RJ, Wilson PW, et al. Incidence of coronary heart disease and lipoprotein cholesterol levels. The Framingham Study. JAMA 1986;256:2835–8.
22. Brunzell JD, Bierman EL. Chylomicronemia syndrome. In: Havel RJ, ed. Lipid disorders, Medical

Clinics of North America. Philadelphia: WB Saunders, 1982;66:455–68.

23. Howard BV. Lipoprotein metabolism in diabetes mellitus. J Lipid Res 1987;28:613–28.

24. Denke MA, Grundy SM. Hypercholesterolemia in elderly persons: resolving the treatment dilemma. Ann Intern Med 1990;112:780–92.

25. Blankenhorn D. Can arteriosclerotic lesions regress? Angiographic evidence in humans. Am J Cardiol 1990;65:41S–3S.

HYPERPIGMENTATION, GENERALIZED

ANNE D. WALLING

SYNONYM: Darkening of Skin Color

BACKGROUND

Hyperpigmentation is a general term for darkening of skin color. *Melanoderma*, although literally meaning "brown skin," is often restricted to increased pigmentation at the site of previous skin inflammation or other lesions. In contrast, *melanosis* is used to describe color change without preceding skin pathology.[1] *Melasma* refers to brown-black discoloration of the head, face, and neck, as in "the mask of pregnancy." The term *chloasma* is frequently used interchangeably with melasma[1,2] but should technically be reserved for discoloration with a greenish tinge.[2] Qualifying adjectives may also be used to describe hyperpigmentation by etiology—for example, *melanotic*, owing to an increase in melanin production without a change in the number of melanocytes; *melanocytic*, in which the number of melanocytes is increased; and *nonmelanotic*, owing to deposition of other dark pigments.[3] *Ceruloderma* ("blue skin") refers to any blue-gray coloration and *xanthoderma* to any yellowing of the skin.[3]

Within the general term of hyperpigmentation, specific clinical conditions are often referred to by eponyms or descriptive terms from Latin or French—for example, acanthosis nigricans (like the coat of a black bear) or café au lait (the color of coffee with cream).

This chapter is restricted to conditions that cause generalized rather than circumscribed darkening of skin. Descriptions of the many causes of patchy hyperpigmentation may be found in textbooks of dermatology.[1,3]

"Normal" human pigmentation is a subjective assessment of skin color based primarily on the race and previous appearance of an individual. Melanin is the principal determinant of skin color, although the perceived visual impact results from the interplay of several potential pigments in the skin and blood vessels.[3,4]

Melanin itself consists of several related complex polymers derived from tyrosine by the action of the copper-dependent enzyme tyrosinase (Fig. 1). This family of pigments is composed of insoluble and virtually nonbiodegradable polymers with the ability to absorb radiation in the range 200 to 2400 nm and thus to protect against damage by nonionizing ultraviolet irradiation. Melanin also has the ability to form biochemical bonds with a number of drugs.[5,6] Melanin is synthesized in a specialized organelle, the melanosome, within melanocytes in the basal layer of the epidermis. Each melanocyte interfaces with a group of from 20 to 36 keratinocytes in a functional epidermal melanin unit.[5,6]

Melanosomes are actively transferred through the dendritic processes of the melanocyte into adjacent keratinocytes (Fig. 2), and the migration of keratinocytes upward through epidermal layers carries pigment to the skin surface. As the keratinocyte moves toward the surface, internal lysosomal enzymes degrade the melanosomes, releasing melanin pigment within the keratinocyte. The color of skin and hair is principally determined by

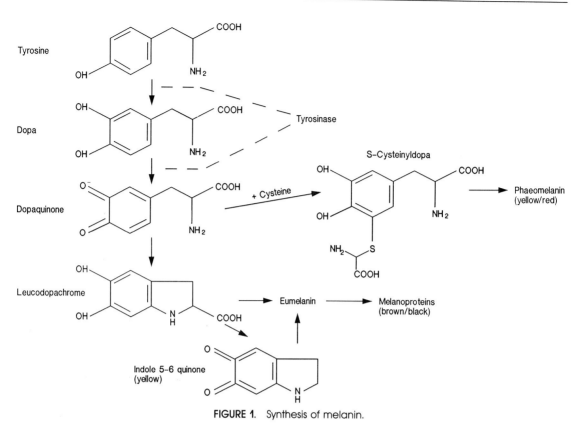

FIGURE 1. Synthesis of melanin.

the amount of melanin pigment in keratinocytes.[5,6] Differences in racial pigmentation result from differences in melanocyte activity and amount of melanin within keratinocytes rather than higher number of melanocytes in dark-skinned races. Melanosomes in white skin are small—about $0.5 \times 0.3 \ \mu m$, compared with $0.6 \times 0.3 \ \mu m$ in oriental and $1.0 \times 0.5 \ \mu m$ in negroid skin.[2] In addition to their larger size, melanosomes in dark skin are more mature and more widely dispersed within the keratinocyte. In white skin, melanosomes tend to aggregate, thus reducing the visual impact.[2,5,6] In an individual, regardless of race, the number of melanocytes varies in different parts of the body from about 900/ cu mm on the trunk to 2400/cu mm on the foreskin.[5,6] Hyperpigmentation results from overactivity of the epidermal melanin unit or, less frequently, from depositions of other dark

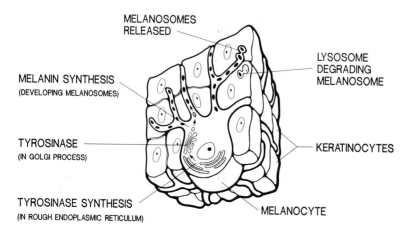

FIGURE 2. Process of skin pigmentation.

TABLE 1. Etiology of Diffuse Hyperpigmentation

Endocrine
  Addison's disease
  Graves' disease
  Cushing's syndrome
  Acromegaly
  Adrenocorticotropin or melanocyte stimulating hormone overproduction
  Estrogen excess
Metabolic
  Biliary cirrhosis
  Renal failure
  Porphyria cutanea tarda
  Hemochromatosis
  Wilson's disease
  Gaucher's disease
  Niemann-Pick disease
Drugs
  Chlorpromazine
  Amiodarone
  Busulphan
  Bleomycin
  5-Fluorouracil
  Minocycline
  Antimalarials
  Estrogens
Toxins
  Mercury
  Silver
  Arsenic
  Gold
  Lead
  Ultraviolet radiation
Nutritional
  Cachexia
  Vitamin deficiency
Neoplastic
  Adenocarcinoma (acanthosis nigricans)
  Disseminated melanoma
Other conditions
  Scleroderma
  Whipple's intestinal lipodystrophy

pigments in the skin. This process may be localized or diffuse but is almost always secondary to one of the many conditions shown in Table 1. Increased brown to black coloration indicates elevated concentrations of melanin in the surface layers of the epidermis. Melanin accumulations in lower epidermal layers and in the dermis may appear blue or gray owing to the light-scattering effect of overlying tissue.[2] Bluish or gray discoloration (ceruloderma) may also be due to deposition of other pigments, especially heavy metals.

HISTORY

As hyperpigmentation can result from so many diverse etiologies (Table 1), the medical history is the key to making an accurate and cost-effective diagnosis in individual cases. Because of the danger of subjective bias, history from friends and family members can also be helpful. The wide variation in color reproduction of photographs limits their usefulness, but they may provide corroborating evidence of increased pigmentation.

The history has two parts: to provide an understanding of the hyperpigmentation and to discover symptoms suggestive of an underlying etiology.

Focused Queries[7]

1. *When was the color change first noted? How quickly is it progressing?*

2. *What color tone (e.g., brown, black, gray, blue, yellow) best describes the pigmentation?*

3. *Are certain areas more severely affected?*

4. *Are mucous membranes involved?*

5. *Does anything, particularly sun exposure, change the intensity of the color change?*

6. *Was the onset of hyperpigmentation associated with any change in light exposure, occupation, diet, drugs, or other factors?*

7. *What symptoms does the patient associate with the color change either locally, such as pruritis, or generally, for example, malaise, nausea, weight loss?*

General Medical History[7]

In addition to asking the patient focused questions concerning his or her present symptoms, it is important to obtain a thorough and complete conventional medical history, including review of systems, previous medical history, family, and social history.[8] A complete review of systems is required to detect any symptom or pattern of symptoms suggestive of a secondary cause of hyperpigmentation (Table 1). This review must include nonspecific items such as weight loss, malaise, and anxiety as well as symptoms more directly linked to a specific body system. Drug and diet history must be included.

A comprehensive previous medical and surgical history is necessary to detect the conditions mentioned in Table 1 and associated/precursor conditions, as well as any condition for which drugs associated with hyperpigmentation may be prescribed. A high index of suspicion is appropriate, and whenever possible, medical records should be obtained to verify the history. For example, the patient may be unaware of potential damage to the adrenal glands during abdominal surgery. Similarly, a personal or family history of diabetes should raise suspicion of hemochromatosis. The prevalence of unrecognized hemochromatosis in diabetics is about 1 per cent, which is two to three times that of the general population,[8] and this condition is inherited as an autosomal recessive linked to the HLA system.

A complete and verified drug history is essential. Family history should include both general questions about morbidity and mortality of close relatives and specific inquiries about those of the conditions in Table 1 that have a familial component and that are possible given the age, sex, life-style, and other characteristics of the patient. Certain of these conditions, particularly Graves' disease and adenocarcinoma, may not have produced hyperpigmentation in the affected relative.

The social history should include documentation of the areas of skin usually exposed to sunlight as well as any exposure to heavy metals, radiation, carcinogens, or etiologic agents for the conditions in Table 1 from occupation or life-style. All historical data should be interpreted in the context of the general characteristics of the patient. With so many diverse possible etiologies, it is important to keep the differential diagnoses ranked by likelihood *in a specific patient;* for example, Addison's and Graves' disease would be highly ranked in a young woman, whereas an older female patient complaining of hyperpigmentation with pruritus might have biliary cirrhosis and renal failure as strong possibilities.

PHYSICAL EXAMINATION

Physical examination has two goals: to document the hyperpigmentation and, as hyperpigmentation is almost always secondary to a pathologic process, to seek signs indicating the etiology.

Confirming Generalized Hyperpigmentation

Whatever the etiology, generalized hyperpigmentation is rarely uniform. Color is accentuated in sun-exposed and traumatized areas such as skin folds and recent scars and over pressure points, particularly elbows. Mucous membranes are frequently also involved except in cases due to sun or other ultraviolet

light exposure. Complete inspection of skin and mucous membranes is important to verify diffuse hyperpigmentation and distinguish this condition from widespread localized increases in color such as those secondary to inflammation.

Inspection with a Wood's lamp accentuates epidermal hyperpigmentation. The use of a Wood's lamp helps to distinguish between true generalized hyperpigmentation and widespread patchy hyperpigmentation such as that secondary to extensive exfoliative dermatitis by showing up the remaining patches of pale, normally pigmented skin between the areas of hyperpigmentation. Wood's lamp also distinguishes between epidermal hyperpigmentation, which it accentuates, and deeper, dermal hyperpigmentation, which is unchanged.[3]

Determining the Etiology

The distribution and characteristics of hyperpigmentation may provide important clues to the etiology, as shown in Table 2.

Acanthosis nigricans is a particular form of generalized hyperpigmentation accompanied by papillomatous hyperplasia of the epidermis, resulting in a velvety appearance. In severe cases, this develops into verrucous patches on exposed or traumatized surfaces. The hyperpigmentation is most marked in skin folds such as the axilla and groin. Acanthosis nigricans should raise suspicion of malignancy, particularly adenocarcinoma of the lung, bowel, or breast,[9] or endocrine disorders such as Cushing's syndrome, acromegaly, or diabetes mellitus.[10]

Exaggeration of normal pigment distribution is seen in Addison's disease, scleroderma, acromegaly, and biliary cirrhosis, whereas that due to conditions of increased estrogenic hormones (including pregnancy) is most pronounced on the face and around the nipples, areolae, external genitalia, and linea alba. Generalized hyperpigmentation that begins in sun-exposed areas is seen in biliary cirrhosis and renal failure.

The many potential causes of hyperpigmentation are diverse and unrelated, requiring thorough physical examination. It is important to be systematic. General appearance and vital signs may give important information such as the tachycardia of Graves' disease, the hypotension of Addison's disease, or wasting from a malignancy. Special attention should be paid to signs associated with those conditions listed in Table 1 that are either supported

TABLE 2. Patterns of Diffuse Hyperpigmentation by Etiology

ETIOLOGY	DOMINANT COLOR	ACCENTUATED AREAS	MUCOUS MEM- BRANES	OTHER SKIN FEATURES	CLINICAL FEATURES
Addison's disease	Brown	Pressure points Trauma sites Previously pigmented areas	Involved	Loss of body hair Longitudinal nail changes	40% have pigment changes
Graves' disease	Brown	Face may be patchy	+/−	Moist, dry, smooth skin Pruritus Pretibial myxedema	70% show pigment changes
Acromegaly	Brown	Addisonian	Involved	Thickening skin, nails Oily skin Hypertrichosis	40% show pigment changes
Biliary cirrhosis	Yellow/ Brown	Exposed areas Creases of palms Face "Masque bilaire"	No	Pruritus Jaundice Hepatic signs	Often presents as pigment change
Hemochromatosis	Bronze or blue/gray	Exposed areas Trauma site	In 25% of cases	Ichthyosis Alopecia Hepatic signs	98% show pigment changes
Porphyria cutanea tarda	Brown or purple/red	Exposed areas	+/−	Hirsutism Atrophy Bullae Pruritus	May be secondary to drug, toxin, or alcohol
Renal failure	Yellow/ Brown	Exposed areas	Involved	Uermic frost Pruritus Nail changes Stomatitis	Common pigment changes
Scleroderma	Brown	Addisonian	Involved	Smooth, tight skin as Raynaud's	May present as skin darkening
Argyria	Blue/gray	Exposed areas	Involved	Nail changes	Intoxication

by history or appropriate for other characteristics of the patient. For example, in an older male smoker, the high degree of suspicion of lung carcinoma would emphasize the respiratory examination, whereas in a nonsmoking woman of the same age who had symptoms of pruritus, special attention would be paid to signs of biliary cirrhosis. Both patients require complete physical examination supported by appropriate laboratory and other diagnostic tests.

DIAGNOSTIC STUDIES

Laboratory tests should be planned to provide confirmatory evidence for the most likely of the differential diagnoses ranked on the history, physical examination, and general characteristics of the patient. Clinical chemistry measurements that have come to be regarded as "routine" such as complete blood count, metabolic profile, liver function tests, thyroid profile, sedimentation rate, and urinalysis may be sufficient to substantiate the diagnosis. These should be performed before more spe-

cific investigations directed toward confirming or excluding a specific etiology.

Similarly, radiologic procedures should be selected based on the ranking of the differential diagnoses. Common procedures such as chest x-ray, mammography, barium studies of the bowel, and computed tomography (CT) of the abdomen may be indicated. Because of the large number of potential diagnoses, many of which share symptoms and historical characteristics, the first-line tests should be performed before subjecting the patient to definitive tests. As many of these—for example, renal or hepatic biopsy—carry potential morbidity, the primary care physician may wish to consult a specialist in dermatology or another subspeciality of internal medicine before referring the patient for a procedure.

ASSESSMENT

Hyperpigmentation is usually a slowly developing process indicating a serious systemic disease (Table 1). The patient's perception of the condition may range from pride in their

TABLE 3.   Causes of Drug-Induced Hyperpigmentation*

DRUG	SKIN COLOR	ACCENTUATED AREAS	MUCOUS MEM-BRANES	OTHER SKIN FEATURES	INCIDENCE
Chlorpromazine (Thorazine)	Blue/gray	Exposed	+/−	−	<15% Patients
Amiodarone (Cordarone)	Gray/purple	Exposed	+/−	−	<75%[12]
Busulfan (Myleran)	Brown	Trunk Neck Face	+/−	Erythema multiforme Atrophy	5–10%
Bleomycin (Blenoxane)	Brown	Over joints Bands on trunk	Involved	Erythema Pruritus Alopecia Striae	50%
Fluorouracil	Brown	Exposed	+/−	Dryness	2–5%
Minocycline (Minocin)	Blue/gray	Scars Lips Palate	Involved	Maculopapular rash	Only in prolonged administration

* (Data from Physicians' desk reference. Oradell, New Jersey: Medical Economics, 1990.)

tanned appearance to disgust and fear. With the possible exception of drug-induced cases—the possibility of which must be considered (see Table 3)[11,12]—the etiology is not immediately apparent. Making the correct diagnosis in generalized hyperpigmentation requires a painstaking approach following the conventional process of history and physical examination. Only by being thorough in these routine matters will the complete set of signs and symptoms be elucidated. Many of the key factors in diagnosis have no apparent connection to the skin changes and will not be volunteered by the patient. Laboratory and other tests should be utilized in a logical sequence based on both the clinical picture and the general characteristics of the patient to confirm the diagnosis. This prudent approach will enhance the chances of making an accurate diagnosis with the least expense and risk for the patient. The doctor-patient relationship built during this process will be important to the following stage of managing a serious or even terminal medical condition.

REFERENCES

1. Lorincz AL. Disturbances of melanin pigmentation. In: Moschella SL, Hurley HJ, eds. Dermatology. 2nd ed. Philadelphia: WB Saunders, 1985:1273–1305.

2. Jimbow M, Jimbow K. Pigmentary disorders in oriental skin. Clin Dermatol 1989;7:11–27.
3. Mosher DB, Fitzpatrick TB, Ortonne JP, Hori Y. Disorders of pigmentation. In: Fitzpatrick TB, Eisen AZ, Wolff K, Freedberg IM, Austen KF, eds. Dermatology in general medicine. 3rd ed. New York: McGraw Hill, 1987:794–876.
4. Epstein JH. Postinflammatory hyperpigmentation. Clin Dermatol 1989;7:55–65.
5. Sober AJ, Fitzpatrick TB. Pathophysiology of melanin pigmentation in man. In: Moschella SL, Hurley HJ, eds. Dermatology. 2nd ed. Philadelphia: WB Saunders, 1985:1261–72.
6. Quevedo WC, Fitzpatrick TB, Szabo G, Jimbow K. Biology of melanocytes. In: Fitzpatrick TB, Eisen AZ, Wolff K, Freedberg IM, Austen KF, eds. Dermatology in general medicine. 3rd ed. New York: McGraw Hill, 1987:224–51.
7. Fitzpatrick TB, Bernhard JD. The structure of skin lesions and fundamentals of diagnosis. In: Fitzpatrick TB, Eisen AZ, Wolff K, Freedberg IM, Austen KF, eds. Dermatology in general medicine. 3rd ed. New York: McGraw Hill, 1987:20–49.
8. Phelps G, Chapman I, Hall P, et al. Prevalence of genetic hemochromatosis among diabetic patients. Lancet 1989; 2:233–4.
9. Flowers FP, Krusinski PA, eds. Dermatology in ambulatory and emergency medicine. Chicago: Year Book Medical Publishers, 1984:193–214.
10. Freinkel RK, Freinkel N. Cutaneous manifestations of endocrine disorders. In: Fitzpatrick TB, Eisen AZ, Wolff K, Freedberg IM, Austen KF, eds. Dermatology in general medicine. 3rd ed. New York: McGraw Hill, 1987:2063–81.
11. Physicians' desk reference. Oradell, New Jersey: Medical Economics, 1990.
12. Rappersberger K, Honigsmann H, Ortel B, Tanew A, Konrad K, Wolff K. Photosensitivity and hyperpigmentation in amiodarone-treated patients. J Invest Dermatol 1989;93:201–9.

HYPERURICEMIA

WORAWIT LOUTHRENOO, KANCHANA BOONSANER, and H. RALPH SCHUMACHER, JR.

SYNONYM: Elevated Serum Uric Acid Level

BACKGROUND

Since serum uric acid is included on most chemical panels, it is quite common for hyperuricemia to be signaled as an abnormal value in patients who may have no previous indication of gout or any other manifestation of urate excess such as nephrolithiasis. This has occasionally led to excessive use of potentially dangerous therapies. In this chapter, we will review the factors that influence handling of elevated uric acid levels, describe some etiologies of hyperuricemia, and present an approach to clinical assessment that will help one identify which patients will need therapy and which therapy may be best in a given setting.

Definition

Hyperuricemia is a physicochemical condition in which the serum uric acid level exceeds the upper limit of an arbitrary normal range, which is epidemiologically defined as the mean serum uric acid value plus two standard deviations. With the specific uricase enzymatic spectrophotometric method, the upper limit of normal has been generally considered to be 7.0 mg/dl in men and 6.0 mg/dl in premenopausal women.[1] The automated colorimetric method gives values about 0.4 to 1.0 mg/dl higher than the specific enzymatic method.[1] Spurious hyperuricemia can occur after ingestion of substances such as aminophylline and coffee, which interfere with readings by the automatic chemical analyzer, or levodopa, which causes confusion with results by the colorimetric analyzer.

Factors Influencing Serum Uric Acid in the General Population

There are many genetic and enviromental factors that can modify or be related to variation of serum uric acid concentration. It is necessary to consider these factors during interpretation of laboratory data in order to make optimal decisions for diagnosis and management of significant hyperuricemia.

Age and Sex

In children, serum uric acid is approximately 3 to 4 mg/dl because of higher renal clearance of uric acid than in adults.[2] This level increases with age until after puberty; the level in normal males rises more than in females and becomes stable at age 20. In females, the level is lower than in males throughout the ages between 20 and 40 years. After menopause, the value rises to be near or equal to that of males. These differences are most likely related to hormonal-induced differences in the renal clearance of uric acid between sexes, as estrogen promotes renal excretion of uric acid.[3]

Body Weight and Body Mass Index

It has been shown in several clinical and population studies that body weight is positively correlated with serum uric acid. Especially when weight is calculated with height to give a body mass index, a significant and independent impact on serum uric acid level has been confirmed. The explanation for this association is not well understood, since it is also found in people who have no complicating factors such as diabetes, hypertension, or hyperlipoproteinemia. Some authors have claimed that obesity is the most common and important predictor of increased serum uric acid.[4,5]

Red Cell Mass

Serum uric acid is also higher in subjects who have higher hemoglobin and hematocrit levels even within the normal range.[4] This may reflect the high turnover rate of red cells releasing uric acid precursors. This possibility is supported by significant hyperuricemia in polycythemia.

Social Status

Studies in different occupations have found an association between high serum uric acid and high social class, academic achievement, intelligence, drive, activities, and leadership. The level of serum uric acid increases in the following order of educational level and professions: high school students, medical students, supervisors, scientists, and executive men.[6] There has been speculation that variation in serum uric acid might have some effect on central nervous system (CNS) function or that mental stress may increase serum uric acid levels. Chronic hyperuricemia in Lesch-Nyhan syndrome is associated with mental retardation.

Race and Genetics

There is evidence that serum uric acids of the Pacific people are higher than in American Caucasians and Europeans. The Maoris in New Zealand and the Polynesians have very high serum uric acid levels.[5]

Environment

Some racial groups who have parts of their population living in different areas have strikingly different serum uric acid levels. The Filipinos who live in the United States have higher serum uric acid levels than those who live in the Philippines. Filipinos appear to inherit a less efficient renal system for excretion of a uric acid load. In the Philippines, this deficiency is often not expressed since most people have a relatively low purine diet that includes large amounts of rice. In the United States, Filipinos consume more meat, which has a high content of purine, and they seem to be unable to compensate for this dietary stress.[7]

Autonomic Nervous System

Some evidence suggests that the parasympathetic system plays a role in renal regulation of uric acid. Anticholinergic agents can increase renal clearance of uric acid in some subjects.[8]

Prevalence

Hyperuricemia as defined is found in at least 5 per cent of asymptomatic Americans.[3] The prevalence of hyperuricemia in different populations around the world ranges between 2.3 and 40 per cent.[5,9] Asymptomatic hyperuricemia is at least four times as frequent as gout. Hyperuricemia is less common in most Asians, especially the Japanese, but more common in the Polynesians and Pacific people.

Formation of Uric Acid

Uric acid is the end product of purine metabolism (see Fig. 1) in humans and some other species that lack uricase, the enzyme that degrades uric acid to allantoin. A purine is a ring compound that is created by fusion of a pyrimidine ring and an imidazole ring. Purines in the human body come from exogenous dietary sources and endogenous purine production. Purine synthesis de novo requires ribose-5-phosphate (R-5-P), an aminosugar, as a backbone substrate and five other precursor products, which are glycine, carbon dioxide, formate, aspartic acid, and glutamine. In the initial step, R-5-P is changed to a higher-energy compound by using a pyrophosphate group of adenosine triphosphate (ATP) and is activated by the enzyme phosphoribosyl pyrophosphate synthetase (PRPP-S) to yield 5-phosphoribosyl-1-pyrophosphate (PRPP). The precursors are then incorporated by using ATP and bicarbonate until a purine ring is formed. The first purine substance formed by this biosynthesis is inosinic acid (IMP). The five resulting purine bases—adenine, guanine, hypoxanthine, xanthine, and uric acid—are then formed. This biosynthesis is regulated by negative feedback of some intermediate products and activated by several enzymes, as shown in Figure 1.

Renal Handling of Uric Acid in Normal Man

The renal control in excretion of uric acid is explained by a four-component system (see Fig. 2).[1,2]

Glomerular Filtration

Plasma uric acid is completely filtered by the glomerulus into the tubules.

Proximal Tubular Reabsorption

When uric acid enters the proximal tubule, almost all of it is reabsorbed by active transport, which is closely linked to the reabsorption of sodium and other components, such as glucose, phosphate, calcium, and bicarbonate. Increasing sodium reabsorption will increase uric acid reabsorption and reduce uric acid clearance. High doses of aspirin also affect the

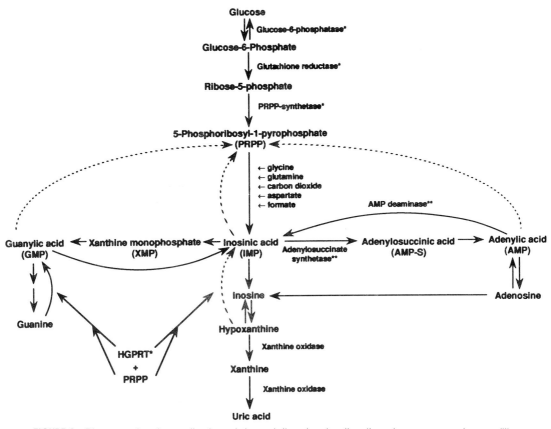

FIGURE 1. Diagram of purine synthesis and degradation showing the sites where enzyme abnormalities are known to cause hyperuricemia (*) and the sites where defects might cause hyperuricemia (**). *HGPRT,* hypoxanthine guanine phosphoribosyl transferase; -----, negative feedback.

proximal tubule and inhibit reabsorption of uric acid.

Tubular Secretion

At the same site in the proximal tubule, uric acid that is reabsorbed is then secreted back against the concentration gradient and electrical potential difference into the tubule by active transport. There is thus bidirectional uric acid transport at the proximal tubule. This tubular secretion is inhibited by low doses of aspirin.

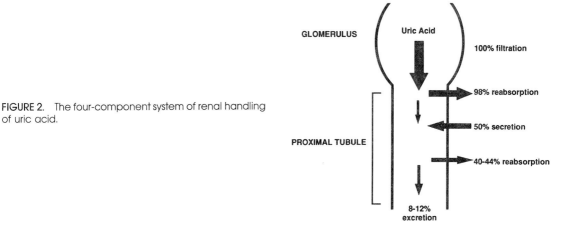

FIGURE 2. The four-component system of renal handling of uric acid.

Postsecretory Reabsorption

When secretory uric acid passes distal to the tubular secretion site, some of it is reabsorbed again. Thus, the net uric acid excretion is around 8 to 12 per cent of the glomerular filtration.

Pathophysiology of Hyperuricemia

The concentration of uric acid in body fluid depends on a balance between purine synthesis plus endogenous purine ingestion and uric acid elimination. Renal excretion is the major route for uric acid disposal. Some uric acid is secreted into the gastrointestinal tract where it is degraded by bacterial uricolysis; however, this is only a small amount. Any mechanism that causes increasing purine intake or synthesis or reduced excretion of uric acid induces hyperuricemia. The most frequent mechanism for hyperuricemia is decrease in renal clearance of uric acid.

ETIOLOGY OF HYPERURICEMIA

Hyperuricemia may be spurious, or it can be due to transient elevation of uric acid from reversible causes such as dehydration, acidosis, hypoxemia, or use of some drugs. These should all be considered before any consideration of giving drug therapy for hyperuricemia. Hyperuricemia can be classified as shown in Table 1.

Idiopathic Hyperuricemia

This is any hyperuricemia for which no primary cause, genetic defect, or physiologic or anatomic abnormalities can be identified. This accounts for approximately 10 per cent of all hyperuricemia. Even in the absence of overt renal disease, there is generally inability to excrete uric acid appropriately for the blood level.

Hyperuricemia Secondary to Identifiable Causes

In this classification, we include hyperuricemia that accompanies, or is the consequence of, definite diseases and medical conditions. These can be grouped by mechanism of hyperuricemia.

TABLE 1.   Etiology of Hyperuricemia

IDIOPATHIC HYPERURICEMIA
HYPERURICEMIA SECONDARY TO IDENTIFIABLE CAUSES
Causes of overproduction of uric acid
  Increased purine synthesis
    Increased PRPP-S activity
    HGPRT deficiency
    Glucose-6-phosphatase deficiency or absence
    Glutathione reductase mutation
    Drugs: nicotinic acid, warfarin, fructose
    Other possible causes: adenylosuccinate synthetase and AMP deaminase abnormalities
  Increased nucleic acid turnover
    Hematologic diseases: myelolymphoproliferative disorders, polycythemia vera, hemoglobinopathies, hemolytic anemia, pernicious anemia
    Neoplastic diseases: carcinomas, sarcomas, lymphomas, leukemia, multiple myeloma
    Hypoxic conditions: respiratory insufficiency, myocardial infarction, and the like
    Drugs and toxins: fructose, ethanol, cytotoxic drugs
    Miscellaneous: psoriasis, sarcoidosis
Causes of underexcretion of uric acid
  Volume depletion
  Acidosis: lactic acidosis, ketoacidosis, betahydroxybutyric acidosis
  Renal diseases: renal failure, Bartter's syndrome, polycystic kidney, lead nephropathy, pre-eclampsia, hypertension
  Endocrine and metabolic diseases: hyperparathyroidism, hypothyroidism, diabetes, hyperlipoproteinemia
  Drugs and toxins: diuretics, low doses of salicylates, ethambutol, pyrazinamide, methoxyflurane, nicotinic acid, ethanol
  Miscellaneous: Down's syndrome
Unknown mechanisms
  Paget's disease, cystinuria

Causes of Overproduction of Uric Acid

INCREASED PURINE SYNTHESIS. This category is caused by inherited enzymatic defects (as shown in Fig. 1) or drugs.

Increased PRPP-S Activity. PRPP-S is the enzyme that activates R-5-P to PRPP. Increase in its activity causes accumulation of PRPP, which is the high-energy substrate used in purine metabolism, and leads to hyperuricemia. This enzyme is coded by deoxyribonucleic acid (DNA) in the X chromosome and transmitted by X-linked dominance.[1,2]

Hypoxanthine Guanine Phosphoribosyl Transferase (HGPRT) Deficiency. HGPRT is an intraerythrocytic enzyme that reconverts guanine and hypoxanthine to guanylic acid (GMP) and IMP, respectively. The latter have a negative feedback function in purine synthesis. This enzyme needs PRPP as a collaborative substrate. Deficiency of this enzyme results in less negative feedback function and accumulation of PRPP, which enhances purine synthesis and leads to hyperuricemia. Complete HGPRT deficiency causes neurologic and behavior disorders and hyperuricemia in early life, which is called Lesch-Nyhan syndrome. In partial HGPRT deficiency, only hyperuricemia and its consequence are present in adolescent and adult life. Deficiency of this enzyme is also X-linked.[1,2]

Glucose-6-Phosphatase Deficiency or Absence. Glucose-6-phosphatase is an enzyme that reconverts glucose-6-phosphate (G-6-P) to glucose again in the glucose metabolism pathway. In purine synthesis, de novo R-5-P is derived from G-6-P. Deficiency of this enzyme increases G-6-P and R-5-P, thus enhancing purine synthesis and causing hyperuricemia. Autosomal recessive transmission is responsible for its deficiency.[2]

Glutathione Reductase Mutation. This mutant enzyme causes an increased rate of synthesis of R-5-P and PRPP, which is followed by hyperuricemia. This has an autosomal mode of inheritance.[1]

Drugs. Nicotinic acid, warfarin, and fructose increase the rate of purine synthesis in the step of PRPP production and cause hyperuricemia.[1]

Other Possible Causes. Alteration of two other enzymes are proposed to be able to cause hyperuricemia by overproduction of uric acid, but human cases have not yet been described. Adenylosuccinate synthetase is an intracellular enzyme that converts IMP to adenylosuccinic acid (AMP-S),which is the intermediate product between IMP and adenylic acid (AMP). Deficiency of this enzyme causes accumulation of IMP that is metabolized to uric acid.[10] Adenosine monophosphate deaminase is an enzyme that reconverts AMP to IMP. This enzyme controls the rate-limiting step in degradation of adenine nucleotide in liver. It normally is 95 per cent inhibited by various metabolites and appears to be the most highly regulated among the various enzymes of purine synthesis. Alterations in this enzyme making it less sensitive to inhibition could cause increased purine catabolism and hyperuricemia.[11]

INCREASED NUCLEIC ACID TURNOVER. This category includes the medical conditions and diseases that have abnormally rapid metabolism of nucleoprotein.

Hematologic Diseases. All diseases that have active bone marrow proliferation can increase cellular turnover rate and cause hyperuricemia. These include myelolympho-proliferative disorders, polycythemia vera, hemoglobinopathies, hemolytic anemia, and pernicious anemia.

Neoplastic Diseases. Malignancies that can cause hyperuricemia include carcinomas, sarcomas, lymphomas, leukemias, and multiple myeloma with its related diseases. The elevation of uric acid is especially high during chemotherapy.

Hypoxic Conditions. Several medical illnesses and conditions that have hypoxemia such as myocardial infarction, respiratory insufficiency, status epilepticus, and acute smoke inhalation will cause accumulation of adenosine diphosphate (ADP), which is usually oxidized to ATP. This excess nonoxidized ADP can be degraded to uric acid.[12]

Drugs and Toxins. Besides increasing the rate of purine synthesis, fructose also induces more rapid degradation of purines. Ethanol increases adenine nucleotide catabolism in the liver, leading to overproduction of uric acid.[1] Intravenous nitroglycerin used for myocardial ischemia can cause hyperuricemia since a significant amount of alcohol is added to the mixture.[13] All cytotoxic drugs destroy cells, thus increasing nucleotide degradation.

Miscellaneous. Some other diseases that have rapid cellular turnover rates, such as psoriasis and sarcoidosis, may be followed by mild elevations of uric acid levels.

Causes of Underexcretion of Uric Acid

VOLUME DEPLETION. Any situations that reduce effective circulatory volume will decrease glomerular filtration rate (GFR) and increase tubular reabsorption of uric acid. Easily eliminated causes are dehydration, salt restriction, and diuretic usage.

ACIDOSIS. Accumulation of lactic acid, ketoacid, and betahydroxybutyric acid inhibits tubular secretion of uric acid. These are found in starvation, alcoholic ingestion, hypoxia, diabetes, and glucose-6-phosphatase deficiency.[12,14]

RENAL DISEASES. Renal parenchymal, renal tubular, and renovascular diseases have associated reductions of GFR and abnormalities in tubular reabsorption and secretion of uric acid. These include chronic renal failure, preeclampsia, Bartter's syndrome, lead nephropathy, and polycystic kidney. Increased renal vascular resistance in hypertension causes decreased renal blood flow, decreased glomerular filtration, and thus less uric acid excretion.[1,2]

ENDOCRINE AND METABOLIC DISEASES. *Hyperpara-thyroidism.* Several mechanisms contribute to hyperuricemia in this disease. Compromised renal function is one of the important associated factors.[14]

Hypothyroidism. Hyperuricemia results at least in part from impaired renal clearance of uric acid. It can also be a complication of common associated defects in hypothyroidism such as obesity, hyperlipidemia, or hypertension.[14]

Diabetes Mellitus. In the prediabetic stage where there is only an impaired glucose tolerance test, the plasma uric acid level tends to be elevated with no clear explanation.[5] In early overt diabetes, the levels come down and seem to have a negative association with blood sugar, possibly at least partially because hyperglycemia enhances uric acid excretion by impairing tubular reabsorption of uric acid. In addition, patients lose body weight and body mass index after the onset of the disease. In long-standing diabetes with renal failure, decreased GFR and metabolic acidosis can aggravate hyperuricemia.

Hyperlipoproteinemia. The relationship between hyperuricemia and hypertriglyceridemia is well established. Up to 80 per cent of hypertriglyceridemic patients have hyperuricemia.[1] A study in a biracial population on Fiji found a correlation between hypercholesterolemia and hyperuricemia.[5] This finding could be in part explained by increased body weight and body mass index, or it may relate to excessive alcohol intake.

Diabetes Insipidus. Vasopressin-resistant diabetes insipidus is characterized by a defect in renal clearance and is accompanied by hyperuricemia.

DRUGS AND TOXINS. Diuretics are one of the most common causes of drug-induced hyperuricemia. The mechanisms for hyperuricemia are increased sodium and fluid excretion inducing volume depletion, increased tubular reabsorption of uric acid (especially with furosemide and ethacrynic acid), and interference with sodium and potassium exchange. Salicylates in low doses up to about 1.5 gm per day (serum level of 5 to 10 mg/dl) impair renal tubular secretion of uric acid. Antituberculous drugs such as ethambutol and pyrazinamide block tubular excretion of uric acid. Nicotinic acid and methoxyflurane also cause hyperuricemia by renal mechanisms. Large amounts of ethanol induce hyperlacticacidemia, suppressing renal excretion of uric acid.[14] Cyclosporin used in renal transplantation induces hyperuricemia by decreasing renal clearance of uric acid; hyperuricemia is exacerbated by concomitant diuretic use.[15] Chronic beryllium disease diminishes renal clearance of uric acid.

MISCELLANEOUS. Hyperuricemia in Down's syndrome is caused by reduced renal urate clearance.[1]

Unknown Mechanisms

Paget's disease and cystinuria have been found to have hyperuricemia associated with them, but mechanisms are obscure. In Paget's disease, there may be purine overproduction or coincidental occurrence of both diseases in older males.

APPROACH TO THE PATIENT WITH HYPERURICEMIA

Focused Queries

In the assessment of a patient with reported hyperuricemia, the following questions should be answered.

1. *Does the patient have "true" and "persistent" hyperuricemia?*
2. *What is the cause of the hyperuricemia? Can it be corrected?*
3. *Is there any evidence of gouty arthritis or other complications of hyperuricemia?*
4. *Does the patient need treatment? If so, what drugs should be considered?*

Does the Patient Have Hyperuricemia?

It is important first to document that the patient has true and persistent hyperuricemia. Most reported levels of hyperuricemia are accurate, but physicians should be aware of the possible causes of spurious and transient elevation of serum uric acid, as suggested earlier. Interpretation of a single serum uric acid level is difficult and can be easily misleading, since various transient factors can affect a single level. Hypotension, hypertension, dehydration, drugs, metabolic acidosis, and ethanol abuse are among the common causes of transient hyperuricemia. Correction of these can bring serum uric acid levels down to normal. If the patient still has hyperuricemia after correction of these potential causes, persistent hyperuricemia is diagnosed. In normal, healthy individuals, serum uric acid levels can vary from day to day.

What Is the Cause Of Hyperuricemia?

Hyperuricemia is a condition, not a disease. When one is faced with a problem of hyperuricemia, secondary causes of hyperuricemia and associated diseases should be determined. Possible causes of hyperuricemia are listed in Table 1. In most instances, hyperuricemia can be better explained by a complete history, physical examination, and common laboratory tests.

History

History taking should include questions such as: Does the patient have any other diseases that are associated with hyperuricemia, for example, hypertension, diabetes mellitus, and/or hyperlipidemia? Was the patient recently taking any alcohol, aspirin, diuretics, or other medicines that can cause hyperuricemia? Is there any history of lead ingestion or poisoning? Is there any history of volume loss, for example, diarrhea or bleeding? Does the patient have bone pain that might suggest Paget's disease of bone or multiple myeloma? Is there any evidence of a complication of hyperuricemia in the past, for example, gouty arthritis or kidney stones? Is there any history of tumor or lymphoreticular malignancy? Family history should include questions for gouty arthritis and kidney stones as well, since some gout is clearly familial.

Physical Examination

Physical examination should begin with general appearance. Is the patient obese? Is the patient hypotensive or volume depleted? Is the patient pale or plethoric? Does the patient have evidence of psoriatic skin lesions? Is there any evidence of lymphoreticular hyperplasia including lymphadenopathy, hepatomegaly, or splenomegaly? Does the patient have evidence of atherosclerosis? Are there any subcutaneous nodules around the joints or the ear that can be gouty tophi or xanthomatous nodules related to hyperlipidemia? Does the patient have proximal muscle weakness that can relate to underlying hyperparathyroidism, hypothyroidism, or diabetes mellitus?

Laboratory Study

Complete blood counts, urine analysis, and routine blood chemistry are the initial steps in working up hyperuricemia. Anemia, polycythemia, and abnormal white blood cells can be clues to an underlying hematologic disease. Microscopic hematuria and proteinuria suggest urinary tract calculi or renal diseases. Hypercalcemia can be a clue for hyperparathyroidism or multiple myeloma. Elevation of alkaline phosphatase can be a clue for Paget's disease of bone. Underlying causes of metabolic acidosis should be sought. Hypokalemic hyperchloremic acidosis suggests renal tubular acidosis and Bartter's syndrome.

A 24-hour urine uric acid excretion determination plays an important role in evaluation of patients with hyperuricemia. The amount of uric acid excreted by the kidney will help as a screen for causes of elevated serum uric acid by finding patients with overproduction (hyperexcretion) and will help in selecting the appropriate hypouricemic agents in patients who may need urate-lowering drug therapy. When performing the 24-hour urine collection, ensuring a sufficient urine volume is the most important step. Patients should have adequate hydration to produce good urine flow before the urine is collected. High purine diets, alcohol, and drugs that can interfere with urinary excretion of uric acid should be stopped at least three to five days prior to the collection. Values of uric acid over 800 mg per day on a normal diet indicate uric acid hyperexcretion. Adequacy of the urine collection can be rechecked by calculation of 24-hour urine creatinine excretion. Daily creatinine excretion is approximately 20 to 25 mg/kg per day in men and 15 to 20 mg/kg per day in women.

Performing a urine uric acid excretion determination in every hyperuricemic patient is not practical, especially if there is an obvious potential factor such as diuretic therapy. If the patient has mild hyperuricemia and does not have a history of kidney stone or other diseases that can cause increased uric acid production, the 24-hour urine uric acid excretion determination may not be necessary. The 24-hour urine uric acid excretion determination should be done in every case when uricosuric agents are being considered to decrease the serum uric acid level.

Is There Any Evidence of Organ Damage or Complications of Hyperuricemia?

If the patient has had hyperuricemia for a long period of time, monosodium urate (MSU) can form crystal deposits in various tissues of the body and can cause organ damage or inflammation. Uric acid crystals can precipitate in the kidney tubules and collecting system. These complications may occur as the following.

Arthritis

Gouty arthritis is the most common complication of hyperuricemia. This is the result of MSU crystal deposits in and around the joints and commonly causes acute arthritic attacks. The incidence of acute gouty attacks seems to correlate with both the serum uric acid level and duration of hyperuricemia. Long-term studies have shown that the annual incidence of acute gouty arthritis is 4.9 per cent if the serum uric acid is 9 mg/dl or more but only 0.1 per cent if the serum uric acid is less than 7 mg/dl.[16] Definitive diagnosis of gouty arthritis requires demonstration of MSU crystals in the synovial fluid (SF). If MSU crystals cannot be identified in an acutely inflamed joint in a patient with hyperuricemia, the diagnosis of gouty arthritis is unlikely, and other possible causes of acute arthritis should be considered. There are cases of gouty arthritis in which MSU crystals are not demonstrated on initial examination by ordinary light and compensated polarized microscopy but can be demonstrated by re-examination of the SF, very prolonged search, concentration of the fluid, repeated examination of SF from other joints, or collection during subsequent attacks. Rare reports have identified MSU crystals visible under electron microscopy that were missed by light microscopy.[17]

Extracellular MSU crystals can be identified in the joints of less than 5 per cent of asymptomatic hyperuricemic patients but can be seen in up to 70 per cent of gouty arthritis patients even during the intercritical period.[18] Thus, between attacks one can get unequivocal evidence of tissue deposition of MSU that favors the diagnosis of gout. Most workers suspect that the few asymptomatic hyperuricemic persons with MSU crystals in SF are those who will later develop clinical gout.

Other forms of arthritis, especially infectious arthritis, can also occur in hyperuricemic patients. Infection can coexist with acute gouty arthritis. Other crystals such as calcium pyrophosphate dihydrate, apatite, and calcium oxalate can present as acute goutlike arthritis, especially in patients with renal failure and hyperuricemia. Arthrocentesis with careful SF analysis and culture will solve these problems. Arthrocentesis should be done on all hyperuricemic patients who have acute arthritis unless there is a clear history of documented recurrent gouty arthritis. Arthrocentesis can also be used as a therapeutic adjunct for acute gouty arthritis.

Nodules

Subcutaneous nodules in a patient with hyperuricemia may be due to gouty tophi. The presence of tophi seems to correlate with the degree and duration of hyperuricemia. The presence of tophi in the absence of a history of gouty arthritis is unusual, but this can be the first sign of gout. Diagnosis of a tophus can be easily made by aspiration of the nodule and careful examination under polarized light microscopy. The presence of fine needle-shaped negatively birefringent crystals confirms the diagnosis. If the aspirate is negative for crystals and a gouty tophus is still suspected, surgical excision of a nodule can be performed. The tissue should be examined freshly for crystals. If tissue is fixed and stained, there may be few crystals; all fixation should be with alcohol, and stains may also need to be alcohol based to prevent dissolution of the crystals. The differential diagnosis of subcutaneous nodules should include xanthomas, nodules of acute rheumatic fever, sebaceous cysts, basal cell carcinoma, nodules of multicentric reticulohistiocytosis, sarcoidosis, lipomas, and rheumatoid nodules. Low titers of rheumatoid factor can be found in 10 to 30 per cent of patients with gouty arthritis.[19] This finding can be misleading to the unaware and erroneously suggest a diagnosis of rheumatoid arthritis if the patient presents with nodules and polyarticular arthritis.

Bone Deposits

Tophi can deposit in bone and cause bony defects in radiographs. Since urate crystals are radiolucent, the defects appear as erosions or osteolytic lesions. Occasionally, tophi are calcified and can be seen as a radiopaque lesion in or adjacent to bone. The presence of a bony tophus is usually associated with subcutaneous tophi on physical examination. The presence of a bony tophus in a patient with asymptomatic hyperuricemia is unusual, and the physician should look for other possible causes of the bony defects. Bone biopsy may be required to rule out infection or tumor.

Nephropathy

Nephropathy is the second most common complication of hyperuricemia. Despite the well-known mechanisms of renal handling of uric acid, the relationship between hyperuricemia and renal failure is difficult to interpret. Nephropathy from hyperuricemia may present in the following forms.

URATE NEPHROPATHY.   This is due to MSU crystal deposition in the renal interstitium, causing chronic inflammation and fibrosis of the renal medulla. This is surprisingly rare. Patients with asymptomatic hyperuricemia who were followed for 8 to 14 years did not develop significant renal failure any more often than the control group.[16,20] Most patients who had deterioration of renal function had other associated diseases such as hypertension, cardiovascular disease, diabetes mellitus, or benign prostatic hypertrophy, as described later.[16] The patients who developed impaired renal function after sustained hyperuricemia over a 20-year period had initial serum uric acids of more than 13 mg/dl in men and more than 10 mg/dl in women.[20] Renal function was not changed in patients who were treated with hypouricemic agents to normalize serum uric acid level when compared with gouty arthritis patients who did not receive the treatment if the initial renal function was normal.[20]

URIC ACID NEPHROPATHY.   This is the result of uric acid crystals obstructing the renal tubules, causing acute renal failure. This condition is unusual in patients with asymptomatic hyperuricemia or even in patients with gout. It usually occurs in patients with malignancy, especially lymphoreticular malignancy, treated with chemotherapy or radiation therapy without allopurinol prophylaxis to cover the rapid cell lysis and increased endogenous uric acid production that occurs. Uric acid nephropathy has also been reported in patients with gouty arthritis or in hyperuricemic patients who have high urine uric acid excretions and nevertheless receive uricosuric agents. Although not totally reliable, determination of a spot urine uric acid : creatinine ratio may be helpful in promptly suggesting this diagnosis. If the ratio is more than 1, this indicates uric acid hyperexcretion through the kidneys, and renal failure is likely to be due to uric acid crystals depositing in renal tubules.[21] Despite the fact that a spot urine uric acid:creatinine ratio can predict urinary uric acid excretion, studies have shown that it does not accurately predict 24-hour urine uric acid excretion because of diurnal variation in urine uric acid excretion.[22]

URIC ACID CALCULI.   The incidence of uric acid calculi is increased in patients with asymptomatic hyperuricemia or gout when compared with the general population. The incidence of calculi seems to be strongly correlated with the degree of hyperuricemia and hyperuricosuria. Fessel[20] found the incidence of urolithiasis to be one stone per 295 patients per year in asymptomatic hyperuricemia, one per 114 patients per year in established gout, and one stone per 852 patients per year in normouricemic subjects. Ts'ai-Fan Yu and Gutman[23] found that if the 24-hour urine uric acid excretion increased from 300 to 495 mg per day to more than 1100 mg per day, the incidence of renal calculi increased from 21 to 50 per cent. Pure uric acid stones are radiolucent and are not seen on plain radiographs. Stones can present before clinical gouty arthritis in up to 40 per cent of cases.[23] If the patient with hyperuricemia has renal colic and microscopic hematuria, uric acid calculi should be considered. The diagnosis should be confirmed by ultrasound or pyelography. Occasionally, radiopaque stones can be seen in a patient with hyperuricemia. In this situation, the patient may have unrelated oxalate stones or a uric acid stone that served as a nidus for calcium deposition. Urine should be filtered to isolate small stones if no definite stones are passed, as analysis of the stone composition will be of value.

TREATMENT- AND ASSOCIATED DISEASE-RELATED NEPHROPATHY.   Most hyperuricemic patients with renal failure have other associated diseases such as hypertension, atherosclerosis, or diabetes mellitus that can deteriorate renal function. In a patient who has a history of arthritic attacks, determine possible intake of nonsteroidal anti-inflammatory drugs (NSAIDS), which can affect renal function as well. NSAIDS cause renal impairment by various mechanisms including decreased renal blood flow caused by decreased renal prostaglandins and by interstitial nephritis.[24]

MANAGEMENT

Treatment of the complications of hyperuricemia, especially gout, nephrolithiasis, and acute uric acid nephropathy, has been widely described in standard textbooks and will not be discussed here. Discussion will be confined to the treatment of isolated hyperuricemia.

If the patient has any correctable causes of hyperuricemia, these should be addressed first. Volume depletion and metabolic acidosis should be corrected. Alcohol consumption should cease or be drastically decreased. Drugs that can cause hyperuricemia should be stopped unless they are absolutely indicated and cannot be replaced by safer alternatives. Hypertension should be controlled without diuretics if possible. Underlying endocrine abnormalities should be corrected. Weight control by a well-balanced, low-calorie diet will decrease exogenous sources of hyperuricemia. Strict purine-free diets are not usually necessary since these can decrease serum uric acid levels only approximately 1 mg/dl. A balanced diet should be 25 to 30 mg/kg ideal body weight, with 15 per cent for protein, 25 to 30 per cent for fat, and the rest for carbohydrate. Especially high purine foods such as yeasts, sweetbreads, brain, kidney, sardines, herring, roe, and meat extracts should be avoided. Severe diet restriction and starvation can cause ketoacidosis and can actually aggravate hyperuricemia.

There is a definite relationship between hyperuricemia or gout and hypertension or coronary heart disease. However, hyperuricemia alone is not generally accepted as a risk factor for atherosclerosis, because most of the studied patients were also overweight and had other risk factors. One recent study has now suggested that hyperuricemia is a risk factor for coronary heart disease independently of obesity.[25] There is no evidence yet, however, that good control of hyperuricemia per se will decrease the risk of coronary heart disease. Further studies will be of interest.

Hyperuricemia is clearly a predisposing factor to articular gout, uric acid stones, and uric acid nephropathy, but the incidence of these complications is relatively low.[16,20] Treatment to prevent gouty arthritis is both more costly and more risky than observing the patient and responding promptly if gout occurs. We feel that there is no reason to treat asymptomatic hyperuricemia in order to prevent gouty arthritis, uric acid stones, or urate nephropathy unless perhaps the patient has the rare sustained and unexplained hyperuricemia over 10 to 12 mg/dl or has urine uric acid excretion over 1000 mg per day since these will increase the risk of urinary uric acid stones.

The development of uric acid stones has a strong correlation with urinary uric acid excretion through the kidney. Treatment may be of value in hyperuricemic patients who have massive excretion of uric acid, especially over 1000 mg per day. If lowering of the serum uric acid is desired in a patient who has uric acid hyperexcretion, uricosuric agents are almost always contraindicated, as they can increase the risk of stones. A xanthine oxidase inhibitor (allopurinol) is the drug of choice. This drug decreases uric acid synthesis, resulting in decreased urine uric acid excretion. The dosage varies between 300 and 600 mg per day.

In a patient with lymphoreticular malignancy who will receive chemotherapy or radiation therapy, measures to prevent acute uric acid nephropathy should be undertaken. These include hydration, aggressive diuresis, alkalinization of the urine to pH above 6.0, and a xanthine oxidase inhibitor prior to the chemotherapy or radiation therapy. The dosage of allopurinol is about 400 to 600 mg per day. This dosage should be adjusted if the patient has renal impairment.

Underinvestigation of persistent hyperuricemia may lead to incorrect diagnosis and undertreatment of complications or associated diseases. In contrast, overtreatment is more common and both increases the cost of overall treatment and increases the risk of drug toxicity. Recent studies have shown that allopurinol is one of the most frequently prescribed drugs[26] and that up to 40 per cent of the prescriptions are without appropriate indication.[27] Cases of severe allopurinol hypersensitivity syndrome causing fever, severe skin reaction, hepatitis, renal failure, and even death are well recognized. Only a minority of these patients received allopurinol appropriately.[28] Acute uric acid nephropathy after uricosuric therapy is well known. Therefore, uricosuric drugs should also be prescribed with caution, generally only in underexcretors with good kidney function and with proven gout and not in asymptomatic hyperuricemia where risks and cost far outweigh any benefit.

REFERENCES

1. Levinson DJ. Clinical gout and the pathogenesis of hyperuricemia. In: McCarty DJ, ed. Arthritis and allied conditions. 11th ed. Philadelphia: Lea & Febiger, 1989:1645–76.
2. Kelley WN, Fox IH. Gout and related disorders of purine metabolism. In: Kelley WN, Harris ED, Ruddy S, Sledge CB, eds. Textbook of rheumatology. 3rd ed. Philadelphia: WB Saunders, 1985:1395–1448.
3. Becker MA. Gout. Pathogenesis of hyperuricemia. In: Schumacher HR, ed. Primer on the rheumatic diseases. 9th ed. Atlanta: Arthritis Foundation, 1988:195–8.
4. Takala J, Anttila S, Gref CG, Isomaki H. Diuretics and hyperuricemia in the elderly. Scand J Rheumatol 1988;17:155–60.
5. Tuomilehto J, Zimmet P, Wolf E, Taylor R, Ram P, King H. Plasma uric acid level and its association with diabetes mellitus and some biologic parameters in a biracial population of Fiji. Am J Epidemiol 1988;127:321–36.

6. Brooks GW, Mueller E. Serum urate concentrations among university professors. Relation to drive, achievement, and leadership. JAMA 1966;195:415–8.

7. Healey LA, Bayani-Sioson PS. A defect in the renal excretion of uric acid in Filipinos. Arthritis Rheum 1971;14:721–6.

8. Postlethwaite AE, Ramsdell CM, Kelley WN. Uricosuric effect of an anticholinergic agent in hyperuricemic subjects. Arch Intern Med 1974;134:270–5,

9. Popert AJ, Hewitt JV. Gout and hyperuricaemia in rural and urban populations. Ann Rheum Dis 1962.21:154–63.

10. Ullman E, Wormsted MA, Cohen MB, Martin DW. Purine oversecretion in cultured murine lymphoma cells deficient in adenylosuccinate synthetase: genetic model for inherited hyperuricemia and gout. Proc Natl Acad Sci USA 1982;79:5127–31.

11. Hers HC, Van den Berghe G. Enzyme defect in primary gout. Lancet 1979;1:585–6.

12. Woolliscroft JO, Colfer H, Fox IH. Hyperuricemia in acute illness. A poor prognostic sign. Am J Med 1982;72:58–62.

13. Shergy WJ, Gilkeson GS, German DC. Acute gouty arthritis and intravenous nitroglycerin. Arch Intern Med 1988;148:2505–6.

14. Smith C. Disorders associated with hyperuricemia. Arthritis Rheum 1975;18:713–9.

15. Lin HY, Rocher LL, McQuillan MA, Palella TD, Fox IH. Hyperuricemia in cyclosporine treated renal allograft recipients: evidence for under excretion of urate [Abstract]. Arthritis Rheum 1988;31(Suppl): S109.

16. Campion EW, Glynn RJ, DeLabry LO. Asymptomatic hyperuricemia. Risks and consequences in the normative aging study. Am J Med 1987;82:421–6.

17. Schumacher HR, Jimenez SA, Gibson T, et al. Acute gouty arthritis without urate crystals identified on initial examination of synovial fluid. Report on nine patients. Arthritis Rheum 1975;18:603–12.

18. Rouault T, Caldwell DS, Holmes EW. Aspiration of the asymptomatic metatarsophalangeal joint in gout patients and hyperuricemic controls. Arthritis Rheum 1982;25:209–12

19. Kozin F, McCarty DJ. Rheumatoid factors in the serum of gouty patients. Arthritis Rheum 1977;20:1559–60.

20. Fessel WJ. Renal outcomes of gout and hyperuricemia. Am J Med 1979;67:74–82.

21. Kelton J, Kelley WN, Holmes EW. A rapid method for the diagnosis of acute uric acid nephropathy. Arch Intern Med 1978;138:612–5.

22. Wortmann RL, Fox IH. Limited value of uric acid to creatinine ratios in estimating uric acid excretion. Ann Intern Med 1980;93:822–5.

23. Yu TF, Gutman AB. Uric acid nephrolithiasis in gout. Predisposing factors. Ann Intern Med 1967;67:1133–48.

24. Clive DM, Stoff JS. Renal syndromes associated with nonsteroidal antiinflammatory drugs. New Engl J Med 1984;310:563–72.

25. Fessel WJ. High uric acid as an indicator for cardiovascular disease: independence from obesity. Am J Med 1980;68:401–4.

26. Rucker TD. The top-selling drug products: how good are they? Am J Hosp Pharm 1980;37:833–7.

27. O'Rourke KS, Romberg GP, Naguwa SM, O'Rourke ME. Allopurinol prescribing in ambulatory patients [Abstract]. Arthritis Rheum 1987;30(Suppl):S108.

28. Singer JZ, Wallace SL. The allopurinol hypersensitivity syndrome. Unnecessary morbidity and mortality. Arthritis Rheum 1986;29:82–7.

HYPOGLYCEMIA

ABBAS E. KITABCHI and MARK J. RUMBAK

SYNONYM: Low Blood Sugar Level

BACKGROUND

Definitions

There seems to be some difficulty in defining the syndrome of hypoglycemia. Some have defined hypoglycemia in the adult as a plasma glucose of less than 40 mg/dl in individuals under the age of 60 and less than 50 mg/dl in individuals over the age of 60. Others have defined it as a level of less than 50 mg/dl regardless of age.[1]

There are two major groups of signs and symptoms associated with hypoglycemia: (1) the adrenergic response, when there is an abrupt decrease in the glucose level (but not necessarily below 50 mg/dl and counter-regulatory release of epinephrine, resulting in the sudden onset of hunger, diaphoresis, weakness, palpitation, and nervousness), and (2) the neuroglycopenic response, which may result in gradual decrease in blood glucose to a level below 40 mg/dl with symptoms of headaches, confusion, slurring speech, neuromuscular symptoms, behavior aberrations, lack of concentration, focal neurologic signs and symptoms, seizures, and coma. Functionally, the neuroglycopenic response is more important than the adrenergic response, as this reflects actual decreased utilization of glucose by the central and peripheral nervous system. The adrenergic response may be absent in patients with diabetes of long duration or individuals on adrenergic blockers. In addition, however, there is also a cholinergic nervous response involving sweating, as this may be abolished by atropine. Similarly, changes in pupillary size and secretion of saliva may occur during hypoglycemia owing to stimulation of the cholinergic nervous system.[1] Therefore, in the definition of hypoglycemia, Whipple's triad may be a practical approach (i.e., hypoglycemia with signs and symptoms that disappear with administration of glucose.)[2]

In healthy postabsorptive individuals, the maintenance of plasma glucose concentration within the normal range is regularly maintained by an orchestration of numerous metabolic pathways. These depend on the supply and demand of glucose and other substrates producing energy[3] (Fig. 1). The availability of fuel is ensured in the fed state by elaboration of the hormone of the fed state, mainly insulin, stimulated by glucose and inhibited by hypoglycemia (Fig. 2A). Adults are able to maintain a normal plasma glucose even when totally deprived of calories for days or weeks owing to the ability of the body to synthesize glucose from noncarbohydrate precursor (gluconeogenesis) and convert glycogen to glucose (glycogenolysis). During the period of starvation, the brain continues to utilize glucose, whereas insulin-sensitive tissues such as muscle, liver, and fat utilize other substrates such as free-fatty acids, ketone bodies, and amino acids.

This altered metabolic pathway is brought about partially by the two major hormones that predominate during starvation (i.e., epinephrine and glucagon)[3] (Fig. 2B).

The brain—and nervous system—consumes half the body's glucose production and has an obligate glucose need but may use ketone bodies during prolonged starvation. As starvation progresses, the plasma glucose level falls, and the brain uses proportionately less glucose until electrophysiologic abnormalities develop. Clinically, these may be asymptomatic, subtle, and finally overt as glucose utilization by the brain diminishes.[4]

In normal individuals, counter-regulatory hormones are activated when plasma glucose levels fall below 50 to 60 mg/dl in an attempt to maintain euglycemia. Prominent among these hormones are epinephrine and glucagon, with cortisol and growth hormone playing ancillary roles[3] (Fig. 3).

Types of Hypoglycemia

There are two types of hypoglycemia, fasting and postprandial.[1] In general, fasting hypoglycemia is associated with neuroglycopenia, whereas postprandial hypoglycemia is more apt to produce adrenergic responses. The etiologies of fasting and postprandial hypoglycemia are shown in Table 1.

With the advent of intensive insulin therapy for type I diabetes, iatrogenic hypoglycemia has become the most common, with high levels of morbidity and the possible potential of mortality.[5] Although fasting hypoglycemia is rare, it portends an ominous sign that requires a careful evaluation and poses the most important diagnostic challenge to clinicians. However, as insulin-induced hypoglycemia is the most common, we will discuss some of the

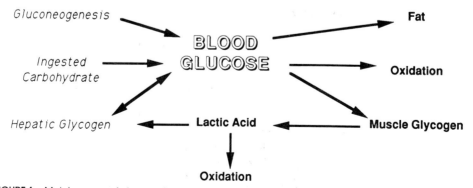

FIGURE 1.   Maintenance of plasma glucose concentration within a narrow normal range by an orchestration of numerous metabolic pathways.

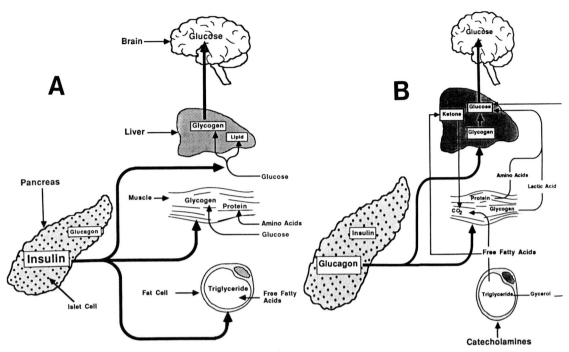

FIGURE 2. Glucose homeostasis during the fed and starved states. Figure 2A shows how the availability of fuel is ensured by the hormone of the fed state, insulin. Figure 2B shows the pathways that come into play during starvation. Glucagon and epinephrine are secreted while insulin is suppressed under normal circumstances. (From Kitabchi AE, Murphy MB. Diabetic ketoacidosis and hyperosmolar hyperglycemic nonketotic coma. Med Clin North Am 1988;72:1545–63. Used with permission.

characteristics of this type of hypoglycemia first, as it would pose very little diagnostic challenge since in most patients the original diagnosis of insulin-dependent diabetes mellitus and history of insulin intake can easily be obtained.

These patients quite frequently present with "severe" hypoglycemia, defined as "that associated with coma or requiring the assistance of another person for reversal." This is be-coming the most common metabolic emergency in the intensively insulin-treated diabetic patient.[6] A survey in one community hospital in Memphis, Tennessee, for three months revealed that 25 per cent of all emergency room visits of patients with diabetes were due to hypoglycemia (Hawkes JM, personal communication). In 10 per cent of patients treated with insulin, the prevalence of severe hypoglycemia is one episode per year.

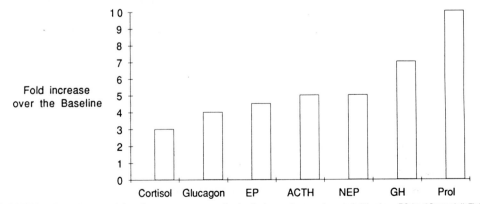

FIGURE 3. Counter-regulatory hormones are activated when glucose levels fall below 50 to 60 mg/dl. This figure shows the relative fold increase over baseline. *EP*, epinephrine; *ACTH*, adrenocorticotropic hormone; *NEP*, norepinephrine; *GH*, growth hormone; *Prol*, prolactin.

TABLE 1. Etiologies of Hypoglycemia

Fasting
  Hypopituitarism (seen only with food deprivation)
  Adrenal insufficiency (seen only with food deprivation)
  Liver pathology (enzymatic or nutritional)
  Alcohol ingestion *and* starvation
  Severe renal failure
  Drug-induced (i.e., insulin, oral hypoglycemic agents, salicylates, beta blockers)
  Retroperitoneal fibrosarcoma
  Insulinoma
  Hypoglucagonemia and hypocatecholinemia (in insulin-dependent diabetes mellitus)
  Somatomedin-induced from tumors
  Insulin receptor antibodies
Postprandial
  Alimentary hypoglycemia (i.e., gastric surgery)
  Functional (idiopathic) hypoglycemia
  Late hypoglycemia (such as one rarely seen in early non-insulin dependent diabetes mellitus)

Thus, hypoglycemia is a cause of, and contributing factor to, death of 3 to 6 per cent of these patients. Mild hypoglycemia may be as frequent as once per week. In patients treated with oral hypoglycemic agents (OHAs), especially chlorpropamide, approximately 4 to 6 per cent may suffer some degree of hypoglycemia and experience severe hypoglycemia as frequently as 0.24 per 100 patient years. In normal subjects, when the blood glucose level reaches mg/dl, insulin secretion is suppressed. This built-in protection is lost in insulin- or OHA-treated diabetics.[5]

In addition, availability and metabolism of insulin depend on a variety of factors, including the site of the injection, degree of absorption, body temperature, presence or absence of insulin antibody, degree of exercise, and so on. These factors by themselves pose additional problems beyond simply lack of substrate (food), increased metabolic activity (severe exercise), or excessive exogenous insulin.[5] Although these findings are most frequent in intensively treated diabetics, type II diabetics—by virtue of their insulin resistance and residual pancreatic reserve—may not exhibit as many hypoglycemic episodes as type I, with the exception of severely debilitated older individuals on long-acting OHAS. Since the most important demanding condition for emergency therapy of hypoglycemia is in intensely treated type I or severely debilitated OHA-treated geriatric patients, we will concentrate on the pathogenesis of drug-induced hypoglycemia.

The normal individual hormonal counter-regulatory responses to hypoglycemia are characterized by increases in epinephrine, cortisol, growth hormone, glucagon suppression of endogenous insulin secretion, and C-peptide (Fig. 3). Recent work by numerous investigators indicates that in type I diabetics there exist certain abnormalities of the counter-regulatory hormones in response to hypoglycemia. This is dependent to a certain degree on the duration of diabetes. For example, a type I diabetic exhibits a limited glucagon response to hypoglycemia about five years after diagnosis. The other secretagogues as amino acids are still able to cause the secretion of glucagon. This abnormality in glucagon secretion does not seem to be related to insulin management, beta-cell function, or nerve dysfunction. As glucagon can no longer adequately counter-regulate hypoglycemia, and autoregulation of insulin secretion is no longer intact, the combined effect of a low glucagon and a high exogenous insulin or OHA results in inhibition of glycogenolysis and gluconeogenesis with persistent hypoglycemia. This may be even more severe in the presence of low epinephrine levels (discussed later). With longer duration of diabetes (greater than 10 years), epinephrine response to hypoglycemia (in addition to decreasing glucagon) also decreases. About 40 per cent of type I diabetics have lost this normal response to hypoglycemia.[5]

Other factors such as growth hormone and cortisol may be impaired in long-standing diabetes. Additionally, the changes in insulin kinetics may alter insulin availability, and inadequate food absorption due to gastroparesis may also contribute in predisposing patients to hypoglycemia. The development of autonomic neuropathy further prevents physiologic recognition of hypoglycemia so that patients may not have adequate warning in order to take adequate food. Therefore, these long-standing diabetics—the phenomenon of the Somogyi effect (i.e., rebound hyperglycemia following a period of hypoglycemia)—may not be observed owing to lack of glucagon and epinephrine. This may result in a state of brittle diabetes (wide swings of hyper- or hypoglycemia). Asymptomatic hypoglycemia is also common if diabetics use beta blockers. In addition, recent studies suggest that with more intensive forms of insulin therapy and better glycemic control, the hypoglycemic threshold for the release of epinephrine in type I diabetics is lowered, and therefore, hypoglycemia without warning signs may be particularly dangerous in the group of well-controlled patients.[5]

HISTORY

The history[2] is probably the most important aspect of the workup since it may save the patient much money and discomfort and the physician hours of searching for causes of hypoglycemia (see the algorithm). The first priority is the establishment of a good rapport between patient and physician, since many of these patients with symptoms of hypoglycemia have become discouraged as they have gone from physician to physician in search of help and in fact do show signs of disability. It is therefore important that careful attention be paid to these patients' histories. For example, a history of diabetes in these patients or a close relative is extremely important. Sweating at night is a subtle way of diagnosing hypoglycemia. If a diagnosis of diabetes has been established, then dietary history and its time relationship to administration of hypoglycemic agents may be important. A detailed history of the signs and symptoms should be obtained, along with the time of occurrence of the hypoglycemia and its relationship to food. It is quite possible that some patients develop symptoms of hypoglycemia in response to certain types of foods (rebound hypoglycemia to high concentration of free sugar or hypoglycemia secondary to high protein in certain patients with insulinoma). Since some patients may not remember the extent and duration of their hypoglycemic episode, a person who is closely associated with the patient may be a more reliable source of history. For example, some patients suffering from hypoglycemia may act quite irrational in the morning, which the spouse may be able to recognize without the patient's being aware of it. Additionally, symptoms of hypoglycemia (adrenergic component) may confuse patients with symptoms of mitral valve prolapse where stress or exercise brings about these changes associated with chest pain. Fasting hypoglycemia may also be further accelerated by exercise.

As part of the history, one needs to establish not only the conditions under which the symptoms appear and what relieves them but, more important, if hypoglycemia was documented. One important aspect of history is to establish if the patient has ever become unconscious or required assistance of other individuals and that such conditions were documented by laboratory diagnosis of low blood glucose in an emergency room setting or by self-monitoring devices. It would also be important to establish if such hypoglycemic symptoms correlated with documented hypoglycemia and were relieved by eating or administration of glucose (Whipple's triad). Therefore, for those patients who complain of frequent bouts of hypoglycemic symptoms, we prescribe a self-monitoring glucose device with which patients can keep records (after directing patients and next of kin in its proper use and recording). This ensures documentation of blood glucose in which the patient may also record additional comments as to the time of day, relationship to food, and the situation (or food) that relieves the hypoglycemia.[6]

PHYSICAL EXAMINATION

Major physical signs due to the adrenergic response are tachycardia, hypertension, nervousness, sweating, fever, and rise of systolic blood pressure with simultaneous fall in the diastolic.[2] Abnormal cardiac rhythms including premature atrial and ventricular contractions have been described. Premature ventricular contractions correlate well with changes in plasma epinephrine levels, which normally increase if the blood glucose falls. Epinephrine may also decrease serum potassium and predispose patients to heart arrhythmias.

Physical findings resulting from the neuroglycopenia include transient aphasia, transient hemiplegia, seizures and postictal states, and peripheral neuropathy. The neuropathy usually is the result of hypoglycemia but on rare occasions may precede these symptoms. It usually involves both the motor and sensory nerves, the motor being the more common. The neuropathy usually is restricted to the proximal muscles but may also involve the distal ones. When the upper extremity is involved, severe distal muscle wasting is common. If objective sensory impairment is found, it is subtle, usually involving decreased vibration and two-point discrimination. Tendon reflexes may be exaggerated or depressed, and fasciculation occasionally occurs. Hypoglycemia may cause a radiculopathy, giving rise to some of the symptoms described earlier.

Additional examination should note body habitus, extent of obesity (which is quite frequent in patients with insulinoma, secondary to food ingestion to combat hypoglycemia), and abdominal girth (i.e., enlarged abdomen in

DIAGNOSTIC ASSESSMENT OF HYPOGLYCEMIA

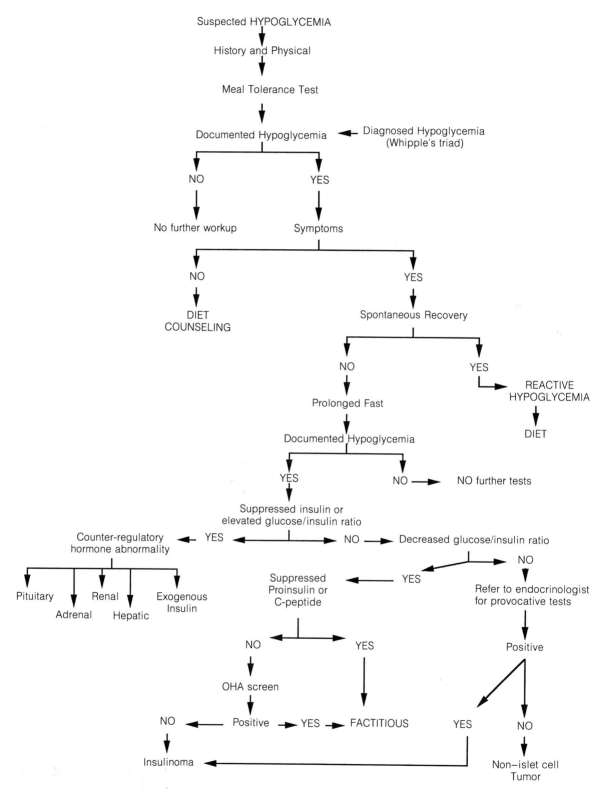

glycogen storage disease; retroperitoneal fibrosarcoma, or any other abdominal mass). Sarcomas anywhere (e.g., chest) may cause significant hypoglycemia but are large enough to be picked up by routine screening. Careful examination for the signs of early diabetic changes in the fundus, autonomic dysfunction (orthostatic hypotension, bradycardia or tachycardia, abnormal response to valsalva), peripheral neuropathy, and microalbuminuria is essential.

DIAGNOSTIC STUDIES

Electrocardiography

With hypoglycemia, angina can occur, especially if the patient has underlying coronary artery disease. The ST segments may therefore be depressed precipitously. There may also be prolongation of the QTc interval and flattening of the T waves. In diabetic autonomic neuropathy, there will be no beat-to-beat variation with respiration (i.e., the R-R interval will not change).

Electroencephalography

There is a good relationship between hypoglycemia and the pattern of the electroencephalogram (EEG). The EEG demonstrates a decreased frequency of alpha waves and increased delta waves. There is also a good correlation between alpha waves and hypoglycemia.

Echocardiography

If a cardiac source for the symptoms and signs is suspected, echocardiography will diagnose mitral valve prolapse and myocardial wall abnormalities.

Computed Tomography (CT)

CT will confirm cerebral or cerebellar tumors, hemorrhage, and especially pituitary tumors.

Chest X-ray

A chest roentgenogram will help to exclude significant tumors and intrathoracic abnomalities.

Blood Count

Owing to the high level of epinephrine, there is a lymphocytosis and, later on, an increase in the neutrophil count. There is also an increase in the hemoglobin and hematocrit.

Plasma Glucose

It is usual to diagnose hypoglycemia when the plasma glucose level is less than 50 mg/dl in adults. This level, however, may be normal in certain conditions.

Insulin

At the time of the hypoglycemic episode, it is very important to measure the plasma insulin level simultaneously. Generally, insulin is decreased during hypoglycemia that is less than 20 μU/ml, but this value may be increased in states of insulin resistance (obesity and polycystic ovarian syndrome) or insulinoma. If insulin has been used for a treatment, for example, in type I diabetics, then the insulin antibody subsequently may interfere with the assay. If heparin is used as anticoagulant, this will decrease binding of insulin to antibody and result in high values. Higher concentrations of heparin, however, will increase insulin binding, resulting in low values. The best anticoagulant to use is ethylenediamine tetraacetic acid (EDTA). Insulins from different species can be distinguished by using species-specific insulin antibodies or by analyzing via high-performance liquid chromatography (HPLC).

C-Peptide

The beta cell of the pancreas produces proinsulin. Proinsulin is cleaved into C-peptide and insulin, and both are therefore secreted in equimolar amounts. Insulin is cleared mainly in the liver and C-peptide by the kidneys. C-peptide can be measured using a radioimmunoassay that is quite sensitive and excludes insulin measurement. If the hypoglycemia is due to exogenously administered insulin, then endogenous insulin production will be decreased, reflected by a low C-peptide level. However, if an insulinoma is the cause of the hypoglycemia (or if an OHA has been ingested), then a high C-peptide level will be found. It should be realized that as the C-peptide is cleared by the kidney, a high C-peptide level is found in renal failure.

Proinsulin

Normally, proinsulin constitutes about 20 per cent of the total fasting insulin level and is the precursor of both insulin and C-peptide. It is easy to separate proinsulin from insulin by means of HPLC. Recently, antibodies to this prohormone have been developed. Again, a high proinsulin level would reflect an endogenous cause (or OHA ingestion) in a patient with hyperinsulinemia, and a low proinsulin level would suggest an exogenous cause.

ASSESSMENT

We prefer to document postprandial hypoglycemia using a standard solid or liquid meal rather than oral glucose tolerance test (OGTT). Documented fasting hypoglycemia at home may be achieved by home glucose monitoring devices, which further strengthens the suspicion and gives impetus for further workup. It is important to measure C-peptide, insulin, and proinsulin (if available) whenever hypoglycemia is documented.

We propose to approach the diagnosis of hypoglycemia via the algorithm presented earlier. Once a meal tolerance has been done, it is important to decide whether hypoglycemia has been documented. If it has not been documented, then no further workup is really necessary. If it has, however, been documented or if hypoglycemia has been previously documented by means of Whipple's triad, then it is important to find out whether the person has symptoms. If the patient does not have symptoms related to hypoglycemia, diet counseling is all that is required. If, however, the patient does have symptoms, it is very important to know whether or not the patient's blood glucose recovered spontaneously from the hypoglycemia. If it did recover spontaneously, the patient will have a diagnosis of reactive hypoglycemia and should be treated with diet. Asymptomatic hypoglycemia may develop in normal individuals who undergo the standard 75-gm OGTT. Alimentary or postgastrectomy hypoglycemia may appear abruptly one to two hours after ingestion of food, which is due to dumping of carbohydrates from the stomach with resultant overstimulation of insulin secretion. The symptoms therefore are primarily adrenergic and subside without food intake.

Idiopathic reactive hypoglycemia is overdiagnosed. It does, however, occur in a small number of patients, and the hypoglycemia is seen three to five hours after a meal. In the odd case, hypoglycemia with a delay seems to be an early precursor of non–insulin-dependent diabetes mellitus, although the connection may be purely coincidental.

Once the serum glucose does not spontaneously recover after a glucose load, then a serious underlying cause must be suspected. The 72-hour fast is the next diagnostic test.

The 72-Hour Fast

Whereas normally insulin secretion is decreased with hypoglycemia, the hypoglycemia in insulinoma or other insulin-producing tumors may lead to variable rates of insulin secretion, as normal pancreatic innervation in these tumors is altered with disruption of autoregulation. Therefore, there is a low glucose-to-insulin ratio during prolonged fasting in insulinemia. Normally, this ratio is greater than 2 and is calculated by the following formula:

$$\frac{\text{Glucose (mg/dl)}}{\text{Insulin } (\mu\text{U/ml})}$$

If a less-than-2 ratio is found with hypoglycemia, this may be either a factitious hypoglycemia due to high exogenous insulin levels or an insulinoma. This test may detect nonreactive (fasting) hypoglycemia. The majority of patients with insulinoma will develop hypoglycemia within the first 24 hours and almost 100 per cent of them by 72 hours. The fast, performed in the hospital, is started after an evening meal that may consist of high glucose, and then only water is allowed to be ingested. C-peptide, insulin, and glucose are determined initially and then every six hours. As soon as the patient develops symptoms, an Accucheck is done. If the glucose level is proved to be down to about 40 mg/dl, then C-peptide, insulin, and formal glucose specimens are drawn. If after the first 24 hours, there are no symptoms, the frequency is increased to every 4 hours for the three tests. A 30-minute exercise period prior to drawing blood may accelerate hypoglycemic events.

Once the patient has been shown to have hypoglycemia, the test is terminated by oral or intravenous carbohydrate. Interpretation of this test for endogenous insulin production is as described earlier (i.e., glucose-to-insulin ratio of less than 2). A good double check is that at the end of the fast ketone should be present in the urine, reflecting starvation. Since insulin is antiketogenic, individuals with insulinoma may not develop ketones. Alternatively, although deprivation of glucose may result in ketosis, ingestion of protein or fat may not increase the extent of ketosis during the fast.

Further Evaluation

If hypoglycemia is not documented after a 72-hour fast, no further tests are indicated, and this patient probably does not have hypoglycemia. If the ratio of glucose to insulin is below 2, the patient should be referred to an endocrinologist for provocative tests, as the case now becomes complicated and there is a lot of controversy regarding these provocative tests. They include a 3-hour intravenous (IV) tolbutamide test in which the patient with insulinoma exhibits hypoglycemia with concomitant large increase in insulin secretion within the first five minutes of injection. Similarly, lack of C-peptide suppression test in response to IV insulin has been used as an indication of insulinoma. Normal autoregulation by negative feedback will lower endogenous insulin (and C-peptide) secretion, but in autonomous insulinoma, insulin secretion will not be suppressed with exogenous insulin. These tests as well as ultrasonography and arteriography may further help in evaluating the location of the insulinoma in the pancreas. If the provocative tests are negative with a positive radiographic workup, then a non–islet cell tumor may be present. Further workup from this point is beyond the scope of this chapter.

Documentation of the hypoglycemia postmeal tolerance test is a clear indication for careful attention to be paid to the insulin level as well as to the ratio of glucose to insulin. If the insulin level is suppressed and there is an increased glucose-to-insulin ratio, then there is some abnormality in the counter-regulatory hormonal system. Careful attention must then be paid to the pituitary, adrenal, renal, and hepatic systems, or perhaps to exogenous insulin.

In addition to pointing to an insulinoma, if high proinsulin or C-peptide level is found in the face of hypoglycemia, it is important to screen for hypoglycemic agents, as they may stimulate proinsulin or C-peptide secretion. If this screen is positive, there is suspicion for factitious hypoglycemia. If it is negative, an insulinoma must be ruled out.

REFERENCES

1. Fields JB. Hypoglycemia. Definition, clinical presentation, classification and laboratory tests. In: Fields JB, ed. Hypoglycemia, endocrinology and metabolism, Medical Clin of North Am. Philadelphia: WB Saunders, 1980;64:27–43.
2. Kitabchi AE, Goodman RC. Hypoglycemia pathophysiology and diagnosis. Hosp Pract 1981;26:45–60.
3. Kitabchi AE, Murphy MB. Diabetic Ketoacidosis and hyperosmolar hyperglycemic nonketotic coma. Medical Clin North Am. Philadelphia: WB Saunders, 1988;72:1545–63.
4. Butler DC, Rizza RA. Regulation of carbohydrate metabolism and response to hypoglycemia. In: Fields JB, ed. Hypoglycemia, endocrinology and metabolism, Medical Clin of North Am. Philadelphia: WB Saunders, 1980;64:1–26.
5. White WH, Skor DA, Cryer DE, Levandoski LA, Vier DM, Santiago JV. Identification of type I diabetic patients at increased risk to hypoglycemia during intensive therapy. N Engl J Med 1983;309:61–6.
6. Fisher KF, Lees JA, Newman JH. Hypoglycemia in hospitalized patients: causes and outcomes. N Engl J Med 1986;315:1245–50.
7. Fajans SS, Floyd JC Jr. Fasting hypoglycemia in adults. N Engl J Med 1976;294:766–79.

HYPOMAGNESEMIA

ROBERT WHANG and KENNETH W. RYDER

SYNONYMS: Magnesium Depletion, Magnesium Deficiency

BACKGROUND

Magnesium (Mg) is the second most common intracellular cation, exceeded only by potassium (K). Because of its predominantly intracellular distribution, like K, serum Mg samples only 1 to 2 per cent of total body content. While methods exist to assess intracellular Mg in skeletal muscle, red cells, lymphocytes, and even buccal mucosal cells, the single most practical and useful method to detect clinical Mg deficiency remains the finding of hypomagnesemia in a patient with an illness known to cause Mg deficiency.[1]

The clinical causes of hypomagnesemia are varied and encompass a wide clinical spectrum.[2] Table 1 lists many of the clinical causes of hypomagnesemia. Note that it is possible to subdivide these into four categories: gastrointestinal, endocrine, renal, and miscellaneous. Gastrointestinal (GI) causes of Mg deficiency result from interruption of nutritional intake coupled with enhanced GI losses of Mg. Examples include alcoholism with substitution of ethyl alcohol for food ("empty calories"), accompanied by nausea, vomiting, and diarrhea, especially in the withdrawal stage.

Additional Mg losses are encountered through enhanced renal Mg losses resulting from alcohol ingestion. Interruption of GI function necessitating prolonged intravenous therapy without Mg replacement, gastric suction, and diarrhea are all recognized as causes of hypomagnesemia. Enhanced losses of Mg resulting from intestinal bypass surgery for obesity, laxative abuse, bulimarexia, short bowel syndrome, and malabsorption constitute other GI causes of hypomagnesemia and Mg depletion.

Endocrine causes of hypomagnesemia include hyperaldosteronism, hyperparathyroidism, hyperthyroidism, and diabetic ketoacidosis. In most instances, enhanced renal losses

coupled with inadequate Mg replacement appear to be the genesis of the hypomagnesemia.

Renal losses of Mg accompany the clinical use of diuretics, antibiotics such as gentamicin, carbenicillin, and ticarcillin, and the chemotherapeutic agent cisplatin. Enhanced renal Mg losses occur with postobstructive diuresis, the diuretic phase of acute tubular necrosis, and hereditary renal Mg wasting and in hypercalcemic states including malignancies.

A group of miscellaneous causes of clinical hypomagnesemia including excessive lactation and exchange transfusion constitute other known causes of clinical Mg depletion and hypomagnesemia.

The frequency of clinical hypomagnesemia in hospitalized patients ranges from 6 to 11 per cent.[2] Patients who are in intensive care units have an even higher frequency of hypomagnesemia, ranging from 7.7 to 20 per cent.[2] These data are based on measurements of serum Mg on a routine basis without relying on clinicians' orders for serum Mg. In clinical practice today, Mg is not routinely included with the serum "electrolyte panel": sodium (Na), K, chloride (Cl), and bicarbonate (HCO_3).

Comparing routine serum Mg determination to Mg determined only on specific physician orders for this analyte, we have learned that physicians identify only about 10 per cent of the hypomagnesemic patients in the hospital. Conversely, routine serum Mg determination is nine times more effective, identifying the other 90 per cent of the hypomagnesemic patients.[3] Thus, hypomagnesemia may represent the single most underdiagnosed electrolyte abnormality in clinical practice today.

HISTORY

Hypomagnesemia per se, on clinical grounds alone, is not easily recognizable. Therefore, the chief complaint and history of present illness may be related to any one of the many clinical conditions associated with hypomagnesemia (Table 1). Of these, alcoholism, use of potent diuretics such as loop

TABLE 1. Clinical Causes of Hypomagnesemia

Gastrointestinal
  Laxative abuse, villous adenoma, adenocarcinoma of the colon, ulcerative colitis, malabsorption states, pancreatic insufficiency with steatorrhea, fistulae, protein-calorie malnutrition, alcoholism, prolonged intravenous therapy without magnesium replacement, anorexia nervosa, bulimarexia
Endocrine
  Hyperaldosteronism
  Hyperparathyroidism
  Hyperthyroidism
  Diabetic ketoacidosis
Renal
  Diuretics
  Alcoholism
  Antibiotics (e.g., gentamicin, carbenicillin, and ticarcillin)
  Cisplatin
  Postobstructive diuresis
  Diuretic phase of acute tubular necrosis
  Hereditary renal magnesium wasting
  Hypercalcemic states including malignancies
Miscellaneous
  Excessive lactation
  Exchange transfusion

blockers, and other medications such as cisplatin and gentamicin may represent the most common clinical conditions associated with hypomagnesemia.

In alcoholic patients, the history may relate to the GI symptoms associated with gastritis or alcoholic diarrhea. These losses of upper and lower GI secretions coupled with inability to eat normally result in hypomagnesemia and Mg deficiency. The renal losses of Mg following alcohol ingestion also contribute overall to the problem of hypomagnesemia in the alcoholic patient.

Neurologic signs and symptoms may dominate the clinical history. Any withdrawing alcoholic who has had a seizure should be considered to be hypomagnesemic as well as possibly having had a "rum fit," subdural hematoma, or hypoglycemia. Ataxia can be another vexing complaint. This may be coupled with recent onset of tremulousness. The patient's family may give a history of lack of concentration and disorientation exhibited by the patient.

Diuretics, especially the loop blockers, are another common cause of hypomagnesemia and Mg deficiency. The history in those patients relates primarily to the reason for diuretic therapy, commonly congestive heart failure. Hypomagnesemia can also cause arrhythmias, both atrial and ventricular. These arrhythmias, when present, include atrial premature contractions, multifocal atrial tachycardia, ventricular premature contractions, ventricular tachycardia, torsade de pointes, and ventricular fibrillation.[4]

Focused Queries

Pertinent questions to be asked a patient suspected to be hypomagnesemic are:

1. *Are you an alcoholic? Have you had seizures since stopping drinking?*
2. *How long have you been on diuretics, especially furosemide (Lasix)? Has the dosage been recently increased?*
3. *Have you had a convulsive seizure?*
4. *Do you have problems with concentration, or has your family noticed that you may be disoriented?*
5. *Do you feel weak and shaky?*
6. *Have you noticed any difficulty in swallowing (dysphagia)?*
7. *Has your vision been poor recently, or have you noticed that your eyes have abnormal movements (nystagmus)?*
8. *Have you noticed any irregularities or fluttering or racing of your heart (arrhythmias)?*

PHYSICAL EXAMINATION

Vital signs that may be helpful in diagnosing hypomagnesemia and Mg depletion include mild to moderate hypertension[5] and tachycardia or arrhythmias. On general examination, the patient may be tremulous, inattentive, or disoriented or may complain of weakness.

Head, Eyes, Ear, Throat

The patient may present with nystagmus.[6] Nystagmus associated with hypomagnesemia can be either in the horizontal or vertical plane.

Cardiac

Arrhythmias, either atrial or ventricular, are associated with hypomagnesemia.[4,7] Tachycardia, including sinus tachycardia, multifocal atrial tachycardia, ventricular tachycardia with or without hypotension, and ventricular fibrillation with hypotension may be seen. Premature contractions, either atrial or ventricular, may also be present on cardiac examination.

Gastrointestinal

Dysphagia may be present and should be checked.[8]

Neurologic Examination

Disorientation, tremulousness, and presence of involuntary movements of the extremities may be present in the hypomagnesemic patient. Nystagmus may be seen on examination of the cranial nerves. A positive Chvostek's, but negative Trousseau's sign, has been reported in hypomagnesemic patients. Deep tendon reflexes may be hyperactive. The hypomagnesemic patient's gait is ataxic. Muscle strength testing is consistent with significant muscle weakness. Finally, severe hypomagnesemia, if uncorrected, can result in generalized grand mal seizures.

DIAGNOSTIC STUDIES

The ordering of a serum Mg determination in patients who are at risk for hypomagnesemia is the most practical approach to diagnosing clinical Mg deficiency. Estimates of the frequency of clinical hypomagnesemia range from 6.9 to 20 per cent in hospitalized patients. Since serum Mg is not routinely included with serum electrolyte panels and is dependent on a specific physician's orders for this analyte, only about 10 per cent of clinical hypomagnesemia is being detected. Fully 90 per cent of hypomagnesemic patients may be undiagnosed if serum Mg is not performed routinely as a part of the patient's electrolyte assessment. Therefore, hypomagnesemia may be the most underdiagnosed serum electrolyte abnormality in clinical practice today.[3]

Clinical Laboratory Tests

Primary Test

The most clinically relevant approach to diagnosing clinical Mg depletion is identification of hypomagnesemia with a clinical condition associated with Mg deficiency (Table 1).

Associated Tests

Until serum Mg is routinely performed, abnormalities in other serum electrolytes that are presently available on a routine basis may assist in identifying hypomagnesemic patients.

Whang et al.[9] reported that hyponatremia was associated with a 23 per cent incidence of hypomagnesemia; hypokalemia, 42 per cent; hypophosphatemia, 29 per cent; and hypocalcemia, 23 per cent. Thus, in the absence of routine serum Mg determination, hypokalemia, hyponatremia, hypophosphatemia, and hypocalcemia should alert the clinician to order a serum Mg because of the high probability of coexisting hypomagnesemia.

False-Negative Tests (Normal Serum Mg Concentration with Mg Deficiency)

A diagnosis of Mg deficiency is based on the finding of hypomagnesemia in patients with clinical conditions known to be associated with depletion of Mg. However, there are exceptions to this rule. Muscle biopsy has provided evidence of intracellular deficits of Mg in the absence of hypomagnesemia. Similarly, lymphocyte and red cell analyses have demonstrated intracellular Mg depletion not necessarily accompanied by hypomagnesemia.

A magnesium tolerance test has been advocated as another means of identifying clinical Mg depletion.[10] In this test, the percentage of intravenous Mg excreted in the urine is measured. The assumption is made that greater amounts of administered Mg will be retained in the Mg-deficient state. Conversely, with sufficient body Mg stores, a significantly greater percentage of intravenous Mg will be excreted by the kidneys. Thus, Ryzen et al. reported that after three weeks of Mg depletion, significant hypomagnesemia ensued and Mg retention increased from 12 to 65 per cent.[10]

False-Positive Tests (Hypomagnesemia Without Mg Deficiency)

When is hypomagnesemia *not* an indicator of Mg deficiency? There are two instances of "spurious" hypomagnesemia. The first is related to significant hypoalbuminemia.[11] Serum Mg determination measures total Mg. Approximately one third of total serum Mg is bound to serum albumin. Therefore, with significant lowering of serum albumin, serum Mg can be lowered without being indicative of Mg depletion. Second, stress may be associated with translocation of extracellular Mg into cells. Recently, Ryzen et al. reported that catecholamine administration resulted in a statistically significant hypomagnesemia, suggesting that hypercatecholaminemia may be the basis for the high incidence of hypomagnesemia in critically (intensive care) ill patients.[12]

ASSESSMENT

Until such time that serum Mg is routinely determined as part of the electrolyte assessment of patients, it is recommended that serum Mg be ordered in the following clinical conditions:

1. Any patient with seizures, alcoholics especially.
2. Any patient with significant atrial and/or ventricular arrhythmias, especially if the patient is an alcoholic or in congestive heart failure and receiving a loop blocking diuretic.
3. Patients with recurrent ventricular tachycardia and/or fibrillation resistant to all conventional therapy.
4. Patients suspected of or suffering from digitalis toxicity.
5. Patients with hypocalcemia, especially alcoholics.
6. Patients in whom hypokalemia is refractory to the usual methods of K repletion.

In each of these clinical situations, it is recommended that serum Mg be ordered to rule out the possibility of undiagnosed hypomagnesemia or untreated Mg depletion. These clinical conditions will be discussed in seriatim.

Clinicians are very quick to recognize in the withdrawing alcoholic who has had seizures the possibility of hypoglycemia, hyponatremia (in beer drinkers—"beer potomania"), hypocalcemia, or delirium tremens. However, because serum Mg is not routinely performed by most laboratories, hypomagnesemia may go undetected. Any patient with significant atrial or ventricular arrhythmia who is being treated with diuretics for congestive heart failure should be investigated for hypomagnesemia. In patients with congestive heart failure, the problem of sudden death may be related in part to undiagnosed and untreated Mg depletion. This is especially pertinent in the patient receiving loop blockers and/or digitalis.

Magnesium deficiency can be associated with both atrial and ventricular arrhythmias. Torsade de pointes is commonly associated with hypomagnesemia, as are ventricular tachycardia and ventricular fibrillation. It should be noted that recurrent ventricular tachycardia and fibrillation refractory to conventional antiarrhythmic therapy may be indicative of coexisting Mg deficiency with or without hypomagnesemia.[13] Treatment with Mg should be considered in patients with refractory and recurrent ventricular arrhythmias. Iseri et al. have demonstrated the frequency with which arrhythmias associated with Mg deficiency occur in hospital intensive care units.[7] Both hypokalemia and hypomagnesemia can contribute to the problem of digitalis toxicity. In patients receiving digoxin, we found that hypokalemia occurred in 9 per cent of cases, whereas 19 per cent of these patients were hypomagnesemic.[14] In another study, we found that 100 per cent of hypokalemic patients were recognized and treated. In contrast, only 38 per cent of hypomagnesemic patients receiving digoxin were diagnosed by their physicians.[15] These observations strongly suggest that clinicians are more skilled in avoiding hypokalemia than hypomagnesemia in patients receiving digoxin. Thus, hypomagnesemia may contribute significantly more to the problem of digitalis toxicity than hypokalemia.

Hypocalcemia refractory to treatment should alert the clinician to undiagnosed hypomagnesemia. There is a problem in calcium homeostasis associated with Mg deficiency. This perturbation results either from decreased parathyroid hormone (PTH) release or from impaired target organ response to PTH.[16] Mg repletion corrects the perturbation and restores serum calcium to normal levels without necessitating calcium supplementation.[17]

Clinicians will periodically encounter perplexing patients in whom hypokalemia is refractory to K repletion.[18] The vast majority of these patients had congestive heart failure, and many were receiving loop diuretics.[19] Obese patients with surgical bypass of the GI tract, burn patients, familial hypokalemic alkalosis with tubulopathy, and Bartter's syndrome have shared in the problem of refractory K repletion due to coexisting hypomagnesemia. More recently, two cancer patients receiving cisplatin were observed to have significant hypokalemia refractory to K repletion. It was only after recognition that cisplatin can cause renal loss not only of K but of Mg as well that hypomagnesemia was detected and treated. Treatment of the coexisting Mg depletion resulted in normalization of the previously refractory hypokalemia.[20] Magnesium deficiency can result in increased fluidity of the cell membrane, decrease in adenosinetriphosphatase (ATPase) activity, decrease in Na-K pump density, increase in intracellular calcium, and accumulation of Na in cells, all of which separately or in concert may be the mechanism or mechanisms underlying the problem related to refractory K repletion.[21]

Thus, it is clear that the problem of hypomagnesemia and Mg depletion is pervasive in the clinical practice of medicine. The clinician will be significantly aided in diagnosing and treating hypomagnesemia when serum Mg is a routine part of the electrolyte assessment of hospitalized patients.

REFERENCES

1. Whang R. Routine serum magnesium determination—a continuing unrecognized need. Magnesium 1987;6:1–4.
2. Whang R. Magnesium deficiency: pathogenesis, prevalence and clinical implications. Am J Med 1987;82(Suppl 3A):24–9.
3. Whang R, Ryder KW. Frequency of hypomagnesemia and hypermagnesemia: requested versus routine. JAMA 1990;263:3063–4.
4. Whang R. Magnesium and potassium interrelationships in cardiac arrhythmias. Magnesium 1986;5:127–33.
5. Whang R, Chrysant S, Dillard B, Smith W, Fryer A. Hypomagnesemia and hypokalemia in 1000 treated ambulatory hypertensive patients. J Am Coll Nutr 1982;1:317–22.
6. Smith WO, Clark RM, Mohr JA, Whang R. Vertical and horizontal nystagmus in magnesium deficiency. South Med J 1980;73:269.
7. Iseri LT, Allen BJ, Brodsky MA. Magnesium therapy of cardiac arrhythmias in critical-care medicine. Magnesium 1989;8:299–306.
8. Hamed IA, Lindeman RD. Dysphagia and vertical nystagmus in magnesium deficiency. Ann Intern Med 1978;89:222–3.
9. Whang R, Oei TO, Aikawa JK, et al. Predictors of clinical hypomagnesemia: hypokalemia, hypophosphatemia, hyponatremia and hypocalcemia. Arch Intern Med 1984;144:1794–6.
10. Ryzen E, Elbaum N, Singer ER, Rude RK. Parenteral magnesium tolerance testing in the evaluation of magnesium deficiency. Magnesium 1985;8:137–47.
11. Kroll MH, Elin RJ. Relationships between magnesium and protein concentrations in serum. Clin Chem 1985;31:224–46.
12. Ryzen E, Servis KL, Rude RK. Effect of intravenous epinephrine on serum magnesium and free intracellular red blood cell magnesium concentrations measured by nuclear magnetic resonance. J Am Coll Nutr 1990;9:114–9.
13. Iseri L, Chung P, Tobis J. Magnesium therapy for intractable ventricular tachyarrhythmias in normomagnesemic patients. West J Med 1983;138:823–8.
14. Whang R, Oei TO, Watanabe A. Frequency of hypomagnesemia in hospitalized patients receiving digitalis. Arch Intern Med 1985;145:655–6.
15. Njinimbam CCG, Ryder KW, Glick SJ, Whang R. Identification and treatment of hypomagnesemia and hypokalemia in patients receiving digoxin. Clin Chem 1990;36:575–6.
16. Freitag JJ, Martin KJ, Conrades MB, et al. Evidence for skeletal resistance to parathyroid hormone in magnesium deficiency. J Clin Invest 1979;64:1238–44.
17. Estep H, Shaw WA, Watlington C, Hobe R, Holland W, Tucker SG. Hypocalcemia due to hypomagnesemia and reversible parathyroid hormone unresponsiveness. J Clin Endocrinol Metab 1969;29:842–8.
18. Whang R, Aikawa JK. Magnesium deficiency and refractoriness to potassium repletion. J Chronic Dis 1977;30:65–8.
19. Whang R, Flink EB, Dyckner T, Wester PO, Aikawa JK, Ryan MP. Magnesium depletion as a cause of refractory potassium repletion. Arch Intern Med 1985;145:1686–9.
20. Rodriguez M, Solanki DL, Whang R. Refractory potassium repletion due to cisplatin induced magnesium depletion. Arch Intern Med 1989;149:2592–4.
21. Whang R, Whang DD. Update: mechanisms by which magnesium modulates intracellular potassium. J Am Coll Nutr 1990;9:84–5.

INSOMNIA

ROBERT N. GOLDEN

SYNONYM: Disorders of Initiating or Maintaining Sleep (DIMS)

BACKGROUND

Insomnia is a common experience. In a national survey, about one third of the population reported that they had experienced insomnia during the past year; 17 per cent of the respondents felt that their insomnia was "serious."[1]

Insomnia is a chief complaint, with many possible causes, and should not be regarded as a specific diagnosis. Insomnia describes the perception of difficulty in falling asleep and/or maintaining sleep over the desired period of time. There are many different diseases that can present with insomnia as a primary symptom. Table 1 lists the general categories under which the various conditions associated with long-term insomnia can be organized. A careful workup, based on a systematic history gathering and the formulation of a differential diagnosis, is essential in order to assess and treat the symptom of insomnia adequately.

When the sleep of patients who feel that they have significant insomnia is studied in a sleep laboratory and compared with that of individuals who report having normal sleep, the objective parameters between the two groups are strikingly similar, with considerable overlap. While a small fraction of insomnia patients do in fact demonstrate fragmented, inefficient sleep and long sleep latencies, the large majority fall asleep as rapidly and demonstrate the same duration and quality of sleep as the rest of the population.[1] Thus, insomnia should be regarded as a subjective experience that is very real and upsetting to many patients and yet often is not accompanied by objective laboratory findings.

There are several important sources of information that should be utilized in evaluating a complaint of insomnia. In addition to obtaining a history from the patient, one should interview the sleep partner, when available. The sleep partner can describe certain phenomena, such as snoring patterns, leg movements, and sleep walking, with more accuracy than the patient. The patient should be asked to keep a prospective sleep diary for one or two weeks, in which he or she records data pertaining to sleep and daytime functioning. The patient should record the time of retiring, estimate of the time it took to fall asleep, awakening and arising times, any periods of the day when he or she felt drowsy, the timing and duration of any naps, and consumption of psychoactive medication or beverages containing alcohol or caffeine. In selected cases of severe chronic insomnia, or for patients for whom a primary sleep disorder such as sleep apnea or nocturnal myoclonus is suggested by the history, referral to a certified sleep laboratory for polysomnographic study should be considered.

HISTORY

History of the Present Illness

The medical history should begin with the patient's chief complaint of the perceived sleep problem. Many patients will focus exclusively on their difficulty in initiating and/or maintaining sleep. It is important to explore also for signs and symptoms of a disorder of excessive somnolence (DOES), since sleepiness during the day often accompanies insomnia and provides an important indicator of the severity of the condition.

The history should cover all the events of a typical night and subsequent day. What time do the patients get into bed? Do they usually read, watch television, do paperwork, and the like, and if so, for how long before turning the lights out? How long does it take them to fall asleep? Do they sleep through the night, or are there awakenings? Do they toss and turn, fall out of bed, or find themselves in another room? Is there a snoring pattern? Do they experience hallucinations as they are falling asleep or waking up? Do they wake up before the alarm clock goes off? Do they linger in bed or promptly get out of bed? Do they wake up feeling refreshed, or are they fatigued immedi-

TABLE 1. Common Conditions Associated with Long-Term Insomnia

PSYCHIATRIC ILLNESS

Adjustment disorder
  Adjustment disorder with anxious mood
  Adjustment disorder with physical complaints
Anxiety disorder
  Generalized anxiety disorder
  Panic disorder
  Post-traumatic stress disorder
Mood disorder
  Bipolar disorder
  Major depression, single episode or recurrent
  Dysthymia
Personality disorder

MEDICAL ILLNESS

Arthritis
Asthma
Brain tumors
Chronic obstructive pulmonary disease
Chronic renal failure
Diabetes mellitus
Endocrine disorder
  Addison's disease
  Cushing's disease
  Thyroid disease
Parkinson's disease
Peptic ulcer disease

DRUGS

Alcohol
Benzodiazepines
Beta blockers
Bronchodilators
Caffeine
Decongestants
Steroids
Stimulants

SLEEP DISORDERS

Psychophysiologic insomnia
Sleep apnea syndrome (obstructive, central, or mixed)
Nocturnal myoclonus
Restless legs syndrome
Disorders of the sleep/wake schedule
  Rapid time zone change ("jet lag") syndrome
  "Work-shift" change in conventional sleep/wake schedule
  Delayed sleep phase syndrome

---

ately after awakening? Do they nap during the day, and if so, how frequently, at what time(s) during the day, and for what duration? Do they fall asleep at very inappropriate times (e.g., while driving a car or while talking to a supervisor at work)? What is their pattern of caffeine and alcohol consumption? Do they sleep better when away from home?

In addition to obtaining a careful history of a typical 24-hour cycle, one should also ask about changes in circadian rhythms that might suggest a disorder of the sleep/wake cycle. Do the patients work on a rotating shift schedule? Do they frequently travel across time zones?

Do they have a pattern of falling asleep and waking up at progressively later times? Do they stay up later and sleep later on weekends than during the week?

Duration of the Complaint

The duration of the insomnia is a critical dimension that can serve as a guide for the evaluation and history gathering. By definition, insomnia can be classified as acute or transient if it has been present for days, short-term if it has lasted for a few weeks, and chronic if it has persisted for months to years.[2]

Patients with acute insomnia often have an identifiable precipitant, such as an acute stress (e.g., hospitalization, acute medical illness) or a change in their sleep schedule (e.g., a work-shift change, air travel across several time zones), and an otherwise normal sleep history. Short-term insomnia also is accompanied by a precipitating stress quite often, which can include a recurrence of a psychiatric illness (e.g., recurrent major depressive episode, panic disorder). With appropriate interventions, such as education in sleep hygiene techniques, behavioral therapy, and in some cases, adjunctive intermittent pharmacotherapy,[3] the treating physician can prevent the development of psychophysiologic insomnia, a common and difficult-to-treat cause of chronic insomnia. The common causes of long-term insomnia also include psychiatric disorders, chronic use of alcohol or other central nervous system depressants, and several specific sleep disorders, including sleep apnea, nocturnal myoclonus, and disorders of the sleep/wake cycle.

Past Medical History

The past medical history should emphasize chronic exposure to drugs and toxic compounds that can impair sleep, including alcohol, sleeping pills, steroids, bronchodilators or decongestants, beta blockers, psychostimulants, thyroid hormones, caffeine, and tobacco. Also, one should inquire about past injuries to the nose or chest wall, which might increase the risk for obstructive sleep apnea.

PHYSICAL EXAMINATION

Physical examination is primarily useful in detecting reversible causes of obstructive sleep apnea, as well as sequellae of the chronic hypo-oxygenation that can be associated with untreated apnea. General examination should note obesity (which increases the risk of sleep apnea) or hypertension (which can result from untreated apnea) when present. Head and neck examination should explore for deviated nasal septa or nasal polyps. Swollen tonsils or excessive soft tissue in the pharynx should be noted. Physical signs of right-sided heart failure, pulmonary hypertension, or renal failure can occur in severe forms of chronic sleep apnea.

aged to fall asleep. The sleep latency, that is, the time that elapses from "lights out" until the first objective evidence of sleep onset on the EEG, is recorded.

Polysomnographic laboratory studies can be obtained in specialized sleep disorders centers. The American Sleep Disorders Association (ASDA) maintains a list of accredited centers throughout the country, which can be obtained by contacting the ASDA (604 Second Avenue, S.W., Rochester, Minnesota 55902).

DIAGNOSTIC STUDIES

In the vast majority of cases, the assessment of insomnia can be completed without laboratory tests. When medical conditions associated with insomnia are suggested by the history and physical examination (e.g., thyroid disease), appropriate blood tests can help rule in or rule out specific diseases. Finally, in selected cases of severe chronic insomnia, or when the diagnosis is questionable, or when the history suggests a specific pathologic sleep disorder such as sleep apnea syndrome, referral to a sleep center for clinical polysomnography can be considered.

A polysomnographic study usually includes the measurement of a number of physiologic variables during sleep, including an electroencephalogram (EEG), chin and bilateral tibialis electromyogram (EMG), electrocardiogram (ECG), chest and abdominal strain gauges for measuring respiratory excursion, oral and nasal thermistors for measuring airflow, and an ear oximeter to gauge oxygenation. With these data, the polysomnographer can determine the "sleep architecture," including the sleep latency and sleep staging, and can detect the presence and severity of specific sleep disorders, such as nocturnal myoclonus or sleep apneas. These studies are usually performed at night, although daytime studies are sometimes appropriate for night-shift workers. At many centers, the patient will first spend a "practice night" at the laboratory in order to begin to accommodate to the new sleep environment; on the second night, the actual study will be conducted.

In cases where it is important to quantify daytime drowsiness, multiple sleep latency tests (MSLTs) can be performed in the laboratory. At five timed intervals over the course of the day, the patient is attached to a polysomnographic recording apparatus and encour-

ASSESSMENT

Psychophysiologic Insomnia

The typical clinical picture of this common cause of chronic insomnia includes hyperarousal in bed, which becomes more fixed over time, daytime fatigue, and night-time awakenings. Usually, patients report that they can fall asleep when they "aren't trying," such as while watching television at night, but when they get into bed, they become fully alert. Often patients will sleep better when they are away from home.[4]

Sleep Apnea

Sleep disruption and frequent awakenings are commonly described in sleep apnea. The patient may also complain of severe daytime fatigue. Also, patients may experience dysphoria, decreased libido, and difficulty with concentration and memory. The sleep partner may report loud snoring with prolonged interruptions. Irritability and personality changes may be observed by family members.[5]

Nocturnal Myoclonus

The patient may report periodic rhythmic leg jerks over the course of the night, with very brief awakenings, but often the patient is unaware of these events. The bed partner can usually provide a description of recurrent episodes of leg kicking in the patient and consequent disruption in both parties' sleep. The patient's bedclothes may be in disarray in the morning.[6] Nocturnal myoclonus may be accompanied by the "restless legs syndrome," characterized by uncomfortable "crawling" feelings, usually in the calf of the leg, that begin when the patient lies down to go to sleep and are relieved by motion, usually walking.

Insomnia Associated with Psychiatric Conditions

Mood and anxiety disorders are often accompanied by insomnia. In the former group of disorders, the insomnia can take the form of difficulty falling asleep and/or midnight or early morning awakenings. In anxiety disorders, the sleep complaint is usually that of difficulty falling asleep. Many other categories of psychiatric illness can be accompanied by insomnia, such as acute exacerbations of schizophrenia, post-traumatic stress disorder, and adjustment disorders. In contrast to psychophysiologic insomnia, sleep does not improve when the patient is away from home, and the severity of the insomnia often covaries with the severity of the underlying psychiatric condition.

Insomnia Associated with Medical Conditions

Several types of medical conditions are associated with insomnia, including endocrinopathies involving the thyroid or adrenal systems, diabetes mellitus, central nervous system neoplasms, chronic obstructive pulmonary disease, hay fever, chronic renal failure, arthritis, and Parkinson's disease. As in the case of insomnia secondary to psychiatric illness, the insomnia does not usually improve when the patient is away from home, and the severity of the insomnia often covaries with the severity of the underlying medical condition.

Managing Insomnia

Insomnia is a very common experience, and while it is rarely, if ever, life-threatening, for some patients it creates very intense anxiety and concern. By following a systematic line of inquiry, the physician usually can identify the underlying cause, leading to an appropriate treatment plan and reassurance for the patient.

REFERENCES

1. Consensus conference. Drugs and insomnia: the use of medications to promote sleep. JAMA 1984;251:2410–4.
2. Carskadon MA, Dement WC, Mitler MM, Guilleminault C, Zarcone VP, Spiegel R. Self-reports versus sleep laboratory findings in 122 drug-free subjects with complaints of chronic insomnia. Am J Psychiatry 1976;133:1382–8.
3. Golden RN, James SP. Insomnia: clinical assessment and management of the patient who can't sleep. Postgrad Med 1988;83:251–8.
4. Mendelson WB. Chronic insomnia. In: Human sleep. New York: Plenum Medical, 1987:323–42.
5. Guilleminault C, Eldridge FL, Dement WC. Insomnia with sleep apnea: a new syndrome. Science 1973;181:856–8.
6. Coleman RM, Pollack CP, Weitzman ED. Periodic movements in sleep (nocturnal myoclonus): relation to sleep disorders. Ann Neurol 1980;8:416–21.

INTERSTITIAL PULMONARY DISEASE

PEADAR G. NOONE and LEONARD SICILIAN

SYNONYMS: Diffuse Infiltrative Lung Disease, Pulmonary Fibrosis, Idiopathic Pulmonary Fibrosis, Interstitial Pneumonitis

BACKGROUND

Interstitial lung diseases comprise a group of inflammatory disorders characterized by diffuse involvement of lung parenchyma as seen on chest radiograph. Although the term interstitial is frequently used, the pathologic process involves not only alveolar septa and interstitium but also the alveolar space, airways, pulmonary microvasculature, and pleura. This results in a characteristic clinical, radiologic, and physiologic picture of dyspnea, diffuse bilateral pulmonary infiltrates on chest radiograph, and restrictive pattern on pulmonary function testing. It is important to remember that in 40 to 60 per cent of cases a specific diagnosis will not be made. Even for many of the others associated with a known disease, a specific "cause" is not known. The former cases are labeled as idiopathic, and names used to describe this condition are idiopathic pulmonary fibrosis (IPF) (in the United States) and cryptogenic fibrosing alveolitis (in the United Kingdom). When histologic subgrouping is possible, the terms usual interstitial pneumonitis (UIP) and desquamative interstitial pneumonitis (DIP) have been used. The latter term applies when desquamation of

alveolar cells, rather than fibrosis, is more prominent. When giant cells predominate, the term giant cell interstitial pneumonitis (GIP) is used, as is lymphocytic interstitial pneumonitis (LIP) when lymphocytes are the principal cells. Finally, bronchiolitis obliterans interstitial pneumonitis (BIP) is used when bronchiolitis obliterans is the major feature on biopsy.[1,2]

There is evidence that some of the subtypes of interstitial pneumonitis may have a better prognosis than others; for example, those with a predominantly cellular infiltrate (DIP, LIP) may be more responsive to steroid therapy and have better survival.[3,4] One should, therefore, attempt to classify the interstitial lung diseases into several subgroups—idiopathic, those with a known associated disease or specific histologic pattern but of unknown etiology, and those having a specific cause (Table 1).

Among interstitial diseases with better defined specific diagnoses, sarcoidosis is the

TABLE 1. Causes of Interstitial Lung Disease—Partial List

ETIOLOGY KNOWN	ETIOLOGY UNKNOWN
Organic dusts	Idiopathic
Farmer's lung	Idiopathic pulmonary fibrosis (IPF)
Bird breeder's lung	IPF associated with the collagen vascular diseases
Mushroom worker's lung	Progressive systemic sclerosis
Humidifier lung	Rheumatoid arthritis
Malt worker's lung	Systemic lupus erythematosus
Inorganic dusts	Sjögren's syndrome
Silica—coal, dust	Polymyositis/dermatomyositis
Silicates—asbestos, talc	Mixed connective tissue disease
Beryllium	Vasculitis and granulomatous disease
Mixed dusts—oxides of iron	Sarcoidosis
Gases, fumes, vapors	Wegener's granulomatosis
Oxygen	Churg-Strauss syndrome (allergic granulomatosis)
Chlorine, sulfur dioxide, ammonia	Polyarteritis nodosa
Oxides of metals—zinc, copper, and the like	Lymphomatoid granulomatosis
Mercury	Inherited disorders
Drugs	Tuberous sclerosis, lymphangioleiomyomatosis
Chemotherapeutic agents	Neurofibromatosis
Bleomycin, busulfan, cyclophosphamide, BCNU*	Familial pulmonary fibrosis
Antibiotics	Hermansky-Pudlak syndrome
Nitrofurantoin, sulfonamides, penicillin	Ankylosing spondylitis
Others	Weber-Christian disease
Phenytoin, gold salts, methysergide, carbamazine	Pulmonary hemorrhagic syndromes
Miscellaneous	Idiopathic pulmonary hemosiderosis
Poisons—paraquat	Goodpasture's syndrome
Radiation	Miscellaneous infiltrative conditions
Postinfectious—especially post-tuberculosis	Associated with gastrointestinal disease
Chronic aspiration pneumonia—lipoid pneumonia	chronic liver disease, celiac disease, ulcerative
HIV-related	colitis, Crohn's disease
Toxic oil syndrome, eosinophilic—myalgic syndrome	Amyloidosis
Secondary to other organ dysfunction	Alveolar proteinosis
Chronic cardiogenic pulmonary edema	Chronic eosinophilic pneumonia
Chronic renal failure	Lymphoma
Lymphangitis carcinomatosis	

* BCNU = Bis-2-chloroethyl-1-nitrosurea

most common disease encountered and has a worldwide distribution. In the United States, it is found particularly among blacks. The incidence is approximately 20 per 100,000 population, and the disease tends to occur more commonly in younger individuals. Although it is a multisystem granulomatous disease, the lungs are affected in greater than 90 per cent of cases. Hence, when symptoms are present, they are usually respiratory, but extrathoracic complaints may be prominent. Genetic factors may play a role, as there are sporadic reports of familial sarcoidosis. An infectious etiology is also possible, based on reports of clustering. To date, however, no etiologic agent or agents have been discovered.[5]

IPF, though less common than sarcoidosis, has an estimated incidence of 3 to 5 per 100,000. It can occur at any age, but the mean age at onset is 50 to 60 years. There appears to be a slight male preponderance. It has been reported with a higher-than-expected frequency in families and in families with an excess of autoimmune disease.[4] Collagen vascular disease can also involve the lung. Pulmonary fibrosis occurs commonly in progressive systemic sclerosis, and at times without the classic skin, gastrointestinal, and renal manifestations, this is known as progressive systemic sclerosis sine scleroderma.[6] Interstitial lung disease occurs in 6 to 13 per cent of patients with systemic lupus erythematosis; the most common pulmonary problems in this condition, however, are pleuritis and pleural effusion.

The most common drug related diffuse pulmonary disease appears to be nitrofurantoin-induced pneumonitis. Swedish reports suggest that it occurs in about 1 per cent of those taking the drug. Of the total reactions to nitrofurantoin, 43 per cent of patients had acute pneumonitis, and 5 per cent had chronic fibrosis.[7] Chemotherapeutic agents, especially bleomycin, are also a well-established cause of infiltrative lung disease.[8]

Asbestos has long been recognized to cause a variety of lung diseases including pulmonary fibrosis, and this is related to fiber type and the duration and degree of exposure.[9] Exposure to a high fraction of inspired oxygen (FiO_2) greater than 0.5 for 48 to 72 hours at sea level is well recognized to cause acute lung injury, which may result in pulmonary fibrosis. This is thought to be related to the cytotoxic effect of free oxygen radicals, particularly on macrophages, capillary endothelial cells, and type I pneumocytes.[10] A variety of other causes for interstitial diseases exist (Table 1), but these will not be discussed in any detail in this section.

Pathogenesis

The initial histologic picture of interstitial lung disease is of acute alveolitis, defined as an accumulation of inflammatory and immune effector cells in the alveoli with resulting inflammation of surrounding structures. This is followed by derangement of the alveolocapillary unit (distortion of alveolar walls due to the presence of inflammatory cells, with edema or granulomas), which then may progress to end-stage fibrosis. At that point, the alveolar structures are no longer recognizable, and there are bands of connective tissue interspersed with the inflammatory and immune effector cells. This has been demonstrated by biopsies in both humans and animal models.[11,12] Alveolitis is potentially reversible, whereas end-stage fibrosis of the parenchyma is not. This, of course, has therapeutic implications, since only early treatment would be expected to work.

What actually stimulates the local aggregation of inflammatory cells and subsequent injury remains unknown in the majority of cases. In certain diseases, however, there is a better understanding of the train of events. The classic example is hypersensitivity pneumonitis due to inhaled antigens as in farmer's lung. Here the antigen concerned is probably one of the family of thermophilic actinomyces, bacteria that proliferate in moldy hay under certain conditions. The antigen or antigens promote the development of humoral type III and cell-mediated type IV immunity, which activate inflammatory cells in the lung. Not all exposed individuals exhibit a response, as several factors—environmental, genetic, and host—presumably play a role.[13] The scenario is thought to be the same in the other interstitial lung diseases, except that the offending agent is unknown and therefore cannot be avoided as with farmers' lung. Therapeutic maneuvers are therefore limited. If the inflammatory process cannot be arrested, eventual repair of the alveolar structures is impossible, and healing by fibrosis takes place.

HISTORY

A careful history is most important in patients with suspected interstitial lung disease and is often more helpful than the physical examination and laboratory studies. Significant historical negatives are as important as positive information. It is wise to assume that the patient will not always volunteer important information and will occasionally underemphasize vital clues.

Dyspnea is generally the cardinal symptom. Its onset, duration, timing and any associated symptoms should be carefully chronicled since the various causes of interstitial lung disease often have quite characteristic features in this regard. A precise smoking history should be obtained since chronic bronchitis or emphysema may contribute to the shortness of breath.

Cough is another common symptom resulting either from the primary condition or from coexistent chronic bronchitis, bronchiectasis, or infection. In the latter case, the cough can be productive. The cough of interstitial disease is most often dry and occurs as a result of triggering irritant receptors in the lung parenchyma.

Wheezing is an unusual symptom in interstitial disease and rarely will be the presenting complaint. However, it can be present in Churg-Strauss syndrome with associated asthma and vasculitis. In chronic eosinophilic pneumonia, wheezing when heard is the result of concomitant asthma.[14]

Hemoptysis is a feature of the hemorrhagic conditions, idiopathic pulmonary hemosiderosis, and Goodpasture's syndrome and can be of alarming proportions. Hemoptysis can also occur in valvular heart disease (particularly mitral stenosis) and acute cardiogenic pulmonary edema. Both the latter entities may mimic an interstitial pulmonary process and should be eliminated before evaluation of lung disease is undertaken.

Pleuritic chest pain may be due to an associated pneumothorax. There is a higher incidence of pneumothorax with infiltrative conditions, especially IPF, histiocytosis X, and lymphangioleiomyomatosis. Pleural involvement is common in the connective tissue diseases, and pleuritic pain unrelated to pneumothorax may accompany systemic lupus erythematosus and rheumatoid arthritis.

Occupational and environmental history may be the most important part of the assessment. The occupational history needs to be taken in careful chronologic order, starting with the patient's first job and including temporary, school, and summer jobs, up to the present day. It must include the patient's own description of the job and work environment.

Time spent in the armed services should be included, since asbestos was widely used during World War II in the shipbuilding and defense industry. In some instances, the spouses of asbestos-exposed individuals developed disease due to exposure to contaminated clothing, and thus the history of exposed family members is important. Obviously, any time spent in the mining or other dusty industries should be detailed. In the agricultural industry, the work environment and potential exposure to toxic or organic fumes and dusts should be clarified. (e.g., thermophilic actinomyces in farmer's lung, oxides of nitrogen in silofiller's disease.)

A detailed drug history should include inquiries about such drugs as nitrofurantoin, chemotherapeutic agents, and amiodarone. Any drug should be regarded as suspect for unexplained diffuse lung disease until proved otherwise.

Extrapulmonary symptoms may be helpful in determining whether underlying systemic disease is the cause of the diffuse infiltrates. Arthralgias, Raynaud's phenomenon, and skin or joint lesions suggest connective tissue diseases such as rheumatoid arthritis, progressive systemic sclerosis, or systemic lupus erythematosus. Nasal symptoms are common in Wegener's granulomatosis. Eye, joint, and skin symptoms or symptoms of hypercalcemia are common in sarcoidosis.

PHYSICAL EXAMINATION

Although the physical examination is often nonspecific, the presence or absence of certain physical signs can prove helpful in the diagnosis. For example, digital clubbing is quite common in IPF and asbestosis. Bilateral dry inspiratory crackles are the rule in diffuse disease. They are notably absent, however, in sarcoidosis and most of the pneumoconioses. Signs such as cyanosis and reduction of chest expansion may be helpful in assessing severity of disease but are nonspecific findings since they may occur in the end-stage of many pulmonary diseases. Signs of cor pulmonale, a loud pulmonary second heart sound, a pulmonary flow murmur, or overt right heart failure may be present in advanced disease but are similarly nonspecific.

A careful examination of skin, bone, joints, and eyes occasionally yields helpful information and may reveal the presence of a systemic disease. A search for a primary malignancy should include careful examination of the thyroid, breasts, and rectum. With a good history and physical examination, the physician can often narrow down the initially quite broad differential diagnosis and proceed with more focused investigations.

DIAGNOSTIC STUDIES

Imaging

The chest radiograph, whether obtained for specific pulmonary complaints or as part of the workup for other diseases, is the usual first clue to the presence of interstitial lung disease. However, it should be borne in mind that the radiograph may be normal about 10 to 15 per cent the time.[15] Once an interstitial pattern has been noted, the distribution and characteristics of the infiltrate can be helpful in the differential diagnosis (Table 2).

Specific diseases have typical radiologic features. For example, pulmonary fibrosis of any type usually will have a reticular (linear) irregular infiltrate, mainly in the lower zones.

TABLE 2.   Common Radiologic Patterns in Interstitial Lung Disease, with Overlap in Some Conditions

Predominantly lower zone reticular
  Pulmonary fibrosis (idiopathic and known)
  Lymphangitis carcinomatosis
  Asbestosis
Diffuse reticular
  Pulmonary fibrosis (idiopathic and known)
  Asbestosis
  Histiocytosis X and related diseases
  Tuberous sclerosis, lymphangioleiomyomatosis
  Neurofibromatosis
  Sarcoidosis
Predominantly upper zone reticulonodular
  Sarcoidosis
  Pneumocystis carinii pneumonia
  Pulmonary edema
Diffuse reticulonodular
  Sarcoidosis
  Histiocytosis X
  Berylliosis
  Pneumocystic carinii pneumonia
Predominantly upper zone nodular
  Silicosis
  Coal workers' pneumoconiosis
  Tuberculosis
  Sarcoidosis
Diffuse nodular
  Tuberculosis—miliary
  Fungal diseases
  Metastatic malignancy
  Sarcoidosis
  Rheumatoid arthritis

Honeycombing suggests end-stage fibrosis. The granulomatous diseases tend to have a nodular or reticulonodular infiltrate that is often predominant in the upper zones.

Old films should be obtained when possible. Subtle or early changes may suggest more chronic, previously unsuspected disease, which is often easier to detect in retrospect. This is particularly important when coexistent carcinoma is suspected. The degree of abnormality on chest radiograph does not necessarily correlate with the symptoms or pathophysiologic derangement. However, it remains a very useful monitor of progression or regression of disease.

Computed tomography (CT) of the chest may be useful in delineating more clearly the distribution of the infiltrates and may show enlarged mediastinal lymph nodes. High-resolution CT scanning of the chest is now being studied as a method of early detection of parenchymal lung disease. Its utility in the diagnosis and management of specific interstitial diseases remains to be seen.[16]

^{67}Ga-citrate is a radioisotope that has increased uptake at sites of inflammation.[11] It was initially proposed as a useful tool to diagnose interstitial lung disease—in particular, sarcoidosis. However, its lack of specificity in this setting has been disappointing. ^{67}Ga scanning can be useful to detect disease where the plain radiograph is normal. This has been most recently seen in *Pneumocystis carinii* pneumonia in human immunodeficiency virus (HIV)-infected patients and has resulted in earlier diagnosis and therapy.[17] It may, therefore, help in decision making, particularly when diffuse lung disease is suspected but presenting symptoms and radiograph changes are not diagnostic.

Pulmonary Function Tests

Pulmonary function tests (PFTs) usually show a "restrictive pattern" but are not diagnostic of a particular pathologic entity. In addition, they do not necessarily correlate with the activity of the inflammatory process. Nevertheless, they are useful to assess the degree of impairment and the progression of that impairment longitudinally, particularly in relation to treatment. PFTs also help to rule out coexisting chronic obstructive lung disease, which may contribute to the presenting symptoms.[18] Minimum testing should include spirometry, static lung volumes, diffusing capacity, and an arterial blood gas at rest. The typical findings of a restrictive pattern are reduced forced vital capacity (FVC), and forced expired volume in one second (FEV$_1$), with a normal FEV$_1$/FVC. Reduced lung volumes—that is, total lung capacity (TLC)—and single breath diffusing capacity for carbon monoxide are also seen.

Monitoring of gas exchange during exercise probably gives the most sensitive estimate of interstitial disease. Either maximal or steady-state exercise will unmask a loss of gas exchange reserve early in disease. These studies are also particularly relevant in the patient who is quite dyspneic in the face of normal or near-normal mechanics, diffusion lung carbon monoxide, and resting blood gases. In more advanced disease, the resting values, of course, will be affected, and severe hypoxemia (PaO$_2$ less than 55 mm Hg) with normal or low carbon dioxide tension (PaCO$_2$ less than 37 mm Hg) may be present. The detection of severe hypoxemia at rest or exercise will also guide the physician in prescribing supplemental oxygen.

Pulmonary function tests, therefore, will not distinguish between reversible and irreversible disease and thus are not helpful in making the decision as to whether or not to treat the patient. However, once that decision is made, PFTs may be helpful in monitoring responses.

Hematologic and biochemical screening can occasionally help make a specific diagnosis. Eosinophilia might suggest chronic eosinophilic pneumonia, for example. More specific immunologic markers should also be sought, and these should, at least, include rheumatoid factor, antinuclear antibodies, and anticentromeric antibodies. The latter is fairly specific for progressive systemic sclerosis. In hypersensitivity pneumonitis, serum precipitins against suspected antigens can be sought. Serum angiotensin converting enzyme is elevated in up to 70 per cent of patients with sarcoidosis. Among the rarer conditions, anti–glomerular basement membrane antibodies are specific for Goodpasture's disease, and recent reports of a specific marker for Wegener's granulomatosis, anticytoplasmic antibodies, seem promising.[19]

Bronchoalveolar Lavage

Bronchoalveolar lavage (BAL) initially promised to be an important new tool in the assessment of the interstitial lung diseases.[20,21] By instilling 100 ml of saline, in 20-ml aliquots,

into a subsegmental bronchus, via a fiberoptic bronchoscope, and reaspirating the fluid, it is possible to recover the inflammatory cells and proteins involved in the alveolitis.[20] In the normal individual, 80 to 90 per cent of the recovered cells are macrophages, 10 per cent are lymphocytes, and the remainder are polymorphonuclear leukocytes. Smoking or coexisting bronchitis or infection will increase the cell yield and alter the differential cell count. In sarcoidosis there is generally a higher percentage of lymphocytes, in particular activated helper lymphocytes, and in IPF, there is a higher proportion of polymorphonuclear cells.[21] Early efforts were made to relate the number and type of cells recovered to the specific diagnosis or to the intensity of alveolitis. However, BAL has not provided a test that could be utilized in everyday practice as a diagnostic tool. Thus, it remains a research tool in the assessment of interstitial lung disease. In contrast, BAL has become the diagnostic procedure of choice for opportunistic infections presenting as diffuse infiltrates in HIV-infected patients. The diagnosis of *Pneumocystis carinii* pneumonia can be made reliably with BAL in over 90 per cent of patients with this disease.[22,23]

Lung Biopsy

Transbronchial lung biopsy via a fiberoptic bronchoscope is extremely useful in the diagnosis of certain diffuse lung diseases. In sarcoidosis, the diagnostic yield can be as high as 90 per cent. The yield in other interstitial diseases, with the exception of widespread carcinomatosis, is lower, since the pieces of tissue are small.[24] When the disease is patchy and architecture is important to establish the diagnosis (IPF, vasculitis, amyloidosis), an open lung biopsy is necessary. Open lung biopsy may also be indicated when the risks of transbronchial biopsy are increased by a coagulopathy or severe hypoxemia. At times, it may be necessary to proceed to open lung biopsy when the tissue obtained at transbronchial biopsy is nonspecific. Such tissue may lie adjacent to an area of malignancy or granulomatous disease.[24]

With a good history, diagnostic chest radiograph, and laboratory studies, a lung biopsy may not be necessary to establish the diagnosis. This is especially true for occupationally related lung disease and chronic eosinophilic pneumonia.[14]

Now that lung and heart transplantation

have become feasible for certain patients as a therapy for end-stage interstitial lung disease, open lung biopsy must be considered carefully.[25] Postbiopsy pleural reaction can make transplant surgery difficult to perform and may therefore eliminate that patient from consideration. Thus, every effort should be made to establish the diagnosis in these individuals without the use of an open lung biopsy. When this is not possible, prior discussion with the transplantation surgeon should be undertaken to establish the best plan of action.

ASSESSMENT

As with other areas in medicine, if the physician follows the maxim that "Common things are common" and approaches the patient with interstitial lung disease in a structured, logical manner, a diagnosis will be apparent in the majority of cases. A brief discussion of the constellation of findings in some of the more common conditions will help illustrate this point.

Idiopathic pulmonary fibrosis should be considered in the older patient who presents with gradually progressive dyspnea. Occasionally, symptoms appear to begin acutely, but the disease may have been chronically present when old radiographs are reviewed. Constitutional symptoms such as fever, fatigue, and myalgia occasionally occur. Nonproductive cough occurs commonly. Clubbing of the digits and bibasilar crackles are the most common physical findings. The chest radiograph shows a linear infiltrate with predominantly basal distribution. Connective tissue diseases associated with IPF may not be obvious until serology suggests a link. The absence of systemic findings should not deter the physician from asking the relevant questions regarding Raynaud's phenomenon, difficulty swallowing, skin lesions, arthritis, etc. Further investigations directed at these diseases, such as barium swallow to detect esophageal motility problems that occur in scleroderma should be considered.

Sarcoidosis classically presents acutely with erythema nodosum, fever, and bilateral hilar adenopathy. However, it is more likely to present as asymptomatic hilar adenopathy on a chest radiograph that has been taken for other reasons. Sarcoidosis also presents as symptomatic or asymptomatic adenopathy with infiltrates or with infiltrates alone. The symmetry of the lymphadenopathy, when present, suggests the diagnosis, but lymphoma can mimic the disease closely, especially when constitutional symptoms occur. Hence, a tissue diagnosis usually with transbronchial lung biopsy should be pursued in all symptomatic cases. Tuberculosis and fungal infections may also cause a similar picture, including the presence of adenopathy. Patients with sarcoidosis are often anergic to skin testing, so that a positive tuberculin or fungal skin test means that culture of sputum or biopsy material is required to establish these infections. A careful physical examination occasionally shows sarcoidos of the skin (nodules, plaques, lupus pernio), and skin biopsy, a less invasive procedure, may provide the diagnosis when lesions are present.

Organic dust diseases or hypersensitivity pneumonitis are suggested by a history of exposure, although this may not necessarily be obvious. The so-called classic history of chest tightness, dyspnea, and interstitial infiltrate pattern six to eight hours following exposure (e.g., to moldy hay) is often not obtained. A more chronic, progressive dyspnea is usually the cardinal complaint. A pattern of improvement at specific times—for example, when on vacation—or, alternatively, worsening of symptoms on exposure to certain items, situations, or pets should alert the physician to the possibility of a hypersensitivity pneumonitis. Positive precipitating antibodies in the blood of these patients will help establish the diagnosis.[13]

Asbestosis is important to diagnose properly because of the medicolegal implications. Most often a history of exposure, along with dyspnea, restrictive PFT pattern, and chest radiograph showing basilar linear irregular infiltrates (similar to IPF), is enough to establish the diagnosis. This is also the case with the other pneumoconioses.

Chronic eosinophilic pneumonia occurs more commonly in middle-aged women. Asthma may predate the diagnosis, and the disease often has severe associated constitutional symptoms. Nasal symptoms occur less frequently than with the rarer eosinophilia-related vasculitis, Wegener's granulomatosis, and Churg-Strauss syndrome. The chest x-ray often shows a peripheral infiltrate. The presence of blood eosinophilia should strongly suggest the diagnosis.

Drug related pulmonary fibrosis, radiation

fibrosis, or oxygen toxicity should all be suggested by an appropriate exposure history. Alveolar proteinosis is often initially diagnosed as a pneumonia, sarcoidosis, hypersensitivity pneumonitis, or tuberculosis. A biopsy specimen is usually the first clue to the nature of the problem. Goodpasture's syndrome may be suggested by the presence of renal disease. The association of chronic iron deficiency anemia with interstitial lung disease should suggest the presence of idiopathic pulmonary hemosiderosis.

Diagnosis

Because of the many and varied diseases included under the heading of interstitial lung disease, the diagnosis may not be obvious even with the most careful attention to detail, in which case a lung biopsy is unavoidable. Occasionally, one of the rarer causes mentioned in Table 1 is found on histology, and obviously no history taking or other special tests would have proved diagnostic. In a similar fashion, one of the more common conditions may be discovered on histologic examination, when an atypical presentation did not initially suggest the diagnosis. The urgency of such a procedure obviously depends on the particular situation. For example, in an HIV-positive patient, or a patient immunosuppressed as a result of chemotherapy, lung infiltrates require prompt evaluation, as a treatable infective cause is most likely. Patients with more chronic disease can be evaluated through a structured workup.

REFERENCES

1. Fishman AP. UIP, DIP and all that. N Engl J Med 1978;298:843–5.
2. Fulmer JD. The interstitial lung diseases. Chest 1982;82:172–8.
3. Carrington BC, Gaensler GA, Coutu RE, FitzGerald MX, Gupta RG. Natural history and treated course of usual and desquamative interstitial pneumonia. N Engl J Med 1978;298:801–9.
4. Turner-Warwick M, Burrows B, Johnson A. Cryptogenic fibrosing alveolitis: clinical features and their influence on survival. Thorax 1980;35:171–80.
5. Fanburg BL, Pitt EA. Sarcoidosis. In: Murray JF, Nadel JA, eds. Textbook of respiratory medicine. Philadelphia: WB Saunders, 1988:1486–1500.
6. Lomeo RM, Cornella RJ, Schabel SI, Silver RM. Progressive systemic sclerosis sine scleroderma presenting as pulmonary interstitial fibrosis. Am J Med 1989;87:525–7.
7. Holmberg L, Boman G, Nottiger LE, Eriksson B, Spross R, Wessling A. Adverse reactions to nitrofurantoin. Analysis of 921 reports. Am J Med 1980;69:733–8.
8. Van Barneveld PWC, Sleijfer D Th, Van Der Mark Th W, et al. Natural history of bleomycin induced pneumonitis. A follow up study. Am Rev Respir Dis 1987;135:48–51.
9. American Thoracic Society. The diagnosis of nonmalignant diseases related to asbestos. Am Rev Respir Dis 1986;134:363–8.
10. Bruce Davis W, Rennard SI, Bitterman PB, Crystal RG. Pulmonary oxygen toxicity. Early reversible changes in human alveolar structures induced by superoxia. N Engl J Med 1983;309:878–83.
11. Crystal RG, Gadek JE, Ferrans VJ, Fulmer JD, Line BR, Hunninghake GW. Interstitial lung disease: current concepts of pathogenesis, staging and therapy. Am J Med 1981;70:542–68.
12. Crystal RG, Bitterman PB, Rennard SI, Hance AJ, Keogh BA. Interstitial lung disease of unknown causes. Disorders characterized by chronic inflammation of the lower respiratory tract [Two parts]. N Engl J Med 1984;310:154–66, 235–44.
13. Burrell R, Rylander R. A critical review of the role of precipitins in hypersensitivity pneumonitis. Eur J Respir Dis 1981;62:332–42.
14. Jederlinic PJ, Sicilian L, Gaensler EA. Chronic eosinophilic pneumonia. A report of 19 cases and a review of the literature. Medicine 1988;63:154–62.
15. Epler GR, McLoud TC, Gaensler EA, Mikus JP, Carrington CB. Normal chest roentgenograms in chronic diffuse infiltrative lung disease. N Engl J Med 1978;298:934–9.
16. Mathieson JR, Mayo JR, Staples CA, Muller NL. Chronic diffuse infiltrative lung disease: comparison of diagnostic accuracy of CT and chest radiography. Radiology 1989;171:111–6.
17. Lewis CD, Hattner RS, Luce JM, Dodek PM, Golden JA, Murray JF. Correlation between gallium lung scans and fiberoptic bronchoscopy in patients with suspected *Pneumocystis carinii* pneumonia and the acquired immune deficiency syndrome. Am Rev Respir Dis 1984;130:1166–9.
18. Keogh BA, Crystal BA. Clinical significance of pulmonary function testing. Pulmonary function testing in interstitial pulmonary disease. What does it tell us? Chest 1980;78:856–65.
19. Harrison DJ, Simpson R, Kharbanda R, Abernethy VE, Nimmo G. Antibodies to neutrophil cytoplasmic antigens in Wegener's granulomatosis and other conditions. Thorax 1989; 44:373–7.
20. Reynolds HY, Fulmer JD, Kazmierowski JA, Roberts WC, Frank MM, Crystal RG. Analysis of cellular and protein content of bronchoalveolar lavage fluid from patients with idiopathic pulmonary fibrosis and chronic hypersensitivity pneumonitis. J Clin Invest 1977;59:165–75.
21. Weinberger SE, Kelman JA, Elson NA, et al. Bronchoalveolar lavage in interstitial lung disease. Ann Intern Med 1987;89:459–66.
22. Stover DE, White DA, Romano PA, Gellene R. Diagnosis of pulmonary disease in acquired immune deficiency syndrome (AIDS). Role of bronchoscopy and bronchoalveolar lavage. Am Rev Respir Dis 1984;130:659–62.
23. Griffiths MH, Kocjan G, Miller RF, Godfrey-Faus-

sett AF. Diagnosis of pulmonary disease in human immunodeficiency virus infection: role of transbronchial biopsy and bronchoalveolar lavage. Thorax 1989; 44:554–8.

24. Wall CP, Gaensler EA, Carrington CB, Hayes JA. Comparison of transbronchial and open lung biop-

sies in chronic infiltrative lung diseases. Am Rev Respir Dis 1981;123:280–5.

25. Grossman RF, Frost A, Zamel N, et al. The Toronto Lung Transplant Group. Results of single lung transplantation for bilateral pulmonary fibrosis. N Engl J Med 1990;322:727–33.

INTESTINAL BLOATING AND GAS

TIMOTHY T. NOSTRANT and JEFFREY L. BARNETT

SYNONYMS: Gaseousness, Flatulence

BACKGROUND

Excess gaseousness is one of the most common gastrointestinal complaints for which patients seek medical advice. Patients may wrongly attribute gastroesophageal reflux, chest pain, biliary colic, abdominal cramps, anorexia, intestinal obstruction, and malabsorption to excessive gas.[1] Many terms such as functional dyspepsia, flatulent dyspepsia, and irritable bowel syndrome have been used to describe the constellation of symptoms that people attribute to a perceived overproduction of intestinal gas. In this chapter, we will review the physiology of intestinal gas production, common clinical gas syndromes, and the diagnostic approach to the patient who complains of gas or bloating.

Gas Composition

The principal intestinal gases are nitrogen, oxygen, hydrogen, carbon dioxide, and methane. These five gases represent 99 per cent of total intestinal gas.[2] The most important factor determining gas composition is the region of intestine sampled. Esophageal or gastric gas is swallowed air and is almost entirely nitrogen and oxygen. The total amount of fasting gas in the stomach is less than 10 ml. Continuous sampling of gas in the small bowel is technically difficult, and reliable volume estimates are not available. In addition to swallowed air, small intestinal carbon dioxide is produced by neutralization of gastric acid by pancreatic bicarbonate. Since each mEq of acid neutralized produces 22.4 ml of carbon dioxide and daily acid secretion approximates 100 mEq, 2 L of carbon dioxide would be added by acid neutralization.[2] Lipolysis of triglycerides and protein digestion would also add carbon dioxide by neutralization of fatty acids and amino acids. Most carbon dioxide produced in the small intestine will be absorbed during small bowel passage and subsequently expired. Carbon dioxide present in flatus is rarely swallowed air or derived from acid neutralization.

Hydrogen and methane are exclusively products of anaerobic fermentation.[3] The principal substrates for this fermentation are dietary carbohydrates, which escape small bowel absorption and enter the colon. Unabsorbed oligosaccharides such as stachyose and raffinose (beans), starches (wheat, corn), fructose, and glycoproteins are common substrates. Hydrogen is present in the gut even in fasting animals, and therefore endogenous substrates must be present. Hydrogen produced is quickly absorbed and appears rapidly in expired air. Primary lactase deficiency is the most common source of excessive fecal hydrogen and serves as the physiologic basis for breath hydrogen testing in patients with lactose intolerance. Hydrogen is almost exclusively produced in the colon unless conditions are present for small intestinal bacterial overgrowth or gastric stasis.

As with hydrogen, methane is exclusively a product of bacterial metabolism. Methane is produced by anaerobic methanogenic bacteria, principally *Methanobrevibacter smithii*. As opposed to hydrogen, methane is produced in only 33 to 41 per cent of healthy North Americans.[4] Methane excretor status is highly correlated to methane excretion in other family members. Methane excretion occurs in 92 per cent of children with parents who excrete methane and in 82 per cent of children whose siblings produce methane.[4] Methane excretion is acquired early in life when the bowel is colonized. High sulfate diets allow growth of methane-producing bacteria. Environmental influences are more important than genetics, since identical twins who were separated at birth did not show complete concordance. Institutionalization with its associated bacterial contamination was associated with a high frequency of methane excretion in the mentally retarded, further supporting the role of the environment in the development of methane excretion.

The gases present in the intestine other than nitrogen, oxygen, hydrogen, carbon dioxide, and methane include the skatoles, mercaptans, and sulfides. These gases, although present in only trace amounts, cause fecal odor since the five principal gases are odorless.

Gas Volume

The volume of gas in the gastrointestinal tract is difficult to measure secondary to gas fluxes during passage and contamination of intestinal gas with expired air during measurement.[1,2] Abdominal plethysmography has shown volumes in the gastrointestinal tract ranging from 30 to 300 ml, with a mean of 115 ml.[1,2] Graded infusions of gas followed by abdominal radiographs have confirmed these results. Levitt, using inert argon gas to "wash out" intestinal gas, showed similar gas volumes in patients compared with normal subjects (176 to 199 ml).[5,6] However, at every level of argon infusion, patients experienced more discomfort, had slower gas transit, and had more retrograde passage of argon from intestine to stomach. Thus, patients with complaints of excess gas appear not to have more gas but to have abnormal motility and an abnormal perception of the amount of gas present.[6] These findings are similar to patients with irritable bowel syndrome, where balloon inflation of the rectum resulted in pain at lower distending volumes and more pain at every level of balloon distension compared with normal controls. Balloon distension of the colon,

stomach, esophagus, and biliary tree reproduced the multiple areas of discomfort commonly experienced by these patients.[7] These findings suggest a generalized sensorimotor dysfunction of the gut in patients with complaints of pain and abnormal gas.

HISTORY

The major goal of the history in patients with complaints of excess gas is to exclude disease processes that produce symptoms/signs that the patient can misinterpret as too much gas. Gastroesophageal acid reflux and peptic ulcer disease commonly mimic gas in the upper gastrointestinal (GI) tract. Substernal burning, noncardiac chest pain, and worsening discomfort after meals or in the supine position suggest a diagnosis of acid reflux. Recent weight gain, introduction of new medications (particularly calcium channel blocking agents, beta blockers, or birth control pills), and dysphagia are additional clues to this diagnosis.[8] Heavy alcohol or tobacco use or excessive use of stimulants such as caffeine decrease lower esophageal sphincter pressure and predispose to acid reflux. Epigastric pain worsened by fasting and relieved by meals may indicate a duodenal ulcer and postprandial symptoms, a gastric ulcer. Surprisingly frequently, peptic ulcer disease fails to present in the "classical" manner and may instead produce atypical symptoms including those attributed to gaseousness. Other clues pointing toward peptic ulcer disease include a family history or past personal history of peptic ulcer disease, smoking, the use of nonsteroidal anti-inflammatory agents, and several chronic diseases such as renal failure, cirrhosis, and pulmonary disease. A history of GI bleeding should be sought, but most bleeding is occult if present. Several medications, especially aspirin and other nonsteroidal anti-inflammatory agents, frequently cause upper abdominal symptoms without endoscopically visible inflammation or ulcer.

An increasingly common cause of upper abdominal bloating, eructation, and "gas" is poor gastric emptying or gastroparesis. Common disease associations include diabetes mellitus, particularly if autonomic neuropathy is present; collagen vascular diseases such as scleroderma; partial gastrectomy with vagotomy; and possibly postviral infection. Onset can be abrupt or insidious. Midepigastric pain and postprandial bloating are common. When present, profound nausea, solid food vomiting, and weight loss should allow differentiation from functional gas syndromes. If a clinical question still exists, a solid phase gastric emptying nuclear scan will usually answer the question.

Malassimilation of nutrients can produce excessive gas if the nutrients reach the large bowel and are metabolized by colonic bacteria. Lactase deficiency is the classic example and is a common problem worldwide. The enzyme lactase breaks the unabsorbable carbohydrate lactose into its component sugars (glucose and galactose), which are then both absorbed in the small bowel. If lactase is congenitally deficient or lost later in life (perhaps after an episode of gastroenteritis), ingested lactose reaches the colon unabsorbed, and subsequent bacterial fermentation produces organic acids, carbon dioxide, and hydrogen, which cause bloating, diarrhea, and flatus.[9] Patients only recognize the association of milk products and gas about one third of the time but will frequently avoid lactose-containing foods subconsciously.[10] Lactose withdrawal will usually confirm the diagnosis and convince patients of the cause for their symptoms. Both malabsorption (mucosal disease) and maldigestion (pancreaticobiliary disease or bacterial overgrowth) can produce excessive flatus and bloating. Differentiation from functional gas syndromes discussed later can be difficult. A history of alcoholism, liver disease, pancreatitis, nutritional problems, and diarrhea should be sought. Weight loss should alert the physician to possible malabsorption, since this is rarely seen in functional gas syndromes. Bulky, foul-smelling stools that float (because of gas content, not fat content) signify fecal fat loss (steatorrhea), particularly if weight loss is present.[11] (Also see article on Steatorrhea.) Diabetes mellitus, scleroderma, post–gastric resection, jejunal diverticulosis, and hypogammaglobulinemia are diseases commonly associated with bacterial overgrowth. All predispose to small bowel bacterial proliferation by causing intestinal stasis or poor bacterial clearance. Bacterial overgrowth produces bloating and gas by allowing fermentation of carbohydrates in the relatively sterile small bowel. Weight loss, diarrhea, peripheral neuropathy (B_{12} deficiency), and a predisposing disease process should warrant evaluation for bacterial overgrowth.

Intestinal obstruction of either the large or small intestine can produce symptoms mimicking excessive gas such as bloating and foul eructations. Acute symptoms with vomiting or evidence of obstruction on abdominal films will not be confused with a functional gas syndrome. The extent of the evaluation in those with chronic symptoms will be highly dependent on the age of the patient. A young patient with no past surgical history, no weight loss, no abdominal pain, and no symptoms/signs consistent with inflammatory bowel disease (i.e., diarrhea, bleeding, arthritis, skin rash, etc.) may require little evaluation until after a therapeutic trial. An elderly patient with a short history of symptoms, history of GI blood loss (melena, bright red bleeding), or abdominal pain may require an extensive evaluation.

Functional Gas Syndromes

Belching/Eructation

Belching may be defined as the retrograde passage of esophageal and/or gastric gas past the upper esophageal sphincter and out the mouth. Belching begins with involuntary relaxation of the lower esophageal sphincter (LES), thus forming a common cavity with the stomach.[12,13] Pressure builds in the esophagus as the air accumulates until either it passes out orally or peristalsis returns the gas to the stomach. Relaxation of the upper esophageal sphincter allows passage of esophageal air. Inability to relax the upper esophageal sphincter may produce severe chest pain secondary to gas accumulation.

Involuntary belching (secondary to gas accumulation) following a meal is a normal occurrence. Factors that reduce LES pressure such as caffeine, onions, tomatoes, coffee, or mints will facilitate belching. The supine position inhibits belching by covering the posteriorly placed gastroesophageal junction with fluid.

The bulk of upper gastrointestinal gas accumulates because of air swallowing (aerophagia). Approximately 2 to 3 ml are trapped in the stomach with each swallow.[1,2] A tiny amount is also ingested with normal inspiration. Gum chewing, multiple meals, hypersalivation, or anxiety will increase the swallowing rate and therefore the volume of gas accumulated. Smoking, loose dentures, rapid eating, and drinking through a straw are also associated with increased aerophagia. Anxious patients may relax their upper esophageal sphincters subconsciously and allow passage of air into the esophagus with each breath. The patient may describe the sensation of gas in the esophagus as fullness, a dull ache, or pressure.

Chronic belching is a voluntary occurrence but is not always easily controlled. These patients swallow before each belch and then release the air before it reaches the stomach. Chronic inflammatory conditions such as gastroesophageal reflux, biliary colic, angina pectoris, or peptic ulcer disease may initiate the belching process. Even after the inflammation heals, belching may become habitual, and the patient perceives belching as indicative of digestive problems.

Since 2 to 3 ml pass into the stomach with each swallow, marked gastric accumulation can occur during meals. When this is associated with marked midepigastric distension in the first 30 minutes after meals, the term magenblase syndrome is used. An enlarged gastric air bubble is noted on abdominal x-ray, and relief of symptoms with belching or nasogastric aspiration of a distended stomach is usually diagnostic. A similar condition known as "gas-bloat syndrome" may occur following fundoplication surgery for gastroesophageal reflux because the tightened gastroesophageal junction prevents expulsion of ingested air. Patients post–total laryngectomy practice a special form of speech that requires swallowing large amounts of air. Obviously, they are also prone to develop symptoms of upper gastrointestinal gaseousness.

Persistent hiccups (singultus) are occasionally associated with chronic eructation. Aerophagia with resultant gastric or esophageal distension may lead to bothersome hiccupping. Chronic hiccups should not be attributed to gaseousness, however, until disease processes involving the gastroesophageal junction such as gastroesophageal reflux disease and carcinoma have been excluded.

Hepatic or Splenic Flexure Syndromes

Trapping of gas in the right and left upper quadrant with distension of the colonic flexure is the presumed mechanism for abdominal pain in patients with the so-called hepatic or splenic flexure syndrome.[14] The posterior location of the flexures facilitates this air trapping. Pain may be referred to the chest, neck, shoulders, or back and is described as a fullness, dull ache, or pressure. Tachycardia has been documented with splenic gas accumulation. A motor disorder of the colon such as irritable bowel syndrome is common, and relief with defecation or enemas is a useful historical point. Relief with eating may occur if

defecation is stimulated by the gastrocolic reflex, and this would help to differentiate one of the flexure syndromes from the magenblase syndrome.

Flatulence

Frequent passage of gas by rectum is a disturbing symptom to the patient but rarely is indicative of serious pathology. Studies of healthy young men have found that flatus is passed an average of 14 times per day, with less than 20 to 25 times considered normal.[15] Since 5 to 100 ml is usually excreted with each passage, up to 2 L per day can be expelled normally.

While gas in the upper GI tract is mainly swallowed air, flatus composition is highly variable and diet dependent. Passage of carbohydrates into the colon will lead to hydrogen and carbon dioxide production in all patients and methane production in some. Poorly absorbed carbohydrates are the usual substrate for the production of colon gas, but physiologic malabsorption of normally well-absorbed carbohydrates such as starches and fructose has become recognized as important. A careful dietary history will usually reveal a high legume diet, milk product usage, or sorbitol/fructose use (sodas, chewing gum). Magnesium-containing antacids, high-fiber products, and lactulose are other important causes of intestinal gas. Anderson et al. have shown that 20 per cent of dietary carbohydrate is not absorbed.[16] Only rice and gluten-free wheat were completely absorbed, whereas flour of whole wheat, oats, potatoes, and corn was partially malabsorbed. Dietary fibers including cellulose, bran, and gums are inefficiently fermented by bacteria and produce much less gas on a weight basis than lactulose, for example.

Carbohydrate malabsorption as a cause for chronic GI complaints is becoming more common because of our frequent use of artificial sweeteners and the increased popularity of high-fiber diets. Even with the development of aspartamate, fructose remains a popular caloric sweetener and is naturally present in a variety of foods as well. Malabsorption of fructose occurs in everyone. Symptoms can be produced in 25 per cent of normal subjects if 15 gm or more of fructose is given. Ravich et al. noted that a majority of healthy individuals developed gas, cramps, and diarrhea after a 50-gm dose of fructose.[17] Rumessen and Hoyer found that patients with irritable bowel syndrome partially malabsorbed even 25 gm of fructose and developed symptoms.[18] Similar findings have been reported with sorbitol, a common chewing gum sweetener. Combinations of fructose and sorbitol increase the malabsorption of fructose presumably by blocking carrier-mediated fructose absorption. Since the mean daily consumption of fructose is greater than 15 gm, fructose may soon be recognized as a common source of intesinal gas.[18]

PHYSICAL EXAMINATION

Physical examination is of limited value in the patient who complains of excess gas. The patient should be examined for weight loss and signs of vitamin deficiency. The emotional state of the patient should be noted, especially with regard to excessive anxiety, hyperventilation, and air swallowing. Abdominal distension should be confirmed as gas by percussion and ascites ruled out by the absence of shifting dullness and a fluid wave. Abdominal ultrasonagraphy may be required to exclude small amounts of free intraperitoneal fluid. A succussion splash, though rarely present, should be examined for to rule out gastric outlet obstruction. Disease processes that are associated with gut dysmotility and bacterial overgrowth can usually be excluded by physical examination. Raynaud's phenomenon and skin tightening are almost universal in patients with GI scleroderma. Differential sweating, stocking/glove sensory loss, and orthostatic hypotension may signal autonomic neuropathy in a patient with diabetes mellitus. Positive test for blood in the stool makes full evaluation of the colon mandatory. Evaluation of the upper GI tract and the small intestine may be required if a source for bleeding is not found in the colon.

DIAGNOSTIC STUDIES

Simple laboratory panels and abdominal x-rays are of assistance in excluding multiple diagnostic possibilities that may be mistaken for one of the functional gas syndromes. A complete blood count, prothrombin time, albumin, protein, calcium, phosphate, alkaline phosphatase, and liver chemistries are of some help in diagnosing diabetes, malignancy, occult mucosal malabsorption, cholestasis, and cirrhosis. Anemia, particularly when macrocytic, may indicate folic acid deficiency, vitamin B_{12} deficiency, or hypothyroidism. Iron deficiency anemia mandates anatomic evaluation of the entire GI tract to rule out a bleeding lesion but may also be a sign of mucosal malabsorption. Pancreatic function tests may be necessary in the patient with gas and clinical maldigestion even if all laboratory tests are normal.

Flat and upright x-rays of the abdomen may suggest intestinal obstruction if dilated bowel loops and air-fluid levels are seen. The presence of an ileus may also suggest a metabolic problem or, rarely, a pseudo-obstruction syndrome. Ascites may also be seen as a ground glass appearance to the x-ray. Coned-down views may detect pancreatic calcifications in the alcoholic patient.

ASSESSMENT

Differential diagnosis in patients with excess abdominal gas can be divided into organic and functional categories. The two most important features in separating these two categories are weight loss and length of symptoms. The absence of weight loss and long-term symptoms are unusual in organic disease. Patient age and emotional state are of major but secondary importance. Chronic anxiety and a young age usually indicate functional disease. An elderly patient with no precipitating factors should undergo full evaluation for organic disease.

In the patient with upper GI gaseousness and pain, structural evaluation to rule out peptic ulcer disease and esophagitis is mandatory. Endoscopy is the most sensitive and specific test and offers gastric biopsy to evaluate for *Helicobacter pylori* infection, although the clinical significance of this organism has yet to be firmly established. In the absence of endoscopically visual inflammation of the esophagus, 24-hour pH monitoring may be required to rule out acid reflux and allow direct correlation of the patient's symptoms with acid in the esophagus. Aspiration of distal duodenal contents should be performed in the patient with acute upper abdominal gas and recent travel to an endemic area for *Giardia lamblia* (outdoor activity in Colorado, upper Michigan, etc). Cultures of upper GI contents to rule out bacterial overgrowth may be required in patients with intestinal stasis secondary to intestinal dysmotility (diabetes mellitus, scleroderma). Small intestinal biopsies should be reserved for those patients with documented malabsorption. Patients with weight loss, nausea, and solid food vomiting should have a solid phase gastric emptying scan to exclude gastroparesis.

Patients with the onset of intestinal gas or bloating more than one hour after meals require small intestinal evaluation. Stricture formation secondary to Crohn's disease may produce pain and gas in a young patient. Unfortunately, except for Crohn's disease, small intestinal x-rays are rarely helpful unless the patient has malabsorption or in the rare cases of jejunal diverticulosis or malignancy. Malabsorption is the major consideration in the patient group with late postprandial gas and bloating. Fecal fat smears while the patient is consuming a high fat diet will usually be positive in the presence of malabsorption, especially if the patient has lost weight. A 72-hour fecal fat determination on a defined diet (100 gm fat per day) is the definitive test for fat malabsorption. If fecal fat levels are greater than 10 gm per 24 hours, then small bowel biopsies are indicated to search for mucosal disease. If biopsies are normal, a test of pancreatic function is indicated. Bacterial overgrowth may occasionally produce mild steatorrhea, but fecal fat is usually normal, and levels greater than 15 gm per 24 hours are rare. Breath hydrogen examination after 50 gm of glucose is the best screening test. High fasting breath hydrogen levels coupled with a rise after glucose ingestion is highly specific (greater than 90 per cent) but not sensitive (76 per cent) for bacterial overgrowth.[19] Direct bacterial cultures of upper intestinal contents with bacterial counts equal to or greater than 10^5 per ml is diagnostic. A therapeutic trial of broad-spectrum oral antibiotics is also a reasonable approach.

Evaluation of the colon for malignancy should depend on the patient's age and symptoms. Intestinal bloating, gas, or flatulence without other signs such as decreased stool frequency, decreased stool caliber, or blood in the stools (overt or occult) is uncommon in the presence of a colon carcinoma. Elderly patients or patients with a strong family history (two or more first-degree family members) with colon cancer warrant closer scrutiny.

After organic disease is excluded, consideration of functional disorders is indicated. Aerophagia can usually be diagnosed in an anxious patient with subconscious air swallowing or in the individual who eats rapidy and gulps air. Eating more slowly with fewer swallows and avoiding gum chewing, smoking, carbonated beverages, and drinking through a straw will be a useful diagnostic trial. X-rays may be helpful if they show gaseous distension of the stomach but are rarely needed.

Lactase deficiency may be more difficult to exclude by history. Lactose intolerance is extremely variable. Many patients with lactose intolerance may not develop symptoms until they ingest more than two glasses of milk a day, whereas some may develop symptoms with much lesser quantities. Confirmation of lactose intolerance by breath hydrogen testing is important in the long-term management of patients with intestinal gas. It is important to confirm a relationship between symptoms and the food producing the symptom. Breath hydrogen tests are performed by obtaining samples of expired air before and at 30-minute intervals for three hours following ingestion of 50 gm of lactose. Such a monitoring period will detect almost all malabsorbers, with 90 per cent detectable in the first two hours. A rise in breath hydrogen of 10 ppm above baseline values is a positive response.[20] A positive response in the first 30 minutes after lactose ingestion may indicate small bowel bacterial overgrowth, especially if there is a secondary peak in breath hydrogen consistent with lactose appearance in the colon.

Splenic and hepatic flexure syndromes should be suspected if pain and bloating occur one to three hours after meals, localized tympany is present, and the particular anatomic distension is present on x-rays. Defecation after enemas will usually produce relief but can increase or shift the abdominal pain if underlying dysmotility is present. Care must be taken to rule out obstructive lesions before this diagnosis is made.

The assessment of flatulence usually rests primarily with the history. In the absence of significant signs or symptoms of organic disease, flatulence is rarely serious by itself. Colonic evaluation is usually not indicated for flatulence alone. Dietary history will usually document heavy ingestion of some poorly absorbed carbohydrate or stimulant. Coffee, caffeine, legumes, onions, or sorbital usage is common. A more complete list of the tendency for various foods to produce flatulence is presented in Table 1. Although rarely done, gas analysis of fecal samples may be extremely helpful. Although rectal passage of swallowed air is uncommon, a gas sample from the rectum showing only nitrogen and oxygen would be diagnostic. Gas samples showing hydrogen, carbon dioxide, and in some cases, methane would prove fermentation of some unabsorbed carbohydrate and

TABLE 1. Foods and Flatus

HIGH FLATUS	MODERATE FLATUS	LOW FLATUS
Dairy products	Potatoes	Meat, fowl, fish
Onions, beans	Pastries	Lettuce, cucumbers
Bagels, pretzels	Eggplant	Broccoli, peppers
Prunes, apricots	Citrus fruits	Avocado, tomato
Carrots, celery	Apples	Zucchini, okra
Bananas, raisins	Bread	Olives, asparagus
Brussels sprouts	Cauliflower	
	Grapes, berries	
	Rice, chips	
	Popcorn, nuts	
	Eggs, gelatin	

dictate a more thorough dietary history and possible exclusion diets.

REFERENCES

1. Levitt MD, Bond JH. Intestinal gas. In: Sleisenger MH, Fordtran JS, eds. Gastrointestinal disease, pathophysiology, diagnosis and treatment. Philadelphia: WB Saunders, 1989:257–62.
2. Levitt MD, Bond JH, Levitt DG. Gastrointestinal gas. In: Johnson LR, ed. Physiology of the gastrointestinal tract. New York: Raven Press, 1981:1301–17.
3. Levitt MD. Production and excretion of hydrogen gas in man. N Engl J Med 1969;281:122–7.
4. Bond JH, Engel RR, Levitt MD. Methane production in man. J Exp Med 1971;133:572–8.
5. Levitt MD. Volume and composition of human intestinal gas determined by means of an intestinal washout technique. N Engl J Med 1971;284:1394–9.
6. Lasser RB, Bond JH, Levitt MD. The role of intestinal gas in functional abdominal pain. N Engl J Med 1975;293:524–6.
7. Moriarity KJ, Dawson AN. Functional abdominal pain: further evidence that the whole gut is affected. Br Med J 1982;284:1670–2.
8. Castell DO. Medical therapy for reflux esophagitis: 1986 and beyond. Ann Intern Med 1986;104:112–6.
9. Liskere P, Aquilar L, Zavala C. Intestinal lactase deficiency and milk drinking capacity in the adult. Am J Clin Nutr 1978;31:1499–1503.
10. Newcomer AD, McGill DB. Irritable bowel syndrome role of lactase deficiency. Mayo Clin Proc 1983;58:339–41.
11. Levitt MD, Duane WC. Floating stools—flatus versus fat. N Engl J Med 1972;286:973–5.
12. Levitt MD, Bond JH. Volume, composition and source of intestinal gas. Gastroenterology 1970;59:921–9.
13. Kahrilas PJ, Dodds WJ, Dent JL, Wyman JB, Hogan WJ, Arndorfer RC. Upper esophageal sphincter function during belching. Gastroenterology 1986;91:133–40.
14. Magarian GJ. Hyperventilation syndromes: infrequently recognized common expressions of anxiety and stress. Medicine 1982;61:219–32.
15. Steggerda FR. Gastrointestinal gas following food consumption. Ann NY Acad Sci 1968;150:57–66.
16. Anderson IH, Levine AS, Levitt MD. Incomplete absorption of the carbohydrate in all purpose wheat flour. N Engl J Med 1981;304:891–2.
17. Ravich WJ, Bayless TM, Thomas M. Fructose: incomplete intestinal absorption in humans. Gastroenterology 1983;84:26–9.
18. Rumessen JJ, Hoyer EG. Functional bowel disease malabsorption and abdominal distress after ingestion of fructose, sorbitol, and fructose-sorbitol mixtures. Gastroenterology 1988;95:694–700.
19. Kerlin P, Wong L. Breath hydrogen testing in bacterial overgrowth of the small intestine. Gastroenterology 1988;95:982–8.
20. Perman JA, Modler S, Barr RG, Rosenthal P. Fasting breath hydrogen concentration: normal values and clinical applications. Gastroenterology 1984;87:1358–63.

INTRACRANIAL INFECTION, ACUTE

GARY L. WILSON

SYNONYMS: Meningitis, Encephalomyelitis, Encephalitis, Brain Abscess/Cerebritis, Suppurative Vascular Disease, Epidural/Subdural Empyema— Depending on Specific Disease Entity

BACKGROUND

The adult patient with possible intracranial infection represents one of the truly difficult diagnoses in acute care medicine. Most of these infections are life-threatening. Prompt diagnosis and correct management are crucial for recovery and prevention of serious sequelae. Yet the variety of clinical presentations produced by these infections is a constant trap for the unwary and may severely test the diagnostic skills of the most astute clinician. The presenting signs and symptoms are almost always nonspecific and lead to a broad differential diagnosis that includes not only diverse infections but many other diseases as well. Presentations with potential infectious etiology include dementia, suspected degenerative disease, psychiatric disease, seizures, stroke, mass lesions, hydrocephalus, and vasculitic disease, as well as classical infectious meningitis. Superimposed on the problems of recognition of clinical presentation is the identification of the infecting organism. Virtually any recognizable pathogenic organism can cause any of several intracranial infectious syndromes. The number of severely immunocompromised patients is increasing, and in this population, complex and unusual intracranial infections may develop. These problems are intensified by the ever-expanding number of diagnostic modalities and therapeutic interventions available. Thus, the clinician must quickly sort out the clinical presentation, rapidly initiate the appropriate diagnostic procedures, and begin the most efficacious therapy—all with alacrity.

The broad categories of acute intracranial infection are listed in Table 1. The definition of *acute* for the purposes of this discussion will be presentation over the course of hours to days. Further, in the interest of space, only the more common entities listed will be discussed.

Since many patients with acute intracranial infection present with life-threatening disease, the initial focus should be on assuring an acceptable physiologic status. Rapid intervention to maintain adequate ventilation and circulation may be needed. Neurologic deterioration suggestive of possible brain stem compression or herniation may require immediate treatment. Seizure activity, hemorrhage, cardiac rhythm disturbances, severe acid-base problems, or serious traumatic injuries may have to be dealt with prior to consideration of intracranial infection.

HISTORY

The first step after assuring no immediate threat to the patient's life is to obtain a detailed history. Often the physician must play detective to obtain crucial pieces of information that will expedite and focus his or her diagnostic efforts. Any and all potential sources of information should be sought. Since acute intracranial infection often impedes the patient's ability to provide information, other sources such as family, friends, medical records, emergency medical personnel, police officers, and previous physicians should be utilized.

Chief Complaint

The patient may present with any number of diverse complaints. These will include fever and chills; nausea and vomiting; stiff or painful neck; headache; photophobia; focal neurologic deficits such as specific weakness, altered sensation or visual complaints; recent onset of behavioral, emotional, or personality changes; or merely altered state of mental functioning. The focus of presenting complaints may also be that of a precipitating infection such as otitis, sinusitis, pneumonia, or nonspecific upper respiratory tract illness.

History of Present Illness

Whatever symptoms the patient presents as his or her chief complaint should be completely explored. Particularly important is a precise chronologic progression of symptoms so that the tempo of clinical evolution is clear. In this regard, questions such as, When were you last completely well? or What was the very first thing you noticed wrong? or What was the very next thing that you noticed? are particularly helpful. Given the crucial nature of the information to be obtained, the broad range of potential processes and etiologies, and the relative subtleness of many key clues, it is absolutely imperative that the physician be as clear and precise as possible in obtaining this history.

TABLE 1. Categories of Acute Intracranial Infections

Meningitis
Encephalomyelitis
Encephalitis
Brain abscess/cerebritis
Suppurative vascular disease
Epidural/subdural empyema

Review of Systems

Once the picture of the presenting complaint is clear, the next step is a careful review of systems to identify associated phenomena that the patient has not thought relevant to his or her presenting illness. General complaints such as night sweats or weight change should be elicited. A careful history of ear, nasal, or pharyngeal problems including dental difficulties should be sought. Symptoms of pulmonary infection including cough and production of sputum may be important. Gastrointestinal complaints such as chronic diarrhea can lead to diagnosis of important associated illnesses. A careful genitourinary history, especially for complaints associated with sexually transmitted diseases (e.g., dysuria, penile discharge, genital ulcers), is necessary. Questions regarding headaches and subtle neurologic or psychoemotional changes should be asked. Problems with joints or movement suggestive of arthralgia or arthritis should be pinpointed. Lastly, the patient should be asked about any skin lesions, rashes, or other cutaneous problems that he or she may have failed to mention earlier.

Past Medical History

Past medical history should include specific questions regarding past cranial surgery or head trauma. Chronic recurrent problems with mastoid, ear, sinus, dental, or pulmonary infections should be sought. A history of cardiovascular disease, particularly that associated with shunting or abnormal heart valves, is important. Chronic medical problems that are immunosuppressive such as diabetes mellitus, cancer (especially hematologic or lymphatic malignancy), and alcohol abuse should be noted. Tuberculosis status, both past exposure and skin test reactivity, may be important. Lastly, a complete list of recent medications is crucial. Especially noteworthy are drugs used to treat recent complaints that the patient may not have thought to mention and cytotoxic agents or corticosteroids that are immunosuppressive.

Social History

Social history may be particularly important in the evaluation of any potential infection, including intracranial. Specific questions should be asked regarding recent travel or exposure to ill persons, animals, birds, insects, and ticks. Outdoor activities that may lead to significant exposure should be sought. Specific questions regarding occupation and hobbies are important in this regard. A sexual history should be obtained, particularly with regard to homosexual activity and multiple sexual partners. Use of illicit (especially intravenous) drugs should be inquired about.

Additional specific pieces of information that may be important in framing a differential diagnosis include the patient's age, the season of the year at time of presentation, and the geographic locality of patient presentation.

PHYSICAL EXAMINATION

Like the history, a careful physical examination, particularly of areas where emphasis may not be normally placed, is important. Again, the search for clues that will allow the narrowing of what is otherwise a dauntingly broad diagnostic differential is the aim.

The mental status examination should be carefully performed, looking for alterations in personality, consciousness, and higher integrative functions. The head, eyes, ears, neck, and throat examination should be evaluated for neck stiffness, evidence of skull trauma, evidence of cerebrospinal fluid (CSF) leak such as otorrhea or rhinorrhea, otitis, sinusitis, and dental or other orapharnygeal infections. Correct performance of Kernig's and Brudzinski's sign maneuvers can be helpful. The presence of a CSF shunt should be noted. The eyes should be evaluated for focal neurologic findings, papilledema, and Roth spots. Chest examination should note the presence of signs suggestive of pulmonary infection or pathologic heart murmurs. Back examination may reveal focal tenderness on percussion suggestive of vertebral osteomyelitis or the presence of a midline dermal sinus. Abdominal examination may note surgical scars, organomegaly, or ascites. Genitourinary examination is necessary especially to evaluate the presence of genital ulcers or other signs of sexually transmitted diseases. The neurologic examination should include an assessment of cranial nerves and cerebellar function. The motor system part of this examination is performed looking for focal weakness. Sensory function examination is also important for determining focal deficits. Deep tendon reflexes should be tested. The joints should be briefly examined for evidence of arthritis. The skin should be carefully and completely evaluated for rashes, ulcers, evidence of bleeding, or lesions consistent with embolic events. A careful search for adenopathy must also be undertaken.

DIAGNOSTIC STUDIES

Although the history and physical examination are crucial elements in focusing the diagnostic evaluation of acute intracranial infections, the laboratory and/or radiology departments are the arenas in which the final steps for confirmation of diagnosis and elucidation of specific etiology occur. These tests can be divided into three major diagnostic categories. The first is initial laboratory and roentgenographic studies, the second is lumbar puncture with diagnostic evaluation of CSF, and the third is radiologic evaluation of integrity of the central nervous system (CNS).

Laboratory

The initial laboratory and x-ray studies to be considered are presented in Table 2. These are particularly useful for evaluating the patient's physiologic status, investigating potential noninfectious causes of various clinical syndromes that may be associated with acute intracranial infection, and identifying peripheral or parameningeal infections that may have precipitated an acute intracranial infection.

Lumbar Puncture

Performance of a lumbar puncture to obtain CSF for diagnostic evaluation is a crucial test in the diagnosis of many intracranial infections.[1,2] There is no absolute contraindication to performing the examination if CSF infection is strongly considered. However, the test is relatively contraindicated in the presence of intracranial hypertension or mass lesions, in

TABLE 2.   Basic Laboratory and Radiologic Studies

Complete blood count with differential
Serum chemistries including electrolytes, glucose, calcium, magnesium, and blood urea nitrogen
Arterial blood gases or arterial saturation by oximetry
Hepatic transaminases
Urinalysis
Chest x-ray
Drug and alcohol screen
Blood cultures and stain/cultures of any local infection site

which case it may precipitate brain stem herniation.[3] The presence of coagulopathy is a somewhat weaker contraindication.

The test provides a measurement of CSF pressure and samples of fluid for laboratory examination. Generally, 8 to 12 ml are removed. The baseline laboratory examination of this fluid should include cell count with differential, protein and glucose determinations, Gram's stain, and bacterial culture.

Antigen tests (e.g., counterimmune electrophoresis or latex agglutination) may be useful in a patient with clinical meningitis and an abnormal CSF, especially if there has been prior antibiotic therapy. However, these are usually no more sensitive than Gram's stain and therefore cannot be justified as a routine on every specimen of CSF processed.[4,5,6] Other studies that have use in special circumstances include nonspecific determinations such as C-reactive protein, lactic acid concentration, and limulus lysate assay.[7,8,9] Although the latter studies have been recommended to help separate bacterial from viral meningitis, they are perhaps more helpful in evaluating postoperative and post-traumatic patients who have an abnormal baseline CSF, which clouds standard interpretation, and who are at risk of meningitis with unusual and difficult-to-treat organisms. Special cultures for fungus and tuberculosis also cannot be justified routinely.[10] Their use should be reserved for special clinical circumstances.

Some practical considerations regarding the use of lumbar puncture include the following:

1.   Since it is impossible to perform all conceivable tests on a single sample, the need for special tests should be governed by clinical impression and other diagnostic findings.

2.   If possible, save and refrigerate 1 to 2 ml from the initial specimen in case further studies are suggested by the results of routine tests or the patient's postprocedure course.

3.   Acquisition of further CSF with another procedure may be useful, both to follow the patient's course and to obtain further tests.

4.   On occasion, large volumes of CSF (10 to 15 ml) are useful for culture, as in the diagnosis of crytococcal or mycobacterial disease.[11] The need for such large volumes must be balanced against the risk of complications.

IMAGING

Diagnostic imaging for intracranial structural evaluation has revolutionized the approach to intracranial infection. Computed tomography (CT) of the head has been a quantum advance in the diagnosis and management of these processes.[12] It remains the standard for evaluation of mass lesions such as abscess or empyema and the evaluation of noninfectious processes such as tumor, hematoma, hemorrhage, and ischemic events. It is also useful to evaluate intracranial shifts and the presence of intracranial edema. To maximize the utility of this test, the radiologist should be fully aware of all diagnostic considerations before its performance. Unless there is a strong contraindication, any CT scan of the head ordered with consideration of potential infection should be done with a contrast infusion. This may allow the recognition of cerebritis that might otherwise be missed, as well as provide information on mass lesions by means of enhancement and decay of enhancement parameters. Efforts should also be made to ensure visualization of the sinuses and mastoid areas on the initial scan. The availability and relative ease of performance of CT scanning have brought early acquisition of anatomic knowledge of great value to clinicians caring for patients with suspected intracranial infection.

Many clinicians now have the availability of magnetic resonance imaging (MRI). While MRI may offer advantages to CT scanning in certain specific subsets of patients with intracranial infection, in general it is less available and more difficult to perform. Therefore, at the present it represents more of an adjunct to CT scanning than a major advancement.[13] MRI is more sensitive than CT in detection of changes of early cerebritis in the evolution of abscess formation; however, patients rarely present at a stage where this is clinically significant. CT scans are also relatively insensitive to the early changes of viral encephalitis; thus, because of its sensitivity to altered water content, MRI is able to detect these changes earlier and is often able to delineate the extent of disease more fully. For example, the characteristic distribution of herpes simplex encephalitis in adults may be delineated by MRI sooner and more completely than with CT scan. MRI may be more sensitive in detecting complications of severe meningitis. It has been shown to be superior in detecting areas of infarction and vascular occlusion such as corticovenous and/or -dural thrombosis. Also, the rare extracerebral pyogenic collection such as epidural and subdural empyemas is more completely visualized and more easily

characterized by MRI than CT. Lastly, MRI may be more sensitive in detecting certain intracranial infections caused by specific opportunistic organisms such as *Toxoplasma* and specific entities such as progressive multifocal leukoencephalopathy. These are especially common in acquired immune deficiency syndrome (AIDS) patients. Currently, it must be remembered, however, that MRI is a new entity with relatively little cumulative and correlative experience. As such, it should rarely be the crucial diagnostic test.

On occasion, other modalities may be useful in the evaluation of intracranial infection. Electroencephalography (EEG) is obviously useful to rule out seizure activity but may be used on occasion to delineate focal pathology such as seen in herpes simplex encephalitis. Radionuclide brain scanning has been used in the past and been shown to have some utility.[14] However, it has now been largely supplanted by more sensitive techniques such as CT scanning and MRI. Rarely, cerebral angiography may be useful.

ASSESSMENT

As previously noted, once the patient is found to be physiologically stable, the physician must act quickly to focus his or her diagnostic approach. The key initial decision is whether the patient is presenting with a process indicative of diffuse meningitic/encephalitic disease or one of focal CNS dysfunction more likely to be an intracranial mass lesion.[15] The bases for answering this crucial question are the history and physical examination. Although further refinement of the data obtained in this initial time frame will be common, a relatively quick decision regarding performing a lumbar puncture or diagnostic imaging study of the CNS is crucial. In patients with evidence of focal neurologic deficits or signs of increased intracranial pressure, a CNS imaging study, usually CT scan, is of paramount importance. The results of this study will answer questions in three areas. First, does the scan provide evidence of a specific infectious diagnosis, for instance, a hyperdense lesion with ring enhancement on contrast infusion characteristic of brain abscess? Second, does the scan provide evidence of an alternative diagnosis such as brain tumor, subarachnoid hemorrhage, intracerebral bleed, and so on? Third, does the study show signs of cerebral edema or intracranial shift, which will mark-

TABLE 3.   Meningitic Syndrome (Neutrophil Predominant CSF)

Common etiologies
  Streptococcus pneumoniae (recurrent disease, trauma)
  Neisseria meningitidis
  Viral (early in course, usually enterovirus)
  Hemophilus influenzae (common in childhood)
Uncommon
  Staphylococcus (instrumentation, neurosurgery)
  Listeria monocytogenes (cellular immune deficits)
  Enterobacteriaceae (neurosurgery)
  Mycobacterium tuberculosis (early in course)
  Fungal (especially *Candida*)

TABLE 5.   Encephalomyelitis Syndrome

Common etiologies
  Togaviruses (St. Louis, Eastern, Western encephalitis)
  Mumps virus
  Herpes virus (simplex, varicella-zoster)
  Enteroviruses
  Orbivirus (Colorado tick fever)
  Rickettsiae (Rocky Mountain Spotted Fever, Typhus)
Uncommon etiologies
  Most causes of meningitis listed in Table 4
  Ehrlichia canis
  Borrelia recurrentis
  Plasmodium falciparum
  Trypanosoma (Chagas' disease)

edly increase the risk of subsequent lumbar puncture? Additionally, data from the scan may provide the rationale for urgent neurosurgical consultation/intervention.

In the patient in whom the initial history and physical examination indicate a more diffuse meningitic/encephalitic process, or in whom the CT scan provides nonspecific or normal results, the lumbar puncture is the diagnostic procedure of choice. Initial studies performed on the spinal fluid obtained have been discussed earlier. White blood cell counts of

TABLE 4.   Meningitis Syndrome (Lymphocyte Predominant CSF)

Common etiologies
  Enterovirus
  Mumps virus
  Noninfectious causes (in total)
    Neoplastic disease
    Drugs (e.g., NSAIDs)* or chemical (e.g., post-myelography arachnoiditis)
    CNS sarcoid
    Rheumatologic disease (e.g., CNS vasculitis)
    "Idiopathic" diseases (Behçet's syndrome, Mollaret's meningitis)
Uncommon etiologies
  Herpes virus (simplex, zoster varicellosus)
  Lymphocytic choriomeningitis virus
  Arbovirus
  Human immunodeficiency virus
  Bacterial meningitis, partially treated
  Parameningeal infection (e.g., brain abscess)
  Remote extracranial infection (e.g., subacute bacterial endocarditis)
  Fungal meningitis (especially cryptococcal, coccidioidal)
  Mycobacterium tuberculosis
  Mycoplasma pneumoniae
  Toxoplasma gondii
  Listeria monocytogenes
  Treponema pallidum (syphilis)
  Leptospira (leptospirosis)
  Borrelia burgdorferi (Lyme disease)
  Amebas (e.g., *Naegleria*)
  Cyst-related disease (e.g., cysticercosis)
  Brucella
  Trichinella spiralis (trichinosis)

* NSAIDS = nonsteroidal anti-inflammatory drugs.

more than 1000 cells/ml or a predominance of neutrophils in the differential count suggest bacterial (or less commonly, tuberculous or fungal) infection.[16] Protein concentrations greater than 150 mg/dl and glucose concentrations less than 30 mg/dl generally confirm a bacterial etiology.[17] However, such infections may be present without these classic findings. Certainly a positive Gram's stain is highly suggestive of bacterial infection, and a positive culture (except in cases of contamination) is virtually pathognomonic of infection. Lymphocytic pleocytosis is more suggestive of a viral meningitis or meningoencephalitis.[18] See Tables 3, 4, and 5 for specific suspected pathogens based on CSF findings and clinical presentation. As noted previously, antigen tests or nonspecific determinations such as C-reactive protein, lactic acid concentration, and limulus lysate assay may be helpful in certain patients with clinical and CSF findings suggestive of meningitis in the presence of complicating factors such as antecedent antibiotic therapy, recent cranial therapy, head trauma, and the like. Only if all the parameters tested are totally normal is it highly unlikely that meningitis or encephalitis exists.

The majority of patients with treatable acute intracranial infections will have their diagnoses confirmed on the basis of these initial studies. Most of these cases will be bacterial meningitis or brain abscesses.[19,20,21] Occasionally, different diagnostic efforts will be required, for example, brain biopsy to confirm herpes simplex encephalitis. In particularly difficult cases, repeating diagnostic efforts such as reviewing the history, re-examining the CSF, and performing follow-up CNS diagnostic imaging studies may be useful. The majority of patients with aseptic meningitis or encephalitis syndromes never come to precise etiologic diagnosis.[21] This is a reflection in part of the fact that specific therapy does not exist for these syndromes, and the diagnostic techniques (e.g., serologic) required are not easily available and do not provide information in a relevant clinical time frame.

The adult patient presenting with signs and symptoms suggestive of intracranial infection is a difficult problem. A rapid, orderly, and efficient approach is critical. A high degree of clinical suspicion, swift use of the diagnostic approaches described here, and the coordinated cooperative efforts of primary care physicians and infectious disease specialists, neurologists, critical care specialists, and neurosurgeons working closely with radiology and the clinical microbiology laboratory are all necessary to minimize the significant morbidity and mortality of these patients.

REFERENCES

1. Marton KI, Gean AD. The spinal tap: a new look at an old test. Ann Intern Med 1986;104:840–8.
2. Leonard JM. Cerebrospinal fluid formula in patients with central nervous system infection. Neurologic Clinics North Am 1986;4:3–12.
3. Garfield J. Management of supratentorial intracranial abscess: a review of 200 cases. Br Med J 1969;2:7–11.
4. Karandanis D, Shulman JA. Recent survey of infectious meningitis in adults: review of laboratory findings in bacterial, tuberculous, and aseptic meningitis. South Med J 1976;69:449–55.
5. Carey RB. Rapid diagnosis of bacterial meningitis by antigen detection. Clin Microbiol Newslett 1983;117–20.
6. Edberg SC. Conventional and molecular techniques for the laboratory diagnosis of infections of the central nervous system. Neurologic Clinics 1986;4:13–39.
7. Peltola HO. C-Reactive protein for rapid monitoring of infections of the central nervous system. Lancet 1982;II:980–2.
8. Ponka A, Ojala K, Teppo AM, Weber ThH. The differential diagnosis of bacterial and aseptic meningitis using cerebrospinal fluid laboratory tests. Infection 1983;11:129–31.
9. Berg B, Gardsell P, Skansberg P. Cerebral fluid lactate in the diagnosis of meningitis. Scand J Infect Dis 1982;14:111–5.
10. Crowson TW, Rich EC, Woolfrey BF, Connelly DP. Overutilization of cultures of CSF for mycobacteria. JAMA 1984;251:70–2.
11. Laboratory diagnosis of mycotic and specific fungal infections. Medical Section of the American Lung Association. Am Rev Respir Dis 1985;132(6):1373–9.
12. Sarwar M, Falkoff G. Radiologic techniques in the diagnosis of CNS infections. Neurologic Clinics North Am 1986;4:41–68.
13. Sze G, Zimmerman RD. The magnetic resonance imaging of infections and inflammatory diseases. Radiol Clin North Am 1988;26:839–59.
14. Cowan RJ, Moody DM. Radionuclide techniques for brain imaging. Neurologic Clinics North Am 1984;2:835–51.
15. Wilson GL. Acute intracranial infection. Emergency Decisions 1986;2(1):7–24.
16. Bolan G, Barza M. Acute bacterial meningitis in children and adults. A perspective. Med Clin North Am 1985;69:231–41.
17. Overturf GD. Pyogenic bacterial infections of the CNS. Neurologic Clinics North Am 1986;4:69–90.
18. Ratzan KR. Viral meningitis. Med Clin North Am 1985;69:399–413.
19. Schlech WF, Ward JI, Band JD, Hightower A, Fraser DW, Broome CV. Bacterial meningitis in the United States, 1978 through 1981. JAMA 1985;253:1749–54.
20. Kaplan K. Brain abscess. Med Clin North Am 1985;69:345–60.
21. Tyler KL. Diagnosis and management of acute viral encephalitis. Semin Neurology 1984;4:480–9.

LIMB PAIN
IN CHILDHOOD

ILONA S. SZER

SYNONYMS: Growing Pain, Nonspecific Limb Pain, Musculoskeletal Pain, Joint Pain

BACKGROUND

Limb pain refers to a subjective discomfort localized in the soft tissues, bones, or joints. It is the third most common pain of childhood, after abdominal pain and headache.[1] Because pain is a personal experience, it is difficult both to define and to quantitate. The differential diagnosis of limb pain in children is extensive and includes: acute and chronic infections, acute and chronic inflammatory conditions, trauma, metabolic and malignant disorders, diseases of abnormal hemostasis and red cell dyscrasia, and psychogenic causes of pain. The terms *acute* and *chronic* usually refer to the period of time during which the symptoms persist; more than six months is often considered chronic. Pains commonly referred to as ''growing pains'' are not associated with objective physical findings, laboratory abnormalities, or decreased level of activity and function. In contrast, psychogenic pain, while also not associated with objective physical findings, is usually associated with a surprising degree of dysfunction.

This chapter will focus on the evaluation of a child with limb pain of persistent or intermittent nature, with particular emphasis on the differentiation of benign pain from pain secondary to infectious, malignant, metabolic, or inflammatory processes.

HISTORY

The history of the present illness begins with the very first time the complaint was noted. The family is encouraged to provide every detail of the story regardless of how irrelevant it seems. For example, it is important to know whether the pain had its onset on awakening or during a biology final. It is imperative to listen carefully and without preconceived notions. The key questions focus on objective observations and impact of the problem on daily function, particularly on school attendance. It is important to focus on the chronicity (months or years) or acuteness (hours or days) of the symptom(s). Refusal to walk serves as a clue to serious underlying disorders and implies bone pain rather than soft tissue or joint pain (children with osteomyelitis and malignancies may have severe periosteal pain, which causes refusal to ambulate). Isolated pain in one anatomic area must be differentiated from diffuse pain or pain associated with other localized or systemic symptoms, the latter providing a clue to multisystem disorders.

Answers to specific questions often provide the physician with the correct diagnosis. For example, pain upon climbing stairs and riding a bicycle is a clue to the patellofemoral syndrome (chondromalacia patellae), whereas pain at the end of the day is reported by children with the benign hypermobility syndrome. Special inquiry should be made about any precipitating events such as trauma leading to fracture, sprain, or sympathetic joint effusion; repetitive physical activity, which often precedes tendinitis or bursitis; upper respiratory tract infection noted prior to the onset of Henoch-Schönlein purpura; streptococcal pharyngitis needed to establish the diagnosis of acute rheumatic fever; dysentery preceding reactive arthritis; and flulike illness as an early manifestation of Lyme disease. Symptoms of rheumatic diseases are sought and include joint swelling, limitation of motion, and stiffness and gelling after periods of inactivity, as well as muscle weakness. Information regarding skin rashes, conjunctival hyperemia or blurred vision, and genitourinary and gastrointestinal symptoms is specifically required.

Constitutional symptoms of fever, weight loss, poor linear growth, and easy fatigability signify the possibility of a chronic inflammatory illness or an occult malignancy. Review of all therapeutic interventions and their success or failure provides important clues to the appropriate diagnosis. For example, pain that responds to salicylate and not to acetaminophen is likely to be inflammatory.

The usual family history is supplemented with focused queries regarding the presence of a rheumatic disease such as systemic lupus erythematosus, rheumatoid arthritis, or spondyloarthropathy, all of which are associated with specific genetic markers and occur more frequently in susceptible individuals. For example, morning low back pain (inflammatory rather than mechanical), conjunctivitis, mouth sores, psoriasis, and inflammatory bowel disease signify HLA-B27–related disorders, whereas Raynaud's phenomenon, malar rash, or family history of frequent miscarriages suggests lupuslike phenomena. Symptoms similar to those of the child are also important.

The social history should include any preceding stressful events, school performance and attendance, and participation in peer-related activities.

The history of present illness sets the stage for a directed physical examination and for laboratory tests and radiographic studies that may be needed.

PHYSICAL EXAMINATION

A thorough physical examination is a cornerstone in the evaluation of a child with musculoskeletal pain. Special attention is paid to the child's general appearance (healthy and thriving or ill and peaked), nutritional status, and appropriate incremental growth. In addition to a thorough general examination of the lymph nodes, heart, lung, and abdomen, the skin is carefully assessed for the presence of rash, nodules, warmth, pigmentation, nail changes, and alopecia. Mucous membranes are examined for ulceration, hyperemia, and dryness. Muscle strength is evaluated functionally (climbing up on the table, rising from a squatting position, doing a sit-up) and according to a standard grading system (Table 1).

The Joint Examination

A detailed examination of the joints and the surrounding soft tissues is of particular importance in the evaluation of musculoskeletal pain. It begins with the observation of gait, followed by inspection of asymmetry, loss of bony contours and landmarks, and presence of atrophy or deformity. Loss of anatomic landmarks without obvious effusion implies synovial thickening seen frequently in children with chronic arthritis. Palpation follows inspection, noting warmth, tenderness to touch, and presence of intra-articular or bursal fluid. In the knee, the presence of a joint effusion may be documented by forcing the fluid from the suprapatellar bursa into the joint, followed by ballotment of the patella (the patella rides up and down over the joint). If bony tenderness is present, it may be possible to distinguish the point tenderness of metaphyseal infection (osteomyelitis) from diffuse periosteal pain of leukemic infiltrates or metastasis (acute leukemia, neuroblastoma, primary bone tumor). Tenderness to the lightest touch, sometimes elicited in children with paucity of physical findings, is often seen in somatoform disorders.

Following palpation, joint range of motion is assessed. There is little reason to memorize the normal range of motion for every joint. Rather, the examiner should test his or her joint as a reminder. Joints may be limited in full range of motion because of irreducible flexion contracture (a hallmark of long-standing chronic synovitis or metabolic conditions presenting in infancy with joint contracture without inflammation) or because of pain (acute arthritis). A child who has neither objective joint swelling nor limitation of motion with pain does not have arthritis.[2] Motion is carefully tested in all planes of movement possible for a given joint and is expressed in degrees of motion achieved. Passive range (the examiner moves the joint) should be assessed if active range (the child moves the joint without assistance) is limited. The joint examination is performed methodically, starting with the neck (flexion, extension, lateral rotation, cervical tilt) and the temporomandibular joints (mouth opening between the incisors of at

---

TABLE 1.   Grading of Muscle Strength

0 or None = No muscle contractility
1 or Trace = Minimal contractility; no motion
2 or Poor = Full range of motion without gravity
3 or Fair = Full range of motion against gravity
4 or Good = Full range of motion against gravity with some resistance
5 or Normal = Full range of motion against gravity and full resistance

least 4 cm), upper and then the lower extremities (shoulder and hip extension; ab- and adduction; internal and external rotation; elbow flexion, extension, pronation, and supination; wrist flexion and extension; lateral and medial deviation; flexion and extension of all finger joints, knees, and ankles; as well as subtalar joint inversion and eversion), ending with examination of the back.

Joint stability (the anterior drawer sign) and both signs of the patellofemoral syndrome (patella apprehension and inhibition signs) are evaluated during the examination of the knee. The anterior drawer sign is performed with the knee held in 25 degrees of flexion. The examiner grasps the femur with one hand and displaces the tibia anteriorly, with the other hand noting the degree of abnormal anterior motion. Patella apprehension sign is considered positive if the patient becomes anxious when the knee cap is pushed laterally off the knee joint (the patient feels apprehensive during the test and worried about patellar dislocation). Patella inhibition is positive when the patient experiences pain upon contracting the quadriceps muscle while the examiner actively inhibits the upward movement of the patella.[3] Hamstring tightness is elicited during straight leg raising with the child supine. During the examination of the foot, palpation of the Achilles tendon and particularly the insertion of the tendon into the calcaneus may elicit tenderness in the enthesis, often found in spondyloarthropathies.

The joint examination would not be complete without the examination of the back. Low back flexion is assessed with the Schober test: While the child stands erect, the examiner measures a 15-cm span (5 cm below and 10 cm above the anatomic landmarks at L5). The same distance is then remeasured while the child bends over to reach his or her toes without bending the knees. Children with decreased low back flexion have a Schober test of less than 21 cm during flexion (less than 6 cm of expansion).

Functional Status

Following the physical examination, the physician must assess the functional status of the patient with several key questions: Is the child functioning normally despite the complaint? If not, is the loss of function proportional to the visible disability? How does the child function in comparison with other children with the same evidence of physical disease?

Children with obvious physical disability must also undergo a full functional assessment: Can the child with arthritis grip a crayon or a toothbrush, tie shoelaces, open bottle caps? Can the child run or skip or climb onto the school bus? Can the adolescent with muscle weakness get in or out of a bathtub, open doors, and carry school books? Answers to these questions provide a logical direction to future interventions, which should begin even before a diagnosis is firmly established.

DIAGNOSTIC STUDIES

Laboratory

The laboratory evaluation of a child with musculoskeletal pain is guided by the findings in the physical examination and the history. If the pain is intermittent in nature, does not affect daily function, has not produced objective findings nor disrupted normal family life, no laboratory testing may be indicated. At times, however, the family or the physician may need reassurance in the form of negative testing, and normal screening laboratory data such as a complete blood count (CBC), erythrocyte sedimentation rate (ESR), and urinalysis serve a useful purpose.

Children whose symptoms are of recent onset, associated with fever and/or rash, may have a viral exanthem, hepatitis, infectious mononucleosis, poststreptococcal syndrome, acute rheumatic fever, Kawasaki disease, erythema nodosum, Henoch-Schönlein purpura, Lyme disease, or serum sickness–like reactions. When considering these diagnoses, supplemental testing logically includes antibody titers to specific viral (hepatitis A and B serology, Epstein-Barr virus profile), bacterial antistreptolysin-O (ASLO) (streptozyme), or spirochetal (*Borrelia burgdorferi*) agents.

Consideration of Kawasaki disease calls for immediate assessment of the coronary arteries with a two-dimensional echocardiogram.

Bacterial infections invading the musculoskeletal system directly present with a sudden onset of fever, severe pain, and inability to ambulate. If the bacterial process invades the joint, the child is unable to tolerate a range of motion examination in addition to having a hot joint effusion with overlying erythema. Consideration of septic arthritis accounts for one of only few indications for arthrocentesis in children. Tuberculosis may cause a monarticular arthritis of insidious onset; purified protein derivative (PPD) with controls should be placed. Osteomyelitis involving the metaphysis often causes a sympathetic effusion with sterile fluid and calls for an emergency bone scan, followed by bone aspiration for identification of the organism. While the majority of children with osteomyelitis have fever, tender and swollen metaphysis, an elevated peripheral white blood cell (WBC) count and ESR, some may not manifest these signs calling for a high index of suspicion. In one study of 79 children with osteomyelitis, the diagnosis was made in only 16 during the initial evaluation of the presenting complaint.[4]

Chronic inflammatory conditions are considered in children who have objective findings of a few weeks' duration, usually affecting several organs. Inflammatory bowel disease may present with musculoskeletal manifestations prior to overt gastrointestinal symptoms; lack of linear growth, anemia, and often an elevated sedimentation rate may be the only early clues. Systemic lupus erythematosus (SLE) should be considered in a young adolescent female with rash and joint pain; these children must fulfill at least 4 of the 11 specified classification criteria for SLE,[5] which include a positive circulating antinuclear antibody (ANA) and a variety of autoimmune and clinical phenomena often associated with complement consumption. Careful assessment of organ function, particularly renal, heart, lung, and the nervous system, is of paramount importance. Dermatomyositis in children is manifest by a facial rash, violaceous hue over swollen upper eyelids (heliotrope), rash over joints (Gottron's nodes), weak proximal muscles, and elevated muscle enzyme levels (creatinine phosphokinase [CPK], aspartate aminotransferase [AST], and aldolase). Juvenile rheumatoid arthritis (JRA) is a diagnosis of exclusion considered in children with persistent arthritis of one or more joints, lasting at least six weeks, in whom all other causes of arthritis have been eliminated.[2] Children with JRA may have systemic onset of the disease (hectic fevers, rash, elevated WBC count and ESR, and anemia), polyarticular onset (symmetric arthritis in multiple joints, mildly elevated WBC and ESR, mild anemia, low positive ANA, and in a small subset of adolescents, a positive rheumatoid factor) or pauciarticular onset (asymmetric arthritis in only a few joints and usually normal laboratory studies). Children with sys-

temic onset JRA undergo extensive evaluations, particularly aimed at ruling out occult infections, malignancies, and inflammatory bowel disease.[6]

Young children with acute leukemia or neuroblastoma may have bone pain as the sole manifestation of the neoplastic process; the WBC is usually low but may be normal, and plain radiographs may or may not point to the bony involvement (periosteal elevation, metaphyseal lines). Careful laboratory evaluation may include a review of the peripheral blood smear for suspicious cells, lactic dehydrogenase (LDH), uric acid, and bone marrow aspirate as well as urinary measurement of vanillylmandelic acid (VMA) and homovanillic acid (HVA). Psychogenic causes of pain should be considered in children who have a chronic history of pain (months or years), multiple yet unremarkable physical and laboratory evaluations, and withdrawal from normal function, particularly school attendance. These children tend to see multiple specialists and undergo exhaustive, often invasive testing and treatments without improvement.[7]

Imaging

Routine radiographs are used to diagnose sequelae of trauma, both spontaneous and induced (child abuse), mechanical causes of pain, including Legg-Calvé-Perthes disease and slipped capital femoral epiphysis, bone tumors (i.e., osteoid osteoma, osteogenic and Ewing sarcoma), and metastasis (neuroblastoma, lymphoma) and to establish a baseline for future management of chronic arthritis. Chest radiographs provide a screening tool in the evaluation of multisystem diseases (SLE, vasculitis, sarcoid, systemic onset JRA with pericarditis) and tuberculosis.

Ultrasound is particularly helpful in the evaluation of soft tissues (bursae, tendons, synovial thickening) and documentation of fluid, particularly in the shoulder and hip joints, which are difficult to assess clinically.[8]

Nuclear imaging studies, such as technetium bone scan, aid in the diagnosis of primary bone diseases (osteomyelitis, diskitis, benign and malignant bone and joint tumors).

Magnetic resonance imaging is of particular use in the evaluation of back pain (sacroiliitis, intraspinal tumors) as well as in the assessment of ligamentous injury in young athletes.

Upper gastrointestinal studies with small bowel follow-through will aid in the diagnosis of inflammatory bowel disease, whereas gallium scans are at times used to diagnose occult lymphoma and abscesses.

ASSESSMENT

To avoid duplication, this section will be limited to the more elusive causes of limb pain in children whose evaluations are largely negative. Both the physical examination and the laboratory studies aid in the diagnosis of underlying disorders that produce objective findings and abnormal laboratory tests. Subjective musculoskeletal pain may be the only manifestation of the following conditions.

Growing pains, the most common form of limb pain in children will be discussed first. These pains usually begin in healthy children between the ages of 3 and 5 years or 8 and 12 years, although they may begin at any time, including infancy and adulthood. The reported prevalence of growing pains is as high as 33.6 per cent of school-aged children. Diagnostic criteria developed by Naish and Apley[9] call for a three-month history of pains that are characteristically intermittent with symptom-free intervals of days, weeks, or months. The pains occur most frequently at the end of the day or awaken the child from sleep. They are usually described as deep within the muscles of calves or thighs, sometimes occurring behind the knees or in the groin, and rarely affecting the upper extremities. In older children, the pains may resemble cramps, creeping sensations, or restless legs. There are no associated objective findings of erythema, swelling, decreased range of motion, limping, or local tenderness. All evaluations, including the physical examination, laboratory tests, and radiographic studies, are within normal limits. Growing pains usually decrease in frequency over a 12- to 24-month period but may rarely recur during adolescence.[10]

Several conditions that result in musculoskeletal pain and paucity of physical findings should be considered in healthy-appearing children before the diagnosis of growing pains is established. Benign hypermobility syndrome is a common entity, encountered more frequently in girls than in boys and particularly in children who excel in gymnastics and ballet. Hypermobile children frequently experience pain at the end of the day. Their pain, unlike growing pains, is localized to the joints and does not interrupt sleep. Documentation of ligamentous laxity (passive apposition of the thumb to the flexor aspect of the forearm,

hyperextension of the finger, elbow, and knee joints) and an otherwise normal physical examination provide the necessary clues to the diagnosis.[11] The patellofemoral syndrome or chondromalacia patellae affects adolescents, particularly girls, and is manifested by medial patellar pain exacerbated by climbing stairs or riding a bicycle. There may be intermittent joint swelling without limitation of motion. The pain can be reproduced during the physical examination by palpating the undersurface of the patella as well as by positive apprehension and inhibition signs, described earlier.[12]

Intermittent nocturnal leg cramps may occur at night in healthy, active children. These are thought to follow vigorous daytime activity and are associated with palpable tight muscles during the painful episodes but not in the pediatrician's office.[13]

Osteoid osteoma, a benign bone tumor, often presents with night-time pain. In contrast to growing pains, this discomfort is usually unilateral (over the tibia or femur) and exquisitely sensitive to salicylate. Physical examination and plain radiographs may be normal or reveal muscle atrophy or osteopenia, respectively. Technetium bone scan is a sensitive diagnostic tool.[14]

Musculoskeletal pain in childhood should always be taken seriously, as it may be the first sign of a serious underlying illness, particularly when the pain is associated with limping or refusal to bear weight. However, the overwhelming majority of children with limb pain who appear healthy and maintain normal function do not have serious disorders and can be diagnosed in the pediatrician's office with the aid of the history, physical examination, and screening laboratory tests.

REFERENCES

1. Oster J. Recurrent abdominal pain, headache and limb pains in children and adolescents. Pediatrics 1972;54:429–31.
2. Brewer EJ Jr, Bass J, Baum J, et al. Current proposed revision of JRA criteria. Arthritis Rheum 1977;20 (Suppl):195–9.
3. Dugdale TW, Barnett PR. Historical background: patellofemoral pain in young people. Orthop Clin North Am 1986;17:211–9.
4. Jacobs JC. Acute osteomyelitis: medical management in children. NY State J Med 1978;78:910–2.
5. Tan EM, Cohen AS, Fries JF, et al. The 1982 revised criteria for the classification of SLE. Arthritis Rheum 1982;25:1271–7.
6. Cassidy JT, Levinson JE, Bass JC, et al. A study of classification criteria for a diagnosis of juvenile

rheumatoid arthritis. Arthritis Rheum 1986;29:274–81.

7. Jacobs JC. The differential diagnosis of arthritis in children. In: Katz M, Stiehm ER, eds. New York: Springer Verlag, 1982:162–8.

8. Goldenstein C, McCauley R, Troy M, Schaller JG, Szer IS. Ultrasonography in the evaluation of wrist swelling in children. J Rheumatol 1989;16:1079–87.

9. Naish JM, Apley J. "Growing pains": a clinical study of nonarthritic limb pains in children. Arch Dis Child 1951;26:134–9.

10. Szer IS. Are those limb pains "growing" pains? Contemp Pediatrics 1989;6:143–8.

11. Biro PB, Gewanter HL, Baum J. The hypermobility syndrome. Pediatrics 1983;72:701–6.

12. Bourne MH, Hazel WA Jr, Scott SG, Sim FH. Anterior knee pain. Mayo Clin Proc 1988;63:482–91.

13. Sontag SJ, Wanner JN. The cause of leg cramps and knee pains: an hypothesis and effective treatment. Med Hypotheses 1988;25:35–41.

14. Orlowski JP, Mercer RD. Osteoid osteoma in children and young adults. Pediatrics 1977;59:526–32.

LYMPHADENOPATHY

MARK A. GETZ and FRANK M. GRAZIANO

SYNONYM: Lymph Node Enlargement

BACKGROUND

An extensive network of lymphoid tissue throughout the body functions to provide an appropriate microenvironment for the maturation of lymphoid stem cells into immunocompetent lymphocytes, to provide a filtration system for foreign antigens, and to act as the center of both humoral and cellular immunity.[1] Both primary and secondary lymphoid organs exist.[2,3] The thymus and bone marrow (the exact anatomic organization of the bone marrow lymphoid organ is not yet known) are primary lymphoid organs and are important in the maturation of immunocompetent lymphocytes. Lymph nodes, spleen, and mucosal-associated lymphoid tissues are secondary lymphoid organs through which circulate the immunocompetent lymphocytes. It is in these secondary lymphoid organs that foreign antigen is filtered and presented to lymphocytes as part of the immune response. In this chapter, we will focus on the lymph node and the processes that alter or enhance its function, leading to lymph node enlargement or lymphadenopathy.

It is estimated that there are in excess of 500 lymph nodes in the body varying in size from less than 1 mm to 1 to 2 cm in diameter.[1,2,3] Excessive production of lymphocytes, plasma cells, monocytes, and reticulum cells in lymph nodes is a feature of many regional and systemic diseases. This increased production of cells and resultant lymph node enlargement may follow exposure to a variety of exogenous and endogenous stimuli and is related to the immune response stimulated in the nodes. Lymph node enlargement confined to one lymph node group or involving contiguous areas in the body is termed regional lymphadenopathy. Generalized lymphadenopathy denotes enlargement of at least two or more noncontiguous lymph node groups in the body.

Lymphadenopathy, of course, is a symptom/physical finding and not a diagnosis. Proliferative abnormalities in lymph nodes leading to enlargement may be broadly categorized into infectious, neoplastic, inflammatory, and miscellaneous causes (Table 1). The degree of lymphoreticular proliferation and enlargement depends on many factors including: the nature, virulence, and degree of the stimulus; the site of entry; and the individual capacity of the host to react to the stimulus. Enlargement of lymph nodes may be accompanied by signs of acute inflammation (reddening of the skin over the node, heat, tenderness), or particularly in the case when the proliferation is slow in development, great enlargement of lymph nodes can occur in the absence of signs of inflammation. Regional syndromes of lymphadenopathy usually reflect pathology in the drainage area of a particular lymph node group, and each region has its own characteristic differential diagnosis. Gen-

TABLE 1. Etiologic Classification of Causes for Lymphadenopathy

INFECTIOUS

Bacterial
  Scarlet fever
  Syphilis
  Brucellosis
  Leptospirosis
  Tuberculosis
  Atypical mycobacterium
  Scrub typhus
Viral
  "Mono syndrome"
    Epstein-Barr virus
    Cytomegalovirus
  Viral hepatitis
  Rubeola
  Rubella
  Human immunodeficiency virus
Parasitic
  Toxoplasmosis
Fungal
  Histoplasmosis

NEOPLASTIC

Malignant lymphoma
  Hodgkin's disease
  Non-Hodgkin's lymphoma
Metastatic adenocarcinoma
Angioimmunoblastic lymphadenopathy
Reticuloendothelioses
Waldenström's macroglobulinemia
Myeloid metaplasia

INFLAMMATORY

Systemic lupus erythematosus
Rheumatoid arthritis
Sjögren's syndrome
Sarcoidosis
Serum sickness

MISCELLANEOUS

Hereditary
  Immunodeficiency diseases
  Lysosomal storage diseases
Hyperthyroidism
Generalized dermatitis
Phenytoin

eralized lymphadenopathy implies an underlying systemic illness.

As a consequence of prior inflammation, enlarged lymph nodes are frequently found when examining children and adolescents. Cervical nodes ranging in size from 0.5 to 1 cm in diameter are almost always palpable in children up to age 12 years. Such nodes have been referred to as "shotty," which has come to mean firm, freely movable, and nontender. In addition to the enlargement of lymph nodes that can be observed in young people, lymphoid tissue in this population also has the ability to respond dramatically to infection. With age, there is a gradual involution of lymphoid tissue, but these nodes do retain the

capacity to enlarge in response to antigenic stimuli. The annual incidence of lymphadenopathy is 0.5 per cent in the primary care setting.[4]

Pathologically, the normal lymph node is generally depicted as having a static structure consisting of cortical and medullary components distributed in a reticular stroma, with secondary cortical reaction or follicular centers encompassed by a prominent collagen capsule. Afferent lymphatic vessels enter through the capsule, emptying into a subcapsular sinus from which lymph flows through the sinusoids of the lymphoid tissue to emerge through the hilus into the efferent lymphatic vessels. Because lymph nodes are continually being stimulated, however, from a dynamic standpoint, lymph nodes have an almost unlimited range of morphologic expression. Even with a single stimulus, the morphologic appearance may vary with age of the individual, prior immunization, immunologic capability of the individual, general nutritional status, and time following the exposure to the stimulus. Thus, interpretation of pathologic changes in lymph node biopsies can often be difficult.

Two basic pathologic changes can be observed in abnormal lymph nodes: inflammatory or neoplastic. Inflammatory responses can be specific to lymph node tissue (reactive hyperplasia) or similar to reactions seen in other tissues (suppuration, necrosis, granulomatous inflammation, etc.). Reactive hyperplasia is further characterized as nodular, paracortical, sinus histiocytosis, or mixed pattern. Atypical lymphoid hyperplasia refers to nodes with features unlike the reactive changes described earlier but yet not diagnostic of malignancy. Neoplastic conditions causing lymphadenopathy are either lymphoma or metastatic cancer. Lymphomas are derived from lymphocytes or mononuclear-phagocytic cells and are classified clinicopathologically as either Hodgkin's lymphoma or non-Hodgkin's lymphoma. Microscopically, the nodal pathology is differentiated from reactive processes by assessment of the architectural effacement, monomorphous proliferation, and cellular atypia of the lymph node.

HISTORY

History of the Present Illness

The medical history should first assess the time course of the illness. What symptom appeared first? How long has the patient noticed the lymph node enlargement? Is it recurrent? Next, symptoms referable to lymph nodes themselves should be determined. Are they painful or tender? Have they been changing in size and over what time period? The patient should then be questioned regarding any systemic symptoms. Has the patient experienced any fever, chills, sweats, weight loss, arthralgias, arthritis, morning stiffness, malaise, dry eyes, dry mouth, pleurisy, skin rash, sore throat, bruising, or cough?

Lymphadenopathy of rapid onset and progression is characteristic of many infectious processes. If localized to one lymph node group, the site of entry of the infectious agent usually can be found in the region drained by the enlarged lymph node. When generalized, the etiology usually is viral, particularly in children and young adults. In such instances, a history of recent exposure to individuals with infections such as infectious mononucleosis, rubella, or hepatitis B is important to obtain. Lymphadenopathy secondary to a malignant disorder may also (at times) be rapid in onset and show rapid progression (e.g., Hodgkin's disease). Slowly progressive lymphadenopathy that is more generalized in distribution and relatively asymptomatic is most characteristic of malignant neoplasms such as lymphoma and chronic lymphocytic leukemia but may also occur in connective tissue disorders (systemic lupus erythematosus [SLE], rheumatoid arthritis) and in chronic inflammatory cutaneous disorders.

Family History

A family history may reveal a genetic link implicating an inherited immunodeficiency disease or lysosomal storage disease.

Past Medical History

Diligent questioning concerning whether the individual is part of a risk group for human immunodeficiency virus (HIV) infection is absolutely imperative in our current times. These risk groups include gays/bisexuals, intravenous drug abusers, spouses/partners of these two groups, those individuals receiving blood products, heterosexuals having frequent sexually transmitted diseases or multiple partners, prostitutes, and newborns of women infected or potentially infected with HIV.[5,6]

Focused Queries

1. *What medications has the patient been taking?* Medications should always be considered as a possible cause for enlarged lymph nodes. Anticonvulsant drugs, particularly phenytoin (Dilantin) and mephenytoin (Mesantoin), are the most frequent offenders.[7] Lymphadenopathy associated with medication is frequently accompanied by symptoms and signs suggestive of a systemic allergic reaction (e.g., skin rash, fever, hepatosplenomegaly, and eosinophilia). The duration of lymphadenopathy after drug exposure is variable, but the node enlargement and other findings usually subside after the drug is discontinued. Pain in lymph nodes with alcohol ingestion has traditionally been characteristic of Hodgkin's disease but has also been reported with sarcoidosis.

2. *Is there a history of contact with animals?* The most common causes of lymphadenopathy secondary to animal exposure are toxoplasmosis (*Toxoplasma gondii*), cat-scratch fever (a gram-negative bacillus with no name), rat-bite fever (*Spirillum minus*), tularemia (*Francisella tularensis*), anthrax (*Bacillus anthracis*), erysipeloid (*Erysipelothrix rhusiopathiae*), and erythema chronicum migrans (Lyme disease, *Borrelia burgdorferi*).

3. *What is the occupation of the individual?* Ulceroglandular lymphadenopathy (a syndrome characterized by the presence of a lesion, usually papulonodular and vesicular, at the site of entrance of the responsible agent and by regional lymphadenopathy that is frequently tender and painful—e.g., cat-scratch fever) is often occupation related (e.g., veterinarians, laboratory workers, farmers, fishermen, butchers). Lymph node enlargement (minimal to moderate) observed most often in the epitrochlear, axillary, or inguinal areas is often seen in manual laborers and is secondary to trauma or minor infections in these individuals. Hilar and mediastinal lymphadenopathy may result from an occupational pulmonary disorder such as silicosis.

PHYSICAL EXAMINATION

General

There are over 60 standard groups of lymph nodes listed by anatomists.[8] On physical examination, however, the clinician generally

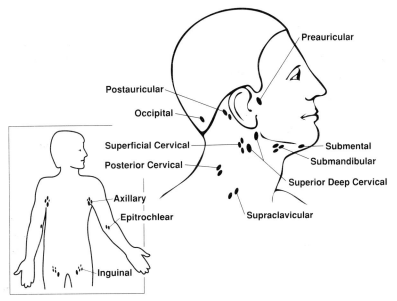

FIGURE 1. Anatomic location of important palpable lymph nodes and lymph node groups in the body.

need only consider the palpable nodes in terms of three regional groups: (1) cervicofacial and supraclavicular, (2) axillary and epitrochlear, and (3) inguinal (Fig. 1). Needless to say, many centrally located node groups lie beyond the reach of physical examination and must be evaluated by radiologic and/or surgical techniques. The standard examination of peripheral lymph nodes requires inspection and palpation (using the middle three fingers) with comparison of lymph node characteristics on both sides of the body. Because of the wide range of causes of lymphadenopathy and the systemic nature of some of the diseases associated with it, a complete physical examination is always necessary.

Focused Examination

Special attention should go to assessing each of the lymph node groups. In recording your findings, five characteristics should routinely be included: (1) location; (2) size, preferably giving the diameter in centimeters; (3) tenderness; (4) degree of fixation—movable, matted, fixed; and (5) texture—hard, soft, firm. Cervical and femoral nodes are usually easily appreciated when enlarged, but more care is required to evaluate for the presence of enlarged epitrochlear, axillary, and supraclavicular nodes. Because of their prognostic significance, it is especially important not to miss supraclavicular nodes. At times, it may be necessary to have the patient perform the Valsalva maneuver to make these nodes more easily palpable.

Generally, any lymph node that is 1 cm or greater in diameter is considered to be enlarged. In certain locations, however, such as the supraclavicular area, a palpable lymph node that is less than 1 cm in diameter is often a significant finding and should be further evaluated. In other areas, such as the superior deep cervical area, lymph nodes 1 cm or more in diameter are a frequent finding, particularly in children and young adults, and are usually of no clinical significance. Lymph node size should not be estimated but rather carefully measured and compared over time.

Besides the mere presence of enlarged lymph nodes, it is necessary to assess their characteristics. Is tenderness present? This usually indicates an acute inflammatory condition, but nodes can be tender in Hodgkin's disease. The character of infectious lymphadenopathy or lymphadenitis is quite variable, depending on the causative organism. Lymphadenitis secondary to bacteria such as *Streptococcus* is usually red, hot, tender, painful, and often fluctuant, whereas that due to other bacteria such as the tubercle bacillus (*Mycobacterium tuberculosis*) may be fluctuant but is often not painful, red, hot, or tender. In most cases of viral-induced lymphadenopathy, the lymph nodes usually are only minimally to moderately enlarged; relatively soft in consistency; and not painful, red, hot, tender, or fluctuant. Are the nodes movable, or fixed and matted? What is their consistency?

Are they firm, rubbery, hard, or fluctuant? Is the surrounding skin involved in an inflammatory process? Is there redness, warmth, or skin breakdown in the area?

Enlarged, flat, and relatively soft lymph nodes are usually non-neoplastic. If biopsied, such lymph node specimens often reveal nonspecific hyperplasia, fibrosis (scarring), fat replacement, or a combination of these changes. Neoplastic infiltration of lymph nodes often produces enlarged, irregular, and rubbery hard nodes, particularly in carcinomatous lymphadenopathy. In lymphoma, the degree of hardness varies depending on the histologic subtype. In Hodgkin's lymphoma, the involved lymph nodes tend to be firmer than in either the low-grade non-Hodgkin's lymphoma or chronic lymphocytic leukemia.

Splenomegaly is often associated with lymphadenopathy. Some disorders producing splenomegaly include: Epstein-Barr virus (EBV) mononucleosis, cytomegalovirus (CMV) infection, secondary syphilis, brucellosis, leptospirosis, salmonellosis, typhoid, paratyphoid, tularemia, listeriosis, diphtheria, rickettsial infection, tuberculosis, rheumatoid arthritis, SLE, lymphoma, hairy-cell leukemia, hypersensitivity reactions, and hyperthyroidism. Having patients lie on their right side while taking a deep breath may facilitate splenic palpation. It should be noted that 3 per cent of normal college freshmen have enlarged spleens.[9]

Important clues to an underlying systemic illness on physical examination include: the presence of fever, skin rash (syphilis, childhood exanthems, SLE, angioimmunoblastic lymphadenopathy, sarcoidosis), evidence of arthritis (rheumatoid arthritis, Sjögren's syndrome, or SLE), thyroid enlargement, exophthalmos, heart murmur, or stigmata of subacute bacterial endocarditis. Throat examination may reveal oral candidiasis or hairy leukoplakia, suggesting the presence of HIV infection. More commonly, throat examination may reveal a gray tonsillar membrane, petechial eruption at the junction of the soft and hard palates, and pharyngeal erythema as an early diagnostic sign of EBV mononucleosis.

DIAGNOSTIC STUDIES

The history and physical examination are important in the diagnosis of lymphadenopathy and should direct one to select the appropriate and minimum number of laboratory studies needed for evaluation of the process. Laboratory examination of individuals with lymph node enlargement, however, is often critical for the appropriate and final diagnosis of lymphadenopathy. For example, in those individuals with enlarged lymph nodes as part of a systemic illness, serologic identification of autoantibodies and/or lymph node biopsy and culture may be helpful or even diagnostic of the underlying disease.

Laboratory

As part of the clinical laboratory data base, a complete blood count (CBC), peripheral smear, sedimentation rate, and blood chemistry tests should first be ordered. The CBC and peripheral smear may give specific clues (such as the atypical lymphocytosis seen in EBV, CMV, or toxoplasmosis) to infection. Eosinophilia may be present in angioimmunoblastic lymphadenopathy, serum sickness, or the pseudolymphoma observed with phenytoin. The anemia of chronic disease or elevated sedimentation rate often reflects an underlying systemic illness. Liver enzyme elevation can signal the presence of EBV, CMV, toxoplasmosis, or leptospirosis.

The ordering of more specific laboratory tests is guided by clues from the history, physical examination, and initial laboratory tests. Helpful tests include: throat culture, monospot test, purified protein derivative (PPD) skin test, HIV serology, Venereal Disease Research Laboratories (VDRL), rheumatoid factor, hepatitis serology, thyroid function tests, angiotensin converting enzyme (ACE) level, and antinuclear antibody (ANA). Blood cultures and serology for EBV, CMV, toxoplasmosis, leptospirosis, or brucellosis may be indicated in special circumstances.

Imaging

Noninvasive diagnostic imaging, such as plain chest x-ray or computed tomography (CT), is used more to assess the extent of lymphadenopathy involving the central lymph node groups than to evaluate its etiology. Still, some clues can be obtained on noninvasive imaging tests. For example, on chest x-ray, mediastinal lymphadenopathy in young people is usually suggestive of malignant disease. The bilateral hilar adenopathy of sarcoidosis is characteristic. Calcification of lymph nodes on chest x-ray implies tuberculosis or histoplasmosis. Abdominal CT is the preferred method for evaluating retroperitoneal lymphadenopathy.

Lymphography (lymphangiogram) is more specific for neoplastic disease than other noninvasive methods and has the advantage of being able to detect abnormal lymph node architecture even before the nodes are enlarged.

Lymph Node Biopsy

Lymph node biopsy is usually necessary to diagnose serious disease. Aspiration of a fluctuant node may yield a diagnosis in infectious suppurative lymphadenitis.[10] Fine-needle aspiration cytology can be useful for diagnosing metastatic carcinoma or melanoma but is less accurate at differentiating lymphoma from benign lymphadenopathy.[10] Excisional node biopsy, however, remains the gold standard.

The diagnostic yield of lymph node biopsy ranges from 37 to 70 per cent.[11,12] The yield in repeat biopsy after an initial nondiagnostic attempt is 25 to 50 per cent, with 20 per cent of these being lymphomas.[12] Patients who develop a lymphoproliferative disorder after initial negative biopsy usually do so in six to eight months.[13,14,15] The yield is increased in patients greater than age 40 with nodes larger than 1 cm. The choice of node for biopsy is also important, with supraclavicular nodes having the highest yield, and inguinal or axillary nodes less often diagnostic.[7,11,12] Culture of lymph node tissue has a low yield (10 per cent) but should be done if infectious disease such as tuberculosis or histoplasmosis is suspected. Care should be taken not to biopsy nodes in patients with clinically obvious EBV mononucleosis, as the pathology is easily confused with malignant lymphoma.

ASSESSMENT

Regional Considerations

In individuals with regional lymphadenopathy, the anatomic location of the enlarged nodes is often helpful in assessing the problem.[16] In most instances, the predilection for a particular lymph node region either is directly related to the entry site of the causative agent or is a consequence of the pattern of drainage of a diseased organ. In addition, specific regional node enlargement in generalized lymphadenopathy can provide clues to its underlying etiology. The clinically important peripheral lymph node groups are those found in the head and neck region, axilla, and epitrochlear and inguinal areas (Fig. 1). Following are some important regional lymph node groups, their drainage sites, and processes associated with enlargement of these nodes.

Head and Neck Nodes

The head and neck lymph nodes are frequently enlarged (Fig. 1). Occipital lymph nodes drain the scalp and back of the head. They enlarge in response to scalp conditions such as pediculosis capitis, ringworm, or acute recurrent folliculitis. Postauricular lymph nodes drain the external auditory meatus, posterior pinnae, and the temporal scalp. Lymph node enlargement in this area is seen with scalp conditions, external otitis, and the Ramsay-Hunt syndrome secondary to herpes zoster. Postauricular nodes enlargement is also seen with rubella but not rubeola. Preauricular nodes filter lymph from the anterior pinnae, external auditory meatus, temporal scalp, lateral eyelids, and palpebral conjunctivae. Factors responsible for enlargement of these lymph nodes are usually easily identified and include squamous cell carcinoma, erysipelas, and herpes zoster ophthalmicus. Conjunctival infection associated with preauricular lymph node enlargement is termed the "oculoglandular syndrome." Submandibular and submental lymph nodes can also be involved in the oculoglandular syndrome because they drain the medial angle of the eye as well as the tongue, lips, and cheeks. Other common etiologies for enlargement of these nodes include dental infections, primary syphilis with an oral chancre, and oral cancer.

The superior deep cervical lymph nodes drain the palatine tonsils and the tongue. Enlargement of these nodes is seen most commonly with pharyngeal or tonsillar infections, but neoplasms involving the tongue or Waldeyer's tonsillar ring must be considered, especially in older adults. The inferior deep cervical lymph nodes receive drainage from the entire head and neck, along with some from the arm and thorax. Because of their wide drainage, infectious and neoplastic processes of all these areas must be considered when enlargement of these nodes is observed. In addition, abdominal neoplasms at times metastasize to the supraclavicular lymph nodes, especially on the left. Superficial cervical lymph nodes lie atop the sternocleidomastoid muscles and receive afferents from the pinnae of the ear and the parotid gland region. In addition to disorders affecting these structures, the superficial cervical nodes are often involved in lymphoma.

Axillary Nodes

The axillary borders form a pyramid with a proximal apex. Lymph nodes are located anteriorly, posteriorly, laterally, centrally, and apically. The anterior lymph nodes drain the mammary glands and the anterior chest, whereas the posterior nodes drain the posterior chest and upper extremity. The lateral nodes drain the upper extremity, and the central and apical nodes receive afferents from the other axillary nodes. The main considerations in axillary node enlargement are upper extremity lesions and breast cancer. It should be noted that infections of the third finger can bypass the axillary nodes and involve the infraclavicular nodes, producing a subpectoral abscess with fever, and shoulder pain with abduction.

Epitrochlear Nodes

Epitrochlear nodes receive afferents from the ulnar one half of the hand. Because the hand is a common site for infectious agent inoculation, epitrochlear lymphadenopathy is common with many infectious diseases. These include streptococcal infection, sporotrichosis, anthrax, erysipelothrix, tularemia, bubonic plague, scrub typhus, rat-bite fever, and cat-scratch disease. In addition, bilateral epitrochlear node enlargement is seen in sarcoidosis and secondary syphilis.

Inguinal Nodes

The inguinal nodes consist of superficial and deep groups. The superficial group drains the upper abdominal wall, genital area (but not the testes or ovaries), gluteal area, and the medial lower extremity. The deep group receives afferents from the posterior and lateral foot, popliteal nodes, and the superficial inguinal nodes. The causes of lymphadenopathy secondary to lesions in the lower limbs are similar to those of the upper limbs.

Sexually transmitted diseases commonly cause inguinal adenopathy. The differential diagnosis includes syphilis, herpes simplex, chancroid lymphogranuloma venereum, and occasionally gonococcal infection. Granuloma inguinale produces a similar picture, but the swelling is not lymph node enlargement but rather subcutaneous granulation tissue.[16]

Generalized Lymphadenopathy

The diagnostic approach to a patient with generalized lymphadenopathy takes into account the patient's risk factors for serious disease, such as malignancy, systemic infection, or systemic inflammatory disease. In assessing individuals with generalized lymphadenopathy, children and adolescents, adults, and patients at risk for HIV infection should be considered separately. (See chapter on Human Immunodeficiency Virus Infection.) Diagnostic options include an observation period (if benign self-limited disease is suspected), a noninvasive workup (i.e., specific laboratory tests, CT), or an invasive workup (lymph node biopsy). High-risk patients will require a more aggressive diagnostic approach, including early biopsy.

A higher incidence of generalized lymphadenopathy is seen in children and adolescents because of the increased amount of lymphoid tissue and the greater responsiveness of this tissue to antigen stimulation. Generalized lymph node enlargement in this age group, therefore, is less likely to represent serious disease. In young patients who are otherwise well, a period of observation from one to four weeks is reasonable. During this observation period, the node size should be measured carefully. Lymph node biopsy should be strongly considered if the node has increased in size after 2 weeks, has not changed in size after 4 to 6 weeks, or is persistently abnormal after 8 to 12 weeks.[13,15,17] Risk factors for more serious disease in children and adolescents incude an abnormal chest x-ray, lymph node size greater than 2.0 cm, night sweats, weight loss, anemia, presence of supraclavicular nodes, or fixed and matted nodes.[13,15]

Worthy of special note in older children, adolescents, and young adults is the "mono syndrome," which is a relatively common process causing lymph node enlargement in these individuals. Noninvasive evaluation for this syndrome should include a peripheral blood smear (50 per cent or more lymphocytes/monocytes and 10 per cent or more atypical lymphocytes) and heterophile antibody (monospot positive two to five weeks into the course of the syndrome). EBV is causative in over 90 per cent of cases of the mono syndrome, and the term infectious mononucleosis should be reserved for these cases.[18] CMV is causative in about 5 to 7 per cent[19] and *Toxoplasma gondii* in less than 1 per cent of such cases.[20] Presence of atypical lymphocytosis and a persistently negative heterophile antibody suggests heterophile-negative EBV, CMV, or *Toxoplasma* infection, and appropriate serology should be obtained.

Evaluation of generalized lymphadenopathy in the adult is similar to that in children and adolescents except that the risk of serious disease is much greater. The strongest predictors of serious disease in the adult are age greater than 40, weight loss, and presence of supraclavicular lymphadenopathy.[7]

Individuals at risk for HIV infection also deserve special consideration. Acute HIV infection can cause lymphadenopathy that may resolve during the following period of asymptomatic infection.[21,22] Later, persistent generalized lymphadenopathy (PGL) develops and is defined as greater than three months of lymph node enlargement in an HIV-positive individual in the absence of any other cause.[23,24] Biopsy of these nodes reveals a characteristic but not specific pathologic picture ranging from florid follicular hyperplasia in the early stages to lymphoid depletion in the later stages.[25] PGL is an early sign of progression of HIV infection to the acquired immunodeficiency syndrome (AIDS). The finding of herpes zoster, thrush, and systemic symptoms (fever, diarrhea, weight loss, night sweats) is much more ominous in suggesting progression of HIV to AIDS. Since the clinical and serologic picture is most often diagnostic for HIV infection and lymph node pathology is not, lymph node biopsy is not generally recommended for diagnosis of HIV disease. However, marked lymph node enlargement or rapidly enlarging lymph nodes during the course of HIV infection should prompt caution, and biopsy should be performed to rule out lymphoma or metastatic Kaposi's sarcoma.

Because of the broad range of possible causes of generalized lymphadenopathy, a thorough clinical evaluation is always necessary. Evidence from this evaluation should lead to specific laboratory tests that may provide the diagnosis. If not, assessment of the patient's risk for serious disease will decide the urgency of more invasive procedures such as lymph node biopsy. Individuals with low risk of serious disease may benefit from a period of observation before subjecting them to invasive procedures.

REFERENCES

1. Butcher EC, Weissman IL. Lymphoid tissue and organs. In: Paul WE, ed. Fundamental immunology. New York: Raven Press, 1984:109–27.
2. Roitt IM, Brostoff J, Male DK. Immunology, Vol 3. 1st ed. St Louis: CV Mosby, 1985:1–39.
3. Chapel H, Haeney M. Essentials of clinical immunology. 1st ed. St Louis: CV Mosby, 1984: 1–36.
4. Allhiser JN, McKnight TA, Shank JC. Lymphadenopathy in family practice. J Fam Pract 1981;12:27–32.
5. Fauci AS, Masur H, Gelmann EP, et al. The acquired immunodeficiency syndrome: an update. Ann Intern Med 1985;102:800–13.
6. Haverkos HW, Edelman R. The epidemiology of acquired immunodeficiency syndrome among heterosexuals. JAMA 1988;260:1922–9.
7. Hess CE. Approach to patients with lymphadenopathy or splenomegaly. In: Thorup OA Jr, ed. Fundamentals of clinical hematology. Philadelphia: WB Saunders, 1987:536–77.
8. Meyers MC. Hematopoietic system. In: Judge RD, Zuidema GD, eds. Physical diagnosis: a physiologic approach to the clinical examination. Boston: Little Brown, 1968:263–75.
9. Ebaugh FGL, McIntyne OR. Palpable spleens: ten years follow up. Ann Intern Med 1979;90: 130–3.
10. Kline TS, Kanhan V, Kline IK. Lymphadenopathy and aspiration biopsy cytology: review of 376 superficial nodes. Cancer 1984;54:1076–81.
11. Doberneck RC. The diagnostic yield of lymph node biopsy. Arch Surg 1983;118:1203–5.
12. Kunitz G. Diagnostic evaluation of lymphadenopathy. In: Stults BM, Dere WH, eds. Practical care of the ambulatory patient. Philadelphia: WB Saunders, 1989:342–50.
13. Kissane JM, Gephardt GN. Lymphadenopathy in childhood: long term follow-up in patients with nondiagnostic lymph node biopsies. Hum Pathol 1974;5:431–9.
14. Saltzstern SL. The fate of patients with nondiagnostic lymph node biopsies. Surgery 1965;58: 659–62.
15. Lake AM, Oski FA. Peripheral lymphadenopathy in childhood: ten years experience with excisional biopsy. Am J Dis Child 1978;132:357–9.
16. Jeghers H, Clark SL, Templeton AC. Lymphadenopathy and disorders of the lymphatics. In: Blacklow RS, ed. MacBryde's signs and symptoms: applied pathologic, physiologic, and clinical interpretation. Philadelphia: JB Lippincott, 1983:467–533.
17. Carithers HA. Lymphadenopathy: a diagnostic enigma. Am J Dis Child 1978;132:353–4.
18. Evans AS. Infectious mononucleosis and related syndromes. Am J Med Sci 1978;276:325–39.
19. Cohen JI, Corey GR. Cytomegalovirus infection in the normal host. Medicine 1985;64:100–14.
20. Krick JA, Remington JS. Toxoplasmosis in the adult—an overview. N Engl J Med 1978;298:550–3.
21. Abrams DI. The pre-AIDS syndrome. Infect Dis Clin North Am 1988;2:343–51.
22. Said JW. AIDS-related lymphadenopathies. Semin Diagnost Pathol 1988;5:365–75.

23. Mathur-Wagh V, Enlow RW, Spigland I, et al. Longitudinal study of persistent generalized lymphadenopathy in homosexual men: relation to acquired immunodeficiency syndrome. Lancet 1984;1:1033–8.
24. Centers for Disease Control. Persistent generalized lymphadenopathy among homosexual males. MMWR (CDC) 1982;31:249–51.
25. Levine AM, Meyer PR, Gill PS, et al. Results of initial lymph node biopsy in homosexual men with generalized lymphadenopathy. J Clin Oncol 1986;4:165–9.

MEDIASTINAL MASS

GLEN A. LILLINGTON and R. STEVEN THARRATT

SYNONYM: Mediastinal Tumor

BACKGROUND

A mediastinal mass is an abnormal localized enlargement or swelling within the mediastinum. In most cases, the mediastinal mass is detected on standard chest roentgenogram; in an occasional instance, the mass is detectable only by computed tomography (CT). In current clinical usage, the term mediastinal tumor is essentially identical in meaning to mediastinal mass. The word *tumor* in this context means "swelling" and does not necessarily connote neoplasia.

Anatomy

The mediastinum lies between the two pleural cavities and is enclosed by the mediastinal parietal pleura on each side.[1] The anterior border is the sternum, the upper margin is the thoracic inlet, and the lower margin is the diaphragm. Although anatomists usually consider that the mediastinum extends posteriorly only as far as the anterior surface of the thoracic spine, most diagnosticians find it clinically useful to include the entire thoracic spine and the paravertebral areas within the boundaries of the posterior mediastinum.[2]

For clinical purposes, the mediastinum can be subdivided into compartments, which have been defined in different ways by different writers.[2] In general, the superior mediastinal compartment is above the level of the aortic arch or the bifurcation of the trachea; below this are the anterior, middle, and posterior compartments. The anterior compartment is anterior to the heart and great vessels; the middle compartment includes the heart and hilar areas; and the posterior compartment includes the retrocardiac area, the spine, and the paraspinal areas. In some classifications, the prespinal retrocardiac area is placed in the middle compartment; in others, the heart is included in the anterior compartment.

As many of the specific mediastinal masses are commonly situated in only a single compartment, determination of the anatomic location of the lesion provides significant aid in differential diagnosis. With the use of CT, it has become apparent that diagnostic precision can be improved even further by the use of seven compartments (Fig. 1) to describe the position of the mass in the mediastinum.[3] The additional three compartments are (1) the anterior diaphragmatic compartment, (2) the middle/posterior diaphragmatic compartment, and (3) a diffuse compartment to include masses that surround several mediastinal structures.

Mediastinal Diseases

Disorders of the mediastinum may be grouped into three categories: pneumomediastinum, mediastinitis, and mediastinal mass.

Pneumomediastinum (mediastinal emphysema) denotes the presence of free air within the mediastinum. The presence of pneumomediastinum is established by standard chest roentgenography; the determination of its etiology and pathogenesis is mainly dependent on correlation with clinical data.

Mediastinitis encompasses several acute or chronic inflammatory processes involving the mediastinal connective tissues. These may be localized or diffuse. Although the chest roent-

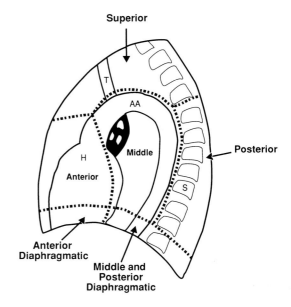

FIGURE 1. Diagram of mediastinal compartments employed with CT studies for the differential diagnosis of mediastinal masses. Mediastinal masses: a system for diagnosis based on computed tomography, by Feigin DS, Padua EM. CT 10(1), pp 11–21. Copyright 1991 by Elsevier Science Publishing Co, Inc.)

genogram may show (1) a localized abscess with an air-fluid interface, (2) areas of mediastinal emphysema, or (3) generalized (diffuse) widening of the mediastinum, there may be no obvious or distinctive roentgen findings. In such cases, the diagnosis is commonly established from the combination of the clinical setting (recent mediastinal surgery, suspected esophageal perforation) and the signs of sepsis. In the diffuse cases, CT shows a diffuse soft tissue density surrounding several organs.[3]

A mediastinal mass (tumor) is a localized enlargement of an area of the mediastinum, usually detectable on standard chest roentgenograms. The remainder of this discussion will be confined to the diagnostic management of mediastinal masses.

Etiology of Mediastinal Masses

The mediastinal contents are anatomically diverse and embryologically complex. Some mediastinal "masses" are merely ectopic normal organs; others are developmental aberrations; and many are manifestations of acquired disease processes, either benign or neoplastic (Table 1).

Except for cardiomegaly (which by clinical tradition is usually excluded from the category of mediastinal masses), the most common cause of a mediastinal mass is lymphadenopathy, either benign or malignant.[2] Lymphadenopathy is usually most prominent in the paratracheal and subcarinal areas but may also involve the anterior and posterior compartments.

Currently, sarcoidosis is the most common benign cause of mediastinal lymphadenopathy, although infectious diseases such as tuberculosis and fungal diseases are prominent etiologic factors in some areas. Extramedullary hematopoiesis is a rare cause of posterior mediastinal adenopathy. Another rare cause is Castleman's disease (angiofollicular lymph node hyperplasia). Malignant mediastinal lymphadenopathy is most commonly due to bronchogenic carcinoma or lymphoma. It may be difficult to differentiate malignant from benign lymphadenopathy by CT or other imaging studies.

Vascular masses within the mediastinum include aneurysms of the aorta and its branches, aneurysms of the main pulmonary arteries, and venous dilatations or congenital abnormalities. Imaging studies employed include thoracic angiography, CT with contrast, and magnetic resonance imaging (MRI).

There is a wide variety of neoplastic masses of the mediastinum. Some of these are benign, but many are malignant. The differentiation of benign from malignant lesions is not always possible with imaging studies.

Cysts of various types may occur in the mediastinum. CT examination will usually detect the cystic nature of the mass and will provide important clues to the etiology. As cystic degeneration can occur in malignant tumors, the presence of a cyst does not guarantee benignity.

TABLE 1. Etiology of Mediastinal Masses

Vascular Masses
  Aneurysms of aorta and branches
  Anomalous venous connections
  Dissecting hematomas
  Ectopic vessels
Endocrine tumors
  Thyroid adenomas
  Thymoma
  Parathyroid adenoma
  Pheochromocytoma
Germ cell tumors
  Dermoid
  Teratoma (benign or malignant)
  Seminoma, embryonal tumor
  Choriocarcinoma
Cystic masses
  Pleuropericardial cyst
  Bronchogenic cyst
  Cystic hygroma
  Enterogenous cyst
Gastrointestinal
  Achalasia
  Enterogenous cyst
  Hiatal hernia
  Pancreatic pseudocyst
Malignant lymphadenopathy
  Bronchogenic carcinoma
  Other metastatic malignancies
  Lymphoma, leukemia
Benign lymphadenopathy
  Tuberculosis
  Fungal infections
  Sarcoidosis
  Castleman's syndrome
  Extramedullary hematopoiesis
Mesenchymal tumors
  Lipoma
  Hemangiopericytoma
  Fibroma, myxoma
  Lymphangioma
Neurogenic masses
  Neurofibroma, schwannoma
  Ganglioneuroma
  Neuroblastoma
  Meningocele
Miscellaneous
  Diaphragmatic hernias
  Mediastinal abscess
  Pericardial fat pads

Gastrointestinal disorders that may present as a mediastinal mass include achalasia with megaesophagus, hiatal hernia, enterogenous cyst, and a pancreatic pseudocyst extending up through the diaphragm into the mediastinum. The diagnosis in the first two is confirmed by barium studies, whereas CT is required for the cystic lesions.

Skeletal disorders that may present as mediastinal masses include paravertebral abscesses, paravertebral hematomas, or bone tumors. Needle biopsy is often indicated in such cases.

Pulmonary lesions adjacent to the mediastinum may simulate mediastinal disease on standard chest roentgenograms. CT will usually permit differentiation.

SYMPTOMS OF MEDIASTINAL MASSES

Most mediastinal masses are asymptomatic. In some instances, however, the presence of the mass gives rise to symptoms or abnormal physical signs that may provide valuable clues to the location and etiology of the mass. The presence of symptoms increases the likelihood that the mass is malignant.

Cough may be due to compression or irritation of the tracheobronchial tree by an adjacent lesion, and dysphagia suggests disease in (or adjacent to) the esophagus. Hoarseness may indicate damage to the recurrent laryngeal nerve. Chest pain in the presence of a mediastinal mass suggests mediastinitis, acute changes within an aneurysm, or direct involvement of the bony thorax by a growing tumor. If mediastinal adenopathy is due to a bronchogenic carcinoma, pulmonary symptoms such as cough and hemoptysis may be noted. Fever and weight loss may be prominent features in mediastinal adenopathies due to lymphoma or to infectious granulomatoses.

In patients with superior vena caval obstruction, particularly those due to fibrosing mediastinitis, standard chest roentgenograms may sometimes appear normal; the presence of symptoms and signs may be the major clue to the presence of the lesion. Symptoms include dizziness and headache, particularly if leaning forward.

Intramediastinal diseases may occasionally result in systemic symptoms or syndromes. Thymic tumors may be accompanied by myasthenia gravis, immunodeficiency syndromes, or even aplastic anemia. Hypertension may be secondary to a mediastinal pheochromocytoma, and a mediastinal parathyroid tumor may be manifested clinically by hypercalcemia or even osteitis fibrosa cystica. Mediastinal adenopathy secondary to small cell bronchogenic carcinoma may be associated with one or more of a number of endocrine or neurologic syndromes.

PHYSICAL SIGNS IN MEDIASTINAL DISEASE

Subcutaneous emphysema in the neck may accompany pneumomediastinum. Cervical lymphadenopathy is often present in patients with mediastinal lymphadenopathy, particularly if lymphoma is present. Murmurs or bruits may accompany aortic aneurysms. The muscle weakness of myasthenia gravis is quite distinctive but is mimicked to some extent by the "pseudomyasthenia" of small cell bronchogenic carcinoma. The signs of superior vena caval obstruction may include swelling and cyanosis of the face, neck, and arms; dilated neck and arm veins; and the appearance of dilated collateral veins on the upper chest wall. In cases of substernal goiter, it may be possible to palpate the lesion in the suprasternal area; characteristically, it moves upward with swallowing. Gynecomastia may be present with certain germ cell tumors of the mediastinum.

IMAGING STUDIES IN MEDIASTINAL DISEASE

Standard Chest Roentgenograms

In most instances, the mediastinal mass is first detected by standard posteroanterior (PA) and lateral chest roentgenograms.[4] The approximate size and location of the mass can be discerned with a moderate degree of assurance in many instances, but it is unusual for the clinician to be able to determine the nature of the lesion from these studies alone.

Significant mediastinal disease may be present in cases in which the standard chest roentgenograms appear entirely normal. In these cases of occult mediastinal disease (Table 2), the possible presence of a mediastinal disorder is suggested by the occurrence of symptoms, by the detection of abnormal physical signs such as superior vena caval obstruction, by evidence of lung disease on the standard chest roentgenograms, or by the presence of an extrathoracic syndrome that may be due to a mediastinal lesion, such as myasthenia gravis, hypogammaglobulinemia, ectopic adrenocorticotropic hormone (ACTH) production, agammaglobulinemia, or aplastic anemia.

Pulmonary or intrapleural processes in paramediastinal locations may simulate mediastinal masses on chest roentgenography. CT will usually resolve such dilemmas, although in some instances, it is difficult to determine if a given mass originated in the mediastinum and then encroached upon the lung, or vice versa.

Standard Tomography

In the study of mediastinal masses, standard tomography has been replaced by CT in virtually all instances.

Thoracic Angiography

Thoracic aortography is a very precise technique for the identification of dissecting hematomas and aneurysms of the thoracic aorta and its branches. Even if the diagnosis is known, angiography may be required for surgical planning. Specialized angiographic studies help in

TABLE 2. Occult Mediastinal Masses: Mediastinal Masses that Are Sometimes Undetectable by Standard Chest Roentgenography

DIAGNOSTIC CLUE	MEDIASTINAL LESION	TEST
Myasthenia gravis	Thymoma	CT
Hypogammaglobulinemia	Thymoma	CT
Aplastic anemia	Thymoma	CT
Ectopic ACTH syndrome	Bronchogenic CA*	CT
SIADH† secretion	Bronchogenic CA	CT
"Chemical" hypertension	Paraganglioma	CT, MIGB
Hyperparathyroidism	Parathyroid adenoma	CT
Bronchogenic carcinoma	Adenopathy	CT
SVC‡ obstruction syndrome	Mediastinitis	CT, venography
SVC obstruction syndrome	Malignancy	CT, venography
Dysphagia	Esophageal lesions	CT, barium
Chylothorax	Thoracic duct disease	CT
Gynecomastia	Germ cell tumor	CT

* CA = carcinoma.
† SIADH = syndrome of inappropriate antidiuretic hormone.
‡ SVC = superior vena cava.

the diagnosis of mediastinal parathyroid tumors.

Superior vena cavagrams confirm the presence and location of superior caval obstruction but do not always indicate the etiology.[5]

Mediastinal Sonography

Sonography has proved useful in the investigation of mediastinal masses in certain locations, particularly parasternal and subcarinal tumors.[6]

Radioisotope Studies

Thyroid scintiscans have a high sensitivity and specificity in demonstrating that a mediastinal mass is a substernal or ectopic goiter.[7] However, CT has replaced thyroid scans to a major extent and is particularly helpful in the detection of intrathoracic thyroid malignancy.[8]

Metaiodobenzylguanide (MIGB) scintigraphy is very sensitive and specific in the detection of mediastinal paraganglioma (pheochromocytoma).[9]

Computed Tomography

CT is now employed in virtually all cases of suspected or proved mediastinal masses (Table 3). There are, however, a few instances in which CT may not be required despite the detection of mediastinal abnormality on the standard chest roentgenograms.[2,3] Examples include pneumomediastinum, apparent vascular lesions (for which MRI or immediate angiography may be more appropriate), an apparent hiatal hernia, patients with dysphagia (for which barium studies may be more appropriate), suspected substernal thyroid (for which radio-iodide thyroid scans might be more appropriate), and some instances of pericardial fat pads.

CT is the most sensitive imaging technique for detecting the presence of mediastinal masses. CT indicates the size and exact location of the lesion and in many instances will provide important clues to the etiology of the mass by determining the density, contour, shape, and the nature of the edge of the lesion and by assessing the effect of the lesion on surrounding structures. The correlations between the CT density and location of the lesion and the possible etiologies are shown in Table 4.

In many instances, CT will provide a specific diagnosis with a high degree of assurance. In other cases, CT will not be diagnostic, but the combination of CT characteristics of the lesion and its location will indicate probable and possible diagnoses and will aid in the selection of further diagnostic studies such as biopsy. The radiologist interpreting the study should enumerate the possible diagnoses, provide an estimate of relative likelihoods, and suggest further investigative procedures.

Needle aspiration biopsy of the mediastinum usually requires CT guidance for needle emplacement.[10]

Magnetic Resonance Imaging

MRI is particularly helpful in the study of mediastinal and hilar blood vessels.[11] It differentiates vessels with flowing blood from solid opacities without the requirement for injection of radiopaque contrast and detects most abnormalities or diseases of the vessels. In addition, MRI appears to be about as effective as CT in the detection of mediastinal/hilar lymphadenopathy.

As adipose tissue appears very dense on MRI, the technique is useful in identifying mediastinal lipomatosis, lipomas, and other tumors that contain fat.

BIOPSY OF MEDIASTINAL MASSES

Needle Aspiration Biopsy

Needle biopsy of mediastinal lesions requires sonographic, fluoroscopic, or CT guidance, the latter being most commonly employed.[12] The procedure is very helpful and accurate in the identification of carcinomatous lymphadenopathies and is less reliable in the identification of lymphomas.[10] Needle aspiration of cystic lesions may confirm the presence of a cystic mass in questionable cases[13] and helps to rule out necrotic degeneration of a malignant tumor as the cause of the cystic appearance.

TABLE 3. Uses of CT in Mediastinal Diseases

1. Detection of occult mediastinal lesions.
2. Investigation of "borderline" abnormalities to determine if a mediastinal mass is present.
3. Determination of the size, shape, and location of a mediastinal mass.
4. Determination of the etiology of a mediastinal mass.
5. Guidance for needle aspiration biopsy of a mediastinal mass.

TABLE 4. Correlation of the Location and CT Density of Mediastinal Masses with the Specific Etiologies

LOCATION	FAT DENSITY	WATER/FLUID DENSITY	SOFT TISSUE DENSITY	VASCULAR DENSITY	MINERAL DENSITY
Anterior compartment	Lipoma	Cystic masses	Thymic masses Teratoma Lymphoma Benign nodes	Anomalous vessels	Teratoma Benign lymph nodes Others
Anterior diaphragmatic compartment	Pericardial fat pad	Pericardial cyst	Morgagni hernia		
Middle compartment	Lipoma	Cysts	Esophageal masses Nodes		Vessels Benign nodes
Middle and posterior diaphragmatic compartment	Omental hernia	Pancreatic pseudocysts	Hiatal hernia Bochdalek hernia		
Superior compartment		Lymphangioma	Thyroid masses Parathyroid mass	Anomalies or tortuosities of vessels	Thyroid masses Vessels
Posterior			Neurogenic tumors Extramedullary hematopoiesis	Aneurysm Dissecting hematoma	Vessels
Diffuse	Lipomatosis		Sclerosing mediastinitis		

(Reprinted by permission of the publisher from Mediastinal masses: a system for diagnosis based on computed tomography, by Feigin DS, Padua EM. CT 10(1), pp 11–21. Copyright 1991 by Elsevier Science Publishing Co, Inc.)

Needle biopsy is most often employed in cases in which thoracotomy would likely be unhelpful or inadvisable.

Mediastinoscopy

Mediastinoscopy is a relatively minor surgical procedure that provides visual and instrumental access to the pretracheal and paratracheal areas and the proximal portion of the right hilum. Although its principal function is the diagnosis of malignant and benign lymphadenopathies in these areas, other lesions in the upper anterior mediastinum may sometimes be biopsied successfully by the mediastinoscopic approach.[14]

In patients with proved bronchogenic carcinoma but without evidence of mediastinal lymphadenopathy on standard chest x-rays, mediastinoscopy is often carried out for staging if CT shows node enlargement.

Access to the left hilum and aortic-pulmonary window is difficult with mediastinoscopy; in such instances, the performance of parasternal mediastinotomy is more efficacious.

Bronchoscopy

Bronchoscopy is particularly helpful in cases of mediastinal adenopathy suspected to be due to bronchogenic carcinoma. The primary tumor mass can usually be visualized and biopsied. In cases of mediastinal lymphadenopathy due to sarcoidosis, blind transbronchoscopic lung biopsy (TBLB) may provide the diagnosis.

In some instances, biopsies of paratracheal mediastinal nodes can be obtained by transtracheal needle aspiration during bronchoscopy. This procedure has been employed most commonly for staging of bronchogenic carcinomas.

Thoracotomy

Open thoracotomy is often required to gain access to mediastinal lesions for biopsy. Resection of the lesion, if indicated, can be carried out during the same procedure. The use of CT and mediastinoscopy often establishes the diagnosis and has reduced the number of diagnostic thoracotomies performed in cases of mediastinal disease.

Thoracotomy carries a small mortality rate and the short-term morbidity of a major surgical procedure.

ASSESSMENT

The main goal of the assessment process in the patient with a known or suspected mediastinal mass is to establish the presence of a lesion and to determine its nature in order to plan a rational therapeutic approach. Diagnostic thoracotomy, which becomes the definitive component of the assessment process in some cases, may also, of course, be therapeutic. A secondary goal of the assessment process is to decrease the number of purely diagnostic thoracotomies.

A suggested approach for diagnostic management of mediastinal masses (see the algorithm) starts with the standard chest roentgenograms. In most cases of mediastinal disease, the probable presence of a mediastinal mass will be apparent; in a few instances, however, the standard chest roentgenograms are normal (or virtually so), and the presence of "occult mediastinal disease" is inferred from the presence of other clinical features (Table 3).

Occult Mediastinal Disease Suspected

The various clinical clues that suggest that a mediastinal process is present despite normal standard chest roentgenograms are listed in Table 3. In virtually all such cases, the next step is to obtain CT studies of the mediastinum. An exception is the patient with dysphagia and normal chest x-rays: In most cases, the appropriate study would be a barium swallow rather than CT.

Abnormal or Suspicious Chest Roentgenograms

Most patients in this category go on to CT examination, but in a few instances, CT may not always be required.

CT Not Required

If the lesion appears to be vascular, the clinician may in some circumstances choose angiography or MRI rather than CT. If the roentgen abnormality is pneumomediastinum or cardiomegaly, CT is usually not necessary or even helpful. A substernal thyroid can often be diagnosed with considerable assurance

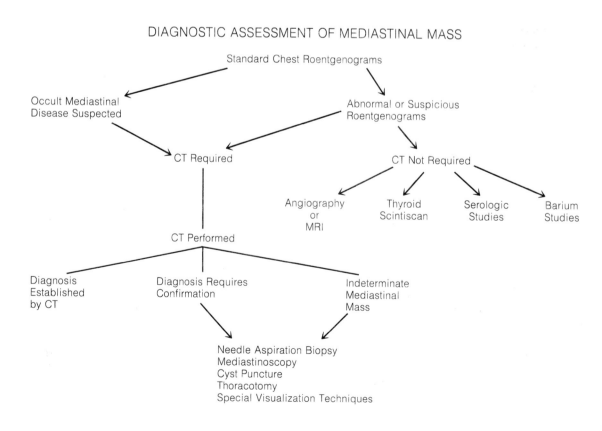

DIAGNOSTIC ASSESSMENT OF MEDIASTINAL MASS

from the standard films and the physical examination; in such cases, a radioactive iodine scintiscan would be chosen by some, whereas others would employ CT. In many instances, an esophageal hiatal hernia can be recognized from the standard films. A clinical diagnosis of mediastinal granulomatous lymphadenopathy due to tuberculosis, coccidioidomycosis, or histoplasmosis can sometimes be made from the clinical history, skin tests, exposure history, serologic studies, and standard roentgen studies; CT may therefore not be required in many such cases. Although some mediastinal lesions (fat pads, pericardial cyst) are sometimes diagnosed from the appearance on standard chest films, CT is advisable for confirmation in most instances.

CT Required

This group includes patients with occult mediastinal lesions and most patients with abnormal or suspicious chest roentgenograms. The CT features employed in the decision process include the size, shape, location, and density of the lesion; the contour and sharpness of the edge; and the relationship to (and effect on) neighboring normal structures. In some cases, the diagnosis will be established by CT; in others, the diagnosis will be strongly suggested, but confirmation will be required; and in still others, the diagnosis will remain obscure after CT.

Diagnosis Established by CT

In many instances, a diagnosis will be established (or confirmed) by CT with sufficient assurance to negate the need for further diagnostic tests. Examples of such lesions include pericardial fat pads, pleuropericardial cyst, some other cystic lesions, hiatal hernia, foramen of Morgagni hernia, lipoma, diffuse lipomatosis, diaphragmatic hernia containing omentum or bowel, pancreatic pseudocyst, aneurysms and other vascular masses, dermoid teratoma containing a tooth, and some thyroid masses. Many of these mediastinal masses will be subjected to therapeutic thoracotomy. In the patient with clinical evidence for mediastinitis, CT may be confirmatory for both localized and diffuse lesions.[15]

Diagnosis Requires Confirmation

The diagnosis of thymoma can be made by CT with considerable assurance, but biopsy is usually required to confirm the diagnosis of thymoma and to identify other thymic tumors that resemble thymoma on imaging studies.[16] CT demonstration of capsular invasion helps determine that the lesion is malignant rather than benign. Thoracotomy is usually employed and is therapeutic as well as diagnostic. Although mediastinal lymphadenopathy can be detected and identified by CT, differentiating benign nodes from malignant nodes is difficult, and determining the specific etiology requires lymph node biopsy. Nodes in the paratracheal areas are best approached by mediastinoscopy or transtracheal aspiration biopsy; transthoracic needle biopsy or exploratory thoracotomy may be employed for lymphadenopathy in the anterior or posterior compartments.

Some cystic masses require needle puncture to determine their nature. The posterior compartment lesions of extramedullary hematopoiesis can be detected by CT and a presumptive diagnosis made from the concurrent hematologic abnormality, but transthoracic needle biopsy is sometimes indicated. On occasion, vascular lesions detected by CT will require angiographic or MRI studies to obtain precise details of the lesion.

Intramediastinal paragangliomas or parathyroid tumors will often be detected by CT, but determination of the nature of the mass depends on specialized clinical and radiologic techniques. Thoracotomy with removal of the lesion is confirmatory.

Indeterminate Mediastinal Mass

This category includes mediastinal masses that are detected by CT but that almost always require other diagnostic studies because CT fails to establish a precise diagnosis with any degree of certainty. Such lesions include teratomas and other germ cell tumors, connective tissue tumors, lymphangiomas, Castleman's disease, neurogenic tumors, enteric and neurenteric cysts, thoracic myelocele, paraganglioma, and parathyroid adenoma.

In some instances, mediastinoscopy or transthoracic needle biopsy will suffice to identify the nature of the mass. In most cases, however, these lesions will require exploratory thoracotomy.

REFERENCES

1. Proto AV. Mediastinal anatomy: emphasis on conventional images with anatomic and computed

tomographic correlations. J Thorac Imag 1987;2(1):1–48.

2. Lillington GA. A diagnostic approach to chest diseases. 3rd ed. Baltimore: Williams & Wilkins, 1987:389–412.

3. Parish JM, Rosenow EC III, Muhm JR. Mediastinal masses: clues to interpretation of radiologic studies. Postgrad Med 1984;76(3):173–86.

4. Feigin DS, Padua EM. Mediastinal masses: a system for diagnosis based on computed tomography. CT 1986;10(1):11–21.

5. Stanford W, Doty DB. The role of venography and surgery in the management of patients with superior vena cava obstruction. Ann Thorac Surg 1986;41:158–63.

6. Wernecke K, Potter R, Peters PE, Koch P. Parasternal mediastinal sonography: sensitivity in the detection of anterior mediastinal and subcarinal tumors. AJR 1988;150:1021–6.

7. Park H-M, Tarver RD, Siddiqui AR, Schauwecker DS, Wellman HN. Efficacy of thyroid scintigraphy in the diagnosis of intrathoracic goiter. AJR 1987;148:527–9.

8. Pearlberg JL, Sandler MA, Talpos GB, Beute GH. Computed tomographic evaluation of intrathoracic thyroid malignancy. Comput Med Imag Graphics 1989;13:411–7.

9. Sheps SG, Brown ML. Localization of mediastinal paragangliomas (pheochromocytoma). Chest 1985;87:807–9.

10. Westcott JL. Percutaneous transthoracic needle biopsy. Radiology 1988;169:593–601.

11. Von Schultess GK, McMurdo K, Tscholakoff D, de Geer G, Gamsu G, Higgins CB. Mediastinal masses: MR imaging. Radiology 1986;158:289–96.

12. Linder J, Olsen GA, Johnson WW. Fine-needle aspiration biopsy of the mediastinum. Am J Med 1986;81:1005–8.

13. Nath PH, Sanders C, Holley HC, McElvein RB. Percutaneous fine needle aspiration in the diagnosis and management of mediastinal cysts in adults. South Med J 1988;81:1225–8.

14. Ferguson MK, Lee E, Skinner DB, Little AG. Selective operative approach for diagnosis and treatment of anterior mediastinal masses. Ann Thorac Surg 1987;44:583–6.

15. Breatnach E, Nath PH, Delany DJ. The role of computed tomography in acute and subacute mediastinitis. Clin Radiol 1986;37:139–45.

16. Batra P, Hermann C, Mulder D. Mediastinal imaging in myasthenia gravis: correlation of chest radiography, CT, MR, and surgical findings. AJR 1987;148:515–9.

MENSTRUAL DYSFUNCTION

GEOFFREY P. REDMOND

SYNONYMS: Amenorrhea, Oligomenorrhea

BACKGROUND

Normal menstruation requires normal anatomy and function of the hypothalamus, pituitary, ovary, adrenal, uterus, and vagina. Actual or perceived abnormalities of menstruation are a frequent reason for women becoming concerned about their health and seeking medical assistance. From the physician's perspective, changes in menstruation may be a helpful clue to the presence of systemic disease. The purpose of this chapter is to enable the physician to evaluate changes in menstrual cyclicity and to evaluate the possibility of systemic medical illness as a causative factor when appropriate.

Alterations in cyclic body functions frequently give rise to great apprehension. Yet few female patients and few physicians, whether male or female, have a clear idea of the normal limits for parameters of the menstrual cycle. Treolar et al.[1] in their landmark study reported on menstrual cycle length and other characteristics in a very large series of normal women. With the exception of the early teens and later middle years, a cycle length of 21 to 40 days is approximately ±2 standard deviations from the mean. A pattern of longer or shorter cycles is suggestive of a potentially significant abnormality, and some degree of investigation should be carried out. If the deviation is present for only one or two cycles, further observation may be all that is required. If normal cycling resumes, workup may not be necessary.

It is obvious that pregnancy and its complications must be considered when there has been any change in the menstrual pattern. In particular, changes in bleeding pattern may be the only early sign of ectopic pregnancy, which may rapidly become emergent. The physician dealing with menstrual disorders must always be alert to this possibility. Readers are referred to standard texts on gynecology for further discussion of this important issue. The discussion in this chapter will assume that pregnancy has been ruled out.

Traditionally, a distinction is made between primary and secondary amenorrhea. However, the causes overlap to a considerable extent. A more useful distinction is between females with primary amenorrhea but otherwise normal secondary sexual development and those in whom no estrogen-related changes have occurred. Thelarche occurs at an average age in American females of about $10\frac{1}{2}$ years and about 6 months later in other populations. If breast development has not started by age $12\frac{1}{2}$ or 13, thorough investigation should be carried out. From an endocrinologic viewpoint, thelarche is as clinically relevant a milestone as menarche. Although most texts suggest 16 years as the upper normal age limit for menarche, this is too old. Age $14\frac{1}{2}$ or 15 is more appropriate, assuming thelarche has occurred. Lack of thelarche should prompt investigation at an earlier age, as just stated. Progressing from thelarche to menarche takes two to two and a half years; a prolonged interval should create concern. However, a female who started thelarche late but whose puberty is progressing only requires observation.

Special concerns relate to menstrual disorders in adolescent females. While it is usually assumed that infrequent or irregular periods in the first year or two after menarche are a normal finding, the limited research available indicates that this is not the case.[2,3] The actual data suggest that oligomenorrhea beginning a year or two after menarche is *more* likely to be persistent than oligomenorrhea beginning later in life. Accordingly, a workup should not be deferred more than a few months even in a very young teenager. If preceded by six or more months of regular menstruation, the onset of oligomenorrhea is highly suggestive of an underlying abnormality.

Teens of both sexes are extremely anxious about the normality of their sexual development. They are quite concerned about even small deviations from the perceived normal, even though such concerns are not always directly expressed. Often, adequate evaluation is omitted because of embarrassment of both patient and physician. Parents may become anxious when these matters are discussed. It is often helpful to clarify that the concerns relate to physical health and are no different than they would be for any other part of the body. Thorough history and physical examination should not be unduly stressful for a teenage girl when carried out by a physician, either female or male, who has acquired comfort in working with teenagers and who is sympathetic to their concerns. It is also important that the mother understand the medical necessity of the evaluation so that she will help enlist her daughter's cooperation. Sometimes adult women also wish to avoid discussion or examination related to the reproductive system. It is misguided to omit these aspects of the history and physical because it is often the unusually modest patient who may fail to mention clinically important alterations in function.

HYPOTHALAMIC-PITUITARY DISORDERS

It is convenient to review causes of menstrual dysfunction in a cephalodcaudad sequence. The first medical disorder to be considered in the woman with oligomenorrhea is neoplasia of the pituitary or suprasellar region. Prolactinomas inhibit menstruation by their increased release of this hormone. Prolactin probably produces cessation of menses by action at the hypothalamic, pituitary, and ovarian levels combined. However, the hypothalamic action is probably most important because recent studies suggest prolactin inhibition can be bypassed by the cyclic administration of gonadotropin releasing hormone (GnRH). Other tumors in this region inhibit menses by their mass effect. We have reported amenorrhea in association with hydrocephalus.[4] Whether this is due to the mild increase in prolactin sometimes found or to hypothalamic dysfunction induced by pressure is uncertain, but the latter explanation appears more likely. Suprasellar tumors in this area may produce other damage because of the expanding mass of the lesion. The most devastating effect is visual loss or blindness resulting from chiasmatic pressure. Accordingly, when an intracranial tumor is suspected as the cause of amenorrhea, computed tomography (CT) or magnetic resonance imaging (MRI) scanning of the region is mandatory. Visual fields are important when a documented lesion is shown; however, normal visual fields do not rule out a tumor in this region. Follicle stimulating hormone (FSH)-secreting tumors produce hypogonadism by their mass effect but may be confused with premature gonadal failure because immunoassayable FSH is elevated. These tumors have been most often described in middle-aged or older males but can occur in women.

Simple measurement of serum prolactin should identify patients with prolactinomas. Because mild elevations of prolactin are common and usually benign, one would like to have a lower limit below which CT scanning is not necessary. Unfortunately, however, our own experience and that of others indicates that quite large tumors may be found even with prolactin levels in the 30s or 40s. Accordingly, when prolactin is elevated, imaging studies must be done. A decision as to whether to perform these studies in the amenorrheic woman with a normal level of prolactin is more difficult. This is not necessary most of the time; however, the presence of other findings or symptoms suggestive of an intracranial lesion should prompt imaging studies, which would include: headaches, visual complaints, seizures, or other changes in central nervous system (CNS) function.

In most cases, medical treatment with the drug bromocriptine is sufficient to produce lowering of the level of prolactin, shrinkage of the tumor, and resumption of menses.[5] Even when field cuts are present, they often reverse with bromocriptine. This drug is also highly effective in inducing ovulation in hyperprolactinemic women. However, the drug can cause dizziness and nausea and is not always well tolerated. Adolescent patients in particular seem to have difficulty with it. At times, birth control pills or other estrogen supplementation is appropriate in spite of the tendency to cause some enlargement in the size of the tumor. The decision to treat women with prolactinomas with oral contraceptives or estrogens should be made by a physician experienced in the evaluation of these conditions. Since tumor expansion is likely to occur in late pregnancy, it is essential that the patient be closely monitored by someone with experience in management of these lesions.

Treatment of other tumors causing amenorrhea is dependent on the location and histopathology of the lesion. In general, estrogen and progestin replacement therapy is appropriate for the amenorrhea.

A variety of other medical illnesses can cause amenorrhea through pituitary damage, including such conditions as histiocytosis X and hemosiderosis.

Stress, weight loss, and exercise can cause amenorrhea, but amenorrhea should not be casually ascribed to these factors. At any point in time, everyone is under stress; most are trying to diet; and many are exercising. The relationship of amenorrhea to severity of stress has been well described in Drew's classic paper.[6] Whether minor stresses, such as traveling or starting college, can cause amenorrhea is unclear.[7,8] If so, only a small minority have menstrual change under these circumstances. The stress required to induce a high incidence of amenorrhea is quite severe. For example, only 23 per cent of nurses interned as prisoners of war in Manila during the Japanese occupation were amenorrheic.

Similarly, weight loss must be substantial—generally to 85 per cent of ideal body weight or a body mass index of less than 18—in order for amenorrhea to result. There is an impression that menses may cease in females with anorexia nervosa before substantial weight loss has occurred. Unquestionably, anorexia nervosa, like malnutrition due to other causes, and other systemic illness cause amenorrhea. As with stress, this is an overused diagnosis. Not all thin or dieting women with amenorrhea have anorexia nervosa. Modest exercise regimens—a few hours a week of running or aerobics—do not cause amenorrhea. Women must run 30 or more miles a week before amenorrhea is likely to occur.

PREMATURE OVARIAN FAILURE

Premature ovarian failure, or early menopause, is probably more common than usually recognized. In this situation, the ovary fails at an unusually early age. The usual cutoff is age 40 or younger, although the average age of menopause in the United States is about 50. The signs and symptoms of premature menopause are identical to those of normal menopause, that is, hot flashes, mood changes, and vaginal dryness. Many such cases are masked because of the common practice of treating amenorrhea with birth control pills without diagnostic evaluation. The patient on the pill will have no menopausal symptoms and will menstruate on a regular basis. Frequently, premature menopause shows itself when birth control pills are discontinued, menses do not return, and hot flashes emerge as a source of patient discomfort. In such cases, of course, it is impossible to know how long the ovarian failure has been present. Premature ovarian failure is one of the causes of amenorrhea that may be associated with significant medical illnesses, and a thorough medical evaluation should be carried out when premature menopause occurs.

The first category is genetic and includes not only the varying forms of gonadal dysgenesis but also a diverse group of syndromes and metabolic errors, for example, galactosemia and 17-alpha-hydroxylase deficiency. The most common form of gonadal dysgenesis is Turner's syndrome with a 45XO karyotype. However, a variety of mosaic forms of gonadal dysgenesis occur, and the associated phenotypic features such as webbing of the neck, short fourth metacarpal, wide-spaced nipples, and short stature may not be present. Indeed, in some women with the mosaic forms, ovulation may occur for months to years before the ovarian defect becomes apparent. For this reason, karyotyping is frequently appropriate in evaluating premature menopause. When there is a fragment of a Y chromosome present, there is a greatly increased risk of ovarian tumors, and prompt gonadectomy should be performed.

Autoimmune oophoritis is another cause of premature menopause. The histopathology is similar to that seen in other forms of autoimmune inflammation, such as Hashimoto's thyroiditis or the insulitis present at the onset of insulin-dependent diabetes. Although the ovarian damage is probably mediated by cellular immunity, there may be measurable autoantibodies against the ovary and adrenal gland. However, short of positive antibodies, there is no sure method of diagnosis other than ovarian biopsy. It is prudent to inform the pathologist of the expected findings since, in our experience, ovarian tissue showing these changes is frequently read as normal when ovarian surgery has been performed for a coexistent condition. Ovarian cysts are quite common in association with autoimmune oophoritis, perhaps because of the intense stimulation of the ovary by the elevated gonadotropins. However, whether there is a true increase in incidence or whether cysts are detected simply because the cessation of ovarian function prompts pelvic examination is uncertain. It is likely that in some affected individuals immunosuppression will permit the occurrence of ovulation. We have reported one such case[9] in which a high dose of methylprednisolone was used. However, there is little work in this area to indicate the risk-benefit issues of this approach to treatment. In the absence of desire for pregnancy, standard replacement with estrogen and progestin is sufficient therapy.

Many other autoimmune diseases have been associated with premature ovarian failure, including Addison's disease, multiple sclerosis, myasthenia gravis, rheumatoid arthritis, and others. For this reason, women with premature menopause should have a thorough medical evaluation, and signs and symptoms suggestive of an underlying autoimmune disorder should be followed up. Occasionally, autoimmune ovarian failure may be associated with other autoimmune conditions that are readily visible on physical examination, notably vitiligo and alopecia areata.

A puzzling cause of ovarian failure is so-called Savage's syndrome in which there are many follicles in the ovary but none mature beyond the primordial stage. The mechanism is thought to be a resistance to gonadotropin actions, but the cause is unknown. Some patients with Savage's syndrome have ovulated while on replacement therapy with conjugated estrogen and medroxyprogesterone acetate. Accordingly, there is some possibility that a patient with Savage's syndrome treated this way may achieve pregnancy. However, the odds that this will occur are low.

The fourth major category of ovarian failure is environmental. The most common causes seen in this country are chemotherapy, notably MOPP (mechlorethamine, Oncovin [vincristine], procarbazine, and prednisone) for Hodgkin's disease and radiotherapy in which the ovary is included in the field. Occasionally, the ovarian dysfunction induced by these agents is temporary, but often permanent ovarian failure occurs. Usually, the medical history makes the cause of ovarian failure evident in these situations.

ANDROGENIC DISORDERS

The group of androgen excess disorders is a very frequent cause of oligomenorrhea. In addition to lack of menstruation, or anovulation, these conditions are also associated with undesirable skin and hair changes and with insulin resistance of varying degrees. The skin changes include persistent or severe acne, hirsutism, and androgenic alopecia. Because these conditions are embarrassing, patients do their best to conceal them. Thus, makeup may partially conceal acne lesions, and bleach, depilatory, plucking, or razor may be used to make unwanted hair less visible. The modified Ferriman-Gallwey scoring system provides a useful checklist of areas on which androgen-dependent hair appears. Androgenic alopecia is the mild variant of male pattern baldness that occurs commonly in women. The anterior hairline is preserved in all but the most severe cases, but this occurs on vertex, crown, and sometimes temples. Any of these physical findings suggest the possibility of androgenic excess as the cause of the menstrual abnormalities.

Use of the term polycystic ovaries for this group of conditions is not very helpful. The biochemical disturbance of excessive androgen secretion or action does not correlate fully with the anatomic change of cysts in the ovary. In particular, the early pubertal ovary contains many small cysts. We have seen several cases in which pelvic ultrasound was performed for pain or other nonendocrine complaint in an adolescent girl who was then wrongly labeled as having polycystic ovaries on the basis of this normal finding. To laypeople, the term cyst is taken to mean tumor, and considerable unnecessary anxiety may be created. Finally, our studies with dexamethasone suppression indicate that assignment of ovarian origin of the elevated androgens is frequently incorrect.

The degree of skin manifestation with androgenic disorders is quite variable and depends as much on the target organ responsiveness as it does on the actual androgen level. Indeed, one of the puzzling features of this group of conditions is the limited correlation between androgen levels and clinical manifestations. Although more than half of women with hirsutism and androgenic alopecia or cystic acne do have elevated androgens, others simply seem to be unusually sensitive to normal levels of circulating androgens.[10] Sometimes androgens are normal in the presence of severe skin manifestations or virilization, and menstrual disturbance may be associated as well. In these situations, it is tempting to speculate that androgens may have been elevated in past years or that they are elevated only at some times during the cycle. If that is the case, one or two random blood levels may

miss the elevation. We are currently studying the changes in androgens during the cycle to clarify this issue.

One of the classic controversies regarding androgen excess has been the relative role of the adrenal and ovary. Our recent study suggests that the majority of women with high androgens have a substantial fall in their level after dexamethasone suppression testing.[11] This does not prove that the adrenal is the source of the elevated androgen but rather that the androgens are being secreted in response to adrenocorticotropic hormone (ACTH) stimulation. We have also confirmed the long-standing clinical assumption that those women with high androgens and menstrual disturbance are more likely to have an ovarian source than those in whom menstruation is normal. Dysfunctional bleeding is less frequently associated with high androgens than is oligoamenorrhea.

Insulin resistance ranging from mild to severe is more common in women with androgenic disorders.[12] In many instances, glucose tolerance testing (GTT) is appropriate for these women. Hemoglobin A_{1C}, unfortunately, is not sensitive enough to serve as a screen for mild adult-onset (type II) diabetes. The presence of acanthosis nigricans may be a clue to a greater degree of insulin resistance. However, some women with this skin change have totally normal GTTs. This lesion consists of hyperpigmentation, thickening with a velvety appearance, and in severe cases, skin tags. Intertriginous areas are affected, especially axillae and the back of the neck. Obesity is a major predisposing risk factor for diabetes in adults. When this is present with androgen excess, screening for noninsulin-dependent diabetes should be considered. A number of studies clearly indicate the presence of hyperinsulinism in women with elevated androgens. We are pursuing the relationship of androgen excess in diabetes in our own studies; however, in our present state of knowledge, it is unclear what factors determine the presence or absence of diabetes in androgenized obese women.

Although obesity is frequently thought to be a feature of Stein-Leventhal syndrome, our own work indicates that the weight of many women with androgenic conditions is normal.[10] We have found, however, that the ovarian contribution to the circulating androgens is greater in obese women, and the adrenal contribution is relatively greater in the more slender women. This appears to contradict the common belief that obesity produces androgenization by increased adrenal activity.

We have compared androgen levels in women with severe acne, hirsutism, and androgenic alopecia.[8] The proportion of elevations of dehydroepiandrosterone sulfate (DHEA-S), testosterone, and androstenedione are similar in all three groups, although a somewhat higher percentage of women with alopecia had normal levels. This may reflect that the group was, on the mean, about six years older.

Age is an important determinant of androgen levels. DHEA-S, in particular, is extremely low in prepubertal girls, rises during the teens and early twenties, and then gradually declines to very low levels in elderly individuals. Changes in testosterone and androstenedione are also correlated with age. Generally, levels of all three androgens are extremely low in postmenopausal women. Some postmenopausal women do have a gradual increase in facial hair, but the cause of this is unknown. Although it has been suggested that it is due to decreased sex hormone binding globulin (SHBG) levels, our experience indicates that free testosterone levels in this group of women are also extremely low. When androgen levels in postmenopausal women are elevated, it is important to do a thorough diagnostic evaluation. We have seen some cases in which the androgens suppress readily with dexamethasone, suggesting the problem is a disturbance in adrenal function. Another cause of postmenopausal hyperandrogenism is thecal cell hyperplasia of the ovaries. It is important to rule out neoplasia as a cause of any elevation in a postmenopausal woman. The response of hair growth to androgens appears to be less in this age group, so hirsutism will be less dramatic at a given androgen level.

A variety of anatomic anomalies can result in amenorrhea. These can be acquired, such as Asherman's syndrome (uterine synechiae from excessive curettage), but are usually congenital. While a transverse vaginal septum and imperforate hymen are primarily gynecologic in their implications, müllerian agenesis (Rokitansky-Kuster-Hauser syndrome) may have associated renal, vertebral, and rib anomalies and deafness. Androgen insensitivity may present as anatomic amenorrhea when an amenorrheic patient is found to lack a uterus and fallopian tubes. Such individuals have an XY karyotype but develop as phenotypic females because they cannot respond to androgens. Gonads must be removed as early as possible because of the risks of virilization and later tumor formation. Congenital steroid biosynthesis abnormalities can result in amenorrhea but present much earlier because of genital ambiguity.

TREATMENT

Treatment of oligomenorrhea is dependent on the particular manifestations of the condition and the goals of the patient. The importance of estrogen replacement in women in whom levels are low is now well accepted.[13] In younger women, a low-dose combination birth control pill is usually the simplest treatment and has the advantage of providing contraception as well. The use of a sequential regimen of estrogen and progesterone is usually preferable in older women but does not provide contraception. The use of a progestin to avoid an increased risk of endometrial cancer is now well documented. This protective effect is dependent on the number of days the progestin is given during each cycle as well as the dose on each day. A variety of schedules are available, and choice depends on the needs of the patient and desirability of monthly withdrawal bleeding. Although birth control pills or other estrogen replacement is probably safe for most women with microprolactinomas, considerable care must be exercised in this situation. The use of bromocriptine (Parlodel) is more specific. Bromocriptine is not effective in oligomenorrhea that is not due to hyperprolactinemia.

The treatment of androgen excess disorders is more complex. If the concern is the skin manifestations of cystic acne, hirsutism, or androgenic alopecia, we have found the most effective approach is to combine an androgen antagonist such as spironolactone or cimetidine with suppression of the elevated androgens. For suppression, we generally employ ultra-low doses of dexamethasone if the source appears to be adrenal. A combination birth control pill—or, in unusual situations, the GnRH analogue leuprolide—is employed when the ovary is the apparent source. Although we have been impressed with the excellent response of acne, hirsutism, and to a somewhat lesser degree, androgenic alopecia, this form of treatment is complex and requires considerable time for the benefits to manifest. Patient motivation and comprehension of the regimen are critical for success.

It is very important to discuss fertility issues in women who present for evaluation of oligomenorrhea. When the goal is conception, treatment is quite different and involves the use of various methods of ovulation induction. It is not unusual for a woman whose real interest is in pregnancy to come for treatment of hirsutism or other manifestations because she has been wrongly advised that pregnancy is totally impossible. In such circumstances, referral to an infertility center is most appropriate.

It is vital to discuss the impact of any other treatment on ovulation. Many women with oligomenorrhea come to believe that they will not become pregnant and do not use effective contraception. Some other treatments for oligomenorrhea, notably bromocriptine and dexamethasone, will increase the probability of ovulation. It is essential that women be warned about this and that effective contraception be provided promptly.

Only a minority of women with menstrual disturbance will be found to have serious underlying medical conditions. However, it is our experience that the majority of women are very grateful to have the problem thoroughly investigated and prefer a thorough approach. Casual reassurance that is not based on complete evaluation is rarely convincing to a concerned patient. The results of the investigation also make possible more accurate counseling regarding the implications of the menstrual disturbance on fertility and other aspects of the woman's health. For this reason, the effort spent on a thorough evaluation of this problem is rewarding to patient and physician alike.

REFERENCES

1. Treolar AE, Boynton RE, Behm BG, Brown BW. Variation of the human menstrual cycle throughout life. Int J Fertil 1967;12:77–126.
2. Southam AL, Richart RM. The prognosis for adolescents with menstrual abnormalities. Am J Obstet Gynecol 1966;94:637–45.
3. Venturoli S, Procu E, Fabbri R, et al. Postmenarchal evolution of endocrine pattern and ovarian aspect in adolescents with menstrual irregularities. Fertil Steril 1987;48:78–85.
4. Redmond GP, Gidwani G, Bay J, Hahn J, Rothner D. Menstrual dysfunction in adolescents with increased intracranial pressure. Pediatr Res 1985;32:310–7.
5. Sisson DA, Sheehan JP, Sheeler LR. The natural history of untreated microprolactinomas. Fertil Steril 1987;48:67–71.
6. Drew FL. The epidemiology of secondary amenorrhea. J Chronic Dis 1961; 14:396–407.
7. Singh KB. Menstrual disorders in college students. Am J Obstet Gynecol 1981;140:299–301.
8. Bachmann GA, Kemmann E. Prevalence of oligomenorrhea and amenorrhea in a college population. Am J Obstet Gynecol 1982;144:98–102.
9. Redmond GP, Gidwani G. Reproductive, endocrine and immunological abnormalities in women with premature menopause. Fertil Steril 1984;43:211–6.
10. Redmond GP, Bergfeld W, Gupta M, et al. Comparison of hormonal abnormalities in women with different manifestations of androgen excess. In: Research in gynecological endocrinology. New York: Parthenon Publishing, 1986.
11. Redmond GP, Gidwani G, Bergfeld W, et al. Regulation of excessive androgen secretion in women: role of ACTH responsive endocrine tissue. Fertil Steril 1987;48(Suppl):82–90.
12. Burghen GA, Givens JR, Kitabchi AE. Correlation of hyperandrogenism with hyperinsulinism in polycystic ovarian disease. J Clin Endocrinol Metab 1980;50:113–6.
13. Speroff L, Glass RH, Kase NG. Clinical gynecological endocrinology and infertility. Baltimore: Williams and Wilkins, 1989.

MYOFASCIAL PAIN

ELLIOTT L. SEMBLE and CHRISTOPHER WISE

SYNONYMS: Trigger Points, Myofascial Pain Syndrome, Myofascial Syndrome

BACKGROUND

Myofascial pain is extremely common and experienced by practically every individual at some time in his or her life. It originates in muscles at localized spots called myofascial trigger points and results in local and referred pain.

Each one of the approximately 500 skeletal muscles in our bodies is at risk for acute or chronic strain. The result of this strain is the development of myofascial trigger points with a characteristic pattern or combinations of patterns of referred pain. Pain is often exacerbated by prolonged immobility and by overexertion of affected muscles. Stretching the affected area, cooling, and compression may also cause referred pain.

A myofascial trigger point may be defined as an area of hyperirritability in a skeletal muscle that is painful with pressure and gives rise to referred pain, tenderness, and autonomic phenomena (e.g., pallor during palpation of a trigger point, followed by reactive hyperemia).[1] Trigger points may be differentiated as being active or latent. Active trigger points cause pain either at rest or in relation to muscular activity. Latent trigger points may demonstrate all the features of an active trigger point except that latent trigger points cause pain only when examined by palpation. Only *active* trigger points are responsible for the pain reported by the patient.[2] Latent trigger points are very common. They affect nearly 50 per cent of the population by early adulthood.[2] Among 200 unselected asymptomatic young adult Air Force recruits, Sola et al.[3] demonstrated focal tenderness in shoulder girdle muscles in 54 per cent of the females and 45 per cent of the males. Referred pain from these trigger points was noted in 5 per cent of these subjects.

Chronic pain centers have reported a high frequency of patients with myofascial trigger points.[2] Some 85 per cent of 283 consecutive admissions to a comprehensive pain center were due to myofascial pain syndromes.[4] Many patients seen in dental clinics may have myofascial trigger points. Fricton et al.[5] found that 164 of 296 (55.4 per cent) patients referred for chronic head and neck pain of at least six months' duration had myofascial pain syndromes as their primary diagnosis.

Myofascial pain syndromes are often seen in general medical practice. Ten per cent of 61 consecutive consultation or follow-up patients for all causes in an internal medicine group practice had trigger points that were responsible for their complaints;[2] 31 per cent of those with pain symptoms were felt to be due to myofascial trigger points.

The severity of myofascial trigger points ranges from painless limitation of motion due to latent trigger points to disabling pain caused by very active trigger points. Although the pain is not life-threatening, patients who have reported other types of severe pain (e.g., pain from myocardial infarction, renal colic, fracture pain) note that trigger point pain can be as intense.[1] The pain experienced from myofascial trigger points is often incapacitating and can adversely affect quality of life.

Although the exact cause(s) of myofascial pain is unknown, myofascial trigger points often present initially as syndromes affecting a single muscle due to acute strain.[6] Occasionally, multiple muscles are activated simultaneously owing to a traumatic event.[7] If repeated episodes of muscular stress occur or perpetuating factors are present, many muscles can be affected over weeks or months owing to chronic muscle strain.

Mechanical stresses perpetuate trigger points in patients with chronic myofascial syndromes. The origin of these physical stresses includes structural abnormalities such as leg length discrepancy, small hemipelvis, long second metatarsal bone, and short upper arms.[9] Leg length discrepancies as little as 6 mm may aggravate myofascial pain after activation of quadratus lumborum trigger points by injury. Patients with a small hemipelvis (i.e., its vertical dimension is short on one side) may develop chronic muscle strain in the quadratus lumborum, scalene, and sternocleidomastoid muscles. The presence of a long second metatarsal bone may perpetuate myofascial pain by overloading muscles in the low back and lower extremities during walking. Shortness of the upper arms in relation to torso height causes stress in the shoulder girdle elevator muscles during sitting and aggravates myofascial pain in the upper trapezius and levator scapulae muscles.

Postural stress may also aggravate trigger points, owing to misfitting furniture, poor sitting and standing posture, or muscle abuse.[1] Prolonged sitting in poorly designed chairs may result in chronic muscle strain. Nonphysiologic positioning at a desk or work surface and head tilting due to poorly adjusted glasses perpetuate muscle stress. Standing correctly avoids the chronic shortening of the pectoral muscles that occurs with a kyphotic, round-shouldered posture. Muscle abuse is caused by improper body mechanics. Movements may be excessively stressful or repetitive, resulting in aggravation of myofascial pain. In addition, lack of movement, especially when a muscle is in a shortened position, may aggravate trigger points. This occurs during sleep or when a muscle cannot be moved through its full range of motion owing to fracture or joint disease.

Psychologic factors including depression and anxiety may perpetuate myofascial pain. Depression and chronic pain are closely associated and result in prolonged inactivity and immobility. Anxiety may be experienced as muscle tension, which causes muscle overload and aggravation of trigger points.

HISTORY

History of Present Illness

The medical history should include data regarding the onset and location of pain. The quality and severity should be noted as well as symptoms associated with the pain. Is the pain aching in quality? Is it dull or intense? Is it deep or superficial? Does it vary in intensity from hour to hour and day to day? Does the pain occur only with activity or is it present at rest?

Other questions that may be pertinent include: Does the patient have poor sleep habits (Moldofsky and Scarisbrick[8] have shown that a primary sleep disturbance may contribute to the pain associated with trigger points)? Is there associated stiffness, weakness, and decreased range of motion of involved muscles (stiffness of muscles is often seen in the morning after arising from bed or after sitting in one position for an extended period of time)? Do cold and inclement weather aggravate symptoms?

Social, Vocational, and Avocational History

What is the patient's job and in what type of leisure activities does he or she participate? Does the patient's job involve prolonged sitting or standing? Are repetitive activities being performed either at home or at work? Is the patient under stress at home or on the job? What are the patient's habits regarding exercise?

Past Medical History

Has the patient suffered any injuries? Is there a previous history of myofascial pain?

Focused Queries

1. *Can you remember the day you were first aware of the pain? What position or movement or what stress or trauma was associated with the onset of pain? What were the specified details of the mechanical stresses associated with the onset of pain? If the pain started after a motor vehicle accident, what was the direction of impact?* The responses to these questions are useful in identifying which muscles are most likely involved in myofascial pain.

2. *Does position or muscular activity affect pain intensity?* Myofascial trigger points develop in muscles subject to repetitive or continuous stress.

3. *Have you been under psychologic stress?* Psychologic factors may perpetuate myofascial pain and result in chronic pain and depression.

4. *Do you have poor sleeping habits?* A primary sleep disturbance is often associated with myofascial pain.[8] Pain may be intensified by sleeping in positions that produce pressure

on myofascial trigger points or cause the involved muscle to remain in a contracted (shortened) position.

5. *Does cold or wet weather exacerbate your pain?* Patients with myofascial trigger points often report that certain climatic conditions aggravate their pain.

PHYSICAL EXAMINATION

The physical examination in a patient with a myofascial pain syndrome has three basic purposes: (1) A general physical examination should exclude visceral processes that might simulate a regional pain syndrome; (2) local articular or periarticular pathology should be sought as a cause for the pain, and (3) trigger points within muscle groups should be sought to confirm the myofascial origin of pain.

General Examination

Referred pain should always be considered in evaluating the patient with myofascial pain. In the upper body, visceral processes can cause pain patterns suggestive of a myofascial process. In the chest wall area, cardiac and esophageal pathology should be considered, and in the shoulder girdle, intrapulmonary or upper abdominal disease may cause referred pain. Abdominal, retroperitoneal, or pelvic pathology can cause pain referred to the low back, hip girdle, or even into the leg. An extensive search for such visceral processes is not necessary in every patient, but a general physical examination should be considered an important part of the evaluation in all patients.

The Joint Examination

Any evaluation of myofascial pain should include a careful examination of the joints and their supporting structures in the region of pain.[9] In the neck, range of motion should be close to normal in a patient with a pure myofascial problem. However, coexistent cervical spondylosis (osteoarthritis) may give rise to diagnostic confusion. When spondylosis is severe, range of motion will usually be limited both actively and passively. Many myofascial syndromes may be accompanied by muscle tightness that limits range of motion. A return to normal motion with gentle passive stretching or successful therapy suggests that a myofascial rather than spondylitic process

was responsible for the majority of the discomfort in this situation.

In the shoulder girdle, the glenohumeral joint should be examined for range of motion. Subtle loss of abduction or internal or external rotation may suggest an intra-articular process or rotator cuff dysfunction. Reproduction of pain with resisted shoulder movement is also very suggestive of rotator cuff pathology. In myofascial shoulder girdle processes, shoulder movement should be normal and pain not reproduced with resisted movements.

Myofascial lumbar and hip girdle syndromes should not be accompanied by fixed limitation of hip movement. As in the cervical region, exacerbations may be accompanied by muscle tightness that limits motion, but this should improve with stretching or therapy. Marked limitation in lumbar or hip movement that does not improve with stretching should suggest a primary arthritic process in the spine, sacroiliac joints, or hip.

Trigger Points

The demonstration of trigger points in muscle groups is essential to the diagnosis of a myofascial pain syndrome.[2,10] As discussed previously, a trigger point is a reproducible spot of exquisite tenderness located within a tight palpable band of muscle fibers. Pressure on such an area will produce a "jump sign" response in the patient and may be associated with a local twitch response in the band of muscle fibers. Palpation of a trigger point will reproduce the pain experienced by the patient. The distribution and quality of the pain reproduced by palpation will be similar to the patient's pain complaints. Trigger points should be distinguished from "tender points," which are areas of tenderness that do not cause a radiation of pain and are more often described in patients with diffuse myofascial pain (fibrositis or fibromyalgia).[2] Trigger points are best examined in a relaxed muscle after passive stretching by the examiner. The tender areas may be rolled under the examining finger while exerting mild to moderate pressure. Tightness in some of these trigger points may result in decreased ability to undergo active or passive stretching, sometimes resulting in an apparent loss of motion in the area being examined. Trigger points may occur in any muscle group in the body. The location of these trigger points and their area of referred pain will dictate the location of the clinical pain syndrome. Common myofascial pain syndromes and their accompanying trigger points may be categorized according to region: for example, head and neck (sternocleidomastoid, masseter, temporalis, etc.), shoulder girdle (trapezius, levator scapulae, supraspinatus, etc.), arm (brachioradialis, etc.), low back (iliocostalis, serratus, quadratus lumborum, glutei, piriformis, etc.), and leg (gastrocnemius, tibialis anterior, etc.).

DIAGNOSTIC STUDIES

Laboratory tests are used to exclude systemic inflammatory or metabolic diseases, local bony or articular processes, or neuromuscular causes of localized pain. Routine blood tests, such as complete blood count, blood chemistry profiles, urinalysis, and erythrocyte sedimentation rate, should all be normal in patients with myofascial pain syndromes. The necessity for such tests in every patient can be debated, and a thorough laboratory evaluation is not necessary in the young healthy patient with nothing in the history or general physical examination to suggest a systemic disease. On the other hand, the patient with a severe and persistent pain refractory to therapy should be looked at more closely for systemic processes and further tests pursued. Radiographs of the area of pain should be normal in patients with myofascial pain. As with laboratory testing, radiographs should be reserved for patients with suspected systemic processes, limitation of motion of a given joint in the area of pain, or persistent pain that does not respond to early therapeutic maneuvers. The use of specialized imaging techniques such as radioisotope scans, computed tomographic scans, and magnetic resonance imaging should be reserved for more complicated patients to exclude alternative diagnoses. Electromyographic and nerve conduction studies should be considered in patients with suspected neuropathic processes. Although some research suggests subtle electromyographic abnormalities of trigger points, it is difficult to apply these findings to clinical use at present. Early muscle biopsy and thermographic studies have suggested nonspecific abnormalities in patients with myofascial pain syndromes but have little use in current medical practice.

ASSESSMENT

A careful history and physical examination in combination with a limited number of laboratory tests should allow the evaluating physician to make a diagnosis of a myofascial pain syndrome in a majority of situations.[11] Although the differential diagnosis of regional pain includes many illnesses, the conditions most often considered should include: systemic illnesses, inflammatory arthritis, osteoarthritis, tendinitis or bursitis, and fibrositis (fibromyalgia) (Table 1).

Systemic Illnesses

As noted earlier, visceral disease with referred pain should be considered in all patients presenting with localized pain syndromes. A careful history and physical examination should rule out the occasional patient with intracranial, cardiopulmonary, or intra- abdominal disease associated with pain in an area suggestive of a myofascial syndrome. Extensive evaluation to exclude systemic disease is certainly not necessary in the typical patient but should be pursued in patients at higher risks for generalized illness, including the elderly, patients with a history of fever, weight loss, ethanol or drug abuse, corticosteroid or immunosuppressive drug therapy, or any symptoms to suggest a cardiopulmonary or intra-abdominal process.

Inflammatory Arthropathies

Examination of peripheral joints may rule out inflammatory musculoskeletal conditions, including rheumatoid arthritis, systemic lupus erythematosus, polymyositis, scleroderma, or crystal-induced arthritis. Occasionally, a patient with rheumatoid arthritis may present with a localized pain syndrome, but later in the course of the illness definite findings of synovitis become evident. In lupus, arthralgias are common but tend to be diffuse rather than localized. Symptoms in polymyositis are usually more diffuse and symmetric and are accompanied by objective muscle weakness. Scleroderma may occur in localized forms that may initially be hard to distinguish from a myofascial syndrome but are characterized by specific cutaneous findings. Crystal-induced arthropathies, such as gout and pseudogout, are more common in peripheral joints and almost always accompanied by obvious warmth and swelling in a joint rather than isolated tenderness in a muscle group. In the young patient with low back pain, sacroiliac involvement from ankylosing spondylitis should be

TABLE 1. Differential Diagnosis of Regional Pain: Common Causes

REGION	ARTICULAR AND PERIARTICULAR SYNDROMES	COMMON MYOFASCIAL SYNDROMES (MUSCLE GROUPS)
Head and neck	Cervical spondylosis Temporomandibular joint derangement Cervical strain	Suboccipital Masseter Temporalis Sternocleidomastoid Posterior cervicals Trapezius (upper)
Shoulder	Rotator cuff tendinitis, bursitis, adhesive capsulitis Arthritis—glenohumoral, acromioclavicular	Trapezius (lower) Infraspinatus Supraspinatus Deltoid Scalenius Rhomboids
Arm	Arthritis—elbow, wrist, hand joints Epicondylitis—medial and lateral elbow Olecranon bursitis Carpal tunnel syndrome Flexor tenosynovitis	Triceps brachii Supinator
Chest wall	Costochondritis Sternoclavicular arthritis	Pectoralis major and minor Sternalis
Low back and hip girdle	Lumbar spondylosis Ankylosing spondylitis with sacroiliitis Lumbar strain Ischial bursitis Trochanteric bursitis	Quadratus lumborum Paraspinals Gluteals Coccygeus Fascia lata Piriformis
Knee and leg	Arthritis—knee, ankle, foot Anserine bursitis Prepatellar bursitis Collateral ligament strain Achilles tendinitis Plantar fasciitis	Rectus femoris Vastus medialis and lateralis Gastrocnemius Soleus

considered, and pelvic radiographs should be ordered to exclude this possibility.

Osteoarthritis

Radiographic findings of osteoarthritis are common in the cervical and lumbar spine, and such findings increase in frequency with age. A large number of patients with these radiographic abnormalities are asymptomatic, and there is disagreement about the pathogenesis of pain. Thus, the relationship of myofascial pain syndromes to osteoarthritis in the cervical and lumbar regions is unclear at present. It is difficult to make a definite diagnosis of a myofascial pain syndrome in a patient with multiple radiographic abnormalities. On the other hand, such a diagnosis may be very useful, as the trigger point may be the major source of pain in many patients. Often the therapeutic response to treatment for myofascial pain is a useful diagnostic tool, and most clinicians think that therapeutic maneuvers used in myofascial pain syndromes may be helpful in patients with cervical and lumbar osteoarthritis.

Tendinitis and Bursitis

The differentiation of myofascial pain syndromes from tendinitis and bursitis can be difficult clinically. In general, a tendinitis or bursitis is a relatively specific syndrome with a well-defined location and localized physical findings. Trigger points causing radiation of pain should typically not be found in tendinitis or bursitis, and areas of tenderness are usually located directly over tendons and bony prominences rather than in muscle groups. In the shoulder, rotator cuff tendinitis will usually cause a pain more in the lateral deltoid region, and examination may demonstrate tenderness as well as pain reproduced by shoulder movements. Myofascial syndromes in the shoulder usually cause pain and trigger points predominantly in the area of the posterior scapulae. Many patients with shoulder girdle pain may seem to have a combination of both tendinitis and myofascial pain, and clinical differentiation is difficult. The "tennis elbow" syndrome causes tenderness over the lateral epicondyle, whereas myofascial pain in this area usually results in tenderness in the more distal muscle

TABLE 2.   Myofascial Pain and Fibrositis (Fibromyalgia): Differentiating Features

	MYOFASCIAL PAIN	FIBROSITIS (FIBROMYALGIA)
Sex distribution	Male = female	Male:female ratio of 1:10
Site of pain	Regional	Widespread; diffuse
Fatigue	Unusual	Common
Sleep disturbance	Common	Very common (80+ %); nonrestorative; with A.M. fatigue
Restricted motion	Common	Unusual
Tender areas	Local "trigger points" in muscle bellies; palpable bands; twitch response; referred pain zone	Widespread "tender points"; characteristic sites, usually at insertion points, sometimes in asymptomatic areas; no referred pain
Response to therapy	Often good response to local injections; "stretch and spray"; often cured	Poor response to local measures; variable response to systemic medications; seldom cured
Natural history	Usually remits with self-limited dysfunction	Chronic pain syndrome with waxing and waning course; chronic low-grade disability; occasional spontaneous remissions

groups. In the low back, bursitis in the sacral and gluteal areas is difficult to define and may well represent myofascial pain syndromes. Tenderness directly over the greater trochanter at the hip, which is a bony prominence, is usually considered a form of bursitis rather than a myofascial pain syndrome. In the knee and lower leg, medial anserine bursitis, prepatellar and infrapatellar bursitis, and medial and lateral collateral ligament strain are characterized by localized pain in these areas rather than in contiguous muscle groups.

Fibrositis (Fibromyalgia)

Fibrositis is a condition characterized by widespread aching in multiple body regions, often with accompanying fatigue and sleep disturbance, and physical examination findings of multiple tender points.[12,13,14] The clinical syndrome of fibrositis is very closely related to regional myofascial pain syndromes, and distinguishing these two conditions may be difficult. Nevertheless, it is clinically useful to make a distinction between fibrositis and regional myofascial pain because of the differences in pain patterns, physical findings, response to therapy, and even pathogenic mechanisms. Features that distinguish these two syndromes are summarized in Table 2. The major point of differentiation is that fibrositis is a more diffuse pain syndrome involving multiple body areas and is characterized by "tender points" rather than "trigger points."[6,15,16] While trigger points can be found in almost any muscle, tender points are located in characteristic periarticular areas that are often the sites of tendon insertions. A diagnosis of fibrositis requires a history of

widespread pain and the demonstration of tender points by digital palpation at 11 of 18 characteristic sites.[14] However, most usually painful. A biopsy may be necessary to differentiate large traumatic ulcers from primary syphilis, tuberculosis, deep-seated fungal infections, and squamous cell carcinoma.

REFERENCES

1. Travell JG, Simons DG. Myofascial pain and dysfunction: the trigger point manual. Baltimore: Williams & Wilkins, 1983:4–6, 103.
2. Simons DG. Myofascial pain syndrome due to trigger points. In: International Rehabilitation Medicine Association monograph series number 1. Cleveland: Rademaker Printing, 1987:3–39.
3. Sola AE, Rodenberger JL, Gettys BB. Incidence of hypersensitive areas in posterior shoulder muscles. Am J Phys Med 1955;34:585–90.
4. Fishbain DA, Goldberg M, Meagher BR, Steele R, Rosomoff H. Male and female chronic pain patients categorized by DSM-111 psychiatric diagnostic criteria. Pain 1986;26:181–97.
5. Fricton JR, Kroening R, Haley D, Siegart R. Myofascial pain syndromes of the head and neck: a review of clinical characteristics of 164 patients. Oral Surg 1985;60:615–23.
6. Simons DG. Fibrositis/fibromyalgia: a form of myofascial trigger points? Am J Med 1986;81 (Suppl 3A):93–8.
7. Baker BA. The muscle trigger: evidence for overload injury? J Neurol Orthop Med Surg 1986;7:36–44.
8. Moldofsky H, Scarisbrick P. Induction of neurasthenic musculoskeletal pain syndrome by selective sleep stage deprivation. Psychosom Med 1976;28:35–44.
9. Wise CM. Introduction and approach to the patient with musculoskeletal complaints. In: Turner RA, Wise CM, eds. Textbook of rheumatology. New York: Medical Examination Publishing Co, 1986:3–35.

10. Campbell SM. Regional myofascial pain syndromes. Rheum Dis Clin North Am 1989;15:31–44.
11. Hench PK. Evaluation and differential diagnosis of fibromyalgia. Approach to diagnosis and management. Rheum Dis Clin North Am 1989;15:19–29.
12. Smythe HA, Moldofsky H. Two contributions to understanding of the "fibrositis" syndrome. Bull Rheum Dis 1977;28:928–31.
13. Goldenberg D. Fibromyalgia syndrome: an emerging but controversial condition. JAMA 1987;257:2782–7.
14. Wolfe F, Smythe HA, Yunus MB, et al. The American College of Rheumatology 1990 criteria for the classification of fibromyalgia. Report of the Multicenter Criteria Committee. Arthritis Rheum 1990;33:160–72.
15. Bennett RM. Fibrositis: evolution of an enigma [editorial]. J Rheumatol 1986;13:676–8.
16. Sheon RP. Regional myofascial pain and the fibrositis syndrome (fibromyalgia). Comp Therapy 1986;12:42–52.

ORAL ULCERS

J. ROBERT NEWLAND

SYNONYMS: Denture Ulcer, Shingles, Trench Mouth, Oral Chancre, Canker Sore

BACKGROUND

Ulcer formation is a common response of oral mucosa to injury. A variety of injurious agents can cause oral ulcers. These agents include trauma, microorganisms, immunologic defects, and malignant neoplasms.

It has been reported that approximately half of all oral ulcers are the result of traumatic injury.[1] The most common forms of trauma affecting oral mucosa are biting injury and denture irritation.

Oral mucosal infections caused by a variety of viral, bacterial, and fungal organisms can present as oral ulcerations. The most common oral ulcers of viral origin are the result of herpes simplex virus infection.[2] Other viral infections that can present as oral ulcers are herpes zoster and herpangina. Acute necrotizing ulcerative gingivitis (ANUG), primary syphilis, and tuberculosis are examples of bacterial infections that cause oral ulcers. Oral ulcers are also a manifestation of deep-seated fungal infections such as histoplasmosis, coccidioidomycosis, and cryptococcosis.

It has been estimated that aphthous ulcers affect approximately 20 percent of the general population.[3] While the precise etiology of aphthous ulcers is unknown, considerable evidence suggests that immunologic mechanisms play a significant role in their development.[4] Oral ulcers are a feature of mucocutaneous diseases such as erythema multiforme, lichen planus, benign mucous membrane pemphigoid, and pemphigus vulgaris. These diseases may also result from immunologic defects.[4]

Squamous cell carcinoma accounts for approximately 95 per cent of all oral malignancies.[5] It originates from the squamous epithelial surface of oral mucosa. Growth of the tumor causes destruction of the epithelium with subsequent ulcer formation.

HISTORY

Age of the Patient

Many oral ulcers show a distinct age predilection. Primary herpetic gingivostomatitis and herpangina are more common in children. ANUG, primary syphilis, aphthous ulcers, and erythema multiforme are encountered most often in young adults. Herpes zoster, tuberculosis, fungal ulcers, lichen planus, benign mucous membrane pemphigoid, pemphigus vulgaris, and squamous cell carcinoma are more common in middle-aged and elderly adults.

Sex of the Patient

The patient's sex can also be an important diagnostic consideration. Men are more likely to suffer from ANUG, erythema multiforme, and squamous cell carcinoma, whereas lichen planus and benign mucous membrane pemphigoid are more common in women.

Focused Queries

A patient who presents with a chief complaint of oral ulcers should be asked the following:

1. *Is there a history of trauma?* The patient may recall a specific incident of trauma related to the onset of the ulcer.
2. *Does the patient wear dentures?* Traumatic ulcers often result from new dentures that have not been properly adjusted or old dentures that are ill-fitting.
3. *Was the ulcer preceded by a blister or swelling?* The patient's description of the ulcer at the time of its onset can be very helpful in formulating a differential diagnosis. Viral ulcers are preceded by vesicles that usually rupture before the patient can be examined. However, the patient may have observed intact vesicles. Oral ulcers associated with erythema multiforme, benign mucous membrane pemphigoid, and pemphigus vulgaris present initially as bullae. Patients with primary syphilis, tuberculosis, fungal ulcers, and squamous cell carcinoma may report that the ulcer was preceded by a swelling.
4. *How long has the ulcer been present?* The duration of the ulcer is also an important diagnostic consideration. Some oral ulcers resolve within two weeks. Examples include small traumatic ulcers, primary herpetic gingivostomatitis, recurrent intraoral herpes, herpangina, and aphthous ulcers. Large traumatic ulcers, herpes zoster, primary syphilis, tuberculosis, fungal ulcers, ulcers associated with some mucocutaneous diseases, and squamous cell carcinoma are all examples of oral ulcers that last for longer than two weeks. In general, persistent ulcers should be biopsied.
5. *Is there a history of recurrence?* Patients with oral ulcers may describe multiple episodes. Oral ulcers that commonly recur include aphthous ulcers, recurrent intraoral herpes, and ulcers associated with mucocutaneous diseases.
6. *Is the ulcer painful?* Pain is probably the most common symptom associated with oral ulcers. Traumatic ulcers, viral ulcers, ANUG, aphthous ulcers, and the mucocutaneous diseases are often acutely painful from their onset. Oral ulcers associated with primary syphilis are usually not painful unless secondarily infected with normal oral flora.

Oral squamous cell carcinoma is usually not painful until late in its clinical course.
7. *Are there any other symptoms?* Patients with ANUG frequently complain of halitosis and gingival bleeding. Intraoral squamous cell carcinoma may be associated with paresthesia. Fever and malaise often accompany primary herpetic gingivostomatitis, herpangina, ANUG, and erythema multiforme.
8. *Has the patient noticed any skin or eye lesions?* Patients with oral ulcers associated with mucocutaneous diseases may also complain of cutaneous or ocular lesions.
9. *Is the patient under stress?* Stress has been implicated as a contributing factor to ANUG, aphthous ulcers, and lichen planus.

Family History

Children are more likely to develop aphthous ulcers if their parents suffer from the same disease, indicating a possible genetic predisposition.[6]

Social History

Patients occasionally describe oral habits that might cause traumatic ulcers. The use of tobacco and/or alcohol greatly increases the risk for oral squamous cell carcinoma.[7] If primary syphilis is suspected, the patient should be asked about recent sexual activity.

Past Medical History

A history of a primary hepatic gingivostomatitis or primary varicella-zoster would be helpful in evaluating the possibility of recurrent intraoral herpes or herpes zoster, respectively. If tuberculosis or a fungal ulcer is suspected, the patient should be asked about previous pulmonary infections. A history of cutaneous or ocular lesions could indicate that an oral ulcer is associated with a mucocutaneous disease.

PHYSICAL EXAMINATION

Extraoral Head and Neck Examination

Examination of the head and neck should include evaluation of the conjunctiva and skin. Conjunctival ulceration and scarring are features of benign mucous membrane pemphigoid. Skin lesions associated with mucocutaneous diseases may be encountered on the face and neck.

The neck should be palpated to determine if enlarged lymph nodes are present. Reactive lymphadenopathy may be associated with traumatic ulcers, ulcers caused by infections, aphthous ulcers, and erythema multiforme. Reactive lymph nodes are usually soft, non-fixed, and tender. Intraoral squamous cell carcinomas often metastasize to lymph nodes in the neck. The involved lymph nodes are usually firm, fixed, and nontender.

Intraoral Examination

Careful examination of the oral mucosa will establish the location, number, size, and appearance of any lesions that might be present.

Some oral ulcers show a distinct predilection for specific anatomic sites. Aphthous ulcers tend to occur on buccal mucosa, labial mucosa, tongue, and soft palate.[8] In contrast, recurrent intraoral herpes usually arises on attached gingiva and hard palate.[9] The lesions of herpangina usually involve the soft palate and faucial pillars.[9] ANUG is localized to the gingival interdental papillae.[10] Buccal mucosa is the most common site for lichen planus,[11] whereas benign mucous membrane pemphigoid arises most often on gingiva.[12] The tongue is the most common intraoral site for squamous cell carcinoma.[5]

The number of ulcers present can also be an important diagnostic consideration. Traumatic ulcers, primary syphilis, tuberculosis, fungal ulcers, and squamous cell carcinoma are usually solitary. Multiple ulcers are characteristic of ANUG, aphthous ulcers, viral ulcers, and the mucocutaneous diseases.

Traumatic ulcers and aphthous ulcers show considerable variation in size, ranging from a few millimeters in diameter to more than a centimeter in diameter. Viral ulcers tend to be small and are often arranged in clusters.[9] Several adjacent viral ulcers may coalesce to form a single large ulcer. The lesions of ANUG begin as small ulcers that subsequently enlarge.[10] Large ulcers, often more than a centimeter in diameter, are characteristic of primary syphilis, tuberculosis, fungal infections, and the mucocutaneous diseases.

The clinical appearance of an oral ulcer is one of the most significant criteria for establishing a differential diagnosis. Small traumatic ulcers, ANUG, viral ulcers, aphthous ulcers, and ulcers associated with mucocutaneous diseases are usually shallow craters with only limited involvement of the underlying submucosa. In contrast, large traumatic ulcers, primary syphilis, tuberculosis, fungal ulcers, and squamous cell carcinoma usually extend deeply into the submucosa and exhibit indurated margins. The presence of intact vesicles suggests a viral etiology,[9] whereas bullae are characteristic of mucocutaneous diseases.[12,13]

DIAGNOSTIC STUDIES

When an oral ulcer cannot be diagnosed solely on the basis of history and clinical features, a variety of laboratory tests may be helpful in establishing an accurate diagnosis.

ANUG can be diagnosed by preparing a smear from an ulcer and examining it with darkfield microscopy. The presence of fusiform bacteria and mobile spirochetes is characteristic. Darkfield microscopy is of limited value in the diagnosis of primary syphilis involving oral mucosa because normal oral flora contains spirochetes that are indistinguishable by darkfield microscopy from *Treponema pallidum*.[14]

The isolation of viral organisms in cell culture or by animal inoculation can be of value in the diagnosis of primary herpetic gingivostomatitis, recurrent intraoral herpes, herpes zoster, and herpangina. *Mycobacterium tuberculosis* can be isolated from an oral ulcer and identified in culture to confirm the diagnosis of tuberculosis.

Cytologic smears stained with Papanicolaou's or Giemsa stain can be helpful in the diagnosis of herpes simplex, herpes zoster, pemphigus vulgaris, and squamous cell carcinoma. Immunohistochemical studies can also be performed on cytologic smears using antisera specific for herpes simplex virus and herpes zoster virus.

Biopsy is one of the most reliable diagnostic tests for establishing the cause of many oral ulcers. A representative biopsy specimen stained with hematoxylin and eosin can be useful in the diagnosis of syphilis, tuberculosis, fungal ulcers, ulcers associated with the mucocutaneous diseases, and squamous cell carcinoma. Specific microorganisms can be demonstrated in biopsy tissue using a variety of special histochemical stains. Examples are Warthin-Starry stain for spirochetes, acid-fast stain for mycobacteria, and periodic acid–Schiff stain for fungal organisms. Immunofluorescent staining using antisera to IgG,

IgM, IgA, C3, and fibrinogen can aid in the diagnosis of mucocutaneous diseases such as lichen planus, benign mucous membrane pemphigoid, and pemphigus vulgaris.[15] Immunohistochemical staining can also be performed on frozen sections of biopsy tissue using specific antisera to herpes simplex virus and varicella-zoster virus.

Other clinical laboratory tests that can also be of value include tuberculosis skin testing and serologic tests for viral infections and syphilis.

ASSESSMENT

Traumatic Ulcers

Traumatic ulcers are probably the most common solitary ulcers affecting oral mucosa. They are usually caused by cheek biting, lip biting, tongue biting, and irritation from ill-fitting dentures (denture ulcer). Any oral mucosal site can be involved; however, traumatic ulcers occur most often on the tongue and buccal mucosa (Fig. 1). Small traumatic ulcers are usually superficial and heal uneventfully within two weeks. Large traumatic ulcers can be more deep-seated and often persist for more than two weeks. Traumatic ulcers are usually painful. A biopsy may be necessary to differentiate large traumatic ulcers from primary syphilis, tuberculosis, deep-seated fungal infections, and squamous cell carcinoma.

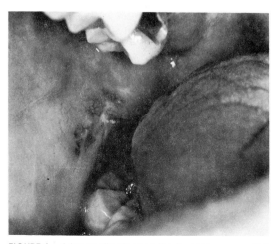

FIGURE 1. A traumatic ulcer on the buccal mucosa. This lesion resulted from cheek-biting injury.

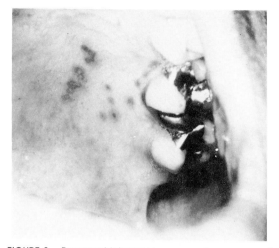

FIGURE 2. Recurrent intraoral herpes on the mucosa of the hard palate. The lesions presented initially as vesicles that ruptured to form a cluster of small painful ulcers.

Viral Ulcers

Viruses that cause oral ulcers include herpes simplex virus, varicella-zoster virus, and group A coxsackieviruses. Oral lesions associated with these viral infections present initially as vesicles that rupture to form small, superficial ulcers. Viral ulcers are often arranged in clusters and are usually very painful.

Herpes simplex virus causes two clinically distinct oral infections, primary herpetic gingivostomatitis and recurrent intraoral herpes.[16] Primary herpetic gingivostomatitis occurs in individuals who have not been previously infected with the virus and is most common in early childhood. The ulcers are preceded by vesicles and can involve any oral mucosal site as well as perioral skin. Fever, malaise, and cervical lymphadenopathy often accompany the onset of oral lesions. The ulcers usually heal within two weeks; however, the virus remains latent in the trigeminal ganglion. Recurrent intraoral herpes result from reactivation of latent herpes simplex virus. It occurs most often in adults and is more common in immunocompromised patients. The ulcers show a distinct predilection for attached gingiva and hard palate (Fig. 2). They usually heal within two weeks; however, multiple recurrences are common. Recurrent intraoral herpes may exhibit a more protracted clinical course in immunocompromised patients.

Intraoral herpes zoster (shingles) results from reactivation of latent varicella-zoster virus in the trigeminal ganglion following a primary infection (chickenpox).[9] The disease occurs most often in older adults and immuno-compromised patients. The lesions present initially as vesicles that rupture to form ulcers arranged in clusters. They involve oral mucosal sites that correspond to the distribution of the infected branch of the trigeminal nerve, and they do not cross the midline. The ulcers are extremely painful and persist for several weeks.

Herpangina is caused by various group A coxsackieviruses.[9] The infection occurs primarily in children and is highly contagious. The oral lesions present as vesicles on the soft palate and faucial pillars. The vesicles rupture to form painful ulcers. Fever, malaise, sore throat, and cervical lymphadenopathy often accompany the onset of oral lesions. The ulcers heal uneventfully within a few days, and recurrences are uncommon.

Bacterial Ulcers

Bacteria that can cause oral ulcers include the "fusospirochetal" bacteria found in dental plaque, *Treponema pallidum,* and *Mycobacterium tuberculosis.*

ANUG, commonly called trench mouth, is a disease caused by anaerobic fusobacteria and spirochetes found in dental plaque. Stress has been implicated as a predisposing factor. ANUG occurs most often in the mouths of young adult males. The infection is characterized by small ulcers that develop on the gingival interdental papillae.[10] They subsequently

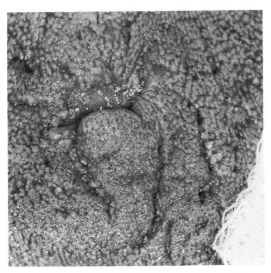

FIGURE 3. Primary syphilis (oral chancre) on the dorsal surface of the tongue. This ulcer had been present for three weeks.

enlarge to destroy the involved papillae and even may spread to adjacent gingival tissue. The ulcers are quite painful, and patients also complain of severe halitosis. Cervical lymphadenopathy may also be present.

The primary lesion of syphilis, called a chancre, develops at the site of inoculation of the causative organism, *Treponema pallidum.* Primary syphilis occurs most often on genital skin and mucosa but can also arise in the mouth (oral chancre). The most common intraoral sites are the lips and tongue.[17] Oral chancres present as large deep-seated ulcers with indurated margins (Fig. 3). They are usually not painful, unless secondarily infected with oral flora. Intraoral chancres tend to persist for several weeks and may be associated with cervical lymphadenopathy. In the absence of positive serology, a biopsy may be necessary to make a definitive diagnosis.

Oral ulcers caused by *Mycobacterium tuberculosis* are usually secondary to pulmonary infection.[18] The microorganisms in contaminated sputum penetrate the oral mucosa at a site of previous trauma and proliferate within the submucosa. The resulting granulomatous reaction produces a deep-seated ulcer with indurated margins. The most common oral mucosal sites for tuberculosis ulcers are tongue, palate, and buccal mucosa. They are usually solitary, painful, and persistent. A biopsy may be needed to differentiate oral tuberculosis from primary syphilis, deep-seated fungal infections, and squamous cell carcinoma.

Fungal Ulcers

Oral mucosal infections caused by *Histoplasma capsulatum, Coccidioides immitis,* and *Cryptococcus neoformans* cause deep-seated indurated ulcers. Like tuberculosis, these ulcers often develop secondary to pulmonary involvement.[19] Proliferation of the fungal organisms within the submucosa causes a granulomatous reaction. Fungal ulcers can arise on any mucosal site, and they are usually painful. A definitive diagnosis often requires a biopsy with histochemical stains for fungal organisms.

Ulcers Secondary to Immunologic Defects

Immunopathologic mechanisms are generally thought to be important in the development of aphthous ulcers and oral ulcers associated with the mucocutaneous diseases erythema multiforme, lichen planus, benign mucous membrane pemphigoid, and pemphigus vulgaris.[4]

Aphthous ulcers, commonly called canker sores, occur most often in young adult women.[8] They are not preceded by vesicles and show a distinct predilection for buccal mucosa, labial mucosa, tongue, and soft palate. Aphthous ulcers range in size from a few millimeters in diameter to more than a centimeter in diameter (Fig. 4). They are frequently multiple. Patients with aphthous ulcers usually complain of severe pain. The ulcers heal uneventfully within two weeks; however, recurrences are common.

The oral lesions of erythema multiforme present initially as bullae that quickly rupture to form large painful ulcers. Any oral mucosal site can be involved; however, hemorrhagic crusting along the vermilion border of the lower lip is characteristic of the disease.[20] Cutaneous lesions present as concentric erythematous rings called "target" or "bull's eye" lesions. Erythema multiforme occurs most often in young adult men. If ocular and genital lesions are present, the patient is suffering from a more severe form of the disease called Stevens-Johnson syndrome.

Interlacing white striations called Wickham's striae are the most common manifestation of intraoral lichen planus.[11] However, ulcers can be associated with the erosive form of the disease. Intraoral lichen planus occurs most often on the buccal mucosa, tongue, and gingiva (Fig. 5). The discomfort associated

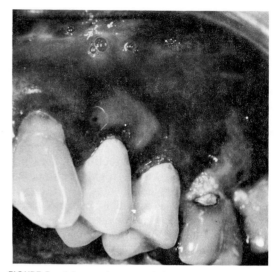

FIGURE 5.   A large ulcer associated with the mucocutaneous disease erosive lichen planus. This patient also had Wickham's striae on her buccal mucosa.

with ulcerated lesions ranges from a burning sensation to severe pain. Lichen planus occurs most often in middle-aged women and displays a protracted clinical course. A biopsy with immunofluorescent studies may be necessary to differentiate erosive lichen planus from benign mucous membrane pemphigoid and pemphigus vulgaris.

Benign mucous membrane pemphigoid is a mucocutaneous disease characterized by oral mucosal, conjunctival, and cutaneous lesions.[12] The oral lesions present initially as bullae that rupture to form large painful ulcers. While any oral mucosal site can be involved, the lesions are encountered most frequently on the gingiva. Benign mucous membrane pemphigoid is a chronic disease that occurs most often in middle-aged women. It can resemble erosive lichen planus and pemphigus vulgaris clinically, and a biopsy with immunofluorescent staining may be required for a definitive diagnosis.

Oral lesions are a common manifestation of pemphigus vulgaris and often precede the onset of cutaneous lesions.[13] They present initially as bullae that rupture to form large painful ulcers. Any oral mucosal site can be involved. Affected oral mucosa exhibits a positive Nikolsky's sign. Pemphigus vulgaris is encountered most often in middle-aged men and is chronic in nature. A biopsy including immunofluorescent studies may be necessary for diagnosis.

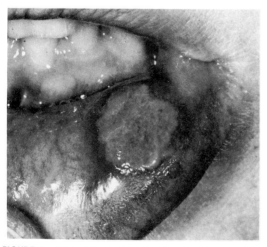

FIGURE 4.   An aphthous ulcer (canker sore) on the lower lip. This ulcer was larger than 1 cm in diameter and very painful.

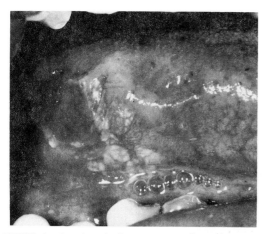

FIGURE 6. An ulcerated squamous cell carcinoma on the posterior tongue of a patient with a history of smoking two packages of cigarettes a day for more than 25 years.

Ulcers Secondary to Malignant Neoplasia

Squamous cell carcinoma is the most common malignant neoplasm affecting the oral cavity.[5] The use of tobacco and alcohol greatly increase the risk of developing intraoral squamous cell carcinoma.[7] Early lesions present clinically as white patches (leukoplakia) or red patches (erythroplakia). If untreated, these lesions develop into ulcerated swellings with indurated borders (Fig. 6). The most common sites of involvement are the tongue, oral floor, and gingiva. Early lesions are usually asymptomatic; however, patients eventually complain of pain and paresthesia. Intraoral squamous cell carcinoma occurs most often in elderly men. A biopsy is essential for diagnosis.

REFERENCES

1. Bouquot JE. Common oral lesions found during a mass screening examination. J Am Dent Assoc 1986;112:50–7.
2. Bottomley WK, Brown RS, Lavigne GJ. A retrospective survey of the oral conditions of 981 patients referred to an oral medicine private practice. J Am Dent Assoc 1990;120:529–33.
3. Rennie JS, Reade DC, Hay KD, Scully C. Recurrent aphthous stomatitis. Br Dent J 1985;159:361–7.
4. Greenspan JS. Immunology of diseases of the oral mucous membrane. In: Stone J, ed. Dermatologic immunology and allergy. St Louis: CV Mosby, 1985:698–706.
5. Silverman S. Epidemiology. In: Silverman S, ed. Oral cancer. New York: American Cancer Society, 1985:2–6.
6. Miller MF, Garfunkel DMD, Rain CA, Ship II. The inheritance of recurrent aphthous stomatitis: observations on susceptibility. Oral Surg Oral Med Oral Pathol 1980;49:409–12.
7. Binnie WH, Rankin KV, Mackenzie IC. Etiology of oral squamous cell carcinoma. J Oral Pathol 1983;12:11–29.
8. Antoon JW, Miller RL. Aphthous ulcers: a review of the literature on etiology, pathogenesis, diagnosis and treatment. J Am Dent Assoc 1980;101:803–8.
9. Eversole R. Clinical virology of the head and neck. Compend Contin Educ Dent 1985;6:298–309.
10. Wood NK, Goaz PW. Differential diagnosis of oral lesions. 3rd ed. St Louis: CV Mosby, 1985:102–4.
11. Scully C, El-Kom M. Lichen planus: review and update on pathogenesis. J Oral Pathol 1985;14:431–58.
12. Manton SL, Scully C. Mucous membrane pemphigoid: an elusive diagnosis. Oral Surg Oral Med Oral Pathol 1988;66:37–40.
13. Kempler DL, Schott TR. Pemphigus vulgaris. J Am Dent Assoc 1980;101:273–5.
14. MacFarlane TW, Samaranayake LP. Clinical oral microbiology. London: Wright, 1989:111.
15. Daniels TE, Quadra-White C. Direct immunofluorescence in oral mucosal disease: a diagnostic analysis of 130 cases. Oral Surg Oral Med Oral Pathol 1981;51:38–47.
16. Scully C. Orofacial herpes simplex virus infections: current concepts in the epidemiology, pathogenesis, and treatment, and disorders in which the virus may be implicated. Oral Surg Oral Med Oral Pathol 1989;68:701–10.
17. Alexander WN. Venereal disease and the dentist. J Acad Gen Dent 1975;23:14–8.
18. Shafer WG, Hine MK, Kevy BM. A textbook of oral pathology. 4th ed. Philadelphia: WB Saunders, 1983:342.
19. Cobb CM, Shultz RE, Brewer JH, Dunlap CL. Chronic pulmonary histoplasmosis with an oral lesion. Oral Surg Oral Med Oral Pathol 1989;67:73–6.
20. Regezi JA, Sciubba JJ. Oral pathology: clinical-pathologic correlations. Philadelphia: WB Saunders, 1989:54.

PAP SMEAR, ABNORMAL

STEVEN H. PURSELL and STANLEY A. GALL

SYNONYMS: Abnormal Pap, Cervical Dysplasia, Cervical Intraepithelial Neoplasia, High-Grade Cervical Intraepithelial Lesions, Low-Grade Cervical Intraepithelial Lesions

BACKGROUND

The Papanicolaou (Pap) smear is one of the single most important advances in the management of cervical cancer. Its true value lies in its use in prevention. Studies have consistently shown that its use decreases the incidence of new invasive cervical cancers in a population with periodic Pap smear evaluations.[1,2] It is simple to perform; relatively easy to interpret; and an inexpensive test, which makes it ideal for use as a screening procedure.

Pap smears are only screening procedures, identifying women who require additional evaluation. The Pap smear is not the definitive test upon which therapy for preinvasive and invasive cervical disease is based.

Anatomy

Premalignant and invasive cervical lesions arise from the squamocolumnar junction, where the squamous epithelium of the cervix abuts the columnar epithelium of the endocervical canal, an abrupt change from one cell type to another. This dynamic interface on the cervix changes over the course of a woman's life in response to her estrogen status. Before the onset of menarche, the junction lies far out on the portio of the cervix. With the onset of menses, the physiologic changes cause the junction to recede across the cervical lip toward the endocervical canal. Pregnancy causes the junction to recede further toward the endocervical canal. Finally, by the premenopausal years, the junction may have receded up into the endocervical canal to such an extent that it can no longer be visualized.

This recession takes place as the columnar cells undergo metaplasia, the conversion of one cell type to another, to become squamous cells. Transformation of cellular architecture offers a protective benefit to the cells. Squamous cells are more resistant to injury and physiologic challenges than are columnar cells. Metaplasia, a normal process, occurs elsewhere in the body and is not considered a premalignant condition.

The active process of metaplasia creates a zone of transformation on the cervical lip where cellular conversion is taking place. This zone, where metabolic activity is increased, is thought to be sensitive to carcinogens, which induce or facilitate the development of dysplastic or premalignant cells.

Several studies have tried to identify factors responsible for the development of cervical neoplasia. Findings suggest an infectious venereal etiology. Recently, human papilloma virus (HPV), and its association with cervical neoplastic changes, has come under intense review.

HPV is one of the most common sexually transmitted diseases. Over 62 subtypes of HPV have been identified, and the virus is found in the nucleus of infected cells, usually as an epimere, separate from the host deoxyribonucleic acid (DNA). HPV subtypes 6, 11, 16, 18, and 31 are frequently found in genital infections. Subtypes 16, 18, and 31 have been associated with upper vaginal and cervical lesions and are thought to be of high malignant potential.[3] Typing of HPV lesions can be accomplished through molecular hybridization techniques. There is evidence suggesting that HPV may be a cocarcinogen in the development of cervical neoplasia.[4] HPV DNA can be found in practically every patient with advanced intraepithelial neoplasia or invasive cancer.[5]

Cervical Dysplasia

The development of cervical cancer represents a progression through a spectrum of pre-

328

malignant changes confined to the epithelium of the cervix. Patients are thought to progress from normal cellular architecture to dysplastic changes that do not penetrate the basement membrane of the epithelium and to invasive carcinoma.

Not all women who develop dysplasia will develop an invasive carcinoma. Occasionally, these lesions will regress spontaneously. Some will also persist as dysplasia without progression to carcinoma. Currently, there is no mechanism to identify those lesions that will not progress. Therefore, all cervical neoplasias should be approached in a uniform manner as though they had the potential to develop into invasive carcinomas.

The World Health Organization monograph on histologic typing of female genital tract tumors characterizes premalignant cervical lesions:[6]

1. *Mild dysplasia.* There is a loss of cellular polarity with enlarged, sometimes irregular nuclei. These changes are confined to the lower one third of the epithelium.

2. *Moderate dysplasia.* This represents an intermediate condition between mild and severe dysplasia. The architectural and nuclei alterations are confined to the lower two thirds of the epithelium.

3. *Severe dysplasia.* The architectural changes and atypia almost fill the depth of the epithelium. The most superficial cells of the epithelium continue to show some level of maturation. Often, only a single layer of flattened cells is present on the surface of the epithelium.

4. *Carcinoma in situ.* This is the most extensive premalignant alteration. The entire epithelium is replaced by cells that demonstrate features of carcinoma. The basement membrane is intact.

Some authors favor a system designated as cervical intraepithelial neoplasia (CIN) that incorporates severe dysplasia and carcinoma in situ into a single entity, CIN III. CIN I corresponds to mild dysplasia, and CIN II corresponds to moderate dysplasia, and so on.

HISTORY

Evaluating the history of a patient with an abnormal Pap smear can be enlightening. Epidemiologic studies have identified certain factors that place the woman at risk for developing cervical neoplasias.[7,8,9] These risks factors include:

1. An early age at the onset of sexual intercourse.
2. Multiple sexual partners.
3. A husband with a history of multiple sexual partners.
4. A husband who was previously married to a woman with cervical cancer.
5. History of sexually transmitted diseases such as Herpes simplex virus (HSV-II) and HPV.

These risk factors all tend to point to the venereal transmission of this disease. Low socioeconomic class and smoking also are found associated with the development of cervical cancer.[10]

Any history of abnormal Pap smears or treatment for premalignant disease of the cervix should be determined. Cervical dysplasia has the potential to recur regardless of the treatment technique. As many as 3 to 5 per cent of the women who have undergone a hysterectomy for carcinoma in situ may demonstrate subsequent abnormal cytology. Women with CIN often will have no symptoms at all. This makes frequent interval screening very important. Authorities debate the timing and frequency of Pap smear testing in asymptomatic women. The American Cancer Society (ACS) recommends that women begin Pap smear evaluations and pelvic examinations when they become sexually active or by age 18, whichever occurs first. After a woman has had three consecutive, normal annual examinations, the Pap smear may be performed less frequently, at the discretion of her physician. The ACS also has indicated that Pap smears after the age of 65 years are less informative in previously normal women.

In contrast, the American College of Obstetricians and Gynecologists (ACOG) continues to recommend annual cytologic screening for most women.[11] The initial screening should be performed on all women by the age of 18 and in those who are sexually active, regardless of age. Most patients with a negative initial evaluation should undergo annual cytologic screening. Low-risk patients—those who begin sexual activity at a later age (after age 18) and who have one sexual partner—have a minimal risk of developing a cervical abnormality within three to five years after two successively negative annual smears. Screening frequency in such cases is arbitrary and may be based on the informed decision of the patient and her physician. Women at increased risk of developing CIN—those who become sexually active at an early age, have multiple sexual partners, have a history of an abnormal Pap smear, or have the presence of HPV—should be screened annually or more often. Although the cost effectiveness of cytologic screening of the vagina in women who have undergone hysterectomy for indications other than cytologic abnormalities has not been fully established, the ACOG recommends Pap smears at minimum intervals of three years.

Women with abnormal Pap smears should be treated appropriately and then evaluated frequently to monitor the effectiveness of the treatment and monitor for recurrence. Many clinicians will examine patients every four months once an abnormality has been detected and treated until two negative Pap smears are obtained on consecutive visits. Thereafter, they will often be examined every six months.

The incidence of cervical dysplasia is not increased by a positive family history of the disease. It does not appear to have a genetic predisposition, and therefore, increased screening among family members of women with this disease is probably not warranted.

PHYSICAL EXAMINATION

The Pap smear is such a simple procedure to perform that the importance of good technique can be overlooked. However, the accuracy of the cytologic diagnosis is related to proper sampling techniques.

The cytologic specimen must be obtained before the bimanual examination. A nonlubricated speculum should be used. The introduction of lubricant into the vagina, whether by speculum or the examiner's fingers, will cause clumping of the exfoliated cells and foul the specimen.

To obtain an adequate specimen, the cervix must be fully visible to the examiner. Blind attempts to sample the cervix are unacceptable.

The endocervix and portio of the cervix should be sampled to provide the most accurate and cost-effective evaluation. Usually, a cotton-tipped swab or a Cytobrush is inserted into the endocervical canal and rotated 720 degrees about the interior of the canal. The specimen is transferred to a clean glass slide by rolling the swab across the surface of the slide

several times to ensure transfer of the cells from all sides of the swab, prevent clumping of the cells, and ensure uniformity of the specimen. The portio of the cervix is then sampled with an Ayre's spatula. The portio is scraped with enough force to obtain cells in a circumferential pattern around the entire surface. The specimen is transferred to a glass slide by rubbing *both* sides of the spatula against the surface of the slide. This ensures transfer of cells from both sides of the spatula. The slides should be placed immediately into fixative to prevent air drying. This will help prevent drying artifacts.

If a large amount of vaginal discharge is present on the cervix, it can be removed gently with a large swab before obtaining the Pap smear. Care should be taken not to wipe away the exfoliated cells that make up the smear. Generally, small amounts of blood or mucus will not obscure the interpretation of the smear and can be left alone. Menses is not a contraindication to obtaining or interpreting a Pap smear.

If the examiner observes a gross lesion on the cervix, a biopsy should be taken in addition to the Pap smear. A Kevorkian biopsy forceps can be used to obtain a small incisional biopsy with little risk of bleeding. The presence of a visible lesion mandates biopsy. The reports in the literature have demonstrated that Pap smears can be negative for cytologic abnormalities even in the presence of a visible cervical cancer.[12]

A thorough bimanual examination should follow the Pap smear. The examiner should try to palpate the uterus and adnexa through the vagina and rectum with the aid of an abdominally placed hand.

DIAGNOSTIC STUDIES

An abnormal Pap smear will identify women who require further evaluation. Since the Pap smear is a screening procedure, it must be followed by further investigation to delineate any abnormality.

Conization

Conization of the cervix has been the standard for histologic evaluation of cervical dysplasia. The procedure requires the surgical excision of a cone-shaped tissue specimen from the cervix that encompasses the squamocolumnar junction and the transformation zone.

The specimen can be sectioned, stained, and examined microscopically. Once the abnormality has been defined, therapy can begin. The cone can be both a diagnostic as well as a therapeutic procedure. The lesion will be removed with the cone specimen and, if no invasion is evident, may be curative in up to 95 per cent of the patients with dysplasia.[13]

Although conization is well tolerated and has a low morbidity rate, it is an outpatient surgical procedure and usually requires regional or general anesthesia. Cervical stenosis, incompetent cervix, and hemorrhage have been reported to complicate this procedure.[14] To minimize the risk, inconvenience, and expense to the patient, many gynecologists have found that the colposcopic evaluation of the cervix is the preferred, first-line evaluation of the abnormal Pap.

Colposcopy

Colposcopy is the direct visual evaluation of the cervix under magnification. Performed in the office without anesthesia, colposcopy is well tolerated, is much less expensive than a cervical conization, and can often provide a definitive histologic diagnosis. A speculum is placed in the patient's vagina to expose the cervix, and a Pap smear is obtained. Next, the cervix is gently swabbed with 3 per cent acetic acid. This will help to remove any mucus that may be present on the cervix and, more important, result in the demarcation of any abnormal vascular patterns present on the cervical epithelium. The cervix is examined with the colposcope under magnification. The use of a green filter will further enhance the vascular pattern.

Colposcopy is particularly helpful in evaluating women during their reproductive years when the squamocolumnar junction is readily accessible for visual inspection. The junction may recede into the endocervical canal in older women where it cannot be seen. CIN will produce subtle changes in the architecture of the cervix along the squamocolumnar junction. The changes are often reflected in the vascular pattern on the surface of the epithelium. The vessels may take on several patterns. Punctation occurs when the vessels are seen on end. Mosaicism occurs when the vessels are seen longitudinally in a random, crossing pattern like a cobblestone street. White epithelium occurs when the surface epithelial cells pile up to form a thick layer over the capillaries, making the epithelium look white rather than pink. There is lack of complete correlation between the degree of cervical dysplasia and the colposcopic pattern. Once an abnormal area is identified with the aid of the colposcope, a biopsy of the area is taken under direct visualization. These colposcopically directed biopsies can then be evaluated histologically. In addition, the endocervical canal should be sampled by an endocervical curettage (ECC) to identify "skip" lesions high in the canal.

Adequate colposcopy can be ensured if certain rules are followed consistently. These rules, formulated to provide reliable information, act as a built-in check for the colposcopist.

1. The squamocolumnar junction must be seen in its entirety. This ensures the whole area at risk for dysplastic change has been evaluated.

2. Any lesion on the cervix must be seen in its entirety. If the lesion extends into the endocervical canal and cannot be seen, then the colposcopist cannot evaluate the abnormality fully. The Pap smear should not be significantly worse than the biopsy. If the pathology of the colposcopically directed biopsy is significantly less than that of the Pap smear, this may indicate that the colposcopist has not sampled the most abnormal area.

3. The colposcopically directed specimen should not demonstrate microinvasive carcinoma. Since the treatment of microinvasive cervical cancer and a frankly invasive cervical cancer is so different and the histologic difference so subtle, final decisions should not be made simply on biopsy specimens.

4. Finally, the ECC should not demonstrate any dysplasias. Should this be positive, an unseen lesion may exist in the endocervical canal that cannot be evaluated adequately by colposcopy alone.

If the criteria for adequate colposcopy cannot be met, the evaluation is "inadequate," and the patient should undergo a cervical conization to provide complete and reliable information for treatment.

Once a histologic diagnosis is made, the appropriate therapy can be chosen and recommended to the patient. A hysterectomy is never the first step in the evaluation of an abnormal Pap smear, even though it eventually may be required.

Pregnancy

An abnormal Pap smear during pregnancy often causes significant concern to the patient and her physician because of the risk to the woman and her fetus. Colposcopic evaluation of the cervix during pregnancy is particularly useful in resolving the concern. It can be performed easily and safely on pregnant women if the ECC is not performed. The minor irritation to the cervix associated with colposcopically directed biopsies does not cause fetal wastage and can provide a definitive diagnosis.

ASSESSMENT

The ACOG has endorsed diagnostic terminology that describes cervical cytology and also is recommended by the American Society of Cytology[11] and the International Academy of Cytology. This is *not* the traditional Papanicolaou classification. The traditional classes I through V lack specificity and precision and should not be part of contemporary cytopathology. The recommended terminology delineates the spectrum of cervical abnormalities including the following categories: (1) unsatisfactory; (2) no abnormal cells; (3) squamous atypia; (4) findings consistent with cervical dysplasia— mild, moderate, and severe; (5) cytologic findings consistent with invasive squamous cell carcinoma; and (6) abnormal cells not specifically categorized.[15]

Any patient with atypia or a more significant abnormality should be considered as a candidate for colposcopic evaluation. Inadequate colposcopy, in turn, requires a conization of the cervix.[15]

The National Cancer Institute recently has reviewed the nomenclature of cervical cytology. In an effort to further standardize the reporting and interpretation of Pap smears, as well as to improve their quality and value as a screening tool, the Bethesda System has been suggested.[16] This system also abandons the traditional Papanicolaou classification. It treats the Pap smear as a medical consultation and provides definitive guidelines for reporting the cytopathology of cervical/vaginal specimens. This system is somewhat cumbersome and so new that it is not yet widely used. Cervical lesions are divided into low- and high-grade squamous intraepithelial lesions (SIL). This division is used to distinguish lesions likely to progress—high-grade SIL—from those whose abnormal appearance may be due to HPV changes and are less likely to progress—low-grade SIL. Although this classification suggests the identification of a high-risk group requiring evaluation and therapy, the low-risk group must not be ignored and assumed to be benign.

Epithelial Cell Abnormalities

The Bethesda System relegates the term atypical cells to those cases in which the cytologic findings are of undetermined significance. It should not be used as a diagnosis for otherwise defined inflammatory, preneoplastic, or neoplastic cellular changes.

Low-grade SIL includes smears with only HPV changes, mild dysplasia alone (CIN I), or the combination of HPV and mild dysplasia (CIN I). High-grade SIL includes the more advanced dysplasias whether or not there are HPV changes present. Therefore, patients with moderate dysplasia (CIN II), severe dysplasia (CIN III), or carcinoma in situ (CIN III) would be included in this category. If cellular changes associated with HPV are present, they would be so noted on the report.

Although the use of low-grade and high-grade SIL is preferred, it is acceptable to include the degree of dysplasia or grade of CIN. Their inclusion will facilitate the transition to the new nomenclature and add to the descriptive value of the information. Pap smears suggestive of invasive lesions would be reported as squamous cell carcinoma.

Treatment

Once the abnormal Pap smear has been fully evaluated by colposcopy or diagnostic conization, therapy can be instituted (see the algorithm). If diagnosis has been made by colposcopy, therapy will often consist of locally ablative treatment that will destroy the abnormal cells present on the cervix. Cryotherapy, a simple and inexpensive method of local destruction, has cure rates ranging from 70 to 80 percent.[17,18] The end of the cervix is frozen with an appropriately tipped cryoprobe. The ice ball formed causes cell death throughout the transformation zone. Abnormal cells as well as some normal stroma and epithelial cells are destroyed. Inflammation causes further destruction. The carbon dioxide laser also can be used to destroy abnormal cells along the transformation zone. Energy from the monochromatic laser is transferred to the tis-

DIAGNOSTIC ASSESSMENT OF AN ABNORMAL PAP SMEAR

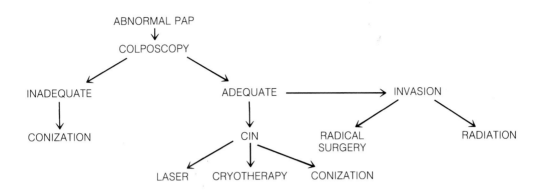

sues causing flash-boiling of the intracellular water with resultant tissue destruction.[19]

A hysterectomy should be undertaken only after establishing the severity of the cervical abnormality by either cone or colposcopy. It is usually reserved for recurrent disease or for women who have completed their child-bearing.

REFERENCES

1. Christopherson WM, Mendez WM, Ahuja EM, Lundin FE Jr, Parker JE. Cervical cancer control in Louisville, Kentucky. Cancer 1970;26:29–38.
2. Canadian Task Force on Cervical Cancer Screening. Cervical cancer screening programs: summary of the 1982 Canadian task force report. Can Med Assoc J 1982;127:581–9.
3. Reid R, Greenberg M, Jenson AB, et al. Sexually transmitted papillomaviral infections. I. The anatomic distribution and pathologic grade of neoplastic lesions associated with different viral types. Am J Obstet Gynecol 1986;156:212–22.
4. Reid R, Fu YS, Herschman BR, et al. Genital warts and cervical cancer. IV. The relationship between aneuploid and polypoid cervical lesions. Am J Obstet Gynecol 1984;150:189–99.
5. Richart RM. Natural history of cervical intraepithelial neoplasia. Clin Obstet Gynecol 1967;10:748–84.
6. World Health Organization. Monograph on the histologic typing of female genital tract tumors. Geneva: WHO, 1975.
7. Catalano LW Jr, Johnson LD. Herpesvirus antibody and carcinoma in situ of the cervix. JAMA 1971;217:447–50.
8. Champion MJ, Singer A, Clarkson PK, McCance DJ. Increased risk of cervical neoplasia in consorts of men with penile condylomata acuminata. Lancet 1985;1:943–6.
9. Fenoglio CM, Ferenczy A. Etiologic factors in cervical neoplasia. Semin Oncol 1982;9:349–72.
10. Trevathan E, Layde P, Webster LA, Adams JB, Benigno BB, Ory H. Cigarette smoking and dysplasia in carcinoma in situ of the uterine cervix. JAMA 1983;250:499–502.
11. American College of Obstetricians and Gynecologists. Cervical cytology: evaluation and management of abnormalities. ACOG Techn Bull 1984;81(Oct).
12. Gad C, Koch F. The limitation of screening effect; a review of cervical disorders of previously screened women. Acta Cytol 1978;22:719–22.
13. Bojerre B, Eliasson G, Linell F, Söderberg H, Sjöberg N-O. Conization as only treatment of carcinoma in situ of the uterine cervix. Am J Obstet Gynecol 1976;125:143–52.
14. Stafl A, Mattingly RF. Cervical intraepithelial neoplasia. In: Mattingly RF, Thompson JD, eds. TeLinde's operative gynecology. 6th edition. Philadelphia: JB Lippincott, 1985:759–79.
15. Van Nagell JR Jr, Gay EC, Powell DF. Cervical intraepithelial neoplasia. In: Van Nagell JR Jr, Barber HRK, eds. Modern concepts of gynecologic oncology. Boston: John Wright-PSG Inc. 1982:21–56.
16. National Cancer Institute. The 1988 Bethesda System for reporting cervical/vaginal cytologic diagnosis. JAMA 1989;262(7):931–4.
17. Creasman WT, Weed JC, Curry SL, Johnston WW, Parker RT. Efficacy of cryosurgical treatment of severe cervical intraepithelial neoplasia. Obstet Gynecol 1973; 41:501–6.
18. Ostergard DR. Cryosurgical treatment of cervical intraepithelial neoplasia. Obstet Gynecol 1980; 56:231–3.
19. Baggish MS. Management of cervical intraepithelial neoplasia by carbon dioxide laser. Obstet Gynecol 1982;60:378–84.

PELVIC MASS IN THE FEMALE PATIENT

THOMAS M. JULIAN and DANIEL A. DUMESIC

SYNONYMS: Pelvic-Abdominal Mass, Pelvic Tumor, Adnexal Mass

BACKGROUND

The best predictors of the etiology of a pelvic mass are the patient's age and the findings on pelvic examination. The most common masses occur in reproductive-age women and are functional cysts of the ovary. In the pre- and postreproductive-age groups, masses are more commonly neoplastic. Physical examination provides a location within the pelvis, helping to determine the organ involved and characteristics that help the examiner determine a plan for further evaluation and treatment.

We will discuss historical and physical findings that best determine the etiology of a pelvic mass in the female and describe useful diagnostic laboratory and imaging studies. It must be remembered that laparoscopy or laparotomy will in most cases be necessary to make the definitive diagnosis. (Also see chapter on Pelvic Pain in Women in *Difficult Diagnosis I.*).

HISTORY

Reproductive Age

Age from a gynecologic standpoint is represented as three groups: prereproductive, reproductive, and postreproductive, with some patients in transition between groups. This broad classification serves as an excellent framework to formulate a diagnostic plan.

Prereproductive

The neonate with a pelvic mass may be asymptomatic or suffer symptoms resulting from abdominal distension. The most common mass in this group is an ovarian cyst caused by elevated circulating gonadotropins. If ultrasonographic evidence confirms an otherwise asymptomatic solitary, unilocular cyst, the mass can be expected to regress as serum gonadotropin levels decline after birth. While no firm guidelines exist, observation may continue several months.[1]

Most childhood female pelvic masses are neoplastic or endocrinologic in origin. Fifty per cent of pelvic masses in childhood are malignant, 40 per cent of abdominal masses in children under the age of two are renal in origin, 2 to 5 per cent of malignant pediatric tumors involve the female reproductive organs, most commonly ovary. Neoplastic ovarian masses will be of germ cell origin in about 80 per cent of cases. Abdominal distension, fullness, and pain are the most common presenting symptoms. Gynecologic symptoms include vaginal bleeding, discharge, or abnormal sexual development. Precocious puberty (secondary sexual characteristics in a female child less than eight years old) may be the first symptom of an endocrinologically active tumor. Other common childhood masses include neuroblastoma, Wilms' tumor, and sacral tumors.[2,3,4]

Reproductive

The functional ovarian cyst is the most common pelvic mass in the reproductive-age group. This gonadotropin-dependent cyst occurs during the follicular (follicle cyst) or luteal (corpus luteum cyst) phase of the menstrual cycle and regresses with normal, cyclic ovarian function. Most of these cysts are less than 30 mm in diameter and asymptomatic. Symptoms consist of pain usually from torsion, intermittent torsion, intracystic bleeding, or rupture of the cyst. Delayed resolution of the corpus luteum may result in delayed menses, late cycle spotting, and pain. This constellation of symptoms represents Halban's syndrome.[5]

The young patient with an outflow obstruction to menses (caused by an imperforate hymen, congenital absence of the vagina, or structural müllerian abnormality) may, when reproductive function begins, retain menstrual blood or mucus and develop a mass from the resulting distension of the noncommunicating vagina or uterus. Symptoms consistent with cyclic hormonal function (breast swelling and tenderness, bloating, irritability, edema, or mood alteration) followed by abdominal cramping and tenderness but without menses suggest outflow obstruction.

Patients in the reproductive-age group are the most likely to acquire sexually transmitted diseases and therefore are prone to salpingitis with the sequelae of tubo-ovarian abscesses and hydrosalpinges. These patients present with a history consistent with an infection: sexually active, multiple sexual partners, recent intercourse, fever, chills, low bilateral abdominal pain, abnormal discharge, malaise, intrauterine device (IUD) use, or bleeding.

Endometriosis, the heterotopic presence of endometrial glands and stroma, is common in this age group. It can produce large, cystic masses of the ovary and adhesion formation involving any pelvic intraperitoneal or retroperitoneal structure. Common symptoms include infertility, progressive dysmenorrhea, dyspareunia, or pelvic pain.

Patients with secondary amenorrhea, irregular menses, obesity, hirsutism, or infertility may be chronically anovulatory with hyperandrogenism secondary to polycystic ovarian disease. In these patients, chronic anovulation results in many small follicle cysts in each ovary causing bilateral enlargement of the ovaries interpreted during examination as a solitary large mass.[6]

Pregnancy is the most common etiology of a pelvic mass associated with amenorrhea. A reproductive-age patient must always be assumed to be pregnant until proved otherwise. Implantation of the fertilized ovum into an area other than that of the uterus is an ectopic pregnancy. (Also see chapter on Ectopic Pregnancy, Suspected.) Ectopic pregnancies most commonly occur in the fallopian tube, causing hemorrhage at the implantation site. Distension of the fallopian tube with blood results in pain and a pelvic mass. Both intra- and extrauterine pregnancy cause amenorrhea, nausea, and breast tenderness.[7]

Patients in the reproductive years develop uterine leiomyomata, approximately 25 and 33 per cent of Caucasian and non-Caucasian women, respectively. These benign neoplastic pelvic masses are most often asymptomatic but may produce vaginal bleeding or abdominal and pelvic pressure. Necrosis of the myoma due to degeneration or torsion may produce pelvic pain.[8]

Postreproductive

When a woman has gone without menstruation for one year after the age of 40 and experiences hot flushes, it is likely she is postreproductive or menopausal. The most common pelvic mass in this group is the uterine leiomyoma as previously described.[9]

Many authorities have long believed that an adnexal mass in the postreproductive patient is malignant until proved otherwise.[10] Women of postreproductive age should not have functional ovarian cysts since folliculogenesis has ceased, nor should they have vaginal bleeding. Hypoestrogenemia results in a reduction in the size of uterine leiomyomata. Leiomyomata that enlarge after menopause are suspect for malignancy, most commonly uterine sarcoma.

Malignant pelvic masses in this age group are most commonly ovarian. The patient may complain of abdominal symptoms such as bloating, dyspepsia, change in bowel habits, or enlargement of the abdomen. This vague symptomatology in conjunction with the rapid growth of the tumor results in 70 per cent of patients having stage III ovarian cancer at the time of initial diagnosis and a 30 per cent five-year survival. The poor prognosis of this disease serves to emphasize the importance of evaluating all pelvic masses in women of postreproductive age.[11,12]

Carcinoma of the cervix and endometrium also may cause vaginal bleeding and usually are localized, respectively, to the cervix or endometrium when diagnosed. Early pelvic malignancies may be asymptomatic. Weight loss, pain, ascites, and edema are symptoms of advanced disease. Postmenopausal bleeding, the classic symptom associated with gynecologic malignancy, seldom occurs with ovarian cancer, the most common malignant pelvic mass in the female.[13]

Nongynecologic Pelvic Mass

Gastrointestinal

Gastrointestinal masses located in the pelvis produce gastrointestinal symptoms like melena, hematochezia, obstipation, constipation, and diarrhea. In the postmenopausal patient, colon cancer should always be considered. A family history of colon cancer or polyposis also increases risk.[14] Inflammatory diseases of the gastrointestinal tract such as regional enteritis, colitis, diverticulitis, and diverticulosis also produce masses, usually a phlegmon palpated on pelvic examination. Lastly, stool in the rectum or sigmoid colon may be confused with a true pelvic mass.

Metastatic Disease

Breast and gastrointestinal cancers may metastasize to the ovary, producing a pelvic mass. Involvement of the ovary, uterus, or pelvic lymph nodes by nonsolid tumors like lymphoma and leukemia also may cause masses. Nonsolid tumors will usually regress with successful chemotherapy of the underlying malignancy; such is seldom the case with solid, metastatic tumors to the ovary.[15]

Urologic Masses

Urologic masses in the pelvis include the asymptomatic pelvic kidney; remnants of the mesonephros (wolffian duct) persisting as a pelvic mass in the vagina, broad ligament or tubal attachments; or a urachal mass, either a fluid-filled remnant or an adenocarcinoma.

Overdistension of the bladder, common in patients with an atonic bladder, may simulate a pelvic mass. Commonly associated historical correlates for bladder atony include the use of psychotropic medications, diabetes, peripheral neuropathy, obstructing uterine myomata, urethral obstruction, a feeling of inability to empty the bladder on voiding, vaginal prolapse, recent pelvic surgery, or urinary tract infection.[16]

PHYSICAL EXAMINATION

The second important diagnostic tool, the physical examination, determines the location and characteristics of the mass. The location and characteristics of a mass can tell an experienced, attentive examiner much about its etiology. First, consider the anatomic location as an examiner would encounter organs during pelvic examination.

Vulva

Masses seen or felt in the vulvar region may be intraperitoneal or extraperitoneal. Vulvar masses are most commonly found in or on the labia and include condylomata, fibromas, leiomyoma, cysts in the canal of Nuck (female hydrocele), sebaceous cysts, and melanoma. Biopsy of these masses is essential for correct diagnosis.

Vagina

Masses within the distal vagina located at the five and seven o'clock positions are Bartholin's gland abscesses or cysts; on the lateral vaginal side walls are remnants of the wolffian duct (Gartner's duct cysts); anteriorly under the urethra are urethrocele and urethral diverticulum; lateral to the urethra are Skene's gland cysts and abscesses; along the anterior wall of the vagina is cystocele; and found posteriorly in the vagina are rectocele and enterocele. Most vaginal masses are benign cysts or prolapsing organs. Solid masses in the vagina require biopsy for diagnosis. The most common solid tumor is condyloma acuminata. Squamous cell carcinoma is the most common adult malignancy, and sarcoma botryoides is the most common malignancy of the prereproductive years.

Cervix

A pelvic mass originating from the cervix may be malignant (squamous cell or adenocarcinoma) or benign (condyloma, polyps, leiomyomas, nabothian cysts). Uncommon cervical tumors that may present as a mass include cervical pregnancy, tuberculosis, or syphilis. Appropriate evaluation requires biopsy and adjunctive laboratory.

Masses Above the Pelvic Diaphragm

Masses above the pelvic diaphragm cannot be directly visualized on physical examination; therefore, the accurate assessment and description of masses from palpation are crucial in making the correct diagnosis. The size, shape, position, consistency, mobility, tenderness, and relationship to other pelvic structures are all important.

The Midline Pelvic Mass

The most common midline pelvic mass is the uterus. The normal size uterus of a reproductive-age woman is about 8 cm long, 6 cm wide, and 5 cm deep. The uterus is most often anteverted and anteflexed. The retroverted, retroflexed uterus may feel larger than it truly is and is often mistaken for a pelvic mass.

Pregnancy is the most common cause of an enlarged uterus. The pregnant uterus is generally symmetrically enlarged, from 6 cm in length to measurable more than 40 cm above the pubic symphysis. Vascular engorgement of the uterus gives the cervix a bluish tinge and a softened consistency to the entire organ. The pregnant uterus is generally mobile on palpation. When the uterus reaches 12 weeks gestation (palpable just above the pubic symphysis), fetal heart tones are audible with a Doppler stethoscope. When the fundal height reaches 20 weeks gestation (palpable at the maternal umbilicus), an obstetrical (DeLee) stethoscope can be used to hear fetal heart tones. Beyond this gestation, the fetal position can be palpated and fetal movement observed through the abdomen.[17]

The second most common midline pelvic mass is the myomatous uterus. Unlike the pregnant uterus, this mass is usually irregular and firm and may be nearly any dimension or shape. While usually nontender, with degeneration from necrosis the uterus may be tender. When the myomatous uterus reaches the size of a 12 week pregnancy, it becomes difficult to differentiate from other pelvic structures by physical examination.

A sarcomatous change may enlarge a myoma rapidly; serial examinations (over one to three months) demonstrating enlargement may be the only diagnostic clue. Carcinoma of the uterine corpus does not usually cause significant enlargement of the uterus.

Ovarian neoplasms also may produce midline masses. Most benign ovarian masses will be cystic, including serous cystadenoma, mucinous cystadenoma, teratoma, endometrioma, and functional cysts. Ovarian malignancy may be contiguous with other pelvic structures, causing adhesion of the uterus, one or both ovaries, and/or bowel. Ovarian malignancy may be solid and/or cystic, with masses characteristically described as irregular, firm, immobile, and nontender. Ovarian carcinomas may produce ascites, causing the abdomen or cul de sac to bulge. Diagnostic paracentesis or culdocentesis for cytology provides diagnostic help.

Other midline masses include the bladder, urachal cysts, and bladder diverticuli. Bladder catheterization can be used to diagnose distension. Masses in the anterior abdominal wall can be confused with a pelvic mass. Stool may be confused with a pelvic mass or can hide a mass by making the examination difficult. Reexamination after an enema can eliminate stool as a confounding variable.

Lateral or Adnexal Pelvic Mass

The laterally located mass is most often ovarian or tubal in origin and commonly called an adnexal mass, the most common being a functional cyst. This cyst is characteristically less than 8 cm in diameter, smooth, unilocular, mobile, and nontender. A functional cyst (follicle cyst or a corpus luteum cyst) should regress spontaneously in one to three menstrual cycles. Observation may be used diagnostically.

Oral contraceptives administered for six weeks as a diagnostic test should suppress all functional cysts. Cysts present after trial suppression are neoplastic and require surgical removal. Recent anecdotal reports suggest that the 35μg estrogen pill may not be as successful at suppressing functional cysts. We recommend the lowest-dose pills not be used as a diagnostic test.[18,19] When a patient already using this low-dose pill presents with a cystic mass, a six-week trial of a higher-dose pill should be considered. For cysts greater than 8 cm in diameter, a trial of suppression is not recommended because the chance of neoplasia is too great.

During pregnancy, the corpus luteum cyst may persist for the first 8 to 12 weeks. Spontaneous regression of this cyst should occur and must be followed using serial ultrasound examination. The rare theca lutein cyst is also a functional cyst of pregnancy. It is bilateral and associated with pregnancies having high level of human chorionic gonadotropin (HCG) such as gestational trophoblastic disease or multifetal gestation. With termination or delivery, theca lutein cysts spontaneously regress.[20]

The pregnant patient with pain, bleeding, and a mass may have an ectopic pregnancy. Confirmation of the location of pregnancy becomes very important in this life-threatening situation. This differentiation relies on ultrasound findings and serum titers of HCG, discussed later in the laboratory and imaging sections.

Adnexal masses include the neoplastic ovarian masses previously discussed as midline masses. Tumors derived from the ovarian capsular epithelium are the most common neoplastic tumors of the ovary in the reproductive- and postreproductive-age woman (serous cystadenoma, mucinous cystadenoma, endometrioma), and those derived from germ cells (teratoma, choriocarcinoma, dysgerminoma, and endodermal sinus tumor) are the most common neoplastic masses in children and young adults.

Parovarian cysts are remnants of the mesonephric or wolffian duct. This embryologic duct becomes the vas deferens and ductus deferens in the male but without testosterone undergoes degeneration in the female. When ductal degeneration is incomplete, remnants exist in the female as hydatid cysts on the fimbria of the fallopian tube or as cysts in the broad ligament. These cysts are almost always benign, smooth, and unilocular on examination.

Masses with Indistinct Descriptions

Not all masses will be either midline or lateral. Some will fill the pelvis and be impossible to assess accurately by examination. Widespread malignancy, infection (bowel or tuboovarian), and endometriosis are all capable of producing hard, fixed, irregular masses associated with almost any constellation of physical findings.

DIAGNOSTIC STUDIES

Adjunctive Laboratory

To begin, a sensitive pregnancy test either qualitative or quantitative should be performed. A Pap smear should be done, but it will seldom be diagnostic, and often too much credence is placed on the normal Pap smear as a means to rule out gynecologic disease.

In the acutely ill patient presenting with pain or fever and a mass, hematocrit, sedimentation rate, white blood cell count, and C-reactive protein are initial screening tests used to confirm the diagnosis of infection. A gram stain from the cervix is helpful in the diagnosis of gonorrhea (positive for gram-negative intracellular diplococci in about half of cases). Cultures for *Neisseria gonorrhoeae* and *Chlamydia* help when an infection is suspected.[21]

Some serologic tumor markers are of great assistance: HCG is a marker for pregnancy or trophoblastic disease. Alpha-fetoprotein (AFP) or carcinoembryonal antigen (CEA) can be used in germ cell tumors and colon cancer, respectively. Serum CA 125 is elevated in multiple gynecologic diseases but is most helpful in the detection of primary and recurrent ovarian cancer.[22]

Imaging

Ultrasound (US) is the best imaging tool to differentiate the functional from the neoplastic cyst. Transvaginal US often produces better images than abdominal US.[23]

Computed tomography (CT) or magnetic resonance imaging (MRI) provides a better assessment of lymph node status, liver integrity, and survey of the other abdominal organs than US; therefore, in cases of suspected malignancy, CT or MRI enhances diagnostic assessment.

Urologic or bowel studies may be of help in selected cases with appropriate symptoms. The routine use of an intravenous pyelogram or barium enema is inefficient diagnostically.[26] Classically, all patients undergoing gynecologic surgery had an intravenous pyelogram. This was seldom helpful except in children with pelvic masses where up to 40 per cent of masses are urologic in origin. Upper and lower intestinal tract imaging or endoscopy should be done when there is an indication from history or examination. Hysterography may be used to aid in the diagnosis of uterine malformation or to outline the uterine cavity separately from a large pelvic mass.

ASSESSMENT

Reproductive age and pelvic examination findings are the most important tools in formulating the differential diagnosis (see the algorithm). Women of reproductive age will usually have benign, cystic masses that result from normal ovarian function. When this is the case, physical examination shows a smooth, round cyst, less than 8 cm in diameter. US demonstrates a unilocular cyst less than 8 cm in diameter with no internal or external excrescences for this mass. It should regress over one or two spontaneous menstrual cycles or may be suppressed with oral contraceptives as a diagnostic test. Women who do not suppress their cyst on this regimen need further evaluation. Patients outside the reproductive-age group or with masses greater than 8 cm, fixed, irregular, or hard usually have a neoplastic mass.

Initial evaluation in the reproductive-age patient should eliminate the possibility of pregnancy or pregnancy-related complica-

DIAGNOSTIC ASSESSMENT OF PELVIC MASS IN A FEMALE PATIENT

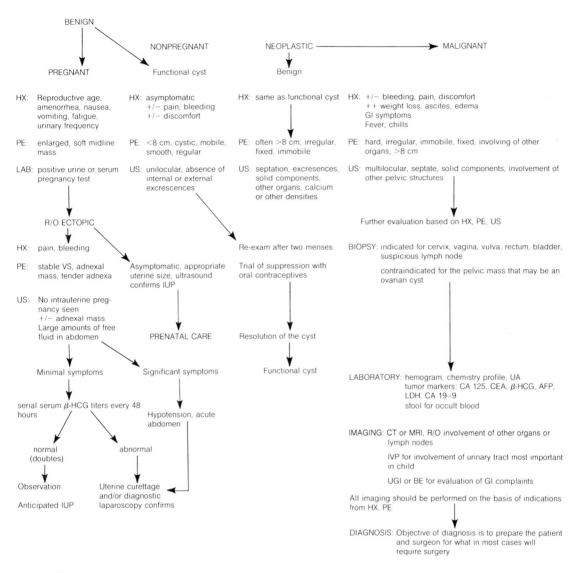

HX = history.
PE = physical examination.
LAB = laboratory.
R/O = to be ruled out as a cause.
US = ultrasound.
GI = gastrointestinal.
IUP = intrauterine pregnancy.
β = HCG = beta subunit of human chorionic gonadotropin.
CEA = carcinoembryonal antigen.
AFP = alpha-fetoprotein.
LDH = lactic dehydrogenase.
CT = computed tomography.
MRI = magnetic resonance imaging.
IVP = intravenous pyelogram.
UGI = upper gastrointestinal.
BE = barium enema.
CA = carcinoma associated antigen.

tions. Amenorrhea, morning nausea, and frequent urination should bring pregnancy to mind. Physical examination demonstrates an enlarged uterus that is mobile, smooth, and nontender. Urine or serum pregnancy tests should be negative. With symptoms of pain or abnormal bleeding, US examination should be done to confirm intrauterine versus extrauterine pregnancy. If no intrauterine pregnancy is seen, serial serum titers of β-hCG should be performed. In normal pregnancy, titers will double every 48 hours.[25] In abortions or ectopic pregnancy, they will not double. Laparoscopy or endometrial sampling is then indicated.

The second most frequent pelvic mass is the functional cyst. When a mass does not meet the criteria for a functional cyst, the objective becomes to differentiate gynecologic from nongynecologic and benign from malignant masses. The patients in the nonreproductive-age groups (pre- or post-reproductive) are at highest risk for both neoplasia and malignancy. Patients who report weight loss, bleeding, edema, ascites, or gastrointestinal or urinary symptoms are at high risk for malignancy, as are patients in which the mass is large (greater than 8 cm), irregularly shaped, hard, solid, fixed, immobile, or bilateral.

Mass lesions of the vulva, vagina, and cervix require biopsy. The decreased survival associated with rupture of a malignant ovarian mass makes biopsy of intra-abdominal masses a poor diagnostic technique. Laparotomy establishes diagnosis and therapy. An enlarged uterus or the uterus with abnormal bleeding requires endometrial biopsy.

Right-sided pelvic masses include a dilated cecum, an appendiceal abscess, an infected Meckel's diverticulum, or regional enteritis. The dilated cecum is usually transient and most common in elderly adults. All these except the dilated cecum have infectious symptoms like pain and fever. The infectious mass is usually fluctuant and fixed when acute but firm, woody, and irregular when chronic.

Gastrointestinal infections are often difficult to differentiate from tubo-ovarian abscesses. On physical examination, however, gynecologic infections demonstrate pus at the cervix or in the mucus of the endocervical canal when sampled with a cotton-tipped applicator and examined on a slide under a microscope. Biopsy of the endometrium is likely to show endometritis when associated with gynecologic infection. Inflammatory bowel diseases will show blood on stool testing and white blood cells on Gram's stain.

The left-sided pelvic mass is of greatest importance in the elderly patient. Sigmoid diverticulosis, diverticulitis, and colon cancer are confused with gynecologic disease. Colonic disease is almost always associated with blood in the stool, making rectal examination an important part of the physical examination.

Sigmoid colon cancer when appreciated on examination as a pelvic mass has a transverse orientation and feels like a hard, tubular mass. The uterus, tubes, and ovaries are usually separate. Diverticular disease as a mass is most often hard, fixed, and tender, with characteristic symptoms.

Most pelvic masses will be gynecologic in origin and functional in nature. In the pre- and postreproductive-age groups, the female pelvic mass is often neoplastic and requires surgery in either the form of laparoscopy or laparotomy for diagnosis and/or therapy. The objective of a thorough diagnostic evaluation is to prepare surgeon and patient for the most likely diagnostic possibilities so that each may participate in optimizing care. Careful history taking, physical examination, and the appropriate selection of laboratory and imaging make this possible.

REFERENCES

1. Edmonds DK. Dewhurst's practical paediatric and adolescent gynecology. 2nd ed. London: Butterworths, 1989:123,423.
2. Carlson JA. Gynecologic neoplasms. Pediatric and adolescent obstetrics and gynecology. New York: Springer Verlag, 1985:124–5.
3. Cancer of the ovary. Washington, DC: American College of Obstetricians and Gynecologists, 1990; ACOG technical bulletin no. 141:6.
4. King DR. Ovarian cysts and tumors. In: Welch KH, Randolph JG, Ravitch MM, O'Neil JA Jr, Rowe MI, eds. Pediatric surgery, Vol 2. 4th ed. Chicago: Yearbook Medical Publishers, 1986:1341–52.
5. Droegemueller W. Benign gynecologic lesions. In: Droegemueller W, Herbst AL, Mishell DL Jr, Stenchever MA, eds. Comprehensive gynecology. St Louis: CV Mosby, 1987:471–2.
6. Chang RJ, de Ziegler D. Polycystic ovarian syndrome. In: Gondos B, Riddick DH, eds. Pathology of infertility. New York: Thieme Medical Publishers, 1986:1443–68.
7. McShane PM, Yeh J. The oviduct and ectopic pregnancy. In: Ryan KJ, Berkowitz R, Barbieri RL. Kistner's gynecology—principles and practice. 5th ed. Chicago: Yearbook Medical Publishers, 1990:232–6.
8. Sloane E. Biology of women. 2nd ed. New York: John Wiley & Sons, 1985:286–8.

9. Weingold AB. Pelvic mass. In: Kase NG, Weingold AB, eds. Principles and practice of gynecology. New York: John Wiley & Sons, 1983:559–60.

10. Barber HRK. Perimenopausal and geriatric gynecology. New York: Macmillan Publishing Company, 1988:179–86.

11. Barber HRK. Manual of Gynecologic oncology. 2nd ed. Philadelphia: JB Lippincott Co, 1989:252–68.

12. Deppe G, Lawrence WD. Cancer of the ovary. In: Gusberg SB, Shingleton HM, Deppe G, eds. Female genital cancer. New York: Churchill Livingstone, Inc, 1988:379–426.

13. Berek JS. Epithelial ovarian cancer. In: Berek JS, Hacker NF, eds. Practical gynecologic oncology. Baltimore: Williams & Wilkins, 1989:327–64.

14. Sterns EE. Clinical thinking in surgery. Norwalk, Connecticut: Appleton & Lange, 1988:88.

15. Gordon AN, Kaufman RH. Sarcoma and lymphoma. In: Gusberg SB, Shingleton HM, Deppe G, eds. Female genital cancer. New York: Churchill Livingstone, Inc, 1988:474–7.

16. Bradley WE. Neurology of micturition. In: Ostergard DR, ed. Gynecologic urology and urodynamics—theory and practice. 2nd ed. Baltimore: Williams & Wilkins, 1985:11–29.

17. Wynn RM. Obstetrics and gynecology: the clinical core. 4th ed. Philadelphia: Lea & Febiger, 1988:80–3.

18. Spanos WJ. Preoperative hormonal therapy of cystic adnexal masses. Am J Obstet Gynecol 1973;116(4):551–4.

19. Speroff L, Glass RH, Kase NG. Steroid contraception. Clinical gynecologic endocrinology and infertility. 4th ed. Baltimore: Williams & Wilkins, 1988:483.

20. Morrow CP, Townsend DE. Tumor-like conditions of the ovary. In: Morrow CP, Townsend DE, eds. Synopsis of gynecologic oncology. 3rd ed. New York: Churchill Livingstone, Inc, 1987:337–40.

21. Ledger WJ. Infections in the female. Philadelphia: Lea & Febiger, 1986:141–53.

22. Malkasian GD Jr, Knapp RC, Lavin PT, et al. Preoperative evaluation of serum CA 125 levels in premenopausal and postmenopausal patients with pelvic masses: discrimination of benign from malignant disease. Am J Obstet Gynecol 1988;159(2):341–6.

23. Fleischer AC. Pelvic masses: endovaginal sonographic appearance. In: Goldstein SR, ed. Endovaginal ultrasound. New York: Alan R Liss, Inc, 1989:27–33.

24. Orr JW Jr. Introduction to pelvic surgery—pre and post-operative care. In: Gusberg SB, Shingleton HM, Deppe G, eds. Female genital cancer. New York: Churchill Livingstone, Inc, 1988:530–1.

25. Romero R, Kadar N, Copel JA, Jeanty P, De Cherney AH, Hobbins JC. The value of serial human chorionic gonadotropin testing as a diagnostic tool in ectopic pregnancy. Am J Obstet Gynecol 1986;155:392–5.

PERICARDITIS

JAMES L. VACEK

SYNONYM: Pericardial Inflammation

BACKGROUND

Pericarditis describes inflammation and/or other ultrastructural changes of the fibroserous membrane surrounding the heart. The pericardium is actually two layers, a fibrous outer layer called the parietal pericardium and an inner serous membrane called the visceral pericardium. The space between these layers is separated by pericardial fluid, which consists of an ultrafiltrate of plasma and which normally may comprise up to 50 ml of fluid. In disease states, the structure and/or function of the pericardium may change, and the amount of pericardial fluid may increase owing to a combination of enhanced production and/or reduced reabsorption. The pericardium is well innervated and very sensitive to pain.

The pericardium provides many important functions. It reduces friction between the beating heart and surrounding structures. It forms a barrier against the spread of infection or inflammation from surrounding structures to the heart. The ligamentous attachments of the heart limit cardiac displacement by extracardiac sources or during changes of position or motion. The pericardium also plays an important role in the regulation of cardiac chamber filling and is an important determinant of the relationship between right- and left-sided cardiac function.

Pericarditis may be caused by a multitude of conditions, as described in Table 1. It is most convenient and also of practical importance to consider pericarditis as being either acute or chronic.[1] Acute pericarditis is clinically much

TABLE 1.   Causes of Pericarditis

Amyloidosis
Anemia (chronic)
Aortic aneurysm/dissection
Chylopericardium
Connective tissue disease (periarteritis nodosa, rheumatoid arthritis, scleroderma, systemic lupus erythematosus)*
Drugs
Familial
Hypercholesterolemia
Idiopathic*
Infectious (bacterial, fungal, parasitic, tuberculosis, viral [Coxsackie A or B, echovirus, several others])*
Inflammatory bowel disease
Malignancy (lungs, breast cancer, lymphoma)*
Myocardial infarction (acute, postinfarction [Dressler's syndrome])*
Multiple myeloma
Myxedema
Pancreatitis
Postpericardiotomy syndrome*
Radiation*
Rheumatic fever (acute)
Sarcoidosis
Trauma (penetrating/nonpenetrating)
Uremia*

* Common causes; others, rarer.

more common and is noted chiefly by the symptoms attendant to pericardial inflammation. Chronic pericarditis is usually the end result of prior inflammatory activity that has resulted in thickening and fibrosis of the pericardium with reduction in the distensibility of this structure. The clinical presentation of chronic pericarditis is dominated by the cardiac hemodynamic alterations that it engenders. There of course may be considerable overlap between these syndromes as a patient progresses from the acute to the chronic stage or has recurrences and remissions of an ongoing or recurrent process.

HISTORY

History of the Present Illness

The most common complaints of patients with acute pericarditis are chest pain followed by dyspnea. The chest pain is precordial and said to be sharp and stabbing. Its severity may vary remarkably both from patient to patient and from time to time for the same patient. It may at times be dull and radiate to the left arm, causing confusion with myocardial ischemia. The presence and intensity of pain are dependent on position, being most severe when the patient is supine and being alleviated when the patient is sitting up and leaning forward. The pain often has dramatic pleuritic components, being exacerbated by deep inspiration, coughing, and swallowing. Patients often have a combined serositis with accompanying inflammation of the pleura, which exacerbates the pleuritic nature of the patient's complaints. Pain with respiration causes dyspnea, which also may be caused by the accumulation of enough pericardial effusion to cause the syndrome of cardiac tamponade. In the setting of cardiac tamponade, accumulation of pericardial fluid limits cardiac chamber distensibility, resulting in higher pulmonary and systemic venous pressures and reduced chamber filling volumes. Cardiac output may fall as stroke volume decreases, resulting in symptoms of hypoperfusion during overt cardiac tamponade.[2] Chronic pericarditis is usually not associated with chest pain. Patients present with symptoms referable to elevated cardiac filling pressures and diminished cardiac output. These symptoms are often easily confused with those of congestive heart failure and include fatigue and exercise intolerance.[3]

When questioning the patient regarding possible pericarditis, it is critical to distinguish acute myocardial ischemia or infarction from acute pericarditis and congestive heart failure from chronic pericarditis. Some aid to diagnosis is given by the clinical presentation of the patient. A young patient with few cardiac risk factors and with the sudden onset of sharp pleuritic chest pain is more likely to have acute pericarditis than the older patient with multiple atherosclerotic risk factors, who has dull, heavy chest discomfort precipitated by exertion. Although a recent viral upper respiratory tract infection may suggest viral pericarditis, it has been reported that a large number of patients presenting with acute myocardial infarction have had a recent antecedent viral respiratory syndrome.

A patient's history regarding maneuvers they have used to relieve their symptoms may also be of significant diagnostic importance. Relief of symptoms with assumption of an upright position, shallow breathing, and use of nonsteroidal anti-inflammatory agents is suggestive of acute pericarditis. A patient whose symptoms are relieved by cessation of exertion and administration of nitrate preparations is giving a history of myocardial ischemia.

Past Medical History

Careful ascertainment of the patient's past medical history is critical in distinguishing pericardial from myocardial disease. Again, assessment of the age and sex of the patient as well as coronary artery disease risk factors is vital in determining the risk of active coronary artery disease. A history of connective tissue disease, malignancy, uremia, or other systemic disease may imply involvement of the pericardium with this process. Recent prior myocardial infarction or cardiac surgery should raise the suspicion of postpericardiotomy syndrome or Dressler's syndrome.[4,5] Likewise, cardiac trauma may cause pericardial or myocardial injury, alone or in combination. Distinguishing primary pulmonary diseases from pericarditis may also be difficult, as pneumonia or pulmonary embolism may cause symptoms similar to acute pericarditis. Each of these syndromes may present with pleuritic chest pain and dyspnea but can usually be distinguished by physical examination, laboratory, electrocardiographic, and radiologic means.

Finally, distinguishing chronic pericarditis from congestive heart failure may be extraordinarily difficult, and it is not uncommon for a patient with chronic pericarditis to have been treated for several years by multiple clinicians for congestive heart failure in the setting of a chronic pericardial constrictive process.

Focused Queries

1. *Is the pain sharp, stabbing, and worse with inspiration?* This helps distinguish from myocardial ischemia.

2. *Has the patient recently had a viral respiratory syndrome?* This suggests a possible viral etiology for pericardial disease.

3. *What other medical problems are present?* This may focus on a specific primary etiology for the pericardial process.

4. *Has recent myocardial infarction, cardiac surgery, or chest trauma occurred?* A positive answer is suggestive of a pericarditis due to one of these insults.

PHYSICAL EXAMINATION

The pericardial friction rub is the sole physical finding that is pathognomonic of acute pericarditis. This sound is heard over the precordium and may be extremely localized. It is scratchy or scraping in character and is mimicked by rubbing two fingers or pieces of leather together close to the ear. This rub may have from one to three components, with two diastolic components corresponding to rapid atrial filling followed by atrial contraction and a ventricular systolic component. This last is the component most usually heard. At times, the rub may be confused with either third or fourth heart sounds, or a cardiac murmur, but usually careful auscultation with attention to timing of the sound and its sonic characteristics allows discernment. This murmur is best heard with the person sitting up and leaning forward and may be heard whether minimal or large amounts of pericardial fluid are present.

The physical findings in cardiac tamponade are dominated by the hemodynamic alterations that are caused.[6] The excess fluid in the pericardial sac causes increase in intrapericardial, and therefore cardiac chamber, diastolic pressures. Increased right ventricular end diastolic and right atrial pressures result in elevation of the jugular venous pressure. The elevated pressure limits early diastolic right atrial filling so that the y descent in the jugular venous pressure wave is attenuated or absent. Decreased left ventricular filling results in a lowered stroke volume, causing hypotension, a narrow pulse pressure, and reflex tachycardia to maintain cardiac output. During inspiration, negative intrathoracic pressure causes obligatory right ventricular filling with subsequent impairment of left ventricular filling. This further drops left ventricular ejection volume, resulting in cyclic inspiratory falls in blood pressure, causing pulsus paradoxus. The heart sounds in a patient with a large pericardial effusion may be muffled owing to the dampening effects of the fluid.

In chronic pericarditis with constriction, the physical findings are also notable for an elevated jugular venous pressure.[7,8] However, with constrictive pericarditis, both the x and y descents are very prominent. Kussmaul's sign may be seen, which is an inspiratory increase in jugular venous pressure. This finding is very rare in cardiac tamponade. Peripheral edema, hepatomegaly, and ascites may be seen owing to the long-standing nature of the process with persistent elevation of jugular venous pressure. Upon auscultation, an early diastolic sound termed a pericardial knock may be appreciated. This sound is usually heard along the left sternal border of the heart and corresponds to the sudden cessation of ventricular filling during diastole. It may be difficult to distinguish from a third heart sound or the opening snap of mitral stenosis.

DIAGNOSTIC STUDIES

There are no diagnostic clinical laboratory findings for either acute or chronic pericarditis. Nonspecific markers of inflammation such as an elevated white blood cell count or erythrocyte sedimentation rate may be noted as well as increased titers of other acute phase reactants. If a systemic process has been the cause of pericarditis, laboratory findings may be seen that are consistent with this diagnosis, such as evidence of uremia, connective tissue disease, or hypothyroidism. Long-standing chronic pericarditis with constriction may result in laboratory findings of hepatic dysfunction.

Noninvasive Cardiac Evaluation

There are few diagnostic features of the history, physical examination, or clinical laboratory evaluation that allow definitive diagnosis of either acute or chronic pericarditis. For pericardial disease, reliance on specific testing modalities is usually important. As will be discussed, although the electrocardiogram and the chest roentgenogram may provide extremely useful information, echocardiography has become the mainstay of diagnosis for pericarditis.

Electrocardiography

The electrocardiogram in acute pericarditis follows a distinct four-stage process (Table 2). Not all four stages are seen in every patient, and in many cases, serial electrocardiographic evaluation is not available to document progression through all phases. The findings of stage I are those considered most typical for acute pericarditis. The ST segment elevation associated with acute pericarditis may be distinguished from that of myocardial infarction by its presence in all leads except AVR and V_1, as opposed to the localized distribution associated with myocardial injury, as well as the other findings in Table 2. In the setting of a large pericardial effusion, the electrocardiogram may demonstrate diffuse low voltage. In

TABLE 2. Electrocardiographic Stages of Acute Pericarditis*

I	ST segment elevation (usually all leads but AVR and V_1; concave upward versus convex upward in myocardial infarction); T waves upright; PR depressed
II	ST segments return to baseline; T waves flatten
III	T waves become inverted
IV	T waves revert to normal (may take weeks to months)

* To further distinguish pericarditis from acute myocardial infarction, examination of serial tracings reveals no loss of R wave voltage or Q wave development.

cases of pericardial tamponade, the phenomenon of electrical alternans may be seen where beat-to-beat alterations in QRS complex amplitude are seen, presumably due to the heart swinging in the distended pericardial sac. Chronic pericarditis has few distinguishing characteristics on the electrocardiogram, although low QRS voltage and nonspecific T wave changes may be seen.

Chest Roentgenography

The chest roentgenogram in acute pericarditis shows no diagnostic features. If a significant amount of pericardial effusion is present, the cardiac silhouette is enlarged and shows configurational changes giving a globular or "water bottle" shape to the heart. Increased space between the two layers of the pericardium may result in separation of pericardial fat lines. Long-standing, chronic pericarditis may be noted on the chest roentgenogram by pericardial calcification, which at times may be extensive.

Echocardiography

Echocardiography[9,10] is presently the gold standard for the diagnosis and follow-up of pericardial effusion. It should be noted that not all episodes of acute pericarditis are accompanied by significant pericardial effusions, so that the absence of a sizable effusion does not rule out the diagnosis of acute pericarditis. Likewise, a significant effusion may be present without symptomatic evidence of pericardial inflammation. Nevertheless, as the major sequela of acute pericarditis is the accumulation of a significant pericardial effusion and potential cardiac tamponade, echocardiography is the usual means of assessment for the presence of pericardial effusion and a qualitative evaluation of its size. Serial echocardiographic studies can be used to monitor the course of an effusion and its response to therapy. Combined M-mode and two-dimensional study can allow sensitive early discernment of pericardial tamponade. Other aspects of the myocardium and pericardium are also assessed by echocardiography, including the presence of masses, thrombi, or fibrinous material in the pericardial cavity.

Cardiac tamponade is diagnosed on echocardiography by the presence of signs indicating elevated pericardial pressures, limitation of cardiac chamber filling, and inspiratory augmentation of right ventricular chamber size at the expense of left ventricular internal dimension. Early diastolic compression of the right ventricle and atrium is considered a sensitive marker for impending cardiac tamponade.[11] As echocardiography is widely available and readily performed even in the most ill of patients, its threshold for use in the patient with suspected pericardial effusion and/or tamponade should be very low.

Chronic pericarditis with constriction is less readily defined by echocardiography. The pericardium may appear thickened, although this does not necessarily imply constriction. Findings that may be seen in pericardial constriction include flattened diastolic ventricular wall motion and abnormal intraventricular septal motion consisting of abrupt posterior motion of the septum in early diastole but are not diagnostic. The inferior vena cava and hepatic veins may be dilated and poorly responsive to forced inspiration, although again these changes are not diagnostic.

Computed Tomography and Magnetic Resonance Imaging

These relatively recent and very expensive imaging techniques are excellent for making the diagnosis of pericardial effusion but offer few advantages over echocardiography in most circumstances. As with echocardiography, there are no specific findings to suggest acute pericarditis in the absence of significant effusion. They may be somewhat more accurate than echocardiography in assessing pericardial thickening and limitation of cardiac motion by a constrictive pericardium.[12] However, the evidence obtained from these studies

in chronic pericarditis with constriction is only supplementary to the patient's clinical signs and symptoms in association with abnormal directly measured hemodynamic parameters.

Cardiac Catheterization

Cardiac catheterization is not necessary in most cases of acute pericarditis. No specific hemodynamic or imaging information is obtained by this technique. For pericardial effusion, echocardiography is superior at making the diagnosis and is far better as a screening test for evidence of hemodynamic compromise. Measurement of intracardiac pressures can confirm a clinical suspicion of cardiac tamponade by yielding elevated and equilibrated diastolic pressures of all the heart chambers. Cardiac catheterization documents elevation of right atrial pressure and its characteristic prominent systolic x descent and diminished or absent diastolic y descent. Right atrial and intrapericardial pressures are by necessity equal in elevation and configuration in the setting of cardiac tamponade. Fluoroscopy and angiography provide no specific benefits in the diagnosis of cardiac tamponade that are not available via echocardiography.

Cardiac catheterization is extremely useful in the evaluation of patients with suspected constrictive pericarditis. The clinical setting is usually of a patient who has signs and symptoms consistent with congestive heart failure but whose systolic cardiac function as measured by echocardiography or other techniques is not consistent with the patient's symptomatology. Cardiac catheterization is most useful in regard to the hemodynamic information it yields in this setting, as angiography has little specific use. Measurement of intracardiac pressures demonstrates equilibration of all intracardiac diastolic pressures, with an elevated right atrial pressure that has prominent x and y descents. This gives a typical *m* or *w* configuration to the right atrial pressure tracing. Both right and left ventricular diastolic pressures show an early diastolic dip followed by a pressure plateau, which has been termed the square root sign. An inspiratory increase in right atrial pressure (Kussmaul's sign) may also be apparent. Careful interpretation of the findings at cardiac catheterization in association with echocardiographic assessment will allow distinguishing constrictive pericarditis from congestive heart failure due to systolic dysfunction or due to diastolic dysfunction associated with restrictive cardiomyopathy.

Pericardiocentesis

Acute pericarditis without evidence of hemodynamic compromise or significant pericardial effusion on echocardiography does not require pericardiocentesis. The presence of a large effusion, even without associated tamponade, is felt by many to be an adequate indication for diagnostic pericardiocentesis. My opinion is that needle pericardiocentesis should be performed only rarely for diagnosis, as the most common causes of acute pericarditis, viral and idiopathic, resolve spontaneously or with anti-inflammatory treatment and rarely progress to tamponade. Pericarditis with effusion that is secondary to other systemic disease processes rarely requires examination for diagnosis, as the primary disease process is usually evident, and in any event, there are few specific diagnostic features of pericardial effusions. In the rare instances where an effusion is persistent without evident diagnosis, limited operative pericardial biopsy with drainage via a subxiphoid window is preferable to needle pericardiocentesis, as diagnostic accuracy is enhanced by the obtaining of tissue. This limited operation appears to be at least as safe as needle pericardiocentesis and, in view of its diagnostic superiority, should be the investigative modality of choice in most settings.[13,14] Although some cardiologists feel that needle pericardiocentesis to evaluate possible neoplastic pericarditis with effusion is appropriate, I would argue again that subxiphoid pericardiectomy provides superior diagnostic results and better long-term control of recurrent effusion.[15] In any event, the diagnosis of a metastatic malignant process made from pericardial effusion rarely alters the clinical course of a patient, as the malignancy is usually widely disseminated at the time of this diagnosis.

Cardiac tamponade may be appropriately treated by either needle pericardiocentesis or operative limited pericardiectomy. Although in certain circumstances needle drainage may allow more rapid control of a patient in severe hemodynamic distress, in most circumstances operating room facilities can be rapidly mobilized to allow expeditious performance of surgery. Again, the opportunity for more complete diagnostic assessment via pericardial biopsy and reduction of the need for repeat needle drainages makes the surgical approach very attractive.

ASSESSMENT

Acute Viral Pericarditis

This, along with idiopathic pericarditis (which may in many cases be caused by an unrecognized viral infection), constitutes the most common cause of acute pericarditis. Onset is usually abrupt, with sharp, stabbing, pleuritic pain, usually distinguishable from the pain of myocardial ischemia or injury. The electrocardiogram commonly confirms the presence of pericardial inflammation and has findings distinguishable from myocardial infarction. A pericardial friction rub consisting of one to three components will be heard upon careful serial physical examination. In the absence of clinical evidence of hemodynamic compromise due to cardiac tamponade, further noninvasive or invasive testing is usually not necessary, although echocardiography is commonly done to assess the presence and volume of pericardial effusion. Acute pericarditis associated with these two syndromes is usually self-limited, without serious sequelae, although treatment with nonsteroidal anti-inflammatory agents will provide prompt relief of symptoms and hasten resolve of pericardial effusion. The use of steroids should be discouraged in this setting.

Pericarditis Associated with Malignancy

It is not uncommon for the first diagnosis of malignancy to be made when a patient presents with the clinical findings of cardiac tamponade and is found to have a large pericardial effusion, which upon evaluation is found to have malignant cells. Typical pericardial pain may be present, although commonly is not, and in the absence of cardiac tamponade, the patient's prognosis is primarily determined by the primary malignancy. However, drainage of the fluid may provide significant symptomatic benefit.

Post–Myocardial Injury Pericarditis

This entity is probably an autoimmune disorder occurring after pericardial injury and/or disruption attendant to myocardial infarction or cardiac surgery.[4,16] Typical pericardial pain may occur within days to several months after the inciting event, and careful taking of the patient's history for characteristics of the pain, physical examination for discernment of a friction rub, and careful analysis of the electrocardiogram usually allow the physician to distinguish these syndromes from acute myocardial infarction or ischemia.

Uremic Pericarditis

This entity may occur either de novo in patients with severe renal insufficiency or during maintenance hemodialysis.[17,18] Typical chest pain is frequently seen, as is a pericardial friction rub in the majority of patients. An associated effusion may be quite large, with progression to cardiac tamponade. The hemodynamic instability associated with a large effusion may complicate the performance of dialysis.

Infectious Pericarditis

Pericarditis may be associated with a variety of pathologic organisms in addition to viruses. Pericarditis due to agents other than viruses is usually not self-limited and requires more aggressive diagnosis and treatment. A high index of suspicion should be maintained in the patient with a known systemic infectious process or with one that is contiguous to the heart. Tuberculous pericarditis was previously the most common cause of chronic constrictive pericarditis.[19] It is still a very common entity in poorly developed nations. Bacterial pericarditis remains a grave medical condition, with high associated mortality.

Radiation-Induced Pericarditis

Patients who have had known exposure of the mediastinum to radiation doses of 400 rads or more are at risk for pericarditis.[20] This is usually an acute fibrinous pericarditis with associated pericardial effusion due to radiation-induced lymphatic and capillary damage. Patients may present as early as one month or as late as several years after mediastinal radiation. Tamponade is not uncommon in this entity, in part because the pericardium often demonstrates a component of constriction with poor distensibility such that even a relatively small amount of pericardial effusion is adequate to restrict cardiac chamber filling.

Drug-Induced Pericarditis

A wide spectrum of drugs has been reported to cause pericarditis. A partial list of the commonly implicated agents is noted in Table 3. During history taking and examination of the patient's prior medical records, a high level of alertness for the prior use of these agents should be maintained in patients suspected of having pericarditis. Diagnosis is extremely important in this setting, as discontinuance of the offending agent usually affords prompt relief.

Traumatic Pericarditis

Penetrating chest trauma that involves the pericardium is an easily recognized cause of pericarditis. Nonpenetrating blunt chest trauma should also be recognized as a cause of pericardial inflammation and possible effusion development, which may occur hours to several weeks after the injury. Other causes of traumatic pericarditis include perforation of the heart at cardiac catheterization, cardiopulmonary resuscitation, esophageal rupture, and cardioversion.

Pericarditis in Association with Connective Tissue Diseases

Almost any connective tissue disease variant may have associated pericarditis as part of its clinical manifestation. Mode of presentation may include acute inflammatory pericarditis, development of large pericardial effusion with possible tamponade, and chronic pericarditis with thickening and constriction. Symptoms and signs consistent with any pericardial syndrome should be carefully monitored for and evaluated in a patient with a known or suspected connective tissue disorder.

Implications of Pericarditis

Pericarditis is a common diagnosis of a disease process with multiple possible etiologies. Patient presentation may vary depending on

TABLE 3.   Drugs That May Cause Pericarditis

Dantrolene	Penicillin
Diphenylhydantoin	Phenylbutazone
Doxorubicin	Procainamide
Hydralazine	Quinidine
Isoniazid	Tetracycline
Methysergide	

the cause of pericardial disease and may present as either an acute or chronic process. Symptoms and signs are due both to direct involvement of pericardial tissue as well as to hemodynamic consequences of the fluid produced by and contained within the pericardial membrane. In most settings, a careful history and physical examination, along with an electrocardiogram and an echocardiogram, serve for initial evaluation of the patient with pericarditis. In the setting of acute pericarditis, these simple, noninvasive diagnostic techniques are usually all that is necessary to define patient status and determine specific therapy. In the setting of chronic pericarditis with suspected pericardial constriction, clinical evaluation and noninvasive assessment will aid in determining the patient in whom invasive evaluation and therapy may be necessary.

REFERENCES

1. Hancock EW. Management of pericardial disease. Mod Concepts Cardiovasc Dis 1979;48:1–6.
2. Reddy PS, Curtiss EI, O'Toole JD, Shaver JA. Cardiac tamponade: hemodynamic observations in man. Circulation 1978;58:265–72.
3. Hirschmann JV. Pericardial constriction. Am Heart J 1978;96:110–22.
4. Dressler W. The post-myocardial-infarction syndrome: a report on forty-four cases. Arch Intern Med 1959;103:28–42.
5. Engle MA, Zabriskie JB, Senterfit LB, Ebert PA. Postpericardiotomy syndrome: a new look at an old condition. Mod Concepts Cardiovasc Dis 1975;44:59–63.
6. Guberman BA, Fowler NO, Engel PJ, Gueron M, Allen JM. Cardiac tamponade in medical patients. Circulation 1981;64:633–40.
7. Blake S. The clinical diagnosis of constrictive pericarditis. Am Heart J 1983;106:432–3.
8. Fowler NO. Constrictive pericarditis: new aspects. Am J Cardiol 1982;50:1014–7.
9. Markiewicz W, Borovik R, Ecker S. Cardiac tamponade in medical patients: treatment and prognosis in the echocardiographic era. Am Heart J 1986;111:1138–42.
10. Schnittger I, Bowden RE, Abrams J, Popp RL. Echocardiography: pericardial thickening and constrictive pericarditis. Am J Cardiol 1978;42:388–95.
11. Engel PJ, Hon H, Fowler NO, Plummer S. Echocardiographic study of right ventricular wall motion in cardiac tamponade. Am J Cardiol 1982;50:1018–21.
12. Sutton FJ, Whitley NO, Applefeld MM. The role of echocardiography and computed tomography in the evaluation of constrictive pericarditis. Am Heart J 1985;109:350–5.
13. Krikorian JG, Hancock EW. Pericardiocentesis. Am J Med 1978;65:808–14.
14. Little AG, Kremser PC, Wade JL, Levett JM, DeMeester TR, Skinner DB. Operation for diagnosis and treatment of pericardial effusions. Surgery 1984;96:738–42.
15. Hawkins JW, Vacek JL. What constitutes definitive therapy of malignant pericardial effusion? "Medical" versus surgical treatment. Am Heart J 1989;118:428–32.
16. Stevenson LW, Child JS, Laks H, Kern L. Incidence and significance of early pericardial effusions after cardiac surgery. Am J Cardiol 1984;54:848–50.
17. Comty CM, Cohen SL, Shapiro FL. Pericarditis in chronic uremia and its sequels. Ann Intern Med 1981;75:173–83.
18. Wray TM, Stone WJ. Uremic pericarditis: a prospective echocardiographic and clinical study. Clin Nephrol 1987;6:195–202.
19. Ortbals DW, Avioli LV. Tuberculous pericarditis. Arch Intern Med 1979;139:231–4.
20. Applefeld MM, Slawson RG, Hall-Craigs M, Green DC, Singleton RT, Wiernik PH. Delayed pericardial disease after radiotherapy. Am J Cardiol 1981;47:210–3.

PHANTOGEUSIA

ROBERT I. HENKIN

SYNONYM: Phantom Taste

BACKGROUND

Phantogeusia is defined as the presence of an unusual, usually unpleasant, oral taste in the absence of food or drink.[1] As a symptom, it is a form of dysgeusia, the general term used to describe any unusual, usually unpleasant, distorted oral taste sensation. As a symptom, it commonly occurs without any antecedant cause, usually in an unsuspecting patient, and no physical change in the oral cavity is evident to account for the symptom. This apparent paradox may be resolved by understanding that the taste system is part of the chemosensory system of the body. As such, changes in body chemistry can alter taste function and can induce several symptoms, including phantogeusia. These changes in body chemistry may result from local or systemic diseases whose symptoms may not be otherwise obvious, the phantom taste being the first, earliest manifestation of the pathology. Thus, occult malignancies, endocrine diseases, or other metabolic diseases can present with phantogeusia as their initial symptom. Phantogeusia may also occur late in the metabolic pathophysiology of a disease or can even occur during treatment of the disease, per se.

Phantogeusia, when severe, may be considered as an atypical form of oral pain.[2] In this sense, it is a very common symptom for which patients often seek medical assistance. However, the complaint coupled with the absence of any physical findings presents one of the difficult problems that physicians face. Although the symptom can be defined or at least limited by words, there is no precise definition of the symptom. Since it is perceived only by the patient and not the observer, it can only be understood by the experience of the physician, who must recognize the history given by the patient. Because of its potential systemic and life-changing portent, the physician would be wise to accept the report of symptom severity of the patient at face value in spite of a negative physical examination, unless there is conclusive evidence to the contrary.

Phantogeusia in itself is not inherently different from the sensation of phantom limb described over 100 years ago in which, following below-the-knee amputation of a leg, patients suffered from sensations in the missing leg, foot, or toe and about 10 per cent complained of pain, burning, or other dysethesias in the amputated area. This symptom, sometimes chronic and severe, usually diminished over time. Although it has been well recognized for many years, it is still mechanistically unclear. Phantogeusia can be distinguished from phantom limb by the obvious lack of a surgical cause for its onset, by its surreptitious appearance commonly without specific etiology, and by its persistence over time.

Phantogeusia must be distinguished from the dysgeusic symptom termed aliageusia,[3] the general reference used to describe unusual, usually unpleasant tastes in the mouth that result directly from the presence of food or drink (Fig. 1). To make matters confusing,

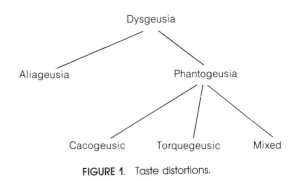

FIGURE 1. Taste distortions.

aliageusia and phantogeusia can occur in the same patient, and the symptoms need to be distinguished since their treatment may differ. To confuse the issue still further, food or drink in the oral cavity can itself taste appropriately but can exacerbate or even initiate the phantogeusia. It is the purpose of this chapter to clarify these confusing issues.

CHARACTERISTICS OF PHANTOGEUSIA

Phantogeusia can be subdivided into three general forms: cacogeusic, in which the taste sensation is either rotten, decayed, foul, or fecal-like;[1] torquegeusic, in which the taste sensation is quite diverse, including either metallic, bitter, chemical, salty, sweet, undescribable, and/or burned tastes;[4] or mixed, that is, containing both torquegeusic and cacogeusic components (Table 1). Torquegeusic components are much more common than cacogeusic components.

Phantogeusia, as a symptom, has been clinically recognized for many years, but it was not until recently that it was formally defined.[1] It usually begins surreptitiously, occurring for a few seconds. This usually does not alarm the patient, who may not even notice this as a change from normal oral sensory status. The symptom may be related by the patient to a sequela of smoking cigarettes or use of other tobacco products. If it occurs only in the morning, it is sometimes thought to be "morning mouth," the sensation of discomfort that can occur following an evening of excessive smoking or excessive intake of ethanol or recreational drugs. If it occurs after meals, it is often related to the "taste" of a "sour stomach" and explained away in this manner. However, if it returns, lasts for longer and

TABLE 1. Types of Phantogeusia

Torquegeusic
Metallic
Bitter
Chemical
Salty
Sweet
Indescribable
Burned
Cacogeusic
Fecal
Spoiled milk
Dead, decayed
Mixed
Two or more distortion   categories

longer periods of time on an increasingly recurrent basis, it cannot be explained away and is recognized as a phantom taste. It can become persistent, occurring all the time without relief, albeit waxing and waning in intensity. It can be so persistent that if the patient awakes from sleep at night, it is present.

The intensity of the phantogeusia can vary from a minor annoyance to a severe, incessant discomfort. It can become so severe, albeit rarely, that it can awaken the patient from sleep at night. With this occurrence, the concept of phantom taste as a type of oral pain may be better understood; this concept is clearer if the symptom is intermittent, of great intensity with sudden onset and offset. Usually, however, onset and offset of the symptom are slow and gradual, the intensity rising to a crescendo and then diminishing. When the onset is sudden, the intensity is usually greater, lasting a shorter period of time than when the onset is slow and gradual.

Usually, the onset and offset are beyond the patient's control without any apparent exacerbant or palliative, beginning and disappearing without obvious cause. The symptom can occur anytime of the day or night, most commonly occurring during the day in two major patterns: (1) beginning in the morning about 10 to 15 minutes after waking from sleep and beginning activity associated with the daily routine, then increasing in intensity during the day and either lasting until bedtime or decreasing slightly at night, or (2) beginning in the afternoon, after lunch, and increasing in intensity and duration as the day wears on, stopping only after the patient goes to sleep.

There is an unusual, relatively uncommon form of phantogeusia that occurs on a cyclic basis, occurring much more frequently in women than men, almost always associated with a similarly distorted phantom smell (phantosmia),[1,5] and relieved by either sleep or a Valsalva maneuver.[6] This relatively infrequent type of phantogeusia has been given the trivial name "cyclic phantogeusia." It is commonly associated with an epileptiform discharge and has been considered a sensory seizure variant and categorized as a partial seizure with simple psychosensory symptomatology.[6]

There are several exacerbants that can activate the phantogeusia. These are commonly acidic foods and drinks such as citrus juices, salad dressings, pickles, or spices used in food preparation. These items activate the phantom taste, although they themselves may not elicit a distorted taste. In this sense, this aspect of phantogeusia must be distinguished from aliageusia in which the food items per se taste foul or chemical. Foods which elicit phantogeusia exacerbate the patient's own oral phantom, which has its own specific, unique character. This distinction can be quite difficult but is very important since treatment for these symptoms can be quite different. In some patients, any food, even bland items, albeit usually spicy ones, can exacerbate the phantogeusia. This exacerbation may cause the patient to avoid eating those foods that induce the phantom. Toothpaste and mouthwashes can also initiate the phantom, although some patients find that these agents can also mask the symptoms. Fatigue, stress, and concern over family or other matters can exacerbate the symptoms, as can exercise.

Palliatives are multiple and diverse. Mouthwashes and toothbrushing are common palliatives, and patients may brush their teeth 5 to 10 times daily to attempt to mask or relieve the taste; however, after rinsing or brushing, much to the displeasure and concern of the patient, the phantogeusia commonly returns at the same level of intensity and with the same characteristics as before these activities. Chewing gum and eating breath mints or candies are common methods used to mask the unpleasant character of the phantogeusia; however, as with toothbrushing, the taste returns after completion of the act. Some patients will chew gum, use breath mints, or eat candy incessantly to attempt to relieve the symptom; patients have been observed to consume 3 to 10 packs of gum or 2 to 4 boxes of breath mints daily. They are rarely observed without gum or mints in their mouth. Some patients find that food, particularly sweets, will temporarily mask the phantogeusia. This causes some patients to gain weight and experience a significant increase in dental cavities in an attempt to control this symptom.

Associated Symptoms

As a corollary, some patients feel their phantogeusia is associated with a bad taste in their mouth that they think others can appreciate, for example halitosis.[7] Some feel that only they themselves can appreciate the phantom, whereas others feel that those around them can perceive their bad breath and are extremely self-conscious about this. With persistent phantogeusia and presumption of halitosis, some patients shun social contact. This is particularly difficult for young men and women during adolescence when patterns of dating and social contact related to the opposite sex are in the process of developing.

Glossopyrosis and/or oropyrosis with burning of the lips, gum, palate, cheeks, and pharynx can accompany the phantogeusia, the patient feeling the burning either as a direct result of the taste or as an associated symptom. Burning is usually localized to the tongue, primarily to the anterior one third of the lingual surface and commonly just to the tongue tip. If symptoms worsen, burning can extend to the blade and posterior portions of the tongue, rarely to the sublingual surface but occasionally to other oral areas. On occasion, patients complain that their teeth feel slimy and/or slippery, that their tongue feels rough, that their saliva feels thick, ropy, and stringy. With extension of the pyrosis to the palate and pharynx, patients may complain of having "dragon's breath," a burning that seems to eructate from their throat into their oral cavity.

Etiology

Phantogeusia can occur as an isolated primary symptom independent of any specific medical etiology, or it can be secondary to a variety of local or systemic medical problems (see Table 2). In this sense, phantogeusia can serve as a diagnostic clue, especially if the symptom is severe and isolated enough to force the patient to seek medical assistance. Phantogeusia can also arise secondary to drug treatment for several disorders[8] (Table 2); antibiotics, antimetabolites, antihypertensives, and many other agents can induce this symptom. These secondary problems, however, are relatively uncommon, albeit medically important, since they are usually treatable and their successful treatment is usually associated with diminution or disappearance of the phantogeusia. However, the vague quality of the phantogeusia, per se, makes its presence difficult to define; its intermittency and/or waxing and waning quality confusing to the physician, who may question its existence; and its relationship to any underlying disease state somewhat nebulous.

Many patients ascribe the onset of the phantogeusia to a local oral or dental problem. Many patients note the beginning of the symptom after symptoms or treatment of periodonitis; after placement of dentures, new or replacement; after placement of a dental amalgam; or after performance of some other dental procedure. Many return to their dentist, sure that their phantogeusia resulted from the dental procedure, but most oral examinations are completely normal and the dentist usually cannot account for the symptom on the basis of the procedure performed. Patients with a metallic phantogeusia question the type of amalgam used for the dental filling and question if some type of "electric current" was initiated by the procedure, particularly if several different materials were used in the past for different fillings. Some patients prevail upon their dentist to remove and replace the amalgam, to remake their dentures using different materials, and in some extreme cases, to remove healthy teeth to attempt to terminate the phantom. In general, these maneuvers are unsuccessful in alleviating the symptom. An example of these findings has been published recently.[9]

Other local oral problems can elicit an unusual oral taste, but the taste is usually short-lived and time locked to the problem. Thus, oral infections of any type, local or general, acute or chronic, including pharyngitis and tonsillitis, may initiate a taste sensation, but this is distinct from a phantom taste. Therapies with oral solutions of various types can elicit local taste responses that may be severe and unpalatable but are usually short-lived. Untreated tooth decay and severe dental

TABLE 2.   Etiologic Factors Producing Phantogeusia in Humans

Infectious disease (oral and systemic)
  Bacterial
  Fungal
  Viral
    Postinfluenza
    Viral hepatitis
  Rickettsial
  Microfilarial
  Luetic
Neurologic disease
  Meningioma, neuroesthisioblastoma, other tumors
  Head trauma
  Cerebral vascular accidents
  Multiple sclerosis
  Myasthenia gravis
  Postcraniotomy
Metabolic disease
  Hypothyroidism
  Addison's disease
  Panhypopituitarism
  Cushing's syndrome
  Cirrhosis of liver
  Gout
  Diabetes mellitus
  Chronic renal failure
Nutritional disease
  Metal deficiences (zinc, copper)
  Vitamin deficiencies (A, B_6, B_{12})
  Protein calorie malnutrition
  Total parenteral nutrition (without adequate trace
    metal replacement)
Drug-induced disease
  Clofibrate
  Cholestyramine
  Antithyroid drugs

Antibiotics
Anticancer agents
Tranquilizers
Amino acid excess (histidine, cysteine)
Adrenal steroids (chronic usage)
H_2 inhibitors (cimetidine)
Other disease processes
  Malabsorption
  Occult, overt carcinoma (lung, gastrointestinal tract,
    ovary)
  Postsurgical procedures (involving and not involving
    nasal area)
  Postlaryngectomy
  Postanesthesia
  Sjögren's syndrome
Local processes involving nasal area
  Infections (bacterial, fungal)
  Granulomatous (sarcoid, Wegener's, midline)
  Allergic rhinitis
  Chronic sinusitis
Environmental processes
  Chemical exposure
    Gases (chlorinated hydrocarbons, sulfur oxides,
      nitrogen oxides, carbon monoxide)
    Metals (mercury, lead, cobalt)
    Liquids (jet fuels, industrial chemicals)
    Tobacco smoke
Physiologic processes
  Pregnancy
Other factors
  Head injury
  X-irradiation (oral, other local or systemic)

plaque can initiate halitosis and specific oral taste sensations; these conditions, after effective treatment, improve clinically, and the associated taste sensations disappear as opposed to the persistent phantogeusia.

Taste sensations from local nasal problems, particularly chronic sinusitis and other chronic nasal infections, may occur and, if the underlying problem is not readily apparent, may be considered a phantom taste. These taste sensations are usually of a different character than observed with phantogeusia, per se, having a medicinal, fetid quality that differs from the fecal-like foul quality of cacogeusic phantogeusia.

Zenker's diverticulum of the pharynx, albeit not strictly an esophageal diverticulum, can retain saliva and food particles, and has been classically considered a relatively common anatomical cause of dysphagia, halitosis and, on occasion, the perception of phantogeusia. Other esophageal conditions associated with dysphagia include an esophageal web in the upper esophagus with multiple eccentric open-ings, or less commonly a web or ring in the terminal esophagus. While these conditions may be associated with dysphagia they are rarely associated with phantogeusia.

Underlying systemic disease, with or without local oral or nasal components, can initiate phantogeusia, as noted earlier (Table 2). As previously noted, the oral symptom may be the earliest component of the symptom complex, and the multiplicity of disease states that can manifest themselves with a phantogeusic component can be most confusing, especially since physical examination of the oral and/or nasal cavities may be completely benign. However, with the concept in mind that these symptom complexes can occur, the astute physician will consider these several factors in the list of differential diagnoses (Table 2).

EFFECTS OF PHANTOGEUSIA

Because of the complexity of these problems, it is easy to dismiss phantogeusia as part of a depressive or psychiatrically oriented illness. Indeed, the presence of the symptom and its peculiar character can lead to a depressive state on the part of patients, since they themselves may be confused by the vagueness of the symptom. As these symptoms interfere with the ability of the patient to eat, to socialize with others, and to lead a normal life, it can contribute to a depressive aspect of daily existence. Some patients, particularly if the taste is intense and persistent, seem to focus on the symptom to the exclusion of other aspects of their life-style and appear to be controlled by the symptom or appear to others to have the symptom control their behavior. While outsiders may feel this behavior bizarre or extreme, these symptoms can become the overriding factor in their lives since they cannot shut themselves off from the intense, persistent, and apparently subjective symptom. Perhaps an example may help to shed a little light on this type of behavior. Many of us have had the occasion to have a dental amalgam fall out of a molar tooth and find that our tongue, on a moment-by-moment basis, seems only to find the hole, which—while our knowledge tells us is small—seems to be "as large as the Carlsbad Caverns." Indeed, the cavity seems to be a yawning chasm that fills the mouth. The neurologic rationale for such an irrational feeling may lie in the large anatomic area and the physiologic importance of the central nervous system representation of the sensory homunculus of the fifth cranial nerve, since the oral portion of this representation is much larger anatomically than the representation of the trunk, arm, or leg. Perhaps it is this central nervous system emphasis on oral sensory input that serves to reinforce the focus on this area to the relative de-emphasis for other sensory inputs from portions of the body of much larger mass. Perhaps this same type of input literally forces some patients to focus on the taste phantom and associated symptoms such as pyrosis and other dysesthesias.

The effect of phantogeusia on personality cannot be underestimated. Whether the physician wishes to believe it or not, the patient with phantogeusia may perceive the oral taste as associated with, or the initiator of, bad breath or halitosis. Patients are fearful of opening their mouths, lest their neighbor recognize their "hidden problem." For some women, this drastically changes their social lives. I have listened to complaints such as, "I can't get close to any man" "I can't kiss anyone" "Everyone thinks that I am cold." Although the fruit of these statements comes from many seeds, it is important for the astute physician to recognize the powerful psychologic importance of the symptom.

STUDY RESULTS

In an effort to describe this putatively vague symptom more accurately, data from all patients with this symptom evaluated at The Taste and Smell Clinic, Washington, D.C. from December 1988 through May 1990 were evaluated. Of a total of 113 consecutive patients evaluated, 49, or 43 per cent, complained of having a phantom taste either as an isolated symptom or associated with another illness. Of these 49 patients, 12 were men and 37 were women, emphasizing that nearly three times as many women as men experience this symptom. Ages of the patients ranged from 18 to 83 years; for women, the age range was 18 to 83 years (mean—51 years); for men, 19 to 79 years (mean—55 years). Thus, as with isolated glossopyrosis, the majority of the patients are either postmenopausal women or middle-aged men. Of the patients, 40 (92 per cent) were Caucasian, 3 (6 per cent) were black, and 1 (2 per cent) was Oriental. Patients were evaluated 2 months to 45 years after the onset of the phantogeusia (mean—4 years). Of the 49 patients evaluated, 14, or 22 per cent, were seen within six months of the onset of their symptom.

The character of the phantogeusia in these patients is described in Table 3. The majority of patients (55 per cent) described their phantogeusia as either metallic, bitter, or some

TABLE 3. Phantogeusia Quality

	NUMBER OF PATIENTS	PERCENTAGE OF PATIENTS
Metallic*	15	31
Metallic/bitter*	2	4
Bitter*	10	20
Chemical*	6	12
Salty*	5	10
Rotten†	5	10
Overly sweet*	2	4
Undefined*	2	4
Sour milk*	1	2
Burned*	1	2

* Torquegeusic qualities—44 (90 per cent).
† Cacogeusic qualities—5 (10 per cent).

combination of these perceptions. Bitter taste sensations were sometimes associated with chemical or metallic tastes, whereas metallic taste sensations were sometimes associated with salty tastes. The remainder of the major taste characteristics were either chemical (consisting of an undefined chemical or a sulfur or minty taste), overly salty, or rotten. Torqueguesic (i.e., associated with chemical, bitter, metallic taste distortions) characteristics were nine times more common then cacogeusic (i.e., associated with rotten, decayed, fecal taste distortions) characteristics (Table 3). This differs from the distribution of these markers observed in aliageusia, in which the cacogeusic markers are almost as common as the torquegeusic ones.

Of the 49 patients with phantogeusia evaluated, 22, or 45 per cent, sought medical assistance for treatment of their phantogeusic symptoms (Table 4) which was their primary complaint. Of these, 19 had idiopathic phantogeusia, for example, phantogeusia of unknown etiology. One patient developed phantogeusia following radiation after surgery for cancer of the colon, and two developed phantogeusia following tonsillectomy. It is of interest to consider the putative relationship between radiation to the lower abdomen and the onset of phantogeusia. Whereas abscopal changes following radiation to distal areas have been associated with hypogeusia,[10] little mention has been made of phantogeusia as a sequela of such radiation. The mechanism whereby radiation to the lower gastrointestinal tract produced a phantom taste—in this case, a bitter phantogeusia—is unclear.

While phantogeusia has been associated with systemic diseases and can serve as an identifying symptom of that disease (see Table 2), the diagnoses associated with phantogeusia in the present study emphasize the common, primary nature of phantogeusia. Most patients with phantogeusia developed the symptom spontaneously, without a known etiologic antecedent, and, hence the symptom fails within the broad spectrum of idiopathic phantogeusia (Table 4). Phantogeusia was also a common complaint of patients whose primary problem was loss of taste and smell following a systemic viral illness, a coryza.[4] Less common was the development of phantogeusia after a head injury, associated with allergic rhinitis, or following tonsillectomy.

Important associated problems also included clinical depression, observed in two patients not as a sequela but either as a clinical diagnosis prior to or concomitant with the onset of the phantogeusia. The associated depression can confuse the physician, particularly since some drugs used in the treatment of depression may improve both the depression and the phantogeusia (see later discussion).

Xerostomia was observed in one patient. The importance of xerostomia relates to the association of xerostomia, xerorhinia, and xerophthalmia within the context of Sjögren's syndrome[11] and its associated taste and smell dysfunctions. In the patient in the present study, the xerostomia preceded the onset of the phantogeusia, although a diagnosis of Sjögren's syndrome was not conclusive since there was neither associated arthritis or other collagen vascular symptoms nor elevation of erythrocyte sedimentation rate nor the presence of serum antinuclear antibodies or rheumatoid factor. In addition, a Schirmer's test was within normal limits.

One patient with phantogeusia had bilateral blepherospasm of unknown etiology, the onset of this symptom closely related in time to the onset of the phantogeusia.

Patients with phantogeusia commonly exhibited hyposmia (loss of smell acuity) or hypogeusia (loss of taste acuity), whether or not they were subjectively aware of these sensory changes (Table 5). Of the 49 patients studied, 40, or 82 per cent, exhibited some form of hyposmia, although only 30 patients complained of smell loss. Of the patients with hyposmia, 26 exhibited the most common form of hyposmia, that is, Type II hyposmia, in which there is a quantitative decrease in either detection or recognition of vapors.[12] Five patients exhibited Type I hyposmia, in which there is an absolute inability to recognize any vapor at

TABLE 4.   Patient Diagnosis

ETIOLOGY	NUMBER OF PATIENTS
Idiopathic phantogeusia	19 (39%)
PIHH*	15 (31)
Head injury	7 (14)
Allergic rhinitis	3 (6)
Postoperative phantogeusia (tonsillectomy)	2 (4)
Carbon monoxide intoxication	1 (2)
Congenital hyposmia	1 (2)
Radiation for cancer (colon)	1 (2)

* PIHH = Post-influenza hyposmia and hypogeusia.

TABLE 5. Taste and Smell Changes Associated with Phantogeusia*

		TASTE				
		Hypogeusia				
Patient number	Ageusia†	Type I	Type II	Type III	Total	Normal
	0	0	16	10	26	23

		SMELL				
		Hyposmia				
Patient number	Anosmia‡	Type I	Type II	Type III	Total	Normal
	1	5	26	8	40	9

		FLAVOR				
Patient number	Absent	Decreased	Distorted	Decreased and Distorted	Total	Normal
	7	21	2	7	37	12

* Number of patients with both taste and smell changes is 24.

† Ageusia is defined as the absence of tastant detection or recognition; Type I hypogeusia, as absence of tastant recognition (usually associated with decreased tastant detection thresholds); Type II, as decreased taste detection and/or recognition thresholds; Type III, as decreased magnitude estimation, with normal detection and recognition thresholds.[12,13]

‡ Anosmia is defined as the absence of vapor detection or recognition; hyposmia, as decreased vapor detection or recognition; Type I, as absence of vapor recognition (usually associated with decreased vapor detection thresholds); Type II, as decreased vapor detection or recognition thresholds; Type III, as decreased magnitude estimation, with normal detection and recognition thresholds.[12,13]

the primary area of olfaction and usually a decrease in ability to detect vapors.[12] Eight patients exhibited Type III hyposmia; that is, normal detection and recognition thresholds are exhibited, but ability to appreciate strength of vapors is significantly impaired. Only one patient exhibited anosmia, the inability to detect or recognize any vapor at the primary or accessory areas of olfaction.[13]

Taste impairments in these patients with phantogeusia were much less frequent than smell impairment, with about half (53 per cent) of the patients exhibiting hypogeusia.[14] As would be expected, about as many patients stated that they had a decreased ability to obtain flavor from food as had hyposmia, with the majority stating they had a decrease in their flavor perception, with some of them noting an associated flavor distortion (Table 5).

Phantosmia was present with the phantogeusia in only 19 (39 per cent) of the patients with phantogeusia (Table 6). The character of the phantosmia was mainly chemical (torquegeusic) or rotten (cacogeusic). As opposed to the relatively infrequent cacogeusic phantogeusic character (Table 3), 32 per cent of the patients with phantogeusia had an associated cacogeusic phantosmia. Of the patients with phantosmia and phantogeusia, 10 (53 per cent) had a phantom smell similar to that of their phantom taste; however, in 9, the phantosmia was different. These patients developed a relatively specific phantogeusia, either metallic, bitter, or metallic and bitter. Of the six patients with metallic phantogeusia, three had a rotten, cacogeusic phantosmia, two had a burned phantosmia; and one had a chemical phantosmia. Of the two patients with a bitter phantogeusia, one had a chemical phantosmia and one had a rotten, cacogeusic phantosmia. The one patient with a metallic and bitter phantogeusia developed an accompanying rotten, cacogeusic phantosmia.

TABLE 6. Phantosmia Associated with Phantogeusia

PHANTOSMIA CHARACTER	PATIENT NUMBER
Chemical	7
Chemical and bitter	1
Rotten	6
Metallic	2
Metallic and salty	1
Burned	2

MECHANISM OF PHANTOGEUSIA

No specific mechanism(s) of onset or perpetuation of phantogeusia has been defined. However, natural history of the symptom suggests that there are several factors, hormonal, neural, neuroendocrine and neurotransmitter, influencing a variety of receptors in the oral cavity and/or the central nervous system, which contribute to the symptom. Since most patients are post-menopausal women or middle-aged men, gonadal hormones have been considered significant contributers to the symptom. However, failure of estrogen and/or progesterone replacement to correct the symptom consistently has lessened dependence upon lack of these hormones a primary factors. However, it is well-established that several peripheral and centrally acting hormones influence taste and smell function[15] so that these substances may play some role, albeit presently unclear, in the generation of this symptom. Other factors which influence this symptom lie in the endogenous cerebrally active GABAnergic system and its agonists, in the dopaminergic system and its antagonists, in the serotinergic system and its antagonists, in calcium channel antagonists, and in the complex interactions of these systems and their effects on their specific receptors in the central nervous system and in the oral cavity.

MANAGING PHANTOGEUSIA

Phantogeusia may be considered an atypical form of pain and, in this context, may be better appreciated as a distinct syndrome. It can be distinguished from trigeminal or postherpetic neuralgia by both history and character. However, if causalgia is the predominant component of these syndromes, it is necessary to consider the taste component of the phantogeusia primary in distinguishing it from the atypical facial pain that may accompany trigeminal or postherpetic neuralgia.

The mechanism(s) by which phantogeusia is initiated is obscure, just as in phantom limb. Whether only taste receptors or, in addition, taste nerves and/or central nervous system projections are involved is not clear. Since treatment with a variety of drugs[16]—some of which act as dopaminergic antagonists[17] (but also as central nervous system calcium channel blockers)—seems to be effective in inhibiting the phantogeusia, regulation of neurotransmitter secretion seems to be a controlling factor that may either initiate or block the development of this symptom. Whether this occurs peripherally, centrally, or at both neural areas, the details of chemical onset and offset of the symptom may offer important clues not only to the evaluation and treatment of this symptom but also to the neurobiology of chemosensation.

REFERENCES

1. Henkin RI. Disorders of taste and smell. JAMA 1971;218:1946.
2. Henkin RI. Taste distortion. JAMA 1981;245:1259.
3. Henkin RI, Raiten DJ. Characterization of patients with type I aliageusia. FASEB J 1990;4:A666–70.
4. Henkin RE, Frazier KB. Torquegeusia: a new, distinct and common form of dysgeusia. FASEB J 1989;3:A338–42.
5. Henkin RI. Phantom odor. Consultant 1987;27:19–25.
6. Potolicchio SJ Jr, Lossing JH, O'Doherty DS, Henkin RI. Partial seizures with simple psychosensory symptomatology (cyclic phantosmia). Clin Res 1986;34:635A–39A.
7. Goldberg RL, Buongiorno PA, Henkin RI. Delusion of halitosis. Psychosomatics 1985;26:326–31.
8. Henkin RI. Drug effects on taste and smell. In: Pradhan SN, Maickel RP, Dutta SN, eds. Pharmacology in Medicine: Principles and Practice. Bethesda, Maryland: SP Press International, Inc., 1986;748–53.
9. Henkin RI Salty and bitter taste. JAMA 1991;265:2253.
10. Mossman KL, Henkin RI. Radiation induced changes in taste acuity in cancer patients. Int J Radiat Oncol Biol Phys 1978;4:663–70.
11. Henkin RI, Talal N, Larson AL, Mattern CFT. Abnormalities of taste and smell in Sjögren's syndrome. Ann Intern Med 1972;76:375–83.
12. Henkin RI. Olfaction in human disease. In: English, GM, ed. Looseleaf Series of Otolaryngology. New York: Harper & Row, 1982: 1–39.
13. Henkin RI. The definition of primary and accessory areas of olfaction as the basis for a classification of decreased olfactory acuity. In: Hayashi TI, ed. Olfaction and Taste II. London: Pergamon Press, 1967;235–52.
14. Henkin RI. Taste in man. In: Harrison D, Hinchcliffe R, eds. Scientific Foundations of Otolaryngology. London: William Heinemann Medical Books Ltd, 1976;468–83.
15. Henkin RI. The role of adrenal corticosteroids in sensory processes. In Blaschko H, Sayers G, and Smith AD eds. Handbook of Physiology, Endocrinology. Washington, DC: Amer Physiol Soc, 1975;(VI):209–30.
16. Henkin RI. Taste and smell disorders. In: Adelman G, ed. Encyclopedia of neuroscience. Boston: Birkhauser, 1987;1185–6.
17. Henkin RI. Hyperosmia and depression following exposure to toxic vapors. JAMA 1990;264:2803.

POLYARTERITIS

LEE D. KAUFMAN

SYNONYMS: Polyarteritis, Polyarteritis Nodosa, Periarteritis Nodosa, Systemic Necrotizing Vasculitis

BACKGROUND

The primary vasculitides comprise a heterogeneous group of idiopathic disorders that have been categorized by different investigators according to the size of vessel involvement, the histologic presence or absence of granulomata, and the spectrum of clinical disease.[1] The distribution of inflammatory vascular disease has been divided in an arbitrary fashion morphologically into small vessel leukocytoclastic vasculitis (often associated with specific drugs, infections, neoplastic disease, or connective tissue diseases), the polyarteritis group of medium-size vessel necrotizing arteritis, and the large vessel diseases of temporal (cranial) arteritis and Takayasu's arteritis[2] (Table 1). This chapter will focus primarily on the clinical disorders associated with small and medium vessel necrotizing vasculitis that include classical polyarteritis nodosa as initially described by Kussmaul and Maier[3] in 1866 as well as the more commonly observed overlap group of systemic necrotizing vasculitis. The little epidemiologic data that exist for these syndromes suggest that they occur with an annual incidence of from 4.6 to 9 per 1 million in England and Minnesota, respectively.[4]

The primary target in the polyarteritis group is the small- to intermediate-size muscular artery.[5] The pathologic findings are characterized by involvement of arterial bifurcation sites with destruction of the media and internal elastic lamella, resulting in the formation of aneurysmal dilatation. A panarteritis often occurs, and the inflammatory infiltrate varies with the age of the lesion. In early acute disease, there is a predominance of polymorphonuclear leukocytes invading the vascular wall with endothelial cell proliferation and fibrinoid necrosis associated with regional ischemia and infarction (Fig. 1). Immunoglobulin (Ig) and complement (C) deposition may occur but are often absent when direct immunofluorescence is accomplished on biopsy specimens. The chronic stages are marked by mononuclear cell infiltrates and ultimately fibrosis. It is important to recognize that a single biopsy sample may reflect the spectrum of both acute and chronic abnormalities.

These pathologic features are similar to those found in experimental and human serum sickness.[6,7] In that pathophysiologic model of systemic vasculitis, circulating immune complexes form in the presence of antigen excess and—depending on their size, charge, and the physical properties of local blood flow—deposit in the vascular wall of small- and medium-size arteries. Vasoactive amines such as histamine may be released from circulating basophils and tissue mast cells by the formation of complement cleavage products known as anaphylatoxins (C3a, C4a, C5a); cell-derived histamine releasing factors (neutrophils, platelets, mononuclear cells); and possibly anti-IgE autoantibodies, which have been identified in connective tissue diseases associated with a vasculopathy.[8] Following the increased permeability mediated by vasoactive substances, these immune complexes gain access to the subendothelial portions of the vascular wall. Neutrophil chemoattractants are then generated from complement (C5a), arachidonic acid (leukotriene B4), mast cells (platelet activating factor), and mononuclear cells (neutrophil activating peptide-1 or interleukin-8 [IL-8]).[5,9] As polymorphonuclear leukocytes infiltrate the lesion and become activated, vascular injury evolves as the result of proteinases (neutrophil collagenase and cathepsins) and toxic oxygen radicals that are released. Cytokines produced by activated T lymphocytes (interferon-γ [IFN-γ]) and monocyte macrophages (interleukin-1 [IL-1] and tumor necrosis factor-α [TNF-α]) play a potentially important role in the regulation of leukocyte–endothelial cell interactions. Specifically, the expression of the endothelial leukocyte adhesion molecule (ELAM-1), which is absent on unstimulated endothelial cells, is induced by both IL-1 and TNF-α.[10] A similar adherence marker re-

TABLE 1.   Classification of the Vasculitides*

POLYARTERITIS NODOSA GROUP

Classic polyarteritis nodosa
Churg-Strauss allergic granulomatosis
Microscopic polyarteritis
Overlap systemic necrotizing vasculitis
Kawasaki disease (childhood polyarteritis)
Localized arteritis
    Appendix
    Gallbladder
    Kidney
    Epididymis
    Uterus

WEGENER'S GRANULOMATOSIS

LARGE VESSEL VASCULITIS

Temporal arteritis
Takayasu's arteritis

HYPERSENSITIVITY (SMALL VESSEL) VASCULITIS

Serum sickness
    Drug (penicillin, sulfonamide, phenytoin, etc.)
    Infection (bacterial, viral, parasitic)
    Foreign protein (passive immunization with heterologous
      gammaglobulin)
Cryoglobulinemia
Henoch-Schönlein purpura
Vasculitis of connective tissue diseases (systemic lupus erythe-
    matosus, rheumatoid arthritis, Sjögren's syndrome)
Behçet's disease
Buerger's disease (thromboangiitis obliterans)
Erythema elevatum diutinum
Hypocomplementemic urticarial vasculitis

* Compiled from references 1, 5, 13, and 26.

ferred to as the intercellular adhesion molecule (ICAM-1), normally present on resting endothelial cells, is upregulated by IL-1, TNF, and IFN-γ.[10] These adherence proteins help to recruit and maintain neutrophils in the vessel wall. In addition, IL-1 decreases the production of plasminogen activator and increases the production of tissue thromboplastin and plasminogen activator inhibitor from endothe-

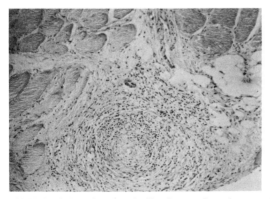

FIGURE 1.   Subacute panarteritis of a medium-size muscular artery. Myofibers are seen surrounding the inflammatory vascular lesion. (Courtesy of Frederick Miller, M.D.)

lial cells, producing a procoagulant effect[11] promoting thrombosis and vascular occlusion.

Although the antigenic stimulus responsible for immune complex vasculitis is unknown in most circumstances, specific clinical associations have been established. There is good evidence for both infectious agents and neoplasia in the development of these disorders. The hepatitis B virus (HBV) has been identified in 30 to 71 per cent[12,13] of patients with classic polyarteritis, and some patients with HBV antigenemia followed prospectively will develop a necrotizing vasculitis.[13] Cytomegalovirus[14] and parvovirus[15] infection have also been associated with vasculitis, and recent studies have identified a necrotizing vasculitis in individuals with the human immunodeficiency virus (HIV).[16] Additional evidence of an infectious agent inducing or "triggering" disease is the onset of a systemic vasculitis following serous otitis media.[17] Hairy-cell leukemia is the best example of neoplastic disease associated with vasculitis, and this may mimic the idiopathic form of classic polyarteritis.[18] Occasional patients with a connective tissue disease such as systemic lupus erythematosus or rheumatoid arthritis will also develop a systemic vasculitis; however, this is the exception and not the rule.[19,20]

CLINICAL FEATURES

The initial clinical manifestations of systemic necrotizing vasculitis are for the most part nonspecific. Fever, fatigue, weight loss, arthralgias (with occasional synovitis), and myalgias occur in one half to two thirds of patients. The relative prevalence of organ system involvement varies with the specific vasculitis syndrome. Contrasting features of the polyarteritis group of systemic vasculitis are shown in Table 2.

Renal involvement occurs in 70 to 100 per cent of patients[5,12] and leads to uremia in up to one half of patients with classic polyarteritis as a result of vasculitis, glomerulonephritis, or the vasculopathy of hypertension. Nephrotic range proteinuria suggests renal vein thrombosis and is not generally due to the glomerular disease associated with the vasculitis. Rarely, spontaneous rupture of a microaneurysm from the renal circulation can occur, leading to flank pain and hypotension.[21] Peripheral neurologic disease develops in 60 to 76 per cent of patients with polyarteritis[12,22] and manifests most often as a polyneuropathy with diffuse paresthesias; however, an isolated cutaneous neuropathy and mononeuritis multiplex (both limited and extensive) are also common.[22] The mononeuritis syndrome often develops over the course of hours to days, is preceded by severe pain in the involved limb, and is usually associated with motor and sensory dysfunction. These deficits may be transient or may remain fixed for months. The peroneal, sural, radial, ulnar, and median nerves are among the most commonly affected peripheral nerves. Cranial neuropathies also occur, most notably involving cranial nerves II, VII, and VIII.[12] Central nervous system disease is seen in 40 per cent of individuals affected by systemic vasculitis and may present with diffuse dysfunction characterized by an encephalopathy or a seizure disorder, or focal abnormalities secondary to a cerebrovascular accident.[22]

Gastrointestinal manifestations are generally the result of a ruptured aneurysm or a small bowel and/or liver infarction related to involvement of the celiac or superior mesenteric vessels. These are seen in 31 to 50 per cent of patients and include severe, usually acute abdominal pain associated with fever, diarrhea, and often upper or lower gastrointestinal bleeding.[20,23] Intra-abdominal bleeding

TABLE 2. Contrasting Features of the Polyarteritis Group of Systemic Vasculitis

	CLASSIC PAN*	MP†	CHURG-STRAUSS‡
Target artery	Small/ medium	Small	Medium
Renal disease	70%	100%	38%
Neurologic disease	80%	30%	63%
Gastrointestinal disease	50%	50%	42%
Pulmonary disease	Absent	50%	100%
Cardiac disease	40%	Absent	40%
Arthralgia/ arthritis	50%	75%	20%
Skin lesions	40%	50%	70%
Oral ulcers	Absent	20%	Absent
HB$_s$Ag§	30%	Absent	Absent
Cryoglobulins	30%	Absent	Absent
ANCA‖	Absent	Present	Absent
Angiography	Micro- aneurysms	Normal	Normal

* PAN = polyarteritis nodosa.
† MP = microscopic polyarteritis.
‡ Churg-Strauss = allergic granulomatosis.
§ HB$_s$Ag = hepatitis B surface antigen.
‖ ANCA = antineutrophil cytoplasmic antibody.

into the peritoneal cavity or occasionally into the liver is associated with signs of peritonitis.[20,24] Pancreatitis, cholecystitis, and appendicitis may also develop.

Cardiac involvement is more common in the juvenile form of polyarteritis (Kawasaki's disease or the mucocutaneous lymph node syndrome) than in adults. This relates primarily to the development of a coronary arteritis. Clinically, myocardial disease with congestive heart failure, frequently complicated by coexisting hypertension, is more prevalent. This is followed by myocardial infarction, pericarditis unrelated to either uremia or ischemic heart disease, and conduction disturbances.[5,12]

Visual abnormalities are an important part of the spectrum of polyarteritis. These are usually related to hypertensive disease, central retinal artery or choroidal vasculitis, and episcleritis. Amaurosis fugax, monocular blindness, and retinal detachment are common sequelae.[5,12]

Skin lesions resemble those seen in the smaller vessel vasculitic syndromes and are important clinical clues to the diagnosis of a systemic vasculitis. These include nonthrombocytopenic petechiae and palpable purpura, urticaria, livedo reticularis, ulcers, and occasionally painful subcutaneous nodules.

Pulmonary involvement has been considered not to be part of classic polyarteritis nodosa. However, the association of pulmonary infiltrates with pre-existing asthma and eosinophilia compose the variant of allergic granulomatosis or the Churg-Strauss syndrome.[5] Furthermore, pulmonary manifestations are not uncommon in the subset of disease referred to as microscopic polyarteritis.[25] Pleural disease is uncommon and should suggest a possible infectious etiology.

DIAGNOSTIC STUDIES

There are no laboratory parameters that are diagnostic of a systemic necrotizing vasculitis. The most common abnormalities include an elevation of the erythrocyte sedimentation rate, a mild to moderate leukocytosis, anemia, thrombocytosis, and urinary findings reflecting the frequent renal involvement. A peripheral eosinophilia is most often found in association with pulmonary involvement (Churg-Strauss variant); however, eosinophilia has been reported to occur in up to one third of patients with classical polyarteritis. The differences are more arbitrary than real,

as overlap between categories is seen. Tests for antinuclear antibody are usually negative. However, rheumatoid factor has been reported to be present in about 40 per cent of individuals. Antibodies to extractable nuclear and cytoplasmic antigens such as Ro (SS-A) and La (SS-B) are rarely found in polyarteritis but may be useful in identifying patients with a systemic vasculitis associated with a connective tissue disease.[26] Elevated levels of von Willebrand factor antigen, synthesized by endothelial cells, have been found in patients with systemic vasculitis and may be useful for following disease activity in certain patients. Recent studies have identified autoantibodies directed against neutrophils in the subset of microscopic polyarteritis as well as the vasculitis of Wegener's granulomatosis.[25,27] These antineutrophil cytoplasmic antibodies have a high specificity for these disorders and are the first serologic markers described that are of diagnostic utility in the differential diagnosis of the vasculitides.

Radiographic studies in patients with systemic necrotizing vasculitis have revealed the presence of saccular or fusiform microaneurysms in up to 80 per cent of cases.[5] The demonstration of aneurysms in the renal vasculature has been from 47 to 60 per cent; in the celiac axis, 50 to 60 per cent; and in the superior mesenteric arteries, 38 per cent.[12,28] It is important to recognize that angiographically demonstrable aneurysms are not pathognomonic of polyarteritis and may also be found in association with intravenous drug abuse, the embolic syndrome of a left atrial myxoma, endocarditis, fibromuscular dysplasia, pseudoxanthoma elasticum, and rarely in connective tissue diseases such as systemic lupus erythematosus.[5] Furthermore, caution should be taken when considering angiography in a patient with suspected vasculitis, as irreversible contrast dye–induced renal dysfunction may develop.[29]

Biopsy material is the most desirable route to establish a diagnosis of systemic vasculitis and should be obtained from the most accessible site in order to minimize morbidity without compromising diagnostic yield. Skin lesions are a useful source when they are present. In patients with neuropathic signs or symptoms, a sural nerve biopsy will reveal an arteritis of the vasa nervorum in the majority of patients.[30] Muscle biopsies are of greatest value when symptomatic tissue is sampled.[22,31] Recent studies have emphasized the usefulness of rectal mucosal biopsies for the diagnosis of systemic vasculitis[32]—a procedure that requires adequate familiarity with the technique so that an appropriately deep sample can be obtained. In most situations, a percutaneous renal biopsy is not useful for establishing a pathologic diagnosis of vasculitis. Furthermore, this procedure may be associated with a significant morbidity, including hemorrhage from a perforated renal artery aneurysm.[5] Testicular involvement occurs in greater than 80 per cent of cases of polyarteritis at autopsy,[5] and necrotizing testicular vasculitis is most often found in polyarteritis.[33] Biopsy appears to be indicated in the presence of testicular swelling or acute epididymitis when vasculitis is suspected.

ASSESSMENT

The Diagnostic and Therapeutic Criteria Committee of the American College of Rheumatology has recently established diagnostic criteria for the classification of polyarteritis.[34] This important study has demonstrated that when at least 3 of the 10 criteria listed in Table 3 are present, the sensitivity and specificity for a diagnosis of polyarteritis are 82.2 and 86.6 per cent, respectively. The sensitivity increases to 83.9 per cent if abdominal angina or bowel perforation is appended as an eleventh criterion. However, this is at the expense of the specificity, which decreases to 84.9 per cent.

There are many syndromes that mimic systemic vasculitis and must be considered in the differential diagnosis of idiopathic polyarteritis. These include some of the infectious diseases previously mentioned such as hepatitis B, HIV, and cytomegalovirus as well as bacterial endocarditis. Disorders associated with thromboembolic phenomena such as cholesterol(athero) emboli and atrial myxomas may also present with digital ischemic lesions, renal disease, and in the case of atheroemboli, eosinophilia.[35] Thrombotic thrombocytopenic purpura, which manifests with fever, renal insufficiency, central nervous system dysfunction, microangiopathic hemolytic anemia, purpura, and occasionally angiographic microaneurysms, also resembles the syndrome of systemic vasculitis.[5] The vasculopathy associated with the antiphospholipid syndrome may also present with cutaneous and visceral lesions that mimic polyarteritis.[36]

The utilization of the new diagnostic criteria in association with a judicious laboratory evaluation will provide the most expeditious pathway to identifying a clinical syndrome consistent with polyarteritis. The antineutrophil cytoplasmic antibody is an important serologic marker that should be sought for in any patient with a suspected systemic vasculitis in view of its specificity. The presence of a systemic disease associated with nephritis and a positive antineutrophil study would be considered sufficient at this time by many investigators to establish a diagnosis of microscopic polyarteritis or Wegener's granulomatosis (disorders with nearly identical renal pathology). A rational approach to tissue biopsy should be pursued from the least to the most

---

TABLE 3. The 1990 Criteria for the Diagnosis
of Polyarteritis Nodosa

1. Weight loss of $\geq$4 kg
2. Livedo reticularis
3. Testicular pain or tenderness (excluding infection and trauma)
4. Myalgias (excluding proximal thoracic and pelvic girdles), weakness or leg tenderness
5. Mononeuropathy or polyneuropathy
6. Diastolic blood pressure >90 mm Hg
7. Elevated blood urea nitrogen (>40 mg%) or creatinine (>1.5 mg%)
8. Hepatitis B surface antigen or antibody
9. Arteriographic demonstration of an aneurysm or occlusion of a visceral artery not related to atherosclerosis or fibromuscular dysplasia
10. Histologic evidence of a polymorphonuclear or mononuclear infiltrate in the wall of a small- or medium-size artery

(From Lightfoot RJ, Michel B, Bloch D, et al. The American College of Rheumatology 1990 criteria for the classification of polyarteritis nodosa. Arthritis Rheum 1990; 33:1088–93.)

invasive site. Skin lesions would be the initial choice for biopsy, if available, followed by a sural nerve biopsy in the presence of neuropathic symptoms or an abnormal electrophysiologic study. Tender or painful muscles (often distal groups) provide a generally high-yield biopsy site. Blind muscle biopsies may also be helpful but are associated with a significant degree of sampling error and are therefore not recommended. Depending on the institutional expertise and availability, a rectal mucosal biopsy would be the next blind site to consider. A renal biopsy remains the last option for histopathologic confirmation and should be pursued only if the etiology of a systemic illness associated with renal disease remains otherwise unclear. In the absence of the ability to confirm a diagnosis by biopsy, an angiographic study should be pursued. This must include both renal arteries, the celiac axis, and the superior mesenteric artery in order to maximize the yield of identifying microaneurysms. The majority of patients with polyarteritis will have multiple aneurysms. The results of angiography should be interpreted with the knowledge that many of the systemic vasculitic syndromes will not have radiographically demonstrable aneurysms (Table 2), and even when present, these aneurysms are not diagnostic of polyarteritis (*vide supra*).

REFERENCES

1. Fauci A, Haynes B, Katz P. The spectrum of vasculitis—clinical, pathologic, immunologic, and therapeutic considerations. Ann Intern Med 1978;89(Pt 1):660–76.
2. Christian C. Vasculitis: genus and species [Editorial]. Ann Intern Med 1984;101:862–3.
3. Kussmaul A, Maier K. Uber eine bischer nicht beschreibene eigenthumliche arterienerkrankung (periarteritis nodosa), die mit morbus brightii und rapid fortschreitender allgemeiner muskellahmung einhergeht. Dtsch Arch Klin Med 1866;1:484–517.
4. Michet C. Epidemiology of vasculitis. Rheum Dis Clin North Am 1990;16:261–8.
5. Cupps T, Fauci A. The vasculitides. In: Smith LJ, ed. Major problems in internal medicine, Vol 21. Philadelphia: WB Saunders, 1981.
6. Bielory L, Gascon P, Lawley T, Young N, Frank M. Human serum sickness: a prospective analysis of 35 patients treated with equine anti-thymocyte globulin for bone marrow failure. Medicine 1988;67:40–57.
7. Cochrane C, Koffler D. Immune complex disease in experimental animals and man. Adv Immunol 1973;16:185–264.
8. Kaufman L, Gruber B, Marchese M, Seibold J. Anti-

9. Baggiolini M, Walz A, Kunkel S. Neutrophil activating peptide-1/interleukin 8, a novel cytokine that activates neutrophils. J Clin Invest 1989;84: 1045–9.
10. Pober J. Cytokine-mediated activation of vascular endothelium: physiology and pathology. Am J Pathol 1988;133:426–33.
11. Bevilacqua M, Schleef R, Gimbrone M, Loskutoff D. Regulation of the fibrinolytic system of cultured human vascular endothelium by interleukin-1. J Clin Invest 1986;78:587–91.
12. Vertzman L. Polyarteritis nodosa. Clin Rheum Dis 1980;6:297–317.
13. Sergent J, Lockshin M, Christian C, Gocke D. Vasculitis with hepatitis B antigenemia—long-term observations in nine patients. Medicine 1976;55:1–18.
14. Doherty M, Bradfield J. Polyarteritis nodosa associated with acute cytomegalovirus infection. Ann Rheum Dis 1981;40:419–21.
15. Li Loong T, Coyle P, Anderson M, Allen G, Connolly J. Human serum parvovirus associated vasculitis. Postgrad Med J 1986;62:493–4.
16. Calabrese L, Estes M, Yen-Lieberman B, et al. Systemic vasculitis in association with human immunodeficiency virus infection. Arthritis Rheum 1989;32:569–76.
17. Sergent J, Christian C. Necrotizing vasculitis after acute serous otitis media. Ann Intern Med 1974;56:412–6.
18. Komadina K, Houk R. Periarteritis nodosa presenting as recurrent pneumonia following splenectomy for hairy cell leukemia. Semin Arthritis Rheum 1989;18:252–7.
19. Scott D, Bacon P, Tribe C. Systemic rheumatoid vasculitis: a clinical and laboratory study of 50 patients. Medicine 1981;60:288–97.
20. Zizic T, Classen J, Stevens M. Acute abdominal complications of systemic lupus erythematosus and polyarteritis nodosa. Am J Med 1982;73:525–31.
21. Smith D, Wernick R. Spontaneous rupture of a renal artery aneurysm in polyarteritis nodosa: critical review of the literature and report of a case. Am J Med 1989;87:464–7.
22. Moore P, Fauci A. Neurologic manifestations of systemic vasculitis: a retrospective and prospective study of the clinicopathologic features and responses to therapy in 25 patients. Am J Med 1981;71:517–24.
23. Camilleri M, Pusey C, Chadwick V, Rees A. Gastrointestinal manifestations of systemic vasculitis. Q J Med 1983;52:141–9.
24. Alleman M, Janssens A, Spoelstra P, Kroon H. Spontaneous intrahepatic hemorrhages in polyarteritis nodosa. Ann Intern Med 1986;105:712–3.
25. Kaufman L, Kaplan A. Microscopic polyarteritis. Hosp Pract 1989;24(June):85–104.
26. Scott G, Skinner R, Bacon P, Maddison P. Precipitating antibodies to nuclear antigens in systemic vasculitis. Clin Exp Immunol 1984;56:601–6.
27. Savage C, Winearls C, Jones S, Marshall P, Lockwood C. Prospective study of radioimmunoassay for antibodies against neutrophil cytoplasm in diagnosis of systemic vasculitis. Lancet 1987; 1:1389–93.
28. Travers R, Allison D, Brettle R, Hughes G. Polyar-

IgE autoantibodies in systemic sclerosis (scleroderma). Ann Rheum Dis 1989;48:201–5.

teritis nodosa: a clinical and angiographic analysis of 17 cases. Semin Arthritis Rheum 1979;8:184–99.

29. Kaur J, Goldberg J, Schrier R. Acute renal failure following arteriography in a patient with polyarteritis nodosa. JAMA 1982;247:833–4.

30. Wees S, Sunwoo I, Oh S. Sural nerve biopsy in systemic necrotizing vasculitis. Am J Med 1981; 71:525–32.

31. Dahlberg P, Lockhart J, Overholt E. Diagnostic studies for systemic necrotizing vasculitis: sensitivity, specificity, and predictive value in patients with multisystem disease. Arch Intern Med 1989;149:161–5.

32. Tribe C, Scott D, Bacon P. Rectal biopsy in the diagnosis of systemic vasculitis. J Clin Pathol 1981;34:843–50.

33. Shurbaji M, Epstein J. Testicular vasculitis: implications for systemic disease. Human Pathol 1988;19:186–9.

34. Lightfoot RJ, Michel B, Bloch D, et al. The American College of Rheumatology 1990 criteria for the classification of polyarteritis nodosa. Arthritis Rheum 1990;33:1088–93.

35. Cappiello R, Espinoza L, Adelman H, Aguilar J, Vasey F, Germain B. Cholesterol embolism: a pseudovasculitic syndrome. Semin Arthritis Rheum 1989;18:240–6.

36. Lie J. Vasculopathy in the antiphospholipid syndrome: thrombosis or vasculitis, or both? J Rheumatol 1989;16:713–5.

POLYARTICULAR ARTHRITIS

LENORE J. BRANCATO and JOEL N. BUXBAUM

SYNONYMS: Arthritis, Joint Pain, Rheumatism

BACKGROUND

It has been estimated that approximately 37 million Americans have some form of arthritis or related disorder. Arthritis is the fourth leading cause of hospitalization of men and the sixth leading cause in women.[1] Data from the National Health Survey of the early 1960s indicated that some 16 million individuals suffered from osteoarthritis (OA), whereas another 2.1 million had classical or definite rheumatoid arthritis (RA). More recent analyses suggest an even higher prevalence of OA. Hence, the need to distinguish between the various inflammatory polyarthritides may be an everyday occurrence for the family practitioner or general internist.

Polyarticular arthritis refers to the inflammation of more than one joint in the course of the same illness. The distinction between polyarticular and monarticular forms of inflammatory joint disease is artificial, since most arthritides that affect multiple joints may also affect a single joint at some time in the patient's disease and at that time must be distinguished from other, primarily monarticular, conditions such as septic or post-traumatic arthritis. Nonetheless, some forms of inflammatory arthritis are more commonly polyarticular, whereas others, during the course of a given episode, usually involve a single joint. More critical in our discussion will be the distinction between true "arthritis," associated with erythema, warmth, pain, and loss of function, and noninflammatory joint involvement, in which the pain, swelling, and loss of function are due to pathophysiologic mechanisms requiring other types of therapeutic intervention. Hence, the distinction between arthritis and arthralgia is more than a semantic exercise.

Inflammatory joint involvement occurs in a variety of clinical settings. It may occur in the course of a systemic inflammatory disease in which the joints are the major affected organ system. RA, Reiter's syndrome, and ankylosing spondylitis (AS) are representative of this type of polyarticular arthritis. In systemic lupus erythematosus (SLE), the joints usually represent a minor target of the systemic inflammatory process. In gout and the related crystal deposition diseases, the joints are the dominant clinically affected organ in a generalized metabolic disorder, whereas OA seems to reflect the sum total of a variety of mechanical, hereditary, and perhaps metabolically determined processes that sometimes result in aggressive inflammatory joint destruction. Each of these is a form of chronic arthritis. However, the initial presentation of any of them may be sudden and must be distinguished from other joint disorders with characteristically acute onsets, notably those with infectious etiologies, which require relatively rapid treatment; those of unknown postinfectious nature, which follow an intrinsically self-limited course; and post-traumatic disorders, in which there may be no history of trauma.

The diagnosis of any of the arthritides is based predominantly on the history and physical examination. Analysis of synovial fluid may be definitive; most other laboratory studies are only supportive but can be extremely useful in following a patient's course. Radiologic examinations are most helpful in determining the extent of disease and, in some cases, provide findings unique enough to be diagnostic.

HISTORY

The age and sex of the patient at the time of presentation help to epidemiologically define the risks of developing a particular form of joint disease. Young women are at greatest risk for developing SLE, whereas young men are the most likely to acquire Reiter's syndrome.[2,3] RA is a disease of young to middle-aged women and middle-aged and older men, whereas OA is predominantly a disease of the elderly.[4,5] Gout is almost the exclusive province of men in midlife and older.[6]

History of the Present Illness

Since pain usually brings the patient to the physician, the question, "Where does it hurt?" is a good place to start. The answer will establish if the disease is polyarticular and the pattern of involvement. It should define if it is symmetric, more likely in RA than OA, and whether it is primarily axial, as in the spondyloarthropathies, or peripheral, as in rheumatoid disease or gout.

The patient's description of a painful joint that is associated with warmth, redness, and swelling will allow the distinction between the arthralgias with associated myalgias found in many viral states and true polyarticular arthritis. Some polyarticular arthritides have a characteristic migratory rather than static pattern of involvement. Acute rheumatic fever and the early arthritis of hepatitis B infection manifest both migratory polyarthralgia and polyarthritis. Migratory joint symptoms are also seen in the gonococcal dermatitis-arthritis syndrome. The transiently involved arthralgic joints frequently yield sterile, mildly inflammatory fluid on joint aspiration, which may be related to the presence of immune complexes rather than persistent infection with the organism.[7]

The temporal pattern of discomfort is also informative, as is the association of inflamed joints with other evidence of systemic inflammatory disease, that is, fever, weight loss, anorexia, weakness, anemia. The latter is consistent with the diagnosis of RA, whereas similar findings coupled with the characteristic vasculitic rash would suggest SLE. In the elderly, the same presentation without the rash might suggest polymyalgia rheumatica or giant cell arteritis. The presence of fever associated with acute polyarthritis does not necessarily direct the diagnosis toward systemic inflammation, since acute polyarticular or monarticular gout and septic arthritis can also produce fever equivalent to that seen in either systemic infection or disseminated immune complex diseases.[8]

Is the joint disease occurring in the course of any other illness or subsequent to any identifiable triggering event? Clearly, its association with any form of serositis, suggesting pleural, pericardial, or peritoneal inflammation, would point toward either rheumatoid disease or lupus. Associated visual disturbances or the description of scalp tenderness raises a suspicion of giant cell arteritis. The occurrence of a recent tick bite and rash preceding or accompanying an oligoarticular arthritis in an individual from an endemic area makes Lyme arthritis a strong possibility.[9] A recent exposure to any of the drugs known to be associated with drug-induced lupus would be suggestive of a relationship with a mild polyarticular arthritis of short duration.[10]

The clinical course of the arthritis should also be established historically. Has it been chronic and unremitting from its inception? Are there acute severe episodes separated by asymptomatic latent periods? The latter pattern is almost unique to gout and pseudogout, although the discrete pattern of the attacks becomes blurred in long-standing chronic disease. Untreated RA and OA may wax and wane, but true symptom-free periods are unusual without therapy.

Family History

Many of the polyarticular arthritides have a hereditary component. While the molecular bases of the inheritance of all forms of arthritis are not known, it has been clearly shown that RA is increased in individuals carrying the major histocompatibility complex (MHC) class 2 antigen DR4 and other related specificities. Similarly, people whose cells express HLA B27 are at increased risk of seronegative spondyloarthropathies.[2,3,4] The genetic predisposition to gout has been clear for almost a century, even though the molecular defect is known only for a minority of cases. It is also apparent that OA is found in families, but even less is known about the specifics of its genetics.

Social History

In the current social milieu, any case of inflammatory polyarthritis, particularly those of abrupt onset occurring in sexually active individuals, must raise the issue of either infectious or noninfectious diseases that have their origin in either heterosexual or homosexual interactions or intravenous drug abuse. Gonococcal arthritis occurring in the course of disseminated infection; Reiter's syndrome appearing after any form of urethritis including gonorrhea, chlamydia, or ureaplasma infection; and the oligoarticular reactive arthritis found in human immunodeficiency virus 1–(HIV 1) infected individuals are all characterized by polyarticular inflammatory disease.[3,6,11] In some cases, the latter has been an early clue to the presence of HIV infection.

Focused Queries

1. *Is there morning stiffness?* RA may be associated with several hours of morning stiffness, sometimes relieved by a hot bath or shower. The degree of disease activity is often proportional to the duration of morning stiffness.[12] OA may cause 10 to 20 minutes of stiffness on arising that usually eases as the patient is up and about.

2. *Does the pain improve or worsen throughout the day?* Individuals with RA tend to improve once the gelling phenomenon of morning stiffness abates, whereas patients with OA feel worse at the end of the day.[13] Patients with AS have improvement in their back discomfort with exercise, but patients with degenerative disk disease or OA of the spine do not.[14]

3. *Are the arthritis attacks recurrent?* Gouty attacks are painful and recurrent, often triggered by specific events such as trauma, alcohol, intercurrent medical diseases, stress, and drugs (diuretics).[15] Pseudogout attacks can be as abrupt and severe as gout but in general are less painful. The acute episodes of both types of crystalline deposition are self-limited, particularly early in the course of the disease.

4. *Is the arthritis monarticular or polyarticular?* Most forms of septic or post-traumatic arthritis are monarticular; however, nongonococcal septic arthritis may be polyarticular 20 to 30 per cent of the time, whereas disseminated gonococcemia may be associated with migratory polyarthritis culminating in one or two dominant septic joints.[7]

5. *Was the arthritis preceded by an acute febrile illness?* If so, infectious arthritides or rheumatic fever may be the cause. If an enteric illness or diarrheal episode preceded the joint pain, stools should be checked for organisms such as *Salmonella, Shigella,* and *Yersinia.* These bacteria may precipitate reactive arthritis in a genetically susceptible host.

6. *Are there associated skin or mucocutaneous lesions?* A history of diagnosed psoriasis in the presence of either peripheral or axial joint complaints is prima facie evidence in favor of a diagnosis of psoriatic arthritis. The activity of the peripheral disease commonly, although not always, mirrors the severity of the skin involvement. The axial disease seems to be more independent in its course. Occasionally, the arthritis will be more apparent than the skin lesions and may even precede the appearance of the plaques. Any arthritis, either axial or peripheral, occurring in the presence of psoriasis should be considered psoriatic, unless other features, such as a single dominant joint or an atypical course, suggest coincidental rheumatoid, septic, or degenerative disease. Gonococcal arthritis is associated with characteristic skin pustules, papules, or vesicles. The mucous membrane lesions of Behçet's disease are extremely painful, whereas those of Reiter's syndrome are painless.[16]

PHYSICAL EXAMINATION

General

Examination of the scalp and hair may reveal alopecia suggestive of SLE or scalp tenderness and a prominent temporal artery consistent with giant cell arteritis. Dryness of the eyes, assessed by inspection or by a Schirmer's test, is present in Sjögren's syndrome, whereas funduscopy will reveal vascular changes seen in SLE or certain types of vasculitis. (Also see chapters on Dry Eye and Polyarteritis.) Cardiac findings can include a pericardial friction rub in RA or SLE, whereas an organic murmur may suggest endocarditis. Conduction abnormalities may be due to rheumatoid nodulosis or Lyme carditis. Auscultation of the lungs may discern the pleuritis seen in SLE or RA or the interstitial fibrosis of scleroderma. Neurologic examination can reveal central nervous system (CNS) dysfunction in SLE, Bell's palsy in Lyme disease, or peripheral nerve abnormalities such as foot drop in systemic vasculitis. The presence or absence of these findings serves to place the polyarticular inflammation in the context of a systemic disease.

Examination of the Skin

A malar rash on sun-exposed skin is characteristic of SLE, whereas a periorbital heliotrope rash is more in keeping with a diagnosis of dermatomyositis. The extensor surfaces of the elbows and knees should be checked for rheumatoid nodules and psoriatic plaques. Generalized skin tightening over the proximal limbs or trunk is found in scleroderma. Nail pitting or dystrophy often accompanies psoriasis. An enlarging macular rash with central clearing may be the first sign of Lyme disease. The presence of a Kaposi's sarcoma lesion in a young person indicates underlying acquired immune deficiency syndrome (AIDS).

The oral mucosa should be inspected for ulcers seen in Reiter's syndrome, Behçet's, or SLE. Examination of the genitalia may also reveal mucocutaneous lesions suggestive of Reiter's syndrome or Behçet's disease.

Rheumatologic Examination

The joint examination begins when the patient enters the physician's office or examining room. Useful information can be obtained from the patient's nutritional state, posture, gait, and habitus. Observations can be made of the patient's ability to get in and out of a chair and his or her capacity to perform activities of daily living such as grooming and feeding.

The specifics of the examination are designed to determine whether the patient has monarticular or polyarticular involvement, true arthritis or arthralgias, acute inflammation or chronic synovitis with deformity, or symmetric or asymmetric joint findings and whether the condition affects primarily peripheral or axial joints. In addition, one can establish if reported weakness is localized and related to an inflamed joint or whether it reflects primary neuromuscular disease with pain secondary to an increased work load. Hence, a systematic approach to examining the joints is imperative. Paired joints are compared with each other and with respect to structural or functional abnormality of the particular joint. Inspection and palpation are followed by assessment of joint range of motion. Each joint should be evaluated for swelling, warmth, tenderness, crepitus, and deformity. Swelling may be caused by intra-articular effusion, synovial thickening, periarticular soft tissue inflammation such as bursitis or tendinitis, or bony overgrowth. Warmth is detected on palpation and facilitated by comparison with the contralateral joint or an adjacent area of skin. Tenderness is elicited by gentle palpation. The observer must differentiate articular from periarticular tenderness. Proper interpretation of tenderness on examination requires adequate relaxation of the muscles and tendons in the area being examined. With true joint involvement, motion of the joint in any direction is apt to be painful, but with primary soft tissue disease, movement in some planes may be possible without pain. Spinal involvement is determined by assessing the degree of lumbar lordosis, measuring flexibility (finger to floor distance), and noting the presence of paraspinal spasm.

Crepitus is the palpable or audible grating or crunching sensation produced by motion of a joint. Crepitus occurs when roughened articular or extra-articular surfaces are rubbed together either by active motion or by manual compression during the course of the examination. Deformity may be due to bone enlargement, articular subluxation, contracture, collapse of bone, or ankylosis.

DIAGNOSTIC STUDIES

Laboratory

For the great majority of patients with polyarthritis, only a few laboratory tests actually aid in the diagnosis. Initial studies should include a complete blood count, erythrocyte sedimentation rate (ESR), a test for rheumatoid factor (RF), and a serum uric acid. These are sufficient to establish the presence of systemic inflammation (elevated ESR), hyperuricemia but not necessarily clinical gout, and the possibility of RA if the RF is present in high titer. Synovial fluid analysis with culture and examination with a polarizing microscope will definitively diagnose septic arthritis, crystal deposition disease, and RA if there is a significant titer of RF in the fluid[17,18] (see Table 1).

A variety of other studies may be required in order to diagnose or eliminate the possibility of other, less common forms of polyarthritis. Blood chemistry tests including serum calcium and alkaline phosphatase (Paget's disease), urinalysis (immune complex nephropathy), throat culture, antistreptolysin-O titer, C-reactive protein, and electrocardiogram (acute rheumatic fever) should be performed, depending on the clinical features of the patient.

If SLE is suspected, an antinuclear antibody assay; serum complement (C) levels, including C3 and C4; a serologic test for syphilis (Venereal Disease Research Laboratories [VDRL]); and a partial thromboplastin time (PTT) may be obtained. The last is a good screen for a circulating lupus anticoagulant, in which case the PTT is prolonged and does not correct with mixing studies.[19] Serum glutamic-oxaloacetic transaminase and hepatitis B antigen and antibody determinations should be checked if exposure to the virus is suspected.

Stool cultures for enteric pathogens should be performed in patients likely to have a reactive arthritis. Blood cultures are often positive in cases of infectious polyarthritis and in cases of subacute bacterial endocarditis accompanied by immune complex polyarthritis. Lyme titers should be sent in patients with an appropriate history and travel to a tick-endemic area. If gonococcal arthritis is suspected, rectal and pharyngeal cultures must be obtained as well as cultures of the cervical or urethral discharge and the inflamed joint.

Joint fluid studies are definitive in diagnos-

TABLE 1.   Synovial Fluid Analysis

	NORMAL	GROUP I Noninflammatory	GROUP II Inflammatory	GROUP III Septic
Volume (knee, in ml)	<3.5	>3.5	>3.5	>3.5
Viscosity	Very high	High	Low	Low
Color	Clear to straw	Straw to xantho-chromic	Xanthochromic to opalescent	Yellow, grayish, or bloody
Clarity	Transparent	Transparent	Slightly cloudy, opaque at times	Turbid to purulent
Mucin clot*	Good	Good	Fair to poor	Poor
White blood cells/cu mm	<200	<2000	2,000–30,000	Usually >100,000 but may be much lower
Percent polys	<25%	<25%	>50%	>75%
Glucose	Nearly equal to blood	Nearly equal to blood	<25, lower than blood	<25, much lower than blood
Culture	Negative	Negative	Negative	Usually positive except in gonococcal arthritis
Diseases	None	Osteoarthritis Trauma Systemic lupus erythematosus Scleroderma Amyloidosis Hemochromatosis Acromegaly	Rheumatoid arthritis Systemic lupus erythematosus Reiter's syndrome Gout Pseudogout Rheumatic fever Psoriatic arthritis	Tuberculous arthritis† Septic arthritis

* Good = tight, ropy mass; fair = softer mass with shreds; poor = friable.
† Culture may be positive; *M. tuberculosis* may be seen in smear.

ing septic and crystal-induced arthritis and amyloid joint involvement. They are less helpful in differentiating other arthritides.

Other Tests

Arthroscopy allows direct visualization of intra-articular structures, biopsy when required, and repair of both ligamentous and cartilage damage. It generally adds little in the diagnosis of polyarticular inflammatory disease. Although OA can be verified by arthroscopy, the clinical diagnosis is usually sufficient unless other complicating disease is suspected. Synovial biopsy via the arthroscope or using a closed needle procedure is most helpful in the assessment of chronic undiagnosed, primarily monarticular, inflammatory arthropathies such as tuberculosis, fungal infections, and sarcoidosis.

Diagnostic Imaging

Routine radiographs of the most severely involved joints and their asymptomatic normal contralateral counterparts should be obtained. They are helpful in assessing the degree of joint damage and aid in making the differential diagnosis. Although radiographic features are often nonspecific, certain combinations of findings are apt to occur in a particular disease.

In RA, osteoporosis may appear early in juxtaarticular areas. Loss of articular cartilage results in symmetric narrowing of the joint space. Bony erosions occur where the articular cartilage ends and the synovial reflection begins. Common sites include the metacarpophalangeal (MCP) and proximal interphalangeal (PIP) joints of the hands, the ulnar styloid, and the metatarsal heads of the feet. In general, irreversible joint changes such as attrition of cartilage or bone erosion take at least three months to appear.

Gouty arthritis can be recognized by the presence of erosions characteristically located in the first metatarsophalangeal joint and the joints of the hand. They typically have an overhanging margin and may cross the joint space—radiographic features that help differentiate them from the erosions of RA.

Calcification of fibrocartilages, particularly the menisci of the knee, intervertebral disks, and the triangular cartilage of the wrist, is typical of pseudogout or calcium pyrophosphate dihydrate (CPPD) deposition disease. Chondrocalcinosis is usually bilateral, but bilateral-

ity is not pathognomonic of CPPD since it may occur with other crystalline deposition diseases.

Joint space narrowing, subchondral bony sclerosis, and osteophyte and cyst formation are the classic changes of OA. Primary OA has a predilection for weight-bearing joints including knees and hips. Inflammatory or erosive OA may occur in the distal joints of the fingers. Clinically, there is prominent soft tissue swelling of the joints, and radiographically, subchondral bony destruction is observed.

Joint space narrowing, erosions, and ankylosis of the distal interphalangeal joints typify psoriatic arthritis. Resorption of the terminal phalanges is common. A characteristic "pencil and cup" deformity may be seen in which the tapered end of the proximal bone of the joint projects into the splayed end of the distal bony surface. New bone deposition near involved joints is characteristic and helps differentiate this arthropathy from RA.

It is often difficult to distinguish axial psoriatic arthritis and Reiter's syndrome because of the overlap of radiographic findings. Typical features of Reiter's syndrome include asymmetric sacroiliitis, severe destruction of pedal joints, and frequent periosteal bone elevation near affected joints. Focal periostitis or reactive new bone formation may persist as cortical irregularity with relatively minimal alteration of the adjacent cartilage space. This, coupled with frequent calcification of the insertions of tendons (so-called enthesopathy), suggests that periarticular structures are prime targets of the inflammatory process.

The radiologic manifestations of infectious arthritis vary with the causative organism, host defense, and duration and efficacy of antibiotic treatment. Untreated, or undertreated, pyogenic arthritis may rapidly progress with rapid bone and cartilage destruction, extensive sequestrum formation, and osteomyelitis. Usually, only one joint is infected unless there is an underlying systemic illness or immunodeficiency. Radiologic features typically occur 8 to 10 days after the onset of symptoms; thus, normal x-rays at the onset of disease do not exclude the diagnosis.

The main role of computed tomography (CT) is the evaluation of the spine, particularly the sacroiliac joints. CT is superior to conventional x-rays in detecting sacroiliitis and is recommended in those cases where findings on plain x-ray are normal but clinical suspicion is high. In one study, the sensitivity of CT was

81 per cent compared with 50 per cent for conventional x-rays, whereas the specificity was similar in both modalities.[20]

The role of magnetic resonance imaging (MRI) in imaging joints is still evolving. MRI's ability to visualize anatomic structures clearly in multiple planes is a clear advantage in assessing the musculoskeletal system. Abnormalities of the cervical spinal cord in RA patients are easily seen on MRI. Preliminary studies suggest a correlation between these anatomic abnormalities and the subsequent risk of developing neurologic sequelae.[21]

ASSESSMENT

Constellations of Findings

The algorithm illustrates the approach to the patient with joint pain.

Infectious Agents

Pyogenic arthritis is usually monarticular and of abrupt onset but may involve more than one joint in 30 per cent of cases. Other syndromes related to infection, including Lyme arthritis, gonococcal arthritis, and musculoskeletal manifestations of subacute bacterial endocarditis, can best be differentiated by type of presentation. Lyme disease may present with arthralgias in early stages and progress to recurrent attacks of oligoarthritis or chronic monarticular involvement, particularly the knee, in later stages. A history of tick exposure or travel to endemic areas may be elicited. Gonococcal arthritis often occurs early in menses. A history of recent sexual exposure may be obtained. Patients present with migratory polyarthralgias, and on examination, tenosynovitis or polyarthritis is common. Musculoskeletal symptoms may precede the diagnosis of endocarditis by weeks. A high index of suspicion and careful search for other extracardiac features are crucial. Patients who are immunosuppressed (on steroids or with HIV infection) are at risk for infection with rare fungal or mycobacterial organisms. Usually, one joint is involved to a greater extent than any other. Infection should also be suspected in patients with known RA who have one or two joints that are recalcitrant to antirheumatic therapy. These unresponsive joints may be infected; hence, diagnostic aspiration is critical in their assessment.[22]

The viral arthritides usually begin with nonspecific symptoms such as fever, fatigue, malaise, sore throat, and myalgias. Arthralgias are more common than true arthritis. A diagnosis of viral arthritis should be considered in postimmunization patients (rubella vaccination) and in those with known exposure during viral epidemics. Joint involvement associated with hepatitis B infection tends to be symmetric, most often involving hands, wrists, elbows, and knees. These symptoms often abate when jaundice ensues.

Acute Inflammatory Polyarthritis

RA, gout, and acute rheumatic fever may present with an abrupt onset. RA is a systemic illness that presents with symmetric small joint involvement. Fever, fatigue, anorexia, and morning stiffness are associated symptoms. Gout usually presents with the abrupt onset of a single severely inflamed joint such as the great toe (podagra); however, in 20 to 30 per cent of cases, particularly those of longstanding, the presentation is polyarticular. The patient may have fever, and the clinical scenario may mimic cellulitis or superficial thrombophlebitis due to inflammation of periarticular structures as well as the joint. In our experience, 20 per cent of hospitalized patients with acute gout have been treated with antibiotics prior to being seen by a rheumatologist, despite giving a history of confirmed gouty episodes.

In contrast to both RA and gout, the arthritis of acute rheumatic fever is migratory, although any number of joints may be involved at one time. Erythema marginatum, fever, subcutaneous nodules, and carditis are associated features. Polymyalgia rheumatica can present with a symmetric synovitis of small joints, usually without effusion, that greatly resembles RA. Morning stiffness may be striking, as is the presence of anemia. Visual disturbances or temporal artery tenderness, particularly in the presence or absence of low-titer RF, make temporal artery biopsy necessary.

Subacute Chronic Polyarthritis

OA or degenerative joint disease involves weight-bearing joints (hips, knees) as well as the cervical and lumbar spine. It tends to occur in the middle-aged and elderly, especially in those that are obese or sedentary. The arthritis tends to be noninflammatory with characteristic pain on weight bearing; however, in some patients, inflammation may be striking, particularly in the hands. Chronic or recurrent gout and pseudogout typically have a polyar-

DIAGNOSTIC ASSESSMENT OF POLYARTICULAR ARTHRITIS

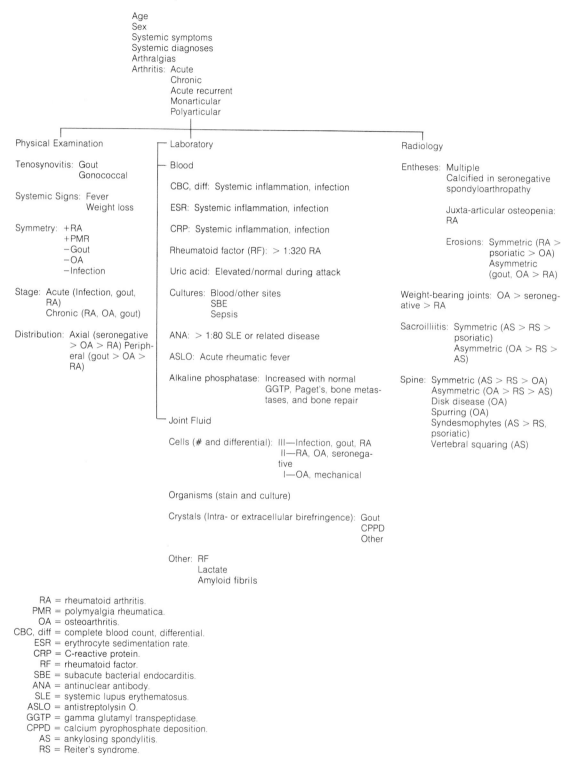

Chief Complaint: Joint Pain

Age
Sex
Systemic symptoms
Systemic diagnoses
Arthralgias
Arthritis: Acute
     Chronic
     Acute recurrent
     Monarticular
     Polyarticular

Physical Examination

Tenosynovitis: Gout
             Gonococcal

Systemic Signs: Fever
             Weight loss

Symmetry: +RA
        +PMR
        −Gout
        −OA
        −Infection

Stage: Acute (Infection, gout,
      RA)
      Chronic (RA, OA, gout)

Distribution: Axial (seronegative
        > OA > RA) Periph-
        eral (gout > OA >
        RA)

Laboratory

Blood

  CBC, diff: Systemic inflammation, infection

  ESR: Systemic inflammation, infection

  CRP: Systemic inflammation, infection

  Rheumatoid factor (RF): > 1:320 RA

  Uric acid: Elevated/normal during attack

  Cultures: Blood/other sites
          SBE
          Sepsis

  ANA: > 1:80 SLE or related disease

  ASLO: Acute rheumatic fever

  Alkaline phosphatase: Increased with normal
          GGTP, Paget's, bone metas-
          tases, and bone repair

Joint Fluid

  Cells (# and differential): III—Infection, gout, RA
                 II—RA, OA, seronega-
                 tive
                 I—OA, mechanical

  Organisms (stain and culture)

  Crystals (Intra- or extracellular birefringence): Gout
                       CPPD
                       Other

Other: RF
      Lactate
      Amyloid fibrils

Radiology

Entheses: Multiple
       Calcified in seronegative
       spondyloarthropathy

       Juxta-articular osteopenia:
       RA

       Erosions: Symmetric (RA >
           psoriatic > OA)
           Asymmetric
           (gout, OA > RA)

Weight-bearing joints: OA > seronegative > RA

Sacroilliitis: Symmetric (AS > RS >
          psoriatic)
          Asymmetric (OA > RS >
          AS)

Spine: Symmetric (AS > RS > OA)
      Asymmetric (OA > RS > AS)
      Disk disease (OA)
      Spurring (OA)
      Syndesmophytes (AS > RS,
      psoriatic)
      Vertebral squaring (AS)

RA = rheumatoid arthritis.
PMR = polymyalgia rheumatica.
OA = osteoarthritis.
CBC, diff = complete blood count, differential.
ESR = erythrocyte sedimentation rate.
CRP = C-reactive protein.
RF = rheumatoid factor.
SBE = subacute bacterial endocarditis.
ANA = antinuclear antibody.
SLE = systemic lupus erythematosus.
ASLO = antistreptolysin O.
GGTP = gamma glutamyl transpeptidase.
CPPD = calcium pyrophosphate deposition.
AS = ankylosing spondylitis.
RS = Reiter's syndrome.

ticular subacute presentation. The latter is often associated with radiographic evidence of chondrocalcinosis. Articular involvement in sarcoid is infrequent but usually occurs when other evidence of disease—such as fever, parotid swelling, and rash—is present.

Seronegative Spondyloarthropathies

Psoriatic arthritis tends to involve the distal interphalangeal (DIP) joints of the hand with psoriatic changes such as pitting and onychodystrophy of the fingernails. Skin and nail changes usually precede articular disease. Reiter's syndrome consists of the classic triad of arthritis, urethritis, and conjunctivitis, but any of the elements may be absent during a particular episode. Urethritis may be misdiagnosed as gonorrhea and treated as such. Reiter's syndrome occurs most commonly in sexually active males but has also been reported in susceptible individuals after epidemic acute diarrheal illness. Mucocutaneous lesions such as balanitis and oral ulcers may be associated findings. Joint disease occurs in the lower extremities, with knee and ankle involvement predominating. Radiographic involvement of the spine and sacroiliac joints is similar in Reiter's and psoriatic axial disease. Complete and partial forms of Reiter's syndrome have been described in patients with HIV disease. Postenteropathic reactive arthritides have joint manifestations similar to those in Reiter's syndrome, and it is possible that the distinction may soon be abandoned. *Salmonella, Campylobacter,* and *Yersinia* are among the known inciting agents.

Crystal-Induced Arthropathy

Chronic polyarthritis may be a manifestation of recurrent gouty attacks in which the urate deposits take the form of soft tissue tophi and synovitis is persistent. The tophi may mimic rheumatoid nodules, but analysis of the chalky tophaceous material under polarized microscopy will reveal the presence of negatively birefringent urate crystals. Pseudogout or chondrocalcinosis may also cause chronic polyarthritis. The chronic synovitis represents an inflammatory response to synovial deposits of calcium pyrophosphate dehydrate crystals. The knee is the most common joint involved. Surgical procedures and severe medical illness such as stroke or myocardial infarction may precipitate attacks in both gout and pseudogout.

Other Collagen Vascular Disorders

Joint disease in SLE is nondeforming and nonerosive arthritis. However, in many lupus patients, polyarthralgias are common without objective joint inflammation. Chronic polyarthritis in other connective tissue diseases, such as scleroderma, polymyositis/dermatomyositis, Behçet's syndrome, and mixed connective tissue disease is usually limited in the extent and severity of the inflammatory changes. These are multisystem disorders with protean manifestations. Thus, articular symptoms must be appreciated in the context of other clinical findings that together will help make the diagnosis.

REFERENCES

1. National Arthritis Advisory Board. Annual report 1987, p 1.
2. Hochberg MC. The incidence of systemic lupus erythematosus in Baltimore, Maryland 1960–1977. Arthritis Rheum 1985;28:80–6.
3. Arnett FC. Reiter's syndrome. Johns Hopkins Med J 1982;150:39–44.
4. Hochberg MC. Adult and juvenile rheumatoid arthritis: current epidemiologic concepts. Epidemiol Rev 1981;3:27–41.
5. Peyron JG. The epidemiology of osteoarthritis. In: Moskowitz RW, Howell DS, Goldberg VM, Mankin HJ, eds. Osteoarthritis diagnosis and management. Philadelphia: WB Saunders, 1984:9–27.
6. Hochberg MC. Epidemiology of the rheumatic diseases. In: Schumacher HR Jr, ed. Primer on the rheumatic diseases. 9th ed. Atlanta: Arthritis Foundation, 1988:48–51.
7. O'Brien JP, Goldenberg DL, Rice PA. Disseminated gonococcal infection: a prospective analysis of 49 patients and a review of pathophysiology and immune mechanisms. Medicine 1983;62:395–406.
8. Lowery GV II, Fan PT, Bluestone R. Polyarticular versus monarticular gout: a prospective, comparative analysis of clinical features. Medicine 1988;67:335–43.
9. Sigal LH. Summary of the first 100 patients seen at a Lyme disease referral center. Am J Med 1990;88:577–81.
10. Lee SL, Chase PH. Drug induced systemic lupus erythematosus: a critical review. Semin Arthritis Rheum 1975;5:83–103.
11. Winchester R, Bernstein DH, Fisher HD, Enlow R, Solomon G. The co-occurrence of Reiter's syndrome and acquired immunodeficiency. Ann Intern Med 1987;106:19–26.
12. Arnett FC, Edworthy SM, Bloch DA. The 1987 revised ARA criteria for classification of rheumatoid arthritis. Arthritis Rheum 1988;31:315–24.
13. Altman R, Asch E, Bloch D, et al. Development of criteria for the classification of osteoarthritis of the knee. Arthritis Rheum 1986;29:1039–49.
14. Calin A, Porta J, Fries JF. The clinical history as a screening test for ankylosing spondylitis. JAMA 1977;237:2613–4.

15. Wordsworth BP, Mowat AG. Rapid development of gouty tophi after diuretic therapy. J Rheumatol 1985;12:376–7.

16. Rogers R. Recurrent aphthous stomatitis: clinical characteristics and evidence for an immunopathogenesis. J Invest Dermatol 1977;69:499–509.

17. Cohen AS, Goldenberg D. Synovial fluid. In: Cohen AS, ed. Laboratory diagnostic procedures in the rheumatic diseases. Orlando: Grune & Stratton Inc, 1985:1–54.

18. Gatter RA. Clinical significance of joint fluid findings. In: A practical handbook of joint fluid analysis. Philadelphia: Lea & Febiger, 1984:71–4.

19. Much JR, Herbst KD, Rapaport SI. Thrombosis in patients with the lupus anticoagulant. Ann Intern Med 1980;92:156–9.

20. Kozin F, Carrera GF, Ryan LM, et al. Computed tomography in the diagnosis of sacroiliitis. Arthritis Rheum 1981;24:1479–85.

21. Aisen AM, Martel W, Ellis JH, et al. Cervical spine involvement in rheumatoid arthritis: MR imaging. Radiology 1987;165:159–63.

22. Gardner GC, Weisman MH. Pyarthrosis in patients with rheumatoid arthritis: a report of 13 cases and a review of the literature from the past 40 years. Am J Med 1990;88:503–11.

POLYCYTHEMIA

GERALD M. SEGAL

SYNONYMS: Erythrocytosis, Erythremia

BACKGROUND

The term *polycythemia* actually means "many cells," but traditionally it has come to be synonymous with *erythrocytosis,* an increase above normal in the concentration of red blood cells. The latter term will be utilized in this chapter because of its greater nosologic precision and to avoid confusion with the disease polycythemia vera. According to common usage, polycythemia is said to be present if the hematocrit (or packed cell volume) exceeds 51 per cent in men or 47 per cent in women. Erythrocytosis may be absolute, due to an increase in total red cell mass, or relative, in which the elevated hematocrit reflects a reduction in plasma volume. The diagnostic approach to unexplained erythrocytosis requires a systematic evaluation based on an understanding of erythropoietic regulation.

Regulation of Erythropoiesis

Red blood cells are, in essence, packets of hemoglobin that survive for an average of 120 days in the circulation. Unless perturbed by disease, the parameters of red cell size, intracellular hemoglobin concentration, and life span are maintained within narrow limits. Accordingly, compensatory increases in the blood hemoglobin concentration in response to tissue hypoxia necessarily entail increases in red blood cell production. The physiologic mediator of this erythropoietic response is the hormone erythropoietin (epo), a 34-kd glycoprotein encoded by a gene on the long arm of chromosome 7.[1] Epo is manufactured by the kidneys and, to a far lesser extent, the liver. In situ hybridization studies with specific molecular probes have identified a subset of cortical interstitial cells as the epo-producing cells in the kidneys. Tissue hypoxia, whether due to anemia, hypoxemia, or impaired release of oxygen from oxyhemoglobin, is detected by a poorly characterized renal "oxygen sensor" (which may utilize a heme-like moiety), stimulating a prompt increase in renal epo production. Serum epo levels, which may vary over two to three orders of magnitude, increase in an exponential fashion in response to reductions in hematocrit.[2]

Epo promotes the growth and differentiation of erythroid progenitor cells after binding to specific cell surface receptors. Epo supports the development of colonies of hemoglobinized erythroblasts from erythroid progenitor cells in vitro; such colonies will not form in cultures of normal marrow or blood cells in the absence of epo. Epo stimulates erythropoiesis in vivo, as reflected by bone marrow erythroid hyperplasia, shortened transit time through the marrow erythroid compartment, absolute reticulocytosis, and increased incorporation of iron into the erythron.[1,3]

HISTORY

History of Present Illness

The medical history should document the time of onset of the erythrocytosis as closely as possible and whether the erythrocytosis has been progressive. Prior hemograms, if available, are particularly informative. The existence of any normal hemograms prior to the onset of erythrocytosis effectively eliminates congenital disorders, such as high-affinity hemoglobins, from consideration. In the absence of past hemograms, the duration of plethora should be determined by questioning the patient and family members or friends. The examiner should inquire about the presence, duration, and severity of headache, dizziness, and visual changes, symptoms that may reflect cerebral vascular engorgement and/or hyperviscosity-induced reduction in cerebral blood flow.

Past Medical History

The patient should be carefully questioned about symptoms of abnormal bleeding and prior thrombotic or hemorrhagic episodes. Any history of cardiovascular or pulmonary disease should be documented.

Habits

The duration and magnitude of smoking and alcohol consumption should be determined.

Family History

A family history of erythrocytosis may suggest the presence of a high-affinity hemoglobin variant or one of the rare familial erythrocytosis syndromes.

Focused Queries

1. *Has itching of the skin, especially with warm showers or baths, become noticeable or bothersome?* Pruritus, particularly aquagenic pruritus, is highly suggestive of polycythemia vera.[4]

2. *Have you noticed that you are not able to eat as much food now before feeling full as you could in the past?* Early satiety may reflect the presence of splenic enlargement, a feature of polycythemia vera.

PHYSICAL EXAMINATION

Patients with absolute erythrocytosis, regardless of the etiology, demonstrate signs of vascular distension including plethora, dilated retinal veins on funduscopic examination, and conjunctival injection. The abdomen should be carefully evaluated for the presence of splenic enlargement, a finding suggestive of polycythemia vera. Findings of chronic cardiopulmonary disease might suggest an etiology for secondary erythrocytosis. Cyanosis in the absence of arterial hypoxemia raises the possibility of methemoglobinemia.

DIAGNOSTIC STUDIES

Essential Laboratory Studies

Hemogram

In addition to documenting the presence of erythrocytosis, the hemogram (including white blood cell differential and platelet counts) may provide important diagnostic clues. Neutrophilic leukocytosis, increased numbers of basophils, and/or thrombocytosis are suggestive of polycythemia vera.[4] The total and differential white cell counts and platelet count are typically normal in secondary erythrocytosis.

Red Cell Mass Determination

The initial step in the diagnostic evaluation of the patient with documented erythrocytosis is to determine whether the erythrocytosis is absolute or relative. In most patients, this involves the measurement of the red cell mass by radioisotope dilution in blood of ^{51}Cr- or ^{99m}Tc-labeled autologous red cells.[5] Red cell mass is most commonly reported in terms of milliliters per kilogram of body weight (for normal males, it is 26 to 32 ml/kg, and for normal females, 23 to 29 ml/kg). It is important to recognize, because of the relative hypovascularity of adipose tissue, that red cell mass values of obese individuals expressed in this manner may be artifactually low. For such patients, the red cell mass is better expressed in terms of the calculated lean body mass or body surface area.[5] In scheduling the red cell mass measurement and interpreting the results, one must also take into account the possibility of coexistent iron deficiency and/or recent blood loss due to hemorrhage or phlebotomy, conditions that would obviously depress the measured red cell mass.

Whether the red cell mass should be measured in all patients with erythrocytosis is controversial. Patients with markedly elevated hematocrits (i.e., equal to or greater than 60 per cent) usually, but not always, have elevated red cell masses. In such patients, if other features of polycythemia vera (see later discussion) are present, it is not necessary to measure the red cell mass. In patients with lesser elevations in hematocrit or who lack other features of polycythemia vera, the red cell mass should be measured directly.

The plasma volume may also be measured with ^{131}I-labeled human serum albumin. However, the distribution of albumin into extravascular compartments introduces technical problems in interpretation, plasma volume is somewhat labile, and normal values are not as well established as for red cell mass.[5] Furthermore, plasma volume measurement usually does not add clinically useful information to that provided by the hematocrit and the red cell mass. Hence, it is seldom, if ever, necessary to measure the plasma volume.

Laboratory Studies in Patients with Absolute Erythrocytosis

Arterial Blood Gases

This study is necessary to determine whether arterial hypoxemia, a cause of secondary erythrocytosis, is present.

Carboxyhemoglobin Determination

This study should be performed in all smokers and in selected nonsmokers with unexplained secondary erythrocytosis. The half-life of carbon monoxide in the blood is three to five hours. Carboxyhemoglobin levels in smokers are lowest upon awakening in the morning and progressively increase during the day. Hence, carboxyhemoglobin levels are best measured in the late afternoon or evening. Normal carboxyhemoglobin levels are 0 to 2 per cent and average 5 to 11 per cent in patients with smokers' polycythemia.[6,7]

Hemoglobin P50 Measurement

The P_{50}, the partial pressure of oxygen at which hemoglobin oxygen saturation is 50 per cent, is a convenient measure of the affinity of hemoglobin for oxygen. The normal P_{50} at 37° C and pH 7.4 is 26 torr (mm Hg). The P_{50} is reduced (i.e., the oxygen affinity of hemoglobin is increased, thereby compromising oxygen unloading in the tissues) with high-affinity hemoglobin variants, carbon monoxide intoxication, and methemoglobinemia.

Serum Vitamin B12, Unsaturated B12-Binding Capacity, and Leukocyte Alkaline Phosphatase Score

These values are frequently elevated in polycythemia vera (see later discussion). However, such elevations are by no means specific since they may also occur in a variety of infectious and inflammatory conditions.

Bone Marrow Biopsy

In polycythemia vera, the bone marrow reveals panmyelosis with erythroid, granulocytic, and megakaryocytic hyperplasia.[4] The bone marrow in patients with secondary erythrocytosis is normal or shows only erythroid hyperplasia.

Serum Epo Level

The serum epo level is characteristically reduced or normal in autonomous erythrocytosis.[8,9,10] Low serum epo levels may also be seen in association with renal disease and, occasionally, with infectious, inflammatory, or neoplastic conditions.[1] In secondary erythrocytosis, the serum epo level is increased but sometimes only intermittently.[8,9] Hence, repeated blood sampling may occasionally be necessary in order to document the elevated serum epo level.

Endogenous (Epo-Independent) Erythroid Colony Growth

Colonies of hemoglobinized erythroblasts will develop in the absence of exogenous epo in cultures of peripheral blood or marrow cells from polycythemia vera patients. This so-called *endogenous* or epo-independent erythroid colony growth is not observed in normal individuals or in patients with secondary or relative erythrocytosis.[10,11] Although originally described in polycythemia vera, it is now clear that endogenous erythroid colony growth is often observed in the other chronic myeloproliferative disorders[11] (see later discussion).

Other Laboratory Studies

The blood chemistry screen may reveal hyperuricemia in polycythemia vera (reflecting increased cell turnover) or, in conjunction with the urinalysis, evidence of renal lesions associated with secondary erythrocytosis (elevated blood urea nitrogen [BUN], creatinine; hematuria). Appropriate diagnostic imaging studies may reveal subclinical splenomegaly, evidence of cardiopulmonary disease, or tumor masses or renal structural abnormalities associated with secondary erythrocytosis.

ASSESSMENT

Based on the measured red cell mass, erythrocytosis may be classified as absolute (i.e., elevated red cell mass) or relative (normal red cell mass). Absolute erythrocytosis may be further classified as autonomous (primary) or secondary (i.e., due to elevated epo levels). Secondary erythrocytosis may be appropriate, owing to increased renal epo elaboration in the setting of generalized tissue hypoxia, or inappropriate, when elevated renal or extrarenal epo production does not reflect generalized tissue hypoxia. Table 1 summarizes the characteristic laboratory findings of relative erythrocytosis, polycythemia vera (the predominant form of autonomous erythrocytosis), and secondary erythrocytosis.

The individual erythrocytosis syndromes will now be discussed.

Relative Erythrocytosis

Relative erythrocytosis refers to chronic elevation of the hematocrit without elevation of the red cell mass above the normal range. Also known as *Gaisböck's syndrome or spurious, stress, pseudo-,* or *benign polycythemia,* relative erythrocytosis is the most prevalent diagnostic entity among patients with elevated hematocrits encountered in clinical practice.[12,13] The major cause of relative erythrocytosis is a chronic reduction in plasma volume. In some patients, the plasma volume is in the low-normal range and coexists with a high-normal red cell mass. In others, the plasma volume is clearly less than normal. A number of authors have described the "typical" patient as an anxious middle-aged male under chronic stress and prone to cardiovascular disease. Many such patients complain of headache, weakness, fatigue, and dizziness, but it is not at all clear whether such symptoms are any more common than among appropriate nonerythrocytotic controls.[12] Relative erythrocytosis has been most convincingly associated with chronic hypertension and smoking, although the mechanisms underlying the plasma volume dysregulation are unknown.[12,13] Chronic diuretic use occasionally results in relative polycythemia. The reported associations of heavy alcohol use or stress with relative polycythemia are not well established. Most patients with relative polycythemia due to a high-normal red cell mass and low-normal plasma volume appear to represent a segment of the normal population; limited data provide no evidence of excess mortality or increased incidence of cardiovascular disease.[12]

Absolute Erythrocytosis—Autonomous

These syndromes are characterized by elevations in the red cell mass due to excessive proliferation of erythroid progenitor cells occurring in the absence of normal physiologic erythropoietic stimuli. The cellular and molec-

TABLE 1. Summary of Major Laboratory Findings in Relative Erythrocytosis, Polycythemia Vera, and Secondary Erythrocytosis*

	RELATIVE ERYTHRO-CYTOSIS	POLYCYTHEMIA VERA	SECONDARY ERYTHROCYTOSIS
Red cell mass	N	↑	↑
Splenomegaly	0	+	0
Neutrophilic leukocytosis	0	+	0
Basophilia	0	+	0
Thrombocytosis	0	+	0
Serum vitamin B_{12}	N	↑	N
$UB_{12}BC$	N	↑	N
LAP score	N	↑	N
Bone marrow	N	Panmyelosis	N, erythroid hyperplasia
Serum epo	N	N, ↓	N, ↑
Endogenous colony growth	0	+	0

* Symbols: N = normal; ↑ = increased; ↓ = decreased; 0 = absent; + = present.

ular mechanisms that underlie this hematopoietic dysregulation are not understood.

Polycythemia Vera

Polycythemia vera, one of the chronic myeloproliferative disorders (which also include chronic myelogenous leukemia, primary thrombocythemia, and agnogenic myeloid metaplasia), is a clonal hemopathy in which red cells, granulocytes, platelets, and B lymphocytes are derived from a single abnormal pluripotent stem cell.[4,14]

Polycythemia vera is diagnosed most often during the sixth or seventh decades of life, but cases have been reported in every age group. Many of the symptoms and signs of this disease are consequences of hypervolemia or hyperviscosity. Vascular distension is manifested as plethora, dilated retinal veins on funduscopic examination, and conjunctival injection. Lethargy, headache, dizziness, tinnitus, and visual disturbances have been attributed to reduction in cerebral blood flow and/or cerebral vascular engorgement. Pruritus, which often is induced or exacerbated by warm baths or showers (*aquagenic pruritus*), occurs in approximately 40 per cent of patients.[4] Gastrointestinal symptoms, particularly dyspepsia or bleeding due to acid-peptic disease; early satiety; and left upper quadrant discomfort from splenic enlargement (a result of expansion of the splenic red cell pool and extramedullary hematopoiesis) are common. Splenomegaly is present in three fourths of patients at diagnosis. Thrombotic and/or hemorrhagic complications related to hyperviscosity, abnormal platelet function, and other uncharacterized pathogenetic factors develop frequently. While deep venous thrombosis, pulmonary embolism, myocardial infarction, and peripheral arterial thrombosis predominate, thromboses of intra-abdominal veins may occur. Indeed, the majority of patients with hepatic vein thrombosis (Budd-Chiari syndrome) either have polycythemia vera or an occult myeloproliferative disorder.[15]

Patients invariably demonstrate an increased red cell mass unless bleeding and/or iron deficiency have supervened. Neutrophilic leukocytosis and thrombocytosis are present in the majority of patients as well. An increased number of basophils, a finding that by itself strongly suggests the possible presence of a myeloproliferative disorder, occurs in approximately two thirds of patients.[4] The leukocyte alkaline phosphatase (LAP) activity of segmented neutrophils, expressed semiquantitatively as an LAP score, is elevated in about 70 per cent of patients. The bone marrow biopsy reveals panmyelosis with erythroid, granulocytic, and megakaryocytic hyperplasia. Marrow iron stores, demonstrated by Prussian blue staining, are usually reduced or absent as a result of mobilization of iron into the erythron and, often, occult blood loss.[4] Serum vitamin B_{12} concentration and unsaturated B_{12}-binding capacity ($UB_{12}BC$) are frequently elevated, reflecting increased serum levels of transcobalamin III, a granulocyte-derived B_{12}-binding protein.[4] Serum epo levels are almost always reduced or normal. Finally, cultures of peripheral blood or marrow cells will demonstrate endogenous (epo-independent) erythroid colony growth.[10,11]

The Polycythemia Vera Study Group (PVSG) developed criteria, listed in Table 2, that have been widely utilized to assist in the diagnosis of polycythemia vera.[16] According to the PVSG criteria, a diagnosis of polycythemia vera is established (1) if all three category A criteria are satisfied or (2) if the first two category A criteria and any two of the category B criteria are satisfied. However, there remains a significant cohort of patients with absolute erythrocytosis who do not satisfy the PVSG criteria for the diagnosis of polycythemia vera yet have no identifiable cause of secondary erythrocytosis; these individuals may account for up to 30 to 40 per cent of erythrocytotic patients seen at referral centers.[10] In such patients, culture of blood or bone marrow cells to look for endogenous erythroid colony growth, measurement of the serum epo level, and bone marrow biopsy are helpful.[4,8,9,10,11,16]

TABLE 2. Polycythemia Vera Study Group Diagnostic Criteria*

CATEGORY A

A1. Increased red cell mass: males, ≥ 36 ml/kg; females, ≥ 32 ml/kg
A2. Arterial oxygen saturation $\geq 92\%$
A3. Splenomegaly

CATEGORY B

B1. Platelet count $\geq 400 \times 10^9/L$
B2. White blood cell count $\geq 12 \times 10^9/L$ (in absence of fever or infection)
B3. LAP score >100 (in absence of fever or infection)
B4. Serum vitamin B_{12} level >900 pg/ml or $UB_{12}BC$ >2200 pg/ml

* The diagnosis of polycythemia vera may be made if all three category A criteria are met or if the first two category A *and* any two category B criteria are met.

Primary Erythrocytosis (Erythremia)

Rare patients have been described with pure erythrocytosis and low or normal serum epo levels who lack other features of polycythemia vera, such as splenomegaly, thrombocytosis, leukocytosis, and basophilia.[8,17] In some cases, erythrocytosis has been noted in family members, suggesting the possibility of genetic transmission. Several of the reported patients demonstrated endogenous erythroid colony growth,[10] although culture studies have not been performed in many of these patients. It is likely that this condition is related to polycythemia vera, and indeed, with extended follow-up, some patients eventually go on to develop classic polycythemia vera.[17]

Secondary Erythrocytosis— Appropriate

These conditions are characterized by an elevation of the red cell mass due to increased renal epo production occurring in the setting of generalized tissue hypoxia.

Erythrocytosis due to Chronic Hypoxemia

High Altitude

Erythrocytosis is an essential component of the adaptive response to living at high altitudes.

Pulmonary Disease

Compensatory erythrocytosis due to chronic arterial oxygen desaturation may be seen in association with chronic lung disease.

Alveolar Hypoventilation

Alveolar hypoventilation associated with sleep apnea syndromes, neuromuscular disease, or structural abnormalities of the thorax may cause secondary erythrocytosis.

Cardiovascular Disease

Erythrocytosis, often severe, may be seen with congenital heart disease with right-to-left shunts. Arterial hypoxemia, probably due to pulmonary arteriovenous shunts, can occur with cirrhosis of the liver and produce secondary erythrocytosis.

Erythrocytosis due to Defective Oxygen Transport

Carbon Monoxide Poisoning

Carbon monoxide binds avidly to hemoglobin, reducing its oxygen-carrying capacity and shifting the hemoglobin oxygen dissociation curve to the left (i.e., increasing the affinity of the remaining vacant oxygen-binding sites). Hence, carbon monoxide reduces oxygen delivery to tissues and can produce secondary erythrocytosis. Chronic carbon monoxide intoxication underlies the development of *smokers' polycythemia*.[6,7] In smokers' polycythemia, an unexplained reduction in plasma volume usually also occurs and, in some patients, is not accompanied by an increase in red cell mass. Occasional reports of erythrocytosis secondary to chronic carbon monoxide poisoning from household or occupational exposure (e.g., from a leaky gas furnace)[18] have also appeared. This diagnosis is suggested by the presence of an elevated blood carboxyhemoglobin level.

Hemoglobinopathies

A number of abnormal hemoglobins with increased oxygen affinity have been described.[19] Patients have lifelong erythrocytosis. These hemoglobinopathies, which result from single amino acid substitutions, are inherited in an autosomal dominant fashion. Only heterozygotes, with approximately equal levels of normal and mutant hemoglobins, have been observed; the homozygous state may be incompatible with life. The appropriate screening test for the presence of a high-affinity hemoglobin is the measurement of the P_{50}, since approximately one-half of the amino acid mutations are electrophoretically silent on standard starch gel hemoglobin electrophoresis.[19]

Methemoglobinemia

Methemoglobin, in which iron is in the oxidized ferric state (Fe^{3+}), may develop in increased levels as a consequence of exposure to certain toxins or drugs, congenital deficiency of NADH (nicotinamide-adenine dinucleotide) diaphorase (which catalyzes the reduction of Fe^{3+} in methemoglobin), or certain hemoglobinopathies (the hemoglobin M variants) (see pp. 623–62 of reference 19). Secondary erythrocytosis occasionally develops, primarily as a result of left shift of the oxygen dissociation curve. Since as little as

1.5 gm/dl of methemoglobin produce visible cyanosis, patients are typically cyanotic.

Secondary Erythrocytosis— Inappropriate

These conditions are characterized by an elevated red cell mass due to increased renal or extrarenal epo production occurring in the absence of generalized tissue hypoxia.

Erythrocytosis due to Renal Disease

Renal vascular disease, presumably as a result of diminished oxygen delivery to the renal oxygen sensor, is a surprisingly uncommon cause of secondary erythrocytosis.[20] This may reflect the parallel reductions in glomerular filtration and tubular metabolic activity that accompany significant reductions in renal blood flow, thereby preventing the development of hypoxia in renal tissue.

Erythrocytosis may develop in association with renal cysts (solitary or polycystic) or hydronephrosis. In the former condition, analysis of cyst fluid has generally revealed high concentrations of epo.[21] The mechanism underlying the elevated epo production remains to be determined but may relate to hypoperfusion of adjacent parenchyma due to pressure from the cyst.

Erythrocytosis After Renal Transplantation

Erythrocytosis due to excessive epo production occurs in approximately 10 per cent of patients after renal transplantation. In most cases, the remaining native kidney appears to be the source of the inappropriate epo production; the mechanism is unknown.[22,23]

Tumor-Associated Erythrocytosis

Erythrocytosis due to ectopic epo production has been reported to develop in association with a variety of neoplasms, most commonly renal cell carcinoma (approximately 1 per cent of affected patients have erythrocytosis), Wilms' tumor, hepatocellular carcinoma, cerebellar hemangioblastomas, and uterine leiomyomas. In cases that have been carefully studied, the tumor cells have been shown to produce epo.[24] Androgen-producing tumors, particularly ovarian arrhenoblastomas, may cause erythrocytosis. Androgens both promote epo production and potentiate the stimulatory effects of epo on erythroid progenitor cells.

Erythrocytosis due to Increased Epo Production of Unknown Cause

An elevated serum epo level and erythrocytosis have occasionally been observed in the absence of conditions known to be associated with secondary erythrocytosis. This rare syndrome, sometimes designated *essential hypererythropoietinemia*, sometimes occurs in family members.[8]

REFERENCES

1. Zanjani ED, Ascensao JL. Erythropoietin. Transfusion 1989:29:46–57.
2. Erslev AJ, Wilson J, Caro J. Erythropoietin titers in anemic, nonuremic patients. J Lab Clin Med 1987;109:429–33.
3. Eschbach JW, Adamson JW. Recombinant human erythropoietin: implications for nephrology. Am J Kidney Dis 1988;11:203–9.
4. Murphy S. Polycythemia vera. In: Williams WJ, Beutler E, Erslev AJ, Lichtman MA, eds. Hematology. 4th ed. New York: McGraw-Hill, 1990:193–202.
5. International Committee for Standardization in Hematology. Recommended methods for measurement of red-cell and plasma volume. J Nucl Med 1980;21:793–800.
6. Smith JR, Landaw SA. Smokers' polycythemia. N Engl J Med 1978;298:6–10.
7. Aitchison R, Russell N. Smoking—a major cause of polycythaemia. J R Soc Med 1988;81:89–91.
8. Erslev AJ, Caro J. Pure erythrocytosis classified according to erythropoietin titers. Am J Med 1984;76:57–61.
9. Cotes PM, Dore CJ, Liu Yin JA, et al. Determination of serum immunoreactive erythropoietin in the investigation of erythrocytosis. N Engl J Med 1986;315:283–7.
10. Lemoine F, Najman A, Baillou C, et al. A prospective study of the value of bone marrow erythroid progenitor cultures in polycythemia. Blood 1986;68:996–1002.
11. Greenberg PL. In vitro culture techniques defining biological abnormalities in the myelodysplastic syndromes and myeloproliferative disorders. Clin Haematol 1986;15:973–93.
12. Weinreb NJ, Shih C-F. Spurious polycythemia. Semin Hematol 1975;12:397–407.
13. Lederle FA. Relative erythrocytosis: an approach to the patient. J Gen Intern Med 1987;2:128–30.
14. Adamson JW, Fialkow PJ, Murphy S, Prchal JF, Steinmann L. Polycythemia vera: stem-cell and probably clonal origin of the disease. N Engl J Med 1976;295:913–6.
15. Valla D, Casadevall N, Lacombe C, et al. Primary myeloproliferative disorder and hepatic vein thrombosis. Ann Intern Med 1985;103:329–34.
16. Berk PD, Goldberg JD, Donovan PB, Fruchtman SM, Berlin NI, Wasserman LR. Therapeutic recommendations in polycythemia vera based on Polycythemia Vera Study Group protocols. Semin Hematol 1986;23:132–43.
17. Najean Y, Triebel F, Dresch C. Pure erythrocytosis:

reappraisal of a study of 51 cases. Am J Hematol 1981;10:129–36.

18. Dimarco AT. Carbon monoxide poisoning presenting as polycythemia. N Engl J Med 1988;319:874.

19. Bunn HF, Forget BG. Hemoglobin: molecular, genetic and clinical aspects. Philadelphia: WB Saunders, 1986:595–622.

20. Hudgson P, Pearce JM, Yeates WK. Renal artery stenosis with hypertension and high haematocrit. Br Med J 1967;1:18–21.

21. Waldmann TA, Rosse WF, Swarm RL. The erythropoiesis-stimulating factors produced by tumors. Ann NY Acad Sci 1968;149:509–15.

22. Wickre CG, Norman DJ, Bennison A, Barry JM, Bennett WM. Postrenal transplant erythrocytosis: a review of 53 patients. Kidney Int 1983;23:731–7.

23. Thevenod F, Radtke HW, Grutzmacher P. Deficient feedback regulation of erythropoiesis in kidney transplant patients with polycythemia. Kidney Int 1983;24:227–32.

24. Da Silva J-L, Lacombe C, Bruneval P. Tumor cells are the site of erythropoietin synthesis in human renal cancers associated with polycythemia. Blood 1990;75:577–82.

PROTEINURIA

BLANCHE M. CHAVERS

SYNONYM: Protein in the Urine

BACKGROUND

Protein normally occurs in the urine in amounts up to 150 mg per day.[1,2] However, this amount is undetectable by usual laboratory screening tests. Sixty per cent of the protein in normal urine comes from plasma proteins, and 40 per cent comes from secretions of the kidney and the urogenital tract.[3] Albumin is the most prominent plasma protein found in normal human urine, and Tamm-Horsfall mucoprotein is the most prominent renal tubular protein. The amount of protein excreted in the urine is determined by two processes: glomerular filtration and protein reabsorption by proximal tubules. The determinants of glomerular filtration include the properties of the plasma proteins such as molecular size, shape, and charge; the integrity of the glomerular capillary wall; the electrostatic charge of the capillary wall; and hemodynamic factors. This process has been reviewed in detail, and abnormalities in glomerular permeability result in glomerular proteinuria.[4] The determinants of tubular proteinuria include decreased reabsorption of low-molecular weight proteins normally present in glomerular filtrate and increased secretion of proteins (e.g., Tamm-Horsfall protein) by injured tubules. Abnormal plasma proteins (e.g., Bence Jones protein) in high concentration may also exceed the tubules' capacity for reabsorption. Other proteins that may be increased in tubular proteinuria include lysozyme, beta-2-microglobulin, retinol binding protein, and kappa and lambda light chains.[5]

The amount of protein excreted in the urine is increased when the patient is in the erect posture in both normal and pathologic states. "Dipstick" (standard qualitative laboratory reagent strip impregnated with dye)-positive proteinuria detected on a random, routine urine sample is quite common in apparently healthy children and adults and may not signify renal disease. Fewer than 1.5 per cent of healthy, asymptomatic adults with dipstick-positive proteinuria will have serious and treatable urinary tract disorders.[6] Transient proteinuria is known to occur with fever, when the patient is standing, during emotional stress, with exposure to cold, following administration of epinephrine, following blood transfusions, and after strenuous exercise.[5] This type of proteinuria may occur intermittently and may last a few days. In a study of 313 consecutive patients admitted to a general hospital through an emergency room, 9.5 per cent of patients had transient proteinuria documented by dipstick and confirmed by the sulfosalicylic acid test.[7] Congestive heart failure was the leading cause of proteinuria in these patients, followed by seizures, pneumonia, and fever. In the majority of these patients, the proteinuria was glomerular in origin and resolved within 10 days.[7] Transient proteinuria associated with congestive heart failure resolves after treatment of the heart failure. A false-positive dipstick reaction may occur in highly alkaline urine samples, during menstruation in females, in urine contaminated by antiseptics (e.g., benzalkonium), and in urine contaminated by bacteria. A false-negative dipstick reaction may occur in patients with increased free immunoglobulin light chains (Bence Jones proteins). The sulfosalicylic acid method may yield false-positive results in patients receiving intravenous radiographic contrast media or certain medications (e.g., tolbutamide, sulfonamide, cephalosporin, penicillin, tolmetin). When persistent (present on three or more urine samples collected at least one week apart), proteinuria requires further patient evaluation. This chapter focuses on the diagnostic approach to persistent proteinuria.

Proteinuria has been recognized as a sign of kidney disease since the early 1800s. Although a urine protein concentration greater than 30 mg/dl is indicative of proteinuria, to make a diagnosis of proteinuria the patient must be excreting 150 mg or more of protein in the urine per day. Estimates of the degree of proteinuria can be made using random urine samples and measuring the urinary protein-to-creatinine ratio,[8,9,10] the urinary albumin-to-creatinine ratio,[11,12,13] the urinary protein concentration,[5] or the urinary albumin concentration.[14] Evaluation of random urine samples collected during normal waking hours is useful for screening and follow-up of proteinuria. Unfortunately, there has been no uniformity in either the assay methods or the units used to express values (e.g., mg/mmol, μg/mg, mg/mg, mg/L), and published normal ranges vary.

The urine specific gravity should also be checked since protein may not be detected in a dilute sample. A timed urine collection is required for quantitation of urinary protein excretion. The most representative results are obtained with 24-hour urine collections. However, patients require detailed instructions on how to obtain the collection properly. Urinary creatinine determination on the same 24-hour sample can help determine the adequacy of the specimen. Multiple (four to six) short-term collections obtained as part of clearance studies will also give reliable results. Normal, age-appropriate values for urinary protein are given in Table 1.

Orthostatic (postural) proteinuria requires special mention. It is glomerular in origin. First-morning voided urine samples are usually negative, with proteinuria developing when the patient assumes an erect posture.[15] Total daily excretion of protein may be large but is usually less than 1 gm per day. It is a common cause of proteinuria in older children (rare before six years of age) and young adults, occurring in 2 to 5 per cent of adolescents, and gradually disappearing during the second decade of life.[16,17] Reportedly, 60 per cent of children and 15 to 60 per cent of young adults presenting with asymptomatic proteinuria will have a pattern of orthostatic proteinuria.[5] Orthostatic proteinuria may be a component of serious renal disease or may occur during the early stages of significant renal disease. Abnormal renal biopsies were present in 8 per cent of patients with orthostatic proteinuria followed for 10 to 20 years.[18] Therefore, it should not be considered a benign disorder until several years have passed.

Other possible causes of proteinuria are listed in Table 2. Disorders affecting the glomerulus and leading to persistent proteinuria in the absence of hematuria include essential

TABLE 1.   Urinary Protein Values

GROUP	mg/24 hours	mg/hour/sq m of sa*	mg/mg of creatinine
Adults			
Normal	<150		<0.2
Severe proteinuria	>3500		>3.5
Children			
Normal		<4	<0.5 (<2 years of age)
			<0.2 (>2 years of age)
Severe proteinuria		>40	>1.5

* SA = body surface area.

(From Striegel J, Michael AF, Chavers BM. Asymptomatic proteinuria: benign disorder or harbinger of disease? Postgrad Med 1988;83:287–94. Copyright by McGraw-Hill, Inc. Reprinted with permission.)

TABLE 2.   Causes of Proteinuria

TRANSIENT

Exercise
Fever
Exposure to cold
Emotional stress
Dehydration
Congestive heart failure
Seizures
Pneumonia
Administration of epinephrine
Following blood or plasma transfusions

ORTHOSTATIC

GLOMERULAR ABNORMALITIES

Primary renal disease
    Idiopathic nephrotic syndrome
    Glomerulonephritis
        Focal segmental glomerulosclerosis
        Membranous
        Membranoproliferative
        Hereditary nephritis
        Most types of glomerulonephritis in association with hematuria
Systemic disease affecting the kidney
    Systemic lupus erythematosus
    Diabetes mellitus
    Amyloidosis
    Hypertension
    Infection (syphilis, malaria, hepatitis B, subacute bacterial endocarditis)
    Toxemia of pregnancy
    Multiple myeloma
    Toxins (mercurials, bismuth, gold, penicillamine, probenecid, trimethadione)

TUBULAR ABNORMALITIES

Congenital diseases
    Polycystic kidney disease
    Medullary cystic disease
    Renal hypoplasia
    Reflux nephropathy
    Obstructive uropathy
    Fanconi's syndrome
Cystinosis
Chronic pyelonephritis
Interstitial nephritis (analgesic abuse, lead, mercury, cadmium, aminoglycosides, ampho-
    tericin B, penicillins, indomethacin, fenoprofen, thiazides, furosemide)
Kidney transplant rejection
Radiation nephritis
Multiple myeloma
Waldenström's macroglobulinemia
Benign monoclonal gammopathy
Leukemia
Renal tuberculosis

hypertension, idiopathic nephrotic syndrome, nephrotic syndrome with focal segmented glomerulosclerosis, amyloidosis, membranous glomerulonephritis, diabetic nephropathy, and pre-eclampsia.[5] The incidence of asymptomatic proteinuria in patients with essential hypertension ranges from 3 to 18 per cent, depending on the method used to detect proteinuria.[19] The most common cause of persistent asymptomatic proteinuria in young children is idiopathic nephrotic syndrome. Other names for this disease include minimal-change nephrotic syndrome, nil lesion nephrotic syndrome, lipoid nephrosis, and steroid-responsive nephrotic syndrome.[20] This disease is most common in children one to six years of age who usually come to the attention of their physician after developing edema. Proteinuria may be present for one to two months before the child is recognized to have edema. The total daily protein excretion is usually greater than 3 gm/1.73 sq m body surface area.[20] These children will also have low serum albumin, low serum IgG levels, and high serum cholesterol concentration. Only 20 per cent of adults presenting with nephrotic syndrome will have idiopathic nephrotic syndrome, compared with 80 to 85 per cent of young children.[20]

Urinary albumin excretion has served as an important indicator of diabetic nephropathy. Approximately 40 per cent of insulin-dependent patients will develop diabetic nephropathy, with the incidence peaking after 15 years of disease.[21] The major manifestations of diabetic nephropathy are albuminuria (greater than 400 mg/24 hours), hypertension, and a reduced glomerular filtration rate. Other types of glomerulonephritis (e.g., membranoproliferative, acute poststreptococcal) and systemic diseases affecting the kidney (e.g., systemic lupus erythematosus) will commonly have red blood cells as well as protein in the urine. Tubular disorders leading to persistent proteinuria include congenital anomalies (e.g., polycystic kidney disease, obstructive uropathy), chronic pyelonephritis, interstitial nephritis, and Fanconi's syndrome. Rare (e.g., familial nephritis with proteinuria alone, factitious)[17,22] causes of proteinuria have also been reported.

HISTORY

History of the Present Illness

The medical history should record the onset of proteinuria and associated symptoms. Most commonly, proteinuria is detected during a routine physical examination for school, athletics, or employment. Patients with asymptomatic proteinuria will not have associated signs or symptoms of disease. It is important to document whether there is fever, vomiting, diarrhea, or other symptoms suggestive of infection or dehydration that might lead to transient proteinuria. Has there been a recent respiratory infection (idiopathic nephrotic syndrome, IgA nephropathy), sore throat, or skin infection (poststreptococcal infection)? Has the patient had fever, facial skin rash, sun sensitivity, hair loss, mouth ulcers, or joint pain suggestive of systemic lupus erythematosus? Has there been an increase in the patient's exercise level or activities? Has the patient been exposed to cold? When was the patient's last menstrual period (a false-positive test may result from blood in the urine of menstruating females)? Has the patient traveled to a tropical area recently (malaria)? Has the patient had protein in the urine in the past? Has there been any change in the patient's voiding pattern (less urine output)? Does the patient have to get up to void during the night (nocturia)? Does the patient have swelling of the ankles? Does the patient complain of rings being too tight? Does the patient have heart disease (congestive heart failure)? Does the patient have any trouble breathing with usual exertion or when lying down (congestive heart failure, pleural effusions due to edema)? Is the patient experiencing a period of stress?

Family History

Have any other family members been sick recently or had a serious health problem in the past? Is there a family history of kidney disease? Is there a family history of deafness? Is there a family history of kidney stones? Is there a family history of bladder or urinary tract infections? Is there a disease or condition that tends to run in the family? Is there a family history of high blood pressure? Is there a family history of diabetes? Is there a family history of cancer? Have there been any stillborn children or children with congenital abnormalities born into the family? Is there a family history of toxemia of pregnancy?

Social and Occupational History

What kind of work does the patient do (or the patient's parent or guardian, if a child)? Do you own your own home or rent? Is the patient under stress at home, on the job, or school? What are some of the patient's activities? In the case of children, does anyone besides the parents care for the child?

Past Medical History

Does the patient have a regular physician? When was the patient last seen by the regular physician? Were there any problems at birth? Has the patient grown normally? Has the patient had this problem or a similar problem in the past? Has the patient had urinary tract infections in the past? Does the patient have a chronic illness? Have there been previous hospitalizations? Has the patient ever been in the armed services? Has the patient ever been turned down for life insurance?

Focused Queries

1. *Has there been any change in the color of the patient's urine?* Most of the glomerulonephritidies have proteinuria and hematuria. The hematuria may be transiently macroscopic, giving the urine a brown or tea color, which could suggest membranoproliferative glomerulonephritis, IgA nephropathy, or hereditary nephritis.

2. *Does the patient have dysuria, urgency, frequency, or back pain?* A positive response to this question would suggest a urinary tract infection or chronic pyelonephritis.

3. *Is the patient taking any medications or pills or been on any in the recent past?* Many medications may lead to glomerular or tubular injury such as gold, penicillamine, phenacetin, probenecid, trimethadione, amphotericin B, gentamicin, and methicillin.

4. *Has the patient noticed any weight loss, swelling of glands, increased tiredness, change in appetite?* These findings may suggest leukemia, lymphoma, or multiple myeloma.

5. *Are your shoes or clothes tight or uncomfortable during the day? Have you noticed any swelling of your eyes when you awaken in the morning?* Positive responses are suggestive of edema. Many glomerular diseases may lead to the development of nephrotic syndrome.

PHYSICAL EXAMINATION

A complete physical examination may reveal whether any systemic abnormality exists. Height and weight should be recorded, especially in children, to evaluate for growth retardation (height and weight below the third percentile for age may suggest chronic renal disease), weight loss, or weight gain. Vital signs should be recorded. The presence of an elevated temperature (equal to or greater than 101° F or 38.3° C) may indicate infection. Low blood pressure may be present in patients with gastroenteritis and/or dehydration, and high blood pressure may be present in patients with renal disease, essential hypertension, and preeclampsia. The criteria of the Second Task Force on Blood Pressure Control in Children should be used in defining hypertension in children.[23] Pulse and respirations should be checked. The skin should be inspected for color (pallor, erythema, cyanosis), turgor (diminished with dehydration), and discrete lesions (e.g., malar erythema in systemic lupus erythematosus, petechiae or purpura in leukemia, impetigo).

The head and neck examination includes examination of the head, eyes, ears, nose, throat, neck, and sinuses. Periorbital edema or swelling of the eyelids may be present in patients with nephrotic syndrome. Microaneurysms may be present on funduscopic evaluation of patients with diabetes mellitus. Arterial narrowing and retinal hemorrhage might be present in patients with hypertension, diabetes mellitus, and systemic lupus erythematosus. Deafness may be present in patients with hereditary nephritis. Facial skin rash and oral mucosal ulceration may be present in patients with systemic lupus erythematosus. Localized adenopathy may be present with pharyngitis or upper respiratory tract infection. Generalized adenopathy might suggest infection or malignancy. Jugular venous distension may suggest heart failure. Examination of the chest may reveal dullness to chest percussion, diminished breath sounds, and/or rales (pleural effusion, pneumonia, pulmonary edema). Cardiac examination may reveal abnormalities of heart rate, rhythm, a murmur, or gallop.

Abdominal distension may be present in patients with ascites. The skin may be tense and shiny. Presacral pitting (edema) may be present. Palpation of the abdomen may reveal an enlarged spleen (systemic lupus erythematosus, leukemia, lymphoma, infectious mononucleosis, amyloidosis, polycystic kidney disease) or liver (lymphoma, leukemia, congestive heart failure, amyloidosis, polycystic kidney disease) or palpable kidneys (polycystic kidney disease, hydronephrosis, renal allograft). Normal kidneys are rarely palpated in an adult or beyond the neonatal period in a child. Costovertebral angle tenderness may occur with pyelonephritis. Scrotal or labial edema may be present in patients with nephrotic syndrome. Bilateral cryptorchidism is common in patients with prune-belly syndrome (obstructive uropathy). Examination of joints may reveal swelling, tenderness, erythema, or deformity (rheumatoid arthritis, systemic lupus erythematosus). Edema of the lower extremities may be present in patients with nephrotic syndrome. Partial lipodystrophy may be present in patients with membranoproliferative glomerulonephritis. A

Bell's palsy may be present in patients with chronic hypertension.

DIAGNOSTIC STUDIES

When proteinuria is detected, it is important to determine whether it is transient, orthostatic, or persistent (see Table 3). Three urine samples should be evaluated at one- to two-week intervals to demonstrate persistent proteinuria. The urine should be evaluated for specific gravity, glucose, blood, erythrocytes, leukocytes, casts, and crystals.

After determining persistence, the proteinuria should be assessed to determine whether it is orthostatic. To screen for orthostatic proteinuria, three urine samples should be obtained within a 24-hour period. Initially, the patient voids in the evening immediately before going to bed (sample 1). A second sample is obtained the next morning before the patient arises (obtained while the patient is supine). A third sample is obtained after the patient has been allowed to ambulate during the day. Urine sample 2 should be negative for protein, and samples 1 and 3 should be positive for protein in patients with orthostatic proteinuria. This test should be repeated at least three times.[17] A split (12-hour recumbent, 12-hour upright) 24-hour urine collection should be obtained to confirm orthostatic proteinuria and to quantitate the total amount. Measurement of creatinine on the same split 24-hour collection allows for calculation of the creatinine clearance and can help determine the adequacy of the collection. The normal range for

creatinine excretion in females is 12 to 24 mg/kg per day and in males 16 to 26 mg/kg per day.[5] Orthostatic proteinuria exceeding 1 gm in a 24-hour collection requires further evaluation.

Other clinical laboratory tests should include a complete blood count, electrolytes, blood urea nitrogen, serum creatinine, urine culture, and in adults, a fasting blood glucose level. Patients with impetigo or a sore throat should have cultures (skin or throat), antistreptolysin O, and antideoxyribonuclease B titers done. Patients with nephrotic range proteinuria should have serum albumin, total protein, cholesterol, and triglyceride levels done.

Specialized tests to be performed based on the patient's history and physical examination include fluorescent antinuclear antibody test (FANA), complement (C3, C4, total complement), serum and urine protein electrophoresis, tuberculin purified protein derivative (PPD), chest radiograph, acid-fast bacillus culture, and serology for hepatitis B or syphilis, if indicated.

Diagnostic imaging to rule out structural abnormalities of the urinary tract should include renal ultrasound, intravenous pyelogram, and a voiding cystourethrogram. A negative urine culture should be obtained before performing a voiding cystourethrogram. Patients with persistent nonorthostatic proteinuria exceeding 1 gm per 24 hours should be referred to a nephrologist for consideration of renal biopsy. Exceptions would include a child with typical clinical features of the idiopathic nephrotic syndrome or a patient with severe congestive heart failure. A renal biopsy is indicated to establish diagnosis in patients with coexistent hypertension, hematuria, persistent hypocomplementemia, impaired renal function, or nephrotic range proteinuria.[24,25]

ASSESSMENT

A careful history and physical examination of the patient who presents with proteinuria may suggest an etiology. Common causes of proteinuria should be considered first unless the patient has signs of glomerulonephritis or a family history of renal disease.

Transient Proteinuria

Common causes of transient proteinuria include fever, strenuous exercise, pneumonia, seizures, gastroenteritis, and congestive heart

---

TABLE 3. Laboratory Evaluation of Significant Persistent Proteinuria

Urinalysis, urine culture
Urine samples in recumbent and upright positions
Quantitation of 24-hour urinary protein excretion
Complete blood count, blood electrolytes, blood urea nitrogen, serum creatinine
Serum albumin, total protein, cholesterol
Serum complement (C3, total complement), antinuclear antibody test
Streptococcal studies (antistreptolysin O, antiDNAase* B titers) if indicated
Serology for hepatitis B, syphilis (if indicated)
PPD, acid-fast bacilli culture, chest x-ray (if indicated)
Serum and urine protein immunoelectrophoresis (if indicated)
Renal ultrasound, intravenous pyelogram, voiding cystourethrogram

* DNAase = deoxyribonuclease.

failure. Transient proteinuria usually resolves within 10 to 14 days or with treatment of the primary disorder. The urine sediment is otherwise unremarkable, and renal function is normal.

Orthostatic Proteinuria

The history and physical examination are normal, renal function is normal, the urine sediment is normal, and the total daily protein excretion is usually less than 1 gm. The patient will only have proteinuria when in an upright position. These patients should be followed at three- to six-month intervals.

Hypertension

Patients with long-standing essential hypertension may develop proteinuria. The total daily protein excretion is usually less than 1 gm. Renal function is usually impaired, but the urine sediment is normal.

Urinary Tract Anomaly

The family history may be positive; the physical examination may reveal short stature, palpable kidneys, or palpable bladder; and renal function is usually impaired. The total daily protein excretion is usually less than 1 gm. Hematuria may be present in patients with polycystic kidney disease. Renal tubular acidosis and anemia may also be present in patients with medullary cystic disease. A renal ultrasound or intravenous pyelogram may show enlarged kidneys with cysts (polycystic kidney disease), small shrunken or scarred kidneys (renal hypoplasia, medullary cystic disease, reflux nephropathy, chronic pyelonephritis), hydronephrosis (obstructive uropathy), or hydroureters (reflux nephropathy). A voiding cystourethrogram will confirm the diagnosis in patients with reflux nephropathy.

Nephrotic Syndrome

A variety of glomerular diseases may cause nephrotic range proteinuria (greater than 3 gm per day). These patients will present with edema, hypoalbuminemia, proteinuria, and hyperlipidemia. Idiopathic nephrotic syndrome should be considered as the probable diagnosis in children one to six years of age who have a previous history of good health, normal blood pressure on physical examina-

tion, normal renal function, and a normal urine sediment. The presence of hematuria, hypertension, or abnormal renal function or failure to respond to steroid treatment would suggest other childhood glomerulonephritidies such as focal segmental glomerulosclerosis (hypertension, impaired renal function, steroid resistance), membranoproliferative glomerulonephritis (partial lipodystrophy, hematuria, low complement), membranous nephropathy (positive hepatitis B serology), poststreptococcal glomerulonephritis (positive throat or skin culture, low complement, elevated antideoxyribonuclease B titer, elevated antistreptolysin O titer). Appropriate additional diagnostic studies should be performed in these children, including a renal biopsy. Congenital nephrotic syndrome is detected within the first month of life.

The glomerulonephritidies that cause nephrotic syndrome in childhood also occur in adults. The differential diagnosis in adults should also include diabetic nephropathy (patient with diabetes for approximately 10 to 15 years); systemic lupus erythematosus, which may cause membranous, membranoproliferative, or proliferative glomerulonephritis (malar skin rash, arthritis, positive antinuclear antibody, low complement, decreased renal function); amyloidosis (large kidneys, decreased renal function, specific abnormalities on renal biopsy); multiple myeloma (bone pain or swelling with lesions present on bone x-ray, elevated serum and urine immunoglobulin fragments); malignancy (lymphoma, leukemia); and toxins (gold or penicillamine in patients with rheumatoid arthritis). A renal biopsy is warranted in all cases except in suspected idiopathic nephrotic syndrome of childhood.

REFERENCES

1. Pesce AJ, First MR. Proteinuria: an integrated review. New York: Marcel Dekker, 1979.
2. Berggard I. Plasma proteins in normal human urine. In: Manuel Y, Revillard JP, Betuel H, eds. Proteins in normal and pathological urine. Baltimore: University Park, 1970:7–19.
3. Hemmingsen L, Skaarup P. The 24-hour excretion of plasma proteins in the urine of apparently healthy subjects. Scand J Clin Lab Invest 1975;35:347–53.
4. Kanwar YS. Biology of disease. Biophysiology of glomerular filtration and proteinuria. Lab Invest 1984;51:7–21.
5. Chavers BM, Vernier RL. Proteinuria and enzymuria. Semin Nephrol 1986;6:371–88.
6. Woolhandler S, Pels RJ, Bor DH, Himmelstein DU,

Lawrence RS. Dipstick urinalysis screening of asymptomatic adults for urinary tract disorders. I. Hematuria and proteinuria. JAMA 1989;262: 1215–9.

7. Reuben DB, Wachtel TJ, Brown PC, Driscoll JL. Transient proteinuria in emergency medical admissions. N Engl J Med 1982;306:1031–3.

8. Ginsberg JM, Chang BS, Matarese RA, Garella S. Use of single voided urine samples to estimate quantitative proteinuria. N Engl J Med 1983;309:1543–6.

9. Lemann J, Doumas BT. Proteinuria in health and disease assessed by measuring the urinary protein/creatinine ratio. Clin Chem 1987;33:297–9.

10. Houser M. Assessment of proteinuria using random urine samples. J Pediatr 1984;104:845–8.

11. Davies AG, Postlethwaite RJ, Price DA, Burn JL, Houlton CA, Fielding BA. Urinary albumin excretion in school children. Arch Dis Child 1984;59:625–30.

12. Houser MT. Characterization of recumbent, ambulatory, and postexercise proteinuria in the adolescent. Pediatr Res 1987;21:442–6.

13. Gatling W, Knight C, Mullee MA, Hill RD. Microalbuminuria in diabetes: a population study of the prevalence and an assessment of three screening tests. Diabetic Med 1988;5:343–7.

14. Watts GF, Morris RW, Khan K, Polak A. Urinary albumin excretion in healthy adult subjects: reference values and some factors affecting their interpretation. Clin Chim Acta 1988;172:191–8.

15. Harrison DA, Rainford DJ, White GA, Cullen SA, Strike PW. Proteinuria—what value is the dipstick? Br J Urol 1989;63:202–8.

16. Striegel J, Michael AF, Chavers BM. Asymptomatic proteinuria: benign disorder or harbinger of disease? Postgrad Med 1988;83:287–94.

17. West CD. Asymptomatic hematuria and proteinuria in children: causes and appropriate diagnostic studies. J Pediatr 1976;89:173–82.

18. Robinson RR. Clinical significance of isolated proteinuria. In: Avram MM, ed. Proteinuria. New York: Plenum Press, 1985:67–79.

19. Samuelson O. Proteinuria as a prognostic factor during long term hypertensive care. Drugs 1988;35(Suppl 5):48–54.

20. Vernier RL. Primary (idiopathic) nephrotic syndrome. In: Holiday MA, Barratt TM, Vernier RL, eds. Pediatric nephrology. Baltimore: Williams & Wilkins, 1987:445–8.

21. Chavers BM, Bilous RW, Ellis EN, Steffes MW, Mauer SM. Glomerular lesions and urinary albumin excretion in type I diabetes without overt proteinuria. N Engl J Med 1989;320:966–70.

22. Mitas JA. Exogenous protein as the cause of nephrotic-range proteinuria. Am J Med 1985;79: 115–8.

23. Report of the Second Task Force on Blood Pressure Control in Children—1987. Pediatrics 1987;79:1–25.

24. Norman ME. An office approach to hematuria and proteinuria. Pediatr Clin North Am 1987;34:545–60.

25. Schoolwerth AC. Hematuria and proteinuria: their causes and consequences. Hosp Pract 1987; 30(Oct):45–62.

RAYNAUD'S PHENOMENON

JOHN P. LAVERY and JEFFREY R. LISSE

SYNONYM: Raynaud's Disease

BACKGROUND

Raynaud's phenomenon (RP), a benign disorder characterized by reversible and intermittent vasospasm of the digital arteries, can be induced either by cold or by emotional stimuli. The vasospasm induces a triphasic color change of pallor, cyanosis, and hyperemia.

The disorder can be classified into either primary or secondary types. When RP occurs as an isolated abnormality without any other definable disorder, it is termed primary RP, or Raynaud's disease. Secondary RP, or simply Raynaud's phenomenon, accompanies another medical condition or disorder. Primary RP accounts for approximately 30 per cent of all cases, and secondary RP, for 70 per cent of cases.[1]

Raynaud's phenomenon affects more women than men (approximately 5:1). In 60 to 90 per cent of cases, primary RP will occur in young women of childbearing age. Secondary RP in women is usually associated with connective tissue disease (CTD) and in men is associated with arteriosclerosis. The exact incidence of RP in the general population is unknown. The prevalence may vary from 3 to 5 per cent of the population[2] but may be as high as 22 per cent in young women.[3]

Most patients have involvement of their fingers—one to four or a combination may be affected at any one time. The toes and feet are both involved in 40 per cent of cases. Other acral parts of the body, such as the earlobes, nose, tongue, and nipples, may also be involved.

Clinically, RP is an easily recognized disorder. Digits, such as the fingers, will undergo a series of vascular and skin color changes in response to cold or emotional stimuli. After exposure, severe vasospasm and constriction of the digital arteries develop. Cessation of the capillary flow causes digital pallor with blanching, and there may be a sensation of coldness. Soon reactive vasodilation of the digital vessel follows, caused by accumulation of ischemic metabolites. Desaturated blood slowly enters the blood vessels with resultant cyanosis of the fingertips, which can be blue-tinged with a sensation of numbness. About 15 to 20 minutes after the initial exposure, the vasoconstriction will usually resolve spontaneously or after rewarming. Saturated arterial blood will then flow from unaffected parts of the blood into cyanotic areas until all the bluish discoloration has disappeared. If there is reactive hyperemia, erythema and pain may be noted.

Early in the course of the disorder, the attacks will be mild and infrequent. Usually, only the most distal two thirds of a digit will be affected. With repeated attacks, more proximal areas will be involved. The duration of attacks will also lengthen with time, and the frequency and severity of the episodes will increase.

HISTORY

Raynaud's phenomenon should be considered in any person who complains of extreme sensitivity to the cold and associated color changes in the fingers. Vasoconstriction of the fingers will occur as a result of normal sympathetic activity in response to cold or emotional stimuli. Many persons will complain of cold sensitivity, but digital color changes will help identify the patients with RP.

The classic triphasic changes of RP—pallor (white), cyanosis (blue), and hyperemia (red)—are seen in only one third of RP cases. There may also be uniphasic (cyanosis) or biphasic (pallor and cyanosis) changes of the digits. Other conditions may mimic RP, but the presence of pallor as a color change is considered the most reliable sign.[4]

The history is often sufficient to establish the diagnosis of RP in patients with easily recognizable color changes. It becomes more difficult to diagnose if changes are not obvious or if the episodes of RP are mild. In these cases, an interviewer will need to ask about activities that may have precipitated an episode. Questions need to be nonleading and deal with activities of daily life that could expose a person either to cold or to emotional stimuli. Activities that may not be obvious to the patient as sources of stimuli may be as simple as handling meat, washing dishes, using the refrigerator or freezer, or working outdoors in the wintertime. Feelings of rage and anxiety may also provoke episodes of RP.

Medications have been noted to either induce or exacerbate RP (Table 1). Every history should include a complete list of medications. Excessive amounts of ergot alkaloids, which may be used in the treatment of migraine headaches, have been reported to precipitate episodes of RP. Beta-adrenergic blocking agents and oral contraceptives, as well as chemotherapeutic agents such as bleomycin and vinblastine, have also been implicated.

A person's work history may be extremely important because RP has been associated with various occupational activities. Persons in industries that use tools and equipment involving high-frequency vibration and repetitive trauma—for example, forestry, logging, mining, meat cutting, dressmaking—are at risk for developing RP. Chemical and physical trauma—for example, crush injuries, frostbite, exposure to vinyl chloride—encountered in the workplace may also increase the risk of RP.[5]

Pain of the arm and shoulder suggest the possibility of a neurovascular compression syndrome. Arm and shoulder pain that is either induced or worsened by elevation may indicate the presence of a thoracic outlet syndrome. Enhancing this suspicion would be arm pain that is induced with activities that involve the arm in different positions such as driving an automobile, typing, combing hair, and sleeping. Neurovascular compression of

TABLE 1. Causes of Associated Diseases in Secondary Raynaud's Phenomenon

CONNECTIVE TISSUE DISEASE (COLLAGEN-VASCULAR DISEASE)

Rheumatoid arthritis
Systemic lupus erythematosus
Dermatomyositis/polymyositis
Mixed connective tissue disease
Diffuse scleroderma
CREST syndrome (calcinosis, Raynaud's, esophageal hypomotility, sclerodactyly, and telangiectasia syndrome)
Necrotizing vasculitis
Takayasu's arteritis
Sjögren's syndrome
Cryoglobulinemia

OCCUPATIONAL

Vibration
Trauma
Vinyl chloride
Lead
Arsenic
Frostbite

HEMATOLOGIC

Multiple myeloma
Lymphoma
Chronic leukemia
Polycythemia vera
Cold agglutinins
Dysproteinemia (Waldenström's macroglobulinemia)
Occult carcinoma
Paroxysmal nocturnal hemoglobinuria
Hypergammaglobulinemia
Hepatitis B

DRUGS (MEDICATIONS)

Beta-adrenergic blockers
Ergot alkaloids
Bromocriptine
Vinblastine
Bleomycin
Cisplatin
Cyclosporine
Oral contraceptives
Recombinant alpha-interferon

ANATOMIC

Carpal tunnel syndrome
Shoulder-hand syndrome
Scalene anticus syndrome
Cervical rib
Arteriosclerosis
Thromboangiitis obliterans
Postembolic or post-thrombotic arterial occlusion (thromboembolic disease)
Reflex sympathetic dystrophy

MISCELLANEOUS

Primary pulmonary hypertension
Acromegaly (with carpal tunnel syndrome)
Previous cold injury (frostbite)
Myxedema
Diabetes mellitus
Fabry's disease
Pheochromocytoma
Adenocarcinoma of the lung

the median nerve may arise with the establishment of wrist pain and finger numbness in a patient with RP.

A careful history may contribute a great deal to the diagnosis of a CTD prompting RP. Complaints of skin tightness and dysphagia indicate scleroderma. The presence of skin rashes and photosensitivity help entertain the possibility of systemic lupus erythematosus (SLE) or mixed CTD. Arthralgias and myalgia accompany SLE as well as polymyositis or dermatomyositis. Sjögren's syndrome may be uncovered from complaints of dry eyes or dry mouth. (Also see chapter on Xerostomia.)

Distinct color changes in the digits after cold or emotional stimuli are enough to establish the diagnosis of RP, but careful attention to the affected patient's history detailing occupational and hobby activities, medications, and various signs of systemic disease will also aid in the diagnosis of a secondary condition.

Focused Queries

1. *Do the fingers change color with cold exposure?* Blanching or pallor is the most reliable color change for the diagnosis of RP. Complaints of coldness and numbness without color changes in the digits are not indicative of RP in which there are specific color changes of the fingers.

2. *What activities or events cause color changes of the fingers?* Because RP is often induced by minimal exposure to the cold, the patient may be unaware of specific causes, like cutting meat, opening the refrigerator door, washing the dishes, going outside in the winter.

3. *Are both hands affected?* The typical patient with primary RP is a young woman with brief episodes of vasospasm in all digits of both hands. A unilateral or asymmetric presentation, especially in an elderly man, may indicate the presence of a local vascular lesion. Further workup may include arteriography of the affected extremity.

4. *Do you have dry eyes or dry mouth? Do you have any skin rashes, aches, pain, or fevers?* Of all patients with RP, approximately 60 per cent will have an associated condition, and 20 per cent will have a CTD.

PHYSICAL EXAMINATION

The physical examination of the patient with RP is often completely normal. Occasionally, the clinician will be fortunate enough to observe an RP episode if the patient has recently left a cool environment. A complete examination should be pursued because many details of CTD or another condition may be uncovered.

The peripheral vascular system should be thoroughly examined for any bruits. Asymmetry of the peripheral pulse or blood pressure suggests a vascular lesion such as the thoracic outlet syndrome. Absence of a radial or peripheral pulse may indicate an arterial embolus or Takayasu's arteritis. Useful maneuvers may include the Adson's test to detect a compression of the superior thoracic aperture and an Allen's test to detect any distal obstruction of the radial or ulnar arteries in the hand.

An examination of the extremities may show signs of an underlying CTD. (Also see chapter on Polyarticular Arthritis.) The hands should be examined thoroughly for any evidence of cutaneous change. The presence of digital ulcers and scarring indicates vasculitis. Smooth and tight shiny fingers with loss of subcutaneous tissue may result from diffuse scleroderma. Telangiectasia and swollen fingers may also indicate scleroderma or one of its traits.[6]

Median nerve compression or the carpal tunnel syndrome is associated with RP and may be detected on examination of the extremities. Sustained flexion of the wrist with resultant tenderness of the fingers in the distribution of the median nerve contributes to this diagnosis in the affected extremity.

Other areas of the body should be examined for signs of an underlying condition such as CTD. The eyelids, face, neck, chest, and the mucous membranes should be inspected for telangiectasia and erythema, which may precede the appearance of SLE, scleroderma, or dermatomyositis. Auscultation of the lungs and heart may show further evidence of an underlying condition. A systolic murmur of the heart may manifest atrial myxoma, a rare cause of RP. Fine crackles on auscultation of the lung suggest interstitial lung disease, which can develop with diffuse scleroderma.

DIAGNOSTIC STUDIES

Each person suspected of RP should undergo a limited battery of laboratory tests to exclude a secondary condition. The tests should include a complete blood count, a Westergren sedimentation rate, cryoglobulins, cold agglutinins, serum protein electrophoresis, a fluorescent antinuclear antibody screen, and a chest radiograph. Further investigation may be indicated based on the findings derived from the history and physical examination and the results of the preliminary laboratory investigation.

Features of RP that suggest the presence of an underlying condition are included in Table 2. The list helps define the indications for a more extensive investigation. A unilateral presentation of RP suggests the presence of a localized vascular lesion. If the patient is an older man or has evidence of tissue necrosis, arteriography of the affected limb should be considered to rule out a correctable abnormality.

Vascular laboratory studies such as the measurement of digital systolic pressures in combination with cold provocation can help identify a vasospastic response. Finger systolic pressure will drop modestly with progressively cooler finger temperatures in an unaffected patient. Finger systolic pressures in the RP patient will drop markedly with progressively cooler finger temperatures, indicating the presence of a cold-induced vasospasm of the digital arteries.[1]

Nail fold capillary microscopy is a useful and noninvasive procedure for identification of CTD in the patient with RP. It can also be a marker to identify the patient with primary RP at risk of developing CTD.[7,8] An ophthalmoscope or a wide-angled microscope can show the capillary loops at the finger nail fold just proximal to the cuticle. Applying immersion oil to this area and adjusting the ophthalmoscope to 40 diopters, one can visualize a row of horizontal and red hairpin-shaped capillary loops. These loops parallel the axis of the finger and in CTD may demonstrate abnormalities in their shape and number. With scleroderma, there may be an extensive avascular

---

TABLE 2. Features Suggesting an Underlying Condition in Raynaud's Phenomenon

RP in children

RP in males or females over the age of 30 years

Sudden onset of disease with rapid progression to necrosis

Unilateral or asymmetric presentation involving one to two fingers

Absence or diminution of arterial pulse in affected extremity

Symptoms of systemic disease (i.e., fever, myalgias, and arthralgias)

area with grossly dilated loops.[9] This examination can contribute a great deal in exposing CTD but cannot accurately discriminate one form from another.

Specific antinuclear antibodies such as the anticentromere antibody (ACA) and the antitopoisomerase antibody (Scl-70) can also contribute a great deal to the diagnosis of CTD in RP patients. Although rarely found in the sera of primary RP patients, ACAs have a remarkable specificity for limited scleroderma. This antibody may be found in 22 per cent of the sera of patients with limited scleroderma and may be a marker for progression from RP to this disease.[10] Antibody Scl-70 may be found in the sera of 43 per cent of patients with diffuse scleroderma and may be associated with an increased risk to develop this disease.[11,12] Rarely are both antibodies found in the sera of the same patient. Other laboratory studies may be useful in the investigation of a secondary condition associated with secondary RP. Nerve conduction studies may be ordered to confirm the diagnosis of median nerve compression. The subcutaneous calcifications of scleroderma may be noted on hand radiographs. A chest radiograph can rule out a cervical rib as an etiology.

ASSESSMENT

Raynaud's phenomenon presents three challenges to the clinician: (1) to differentiate RP from other cold-induced vasospastic disorders; (2) to distinguish primary RP from secondary RP; and (3) to identify patients with primary RP that may progress to CTD.

Other Cold-Induced Vasospastic Disorders

As previously mentioned, the diagnosis of RP should be based on a history of well-demarcated color changes of the digits. It can be confused with other cold-induced vasospastic disorders of the skin. These disorders include livedo reticularis, acrocyanosis, thromboangiitis obliterans, and chilblains.[13]

Persons affected with livedo reticularis, a vasospastic condition characterized by cyanotic mottling of the skin in the hands, feet, arms, legs, and the lower trunk, will complain of coldness, numbness, dull aching, and sometimes paresthesias of the lower extremities. The cyanosis may intensify with cold exposure, but unlike RP, livedo reticularis causes no pain and occurs on parts of the body other than the extremities.

Acrocyanosis is a benign but uncommon disorder often confused with RP. There is excessive perspiration and cyanosis of the fingers, hands, toes, and feet upon cold exposure. It is similar to RP in that young women are affected, and it can also be induced by emotional stimuli. Unlike RP, the cyanotic changes will persist after rewarming.

Thromboangiitis obliterans, or Buerger's disease, is segmental disease of the large- and medium-size arteries. Persons complain of numbness, and almost 50 per cent will experience a triphasic color change of the digits with cold exposure. There can be hand claudication and bilateral fingertip ulceration. The reduction of the ulnar and radial pulses helps distinguish it from RP.

Chilblains, or perniosis, a vasculitic disorder that can be confused with RP, develops with prolonged cold exposure usually just above the freezing point. Pruritus and erythema develop in the extremities, and small ulcerations may develop.[13]

Distinguishing Primary from Secondary RP

The second challenge for the clinician is to distinguish primary RP from secondary RP. Approximately 70 per cent of all RP patients will have an associated condition.[1] This may appear easy, but the differential diagnosis for secondary RP is lengthy.

Typically, the person with primary RP will be a young woman with a very mild presentation. Usually, all the digits of both hands are involved, and the frequency of attacks can be greater than 10 per day. Primary RP has also been associated with vasospasm of other parts of the body such as variant angina and migraine headaches. Rarely is there any digital ischemia.

Secondary RP differs from primary RP in that patients are usually older. The severity of attacks are stronger and may involve only one to two digits at a time.

Primary RP That Progresses to CDT

Connective tissue disease will account for approximately 20 per cent of all RP cases. Another 3 to 8 per cent of primary cases of RP will eventually develop CTD. RP is the presenting sign of many CTDs preceding the appearance of other signs of systemic disease by months and even years.[14]

Usually, an observation period of approximately two years is required to eliminate the possibility of a CTD arising in the primary RP patient after the appearance of RP. The exception is limited scleroderma, especially the CREST variant (calcinosis, Raynaud's, esophageal hypomotility, sclerodactyly, and telangiectasia). RP may precede other manifestations of CREST by years, and in this subset of scleroderma patients, the two-year period may not be valid.[15]

Raynaud's phenomenon may be the presenting sign of diffuse scleroderma in 80 per cent of cases. Usually, RP will shortly precede or occur at the time of onset in most. Almost 90 per cent of scleroderma patients will have RP sometime during the course of their disease.[14] Normally, the episodes of RP in scleroderma patients will be more severe with a prolonged cyanotic phase.

Fifteen per cent of patients with SLE will have RP as a presenting sign of the disease. It may precede the appearance of the disease by years and occurs with the presence of cryoglobulins. Corticosteroids may resolve the appearance of RP. Approximately 25 per cent of all SLE patients will develop RP during the course of this disease.

RP may develop in other CTDs. The prevalence of RP in mixed CTD is approximately 25 per cent and in polymyositis (and dermatomyositis) is approximately 20 per cent.

The prognosis for RP generally is that of the underlying disease associated with it. The prognosis for primary RP is good. The severity of attacks in primary RP will remain stable in approximately 50 per cent of patients. The attacks will eventually cease in 16 per cent of cases and worsen in 33 per cent of cases. Less than 1 per cent of all cases will result in any form of permanent ischemia such as digital ulcers.

REFERENCES

1. Porter JM. Raynaud's syndrome. In: Sabiston DC, ed. Textbook of surgery. Biological basis of modern surgical practice. Philadelphia: WB Saunders, 1986:1925–33.
2. Maricq HR, Keil JE, LeRoy EC. Prevalence of Raynaud phenomenon in the general population. J Chronic Dis 1986;39:423–7.
3. Olsen N, Nielsen SC. Prevalence of primary Raynaud phenomenon in young females. Scand J Clin Lab Invest 1978;37:761–76.
4. Campbell PM, LeRoy EC. Raynaud's phenomenon. Semin Arthritis Rheum 1986;16:92–103.
5. Cherniack MG. Raynaud's phenomenon of occupational origin. JAMA 1990;150:519–22.
6. Priollet P, Vayssairat M, Housset E. How to classify Raynaud's phenomenon. Am J Med 1987;83:494–8.
7. Harper FE, Maricq HR, Turner RE, Lidman RW, LeRoy EC. A prospective study of Raynaud phenomenon and early connective tissue disease. Am J Med 1982;72:883–8.
8. Fitzgerald O, Hess EV, O'Connor GT, Spencer-Green G. Prospective study of the evolution of Raynaud's phenomenon. Am J Med 1988;84:718–26.
9. Maricq HR. Widefield capillary microscopy. Arthritis Rheum 1981;24:1159–65.
10. Steen VD, Powell DL, Medsger TA. Clinical correlations and prognosis based on serum autoantibodies in patients with systemic sclerosis. Arthritis Rheum 1988;31:196–203.
11. Sarkozi J, Bookman AAM, Lee P, Keystone EC, Fritzler MJ. Significance of anticentromere antibody in idiopathic Raynaud's syndrome. Am J Med 1987;83:893–8.
12. Kallenberg CGM, Wouda AA, Hoet MH, Van Venrooij WJ. Development of connective tissue disease in patients presenting with Raynaud's phenomenon: a six-year follow-up with emphasis on the predictive value of antinuclear antibodies as detected by immunoblotting. Ann Rheum Dis 1988;47:634–41.
13. Page EH, Shear NH. Temperature-dependent skin disorders. J Am Acad Dermatol 1988;18:1003–18.
14. Belch JF. Raynaud's phenomenon. Curr Opin Rheumatol 1989;1:490–8.
15. Gerbracht DD, Steen VD, Ziegler GL, Medsger TA Jr, Rodnan GP. Evolution of primary Raynaud's phenomenon (Raynaud's disease) to connective tissue disease. Arthritis Rheum 1985;28:87–92.

SCROTAL PAIN

ANGELO S. PAOLA, S. ALI KHAN, and LOUISE FERRAROTTO

SYNONYMS: Orchialgia, Testicular Pain

BACKGROUND

Scrotal pain is a symptom that implies intrascrotal discomfort or pain. It may be described by the patient as discomfort in the inguinal area, also termed groin pain or inguinal pain.[1] The significance of scrotal pain cannot be overemphasized. In the acute stage, early and accurate diagnosis can prevent testicular loss. In chronic scrotal pain, diagnosis and treatment may allow the patient to return to gainful activity.[2] In this chapter, we will review the anatomy and innervation of the inguinal and scrotal areas. We will then discuss the differential diagnosis of scrotal pain and methods of diagnosis, and review in detail the more common causes of scrotal pain.

Anatomy

To formulate a differential diagnosis of scrotal pain, one must be familiar with the structures present in the inguinal canal and scrotum because pathology in these structures can lead to pain or discomfort. As shown in Figure 1, the inguinal canal is the oblique passage taken through the lower abdominal wall by the testis and cord (the round ligament in the female). The canal passes downward and medially from internal to external inguinal rings and lies parallel to and above the inguinal ligament. From the outside inward, its anterior relations are the skin, the superficial fascia, the external oblique aponeurosis covering its entire length, and the internal oblique covering its lateral one third. The conjoint tendon forms its posterior wall medially, and the transversalis fascia constitutes the border laterally. Its roof is formed by the arch of the lowest fibers of the internal oblique and transversus abdominis muscles. Inferiorly, the canal is bordered by the inguinal ligament.[3]

The inguinal canal transmits the spermatic cord and the ilioinguinal nerve in males and the round ligament and ilioinguinal nerve in females.[3]

As shown in Figure 2, the spermatic cord comprises three layers of fascia, three arteries, three nerves, and three additional structures. The three fascial layers are the external spermatic fascia (from the external oblique aponeurosis), the cremasteric fascia (from the internal oblique aponeurosis), and the internal spermatic fascia (from the transversalis fascia). The three arteries of the spermatic cord are the testicular artery (from the aorta), the cremasteric (from the inferior epigastric artery), and the deferential artery (from the inferior vesical). The three nerves include the nerve to the cremaster (from the genitofemoral nerve), the ilioinguinal nerve, and sympathetic fibers. Finally, the three additional structures in the spermatic cord are the pampiniform plexus of veins, the vas deferens, and lymphatics draining the testicle.[3]

The scrotum is a biseptate pouch containing the testis, epididymis, and lower part of the spermatic cord. Deep to the scrotal skin lies the subcutaneous areolar tissue, containing no fat in adults but containing the involuntary dartos muscle. Because the subcutaneous tissue is continuous with the superficial fascia of the abdominal wall and perineum, extravasation of urine or blood deep to this plane will gravitate into the scrotum. The structures normally present in the scrotum include those traversing the inguinal canal. Deep to the scrotal skin and subcutaneous tissue (dartos fascia) lies the external spermatic fascia over the cremasteric fascia and internal spermatic fascia from without inward. Anteriorly, the testis is covered by the parietal and visceral layers of the tunica vaginalis (the remnant of the processus vaginalis). Posterolaterally, the testis is bordered by the epididymis, composed of a head, body, and tail leading to the vas deferens. The epididymis is also covered by tunica vaginalis, except at its posterior margin. Also located in this area are the testicular and deferential arteries, nerves to these structures (discussed later in this chapter), testicular veins, and lymphatics.[3] At their upper

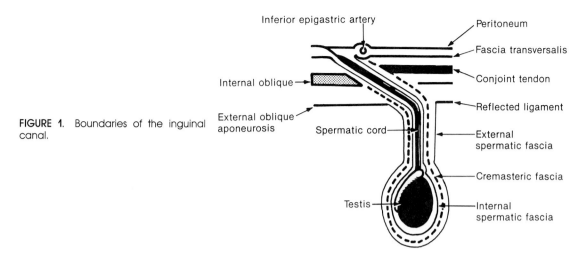

FIGURE 1. Boundaries of the inguinal canal.

poles, both the testis and epididymis contain appendages—small, stalked bodies that are remnants of embryologic structures. The appendix testis is the remnant of the paramesonephric duct, and the appendix epididymis is a remnant of the mesonephros. Their clinical importance is that they are both capable of undergoing torsion, thus simulating testicular torsion.[3]

The testis is covered by a white fibrous capsule, the tunica albuginea. Each testis is divided by septations into 200 to 300 lobules containing one to three seminiferous tubules that anastomose into a posterior plexus called the rete testis. These structures combine to form the efferent ductules leading to the epididymis.[3]

Nerve Supply

Pathology in an organ can be perceived as pain in the vicinity of that organ or at a distant site based on the nerve supply of that structure, that is, referred pain.[4] Therefore, in cases of scrotal pain, one must evaluate not only the structures present in the scrotum and inguinal canal but also the organs that share the same nerves supplying the scrotum and spermatic cord. Consequently, to establish a complete differential diagnosis in evaluation of scrotal pain, one must have a basic knowledge of the nerve supply of the structures in the scrotum and spermatic cord.

As shown in Table 1, most structures in the scrotum and spermatic cord receive their in-

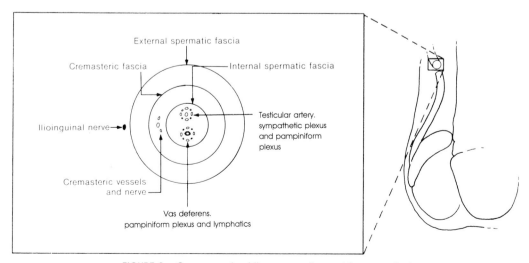

FIGURE 2. Components of the spermatic cord (cross section).

TABLE 1. Scrotal and Cord Structures and Their Nerve Supply

STRUCTURE	NERVE SUPPLY
Scrotal skin	Anterior one third of T_{12}-L_1 segments of spinal cord through ilioinguinal nerve and genital branch of genitofemoral nerve Posterior two thirds of S_2-S_3 segments of spinal cord through scrotal branches of pudendal nerve and perineal branch of posterior cutaneous nerve of thigh
Dartos muscle/fascia	Sympathetic fibers passing through genital branch of genitofemoral nerve
External spermatic fascia	T_{12}-L_1 segments of spinal cord through ilioinguinal nerve
Cremasteric muscle/fascia	L_1 segment of spinal cord through genital branch of genitofemoral nerve
Internal spermatic fascia	T_{12}-L_1 segments of spinal cord through ilioinguinal nerve
Tunica vaginalis testis	L_1 segment of spinal cord through genital branch of genitofemoral nerve
Tunica albuginea	T_9-T_{11} segments of spinal cord through sympathetic fibers that accompany the testicular artery
Seminiferous tubules	No sensory innervation
Epididymis/vas deferens	T_{11}-L_1 segments of spinal cord through sympathetic and afferent fibers that accompany the spermatic vessels

nervation from the T_{12}-L_1 segments of the spinal cord through the ilioinguinal and genitofemoral nerves. These structures include the scrotal skin (which also receives innervation from the scrotal branches of the pudendal nerve and the posterior cutaneous nerve of the thigh), dartos fascia, three layers of spermatic fascia, and the tunica vaginalis testis. Therefore, pathology in these structures, or any disease process causing distortion of the tissues in the area of these structures, will be sensed as pain or discomfort in the scrotum or inguinal area. The same is true of the epididymis and vas deferens, which receive their innervation from the T_{11}-L_1 segments of the spinal cord through sympathetic and afferent fibers that accompany the spermatic and deferential vessels.[5]

Because the testis develops in the posterior abdominal wall (at the level of the kidney) and then migrates down into the scrotum, it receives its nerve supply from the T_9-T_{11} segments of the spinal cord through sympathetic fibers passing through the renal and aortic plexuses, then accompanying the testicular artery into the scrotum. The similar origin of the testicular and renal nerves and the possibility of connections between the testicular and intestinal plexuses may readily explain common referred pain syndromes: that is, distension of the upper ureter (supplied by T_{10}) can cause "testicular pain," and pathology in the testicle may lead to flank pain, abdominal pain, or nausea.[5]

In summary, pain perceived by the patient as originating in the scrotum is usually caused by stimulation of the tunica vaginalis, epididymis, cord coverings, or scrotal skin, whereas pain arising from pathology in the testis itself (including the tunica albuginea) will be perceived in the distribution of T_{10} as abdominal pain or nausea. Furthermore, because of the shared innervation of the testes, kidney, and upper urinary tract, the referral pattern for pain of renal or upper ureteral origin includes the flank, anterior abdominal wall, and testicles. Therefore, pathology in the retroperitoneal area in the distribution of T_9-T_{11} must be considered in the differential diagnosis of scrotal pain.[4,5]

DIFFERENTIAL DIAGNOSIS

Review of the nerve supply of the inguinal and scrotal structures clearly shows that an evaluation of scrotal pain must include consideration of pathology in the retroperitoneum, inguinal canal, and scrotum in the differential diagnosis.

Table 2 shows numerous causes of scrotal pain that can be divided into three main categories: retroperitoneal, inguinal, and scrotal.

Some of the more common retroperitoneal causes of scrotal pain (referred pain) include: upper ureteral obstruction (calculus, ureteropelvic junction [UPJ] obstruction, clot), intervertebral disk protrusion, retroperitoneal fibrosis, neuropathy syndrome (i.e., acquired immune deficiency syndrome [AIDS], diabetes mellitus, herpes zoster), and synovial cysts of the T_{12}-L_1 segments. Rare retroperitoneal causes include: ruptured abdominal aortic aneurysm, common iliac artery aneurysm, perforated duodenal ulcer, perforation of stomach or colon into the retroperitoneal space, sacroiliitis, and extramedullary intraspinal tumors such as neurofibroma, meningioma, or ependymoma.[6]

TABLE 2.   Causes of Scrotal Pain

RETROPERITONEAL

Upper ureteral obstruction (stone, clot, tumor, uretero-
pelvic junction obstruction)*
Intervertebral disk producing orchitis
Neuropathy (diabetes, herpes, AIDS)
Sacral stenosis
Synovial cysts (T_{10}-L_1)
Ruptured abdominal aortic aneurysm
Iliac artery aneurysm
Perforated duodenal ulcer
Perforated stomach
Perforated colon (colonoscopy)
Perforated trachea
Sacroiliitis secondary to brucellosis
Hematoma secondary to percutaneous liver biopsy
Retroperitoneal fibrosis
Extramedullary spinal tumors (e.g., neurofibroma,
meningioma, ependymoma)

INGUINAL

Incarcerated inguinal hernias
Perforated appendix in an inguinal hernia
Entrapment syndrome after herniorrhaphy
Epilepsy (cremaster spasm)
Hematoma secondary to trauma
Inguinoscrotal mass (e.g., tumor in testis)
Neuropathy (diabetes, herpes, AIDS)

SCROTAL

Intratesticular
    Testicular tumor
    Testicular trauma (e.g., gunshot wound, blunt trauma)
    Orchitis (viral mumps, EBV, coxsackie B, rubella,
    bacterial)
    Constrictive albuginitis
Extratesticular
    Torsion (spermatic cord, testicular appendages)
    Epididymitis

Inguinal hernia with scrotal extension
Hydrocele (infected or uninfected; meconium hydro-
cele)
Varicocele
Spermatic granuloma
Postvasectomy syndrome secondary to epididymal
congestion, nerve entrapment, or spermatic granu-
loma
Trauma
Foreign body
Fournier's gangrene
Tumors of cord or scrotal skin (benign or malignant)
Neuropathy (diabetes, herpes, AIDS)
Seminal congestion (e.g., postvasectomy, masturba-
tion interruptus)
Epilepsy (secondary to cremaster spasm)
Fat necrosis of scrotum (scrotal panniculitis)
Vasculitis (e.g., Henoch-Schönlein purpura, SLE)
Idiopathic scrotal edema
Torsion of vermiform appendix in a scrotal hernia
Abdominal catheter migration into scrotum (ventri-
cula-peritoneal shunt, Tenckhoff)
Granulomatous disease (e.g., talc granuloma, tubercu-
losis)
Leukemic infiltration of testis or cord
Scrotal tumors (e.g., basal cell carcinoma, squamous
cell carcinoma, melanoma, rhabdomyosarcoma)
Thrombosis of pampiniform plexus
Infectious disease (e.g., syphilis, tuberculosis, filaria-
sis, brucellosis, falciparum malaria)
Dracunculosis, elephantiasis, tick bite, salmonella,
schistosomiasis, black widow spider, brown recluse
spider, funiculitis
Torsion of cavernous lymphangioma
Ectopic tissue (e.g., adrenal tissue, splenic tissue)

DRUGS

Desipramine, Ionidamine, Mazindol, Vasopressin

Inguinal causes of scrotal pain include: incarcerated inguinal hernias, seminal vesiculitis, cremasteric spasm, entrapment syndrome secondary to herniorrhaphy, and the rarer perforated appendix in an inguinal hernia or nephroblastoma in an ovotestis.[7]

Pain from scrotal pathology can have either intratesticular or extratesticular causes. Because of the pattern of testicular nerve supply, intratesticular pathology leads to discomfort or pain in the flank or abdomen with occasional nausea secondary to stimulation of nerves in the distribution of T_9-T_{11}. However, if the pathologic process involves the tunica vaginalis testis or epididymis, the discomfort will also be perceived to originate in the scrotum. The more common intratesticular causes of scrotal pain include: trauma, tumor, orchitis (viral or bacterial), and constrictive albuginitis. Extratesticular scrotal pain has been noted or associated with epididymitis, torsion of the spermatic cord, hydrocele, varicocele, torsion of testicular appendages, viral syndrome (i.e., mumps, Epstein-Barr virus [EBV]), bacterial infection (such as tuberculosis), hematoma, foreign bodies, fat necrosis, epilepsy, vasculitis syndromes, leukemic infiltration, trauma, postvasectomy pain (secondary to congestion, spermatic granuloma, or nerve entrapment), scrotal edema, ectopic splenic or adrenal tissue, and scrotal tumors (i.e., basal cell carcinoma, squamous cell carcinoma, melanoma, or rhabdomyosarcoma).[6,8]

Several drugs have also been reported to cause scrotal pain secondary to either nervous stimulation or vasoconstriction with resultant ischemia. These drugs include desipramine, lonidamine (a cancer chemotherapeutic agent), mazindol (used in appetite suppression), and vasopressin.

HISTORY

As with all disease processes, an accurate diagnosis of scrotal pain depends on a thorough history, a focused physical examination, and several laboratory and imaging studies.

Aspects in the patient's history that may be helpful in localizing the cause of scrotal pain include age, associated symptoms, and past medical history.

Torsion of the spermatic cord or testicular appendages is uncommon after the teen years. Unfortunately, epididymitis is common in the preadolescent and adolescent age groups. Thrombosis of the spermatic vein is most common in childhood, and Henoch-Schönlein purpura is most common between the ages of four and seven. Fat necrosis of the scrotum tends to occur in overweight prepubertal boys after cold exposure or minor trauma before puberty. Viral orchitis, on the other hand, is exceedingly rare before puberty. Testicular tumors tend to occur between the ages of 18 and 40 years. Finally, aneurysms, peptic ulcer disease, and other causes of scrotal pain tend to occur in adults.

Irritative voiding symptoms in patients with testicular pain and swelling occur more frequently in epididymitis than in torsion. Hematuria in a patient with scrotal pain may be an indication of referred pain secondary to calculi or tumor in the upper urinary tract. Flank or back pain may also indicate a retroperitoneal cause of pain.

Past medical history can provide valuable clues in the evaluation of scrotal pain. History of abdominal aortic aneurysm, peptic ulcer disease, recent colonoscopy, vasculitic diseases (i.e., systemic lupus erythematosus [SLE], rheumatoid arthritis, Henoch-Schönlein purpura), AIDS, diabetes mellitus, epilepsy, recent trauma, renal calculi, and use of certain drugs all may cause scrotal pain. Prior herniorrhaphy or vasectomy can also be responsible for scrotal pain through nerve entrapment or seminal congestion. A history of recent urethral instrumentation in a patient with new onset of scrotal pain and swelling is suspect for epididymitis. Finally, although it must be a diagnosis of exclusion, a psychosomatic etiology must be considered in patients with no abnormal physical findings and a history of psychiatric disorders or drug seeking.

PHYSICAL EXAMINATION

The physical examination in patients with scrotal pain may help localize the source because pain referred from the retroperitoneal and inguinal areas usually elicits no local tenderness—that is, usually no obvious scrotal pathology is immediately obvious. On the other hand, local causes of scrotal pain usually result in tenderness to palpation or other signs of local irritation. Intratesticular disease can also be referred to the abdomen, however, resulting in abdominal pain and nausea and may even be confused with acute appendicitis. Palpation of the kidneys must be part of every abdominal examination. If flank pain is present, costovertebral angle tenderness should be elicited. In patients suspected to have varicocoel or hernia, physical examination of the male genitalia should be performed with the patient in both the supine and standing positions. Inspection and palpation will distinguish most disorders of the male external genitalia. The prepuce should be retracted to reveal the coronal sulcus and the frenulum. Any lesions should be palpated for induration and tenderness. The physician should then palpate the length of the shaft from the penoscrotal junction to the meatus, feeling for nodules and plaques. Finally, the glans should be compressed anteroposteriorly between the thumb and forefinger to open and inspect the external meatus. Any discharge should be examined under a microscope. Cultures should be performed for *Neisseria gonorrhoeae* and *Chlamydia trachomatis*.[9]

The scrotum and its contents are examined by inspection, palpation, and transillumination. Auscultation of the scrotum may yield peristaltic sounds from a loop of herniated gut. Using the thumb and forefinger of both hands to hold the structure of interest, the physician should examine in sequential order: (1) the testis, (2) tunica vaginalis, (3) epididymis, (4) vas deferens and spermatic cord, (5) inguinal area, and (6) inguinal lymph nodes.[9] Some physical findings that may prove useful in evaluation of scrotal pain are: the cremasteric reflex, Prehn's sign, the blue scrotum sign of Bryant, and pneumoscrotum (air in the scrotum).

The cremasteric reflex (retraction of the scrotum and spermatic cord with stimulation of the ipsilateral thigh area), mediated by the genitofemoral nerve, has been reported to be present in 100 per cent of patients with proven epididymo-orchitis and to be absent in approximately 97 per cent of patients with testicular torsion.[10] In addition, early in torsion, the epididymis may be felt in the anterior position, although swelling may later render the distinction between testis and epididymis impossible. Prehn's sign (relief of pain with gentle elevation of the scrotum) tends to be present in cases of epididymo-orchitis and to be absent in cases of torsion of the spermatic cord.

The sign of Bryant (bluish discoloration of the scrotum) has been reported in cases of ruptured abdominal aortic or common iliac artery aneurysms.[11] Pneumoscrotum has been noted with perforation of the trachea, stomach, duodenum, or colon with resultant air dissecting beneath fascial planes into the scrotum.[12] Finally, any scrotal lesions must raise the possibility of an infectious etiology of the pain (i.e., herpes, tick bites, filariasis, salmonella abscess, schistosomiasis, brucellosis). Of course, geographic location is also an important consideration in these conditions; diseases such as dracunculosis, filariasis, bilharziasis, malaria, and actinomycosis are more common in tropical areas.

DIAGNOSTIC STUDIES

Laboratory

Few laboratory studies can add information in evaluation of scrotal pain. White blood cell count tends to be nonspecific because it may be elevated in both torsion and epididymitis and in many other conditions that cause scrotal pain. Pyuria and bacteriuria evidenced by urinalysis are more consistent with epididymitis if local inflammation is present. Hematuria may indicate an upper tract lesion with referred pain, that is, renal or ureteral calculus. If a testicular tumor is suspected, serum tumor markers, such as the beta subunit of human chorionic gonadotropin (β-HCG) or alpha-fetoprotein, should be obtained. Fasting serum glucose levels can be used to rule out suspected diabetic neuropathy.

Radiologic

Diagnostic tests that may be helpful include computed tomography (CT) scanning, magnetic resonance imaging (MRI), ultrasonography, and radioisotopic scans. In cases with a suspected retroperitoneal etiology, CT scan and MRI are the preferable diagnostic procedures; however, ultrasonic evaluation can be of benefit, such as in cases of hydronephrosis or renal calculi. If UPJ obstruction is suspected, the furosemide (Lasix) renal scan is the most appropriate for diagnosis. Inguinal pathology can best be visualized by CT scan. Scrotal disorders are best evaluated by either ultrasonography or radioisotope scrotal scans, especially if the scans are obtained early in the course of disease.[13]

In cases of acute scrotal pain, the resultant findings must be interpreted with respect to the information obtained in the clinical context of history and physical examination. If the diagnosis is still unclear, clinical judgment must be used to determine whether diagnostic surgical exploration is necessary. When torsion cannot be ruled out with certainty, scrotal exploration should be performed to attempt testicular salvage.

COMMON CAUSES OF SCROTAL PAIN

The causes of scrotal pain are many and varied. An in-depth review of the more common causes follows (Fig. 3).

Testicular Torsion

In a patient with a painful scrotal mass, the diagnosis that must be made promptly is testicular torsion, because infarction (secondary to loss of testicular blood supply) will usually occur unless the patient is treated within four to six hours. Torsion is usually a prepubertal disorder in which the testis rotates on its long axis within the tunica vaginalis. The initiating factor has been suggested to be spasm of the cremaster muscle, causing the patient's testis to rotate away from the midline, resulting in vascular compromise of the testis.

The patient with testicular torsion generally has severe unilateral orchialgia, scrotal skin erythema, nausea, lower abdominal discomfort, or pain. Physical examination shows a swollen, tender testicle. Lifting the testicle above the symphysis pubis may increase the pain (in contrast to the pain, this manuever provides relief in inflammatory conditions—Prehn's sign). Rabinowitz[10] reported that the cremasteric reflex was present in 100 per cent of patients with proven epididymitis and absent in approximately 97 per cent of patients with torsion. The examination may be quickly diagnostic if the epididymis can be felt in the anterior position; swelling later may render the distinction between testis and epididymis impossible. In such circumstances, the physician must resort to either imaging procedures or surgical exploration. Nuclear testicular scanning, with ^{99}Tc-pertechnetate as the tracer, should be immediately performed. A rotated testis may exhibit an area of decreased

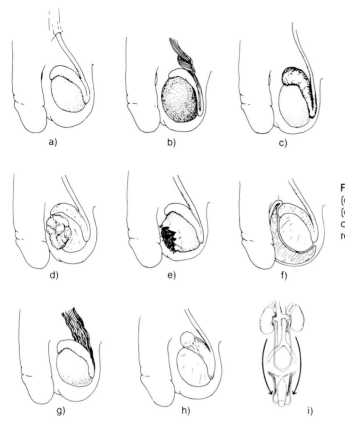

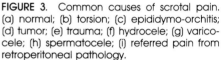

FIGURE 3. Common causes of scrotal pain. (a) normal; (b) torsion; (c) epididymo-orchitis; (d) tumor; (e) trauma; (f) hydrocele; (g) varicocele; (h) spermatocele; (i) referred pain from retroperitoneal pathology.

perfusion, whereas an inflamed testicle (i.e., epididymitis) may demonstrate increased uptake secondary to the increased capillary permeability and the hyperemia that accompanies the inflammatory process. The accuracy of the scan has been reported to vary between 86 and 100 per cent. The scan must be interpreted in terms of the clinical presentation, however, because an area of decreased uptake may represent not only torsion but also a scrotal wall or testicular hematoma, an abscess, hydrocele, or a necrotic tumor. Testicular tumors that are not necrotic also may demonstrate slightly increased perfusion.[14] Doppler flow studies have been shown to be of little additional benefit in the diagnosis of testicular torsion.[15]

Torsion of Testicular and Epididymal Appendages

The appendix testis and the appendix epididymis may undergo torsion, which leads to inflammation followed by ischemic necrosis. This condition is rare after the teen years. It is characterized by onset of testicular pain with swelling of the testicle and scrotum. Early in the condition, a small, tender lump may be felt at the upper aspect of the testis or epididymis. Occasionally, this lump will appear blue when the skin is held taut over the mass (blue dot sign). Testicular scan will tend to be negative for torsion of the cord early in the course of appendicular torsion. However, because examination usually occurs when the entire testicle and scrotum are swollen and tender, differentiating between this condition and torsion of the spermatic cord is often difficult. In such patients, immediate surgical exploration is indicated. If, however, physical examination results in an unequivocal diagnosis of torsion of an appendage, conservative management will suffice; pain and swelling usually subside in five to seven days (see p. 595 of reference).[13]

Epididymitis

Acute epididymitis is a cellulitis of the epididymis. The inflammation usually begins in the vas deferens. Epididymitis generally occurs in the setting of pre-existing prostatitis, after prostatectomy, or after urethral catheterization. It is also believed to be caused by retrograde spread of organisms down the vas deferens from the urethra. The patient usually has scrotal pain and swelling, dysuria, and usually, fever (as high as 104° F). Physical examination shows an enlarged, tender epididymis, which if examined early may be discrete from the testis. Later, with testicular swelling, the two may become a single mass. The inflammatory process may even extend along the spermatic cord into the inguinal area. The cremasteric reflex is a valuable clinical tool in evaluation of the acute scrotum because its presence tends to rule out testicular torsion and its absence increases the suspicion of torsion. Laboratory tests may show leukocytosis, which is nonspecific, and urinalysis may show pyuria, which is usually absent in torsion. Nuclear scanning may be helpful in distinguishing epididymitis from torsion early in the course of the inflammatory process.

Orchitis

Acute orchitis, in contrast to epididymitis, is an isolated inflammation of the testicle itself. Unlike torsion, orchitis occurs mostly in postpubertal males. Mumps is the most common cause of orchitis, although the syndrome may be caused by other organisms, including echovirus, lymphocytic choriomeningitis virus, arbovirus, coxsackie B virus, EBV, rubella virus, and several bacteria. The patient has pain and swelling of the testis and scrotum because the peritesticular structures are usually involved in the inflammatory process. Discomfort will also usually be noted in the inguinal region and lower abdominal area, with nausea and possibly vomiting. Mumps-related orchitis usually develops several days after the appearance of parotitis. Patients have no urinary tract complaints. There may be high fever, and a reactive hydrocele may develop. In two thirds of patients, the process is unilateral, whereas in the remaining one third the orchitis is bilateral. Laboratory examination may show leukocytosis with increased lymphocyte count, but the urinalysis is usually normal.

In 24 to 30 per cent of patients, the involved testis will be unable to function as a result of the inflammatory process. Indeed, viral orchitis is the most common cause of acquired testicular failure in the adult. Testicular atrophy is usually noted about one to two months after the inflammatory process resolves.[14]

Testicular Tumors

Approximately 40 per cent of testicular tumors initially cause scrotal pain, which may be related to internal hemorrhage with sudden distension of the tunica albuginea and involvement of peritesticular structures. The patient's history and physical examination should make it possible to distinguish this etiology from the other causes of orchialgia. In doubtful cases, testicular ultrasound and tumor markers may be helpful. If a testicular tumor cannot be ruled out, surgical exploration is indicated.

Trauma

Testicular trauma is most often confused with acute epididymitis; it is best differentiated on the basis of the history and by the absence of pyuria. Because exploration is performed in most cases of penetrating trauma, blunt trauma to the scrotum usually presents the most common diagnostic problems. Blunt scrotal trauma may result in hematoma of the scrotal layers, hematocele, rupture of the tunica albuginea, and/or strictly intratesticular hematoma. Because rupture of the tunica albuginea and large hematoceles are the only conditions that require surgical exploration, whereas other conditions are treated conservatively, distinction among the aforementioned types of injuries is important. Ultrasound is a valuable tool. Few testicular tumors are discovered incidentally after minor scrotal trauma in which ultrasound shows minor intratesticular hematomas. Therefore, patients with a history of minor scrotal trauma and an intratesticular hematoma on ultrasonic evaluation should undergo close follow-up; if the sonographic appearance does not change after three to four weeks, further evaluation should be considered (e.g., tumor markers, CT scan of abdomen).[16]

Inguinal Hernia

An inguinal hernia usually appears as a bulge in the inguinal region that may extend into the scrotum. It may be intermittent and is usually painless. It may cause intermittent scrotal pain either by impinging on the nerve supply of the scrotal structures or by the inflammatory process that results when incarceration occurs. In the former situation, the patient will usually complain of a dull ache or pain in the scrotum that is exacerbated with long periods of standing or straining and that resolves with supination. Physical examination elicits no associated symptoms or significant findings. Incarceration of an inguinal hernia usually presents either a painful, tender inguinal or scrotal swelling or both. Nausea, vomiting, and abdominal distension may be present. The inflammatory process may result in vascular compromise of the ipsilateral testicle and scrotal contents, causing additional scrotal pain. In this instance, late testicular atrophy will be observed. If an inguinal hernia cannot be reduced manually, immediate surgical repair is indicated since a high risk of strangulation of the inguinal hernia is associated with incarceration. In patients with a history of inguinal hernia repair and ipsilateral scrotal pain since surgery, entrapment of the ilioinguinal nerve in the surgical repair should be considered as a possible etiology of the pain.

Hydrocele

A hydrocele is an accumulation of serous fluid in the cavity of the tunica vaginalis, usually beginning as a nontender scrotal mass. It may sometimes cause a dull ache in the scrotum as a result of distension of the tunica vaginalis and stimulation of the nerves supplying this area. This may also occur secondary to inflammation associated with an infected hydrocele. Examination usually shows a pear-shaped nontender mass that transilluminates and is located anterior to the testis and epididymis, which it sometimes obscures. Cremasteric hypertrophy may also occur, owing to the increased weight of the scrotal contents. Hydroceles may be classified as either primary (idiopathic) or secondary. The most common causes of secondary hydroceles are epididymitis, mumps orchitis, trauma, and tuberculosis. Acute pain in the existing hydrocele can be caused by infection, trauma, hemorrhage, or spasm of the dartos muscle.

Ten per cent of testicular tumors may be present with an acute secondary hydrocele. In patients with a patent processus vaginalis, the mass may be intermittent, which changes with position. This condition should be distinguished from indirect inguinal hernia, which may also be positional. In the latter case, however, the swelling does not transilluminate, usually gives an impulse on coughing, and is not limited above. In cases of inguinal hernia, bowel sounds sometimes can be heard over the scrotum. Ultrasound may be used to confirm the diagnosis and to define the inguinal extent of the hydrocele.

Hematocele

A hematocele is a collection of blood in the tunica vaginalis. The bleeding usually results from trauma or underlying malignant disease. Hematoceles have also been associated with torsion of the testis, hemorrhagic diseases, and aberrant splenic tissue. In the acute phase, the mass has the same physical signs as a hydrocele except that it is not translucent and is usually tender. Ultrasound may be used to distinguish simple hematocele from ruptured tunica albuginea or testicular tumor early on. When the blood clots and the mass hardens, however, a chronic hematocele is indistinguishable from a syphilitic gumma or testicular tumor, even with ultrasound.

Varicocele

Varicocele is characterized by dilatation of the pampiniform plexus of veins above the testis that is believed to be caused by stasis and incompetence of valves in the internal spermatic vein. Varicocele commonly occurs on the left side and, if symptomatic, usually results in vague scrotal heaviness, ache, or discomfort, particularly after physical exercise. Pain is believed to be secondary to compression of the scrotal tissues by the dilated vessels as well as spasm of hypertrophied muscle cremasteric fibers due to increased weight of scrotal contents. Varicoceles rarely occur in younger children and usually are first noted at age 10 years and with increasing incidence through puberty. Their clinical importance is twofold. First, sudden onset of varicocele in older men should raise the suspicion of renal cell carcinoma with renal vein occlusion by tumor thrombus. Second, varicoceles have been associated with infertility, chronic scrotal pain, or both. Physical examination must be performed with the patient standing to show the dilated vessels, which typically feel like a "bag of worms," especially when the patient performs the Valsalva maneuver. In a patient with chronic scrotal pain without obvious scrotal abnormality, a scrotal ultrasound and/or Doppler examination may be useful in determining whether a varicocele exists.[17]

Henoch-Schönlein Purpura

Henoch-Schönlein purpura is the most common systemic vasculitis of childhood, typically occurring between the ages of four and seven years, and is more common in boys. It is characterized by an acute inflammatory process of unknown etiology that produces a vasculitis of the capillaries, arterioles, and venules. This process may involve the scrotum or testicles in up to one third of all patients.

A maculopapular rash characteristically appears first, tending to be more prominent over the lower extremities and buttocks usually before the genitals become involved. Acute scrotal swelling, pain, and tenderness may be noted with the rash. If the vasculitis involves the testis, epididymis, or cord structures, and if sufficient swelling develops, differentiation from torsion can be difficult. In such patients, a radioisotope scrotal scan demonstrating hyperemia is the most accurate diagnostic test to rule out torsion.[17]

Neuropathy

As indicated in Table 2, several conditions result in scrotal pain owing to neuropathy involving the innervation of the scrotal structures. These include diabetes mellitus, herpes (genital, zoster, or both), and AIDS. The diagnosis is usually one of exclusion in a patient with a history of these conditions and no obvious scrotal pathology shown by physical examination.

Postvasectomy Syndrome

Patients who have undergone vasectomy may have scrotal pain that fails to resolve after the surgical wounds have healed. The etiology of the pain includes nerve entrapment during surgery, spermatic granuloma, and epididymal congestion due to continued sperm production. Such patients initially may have sharp pain or a dull ache in the scrotum. Except in spermatic granuloma, which may clinically present as a tender scrotal mass separate from the testicle, the physical examination usually shows no abnormality. Scrotal ultrasound may reveal spermatic granuloma. Surgical removal may be necessary in cases of spermatic granuloma, whereas pain clinic evaluation or microsurgical denervation of the spermatic cord may be required for nerve entrapment or epididymal congestion.[2,18]

Referred Pain

Stimulation of nerves that also send branches to the testis (i.e., in the distribution of T_9-T_{11}) may also result in pain or discomfort perceived by the patient to arise in the scrotum or testicle. Some of the conditions that have been reported to result in pain referred to the scrotum include: upper ureteral obstruction from calculus, clot, tumor, or UPJ obstruction; intervertebral disk protrusion; neuropathy; ruptured abdominal aortic aneurysm; perforation of the gastrointestinal tract into the retroperitoneal space; retroperitoneal fibrosis; and extramedullary spinal tumors (see Table 2).

In the case of upper ureteral obstruction resulting from stone, clot, or tumor, the patient usually complains of renal colic, with pain radiating to the ipsilateral groin or scrotum. Nausea or vomiting may also be present. A prior history of renal calculus may be suggestive. Physical examination is usually nonspecific. Urinalysis will typically reveal hematuria. Intravenous pyelogram and ultrasound will usually be diagnostic.

After diuresis, scrotal pain caused by UPJ obstruction will usually worsen because of increased fluid intake. Physical examination is nondiagnostic, as is urinalysis. If UPJ obstruction is suspected, the preferred diagnostic procedure is the lasix renal scan.

Intervertebral disk protrusion as the cause of scrotal pain may be suggested by a history of low back pain and radiation of pain down the posterior aspect of the thigh. Physical examination may elicit pain on straight leg raising or evidence of weakness in the lower extremities. CT scan, myelogram, or MRI may aid in diagnosis.

Rupture of abdominal aortic aneurysm can result in scrotal pain and may be suggested by a history of abdominal aortic aneurysm in patients with acute onset of abdominal and scrotal pain. Physical examination may show hypotension and shock as well as abdominal distension and bluish discoloration of the scrotum (blue scrotal sign of Bryant).[11] The pressure of an aneurysm on peripheral nerves may also be responsible for scrotal pain, however, without evidence of intrascrotal pathology.

Finally, in patients with a history of new onset of scrotal pain and the finding of pneumoscrotum, the differential diagnosis includes perforated duodenal ulcer, perforation of the stomach, perforation of the colon into the retroperitoneum, and perforation of the trachea. In most cases of suspected retroperitoneal etiology of scrotal pain, CT scan or ultrasound usually aids in the diagnostic evaluation.

MANAGING SCROTAL PAIN

A basic knowledge of the anatomy and nerve supply of the inguinal and scrotal areas is necessary to guide physicians in evaluating scrotal pain. Based on the history, physical examination, laboratory, and imaging studies, the possible etiologies should be divided into retroperitoneal, inguinal, or scrotal origins. Using this classification, and with the knowledge of the more common causes of scrotal pain, the physician may or may not decide to perform other diagnostic radiologic procedures. Finally, when no organic cause is present, the scrotal pain is usually called chronic orchialgia and may respond to pain clinic treatment or microsurgical denervation of the spermatic cord.

REFERENCES

1. Morgan RJ, Parry JR. Scrotal pain. Postgrad Med J 1986;63:521–3.
2. Devine CJ, Schellhammer PF. The use of microsurgical denervation of the spermatic cord for orchialgia. Trans Am Assoc of Genitourin Surg 1979;70:149–51.
3. Ellis H. Clinical anatomy. 6th ed. Blackwell Scientific Publications, 1977:65–7, 126–8.
4. Goldberg SD, Witchell SJ. Right testicular pain: unusual presentation of obstruction of the ureteropelvic junction. Canadian J Surg 1988;31:246–7.
5. Johnson AD. The testis, Vol I. New York: Academic Press, 1970:47–97.
6. Ellis H. Testicular pain. In: French's index of differential diagnosis. 12th ed. Bristol, England: Wright Publishing, 1985:833–9.
7. Wantz GE. Complications of inguinal hernia repair. Surg Clin North Am 1984;64:287–98.
8. Selikowitz SM, Schned AR. A late post-vasectomy syndrome. J Urol 1985;134:494–7.
9. DeGowin EL, DeGowin RL. Bedside diagnostic examination. 4th ed. New York: Macmillan Publishing, 1981:591–615.
10. Rabinowitz R. The importance of the cremasteric reflex in acute scrotal swellings in children. J Urol 1984;132:89–90.
11. Ratzan RM, Donaldson MC, Foster JH, Walzak MP. The blue scrotum sign of Bryant: a diagnostic clue to ruptured abdominal aortic aneurysm. J Emerg Med 1987;5(4):323–9.
12. Redman JF, Pahls WL. Pneumoscrotum following tracheal intubation. J Urol 1985;133(June):1056–7.
13. Tanagho EA, McAninch JW. General urology. 12th ed. Norwalk, Connecticut: Appleton and Lange, 1988:57–109.
14. Paola AS, Khan SA. Clinical evaluation of scrotal masses: an overview. Hosp Pract 1989;24(Mar.):255–64.
15. Haynes BE. Doppler ultrasound failure in testicular torsion. Ann Emerg Med 1984;13:1103–7.
16. Kratzik CH, Hainz A, Donner G. Has ultrasound influenced the therapy concept of blunt scrotal trauma? J Urol 1989;142;1243–5.
17. McCollough DL. Difficult diagnoses in urology. Churchill Livingstone, 1988:23–35.
18. McCormick M, Lapoint S. Physiologic consequences and complications of vasectomy. Can Med Assoc J 1988;138:223–5.

SECONDARY HYPERTENSION

RICHARD M. SLATAPER and GEORGE L. BAKRIS

SYNONYMS: Nonessential Hypertension, Nonprimary Hypertension

BACKGROUND

Hypertension in adults is defined as an arterial pressure of greater than 140/90 mm Hg, whereas in persons under 18 years of age, the arterial pressure must be higher than the 95th percentile for that age; both groups require three separate measurements before diagnostic confirmation.[1,2] Approximately 20 per cent of adults and 3 per cent of children, or 60 million persons, in the United States have hypertension.[1,2] Secondary hypertension, however, only accounts for about 5 to 10 per cent of these cases. Identifying patients with secondary hypertension facilitates treatment, can reduce long-term medical costs, and selects patients (1 to 2 per cent of all cases) for whom surgery may effect a cure. Table 1 summarizes the secondary causes of hypertension.

This chapter discusses some of the more common forms of secondary hypertension with emphasis on their identification by history, physical examination, and diagnostic evaluation. It also reviews the frequency of various physical findings as well as laboratory parameters for specific causes of secondary hypertension.

HISTORY

The History of the Present Illness

The medical history should include the following information: date when hypertension was first noted; associated symptoms such as headache, blurred vision, and abdominal pain; and neurologic symptoms such as loss of sensation or motor function in any of the extremities, nervousness, and so on. Other findings that may prompt thoughts of secondary hypertension include muscle weakness or cramping. Race and sex should also be noted, since secondary causes of hypertension occur with slightly greater frequency in white females and are uncommon in blacks, with the exception of renal vascular causes.[3,4] Furthermore, a review of current medication consumption (e.g., prostaglandin antagonists such as aspirin or nonsteroidal anti-inflammatory agents, diet preparations such as phenylpropanolamine, decongestants such as phenylephrine, or birth control pills) as well as any new onset or increase of previous alcohol consumption should be sought. Questions associated with stress factors in a person's life, whether work or family related, must be asked. These factors may result in a disruption of eating and sleeping patterns as well as precipitate an increase in alcohol and/or drug (amphetamines, cocaine, caffeine, tobacco, etc.) consumption, all of which are known to increase arterial pressure.[3,4,5,6,7,8]

Family History

A family history of essential hypertension does not eliminate the possibility of secondary hypertension. Renal artery stenosis secondary to fibromuscular dysplasia, for example, is more common in middle-aged women (30 to 50 years) and generally seen in those with a family history of fibromuscular dysplasia.[9] Multiple endocrine adenomatosis (MEA) syndromes, which are genetic conditions associated with a number of simultaneous hormonal abnormalities, are associated with pheochromocytoma and hyperparathyroidism, both of which are known to increase blood pressure.[10] Lastly, polycystic kidney disease is a genetic disorder that has hypertension as an initial manifestation.[11] A number of other genetic diseases associated with hypertension are summarized in Table 2.

TABLE 1. Causes of Secondary Forms of Hypertension*

SYSTOLIC AND DIASTOLIC HYPERTENSION	APPROXIMATE INCIDENCE (%)
More common	
Renal vascular disease	5–10
Estrogen-induced hypertension	3–5
Primary aldosteronism	2–4
Pheochromocytoma	<1
Drug-induced (corticosteroids, non-steroidal anti-inflammatory agents, sympathomimetics, cocaine, etc.)	<1
Less common causes	
Renal parenchymal disease	<0.5
Renin secreting tumors	<0.5
Syndromes of mineralocorticoid excess	
Overproduction of 11-deoxycorti-costerone,† 18-hydroxy DOC, and other mineralocorticoids without accompanying defects in steroid synthesis	<0.5
Congenital adrenal hyperplasia	<0.5
Black licorice ingestion (glycyrrhizic acid)	<0.5
Coarctation of the aorta	<0.5
Cushing's syndrome	<0.5
Hyperparathyroidism	<0.5
Acromegaly	<0.5

* No definitive studies exist assessing the incidence of these secondary forms of hypertension in unselected populations. Thus, these data are based on small, selected samples and may be artificially skewed than suspected.
† DOC = deoxycorticosterone.

Focused Queries

1. *Is there a previous history of intra-abdominal or peripheral vascular surgeries for aneurysms or claudication symptoms?*

2. *Does the patient have an abrupt onset of headaches, palpitations, or diaphoresis?* Pheochromocytoma may present with this clinical picture; however, it is usual to have none or only one of these symptoms on initial presentation.[12]

TABLE 2. Genetic Conditions Commonly Associated with Hypertension

Polycystic kidney disease
Fibromuscular dysplasia
Neurofibromatosis
Multiple endocrine adenomatosis (MEA)
Tuberous sclerosis
Wilms' tumor
Fabry's disease (angiokeratoma corporis diffusum)
Renal tubular acidosis with nephrocalcinosis
Congenital adrenal hyperplasia
Pseudoxanthoma elasticum
Acute intermittent porphyria
Familial dysautonomia

3. *Is there a history of an abrupt blood pressure reduction and/or renal failure secondary to angiotensin converting enzyme inhibitors?* If so, this should prompt the thought of renal artery stenosis, since this scenario has been described in patients with this disorder.[13]

4. *Has there been excessive weight gain and increased hair growth over the past few months?* This would prompt the thought of an adrenal cortical tumor.[12]

5. *Is there a family history of polycystic kidney disease, renal failure, or cancer associated with hypertension that required surgery?* Polycystic kidney disease is associated with hypertension and is frequently the earliest associated finding.[11]

6. *Has there been a recent increase or difficulty in controlling previously stable arterial pressure?* Previously well-controlled essential hypertension that now requires maximum doses of three and four medications indicates a secondary form of hypertension, usually renal artery stenosis.[13]

PHYSICAL EXAMINATION

It is imperative that the blood pressure be taken correctly. Cuff size, patient position, and nonstandard technique are all common sources of error.[7,14] The following techniques must be followed for correct blood pressure recording: (1) In order to transmit the pressure evenly to the brachial artery, the cuff width must be two thirds the length between the patient's shoulder and elbow (short, narrow, or loose cuffs lead to falsely elevated readings); (2) the patient's arm should be passively supported, with the cuff at the level of the heart (if the patient supports his or her own arm, the sustained muscular contraction may raise the diastolic pressure as much as 10 per cent; a 13.6-cm difference between arterial cuff level and cardiac level produces a blood pressure error of 10 mm); (3) the cuff should be inflated to about 30 mm Hg above the pressure at which the palpable brachial artery pulse disappears.[7,14] The first Korotkoff sound heard while the cuff pressure is gradually decreasing signals the systolic pressure. If an auscultatory gap is heard, this should be noted to prevent intraobserver discrepancy. As the cuff continues to deflate, the Korotkoff sounds become muffled, and this is generally considered to be the diastolic pressure. In some patients, the muffling point and the disappearance point are farther apart. Occasionally, as in aortic regurgitation, the sounds never disappear. These variations should also be noted. Both blood pressures and pulse measurements should be assessed in both bare arms in the standing and supine positions. An orthostatic drop (defined as greater than a 20-mm drop in systolic pressure or 10-mm drop in diastolic pressure) is suggestive of pheochromocytoma.[12] This drop may normally be present, however, in the elderly population or patients with either diabetes or dehydration. Decreased or absent femoral pulses and/or popliteal blood pressures signify coarctation of the aorta or severe atherosclerosis, which may be associated with a renal arterial lesion.[4,7,9] Continuous periumbilical, abdominal bruit radiating to either flank is consistent with renal artery stenosis.[9] Bilaterally enlarged or palpable kidneys, either on physical examination or by diagnostic procedure, are suggestive of polycystic kidney disease.[11] The funduscopic examination is not useful for distinguishing patients with secondary causes of hypertension.[4,7] Mucosal neurofibromas on the skin are associated either with the diagnosis of von Recklinghausen's disease or with an MEA III syndrome.[10,12] The presence of embolic phenomena, best seen in the area of the toes or lower extremities, represents cholesterol emboli and usually signifies peripheral vascular disease and a higher-than-usual incidence of renal artery stenosis.[15] Abdominal striae, moon facies, and truncal obesity are signs that accompany Cushing's syndrome, whereas prognathism and facial coarsening are seen in acromegaly, both of which are associated with hypertension.[8,16]

DIAGNOSTIC STUDIES

General laboratory screening evaluation should be performed in all patients with hypertension and should include: a urinalysis, electrocardiogram, blood urea nitrogen (BUN), creatinine, sodium, potassium, chloride, bicarbonate, calcium, blood sugar, uric acid, complete blood count, and chest x-ray. These tests will help rule out most secondary causes of hypertension.[4,7,9] Depending on the history and physical examination, other tests that may be useful include: urinary vanillylmandelic acid (VMA) and total metanephrines (metanephrine plus normetanephrine), plasma cortisol, and plasma catecholamines, as well as supine and standing plasma renin and aldosterone measurements.

ASSESSMENT

Renovascular Hypertension

Renovascular hypertension (RVH) results from a renal artery narrowing significant enough to stimulate an increased secretion of renin from the affected kidney ("pressor kidney"). Available estimates suggest that 0.5 per cent of all hypertensives have RVH.[9] However, this number increases to 25 to 30 per cent of hypertensives who are referred to tertiary care centers for evaluation.[9] Atherosclerotic renal lesions account for approximately 67 per cent of patients with RVH and are typically seen in men over the age of 50, whereas the remaining 33 per cent are accounted for by fibromuscular dysplasia, a condition seen in females (age 30 to 50) and rarely in blacks.

There are no specific symptoms associated with RVH except the rare history of sudden flank pain secondary to trauma, or an embolus followed by the appearance of moderate to severe hypertension may be noted.[17] Nocturia may also occur in 25 to 40 per cent of patients with RVH.[7,17] The single best predictor of RVH is a continuous flank bruit, which occurs in 50 to 60 per cent of patients.[17] Clinical clues suggesting renal vascular hypertension are summarized in Table 3.

The following laboratory abnormalities should increase your suspicion of renal vascular hypertension: increased BUN and creatinine from renal insufficiency, if both renal arteries are involved; hypokalemia from secondary aldosteronism; or microscopic proteinuria and hematuria from renal ischemia. See the algorithm illustrating the workup of patients suspected of having RVH.

TABLE 3. Symptoms Raising Suspicion of Renovascular Hypertension

A continuous subcostal or flank bruit
Accelerated or malignant hypertension
Hypertension refractory to appropriate three-drug regimen
Unilateral small kidney discovered by any clinical study
Sudden development or worsening of hypertension at any age
Hypertension and unexplained renal dysfunction
Sudden worsening of renal function in a hypertensive patient in the absence of other obvious causes (i.e., interstitial nephritis, obstruction, etc.)
Sudden impairment in renal function (within 72 hours) in response to angiotensin converting enzyme inhibitor
Presence of moderate to severe hypertension with peripheral vascular and coronary disease

DIAGNOSTIC ASSESSMENT OF RENOVASCULAR HYPERTENSION

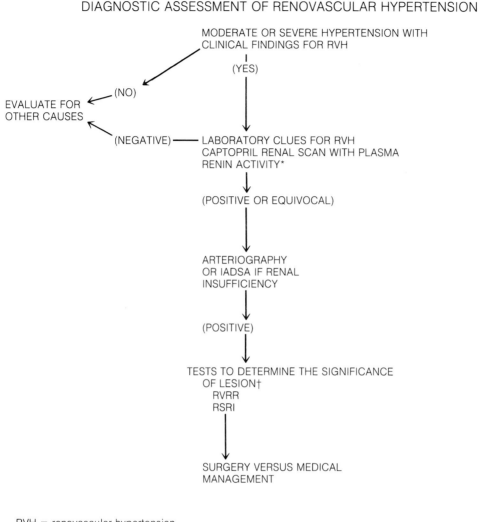

MODERATE OR SEVERE HYPERTENSION WITH
CLINICAL FINDINGS FOR RVH

(YES)

(NO)

EVALUATE FOR
OTHER CAUSES

(NEGATIVE) —— LABORATORY CLUES FOR RVH
CAPTOPRIL RENAL SCAN WITH PLASMA
RENIN ACTIVITY*

(POSITIVE OR EQUIVOCAL)

ARTERIOGRAPHY
OR IADSA IF RENAL
INSUFFICIENCY

(POSITIVE)

TESTS TO DETERMINE THE SIGNIFICANCE
OF LESION†
RVRR
RSRI

SURGERY VERSUS MEDICAL
MANAGEMENT

RVH = renovascular hypertension.
IADSA = intra-arterial digital subtraction angiography.
RVRR = renal vein renin ratio
RSRI = renal to systemic renin index.

* See references 19, 20, 21.
† These tests are recommended to assess hemodynamic significance of a renal arterial lesion.[9]

Diagnostic Tests

Intravenous pyelography and rapid sequence intravenous urography have no place in the routine evaluation of RVH. Studies have shown 20 to 30 per cent false-positive and false-negative rates utilizing these studies.[18] Renal ultrasound and renal tomograms are useful in demonstrating differences in renal size but provide no direct information concerning function or evidence for renal arterial stenosis.[9] Changes in renal size and function, however, are better indicators than blood pressure measurements for progression of renal arterial stenosis.[9]

Conventional triple renal isotope scans have limited usefulness as a screening procedure for assessing renal vascular disease. Although a comparison of renal scans in the presence and absence of captopril has increased the accuracy of this test, no correlation studies with renal arteriography have been performed to assess its accuracy.[9] Furthermore, casual measurement of peripheral plasma renin activity alone has been used as a screening test for

RVH with disappointing results. However, when done under stringent criteria, a significant change in *both* plasma renin activity and renal blood flow by renal scintigraphy, following administration of captopril, is a useful screening test.[19,20,21]

Various forms of angiography remain the most useful visualization techniques for the renal vessels. Two forms of digital subtraction angiography (DSA) are used for diagnostic evaluation. Intravenous DSA requires more contrast and provides suboptimal visualization of the renal arteries but is less invasive than arterial studies. Recent studies, however, suggest it as a good screening test for patients in a high-risk group (e.g., history of claudication, angina, and hypertension) for renal vascular disease.[9,22] Conversely, intra-arterial DSA requires less contrast compared with standard arteriography and provides equivalent visualization. Hence, it is the visualization technique recommended when renal insufficiency is present;[9] however, renal arteriography remains the gold standard for diagnosis of renal vascular lesions. Hemodynamically significant lesions typically include a stenosis of at least 75 per cent with poststenotic dilatation as well as the presence of collateral renal vessels. The functional significance of a given lesion is determined by obtaining renal vein renins from both renal veins and inferior vena cava following captopril administration.[9] A ratio of 1.5:1 of affected to unaffected kidney predicts surgical improvement in 90 per cent of the cases.[4,9]

Pheochromocytoma

Pheochromocytomas are catecholamine releasing tumors that arise from chromaffin cells of the adrenergic nervous system and primarily (85 per cent) secrete norepinephrine, with the remainder secreting epinephrine.[12] Ninety per cent of these tumors are found in the adrenal glands, with the remaining 10 per cent being extra-adrenal (i.e., abdominal, thoracic, or pelvic), bilateral and more common in children (35 per cent of pediatric cases) and those individuals with genetic disorders (i.e., MEA syndromes II and III).[10,12]

Hypertension in affected individuals may be sustained, paroxysmal, or both.[12] About 75 per cent of patients experience one or more paroxysms weekly, whereas the rest have one or more daily. Attacks may occur as rarely as once every few months or as often as 25 times daily and may persist for less than a minute to a week.[12] The most common symptoms during attacks include headaches, palpitations, diaphoresis, anxiety, and a fine tremor.[4,12] In children, visual complaints, nausea, vomiting, weight loss, polydypsia, polyuria, and seizures are more common than in adults.[12] In pregnancy, pheochromocytoma may mimic eclampsia or pre-eclampsia and is associated with a 50 per cent maternal fetal mortality if undiagnosed.[12]

Patients should be screened for pheochromocytoma if hypertension and at least three or more of the following signs or symptoms are present: headaches (severe), excessive sweating, palpitations and/or tachycardia, anxiety or nervousness, tremulousness, nausea and vomiting associated with paroxysms of hypertension, as well as weakness, fatigue, and prostration. In addition, grade III or IV retinopathy of unknown cause, weight loss, hyperglycemia, hypermetabolism without hyperthyroidism, or a cardiomyopathy should all prompt an evaluation for pheochromocytoma. Physical findings observed in patients with pheochromocytoma include: hypertension induced by physical maneuvers such as exercise and significant orthostatic hypotension with standing; a marked pressor response with induction of anesthesia; hyperhidrosis; dilated pupils; hand tremor; and fever as well as an increase in body temperature of approximately 1° F.[12]

Diagnostic Tests

Laboratory abnormalities sometimes present in pheochromocytoma are listed in Table 4. If the biochemical evaluation for pheochromocytoma is positive, the best test for visualization of the tumor is a computed tomography (CT) scan of the adrenal glands.[12] This will visualize over 95 per cent of these tumors. However, in the face of a normal CT scan and biochemical evidence suggesting pheochromocytoma, an ^{131}I-metaiodobenzguanidine (^{131}I-MIBG) scan should be done. ^{131}I-MIBG concentrates in the adrenergic vesicles and thus has a strong propensity to accumulate in pheochromocytomas, which may be extra-adrenal as well as adrenal. Furthermore, scintigraphic imaging with ^{131}I-MIBG seems to be a sensitive and specific method for both diagnosis and localization of pheochromocytomas that may be too small to be visualized by CT scan (less than 1 cm).[12]

TABLE 4.   Laboratory Findings Occasionally Present in Pheochromocytoma*

FINDING	CORRELATION WITH DISEASE (%)
Elevated plasma catecholamines	60
Elevated urinary *total* metanephrines and VMA	98
Impaired glucose tolerance	10
Elevated basal metabolic rate	25
Decreased plasma and/or total blood volume	30
Increased blood urea nitrogen (<60 mg/dl) without increase in serum creatinine	80

Increased plasma renin and aldosterone (when associated with renal artery stenosis)
Association with MEA syndromes
  Hyperparathyroidism
    Increased serum calcium, serum parathyroid hormone, and urinary phosphate
  Medullary thyroid carcinoma
    Increased serum thyrocalcitonin, serum serotonin, urinary 5-HIAA,† and serum prostaglandins

* Table compiled from references 4, 10, 13.
† 5-HIAA = 5-hydroxyindoleacetic acid.

DIAGNOSTIC ASSESSMENT OF PHEOCHROMOCYTOMA

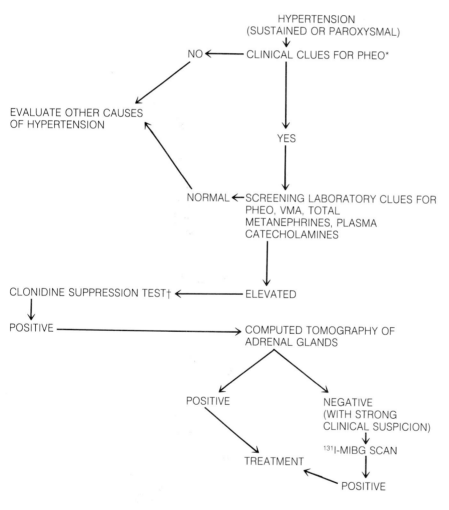

PHEO = pheochromocytoma.
VMA = vanillylmandelic acid (urinary).
131I-MIBG = 131I-metaiodobenzguanidine.

* See text for signs and symptoms.
† See reference 25.

DIAGNOSTIC ASSESSMENT OF PRIMARY ALDOSTERONISM

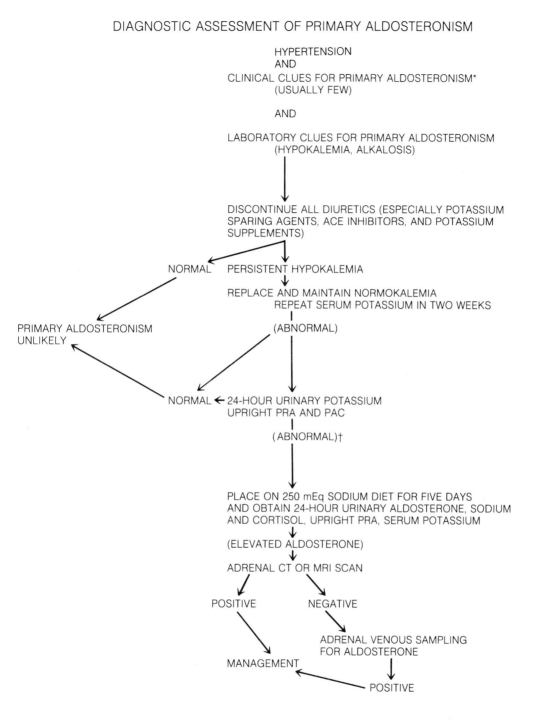

ACE = angiotensin converting enzyme.
PRA = plasma renin activity.
PAC = plasma aldosterone concentration.
 CT = computed tomography.
MRI = magnetic resonance imaging.

 * Normokalemia should not exclude consideration of primary aldosteronism since about one third of patients may present with normal potassiums.
 † PRA less than 3.0 ng/ml per hour and PAC:PRA ratio greater than 20 with or without inappropriate kaliuresis and low serum potassium.

See the algorithm on the general approach to the evaluation of a patient with suspected pheochromocytoma.

Primary Aldosteronism

Primary aldosteronism is a syndrome of aldosterone oversecretion from the adrenal cortex characterized by hypertension, increased aldosterone secretion, suppressed plasma renin, and hypokalemia. The syndrome is usually caused by either a unilateral aldosterone producing adrenal adenoma (Conn's disease) or a bilateral adrenal hyperplasia and rarely by an adrenal cortical carcinoma. Approximately 65 per cent of patients with primary aldosteronism have unilateral adrenal adenomas. The average-sized adenoma measures roughly 1.8 cm and occurs primarily in women, with a peak incidence between the third to sixth decade.[4,23,24]

Unprovoked hypokalemia in a hypertensive patient is characteristic of primary aldosteronism.[24] Clinical symptoms and signs are few; however, when present, they are usually due to hypokalemia. Some clinical signs and symptoms include: muscle cramps, weakness, polyuria, polydypsia, headaches, palpitations, occasional chest pain, and glucose intolerance; occasionally, Chvostek's and Trousseau's signs are noted if alkalosis is severe.[4,24] The mechanism of these latter two signs is the increase in plasma pH binds more ionized calcium to albumin and hence gives a relative hypocalcemia in the face of normal plasma calcium.

Before proceeding with an evaluation, one must exclude all other causes of hypokalemia. These include: diuretics (the most common cause in hypertensives), vomiting, diarrhea, estrogens, exogenous steroids, laxatives, renal artery stenosis, Cushing's syndrome, metabolic acidosis, chronic liver disease, and volume depletion. Note, however, that up to 35 per cent of patients with primary aldosteronism are normokalemic due to a low sodium diet.

The laboratory abnormalities that should prompt the thought of primary aldosteronism include: hypomagnesemia, mild hypernatremia, hypokalemia, and mild metabolic alkalosis. In addition, electrocardiographic findings may reveal mild left ventricular hypertrophy with prolonged ST segment and T wave inversions with occasional U waves; however, findings may be entirely normal.[4,24]

Diagnostic Tests

The biochemical diagnosis of primary aldosteronism is best achieved by demonstration of an elevated urinary aldosterone and failure of suppression of plasma aldosterone in the face of saline loading.[4] The patient should have an adequate plasma potassium level and be on a sodium-rich diet for at least five days prior to the collection of a 24-hour urine specimen for aldosterone.

If a diagnosis is suspected on biochemical grounds, a CT scan of the adrenals is the procedure of choice. If adrenal masses are not visualized, then adrenal vein sampling for aldosterone and renin is warranted to try to localize the process.[24] Other procedures are also available for this localization but are less reliable.[4,25] See the algorithm for the evaluation of patients with suspected primary aldosteronism.

Estrogen-Induced Hypertension

The increased use of estrogen preparations—for contraception, osteoporosis, and the like—has contributed to an increased incidence in hypertension in the female population.[4] These agents increase arterial pressure in a dose-dependent fashion through increased production of angiotensinogen with subsequent increases in angiotensin II and aldosterone.[4] The diagnosis is generally made by history, since there are no associated signs or symptoms of estrogen ingestion that relate to hypertension.

REFERENCES

1. The Joint National Committee on the Detection, Evaluation and Treatment of High Blood Pressure. The 1988 report of the Joint National Committee on the Detection, Evaluation and Treatment of High Blood Pressure. Arch Intern Med 1988;148:1023–8.
2. Londe S, Goldring D. High blood pressure in children: problems and guidelines for evaluation and treatment. Am J Cardiol 1976;4:650–8.
3. Page LB. Epidemiology of hypertension. In: Genest J, Kuchel O, Hamet P, Cantin M, eds. Hypertension. New York: McGraw-Hill, 1983:683–99.
4. Weinberger MH. Systemic hypertension. In: Kelley WN, ed. Textbook of internal medicine. Philadelphia: JB Lippincott, 1989:268–83.
5. Criqui MH, Langer RD, Reed DM. Dietary alcohol, calcium and potassium: independent and combined effects on blood pressure. Circulation 1989; 80:609–14.
6. Ylitalo P, Pitkajarvi T, Metsa-Ketela T, Vapaatalo

H. The effect of inhibition of prostaglandin synthesis on plasma renin activity and blood pressure in hypertension. Prostaglandins Med 1978;1: 479–88.

7. Strong CG, Northcutt RC, Shep SG. Clinical examination and investigation of the hypertensive patient. In: Genest J, Kuchel O, Hamet P, Cantin M, eds. Hypertension. New York: McGraw-Hill, 1983:700–21.

8. Lamberts SW, Kiijn JG, DeJong FH, Birkehage JC. Hormone secretion in alcohol-induced pseudo Cushing's syndrome: differential diagnosis with Cushing's disease. JAMA 1979;242:1640–3.

9. Working Group on Renovascular Hypertension. Detection, evaluation, and treatment of renovascular hypertension. Arch Intern Med 1987;147: 820–9.

10. Khairi MR, Dexter RN, Burzynski NJ, Johnston CC Jr. Mucosal neuroma, pheochromocytoma and medullary thyroid carcinoma: multiple endocrine neoplasia, type 3. Medicine 1975;54:89–112.

11. Nash DA Jr. Hypertension in polycystic kidney disease without renal failure. Arch Intern Med 1977; 137:1571–5.

12. Manger WM, Gifford RW, Hoffman BB. Pheochromocytoma: a clinical and experimental overview. Curr Prob Cancer 1985;9:5–89.

13. Mimran A. Renal function in hypertension. Am J Med 1988;84(Suppl 1B):69–75.

14. Bates B. Examination of peripheral pulses and arterial pressure. In: Bates B, ed. A guide to physical examination and history taking. Philadelphia: JB Lippincott, 1987:264–5.

15. Juergens JL, Barker NW, Hines EA Jr. Arteriosclerosis obliterans: review of 570 cases with special reference to pathogenic and prognostic factors. Circulation 1960;21:188–96.

16. Melmed S. Acromegaly. N Engl J Med 1990;322:966–76.

17. Genest J, Cartier P, Roy P, et al. Renovascular hypertension. In: Genest J. Kuchel O, Hamet P, Cantin M, eds. Hypertension. New York: McGraw-Hill, 1983:1007–34.

18. Grim CE, Luft FC, Weinberger MA, Grim CM. Sensitivity and specificity of screening tests for renal vascular hypertension. Ann Intern Med 1979;91: 617–22.

19. Sfakianakis GN, Bourgoignie JJ, Jaffe D, Kyriakides G, Stable-Perez E, Duncan RC. Single dose captopril scintigraphy in the diagnosis of renovascular hypertension. J Nucl Med 1987;28:1383–92.

20. Muller FB, Sealey JE, Case DB, et al. The captopril test for identifying renovascular disease in hypertensive patients. Am J Med 1986;80:633–44.

21. McCarthy JE, Weder AB. The captopril test and renovascular hypertension. Arch Intern Med 1990;150:493–95.

22. Svetkey LP, Himmelstein SI, Dunnick R, et al. Prospective analysis of strategies for diagnosing renovascular hypertension. Hypertension 1989; 14:247–57.

23. Bravo EL, Tarau RC, Dustan HP, et al. The changing clinical picture of primary aldosteronism. Am J Med 1983;74:641–51.

24. Young WF, Hogan MJ, Klee GC, Grant CS, van Heerden JA. Primary aldosteronism: diagnosis and treatment. Mayo Clin Proc 1990;65:96–110.

25. Bravo EL, Tarazi RC, Fouad FM, Vidt DG, Gifford RW. Clonidine suppression test. N Engl J Med 1981;305:623–6.

SEIZURES IN CHILDHOOD

DANIEL K. MILES and GREGORY L. HOLMES

SYNONYMS: Convulsions, Fits, Spasms

BACKGROUND

A seizure is a "sudden, involuntary, time-limited alteration in behavior including change in motor activity, autonomic function, consciousness, or sensation secondary to an abnormal discharge of neurons in the central nervous system."[1] Seizures are not specific disease processes but rather manifestations of cerebral dysfunction. Epilepsy is the condition of recurrent unprovoked seizures.

A study by Hauser and Kurland revealed a bimodal peak in the incidence of epilepsy in a Minnesota county, with highest rates seen in the first year of life and after age 55 years.[2] Seizures are common in childhood; from 3 to 5 per cent of all children will have at least a single seizure by the age of five years. Fortunately, most of these are provoked by a febrile illness and therefore do not constitute epilepsy.

Depending on the underlying etiology and extent of a cerebral insult, seizure activity will have variable clinical and electroencephalographic (EEG) manifestations. These electroclinical events run the spectrum from a momentary blank stare and unresponsiveness associated with generalized 3-Hz spike and wave discharges seen in simple absence seizures to a more prolonged complex partial seizure with secondary generalization in which a sense of "déjà vu" is followed by focal clonic activity that gradually spreads to involve the entire body, accompanied by loss of consciousness and during which the EEG shows focal epileptiform discharges that spread to the opposite hemisphere.

To foster a neurophysiologic approach to seizure description, the International League Against Epilepsy (ILAE) formulated the international classification of epileptic seizures based on: (1) clinical manifestations of the seizure, (2) ictal (during the seizure) EEG patterns, and (3) interictal (between seizures) EEG abnormalities. Most recently revised in 1981, this classification schema can be seen in Table 1. Seizures are either partial or generalized, and the former may secondarily generalize. Partial seizures, which may involve motor, sensory, autonomic, or psychic symptoms, are localized to one area of the brain and are further categorized as simple or complex, depending on whether consciousness is impaired. Generalized seizures, by definition, involve both hemispheres, and consciousness is impaired. The classification not only provides a systematic and unified manner by which

TABLE 2.   Etiologies of Seizures, by Age

Neonatal
  Perinatal asphyxia
  Intracranial hemorrhage
  CNS* infection
  CNS malformations
  Hypocalcemia
  Hypomagnesemia
  Hypoglycemia
  Inborn errors of metabolism
  Drug withdrawal
  Idiopathic
Infancy
  Chronic condition from the neonatal period
  CNS infection
  Cerebrovascular accident (arterial occlusion and
    venous thrombosis)
  Inborn errors of metabolism
  Trauma
  Degenerative disorders
  Idiopathic
Childhood and adolescence
  CNS infection
  Trauma
  Tumor
  Degenerative disorder
  Cerebrovascular malformation
  Idiopathic

* CNS = central nervous system.

physicians can categorize seizures but additionally aids in determining the antiepileptic drug of choice for a particular patient.

The principal diagnoses of patients with seizures vary with age, the widest range of possibilities being seen in the neonatal group, with perinatal hypoxia-ischemia being the most common etiology. Infancy and childhood seizures are most likely related to infectious processes and toxins, whereas in adults identifiable intracranial lesions secondary to cerebrovascular accidents, trauma, and tumor are most frequently the cause. Other etiologies, including those that are idiopathic, are possible in all age groups. A listing of etiologies is found in Table 2.

TABLE 1.   Classification of Epileptic Seizures

Partial seizures—seizures begin locally
  Simple—without impairment of consciousness
    May include motor symptoms, special sensory or
      somatosensory symptoms, autonomic symptoms,
      or psychic symptoms
  Complex—with impairment of consciousness
    Simple partial onset followed by impairment of
      consciousness
    Impaired consciousness at onset
  Secondarily generalized—partial onset evolving to
    generalized tonic—clonic seizures
Generalized seizures—bilaterally symmetric and without
  local onset
  Absence
  Myoclonic
  Clonic
  Tonic
  Tonic-clonic
  Atonic
Unclassified epileptic seizures—seizures that cannot be
  classified because of inadequate or incomplete data
Status epilepticus

(Modified from: Commission on the Classification and Terminology of the International League Against Epilepsy. Proposal for revised clinical and electroencephalographic classification of epileptic seizures. Epilepsia 1981;22:489–501.)

HISTORY

Since most seizures are not witnessed by the physician, the history represents the initial step in determining whether or not the event was in fact a seizure and, if so, what type. Obtaining as precise and as detailed a description of the event as possible should be the major goal of the physician while taking the patient's history. In addition to learning what the patient did during the ictal period, the patient's activities both prior to and after the seizure must be reviewed.

Whether or not prodromal irritability or uneasiness was noted, as well as if the patient experienced an aura, should be determined. An aura is a simple partial seizure and allows the clinician to determine where the onset of the seizure occurs. In children, auras can be quite varied and consist of fear; abnormal sensation in the mouth, throat, or abdomen; visual or auditory hallucinations; and disturbances of memory such as "déjà vu" or "jamais vu."

Any relationship between the occurrence of the seizure and physiologic states, such as arousal from sleep or onset of menses, needs to be established. Other areas of questioning involve excluding the possibilities that the seizure was induced by hyperventilation, perhaps associated with physical exertion, or photic stimulation that might take place while in a moving vehicle or looking at a television screen or computer terminal. Other circumstances that can cause seizure activity and require exclusion include: antecedent head trauma, any manifestation of encephalopathic processes, and simple febrile illnesses. Lastly, whether or not similar events have been noted previously should be addressed.

With regard to the event itself, what was first noted, if in fact the event was witnessed, needs to be determined. The patient's level of consciousness—that is, ability to interact with his or her environment properly—should be assessed. Inability to respond appropriately during a seizure suggests a complex partial or absence seizure. The presence or absence of motor activity requires investigation. Tonic, clonic, myoclonic, and atonic seizure activity should be described, with particular attention paid to any lateralizing features. Knowing the sequence of ictal manifestations, including the manner in which convulsive activity may have spread from one area of the body to another, also helps characterize the seizure. Incontinence of bowel or bladder and the presence of oral lacerations provide a sense of the seizure's intensity. Knowledge of the duration and frequency of the seizures—if more than one has been noted—aids in the classification and, subsequently, the treatment of the seizure. For instance, periods of detachment or unresponsiveness with or without automatisms could be due either to absence seizures, which are usually less than 30 seconds in duration but may occur hundreds of times a day, or to complex partial seizures, which typically last longer than 30 seconds and take place only several times a day.

Following the seizure, was the patient lethargic, or did he or she return to his or her baseline status quickly? Was there note of any weakness, a Todd's paralysis, at the conclusion of the seizure? A Todd's paralysis usually indicates that the seizure began in the contralateral motor strip. Amnesia for the event may be the only indication of an impairment of the patient's consciousness. The child should be questioned about the event, since he or she may provide useful information regarding an aura and impairment of consciousness.

Past Medical History

Upon obtaining the history of the seizure, the remainder of the patient's medical history should be reviewed. In particular, the perinatal and developmental histories will be of assistance in determining whether the etiology of the seizure is more likely to be congenital or acquired. Other areas needing discussion are head trauma, medications, and immunizations.

Family History

Eliciting a history of seizures in relatives may be critical in making an accurate assessment. Such a history would lend credence to the possible diagnosis of a primary (idiopathic) seizure disorder. The diagnosis of various inherited neurologic disorders that manifest seizures is made easier by obtaining a positive family history. A distinction between seizures related to acquired deficits later in life (secondary epilepsy), such as those associated with stroke or focal trauma, and those that are idiopathic must be made. A family history of mental retardation or psychiatric problems might be consistent with the diagnosis of an inherited disorder.

PHYSICAL EXAMINATION

General Examination

In that a seizure most frequently represents a manifestation of an underlying process and only rarely alters the patient's examination during the interictal period, the goal of the examination is to uncover evidence of particular disease processes that cause seizures.

Growth parameters should always be obtained. Recognition of microcephaly may lead to the diagnosis of an intrauterine infection; macrocephaly may be the result of hydrocephalus or a storage disorder. Overall growth retardation may be an indicator of a chronic disease process. Inspection and auscultation of the head should be performed as checks for evidence of trauma and intracranial bruits associated with cerebral vascular malformations, respectively.

Other portions of the physical to be concentrated on include examination of the abdomen, spine, skin, and extremities. Organomegaly may be secondary to a storage disorder, and abnormalities of the spine can be indicative of a neural tube defect with an intracranial component. Gross inspection of the skin, which is facilitated with a Wood's lamp, may reveal dermatologic abnormalities associated with various phakomatoses including: axillary freckling and café au lait spots (neurofibromatosis); port-wine stains (Sturge-Weber syndrome); and adenoma sebaceum, ash leaf spots, and shagreen patches (tuberous sclerosis). Asymmetries of the hands and feet, as well as the face, suggest lateralized cerebral injury.

Neurologic Examination

Although most often normal in a patient with seizures, the neurologic examination serves a dual purpose: It should be a search both for signs implicating an underlying etiology of the seizure activity and for findings that localize the seizure focus. The interictal neurologic examination may be less rewarding than an ictal or immediately postictal examination, but a thorough investigation can provide useful information.

Lateralizing features of the examination, such as a hemiparesis, aid in evaluation of a seizure focus, but certain findings may be even more localizing, as in the case of a superior quadrant visual field defect—the former implicating the contralateral hemisphere, the latter incriminating the temporal lobe of the contralateral hemisphere.

Other findings must be carefully evaluated for their significance. Memory deficits noted on the mental status examination may either be related to the location of the lesion that underlies the seizure or be a secondary effect of the seizure itself. Subsequently, caution must be used in attributing localizing significance to certain findings. Those findings that are without localizing significance are still of diagnostic importance. Mental retardation, diffuse hypertonicity, and hyper-reflexia do not necessarily aid in determining a seizure focus, but they do suggest a secondary seizure disorder as opposed to a primary or idiopathic disorder.

Funduscopy is a part of the examination that can be quite revealing. The discovery of retinal hemorrhages must lead to the consideration of a subdural hematoma, whereas recognition of a cherry red spot raises interest in certain storage disorders. Funduscopy that reveals changes consistent with chorioretinitis aids in the realization that a patient experienced an intrauterine infection. The presence of papilledema requires urgent evaluation for increased intracranial pressure.

The evaluation of someone suspected of having had an absence seizure is not complete without hyperventilating the patient. Witnessing the abrupt cessation of hyperventilation associated with unresponsiveness and a blank stare confirms the diagnosis even prior to an EEG having been done. With the much greater availability of neuroimaging, transillumination of an infant's head with a Chun-gun is less frequently necessary but can be used to detect cystic changes or other cerebral malformations.

In the event that a seizure is witnessed, the observer should pay particular attention to the initial ictal change, whether it be impairment of consciousness, the patient describing an aura, or motor activity. The type (tonic, clonic, etc.) and distribution of motor activity should be noted. Responsiveness and memory can be tested with simple commands and a phrase or a color to be recalled after the conclusion of the seizure. Finally, evaluation of the patient for postictal deficits needs to be performed.

DIAGNOSTIC STUDIES

Laboratory

While usually of low yield in a patient who is otherwise healthy, we recommend a complete blood count with differential and platelet count, electrolytes, glucose, calcium, and tests of liver and renal function be performed following an initial seizure. This battery of tests may reveal various chemical imbalances or indication of an infectious process as well as provide the clinician with baseline studies of hepatic and renal function in the event anti-epileptic medications are started. Other studies may be warranted, depending on underlying etiologies that are suggested by findings on examination or aspects of the history. A lumbar puncture is indicated if there is evidence of a central nervous system infection or other specific processes associated with characteristic cerebrospinal fluid changes.

If there is a consideration of pseudoseizures, a serum prolactin level should be drawn within 20 minutes after the event and should be compared with another level drawn at the same time on another day. Prolactin levels are elevated after complex partial and generalized seizures.[3]

Neuroimaging

Cranial computed tomography or magnetic resonance imaging is recommended (the latter preferred, if available) in all cases of unexplained seizures, partial or generalized, with the exception of clearly primary generalized seizures (e.g., absence seizures). It should be recognized that many seizures that appear generalized from onset are, in fact, partial seizures with rapid generalization.

Electroencephalography

The ability to distinguish between epileptic and nonepileptic seizures, to aid in the diagnosis of particular seizure types, and to assist in the recognition of characteristic patterns of specific epileptic syndromes makes electroencephalography the most informative laboratory procedure in the evaluation of the seizure patient. It must be remembered, however, that seizures and epilepsy are clinical diagnoses. In fact, 2 per cent of the population[4] and 3 per cent of children[5] have abnormal epileptiform activity in their EEGs but never experience seizures.

It is generally agreed that because the study is not invasive, benign, and relatively inexpensive, it is reasonable to obtain an EEG on any patient who has had or is suspected of having had a seizure. This provides a baseline study for comparison and should be obtained as soon as possible after a seizure. Although spikes may be suppressed and postictal slowing may be seen for up to a week, if the slowing is focal, this may be an important finding, as it may be indicative of focal pathology. It should be realized that although the initiation of antiepileptic drug therapy may change the EEG, it will usually not eradicate the seizure focus.[6]

ASSESSMENT

Numerous forms of nonepileptic, episodic phenomena exist and should be considered prior to making the diagnosis of an epileptic seizure. The misdiagnosis of one of these events places great stress on the patient and the patient's family, stigmatizes the child, and may in fact lead to the patient's being unnecessarily exposed to antiepileptic drugs and their potential toxic side effects. If the physician is uncertain about the diagnosis, it is preferable to wait for a second event before concluding the child has seizures. Briefly, some of the more frequently encountered nonepileptic activities will be described.

Differential Diagnosis

Breath Holding

Seen at any time from the neonatal period through six years of life, breath holding is most frequently noted between 6 and 18 months. Typically, the spells are brought on by surprise, fright, mild injury, or even frustration and begin with the child crying. Apnea and cyanosis follow, leading to loss of consciousness. With the onset of unconsciousness, muscle tone is lost and the child remains limp until normal breathing is restored. If significant hypoxia results, opisthotonic posturing or clonic jerks may occur. During these events, EEGs reveal high-amplitude delta waves as consciousness is lost, and isoelectric tracings correlate with the opisthotonic and clonic activity.[7] Upon restoration of regular respiration, the patient rapidly regains consciousness without the lethargy and confusion commonly seen after a generalized seizure.

Pallid Infantile Syncope

Brief periods of vagal-mediated asystole result in cerebral hypoperfusion accompanied by pallor, cold sweats, and loss of consciousness. Less commonly seen than the cyanotic breath-holding spells, pallid infantile syncope most usually occurs between the ages of 12 and 18 months. The diagnosis can be confirmed using ocular compression while monitoring electrocardiogram (ECG) and EEG. Susceptible individuals experience severe bradycardia and asystole associated with EEG slowing and loss of consciousness when ocular compression is applied. The diagnosis usually can be made, however, by history. Once again, if sufficient hypoxia ensues, opisthotonic or convulsive activity may occur.

Syncope

Another vagal-mediated event, syncope, is ultimately related to cerebral hypoxia, too. The loss of consciousness related to syncope is a gradual process and is often associated with lightheadedness, blurred vision, and vertigo. This entity is a major consideration in the school-age child who has lost consciousness. (Also see chapter on Syncope in *Difficult Diagnosis I*.)

Cardiac Arrhythymias

Asystole, paroxysmal ventricular and atrial tachycardia, and the prolonged Q-T syndrome may result in loss of consciousness that can be mistaken for seizure activity.

Shuddering Attacks

Consisting of rapid tremors of the head, trunk, arms, and legs, shuddering or shivering attacks may be mistaken for seizures. Seen as early as four months of age, the episodes last only seconds and may occur hundreds of times a day. The attacks have no correlation with epileptiform activity on EEG and are benign.

Movement Disorders

Paroxysmal choreoathetosis (both dystonic and kinesiogenic forms), motor tics, and spasmus nutans are all disorders of episodic motor dyscontrol without epileptic correlate. Paroxysmal choreoathetosis is a rare disorder in which episodic attacks of severe dystonia and/or choreoathetosis occur. The triad of head nodding, head tilt, and nystagmus make up the syndrome of spasmus nutans that often has its onset between the ages of 4 to 12 months and usually remits spontaneously one to two years after onset. (Also see chapter on Athetosis.)

Parasomnias

Parasomnias, benign episodic events that occur during sleep, should be recognized as nonepileptic in nature. The forms of this type of disorder that are most frequently seen are night terrors, also known as pavor nocturnus, and sleepwalking. Night terrors, usually seen in patients aged 4 to 12 years, typically occur during the first several hours of sleep and are characterized by the child screaming and

crying inconsolably, appearing frightened, diaphoretic, and tachypneic. After the episode, the patient has no recall of the event. In contrast, nightmares occur later at night, and details of the event are vividly recalled. Somnambulism, like pavor nocturnus, occurs in stages 3 and 4 of sleep, usually during the first hours of sleep. Semipurposeful activity and talking may take place. Attempts to elicit a response from the child are either unsuccessful or result in mumbling by the patient.

Migraine

Migraines may be very difficult to distinguish from seizures; in fact, both may occur in the same patient. Most confusing are those patients with migraine auras (scintillating scotomata, perceptual distortions, paresthesia, aphasia, hemiparesis, ophthalmoplegia, weakness, etc.) that are unaccompanied by headache. While acute confusional states associated with migraines may require an EEG to distinguish them with certainty from seizures, a family history of migraine is very helpful in making the distinction. More easily recognized differences include the fact that automatisms—tonic, clonic, and myoclonic motor activity—are rarely, if ever, seen in migraines.

Hyperventilation

Most often diagnosed in adolescents and young adults, hyperventilation can precipitate neurologic, cardiovascular, respiratory, gastrointestinal, and musculoskeletal symptoms.[8] Lightheadedness, depersonalization, blurred vision, anxiety, and loss of consciousness may be reported. Hyperventilation attacks are usually brought on by stress, anxiety, and emotional factors. The symptoms that have been described are relieved by rebreathing exhaled air.

Psychogenic Seizures

Also referred to as "pseudoseizures," these are involuntary, episodic behaviors that resemble seizures but are nonepileptic in nature. Reported in patients ranging from preschool age to midseventies, they are reported most commonly in adolescents and young adults, with a 3:1 female-to-male ratio.[9] Classically characterized by uncoordinated, asynchronous movements of the extremities, pelvic thrusting, and side-to-side movements of the head, psychogenic seizure is the most difficult differential diagnosis to be made from seizures. Further compounding the problem is the fact that many patients with nonepileptic seizures do in fact have epilepsy. As previously mentioned, serum prolactin levels can be used to aid in distinguishing psychogenic from epileptic seizures, but it is video-EEG that provides the best means to do so.

Epileptic Syndromes

Once a paroxysmal event has been diagnosed as an epileptic seizure, as opposed to any of the other nonepileptic events previously described, the seizure type should be determined, and the physician's energy should be directed toward recognizing any of various childhood epileptic syndromes. By being able to classify the child's disorder in such a way, the patient can be given a more definite prognosis, often reassuringly benign, and the antiepileptic drug of choice for the particular syndrome can be determined. The following are some of the more frequently encountered epileptic syndromes of childhood.

Febrile Seizures

Age-related febrile seizures constitute one of the most common neurologic disorders in pediatrics. A febrile seizure is "an event in infancy or childhood that occurs between 3 months and 5 years of age, associated with a fever but without evidence of intracranial infection or defined cause."[10] Characterized by brief, almost always generalized seizures, the vast majority are uncomplicated, but there are those that are prolonged and followed by transient or permanent neurologic sequelae. A tendency to recurrence is noted in approximately one third of those affected. A slight increase in the risk of developing epilepsy is noted in these patients, as compared with the general population, 2.0 per cent and 0.5 per cent, respectively.[11] This risk is higher if the child has a focal seizure, more than one seizure in a 24-hour period, or a seizure lasting longer than 15 minutes. Prolonged antiepileptic drug therapy is rarely recommended. Neuropsychologic testing of patients with febrile seizures and their sibling controls showed no significant difference. This condition is a relatively benign disorder of early chidhood.

Infantile Spasms

With onset peaking between four and seven months, the triad of myoclonic seizures, hypsarrhythmic EEG, and mental retardation (West's syndrome) is an epileptic syndrome unique to childhood. Frequently occurring in clusters, with varying intensity and frequency, spasms are brief and may be missed by a casual observer. They may be flexor, extensor, or mixed myoclonic seizures. The etiology of the syndrome is either cryptogenic or symptomatic. Those patients with spasms of cryptogenic etiology and normal development prior to onset of spasms have the better prognosis, as do those who receive early therapy with adrenocorticotropic hormone (ACTH) or steroids. Atypical forms, associated with early or late onset and a lack of one of the three components of the triad, do exist. As suggested, ACTH and steroids are the treatment of choice.

Lennox-Gastaut Syndrome

Manifested by a mixed seizure disorder (including atypical absences and tonic, atonic, and myoclonic as well as generalized tonic-clonic seizures) that is often intractable to medical therapy, intellectual impairment, and a characteristic EEG pattern, the Lennox-Gastaut syndrome holds a very poor prognosis. The natural course of the syndrome is such that the frequency of atonic, myoclonic, and atypical absence seizures decreases with age, only to be replaced by an increase in generalized tonic-clonic seizures and new onset of partial seizures.[12] Because of the variability of seizure types in this syndrome, antiepileptic therapy must be individualized. The great difficulty in gaining control of these seizures frequently results in polypharmacologic therapy and its recognized complications.

Childhood Absence Epilepsy

Thought by many to be synonymous with petit mal epilepsy, this syndrome is characterized by absence seizures in otherwise normal children. Usually lasting less than 15 seconds and rarely with a duration greater than 30 seconds, the hallmark of these seizures is an abrupt onset, without an aura, of suppression of mental functions, usually to the point of complete abolition of awareness, responsiveness, and memory.

Typical absence seizures represent a primary generalized seizure and constitute the predominant seizure type in 15 to 20 per cent of children with epilepsy.[13] A "simple" absence, or petit mal seizure, as just described (consisting solely of staring with cessation of activities) represents less than 10 per cent of patients with typical absences, according to one study.[14] The vast majority of typical absences are considered "complex" in that they are associated with changes in tone, automatisms, and autonomic phenomena. EEG tracings reveal the paroxysmal onset of generalized symmetric spike or polyspike-and-slow-wave complexes classically seen at a frequency of 3 Hz, but with a range from 2.5 to 3.5 Hz.

Typical seizures have a favorable prognosis, quite often remitting by adolescence, but those affected are at risk for developing generalized tonic-clonic seizures at the time absences cease. The drugs of choice are ethosuximide, valproate, and clonazepam.

Benign Rolandic Epilepsy (Benign Childhood Epilepsy with Centrotemporal Spikes, Benign Sylvian Epilepsy)

As is apparent from the several eponyms listed above, the syndrome takes its names from the characteristic involvement of seizure activity in the lower portion of the rolandic gyrus. A variation in seizure type is noted between nocturnal and diurnal events. While seizures in the waking state are typically restricted to one side of the body with tonic, clonic, or tonic-clonic activity most prominently involving the face, nocturnal seizures quite frequently generalize. Inherited in an autosomal dominant manner, the centrotemporal spike pattern has a variable penetrance, with only 25 per cent of patients with the EEG trait developing seizures. Aside from the centrotemporal spikes, the EEG is normal. Almost always controlled with a single antiepileptic agent, the seizures invariably resolve by the age of 15 to 16.

MANAGING SEIZURES IN CHILDHOOD

These epileptic syndromes represent but a few of the many entities encountered by those caring for the pediatric patient with seizures. Less common syndromes have been omitted owing to space constraints. The physician managing a patient with seizures must obtain a sufficiently detailed history and perform a thorough examination so that with the addi-tional information provided by neuroimaging and EEG the seizure type and, if appropriate, the epileptic syndrome can be determined. It is only then that an accurate prognosis and proper therapy can be provided.

REFERENCES

1. Holmes GL. Diagnosis and management of seizures in children. 1st ed. Philadelphia: WB Saunders Co, 1987:1.
2. Hauser WA, Kurland LT. The epidemiology of epilepsy in Rochester, Minnesota, 1935 through 1967. Epilepsia 1975;16:1–66.
3. Pritchard PB III, Wannamaker BB, Sagel J, Daniel CM. Serum prolactin and cortisol levels in evaluation of pseudoepileptic seizures. Ann Neurol 1985;18:87–9.
4. Cavazzuti GB, Capella L, Nalin A. Longitudinal study of epileptiform EEG patterns in normal children. Epilepsia 1980;21:43–55.
5. Zivin L, Ajmone-Marsan C. Incidence and prognostic significance of "epileptiform" activity in the EEG of non-epileptic subjects. Brain 1968;91:751–78.
6. McIntyre HB, Goldberg AS. The knowledgeable use of EEG in seizure disorders. Semin Neurol 1981;1:77–80.
7. Engel J Jr. Seizures and epilepsy. 1st ed. Philadelphia: FA Davis Co, 1989:343.
8. Riley TL. Syncope and hyperventilation. In: Riley TL, Roy A, eds. Pseudoseizures. Baltimore: Williams & Wilkins, 1982:34–61.
9. Lesser RP. Psychogenic seizures. In: Pedley TA, Meldrum BS, eds. Recent advances in epilepsy, Vol 2. New York: Churchill Livingstone, Inc, 1985:273–96.
10. Consensus statement on febrile seizures. In: Nelson KB, Ellenberg JH, eds. Febrile seizures. New York: Raven Press, 1981:301–6.
11. Nelson KB, Ellenberg JH. Predictors of epilepsy in children who have experienced febrile seizures. N Engl J Med 1976;295:1029–33.
12. Dreifuss FE. Lennox-Gastaut syndrome. In: Dreifuss FE, ed. Pediatric epileptology. Boston: John Wright, 1983:121–7.
13. Dalby MA. Epilepsy and 3 per second spike and wave rhythms: a clinical, electroencephalographic and prognostic analysis of 346 patients. Acta Scand Neurol 1969;45(Suppl):183.
14. Penry JK, Porter RJ, Dreifuss FE. Simultaneous recording of absence seizures with videotape and electroencephalography. A study of 374 seizures in 48 patients. Brain 1975;98:427–40.

SILENT MYOCARDIAL ISCHEMIA

PASCAL NICOD and FRANÇOIS RICOU

SYNONYMS: Painless, Asymptomatic, Clinically Unrecognized, Inapparent Myocardial Ischemia

BACKGROUND

Coronary artery disease is currently the leading cause of death in the United States. Every year, approximately 550,000 deaths, of which 50 per cent are sudden, are attributable to coronary atherosclerosis. Several facts show that unrecognized or asymptomatic coronary artery disease is the cause of a high percentage of these deaths:

1. About 25 per cent of patients experiencing sudden death have no previous history of cardiac disease, yet the presence of an old myocardial infarction and extensive coronary artery disease are found in over 75 per cent of victims of sudden death.[1]

2. Myocardial infarction can occur in the absence of symptoms. In the Framingham Study involving 5127 participants, 708 myocardial infarctions occurred over 30 years. Of those, 25 per cent were "silent" and discovered fortuitously by standard electrocardiographic criteria during routine follow-up visits. Furthermore, silent infarctions were almost as likely as symptomatic infarctions to cause cardiac complications such as death or cardiac failure. Within 10 years of follow-up, cardiovascular death occurred in 26 per cent of male patients with either silent or symptomatic myocardial infarctions.[2]

3. The development of several noninvasive methods of detecting the presence of myocardial ischemia (such as stress testing with or without radionuclide studies, ambulatory electrocardiographic monitoring) has allowed the identification of patients with some evidence of myocardial ischemia in absence of symptoms (so-called silent myocardial isch-

emia). There is growing evidence that such patients have a prognosis similar to patients with angina and are at increased risk for cardiac complications including death.[3]

Our chapter will only focus on patients with silent myocardial ischemia.

Classification

According to Cohn and Kannel,[3] patients with silent myocardial ischemia can be classified into three groups:

Group 1. Patients with evidence of intermittent myocardial ischemia who never have symptoms.
Group 2. Patients with evidence of intermittent myocardial ischemia who have symptoms with some ischemic episodes but not with others.
Group 3. Patients with previous myocardial infarction who present intermittent myocardial ischemia but no symptoms.

These three groups have recently been the subject of intense investigation. They have in common the occurrence of painless myocardial ischemia and an increased incidence of subsequent cardiac complications including death.

Mechanism of Silent Myocardial Ischemia

Myocardial ischemia, in general, is triggered either by increased myocardial oxygen demand in the presence of limited coronary reserve (due to coronary artery disease) or by decreased myocardial blood supply. The role of decreased myocardial blood supply, due presumably to coronary vasoconstriction, has been first suggested by studies using ambulatory electrocardiographic monitoring. It has been shown that significant electrocardiographic ST segment depression, suggesting ischemia, can occur daily in patients with known coronary artery disease, in absence of significant increases in heart rate, which is one of the major components of myocardial oxygen demand.[4,5] Similar findings were made following smoking[6] and mental stress,[7] suggesting intermittent vasoconstriction and decreased myocardial blood supply. Angiographic and hemodynamic studies have confirmed the presence of vasoconstriction during exercise,[8,9] smoking,[10] or exposure to cold.[11] Such vasoconstriction can be due to sympathetic stimulation or, as more recently suggested, an abnormal endothelium-dependent coronary dilation in atherosclerotic coronary artery disease.[12]

On the other hand, increased myocardial oxygen demand has been suggested by others as a cause of intermittent silent or symptomatic myocardial ischemia. In these studies, myocardial ischemia was often preceded by slight increases in heart rate and was mostly seen in the early morning hours, paralleling the circadian increase in heart rate and blood pressure.[13,14,15]

It is very likely, however, that both mechanisms of ischemia are present in patients and that one mechanism may predominant in some patients or even in the same patient at various times during the day. For example, it has been demonstrated that an increase in heart rate may cause ischemia in the morning but that the same increase may not result in ischemia in the evening, suggesting increased coronary vasoconstriction in the morning hours.[14]

Whether painful or silent, it is likely that myocardial ischemia is triggered by similar mechanisms. Indeed, in patients with myocardial ischemia during ambulatory electrocardiographic monitoring, both silent and painful manifestations of ischemia seem to be triggered by similar increases in heart rates and to occur at the same time and during similar daily activities. Furthermore, both silent and painful ischemia respond to similar treatments, suggesting common pathophysiologic mechanisms.[15,16,17]

There are at least three possible causes for the absence of pain during myocardial ischemia. First, the pain threshold may be higher in patients with silent ischemia. This hypothesis is supported by findings of Droste and Roskamm.[18] In their study, patients with silent ischemia had a higher threshold to other painful stimuli such as electrical pain, cold, or tourniquet. Second, myocardial ischemia may be less severe when silent. This hypothesis is supported by findings of shorter duration of ST segment depression and less evidence of left ventricular dysfunction during painless ischemia.[19,20] However, this hypothesis is controversial. And third, previous myocardial infarction may cause autonomic denervation due to scarring and result in areas of myocardium insensitive to painful stimuli.[21]

Prognosis

Numerous studies have shown that prognosis is altered by the presence of symptomatic as well as painless myocardial ischemia. We will review some of these studies in the three groups.

Group 1

Studies on patients with totally silent ischemia have always used treadmill testing as screening test except for one Swedish study that used ambulatory electrocardiographic monitoring. In the Seattle Heart Watch study[22] including more than 4000 persons with no history of heart disease, patients with abnormal treadmill tests and any risk factor such as hypertension, hypercholesterolemia, diabetes, or smoking had a six-year survival of 76 per cent, compared to 98 per cent for those with normal tests. Similar findings were confirmed in several other epidemiologic studies of asymptomatic persons.[23,24,25] In these studies, the presence of an abnormal exercise test increased the risk of cardiac complications such as angina, myocardial infarction, and death. However, it is important to remember that even though the relative risk of cardiac events is increased by severalfold in asymptomatic patients with abnormal exercise tests, the predictive value of an abnormal test for the occurrence of cardiac events remains low. The result of each test should be interpreted with caution and individualized. As will be discussed later, in a population with a low likelihood of having coronary artery disease, an abnormal exercise test is more likely to be a false-positive. Therefore, in a given patient, the predictive value of an abnormal exercise test for detection of coronary artery disease and cardiac events is increased by the presence of associated risk factors for coronary artery disease, by the presence of associated thallium scintigraphic defects, and by an abnormal exercise test in a patient with previously normal tests.

In the only epidemiologic study from Sweden using 24-hour ambulatory electrocardiographic monitoring,[26] patients with transient asymptomatic ST segment depression had a 14 per cent risk of death within 43 months, compared with 7 per cent in patients with a normal study.

In patients with abnormal exercise tests and documented coronary artery disease using coronary angiography, cardiac events are more commonly seen in the follow-up, as a majority of patients with false-positive exercise tests are not included. In the U.S. Air Force School of Aerospace Medicine study, Hickman et al. found 78 asymptomatic men with abnormal exercise tests and coronary artery disease documented by angiography.[27] Of those, 22 developed overt signs of coronary disease such as angina, myocardial infarction, and death in a follow-up extending up to 90 months. These findings were confirmed in other reports. Furthermore, in the Coronary Artery Surgery Study (CASS) Registry,[28,29] it has been shown that in a population of asymptomatic patients the presence of left main or three vessel coronary artery disease, particularly when associated with decreased left ventricular ejection fraction, is associated with decreased survival and merits consideration for revascularization.

Group 2

Similar findings have been made in patients with symptoms during some ischemic episodes but not with others.

STABLE ANGINA. In a study of stable angina by Rocco et al.,[30] the presence of ischemia on a 24-hour ambulatory electrocardiographic monitoring was associated with a high incidence of cardiac events, including death, myocardial infarction, and unstable angina in a group of 86 patients with abnormal treadmill tests and angiographically proven coronary artery disease in 67 of them. Interestingly, only 14 per cent of the ischemic episodes were symptomatic. Similar findings were reported by others, suggesting that the "ischemic burden," even painless, may affect prognosis in patients with documented coronary artery disease. It remains to be shown, however, in larger series of patients if the presence of repeated ambulatory ischemia, often silent, is independently associated with poor prognosis, once several exercise parameters, clinical factors, and angiographic data are taken into consideration.

UNSTABLE ANGINA. Several studies have shown that the persistence of intermittent ST segment depression, often painless, in patients following admission for unstable angina is associated with a high occurrence rate of deaths, myocardial infarction, and presence of severe coronary artery stenosis.[31,32] Similar poor outcome has been shown to occur in patients with abnormal predischarge exercise tests. The relative value of exercise testing and ambulatory electrocardiographic monitoring in predicting events is, as for patients with stable angina, unknown.

Group 3

Following myocardial infarction, multiple studies in patients have shown that the presence of ischemia during exercise testing or ambulatory electrocardiographic monitoring is associated with high subsequent incidence of cardiac complications, including death. Theroux et al.[33] first reported that in the year following the infarct cardiac mortality was 27 per cent in patients following myocardial infarction who had a greater than 1 mm of ST segment depression during exercise but only 2.1 per cent in those with a normal test. This was confirmed by several studies, some of which had associated thallium scintigraphy or radionuclide ventriculography. Interestingly, in these studies, about 50 per cent of patients were asymptomatic despite an abnormal exercise response.

In a study using ambulatory electrocardiography monitoring in high-risk postinfarction patients, Gottlieb et al.[34] showed that the presence of transient ST segment depression was associated with a 40 per cent incidence of reinfarction or death, compared with 11 per cent in patients with negative studies in the year following infarction. Twenty-eight of the 30 patients with ST depression had no symptoms during the test. Furthermore, those changes were the most important factor of mortality, independently of age, type of infarction, symptoms of cardiac failure, or left ventricular ejection fraction. Again, the relative value of exercise testing and ambulatory electrocardiographic monitoring is not known.

HISTORY

The clinical evaluation of patients with possible silent myocardial ischemia is similar to that of patients with overt symptoms. Risk factors for coronary artery disease should be carefully evaluated because in patients without overt symptoms risk factors may lead to suspicion of coronary artery disease:

1. Hyperlipidemia (hypercholesterolemia with low HDL : LDL [high-density lipoprotein to low-density lipoprotein] ratio).
2. Smoking.
3. Hypertension (both systolic and diastolic).
4. Family history of premature coronary artery disease (before the age of 50).
5. Obesity and distribution of fat (a central distribution of fat, with a high waist-to-hip ratio, is associated with increased risk of coronary artery disease).
6. Diabetes mellitus (in which the prevalence of silent myocardial ischemia is higher than in the general population).
7. Sedentary life.
8. Stress.

A careful history of symptoms can identify patients with mild symptoms, atypical radiation of the pain, and angina "equivalents," such as intermittent dyspnea, faintness, or belching. Angina can present as a vague pressure sensation or fullness in the chest. It can cause pain in the left or right arm or in both arms. Epigastric discomfort and neck or jaw pains are not uncommon.

PHYSICAL EXAMINATION

A number of signs are associated with the presence of coronary artery disease, whether symptomatic or not. These include:

1. Signs of hypercholesterolemia, such as arcus senilis, xanthelasma, and xanthomas.
2. Elevated blood pressure.
3. Presence of carotid or peripheral arterial disease (absence of pulse or presence of bruits).
4. Presence of a precordial dyskinetic bulge on palpation in patients with previous myocardial infarction.
5. Loud S_4 on auscultation, in absence of left ventricular hypertrophy; intermittent paradoxical splitting of S_2; intermittent mitral regurgitation with early, late, or holosystolic apical murmurs.
6. Diagonal earlobe crease, except in American Indians and Orientals.

DIAGNOSTIC STUDIES

Electrocardiogram

Except during episodes of ischemia, resting electrocardiogram (ECG) is of little help in the evaluation of a patient with suspected silent ischemia. Minor ST-T segment abnormalities are common in patients with coronary artery disease but lack specificity. Conduction disturbances such as left bundle branch block or left anterior fascicular block have also been more frequently found in patients with coronary artery disease but are also nonspecific. On the other hand, the presence of Q waves, particularly if new, strongly suggests the presence of coronary artery disease.

Exercise Testing

Exercise testing, as discussed previously, has been shown to be valuable in identifying high-risk patients for coronary events, even in absence of symptoms. In absence of symptoms, the predictive value of exercise testing is, however, highly dependent on the prevalence of coronary artery disease in the population tested. For instance, a positive exercise test in a 20-year-old man with no known risk factors is likely to be a false-positive; in a 55-year-old long-standing smoker, a similar result would make the presence of coronary artery disease highly likely. Thus, the result of exercise testing should be interpreted in light of clinical presentation.

The following exercise parameters can be used to identify patients at particularly high risk for coronary artery disease and cardiac events and therefore may increase the specificity of the test even in absence of symptoms: occurrence of ST depression and/or chest pain at low work load or low heart rate; severe ST depression (greater than 2 mm), particularly if occurring early during exercise; and exercise-induced fall in blood pressure

Thallium scintigraphy or radionuclide ventriculography performed during exercise increases the sensitivity and specificity of exercise tests and is useful in patients suspected of false-positive electrocardiographic exercise responses. High-risk patients can be identified with the following criteria: thallium scintigraphy—presence of multiple or large reversible defects, increased lung uptake (due to an increase in left ventricular filling pressure during exercise); and radionuclide ventriculography—greater than 10 per cent decrease in left ventricular ejection fraction at peak exercise.

Ambulatory Electrocardiographic Monitoring

As discussed previously, the presence of transient ST segment depression in daily life has been associated with an increased incidence of cardiac events and death in various populations. Technical aspects of ambulatory electrocardiographic monitoring are important and well described in other reviews.[3] As for exercise testing, it should be remembered that the predictive value of ST segment is much lower in patients with low likelihood of coronary artery disease.

Which patients should undergo ambulatory electrocardiographic monitoring is still unclear. Furthermore, the relative value of this test compared with exercise testing in various groups of patients is still unclear. Patients unable to undergo exercise testing because of physical disability or functional capacity may be candidates for ambulatory electrocardiographic monitoring.

ASSESSMENT

Assessment of patients with silent myocardial ischemia depends on the clinical presentation.

Group 1

Asymptomatic persons should be screened early in life for risk factors, especially in the presence of a family history of coronary artery disease. If present, these factors need to be controlled—first by changing life-style and habits (such as exercise, diet, and smoking). Patients with overt hypercholesterolemia or hypertension should be considered for medical treatment. Exercise testing should probably be done in men above 40 years and in women above 45 years if risk factors for coronary artery disease are identified. If the exercise test is abnormal, the patients can be followed medically, but those with marked abnormalities during the test should be referred for cardiac catheterization. Patients with low likelihood of coronary artery disease and abnormal exercise test should undergo exercise testing coupled with radionuclide study.

If abnormal, the patient should be treated medically or referred for cardiac catheterization.

The place of ambulatory electrocardiographic monitoring in such patients is not yet well defined, as it has not proved to add additional information to what is learned from exercise testing. Because exercise testing is easier to perform, it remains the test of choice in patients suspected to have coronary artery disease.

Group 2

Stable Angina

Exercise testing is useful to confirm the diagnosis of angina and to identify a high-risk group with marked changes during the test. The scheme, then, is similar as for group 1: follow medically or refer high-risk patients for cardiac catheterization.

Again, the relative predictive value of ambulatory electrocardiographic monitoring compared with exercise testing is still unclear. Therefore, it is currently not used routinely. Some patients unable physically to undergo exercise testing may be candidates for monitoring.

Unstable Angina

Patients admitted for unstable angina should be closely monitored for signs of recurring myocardial ischemia. These signs include: (1) recurrent angina or (2) electrocardiographic evidence of myocardial ischemia, even painless, during either low-grade exercise testing (performed on day 3 or 4 in pain-free patients) or ambulatory electrocardiographic monitoring. Any patients with recurrent myocardial ischemia should undergo cardiac catheterization. Again, whether ambulatory electrocardiographic recording adds useful information to what is learned for exercise testing is not known. Exercise testing is currently used more commonly except in disabled patients.

Group 3

The management of patients following myocardial infarction with evidence of symptomatic or painless ischemia is similar to that of patients with unstable angina. Any patient with recurrent sign of ischemia should be promptly referred for cardiac catheterization. Generally, low-grade exercise testing is recommended at day 8 to 10 following infarction in pain-free patients, and ST change is considered a marker of residual ischemia, even in absence of symptoms. Ambulatory electrocardiographic recording is usually reserved for disabled patients, as its independent value, compared with exercise testing, is not yet known.

REFERENCES

1. Myerburg RJ, Castellanos A. Cardiac arrest and sudden cardiac death. In: Braunwald ME, ed. Heart disease. Philadelphia: WB Saunders Co, 1988:742–77.
2. Kannel WB, Abbott RD. Incidence and prognosis of unrecognized myocardial infarction: an update on the Framingham Study. N Engl J Med 1984;311:1144–7.
3. Cohn PF, Kannel WB. Recognition, pathogenesis, and management options in silent coronary artery disease. Circulation 1987;75(2):1–54.
4. Schang SJ Jr, Pepine CJ. Transient asymptomatic ST-segment depression during daily activity. Am J Cardiol 1977;39;396–402.
5. Deanfield JE, Selwyn AP, Chierchia S, et al. Myocardial ischemia during daily life in patients with stable angina: its relation to symptoms and heart rate changes. Lancet 1983;2:753–8.
6. Deanfield JE, Shea MJ Wilson RA, Horlock P, de Landsheere CM, Selwyn AP. Direct effects of smoking on the heart: silent ischemic disturbances of coronary flow. Am J Cardiol 1988;57:1005–9.
7. Deanfield JE, Kensett M, Wilson RA, et al. Silent myocardial ischemia due to mental stress. Lancet 1984;2:1001–4.
8. Brown BG, Lee AB, Bolson EL, Dodge HT. Reflex constriction of significant coronary stenosis as a mechanism contributing to ischemic left ventricular dysfunction during isometric exercise. Circulation 1984;70:18–24.
9. Gage JE, Hess OM, Murakami T, Ritter M, Grimm J, Krayenbuehl HP. Vasoconstriction of stenotic coronary arteries during dynamic exercise in patients with classic angina pectoris: reversibility by nitroglycerin. Circulation 1986;73:865–76.
10. Nicod P, Rehr R, Winniford MD, Campbell WB, Firth BG, Hillis LD. Acute systemic and coronary hemodynamic and serologic responses to cigarette smoking in long-term smokers with atherosclerotic coronary artery disease. J Am Coll Cardiol 1984;4:964–71.
11. Gordon JB, Ganz P, Nabel EG, et al. Atherosclerosis influences the vasomotor response of epicardial coronary arteries to exercise. J Clin Invest 1989;83:1946–52.
12. Ludmer P, Selwyn A, Shook T, Mudge G, Alexander R, Ganz P. Paradoxical vasoconstriction induced by acetylcholine in atherosclerotic coronary arteries. N Engl J Med 1986;315:1046–51.
13. Davies AB, Bala Subramanian V, Cashman PM, Raftery EB. Simultaneous recording of continuous arterial pressure, heart rate, and ST-segment in ambulant patients with stable angina. Br Heart J 1983;50:85–91.
14. Rocco MB, Barry J, Campbell S, et al. Circadian variation of transient myocardial ischemia in pa-tients with coronary artery disease. Circulation 1987;75:395–400.
15. Mulcahy D, Cunningham D, Crean P, et al. Circadian variation of total ischemia burden and its alteration with anti-anginal agents. Lancet 1988;2:755–9.
16. Imperi GA, Lambert CR, Coy K, Lopez L, Pepine CJ. Effects of titrated metoprolol on silent myocardial ischemia in ambulatory patients with coronary artery disease. Am J Cardiol 1987;60:519–24.
17. Cohn PF, Lawson WE. Effects of long-acting propranolol on AM and PM peaks in silent myocardial ischemia. Am J Cardiol 1989;63:872–3.
18. Droste C, Roskamm H. Experimental pain measurement in patients with asymptomatic myocardial ischemia. J Am Coll Cardiol 1983;1:940–5.
19. Cecchi AC, Dovellini EV, Marchi F, Pucci P, Santoro GM, Fazzini PF. Silent myocardial ischemia during ambulatory electrocardiographic monitoring in patients with effort angina. J Am Coll Cardiol 1983;1:934–9.
20. Chierchia S, Lazzari M, Freedman B, Brunelli C, Maseri A. Impairment of myocardial perfusion and function during painless myocardial ischemia. J Am Coll Cardiol 1983;1:924–30.
21. Inoue H, Skals B, Zipes D. Effects of ischemia on cardiac afferent sympathetic and vagal reflexes in dog. Am J Physiol 1988;255:425–35.
22. Bruce RA, Hossack KF, DeRouen TA, Hofer V. Enhanced risk assessment for primary coronary heart disease events by maximal exercise testing: 10 years' experience of Seattle Heart Watch. J Am Coll Cardiol 1983;2:565–73.
23. Allen WH, Aronow SW, Goodman P, Stinson P. Five year follow-up of maximal treadmill test in asymptomatic men and women. Circulation 1980;62:522–7.
24. Giagnoni E, Secchi MB, Wu SC, et al. Prognostic value of exercise EKG testing in asymptomatic normotensive subjects: a prospective matched study. N Engl J Med 1983;309:1085–9.
25. Gordon DJ, Ekelund LG, Karon JM, et al. Predictive value of the exercise test for mortality in North American men: the Lipid Research Clinics Mortality Follow-Up Study. Circulation 1986;74:252–61.
26. Hedsblad B, Juul-Moller S, Svensson K, et al. Increased mortality in men with ST-segment depression during 24 h ambulatory long term ECG recording: results from prospective population study "Men born in 1914," from Malmo, Sweden. Eur Heart J 1989;10:149–58.
27. Hickman JR Jr, Uhl GS, Cook RL, Engel PH, Hopkirk A. A natural history study of asymptomatic coronary disease [Abstract]. Am J Cardiol 1980;45:422.
28. Taylor HA, Deumite NJ, Chaitman BR, Davis KB, Killip T, Rogers WJ. Asymptomatic left main coronary artery disease in the Coronary Artery Surgery Study (CASS) Registry. Circulation 1989;79:1171–9.
29. Weiner DA, Ryan TJ, McCabe CH, et al. Comparison of coronary artery bypass surgery and medical therapy in patients with exercise-induced silent myocardial ischemia: a report from the Coronary Artery Surgery Study (CASS) Registry. J Am Coll Cardiol 1988;12:595–9.
30. Rocco MB, Nabel EG, Campbell S, et al. Prognostic

importance of myocardial ischemia detected by ambulatory monitoring in patients with coronary disease. Circulation 1988;78:877–84.

31. Gottlieb SO, Weisfeldt ML, Ouyang P, Mellits ED, Gerstenblith G. Silent ischemia predicts infarction and death during two year follow-up of unstable angina. J Am Coll Cardiol 1987;10:756–60.

32. Nademanee K, Intarachot V, Josephson MA, Rieders D, Mody FV, Singh BN. Prognostic significance of silent myocardial ischemia in patients with unstable angina. J Am Coll Cardiol 1987;10:1–9.

33. Theroux P, Waters D, Halphen C, Debaisieux J, Mizgala H: Prognostic value of exercise testing soon after myocardial infarction. N Engl J Med 1979;301:341–5.

34. Gottlieb S, Achuff S, et al. Silent ischemia on Holter monitoring predicts mortality in high-risk post-infarction patients. JAMA 1988;259:1030–5.

SLEEPINESS, EXCESSIVE

ROCCO L. MANFREDI and JOYCE D. KALES

SYNONYMS: Daytime Sleepiness, Prolonged Sleep

BACKGROUND

Excessive daytime sleepiness is a relatively common symptom of various conditions. As a result of more sophisticated diagnostic information provided by the sleep laboratory, the generic term hypersomnia currently is less often used. Instead, most specialists consider three specific diagnoses that present with excessive sleepiness or hypersomnia as their primary symptom: narcolepsy, hypersomnia, and sleep apnea.[1–6] Narcolepsy is characterized by periods of irresistible sleep of brief duration and often by certain auxiliary symptoms. Hypersomnia is distinguished by periods of excessive sleepiness that are relatively more resistible but longer in duration and by the absence of auxiliary symptoms. Patients with sleep apnea characteristically present with a history of excessive daytime sleepiness, sleep attacks, and repetitive nocturnal breath cessations associated with very loud snoring and gasping sounds.

All these disorders cause the patients significant inconvenience and distress; and sleep apnea, in particular, results in serious and often life-threatening sequelae. Most often, these disorders can be differentiated based on the patient's history and current symptoms.

The prevalence of narcolepsy is about 1 in 1000, with men and women being equally affected.[4,6] The initial symptoms, which are usually excessive sleepiness and sleep attacks, most often have their onset during late childhood or early adolescence. It typically begins before the age of 25 years and has a chronic clinical course without major remissions.

Dysfunction within the dopaminergic system probably plays an important role in the symptoms of narcolepsy. In addition, the sleep attacks and certain of the auxiliary symptoms of narcolepsy have been attributed to the neurophysiologic mechanisms that govern rapid eye movement (REM) sleep, specifically, the interaction of the lower brain stem centers during REM sleep.[7] Electroencephalographic (EEG) patterns of arousal, REM bursts, autonomic irregularity, myoclonic twitches, and ponto-geniculo-occipital spikes are a result of the nucleus reticularis pontis caudalis stimulating an ascending activating system. Conversely, areflexia and loss of muscle tone are a result of the locus ceruleus triggering a descending inhibitory system.

The onset of narcolepsy, in certain cases, has been associated with specific neuropathologic diseases, including brain trauma and brain tumors.[4] Epilepsy, however, has not been shown to be etiologic in narcolepsy.

Abnormalities in circadian rhythms have also been identified among narcoleptic patients. This is reflected both clinically and polygraphically by their disturbed nocturnal sleep and abnormal timing of REM sleep.[6] Nonetheless, the exact nature and extent of the chronobiologic disturbance in narcolepsy have not yet been determined. Recent studies have reported an abnormal 24-hour rhythm of core temperature in narcoleptics,[8] higher nocturnal temperatures, and an earlier occurrence of their temperature minimum compared with control subjects, and normal nocturnal dampening of ultradian rhythms of daytime vigilance may be lost in narcolepsy.

About 5 per 1000 of the population are estimated to be affected by the condition of hypersomnia, with a slight male predominance.[4] Most often, the condition develops in puberty and then remains fairly consistent throughout life without major remission. The etiology of hypersomnia will vary according to whether the condition is idiopathic, secondary, or periodic. Several studies have shown a familial incidence of idiopathic hypersomnia.[4,5,9] Analysis of family history data indicates a close link between narcolepsy and hypersomnia along the lines of a two-threshold multifactorial mode of inheritance.[5,10]

Abnormalities in three neurotransmitter systems—serotonergic, cholinergic, and dopaminergic—may be involved with hypersomnia. For example, increased levels of 3,4-dihydroxyphenylacetic acid and homovanillic acid (HVA), which suggest increased dopamine turnover, have been demonstrated as well as decreased indolamine (tryptamine) metabolism in hypersomniac patients.[11] Although hypersomnia may be caused by a variety of lesions, their common characteristic is an interruption of the ascending reticular pathways. Secondary hypersomnia is clearly related to neurologic factors, as arousing and activating systems in the brain are largely concentrated in the junction between the rostral midbrain and the posterior diencephalon.[12] Destruction is always followed by deep coma, and the patient is unarousable, both clinically and electroencephalographically (cerveau isolé). Specific conditions resulting in hypersomnia include head injuries with or without hemorrhage, cerebrovascular insufficiency, brain tumors and other expansive lesions, and in rare cases, other brain syndromes (e.g., Kearns-Sayre syndrome).[4,11]

Medical causes of hypersomnia include metabolic disorders, conditions leading to brain hypoxia, and various toxic influences. Metabolic disorders include hepatic encephalopathy, renal insufficiency, hypoglycemia, and adrenal insufficiency.[4,11] Conditions leading to brain hypoxia are most often secondary to severe cardiovascular insufficiency, anemia, or pulmonary disease. Finally, intoxication with certain industrial poisons (e.g., methylchloride and trichlorethylene) and various medications (such as hypnotics, anxiolytics, and antihistamines) may also lead to hypersomnia.[4]

Secondary hypersomnia is often a result of significant life stress events and psychiatric disorders, especially affective illness. It has also been demonstrated in patients with bipolar disorders and among young depressed patients.[13]

Understanding of the nature of periodic hypersomnias remains incomplete. Most research supports the concept of pathophysiologic dysfunction in the mesodiencephalic region, particularly of the hypothalamus and limbic areas.[4,11] Fluctuations of the condition with the menstrual cycle has suggested a hormonal cause; diffuse paroxysmal slowing on the EEG of some patients suggests a seizure disorder.

Sleep apnea is characterized as central, obstructive (peripheral), or mixed[1-3] (see Table 1). In central apnea, thoracic and abdominal respiratory effort is absent, whereas in obstructive apnea primary respiratory efforts persist but are rendered ineffective by upper airway blockage. In mixed apnea, the episode begins with the absence of respiratory effort followed by upper airway obstruction. Of

TABLE 1.   Clinical Characteristics of Sleep Apnea

TYPE OF APNEA	CLINICAL MANIFESTATIONS
Obstructive	History of snoring and typical intermittent snorting and gasping sounds
	Nocturnal breath cessations observable by bed partner and often perceived by the patient
	Excessive daytime sleepiness and sleep attacks
	Nocturnal body movements, excessive sweating, nocturnal enuresis, loss of libido, morning headaches, obesity, cognitive impairment
	Hypertension and other cardiovascular complications
Central	History of snoring uncharacteristic
	Nocturnal breath cessations often reported
	Usually excessive daytime sleepiness and at times complaints of insomnia

(From Kales A, Vela-Bueno A, Kales JD. Sleep disorders: sleep apnea and narcolepsy. Ann Intern Med 1987;106:434–43.)

these types, obstructive sleep apnea is by far the commonest. (Also see chapter on Sleep Apnea in *Difficult Medical Management,* WB Saunders Co., 1991.)

The disorder of sleep apnea is more prevalent in men[2,3] and in persons with certain major health problems and often may be associated with obesity and hypertension.[7,12,14,15] The condition is seldom seen in normal persons, although there is an age-related increase in the prevalence of mild sleep apneic activity.[16] Symptoms are typically manifest before the age of 40, and the appearance tends to cluster within a few years.

Much speculation about the exact pathogenesis of sleep apnea exists. Genetics appear to play a role in at least some patients. Common snoring and obstructive sleep apnea may actually belong to the same pathophysiologic continuum.[17] Pathophysiologically, obstruction during inspiration is considered to result from failure of contraction of either the pharyngeal muscles or the muscles that hold the tongue forward. As a result of continued diaphragmatic contraction, subatmospheric pressure is generated and the flaccid pharyngeal wall is sucked inward.[6] Finally, obstructive and mixed sleep apnea may be caused by an instability of respiratory control during sleep.

Certain hormonal factors have also been linked with sleep apnea. Hypothyroidism may result in obesity, infiltration of the tongue and upper airway with myxomatous tissue, and abnormalities in control of breathing that contribute to apneas.[2,6] Furthermore, disordered breathing and oxygen desaturation are common among women after menopause, probably secondary to the loss of the respiratory stimulating effects of the progestational hormones.[18,19] In men, the presence of testosterone may predispose them to obstructive sleep apnea.[19]

Anatomically, patients with sleep apnea have been found to demonstrate smaller pharyngeal areas than those found in controls.[6] Occasionally, gross anatomic factors such as mandibular malformation, micrognathia, tonsillar and adenoidal hypertrophy, nasal septal deviation, nasal obstruction, acromegaly, vocal cord paralysis, or glottal web play a major contributory role.

Alcohol ingestion, sleep deprivation, and use of central nervous system (CNS) depressants have been shown to increase the number and severity of sleep apneic events in both patients with sleep apnea and normal controls.[6]

HISTORY

A general medical history and physical examination, drug history, a thorough psychiatric history, and a comprehensive sleep history[20] are essential components in the evaluation of excessive sleepiness. The sleep history must first define the specific problem. For example, the physician must determine whether a complaint of daytime tiredness, fatigue, or sleepiness is associated with insomnia or represents the excessive daytime sleepiness associated with narcolepsy, hypersomnia, or sleep apnea. The physician should also determine the onset of the disorder and assess its clinical course.

It is often helpful to evaluate sleep/wakefulness patterns on a 24-hour, seven-day-a-week basis rather than simply evaluating the nocturnal sleep period.[20] The patient's bed partner can often provide important information that cannot be elicited directly from the patient. Sleep apnea cannot be adequately evaluated without information from the bed partner or family. For example, when evaluating a complaint of daytime sleepiness, the physician should ask the bed partner if the patient's sleep time includes periodic snoring sounds with intervals of more than 10 to 15 seconds; such symptoms indicate the possibility of obstructive sleep apnea.

Because numerous medications affect sleep in various ways, a thorough drug history is essential when evaluating the patient with excessive sleepiness.[20] For example, a number of pharmacologic agents such as stimulant drugs, steroids, theophylline preparations, and some antidepressants and beta-adrenergic blockers, as well as current and past use of hypnotic drugs, have been found to disturb sleep at night, resulting in excessive sleepiness during the day. Drinking large quantities of coffee or cola close to bedtime as well as smoking cigarettes and consuming alcohol have also been shown to disturb sleep. Conversely, excessive daytime sleepiness may result from inappropriate dosages or scheduling of certain CNS depressants and sedating antidepressants.

The classic symptoms of narcolepsy include excessive daytime sleepiness and irresistible sleep attacks most often occurring in conjunction with one or more of three auxiliary symptoms: cataplexy, sleep paralysis, and hypnagogic hallucinations.[4,6,20] Sleep attacks are often precipitated by sedentary, monotonous situations, such as watching television, reading, or driving; they last from a few seconds to half an hour. The narcoleptic often experiences a sleep attack at work, during a conversation, or under other circumstances that ordinarily are considered to be stimulating. (Also see chapter on Narcolepsy in *Difficult Medical Management,* WB Saunders Co., 1991.)

About 70 to 80 per cent of narcoleptics will also report cataplexy. Patients who have this symptom report a brief (lasting a few seconds to two minutes), sudden loss of muscle control that may cause them to collapse while remaining conscious.[4,5,6,20] This often occurs in relation to strong emotional experiences, such as laughter, surprise, or anger. Milder episodes involve only slight knee buckling or drooping of the head or jaw. Many narcoleptic patients develop a flat affect and generalized inexpressiveness, probably in an attempt to control the emotions that could trigger a cataplectic attack. About one fourth to one half of narcoleptics will report sleep paralysis or hypnagogic hallucinations. During sleep paralysis, there is a temporary loss of muscle tone and an inability to move. Hypnagogic hallucinations are vivid, formed hallucinatory perceptions (usually visual or auditory) that occur particularly while falling asleep. Both symptoms occur during the period of transition between wakefulness and sleep and last only for a minute or less. Infrequent episodes of sleep paralysis or hypnagogic hallucinations may occur even in normal persons, but in patients with narcolepsy they may occur far more frequently, up to several times in a week. Patients with narcolepsy may report complex automatic behavior that may last up to several hours. During periods of altered consciousness, patients may continue to speak, write, drive, and perform other activities in an impaired, mechanical fashion. Subsequently, they are typically amnestic for the event.

Recurrent, lengthy periods of excessive sleepiness are characteristic of hypersomnia.[4,6] The nap itself tends to last several hours, and usually the patient awakens feeling unrefreshed. Nighttime sleep is typically prolonged, often lasting up to several days, and rarely is interrupted by awakenings. Patients typically fall asleep at night extremely quickly, that is, within a few seconds. Difficulty with awakening in the morning and sleep

drunkenness, a rather prolonged state of confusion on awakening, are common complaints. Long periods of intense sleepiness may also occur; in some cases, it is more or less permanent.[4,6] Often, the symptom is only alleviated by movement, exercise, stimulating activities, or caffeinated beverages. Eating during monotonous activities is commonly reported to exacerbate sleepiness.

Clinically, hypersomnia is suspected whenever the complaint of constant and persistent daytime sleepiness is discovered in the absence of the auxiliary symptoms of narcolepsy or loud nocturnal snoring. When excessive sleepiness is secondary to mental disorders, sleep is not only prolonged but also restless and generally disturbed; patients often feel worse on arising in the morning, but they do not present with the confusion that is characteristic of sleep drunkenness.

The Kleine-Levin syndrome is a rare disorder that occurs usually during adolescence, with a strong male predominance.[4,11] It is characterized by periodic hypersomnia associated with hyperphagia. The attacks occur two to three times a year, with each episode lasting for periods of two to three weeks. Typically, the patient sleeps for extended periods of time, arising from bed only to eat or excrete. Often, the eating periods resemble binge episodes. The attacks are usually associated with irritability, aggression, or dysphoria and may be followed by periods of increased sexual drive.

Excessive daytime sleepiness is also a characteristic symptom of obstructive sleep apnea. In addition, patients present with sleep attacks and repetitive nocturnal breath cessations associated with very loud snoring and gasping sounds.[1,2] Respiratory pauses, which may last from 10 seconds to more than a minute, are followed by intermittent snorting sounds lasting 2 to 4 seconds, which occur as the airway begins to open. In contrast, the common snoring of persons without sleep apnea is softer, fluctuates in intensity, and is continuous, without any interruptions of appreciable duration. In a large group of patients with severe obstructive sleep apnea, snoring was generally reported to be the first manifestation of this condition, starting in more than half of the sample at or before age 20.[21] In most patients, the bed partner or roommate observes periods of breath cessation followed by snorting and gasping.[2,6,20,21] However, some patients with sleep apnea are aware of having nighttime respiratory difficulty, which they may experience as a choking sensation. Excessive body movements during sleep, sweating, secondary enuresis, sexual dysfunction, and early morning headaches are additional symptoms that may occur.[2,21]

Although patients with obstructive sleep apnea easily fall asleep, their nocturnal sleep is very disrupted. At the end of each repetitive respiratory pause, there is a very short-lasting arousal (probably related to hypercapnia), and then resumption of breathing ensues. Despite these repetitive brief arousals, generally the patient does not awaken fully. Thus, although their sleep is extremely disturbed, apneic patients almost always complain of daytime sleepiness rather than insomnia.

PHYSICAL EXAMINATION

A comprehensive medical history and a thorough physical examination should be included in every sleep patient's evaluation. Careful reassessment of the patient's previous diagnoses is warranted because they may have been inaccurate. A thorough psychiatric evaluation is also essential for cases of hypersomnia.

Narcolepsy has sometimes been misdiagnosed as hypothyroidism, hypoglycemia, epilepsy, myasthenia gravis, or multiple sclerosis.[4,6,11] Independent cataplexy, or cataplexy that precedes the onset of other symptoms, may be mistaken for drop attacks, which are actually due to brain stem vascular insufficiency. In the rare case that positive findings are demonstrated on the neurologic examination, a more thorough workup for structural brain lesions is recommended. The medical history for hypersomnia focuses on previous conditions or injuries that may have a bearing on the current symptoms, such as head injuries, organic brain disease, and exposure to toxins.

The physical examination of patients with suspected sleep apnea should include a thorough otorhinolaryngologic evaluation. Patients often present with moderate hypertension and obesity; in half the cases of severe obstructive sleep apnea, the age of onset of these two conditions precedes that of daytime sleepiness by at least one year.[21] Systemic hypertension is a common consequence of obstructive sleep apnea.[17] Pulmonary hypertension, when present, has been found to relate to increases in pulmonary wedge pressures. The hypoxia and carbon dioxide retention associ-ated with the nocturnal apneic events may contribute to the eventual development of polycythemia and the cardiovascular complications of pulmonary hypertension, cardiomegaly, right-sided heart failure, and persistent cardiac dysrhythmias.[1]

Cognitive impairment may also result from severe obstructive sleep apneas. This may be manifested by a general slowing of thought processes, reduced attention span, memory impairment (especially for recent events), and visual-perceptual difficulties.[22] Also, a high level of psychologic distress with frequent and marked disruption of psychosocial functioning may occur.

DIAGNOSTIC STUDIES

HLA antigen markers have been identified in both narcolepsy and hypersomnia. A recent study showed a prevalence of HLA-DR2 of 100 per cent in narcoleptic patients,[9] although more recent studies could not support this high prevalence. Investigators postulate that the disorder results from a gene-transmitted defect of a neurotransmitter or receptor factor. Studies of HLA antigens in hypersomnia have demonstrated an association of the condition with HLA-Cw2.[9] The absence of HLA-DR2 in hypersomnolent patients clearly demonstrates that despite their heredofamilial link narcolepsy and hypersomnia are two distinct entities.

A psychiatric evaluation for hypersomnia focuses on current mental status and past history of affective disturbance.[4,20,23] Ancillary studies, including psychologic testing such as the Minnesota Multiphasic Personality Inventory (MMPI), Rorschach inkblot technique, and other projective psychological tests, are helpful to rule out emotional factors contributing to the patient's condition. MMPI studies reveal greater psychopathologic findings among narcoleptics than hypersomniacs.[6] When present in hypersomniacs, the depression is usually atypical and therefore difficult to diagnose. More often, it represents the depressive phase of a bipolar disorder.[24]

If indicated by the history or by findings on the physical or neurologic examinations, other ancillary laboratory studies can be helpful in individual cases of suspected narcolepsy and hypersomnia. These include skull radiographs, brain computed tomography (CT) and magnetic resonance imaging (MRI) scans, cerebrospinal fluid (CSF) analysis, and other clinical laboratory tests for endocrine, hepatic, and renal functions.

In the evaluation of sleep apnea, a chest roentgenogram, electrocardiogram, and hematocrit are recommended.[21] The 24-hour electrocardiographic monitor is useful because nocturnal dysrhythmias can occur and sleep-associated bradytachycardia is a feature of this disorder. In addition, a complete blood count (CBC) to assess for polycythemia and a thyroid panel to rule out hypothyroidism as an etiology are generally recommended. Sleep laboratory diagnostic studies are necessary whenever sleep apnea is suspected and when the diagnosis of narcolepsy is in doubt because of an absence of the auxiliary symptoms, particularly cataplexy.

Sleep-onset REM periods occur almost invariably in narcoleptics who have cataplexy. The presence of a short sleep latency (less than 5 minutes) or a REM onset of less than 10 minutes on either of two one-hour daytime naps was shown to reach a diagnostic sensitivity of 84 per cent and a specificity of 80 per cent in 50 patients with narcolepsy and cataplexy.[25] Multiple daytime nap recordings may demonstrate either sleep-onset REM periods or extremely short sleep latencies.

Normal sleep patterns and distribution of sleep stages are characteristic of the polysomnographic studies of hypersomniac patients.[4] The disrupted sleep typically seen in narcolepsy is not found in hypersomnia. In addition, the sleep of the hypersomniac patient is longer and more consolidated. In most cases, the clinical EEG should be carefully evaluated for the presence of seizure activity or other abnormalities.

Regarding sleep apnea, a thorough sleep laboratory evaluation with recording of respiration and monitoring of ear oximetry is necessary to confirm the diagnosis and determine the type (central, obstructive, or mixed) and severity (number and duration of nightly episodes and lowest oxygen saturation) of the condition. Because surgery is often recommended when obstructive apnea is severe, sleep laboratory data must be accurate and complete before the treatment decision is made. The repetitive breath cessations that are characteristic of the disorder also cause marked disruption of sleep stage patterns; deep sleep (stages 3 and 4) is significantly reduced or entirely absent, whereas the amount of lighter sleep (stages 1 and 2) is considerably increased.[1,2] In fact, the sleep cycle may be so disrupted that periods of REM sleep may occur at sleep onset rather than after 70 to 90 minutes of non-REM sleep, which is the normal pattern. The percentage of REM sleep usually approximates normal levels, but its distribution is more fragmented. Usually, the longest and most severe episodes of apnea occur during REM sleep.

ASSESSMENT

In most cases, the differential diagnosis of narcolepsy is easily made from hypersomnia and sleep apnea (Table 2) by obtaining a history of one or more of the auxiliary symptoms that usually accompany the sleep attacks of this disorder. As mentioned before, when auxiliary symptoms are not present, sleep labora-

TABLE 2. Differentiation Among Disorders of Excessive Sleep

CHARACTERISTIC	NARCOLEPSY	IDIOPATHIC HYPERSOMNIA	PSYCHOGENIC HYPERSOMNIA	OBSTRUCTIVE SLEEP APNEA
Sleepiness	Paroxysmal	Constant	Variable	Varies with severity
Sleep attacks	Relatively brief and irresistible	Prolonged and rather resistible	May be present and rather resistible	May be present and resistible
Auxiliary symptoms	Present	Absent	Absent	Absent
Nocturnal sleep	Disrupted	Prolonged	Variable	Interrupted
Sleep drunkenness	Absent	Often present	Absent	Some confusion
Usual onset	Adolescence	Variable	Variable	Middle age
Hereditary factors	Present	Present	Absent	Possible
Psychopathology	Secondary	Secondary?	Primary	Secondary
Loud snorting, breath cessation	Absent	Absent	Absent	Present

(From Manfredi RL, Brennan RW, Cadieux RJ. Disorders of excessive sleepiness: narcolepsy and hypersomnia. Semin Neurol 1987;7:250–8.)

tory studies (multiple sleep latency test) can be most helpful.

Hypersomnia is a disorder of excessive diurnal and nocturnal sleep.[4,11] In contrast to narcolepsy, the excessive daytime somnolence in hypersomnia is less paroxysmal and more prolonged, and there are no auxiliary symptoms. Furthermore, the nocturnal sleep of the hypersomniac is less disrupted than in the narcoleptic. Finally, the hypersomniac often awakens with sleep drunkenness, which is not typical of narcolepsy.

In sleep apnea, reports from the bed partner for the presence of snoring with interrupted nocturnal breathing are important. The physician thus determines if there are frequent periods of interrupted nocturnal breathing associated with snoring, gasping, gurgling, choking, periodic loud snorting, or morning headaches. If this history from the bed partner is positive, then, as previously indicated, sleep laboratory testing is necessary to confirm the diagnosis of sleep apnea.

REFERENCES

1. Lugaresi E, Coccagna G, Mantovani M. Hypersomnia with periodic apneas. In: Weitzman ED, ed. Advances in sleep research, Vol 4. New York: Spectrum Publications, 1978.
2. Guilleminault C, Dement WC, eds. Sleep apnea syndromes. New York: Alan R Liss, Inc, 1978.
3. Block AJ, Boysen PG, Wynne JW, Hunt LA. Sleep apnea, hypopnea and oxygen saturation in normal subjects: a strong male predominance. N Engl J Med 1979;300:513–7.
4. Roth B. Narcolepsy and hypersomnia. Prague: Avicenum-Czechloslovak Medical Press. (Revised and edited by R Broughton, Basel: S Karger, 1980.)
5. Kales A, Cadieux RJ, Soldatos CR, et al. Narcolepsy-cataplexy: I. clinical and electrophysiologic characteristics. Arch Neurol 1982;39:164–8.
6. Kales A, Vela-Bueno A, Kales JD. Sleep disorders: sleep apnea and narcolepsy. Ann Intern Med 1987;106:434–43.
7. Broughton R. Neurology and sleep research. Can Psychiatr Assoc J 1971;16:283–93.
8. Mosko SS, Holowach JB, Sassin JF. The 24-hour rhythm of core temperature in narcolepsy. Sleep 1983;6:137–46.
9. Poirier G, Montplaisir J, Decary F, Momege D, Lebrun A. HLA antigens in narcolepsy and idiopathic central nervous system hypersomnolence. Sleep 1986;9:153–8.
10. Leckman JF, Gershon ES. A genetic model of narcolepsy. Br J Psychiatry 1976;128:276–9.
11. Manfredi RL, Brennan RW, Cadieux RJ. Disorders of excessive sleepiness: narcolepsy and hypersomnia. Semin Neurol 1987;7:250–8.
12. Bricolo A. Neurosurgical exploration and neurological pathology as a means for investigating human sleep seminology and mechanisms. In: Lairy GC, Salzarulo P, eds. The experimental study of human sleep: methodological problems. Amsterdam: Elsevier Science Publishing Co, 1975.
13. Hawkins DR, Taub JM, Van de Castle R. Extended sleep (hypersomnia) in young depressed patients. Am J Psychiatry 1985;142:905–10.
14. Kales A, Bixler EO, Cadieux RJ, et al. Sleep apnea in a hypertensive population. Lancet 1984;2:1005–8.
15. Lavie P, Ben-Yosef R, Rubin AE. Prevalence of sleep apnea syndrome among patients with essential hypertension. Am Heart J 1984;108:373–6.
16. Bixler EO, Kales A, Cadieux RJ, Vela-Bueno A, Jacoby JA, Soldatos CR. Sleep apneic activity in older healthy subjects. J Appl Physiol 1985;58:1597–601.
17. Lugaresi E, Coccagna G, Cirignotta F. Snoring and its clinical implications. In: Guilleminault C, Dement WC, eds. Sleep apnea syndromes. New York: Alan R Liss, Inc, 1978:13–21.
18. Block AJ, Wynne JW, Boysen PG. Sleep-disordered breathing and nocturnal oxygen desaturation in postmenopausal women. Am J Med 1980;69:75–9.
19. Sandblom RE, Matsumoto AM, Schoene RB, et al. Obstructive sleep apnea syndrome induced by testosterone administration. N Engl J Med 1983;308:508–10.
20. Kales A, Soldatos CR, Kales JD. Taking a sleep history. Am Fam Physician 1980;22:101–8.
21. Kales A, Cadieux RJ, Bixler EO, et al. Severe obstructive sleep apnea—I: onset, clinical course, and characteristics. J Chronic Dis 1985;38:419–25.
22. Kales A, Caldwell AB, Cadieux RJ, Vela-Bueno A, Ruch LG, Mayes SD. Severe obstructive sleep apnea—II: associated psychopathology and psychosocial consequences. J Chronic Dis 1985;38:427–34.
23. Guilleminault C, Faull KF. Sleepiness in nonnarcoleptic, non-sleep apneic EDS patients: the idiopathic CNS hypersomnolence. Sleep 1982;5 (Suppl):175–81.
24. Kupfer DJ, Himmelhock JM, Schwartzburg M, Anderson C, Byck R, Detre TP. Hypersomnia in manic-depressive disease. Dis Nerv Syst 1972;33:720–4.
25. Kales A, Bixler EO, Soldatos CR, Cadieux RJ, Manfredi R, Vela-Bueno A. Narcolepsy/cataplexy. IV: Diagnostic value of daytime nap recordings. Acta Neurol Scand 1987;75:223–30.

STEATORRHEA

INGRAM M. ROBERTS

SYNONYM: Excessive Fat in the Stool

BACKGROUND

Steatorrhea (roughly translated from the Greek as "flow of tallow") refers to the passage of large amounts of fat (more precisely, lipid) in the stool. The presence of steatorrhea is usually indicative of malabsorption, although there are several conditions that produce physiologic steatorrhea.

Steatorrhea is considered to be the "hallmark" of malabsorption. Lipid digestion is usually extremely efficient in health. In fact, dietary triglyceride is responsible for 95 per cent of ingested lipid, with cholesterol esters, phospholipids, lipovitamin esters, and cholesterol composing the remaining 5 per cent. Although there are endogenous sources of lipid (30 gm per day), including dead bacteria, desquamated cells, and biliary lipid, these compounds are largely reabsorbed in the distal small bowel.[1] Virtually all the dietary triglyceride is absorbed in health. The 5 to 7 per cent of lipid that is not absorbed is thought to come from nontriglyceride sources and usually represents a normal fecal fat content.

Steatorrhea can lead to the loss of the highest dietary source of calories (fat contains 9 kcal/gm in contrast to 4 kcal/gm for carbohydrate and protein). In addition, deficiency of essential fatty acids, such as linoleic (18:2) and arachidonic (20:4) acids, may occur. Essential fatty acids are the precursors for prostaglandins, thromboxanes, leukotrienes, and other biologically active compounds. Oral or intravenous supplementation with essential fatty acids has been successful in restoring serum essential fatty acid levels toward normal in some patients with malabsorption.

Selected patients with malabsorption may develop fat-soluble vitamin deficiencies. In a similar situation to essential fatty acid deficiency, serum vitamin levels do not correlate well with the absolute degree of steatorrhea. Syndromes that may result include hypo- coagulable state (vitamin K deficiency), osteomalacia (vitamin D deficiency), neurologic abnormalities (vitamin E deficiency), and night blindness (vitamin A deficiency).

HISTORY

Unfortunately, the medical history is often not very helpful in suspecting the presence of steatorrhea. The classical presence of "frothy, floating, foul-smelling" stools is actually not a reliable indication of steatorrhea, as stools float due to their gas content, not to their fat content. Inquiries concerning documented weight loss and diarrhea are, however, important questions to ask in history taking and should lead one to suspect the presence of malabsorption. Patients may notice that they are losing weight despite the fact that their appetites remain good. Interestingly, many patients with steatorrhea, particularly those with pancreatic insufficiency, do not complain of diarrhea. More objective evidence is therefore required in order to establish a definite diagnosis of steatorrhea (see Diagnostic Studies).

Focused Queries

Focused queries that may suggest the presence of steatorrhea are:

1. *Is there a history of abdominal surgery (adhesions, bowel resection, blind loop)?*
2. *Is there a history of bleeding problems (vitamin K deficiency)?*
3. *Is there a history of night blindness (vitamin A deficiency)?*
4. *Is there a history of tetany, muscle spasm, or neurologic disease (vitamin D deficiency and/or hypocalcemia, vitamin E deficiency, vitamin B_{12} deficiency, hypomagnesemia)?*
5. *Is there a history of anemia (iron, folate, or B_{12} deficiency)?*
6. *Is there a history of bone disease (vitamin D or calcium deficiency)?*

TABLE 1. Physical Findings and Signs Associated with Malabsorption

Trousseau's sign, Chvostek's sign—hypocalcemia, hypomagnesemia
Romberg's sign, diminished position and vibration sense—vitamin B_{12} deficiency
Cheilosis and glossitis—iron, folate, and B_{12} deficiencies
Lymphedema—intestinal lymphangiectasia
Edema or anasarca—severe hypoproteinemia
Ecchymoses—vitamin K deficiency
Hyperkeratosis—vitamin A deficiency

7. *Is there a history of skin rash (essential fatty acid, zinc, or niacin deficiency)?*
8. *Is there a history of weight loss?*
9. *Is there a history of diarrhea?*

PHYSICAL EXAMINATION

In similar fashion to medical history, the physical examination is usually not remarkable for signs of a "full-blown" malabsorption syndrome such as cachexia, muscle wasting, peripheral edema, and anasarca. Some of the signs that may be seen on physical examination are shown in Table 1. Mild to moderate abdominal distension may be present, but most patients do not complain of severe abdominal pain. Borborygmi may be heard, and occasionally there may be visible peristalsis. The abdomen is not usually particularly tender in malabsorption syndromes. Grossly bloody stool is unusual in malabsorption syndromes, with the exception of Crohn's disease, and often implies that colonic disease is the source for diarrhea.

DIAGNOSTIC STUDIES

The key screening test for the presence of malabsorption remains the Sudan stain.[2,3,4,5] The qualitative stool fat determination using the Sudan stain is 100 per cent sensitive and 96 per cent specific as a screening test for steatorrhea.[3,4] The ^{14}C-triolein breath test has been reported to have 100 per cent sensitivity and 96 per cent specificity[6] but uses radioisotopes and is not available in most laboratories. Other tests (such as carotene, cholesterol, albumin, etc.) lack the proper sensitivity and specificity for routine use. Another test that could be rapidly performed, but has yet to gain widespread popularity, is the steatocrit.[7] This test uses an aliquot of homogenized stool, capillary microhematocrit tubes, and a hematocrit microcentrifuge to determine quickly the percentage of fat in a stool specimen. After centrifugation for 15 minutes at 15,000 rpm per minute, the tubes are viewed vertically. Three layers (a basal solid layer, an intermediate liquid layer, and an upper fatty layer) are usually seen. The steatocrit is equal to the length of the fatty layer/length of the fatty layer plus the solid layer expressed as a percentage. Normal values for steatocrit were below 4 per cent, and the correlation with fecal fat excretion was high (r = 0.93) in one study.[7] In theory, the Sudan stain or steatocrit determination could be performed rapidly and made available on most hospital ward laboratories.

The definitive test for the diagnosis of malabsorption is the 72-hour quantitative stool collection for fecal fat.[8] There are several situations when fecal fat excretion is increased under physiologic conditions: (1) on extremely high-fiber diets (100 gm per day fiber),[9] (2) when dietary fat is ingested in a form such as whole peanuts,[10] and (3) in the neonatal period when intraluminal levels of pancreatic lipase and bile salts are reduced.[11] Excluding these three situations, the finding of a coefficient of fat absorption less than 93 per cent confirms steatorrhea secondary to malabsorption. It is extremely important that the patient ingest a 100 gm per day fat diet during the three-day period of the fecal fat collection to ensure best results. A high fecal fat concentration (fecal fat/fecal weight × 100) has been suggested by some investigators to be associated commonly with pancreatic disease.[12] Unfortunately, other studies have demonstrated that fecal fat concentration lacks sufficient sensitivity and specificity to differentiate clearly pancreatic causes of steatorrhea from mucosal diseases (see Assessment).[13,14,15]

ASSESSMENT

The evaluation of the patient with malabsorption should follow a clear sequence of screening and diagnostic testing that reveals the correct etiology for the patient's condition. As discussed earlier, the typical history and physical findings suggestive of malabsorption are often not found. The clinician must suspect the presence of malabsorption and determine objectively whether evidence for malabsorption exists.

As a myriad of conditions may cause malabsorption, the precise diagnosis should always be elucidated before the proper medical man-

DIAGNOSTIC ASSESSMENT OF SUSPECTED MALABSORPTION

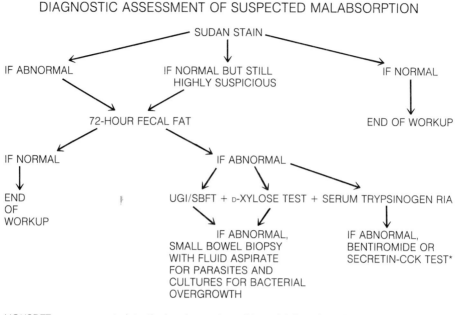

UGI/SBFT = upper gastrointestinal series and small bowel follow-through.
RIA = radioimmunoassay.
CCK = cholecystokinin.
* Not necessary if pancreatic calcifications are present on abdominal flat plate.

agement can be instituted. In most disorders, fat, carbohydrate, and protein malabsorption occur concomitantly. However, enterokinase deficiency or protein-losing enteropathy may produce only protein malabsorption. Congenital lipase or colipase deficiency and abetalipoproteinemia may produce only fat malabsorption. Finally, disaccharidase deficiencies (lactase, sucrase-isomaltase, or trehalase) or transport abnormalities (glucose-galactose or fructose) may lead to malabsorption of carbohydrates alone.

Once the presence of steatorrhea is confirmed, one should determine whether malabsorption is caused by abnormalities of intraluminal digestion or by disease of the intestinal mucosa. To differentiate between these possibilities, the workup follows an algorithm. An upper gastrointestinal series and small bowel follow-through (UGI/SBFT) may reveal anatomic abnormalities such as jejunal diverticuli, show the abnormal mucosal pattern (thickening of the folds, dilatation, segmentation, etc.) found with many malabsorption syndromes, or reveal the "string sign" narrowing seen in Crohn's disease. In addition, a flat plate of the abdomen may show pancreatic calcifications, which are diagnostic for chronic pancreatitis.

The D-xylose test is an excellent method to determine if mucosal absorptive integrity is intact.[16] D-Xylose is a pentose sugar that is absorbed from the small bowel via the same transport mechanism as glucose and excreted unchanged in the urine. The usual dose is 25 gm by mouth after an overnight fast, with urine collection for five hours. Normal urinary excretion of D-xylose should be greater than 5 gm. Measurement of the one-hour serum D-xylose yields a higher sensitivity and specificity than the five-hour urine collection. Normal serum level should be greater than 20 mg/dl. Low values for D-xylose are seen in diseases of the intestinal mucosa or bacterial overgrowth (due to ingestion of xylose by the bacteria), whereas normal values are consistent with pancreatic insufficiency.

The serum trypsinogen radioimmunoassay (RIA) is specific for the diagnosis of chronic pancreatitis if the trypsinogen value is less than 10 ng/ml. Nonpancreatic causes for malabsorption almost always give a normal serum trypsinogen (10 to 75 ng/ml). If steatorrhea and a low serum trypsinogen are found, the diagnosis of chronic pancreatitis is virtually assured.[17,18]

When the D-xylose test and UGI/SBFT are abnormal, a small bowel biopsy should be obtained for histologic diagnosis. Grasp forceps biopsies taken from the distal duodenum via the endoscope may be oriented properly for diagnostic interpretation like the larger biopsies acquired with a Quinton-Rubin tube.[19] The small bowel biopsy is diagnostic in diseases such as Whipple's disease, abetalipoproteinemia, lymphoma, lymphangiectasia, parasitic infections, eosinophilic enteritis, amyloidosis, immunodeficiency syndromes, mastocytosis, and Crohn's disease. Although not diagnostic, the biopsy may suggest the presence of celiac sprue, tropical sprue, bacterial overgrowth, and radiation enteritis. The small bowel biopsy is normal in pancreatic insufficiency and postgastrectomy malabsorption, which do not involve the intestinal mucosa.

A normal D-xylose test and a low serum trypsinogen are characteristic of chronic pancreatitis. Pancreatic calcifications on abdominal flat plate secures the diagnosis, and further studies need not be performed. If calcifications are absent, the bentiromide test, a "tubeless" test of pancreatic function, or a direct pancreatic stimulation test with secretin or secretin-cholecystokinin (CCK) should be performed. Bentiromide (Chymex) is N-benzoyl-L-tyrosyl-para-aminobenzoic acid. Pancreatic chymotrypsin cleaves this tripeptide in the intestinal lumen, liberating para-aminobenzoic acid (PABA). PABA is absorbed by the intestine, conjugated by the liver, and excreted in the urine. The dose is 500 mg given orally, followed by urine collection for five hours, as in the D-xylose test. The presence of certain drugs (thiazides, chloramphenicol, sulfonamides, acetaminophen, phenacetin, sunscreens, and "caine" anesthetics) may result in false-negative tests.

Pancreatic function testing with pharmacologic doses of intravenous CCK and secretin, or secretin alone, is the most sensitive and specific test for diagnosing chronic pancreatitis. As this procedure necessitates small bowel intubation, collection of intestinal content, and analysis for bicarbonate and enzymes (trypsin, lipase, or amylase), it has not achieved widespread popularity in this country. Bicarbonate concentrations less than 70 mEq/L and secretion volume less than 2 ml/kg body weight per hour are abnormal values.

Patients may have malabsorption in association with intestinal motility disorders (scleroderma, intestinal pseudo-obstruction, etc.), intestinal surgery, or anatomic abnormalities (small intestinal diverticuli). In these instances, the diagnosis of bacterial overgrowth should be considered. Patients with overgrowth (greater than 10^6 organisms/ml intestinal content) may have positive D-xylose tests secondary to ingestion of the sugar by bacteria. The small bowel biopsy is often nonspecifically abnormal (partially blunted villi, increased inflammatory cells in the lamina propria). Pancreatic function is normal in these patients. Tests for bacterial overgrowth include culture of intestinal content for aerobic and anaerobic bacteria, the Schilling test, the bile acid breath test, the ^{14}C-xylose breath test, the lactulose breath hydrogen test, and the fasting breath hydrogen determination.[20,21,22] The Schilling test performed before and repeated after administration of antibiotics is available at most medical centers. It remains the most useful adjunct to direct culture of intestinal fluid for aerobes and anaerobes. The bile acid and ^{14}C-xylose breath tests measure $^{14}CO_2$ excreted in breath as a result of bacterial deconjugation of cholyl-glycine-1-^{14}C and metabolism of ^{14}C-xylose, respectively.[21,22] Although breath tests have been found to be highly sensitive and specific for the diagnosis of bacterial overgrowth, they are routinely available at only a few selected institutions. Gas chromatography of volatile fatty acids in jejunal aspirates has recently been reported to have a 100 per cent specificity for the presence of bacterial overgrowth.[23] Finally, the intestinal clearance of alpha-1-antitrypsin has replaced radiolabeled albumin turnover as the test of choice for diagnosing protein-losing enteropathy. An abnormal study strongly suggests protein-losing enteropathy as a cause for malabsorption.

REFERENCES

1. Patton JS. Gastrointestinal lipid digestion. In: Johnson LR, ed. Physiology of the gastrointestinal tract, Vol 2. New York: Raven Press, 1981:1123–46.
2. Drummey GD, Benson JA Jr, Jones CM. Microscopic examination of the stool for steatorrhea. N Engl J Med 1961;264:85–7.
3. Luk GD. Qualitative fecal fat by light microscopy: a sensitive and specific screening test for steatorrhea and pancreatic insufficiency [Abstract]. Gastroenterology 1979;76:1189.
4. Simko V. Fecal fat microscopy: acceptable predictive value in screening for steatorrhea. Am J Gastroenterol 1981;75:204–8.
5. Khouri MR, Huang G, Shiau YF. Sudan stain of fecal fat: new insight into an old test. Gastroenterology 1989;96:421–7.
6. Newcomer AG, Hofmann AF, DiMagno EP, Thomas PJ, Carlson GL. Triolein breath test: sen-

sitive and specific test for fat malabsorption. Gastroenterology 1979;76:6–13.

7. Colombo C, Maiavacca R, Ronchi M, Consalvo E, Amoretti M, Giunta A. The steatocrit: a simple method for monitoring fat malabsorption in patients with cystic fibrosis. J Pediatr Gastroenterol Nutr 1987;6:926–30.

8. Van de Kamer JH, ten bokkel Huinink H, Weyers HA. Rapid method for the determination of fat in feces. J Biol Chem 1949;177:347–55.

9. Levine AS, Silvis SE. Steatorrhea due to high dietary fiber [Abstract]. Gastroenterology 1979;76:1183.

10. Levine AS, Silvis SE. Absorption of whole peanuts, peanut oil and peanut butter. N Engl J Med 1980;303:917–8.

11. Finley AJ, Davidson M. Bile acid excretion and patterns of fatty acid absorption in formula-fed premature infants. Pediatrics 1980;65:132–8.

12. Bo-Linn GW, Fordtran JS. Fecal fat concentration in patients with steatorrhea. Gastroenterology 1984;87:319–22.

13. Roberts IM, Poturich C, Wald A. Utility of fecal fat concentration as a screening test in pancreatic insufficiency. Dig Dis Sci 1986;31:1021–4.

14. Lembcke B, Grimm K, Lankisch PG. Raised fecal fat concentration is not a valid indicator of pancreatic steatorrhea. Am J Gastroenterol 1987;82:526–31.

15. Bai JC, Andrush A, Matelo G, et al. Fecal fat concentration in the differential diagnosis of steatorrhea. Am J Gastroenterol 1989;84:27–30.

16. Haeney MR, Culank LS, Montgomery RD, Sammons HG. Evaluation of xylose absorption as measured in blood and urine: a one-hour blood xylose screening test in malabsorption. Gastroenterology 1978;75:393–400.

17. Jacobson DG, Currington C, Connery K, Toskes PP. Trypsin-like immunoreactivity as a test for pancreatic insufficiency. N Engl J Med 1985;310:1307–9.

18. Steinberg WM, Anderson KK. Serum trypsinogen in diagnosis of chronic pancreatitis. Dig Dis Sci 1984;29:988–93.

19. Achkar EA, Carey WD, Petras R, Sivak MV, Revta R. Comparison of suction capsule and endoscopic biopsy of small bowel mucosa. Gastrointest Endosc 1986;32:278–81.

20. Farivar S, Fromm H, Schindler D, Schmidt F. Sensitivity of bile acid breath test in the diagnosis of bacterial overgrowth in the small intestine with and without the stagnant (blind) loop syndrome. Dig Dis Sci 1979;24:33–40.

21. King CE, Toskes PP. Comparison of the 1-gram [^{14}C] xylose, 10-gram lactulose-H_2, and 80-gram glucose-H_2 breath tests in patients with small intestinal bacterial overgrowth. Gastroenterology 1986;91:1447–51.

22. Fromm H, Hofmann AF. Breath test for altered bile acid metabolism. Lancet 1971;ii:621.

23. Corazza GR, Menozzi MG, Strocchi A, et al. The diagnosis of small bowel bacterial overgrowth: reliability of jejunal culture and inadequacy of breath hydrogen testing. Gastroenterology 1990;98:302–9.

STRIDOR

RONALD A. STILLER and MARK H. SANDERS

SYNONYM: Upper Airway Obstruction

BACKGROUND

Stridor is best described as a loud, distinctive musical sound of constant pitch most commonly heard during inspiration.[1] The importance of stridor is that it is often associated with advanced upper airway obstruction, usually in the supraglottic airway, the larynx, or extrathoracic trachea and may portend airway occlusion with catastrophic results. While most clinicians believe they can readily recognize stridor, the sign may be incorrectly interpreted as wheezing due to bronchospasm, and the presence of an obstructing lesion in the upper airway may be overlooked.[2]

Because of the significant morbidity and mortality associated with upper airway obstruction, it is imperative that physicians and other health care professionals have both the ability to recognize the presence of an obstructing lesion and the skills to manage it successfully. In the discussion that follows, the various causes of upper airway obstruction and the changes that result in the production of stridor will be reviewed. A general understanding of this process will lead to increased awareness of the potential for serious upper airway obstruction. Furthermore, it is hoped that the information provided in this chapter will facilitate the management of patients with upper airway obstruction and stridor and will increase the likelihood of a successful outcome.

Etiologies of Upper Airway Obstruction and Stridor

A review of the literature will reveal a multitude of case reports that document the numerous potential causes of stridor (Table 1). The thread that links each of these clinical scenarios is the presence of upper airway obstruction. Some of the more common etiologies of upper airway obstruction and stridor will be discussed.

Foreign Body Aspiration

Foreign body aspiration is among the leading causes of fatal injury in infants and children and a frequent cause of upper airway obstruction and stridor in adults.[3] The "café coronary" occurs following the aspiration of partially chewed food that subsequently becomes lodged in the upper airway. This most frequently occurs in the setting of excessive alcohol consumption, poor chewing habits, or patients wearing dentures.[4] Among children, aspirated material is most often organic matter. This can pose a particular problem since the aspirated material may absorb secretions and swell, thus worsening the obstruction. In addition, organic matter is frequently radiolucent, which makes x-ray localization of the obstruction somewhat more problematic.[5]

TABLE 1.   Common Causes of Upper Airway Obstruction

Amyloid
Congenital abnormalities
Edema
    Angioedema
    Chemical injury
    Hypersensitivity reactions
    Thermal injury
    Trauma
Foreign body
Goiter
Granulomatous disease
Infection
    Croup
    Diphtheria
    Epiglottitis
    Infectious mononucleosis
    Retropharyngeal abscess
Malignancy
Tonsillar/adenoid hypertrophy
Vocal cord paralysis

Upper Airway Infection

Infection represents the most common etiology of upper airway obstruction among pediatric patients and, while less frequent in older patients, should always be considered when evaluating adults for upper airway obstruction.[5] Viral laryngotracheobronchitis, or croup, may be caused by a number of different viruses, most commonly parainfluenza or respiratory syncytial virus, and may progress to the point of significant upper airway obstruction and stridor due to subglottic edema.[6] Croup is most frequent in children from three months to three years of age and is twice as common in males. The incidence of infection varies seasonally and is greatest from late fall through early spring. In the stridorous patient with croup, onset of symptoms is usually gradual and preceded by a viral prodrome.[7]

This syndrome is to be distinguished from that of bacterial epiglottitis, which represents a true medical emergency owing to its considerable potential for complete airway obstruction.[8] While epiglottitis is usually seen in children between the ages of two and seven, it also has been well described in adults.[9] Epiglottitis, like croup, is more common in males; however, there is no seasonal variation in incidence. Unlike croup, the onset of symptoms can be quite rapid, often occurring over the course of only a few hours, with no prodromal complaints. Patients may complain of severe sore throat, dysphagia, and dyspnea and appear quite ill. *Hemophilus influenzae,* type B, the microorganism most commonly associated with epiglottitis, is frequently identified in blood cultures from affected patients.[4,7] Other pathogens that have been implicated as etiologic agents include *Streptococcus pneumoniae, Staphylococcus aureus, H. parainfluenzae,* and parainfluenza virus. If the diagnosis is unsuspected, the mortality rate from epiglottitis may exceed 50 per cent; even with current standards of antimicrobial therapy, mortality may still reach 2 to 5 per cent.[7] (Also see Laryngotracheobronchitis, Bacterial Tracheitis, and Epiglottitis in Difficult Medical Management, WB Saunders Co, 1991).

In addition to croup and epiglottitis, any number of other upper airway infections may progress to obstruction and stridor owing to abscess formation or edema. Abscess formation may occur in the peritonsillar, laryngeal, or retropharyngeal regions. Most often, this occurs either in the setting of streptococcal infection or as a result of secondary infection of previously traumatized soft tissue, particularly in the larynx and subglottis.[4] Retropharyngeal abscesses are more common in children and are often associated with infections of the middle ear or sinuses. Uncontrolled infection in this region may spread to the mediastinum with fatal consequences.[4,10]

Other infections of the upper airway with the potential to cause obstruction and stridor include diphtheria and infectious mononucleosis. Diphtheria is caused by the exotoxin-producing *Corynebacterium diphtheriae,* which causes the formation of an inflammatory pseudomembrane in the superficial mucosa of the upper airway. Infectious mononucleosis is most frequently associated with Epstein-Barr virus infection and may be complicated by the presence of massive, obstructing edema and lymphoid tissue enlargement within the upper airway.[11]

Trauma

Trauma to the upper airway is yet another potential cause of upper airway obstruction and stridor. Iatrogenic injury to the glottis or subglottic region, which leads to airway obstruction either by fibrous web formation or by disruption of supporting structures within the upper airway, may occur in intensive care unit (ICU) patients following endotracheal intubation or tracheostomy.[12,13] Upper airway injury and impending obstruction should be suspected in any patient with penetrating trauma to the soft tissues surrounding the upper airway.[14] Severe hemorrhage due to tearing of regional blood vessels may cause airway obstruction following aspiration of blood or the formation of a hematoma, which either obstructs the airway lumen or, alternatively, causes extrinsic compression of the airway.

Blunt trauma to the structures of the upper airway most commonly occurs in the setting of motor vehicle accidents but can also be seen in participants in contact sports, assault victims, and battered children. As a result of inertial forces associated with head-on motor vehicle collisions, the victim is propelled forward despite sudden deceleration of the vehicle. The neck becomes hyperextended and exposes the upper airway to injury upon impact with either the steering wheel or dashboard. This sequence of events can lead to increased shear stresses on the soft tissues surrounding the upper airway; lacerations and contusions of the airway itself; and fractures, crushing, or total avulsion of cartilaginous supporting structures. Subsequently, obstruc-

tion may occur as airway caliber is reduced secondary to loss of cartilaginous support, the onset of submucosal edema, or hemorrhage.[4,15]

Fire victims, particularly those exposed within an enclosed space, also are at increased risk for upper airway obstruction. Direct heat to the upper airway can produce immediate injury to the mucosa, causing edema, erythema, and ulceration. Frequently, symptoms of respiratory insufficiency develop after a period of relative stability since mucosal changes within the airway occur 12 to 36 hours postexposure. These changes are usually self-limited and gradually resolve over the course of three to four days.[16,17]

Tumors

In contrast to the acute type of presentation described above, patients also may come to medical attention with more chronic complaints of upper airway obstruction and no obvious precipitating cause. This may be seen particularly in the setting of either benign or malignant tumors of the pharynx, larynx, base of the tongue, or trachea. The onset of signs and symptoms may be both gradual and variable. However, if left untreated, patients may eventually progress to complete airway occlusion. Pathologic changes may develop secondary to the spread of carcinomas of the upper airway or of the relatively rare tracheobronchial gland tumors (e.g., adenoid cystic carcinoma, mucous gland adenoma, mucoepidermoid carcinoma, etc.). Some nonmalignant lesions that may cause chronic upper airway obstruction include glottic and supraglottic retention cysts; pedunculated polyps, which may result in intermittent airway obstruction; hemangiomas, particularly in infants; and viral laryngotracheal papillomatosis.[4,6]

Whatever the etiology, it cannot be overemphasized that the presence of stridor mandates prompt patient assessment in conjunction with physicians skilled in airway management who can assist in evaluating the severity of the obstruction and institute proper therapy when necessary.

Mechanism of Stridor

Acoustically, stridor can be described as a monophonic wheeze. Its presence implies significant airway narrowing, and it is this reduction in airway caliber that accounts for the production of the sound, since wheezes are produced when airway diameter is reduced to

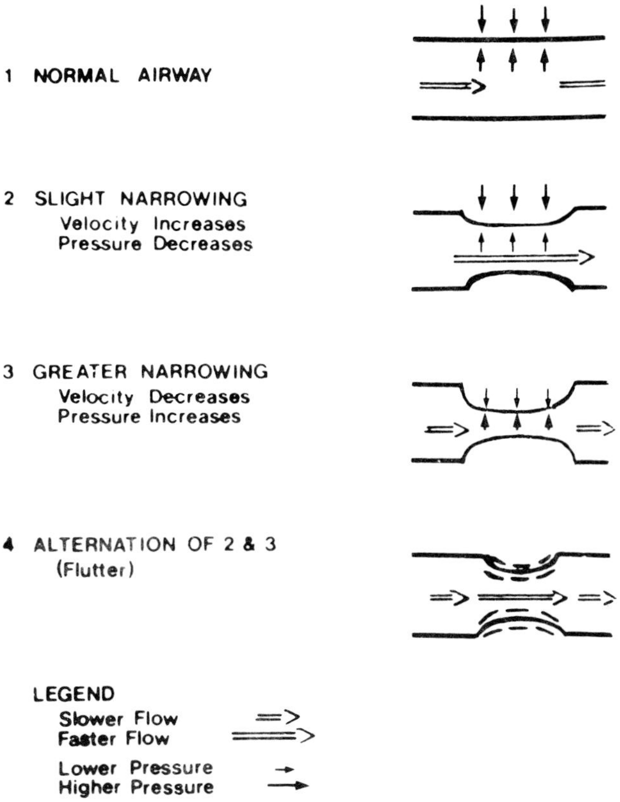

1 NORMAL AIRWAY

FIGURE 1. The stability of the airway wall depends on a balance of internal and external airway pressures as well as on the mechanical properties of the airway wall (1). When narrowing of the airway occurs, the velocity of flow through the point of constriction must increase if the mass of air moved is to remain constant. According to Bernoulli's principle, the increase in air velocity is associated with a decrease in air pressure at the point of constriction. This increases the transmural pressure gradient, thus allowing the airway to be further compressed. (2). Extreme reduction in luminal diameter may cause the pressure inside the airway to increase, thus reopening the lumen (3). Under the appropriate conditions, the airway wall may flutter or vibrate, thus producing a continuous sound whose amplitude, pitch, and duration depend on the velocity of airflow and the mechanical properties of the airway wall. (From Hollingsworth HM. Wheezing and stridor. Clin Chest Med 1987;8(2): 231–40. Reprinted with permission of WB Saunders Co.)

2 SLIGHT NARROWING
   Velocity Increases
   Pressure Decreases

3 GREATER NARROWING
   Velocity Decreases
   Pressure Increases

4 ALTERNATION OF 2 & 3
   (Flutter)

LEGEND
   Slower Flow   =>
   Faster Flow   ===>
   Lower Pressure   →
   Higher Pressure   ⟶

the point that opposite walls nearly touch (Fig. 1). In fact, Geffin et al. have proposed that the presence of stridor indicates an airway diameter of less than 5 mm.[13] Air turbulence, due to the increased velocity of airflow through the narrowed airway at the point of obstruction, promotes vibration of airway walls, similar to the reed of a woodwind instrument, thus producing a musical note. The velocity of air movement, the airway diameter, as well as the mass and elasticity of airway walls all contribute to determining the frequency of vibration and thus the pitch of the wheeze.[18] Since stridor and wheezing are both produced by this mechanism, it is not surprising that the two sounds have similar sound frequencies by acoustic analysis.[2]

The best way to distinguish clinically between stridor and wheezing is to determine the specific location and timing of these respiratory sounds. Wheezing, which is caused by intrathoracic airway obstruction (e.g., bronchospasm), is heard best over the chest wall during the expiratory phase of the respiratory cycle. Stridor, on the other hand, is an extrathoracic upper airway phenomenon and is

FIGURE 2. Airway dynamics associated with a variable extrathoracic obstruction. During forced expiration, the pressure within the extrathoracic trachea (P_{tr}) is greater than extratracheal or atmospheric pressure (P_{atm}). This transmural pressure difference results in increased luminal diameter of the airway. During forced inspiration, P_{atm} exceeds P_{tr}, airway diameter is reduced, and the effect of the obstruction is enhanced. (From Kryger M, Bode F, Antic R, Anthonisen N. Diagnosis of obstruction of the upper and central airways. Am J Med 1976;61:85–92. Reprinted with permission of Cahners Publishing Co.)

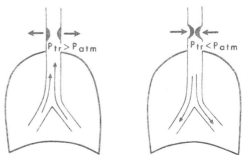

expiration   inspiration

$P_{tr} > P_{atm}$ $P_{tr} < P_{atm}$

loudest over the neck during inspiration.[2] The reasons for these differences become clear when one considers the changes in airway transmural pressure gradients that occur during the respiratory cycle. During forced inspiration, pleural pressure becomes negative relative to atmospheric pressure (P_{atm}) by virtue of the increased capacity of the pleural space following contraction of the muscles of inspiration. This subatmospheric pleural pressure is transmitted to the upper airways and extrathoracic trachea (designated here as P_{tr}), and a transmural pressure gradient ($P_{atm} - P_{tr}$) develops. Under conditions of normal caliber and compliance in the upper airway (i.e., extrathoracic trachea, larynx, and supraglottic space), the pressure gradient across the airway wall during maximal inspiration is minimal. No significant airway narrowing occurs, and ambient air readily flows down the pressure gradient ($P_{atm} - P_{tr}$) into the lungs. In contrast, in the presence of an upper airway obstruction, different forces are present that increase the transmural pressure gradient and worsen the degree of obstruction. As shown in Figure 2, the presence of an upper airway obstruction reduces the luminal diameter of the airway in the region of the obstruction. Recalling that airway resistance is inversely proportional to the radius raised to the fourth power, it can be readily appreciated that a decrease in airway diameter can result in a substantial increase in airway resistance. In order to maintain movement of the same volume of air at comparable flows to that of the normal airway despite the elevated resistance due to airway obstruction, intraluminal pressure, P_{tr}, becomes even more negative relative to P_{atm}. The resulting increase in the transmural airway pressure ($P_{atm} - P_{tr}$) further narrows the

already compromised airway and limits the inspiratory airflow even further. When the intraluminal diameter becomes critically narrowed, aerodynamic conditions favor the production of stridor.[19,20] This limitation in airflow during inspiration is termed variable extrathoracic obstruction. The term variable implies that the magnitude of the obstruction varies with the phase of the breathing cycle. On the other hand, during expiration, in the presence of a variable intrathoracic obstruction, pleural pressure (P_{pl}) exceeds P_{atm} during expiration. This expiratory transmural pressure gradient ($P_{pl} - P_{atm}$) causes increased obstruction of the intrathoracic airways, thus producing an expiratory wheeze (Fig. 3). Should an obstructing lesion in the airway progress to the point where it is unaffected by the respiratory cycle—that is, airway caliber is unchanged during either expiration or inspiration—the obstruction is termed fixed, and stridor may be heard during both phases of the respiratory cycle.

HISTORY

Stridor represents a potential medical emergency. Therefore, initial questions should be directed toward assessing the severity of respiratory distress and its rate of progression in order to determine the need for intervention. Once a decision has been reached concerning the need for airway protection, an attempt should be made to identify the cause of airway obstruction: for example, food or foreign body aspiration, which may be associated with intemperate alcohol consumption, seizure disorder, or neuromuscular disease; trauma to the head or neck; recent exposure to fire or toxic

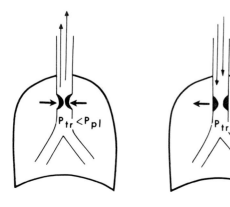

expiration   inspiration

FIGURE 3. Airway dynamics associated with a variable intrathoracic obstruction. During forced expiration, pleural pressure (P_{pl}) exceeds P_{tr} of the intrathoracic trachea, which results in a reduction in airway diameter. Thus, intrathoracic airway obstruction is enhanced with expiration. During forced inspiration, P_{tr} becomes greater than P_{pl}, and the obstruction is relieved. (From Kryger M, Bode F, Antic R, Anthonisen N. Diagnosis of obstruction of the upper and central airways. Am J Med 1976;61:85–92. Reprinted with permission of Cahners Publishing Co.)

fumes; other pertinent history such as allergies or anaphylaxis.

Other areas of inquiry that should be pursued, particularly in children, relate to infection within the upper airway. Patients with viral laryngotracheobronchitis, or croup, often report several days of progressive symptoms of upper respiratory tract infection, including mild temperature elevation, coryza, and a "brassy" or "barking" (i.e., the "bark" of a seal) cough. On the other hand, in epiglottitis the appearance of symptoms can be quite rapid, often occurring over the course of a few hours. Patients may complain of malaise, severe sore throat, dysphagia, and dyspnea. It is noteworthy that significant cough is frequently absent in patients with epiglottitis.[7] Any number of other upper airway infections may progress to obstruction and stridor owing to edema or abscess formation; however, in these cases, the history is often nonspecific and further evaluation is necessary.

As noted above, stridor may also have a more insidious onset. In patients with stridor and no obvious cause, a history consistent with progressive, chronic upper airway obstruction may be obtained. Initially, patients may complain of dyspnea, particularly on exertion, when increased inspiratory effort increases the pressure gradient across the wall of the trachea, thus worsening the obstruction. Reports of stridor at rest often signify severe upper airway obstruction, which will demand immediate attention. Other signs and symptoms of obstruction secondary to tumor include hoarseness due to recurrent laryngeal nerve dysfunction from tumor invasion, orthopnea or positional dyspnea as the obstructing lesion encroaches on the airway with changes in patient position, and stridor as the airway narrows critically as a result of bilateral vocal cord dysfunction and/or intraluminal tumor spread. In the absence of other specific medical history, the physician must rely on further evaluation by physical examination, radiographic testing, and visualization of the involved area to arrive at an etiology for the upper airway obstruction.

PHYSICAL EXAMINATION

Even before considering the clinical history, determining the need for immediate airway protection must be the first priority when evaluating a patient who presents with stridor. In this context, the physical examination initially should be directed toward providing information concerning the degree of respiratory distress and the best means of managing the patient's airway. The examining physician should listen to the stridorous patient at the bedside in order to assess the nature and severity of upper airway obstruction. Particular note should be made of the quality and timing of stridor with respect to respiration: Is stridor heard only with forced inspiratory maneuvers or can it be appreciated during quiet breathing? Is stridor present only during inspiration or during both inspiration and expiration? Observing the patient for signs of tachypnea, chest wall retractions, cyanosis, agitation, lethargy, or stupor may allow the physician to appreciate the degree of respiratory impairment and to anticipate impending respiratory failure. One may also observe the characteristic pose of the patient with epiglottitis and respiratory distress: The individual sits upright, leaning slightly forward with mouth open and tongue protruding, often drooling oral secretions that cannot be swallowed.[7] Other relevant clinical findings that may be seen in these patients include fever, hoarseness, and tenderness and swelling of the neck.

Rapid examination of the trauma victim with stridor may reveal the etiology of the obstruction while providing information concerning the severity of respiratory distress. The presence of facial, mandibular, or cervical spinal fractures may result in upper airway obstruction from edema, displacement of upper airway structures, and hemorrhage. Laryngeal trauma may be suspected if there is loss of the laryngeal prominence, pain with cough or swallowing, dysphonia, aphonia, or subcutaneous air over the neck and chest.[15,21]

The upper airway of the victims of fire should be visualized for signs of mucosal edema and inflammation when thermal injury to the pharyngeal mucosa is suspected.[16,17] These patients may be noted to have facial or upper body burns, singed nasal hairs, oropharyngeal erythema, edema, bullae, and carbonaceous deposits within the oropharynx.

Finally, since stridor may be confused with wheezing due to bronchospasm, auscultation over the neck and chest can be useful in patients with obstructive airways disease. In general, stridor is heard best during inspiration over the neck rather than the chest, whereas wheezing due to peripheral airways obstruction is best heard over the chest during expiration and is either absent or considerably reduced during inspiration.[2]

FURTHER ASSESSMENT OF PATIENTS WITH STRIDOR

Arterial Blood Gases

As we have indicated, the first priority of the physician assessing a patient with stridor is to determine the need for emergency airway protection. Arterial blood gases (ABGs) obtained at the time of presentation and periodically thereafter are a useful adjunct to patient evaluation since they are a relatively specific indicator of abnormalities of gas exchange. The presence of hypoxemia and hypercarbia suggest impending respiratory decompensation and should be promptly treated with endotracheal intubation or, if necessary, tracheostomy. Ideally, this evaluation is best carried out where physicians skilled in airway management are available to assist with the problem patient.

X-Rays

Once the patient with stridor is judged to be stable, roentgenographs of the chest and neck may be obtained to assist in determining the nature and location of the obstructing lesion. It should be noted, however, that conventional roentgenographic studies of the chest may be of only limited utility. While aspirated foreign bodies may be identified by the standard chest roentgenograph, they are frequently radiolucent and cannot be located radiographically.[7] In addition, obstructing lesions may be responsible for variable findings on chest x-ray. For example, plain films of the chest may reveal normal lung volumes, volume loss due to atelectasis distal to the obstruction, or hyperinflation if the obstruction behaves like a ball valve, causing air trapping during expiration.

Nevertheless, x-rays should be routinely obtained since they can be quite helpful in specific circumstances. Careful inspection of neck and chest films, particularly in the lateral projection, may reveal distension of the upper airway proximal to the obstruction and/or narrowing of the tracheal air column, thus suggesting the site of the obstruction. X-rays of the soft tissues of the neck may be of value if stridor is secondary to upper airway infection. The findings associated with acute epiglottitis are well described and include marked thickening of the epiglottis, aryepiglottic folds, uvula, and retropharyngeal tissues.[22] Other etiologies of upper airway obstruction (e.g., hemorrhage, abscess formation, inflammatory edema) also may account for abnormalities in the soft tissues of the retropharyngeal region that can be identified roentgenographically. In our experience, conventional tomography has been an excellent means of delineating obstructing mass lesions in the extrathoracic trachea, although—according to some investigators—computed tomography (CT) is the preferred study for obtaining information concerning the severity of airway narrowing caused by tracheal neoplasms.[23]

Pulmonary Function Tests

In stable patients with upper airway obstruction and stridor, pulmonary function tests (PFTs) may have diagnostic and therapeutic implications owing to their ability to determine whether an obstruction is extrathoracic or intrathoracic in location and to define the obstruction as being fixed or variable. For example, in patients who have been mistakenly, and unsuccessfully, treated for chronic obstructive intrathoracic airways disease, the maximal flow-volume loop has revealed the presence of upper airway obstruction. In patients with variable extrathoracic obstruction, the ratio of FIF_{50} to FEF_{50} (i.e., the forced inspiratory flow at 50 per cent vital capacity divided by the forced expiratory flow at 50 per cent vital capacity) is greater than 1. This occurs because of the limitation in maximal inspiratory airflow, which is represented as a plateauing of the inspiratory limb of the flow-volume loop (Fig. 4). In the setting of a variable intrathoracic lesion, airflow limitation occurs during maximal expiration, and the expiratory limb of the flow-volume loop plateaus. On the other hand, when the obstructing lesion becomes so severe as to be unaffected by the phase of the respiratory cycle, it is termed fixed, and the plateau is seen during both inspiration and expiration (Fig. 5). Finally, a reduction in maximal voluntary ventilation (MVV) in the setting of a normal or near-normal FEV_1 (forced expiratory volume in one second) also suggests the presence of upper airway obstruction.[7,8]

Visualization

Direct visualization of the upper airway, larynx, and trachea by laryngoscopy or by bronchoscopy represents the "gold standard" with

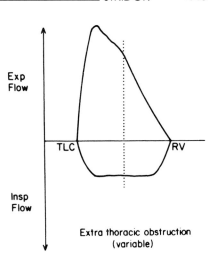

FIGURE 4. Flow-volume loop in variable extrathoracic obstruction. A plateau can be seen in the inspiratory phase of the respiratory cycle. (From Kryger M, Bode F, Antic R, Anthonisen N. Diagnosis of obstruction of the upper and central airways. Am J Med 1976;61:85–92. Reprinted with permission of Cahners Publishing Co.)

respect to diagnosis in the patient with stridor. In this manner, the specific nature and location of the obstruction can be demonstrated, biopsies can be obtained, aspirated foreign bodies can be removed, and when necessary, palliative therapy can be administered by such modalities as laser and brachytherapy. The primary care physician may also attempt to visualize the posterior oropharynx when a patient presents with pharyngitis, hoarseness, and complaints that suggest upper respiratory tract infection. Indeed, the diagnosis of epiglottitis can be confirmed if an edematous, friable, ''cherry red'' epiglottis is seen.[7] The examiner should keep in mind, however, that instrumentation of the oropharynx in the setting of epiglottitis, or any obstructing lesion, may provoke complete airway obstruction. For this reason, if upper airway obstruction is suspected, patients should be examined in a treatment setting in which the necessary equipment and personnel skilled in airway management are readily available.

MANAGING STRIDOR

Stridor is a clinical sign of mechanical dysfunction within the upper airway. This dysfunction may be due to inflammation and edema secondary to infection or trauma, aspiration of a foreign body, or a progressively enlarging mass lesion. The management of stridor is, therefore, ultimately directed toward the recognition and treatment of the underlying process. However, as we have attempted to emphasize throughout the course of this discussion, the first priority of the physician in the assessment of a patient with stridor is to determine the severity of respiratory distress and the need for emergency airway protection. Once the patient has been judged to be stable, a systematic evaluation of the upper airway, using the approach outlined here in conjunction with the appropriate subspecialists, may be employed to determine both the etiology of the obstruction and the appropriate therapy.

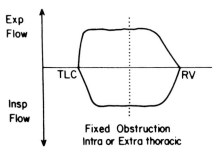

FIGURE 5. Flow-volume loop in fixed obstruction. A plateau in air flow can be seen during both inspiration and expiration. (From Kryger M, Bode F, Antic R, Anthonisen N. Diagnosis of obstruction of the upper and central airways. Am J Med 1976;61:85–92. Reprinted with permission of Cahners Publishing Co.)

REFERENCES

1. Forgacs P. The functional basis of pulmonary sounds. Chest 1978;73:399–405.
2. Baughman RP, Lowdon RG. Stridor: differentiation from asthma or upper airway noise. Am Rev Respir Dis 1989;139:1407–9.
3. Cohen SR, Hubert WI, Lewis GB, Geller KA. Foreign bodies in the airway. Five year retrospective study with special reference to management. Ann Otol Rhinol Laryngol 1980;89:437–42.
4. Leo JD, Simon RR. Upper airway obstruction and procedures and techniques in airway management. In: Brenner BE, ed. Comprehensive management of respiratory emergencies. Rockville: Aspen Systems Corp, 1985:1–31.
5. Maze A, Bloch E. Stridor in pediatric patients. Anesthesiology 1979;50:132–45.
6. Stool SE. Stridor. Int Anesthesiol Clin 1988;26:19–26.
7. Brooks JG. Upper airway obstruction. In: Sahn SA, ed. Pulmonary emergencies. New York: Churchill Livingstone, Inc, 1982:61–72.
8. Bass JW, Steele RW, Wiebe RA. Acute epiglottitis. A surgical emergency. JAMA 1974;229:671–5.
9. Khilanani U, Khatib R. Acute epiglottitis in adults. Am J Med Sci 1984;287:65–70.
10. Henley-Cohn J, Boles R, Weisberger E, Ballantyne J. Upper airway obstruction due to coccidioidomycosis. Laryngoscope 1978;89:355–60.
11. Wolfe JA, Rowe LD. Upper airway obstruction in infectious mononucleosis. Ann Otol Rhinol Laryngol 1980;89:430–3.
12. Rashkin MC, Davis T. Acute complications of endotracheal intubation: relationship to reintubation, route, urgency, and duration. Chest 1986;89:165–7.
13. Geffin B, Grillo H, Cooper JD, Pontoppidan H. Stenosis following tracheostomy for respiratory care. JAMA 1971;216:1984–8.
14. Urschel HC Jr, Razzuk MA. Management of acute traumatic injuries of tracheobronchial tree. Surg Gynecol Obstet 1973;136:113–7.
15. Gallia LJ. Laryngotracheal trauma. In: Blaisdell FW, Trunkey DD, eds. Trauma management, Cervicothoracic trauma. New York: Thieme Medical Publishers, Inc, 1986;3:117–28.
16. Cahalane M, Demling RH. Early respiratory abnormalities from smoke inhalation. JAMA 1984;251:771–3.
17. Herndon DN, Thompson PB, Traber DL. Pulmonary injury in burned patients. Crit Care Clin 1985;1(1):79–96.
18. Hollingsworth HM. Wheezing and stridor. Clin Chest Med 1987;8(2):231–40.
19. Kryger M, Bode F, Antic R, Anthonisen N. Diagnosis of obstruction of the upper and central airways. Am J Med 1976;61:85–92.
20. Miller RD, Hyatt RE. Evaluation of obstructing lesions of the trachea and larynx by flow-volume loops. Am Rev Respir Dis 1973;108:475–81.
21. Boster SR, Martinez SA. Acute upper airway obstruction in the adult. 2. Causative events. Postgrad Med 1982;72:61–7.
22. Schabel SI, Katzberg RW, Burgener FA. Acute inflammation of epiglottitis and supraglottic structures in adults. Radiology 1977;122:601–4.
23. Fraser RG, Paré JAP, Paré PD, Fraser RS, Genereux GP. Diseases of the airways. In: Diagnosis of diseases of the chest. 3rd ed. Philadelphia: WB Saunders Co, 1990;1972–2003.

SYSTOLIC MURMURS

JAMES M. HAGAR and ROBERT A. KLONER

SYNONYMS: Include Systolic Ejection Murmurs, Holosystolic Murmurs, Functional Murmurs

BACKGROUND

Evaluating the patient with a systolic murmur is among the most common clinical problems encountered in everyday practice. On one hand, systolic murmurs are common in healthy patients and are usually not associated with cardiac pathology. On the other hand, the finding of a murmur is not infrequently a sign of serious cardiac disease. When examination is hasty or incomplete, the examiner is left uncertain how to proceed. This may lead the clinician to overlook serious cardiac disease or to overuse noninvasive imaging modalities such as echocardiography. Furthermore, the results of such tests may actually be misleading if not viewed in light of the patient's whole clinical picture.

The evaluation of systolic murmurs begins at the bedside. A careful history and physical examination constitute the cornerstone of assessment and can diagnose most murmurs with a great deal of accuracy. From this process, a single diagnosis or differential diagnosis is made. Further tests then serve to confirm or rule out specific pathologic entities and provide information as to their extent and severity.

HISTORY

The cardiac history in a patient with a systolic murmur will reveal if there is previous heart disease or symptoms attributable to cardiac pathology. Essential aspects of the history that should be sought in all cases are described here.

Previous Heart Murmur or Congenital Disease

Most murmurs heard in childhood are functional or "innocent" murmurs, the frequency of which decreases with age. Patients with congenital or valvular heart disease often have a previous history of an audible murmur, however. Prior diagnostic evaluation, including cardiac catheterization, may have been performed. The patient with suspected congenital disease should be asked about a history of cyanosis, previous corrective or palliative surgery, growth in childhood, and exercise capacity.

The most common forms of congenital heart disease (not including mitral valve prolapse) are shown in Table 1, listed according to their frequency of occurrence. Many of these such as ventricular septal defect and patent ductus arteriosus are easily detected in infancy and childhood and may improve or resolve with age. Some congenital abnormalities such as bicuspid aortic valve are not diagnosed in childhood because they produce no findings until adulthood. Others, such as atrial septal defect, have few physical signs or findings, which are easily overlooked.

TABLE 1.   Most Frequent Congenital Cardiac Disorders

Bicuspid aortic valve
Ventricular septal defect
Atrial septal defect
Patent ductus arteriosus
Pulmonic stenosis
Aortic coarctation
Aortic stenosis
Tetralogy of Fallot

History of Rheumatic Fever

Patients with rheumatic heart disease frequently give a history of acute rheumatic fever. When occurring in childhood, the classic features of polyarthritis, fever, carditis, chorea, subcutaneous nodules, and erythema marginatum are usually present, and standard diagnostic criteria can be applied.[1] However, rheumatic fever in adults does not usually present in a typical fashion,[2] and many patients with rheumatic valvular disease cannot give a history of rheumatic fever. Conversely, a history of rheumatic fever does not necessarily indicate that valvular disease is present. The mitral valve is most frequently affected. If aortic valve stenosis or regurgitation is present, mitral valve disease is virtually always present as well.

Dyspnea

Dyspnea of cardiac origin, either with rest or exertion, usually indicates increased pulmonary venous pressure. Exertional dyspnea is often the earliest symptom of cardiac pathology or impaired ventricular function and may be subtle or ignored by the patient, particularly in mitral stenosis. Dyspnea at rest indicates persistently elevated pulmonary venous pressures and cardiac decompensation.

Orthopnea or paroxysmal nocturnal dyspnea (PND) indicates increased pulmonary venous pressure at rest leading to interstitial pulmonary edema. True PND occurs several hours after laying down and is relieved by sitting or standing up, distinguishing it from oropharyngeal and pulmonary disorders which may wake a patient from sleep. Cough is frequently the most prominent symptom. Sputum production is scant but may be pink and frothy if pulmonary edema is present. Severe bronchospasm may occur, and cases of congestive heart failure resembling asthma are not uncommon. Hemoptysis is usually due to pulmonary disease but can also occur in mitral stenosis and congenital heart disease complicated by the Eisenmenger reaction.

Chest Pain

Angina pectoris is most commonly due to coronary artery disease. The chest pain is pressurelike, has an exertional component, and does not vary with position or respiration. Other conditions that increase myocardial oxygen demand or reduce the blood supply to the myocardium can also lead to angina, most notably aortic stenosis and hypertrophic cardiomyopathy. Mitral regurgitation may be present in coronary artery disease, resulting from ventricular dilatation and dysfunction or papillary muscle dysfunction; in the latter case, the murmur of mitral regurgitation may become more pronounced during angina. Mitral valve prolapse syndrome is frequently associated with chest pain, but its features are often atypical of angina. (Also see chapter on Chest Pain, Acute.)

Edema

Edema of cardiac origin results from elevation of central venous and right atrial pressure, usually due to right ventricular or biventricular heart failure. This leads to bilateral pretibial edema, which worsens with upright posture and improves with recumbency, or to presacral edema in the bed-bound patient. When due to left heart failure, symptoms of dyspnea are invariably present as well. A tricuspid regurgitation murmur is commonly found when there is right heart failure and peripheral edema. Cardiac edema must be distinguished from edema due to nephrotic syndrome, liver disease, or venous insufficiency.

Cyanosis

A history of cyanosis is always a sign of serious cardiac or pulmonary disease. Cyano-

TABLE 2.   Cardiovascular Examination

General appearance
Vital signs
Skin and extremities
Jugular venous pulsations
  Jugular venous pressure
  Jugular venous wave form
Arterial pulses
  Upstroke
  Amplitude
Cardiac palpation
  Apical impulse
  Abnormal pulsations
  Thrills
Cardiac auscultation
  First and second sounds and splitting
  Murmurs
    Location
    Timing and duration
    Quality
    Intensity
    Radiation
    Variation with respiration
    Variation with position and maneuvers
  Extra sounds—clicks, gallops

sis may be central, involving the face, lips, and mucous membranes, or it may be peripheral, involving only the extremities. Central cyanosis indicates desaturation of arterial blood hemoglobin, due either to pulmonary disease or to shunting of venous blood into the arterial circulation. Peripheral cyanosis indicates inadequate flow of oxygenated blood to the extremities, owing to severely reduced cardiac output or to arterial occlusive disease.

A history of cyanosis soon after birth is sometimes elicited; a right to left or bidirectional shunt is indicated by this. Cyanosis developing in adulthood may be the result of a left- to right-sided shunt leading to pulmonary vascular disease and shunt reversal, known as the Eisenmenger reaction. (Also see chapter on Cyanosis in *Difficult Diagnosis I.*)

PHYSICAL EXAMINATION

A thorough cardiovascular examination is not limited to cardiac auscultation. Essential anatomic and hemodynamic information is obtained from examination of the arterial and venous pulses, extremities, and precordial palpation. The techniques of cardiac examination and normal findings are reviewed elsewhere.[3,4] The following elements compose a complete cardiovascular examination (Table 2).

General

General appearance may provide a clue to an underlying cardiac diagnosis. Anemia, hyperthyroidism, Marfan's syndrome, and other systemic disorders may be suspected. Body habitus and chest wall configuration should be noted. The presence of marked obesity or obstructive lung disease may make cardiac examination difficult, whereas unusually loud functional murmurs are common in patients with thoracic deformities such as severe scoliosis and pectus excavatum.

Skin and Extremities

Cyanosis can be either central or peripheral, as already noted. For cyanosis to be visible, greater than 3 gm/dl of desaturated hemoglobin must be present in the circulation; cyanosis is thus evident with lesser degrees of desaturation when polycythemia is present. Digital clubbing is frequently found when central cyanosis is long-standing. Clubbing without cyanosis occurs in infective endocarditis but is also found in pulmonary disease and gastrointestinal disorders.

Edema indicates increased right atrial pressure and accumulation of fluid in interstitial spaces. Several liters of extracellular fluid excess are usually present before edema detectable by palpation occurs. When edema is due to noncardiac causes, jugular venous pressure is not elevated. In renal disease, anasarca and facial edema are unusually prominent; in liver disease, ascites is more prominent than in cardiac disorders; if due to venous insufficiency, edema is often asymmetric, and other signs of venous stasis are evident.

Jugular Venous Pulsations

Examination of the internal jugular venous column and its contour allows the right atrial pressure to be estimated and provides information about right heart function. Jugular pulsations can be distinguished from transmitted arterial pulsations by palpation (venous pulsations are not palpable and are abolished with this maneuver).

Since the right atrium lies 5 cm beneath the sternal angle, right atrial pressure can be estimated in this way, taking patient position into account. A jugular venous pressure of 10 cm H_2O (water) or greater indicates right heart failure or hypervolemia. When latent right ventricular dysfunction is present, pressure over the abdomen or liver may elicit hepatojugular reflux, a sustained rise in the level of the jugular venous pressure (which normally should return to baseline within a few beats). When right atrial pressure is chronically elevated, the liver is enlarged and tender to palpation owing to passive congestion. When moderate to severe tricuspid insufficiency is present, pronounced elevation of systolic V waves is seen in the jugular pulse, coinciding with palpable liver pulsations.

Arterial Pulse Contour

Examination of the arterial pulse provides information about left ventricular ejection and the peripheral circulation. Asymmetry of the pulses may indicate occlusive vascular disease of an extremity. When lower extremity pulses are decreased and delayed with respect to the upper extremities, aortic coarctation is suggested. The contour of the pulse is best examined from a central site, either the carotid or brachial arteries. Both its upstroke (rate of rise) and amplitude (volume) should be noted.

The upstroke relates to the force of ejection of blood from the left ventricle and the compliance of the great vessels. Delayed upstroke is a hallmark of aortic stenosis, although if the aorta is noncompliant owing to aging or atherosclerosis, upstroke may appear relatively normal. The briskness of the upstroke is increased with normal amplitude in severe mitral regurgitation, ventricular septal defect, and hypertrophic cardiomyopathy. Upstroke is increased with increased amplitude in chronic aortic insufficiency, chronic hypertension, and hyperdynamic states.

The amplitude of the pulse correlates with the volume of blood ejected with each beat. It is decreased in congestive heart failure, severe aortic stenosis, and low output states, and it is increased in aortic insufficiency, hyperdynamic states, and patent ductus arteriosus. The wave may have a bisferiens quality, with two distinct systolic peaks, in aortic insufficiency and hypertrophic obstructive cardiomyopathy. It may alternate in intensity between beats, indicating severe left ventricular dysfunction.

Cardiac Palpation

Palpation of the cardiac impulse, frequently overlooked, can give a great deal of information about cardiac function, chamber size, and hemodynamics not available with auscultation. The apical impulse is usually the only cardiac pulsation detected in normal subjects and is best appreciated in the left lateral decubitus posture. Normally, it is found medial to the midclavicular line in the fifth interspace and encompasses an area one inch square. Displacement of the impulse downward and laterally indicates left ventricular dilatation; left ventricular hypertrophy alone causes only slight lateral displacement. Enlargement of the impulse with a sustained quality or a heave indicates left ventricular dysfunction. The impulse will be abnormally forceful if there is increased volume of left ventricular ejection, as in mitral or aortic insufficiency, ventricular septal defect, or high output states. It will be both forceful and sustained if aortic stenosis or hypertrophic obstructive cardiomyopathy is present.

Other cardiac impulses should be sought. A right ventricular lift at the lower left sternal border indicates significant right ventricular volume or pressure overload. A palpable second heart sound in the pulmonic area reliably indicates severe pulmonary hypertension; a pulmonary artery pulsation may be palpated in the same area under conditions of increased pulmonary flow or pressure. Third or fourth heart sounds are often palpable, and loud systolic murmurs palpable as a thrill.

Cardiac Auscultation

Auscultation of the heart is central to the differentiation of systolic murmurs. However, the characteristics of the murmur alone do not constitute adequate cardiac auscultation. It is careful attention to the first and second heart sounds, extra sounds, and cardiac impulses that provides the additional information needed to distinguish functional from pathologic murmurs.

The first sound (S_1) is generated from mitral and tricuspid valve closure. It is increased when the ventricular force of contraction is increased, as with hyperdynamic states, and when the mitral valve remains open at onset of ventricular contraction, as with rheumatic mitral stenosis and short P-R interval. It is diminished in congestive heart failure, myocardial infarction, when the mitral valve leaflets are immobile, and when the mitral valve is closed at the onset of systole, as in severe aortic insufficiency.

The second sound (S_2) consists of the closure sounds of the aortic (A_2) and pulmonic valves (P_2). P_2 is normally only heard in the pulmonic area and middle left sternal border; if heard at the apex, it is abnormally accentuated. A_2 is increased with systemic hypertension and aortic dilatation and decreased in aortic stenosis. P_2 is decreased in pulmonic stenosis and increased when there is pulmonary hypertension or increased pulmonary flow.

Inspiratory splitting of S_2 is one of the most valuable parts of the cardiac examination. Splitting arises because pulmonic valve closure normally occurs after aortic valve closure. The separation of A_2 and P_2 increases with inspiration ("physiologic" splitting), which increases blood flow into the right heart and prolongs right ventricular ejection. The magnitude of this respiratory variation decreases with age and with pulmonary hypertension. Widened but physiologic splitting occurs when pulmonic closure is delayed (delayed right ventricular activation or prolonged mechanical systole) or left ventricular mechanical systole is shortened (Table 3). Splitting is reversed (paradoxical) when aortic closure is delayed (delayed left ventricular ac-

tivation or prolonged mechanical systole) or pulmonic closure occurs early. Splitting is fixed if respiratory changes in blood flow are transmitted to both ventricles, as in atrial septal defect, and when widening or reversal of splitting is extreme.

Third and fourth heart sounds may arise from either ventricle. The third sound corresponds to rapid ventricular filling in early diastole and is a normal finding in children and young adults. It is found in conditions of increased flow (valvular regurgitation, hyperdynamic states, and shunts) and ventricular

TABLE 3. Abnormal Splitting of the Second Heart Sound

Widened splitting
  Right bundle branch block
  Pulmonic stenosis (mild or moderate)
  Mitral regurgitation
  Ventricular septal defect
Fixed splitting
  Atrial septal defect
  Pulmonic stenosis (severe)
  Right bundle branch block with ventricular dysfunction
Reversed splitting
  Aortic stenosis
  Severe aortic insufficiency
  Hypertrophic obstructive cardiomyopathy
  Left bundle branch block
  Right ventricular pacemaker
  Patent ductus arteriosus
  Acute myocardial ischemia

TABLE 4. Etiology of Systolic Murmurs

Systolic ejection type
  Aortic outflow
    Aortic stenosis
    Aortic sclerosis
    Hypertrophic obstructive cardiomyopathy
    Aortic coarctation
  Pulmonic outflow
    Pulmonic stenosis
    Infundibular stenosis
    Atrial septal defect
  Functional murmur
  Others
    Mitral prolapse (mid- or late systolic)
    Hyperdynamic states—pregnancy, hyperthyroidism, fever, anemia, exercise
    Vascular bruits
Holosystolic
  Mitral regurgitation
  Tricuspid regurgitation
  Ventricular septal defect
Continuous
  Patent ductus arteriosus
  Arteriovenous fistula
  Ruptured sinus of Valsalva aneurysm
  Venous hum

TABLE 5. Dynamic Cardiac Auscultation

Hemodynamic Effect	STANDING ↓ Venous Return ↑ Heart Rate	VALSALVA ↓ Venous Return ↓ Cardiac Output	POST-PVC* ↑ Venous Return ↑ Contractility	HANDGRIP ↑ Blood Pressure ↑ Heart Rate ↑ Cardiac Output	AMYL NITRITE ↓ Blood Pressure ↑ Heart Rate ↑ Cardiac Output
Hypertrophic cardiomyopathy	↑	↑	↑	↓	↑
Aortic stenosis	↓	↓	↑	↓	↑
Mitral regurgitation	↓	↓	NC†	↑	↓
Ventricular septal defect			NC	↑	↓
Tricuspid regurgitation	↓	↓	NC		↑
Pulmonic stenosis	↓	↓	↑	↑	↑
Mitral prolapse					
Click	←	←	NC	←	NC
Murmur	↑	NC	NC	↑	↑

↑ = increases murmur.
← = occurs earlier.
↓ = decreases murmur.
* PVC = Premature ventricular contractions.
† NC = no change.

dilatation or dysfunction. The fourth heart sound corresponds to atrial contraction. It occurs when the contribution of atrial systole to ventricular filling is increased, indicating decreased ventricular compliance (as in ventricular hypertrophy, myocardial ischemia, and acute valvular disease).

In auscultation of cardiac murmurs, it is routine to describe a murmur in terms of its location, timing and duration, quality, intensity, and pattern of radiation. A systolic ejection-type murmur does not begin immediately after the first sound. It then has a crescendo-decrescendo pattern, and ends before the second sound. A holosystolic murmur is present throughout all of systole. The timing (systolic, diastolic, continuous) and duration (systolic ejection, holosystolic) of any murmur allow it to be classified as shown in Table 4.

Dynamic Auscultation

Whether a systolic murmur varies with respiration should be noted in all cases. Murmurs arising within right heart chambers increase with inspiration and decrease with expiration, owing to an inspiratory increase in blood flow through the right heart. This respiratory variation particularly aids in the diagnosis of tricuspid regurgitation, known as Carvallo's sign.

Other dynamic maneuvers, shown in Table 5, are useful in particular settings.[5,6] The strain phase of the Valsalva maneuver, which decreases venous return and increases both af-

terload and contractility, causes most systolic murmurs to decrease, with the notable exception of mitral prolapse and hypertrophic obstructive cardiomyopathy, which increase. Standing from a squatting position, by decreasing venous return, has a similar effect.

DIAGNOSTIC STUDIES

Electrocardiogram

A normal electrocardiogram is the expected finding in a patient judged to have an innocent murmur. For example, a conduction abnormality or right ventricular hypertrophy in a patient with an "innocent" pulmonic murmur might lead to the diagnosis of atrial septal defect or pulmonic stenosis. Lack of an abnormal finding, such as left ventricular hypertrophy in aortic stenosis, would tend to make severe disease unlikely. In general, the pattern of atrial or ventricular hypertrophy or conduction abnormalities coincides with the known pathophysiology and severity of the suspected disease. However, the electrocardiogram is relatively nonspecific and does not give the precise anatomic information that echocardiography is capable of supplying.

Echocardiography

Two-dimensional and Doppler echocardiography is the single most useful tool for noninvasive cardiac evaluation in patients suspected of having valvular or congenital heart disease.[7] Two-dimensional and M-mode echocardiography provides detailed anatomic information regarding chamber dimension, wall thickness, and valvular morphology, and a technically adequate study can accurately diagnose nearly all the common conditions causing systolic murmurs. Pulse and continuous wave Doppler echocardiography, and more recently color flow mapping, add an additional physiologic dimension to the echocardiographic study. This allows the size of stenotic valvular lesions to be measured with reasonable accuracy, whereas valvular regurgitation and shunt flow can be estimated semiquantitatively. A detailed discussion of the technique is beyond the scope of this chapter.

Although extremely useful and noninvasive, overuse of echocardiography has potential drawbacks. Findings such as mild aortic and mitral insufficiency,[8] patent foramen ovale, or mitral prolapse are not infrequent in healthy individuals and may lead to unnecessary concern or treatment. Reasonable attention to physical diagnosis will lead to appropriate referral to echocardiography of patients in whom significant pathology is suspected or cannot be ruled out.

Cardiac Catheterization

Although the advent of echocardiography had made cardiac catheterization unnecessary in many cases of valvular and congenital heart disease, it still has an important role. Coronary arteriography is necessary in middle-aged and elderly patients undergoing surgery for valvular heart disease, particularly aortic stenosis. Catheterization can accurately measure shunt flow, pulmonary pressure, valve area, and valvular regurgitation. It may be necessary when the clinical picture suggests that echocardiography has over- or underestimated the extent of disease, when multiple abnormalities are suspected, or when indications for surgical intervention are in question. Furthermore, cardiac catheterization increasingly offers the potential for therapeutic intervention.

ASSESSMENT

Classification of Systolic Murmurs

All systolic murmurs can be placed in one of three categories, the essential first step in their assessment. Murmurs are either "systolic ejection" type (also called midsystolic, "crescendo-decrescendo," or "diamond-shaped"), holosystolic, or continuous ("machinery" murmur). The most common causes of each type of systolic murmur are listed in Table 4.

An ejection murmur arises from the flow of blood through the aortic or pulmonic valves or in the respective outflow tracts. Because a pressure difference does not exist between the chambers at all times during systole (because of isovolumic contraction and relaxation periods), the ejection murmur begins some time after the first sound, increases to a peak, and ends before semilunar valve closure and the second heart sound. This pattern is illustrated in Figure 1A for aortic stenosis.

Holosystolic murmurs are caused by flow of blood from a higher to a lower pressure chamber when a pressure difference exists throughout all of systole. As a result, the murmur begins immediately with the first sound and continues right up to the second sound. This is illustrated in Figure 1B for mitral regurgitation.

Continuous murmurs can arise only when blood flows from a higher to a lower pressure chamber throughout the entire cardiac cycle. This occurs when there is an anomalous connection between a great vessel and a lower pressure chamber as in patent ductus arteriosus, rupture of a sinus of Valsalva aneurysm into the right atrium, or arteriovenous fistula. Continuous murmurs also occur with severe pulmonary artery stenosis or aortic coarctation.

Aortic Ejection Murmurs

Ejection murmurs localized to the aortic area, often radiating to the carotids, become increasingly frequent with age. They may arise from a thickened or stenotic aortic valve, a dilated or atherosclerotic aortic root, or the left ventricular outflow tract. Determining the etiology and hemodynamic significance of an aortic murmur is a common reason for cardiac evaluation.

Three entities, valvular aortic stenosis, hypertrophic cardiomyopathy, and nonobstructive aortic valve thickening or root dilatation known commonly as "aortic sclerosis," are the major causes of such murmurs in adults. Each can be diagnosed and distinguished from the others with reasonable certainty by physical examination.

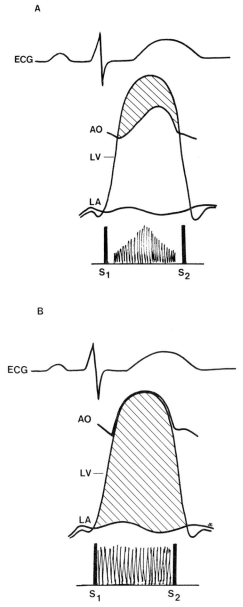

A

ECG

AO

LV

LA

S_1 S_2

B

ECG

AO

LV

LA

S_1 S_2

FIGURE 1. Genesis of holosystolic and systolic ejection murmurs. *A,* In aortic stenosis, an example of an ejection-type murmur, a significant gradient between ventricle and aorta exists only during ejection, which increases, then decreases before A_2. *B,* In mitral regurgitation, an example of a holosystolic murmur, a pressure difference exists between left ventricle and left atrium immediately upon mitral closure and persists up to or beyond aortic valve closure.

Hemodynamically significant aortic stenosis is characterized by a long, ejection-type murmur that radiates to the carotids, often with a palpable thrill. The murmur peaks later when more severe stenosis is present. Radiation to the apex may occur, causing diagnostic confu-

sion, but the murmur is not heard well in the axilla. A_2 is nearly always diminished in intensity with narrowed (or reversed) splitting if significant stenosis is present. An early systolic ejection click may be present with a congenitally stenotic or bicuspid valve but not in rheumatic or degenerative stenosis. The carotids have delayed upstroke and often are of small volume. The apical impulse is usually sustained and forceful but may not be if left ventricular dysfunction is present. Left ventricular hypertrophy is usually present on electrocardiogram. This constellation of findings together suggest that aortic obstruction is significant. If there is no significant obstruction to flow, the pulse contour S_2 and apical impulse are normal. In this case, the murmur is a functional aortic murmur, which may or may not be associated with thickening or calcification of the aortic valve (aortic "sclerosis"). When necessary, aortic stenosis can be distinguished from mitral regurgitation by its accentuation after an extrasystole and following amyl nitrite inhalation. Doppler echocardiography is extremely useful to measure transaortic gradient and calculate aortic valve area.

Hypertrophic obstructive cardiomyopathy may superficially resemble aortic stenosis, but careful examination will suggest its presence. The apical impulse is forceful and sustained, as in valvular aortic stenosis. However, the arterial pulse has an abnormally brisk upstroke, since initial left ventricular ejection is forceful, and A_2 is not reduced. The murmur is usually best heard at the lower left sternal border rather than the aortic area and rarely radiates into the carotids. Standing from a squat and Valsalva maneuver classically increase the murmur if dynamic outflow obstruction is present,[9] further distinguishing it from valvular aortic stenosis. Mitral regurgitation is frequently present as well. The electrocardiogram typically shows severe left ventricular hypertrophy and abnormally large Q waves. Two-dimensional echocardiography readily demonstrates asymmetric septal hypertrophy with systolic anterior motion of the anterior mitral valve leaflet. Doppler examination can localize the outflow tract obstruction to the subvalvular region rather than the aortic valve itself.

Functional Murmurs

The most common type of murmur is a functional or "innocent" ejection murmur unassociated with valvular pathology. This murmur is soft (usually grade I or II), is short in duration, and does not radiate. Cardiac examination is otherwise normal. The murmur arises in the aortic[10] or pulmonic outflow tract. It is frequent in the young and develops or increases in intensity during hyperdynamic states such as pregnancy, anemia, fever, and hyperthyroidism.

Pulmonic Ejection Murmurs

Ejection murmurs arising in the right ventricle and pulmonic outflow tract are heard best at the upper and middle left sternal border and are not heard in the carotids or axilla. Atrial septal defect and valvular pulmonic stenosis produce murmurs of this type, which must be distinguished from innocent flow murmurs.

The murmur in atrial septal defect arises from the increased flow in the pulmonary outflow tract; flow across the defect is silent. Thus, the murmur may resemble an innocent flow murmur. However, fixed splitting of S_2 is present if a significant shunt exists. A right ventricular lift may also be present, and P_2 is usually increased. Electrocardiogram will have right axis deviation, right ventricular hypertrophy, or conduction abnormalities.

Moderate or severe pulmonic stenosis is easily differentiated from a functional murmur. A sustained right ventricular lift is present, and there may be a thrill in the pulmonic area. The P_2 is diminished, and splitting is widened or fixed. An early systolic click is often heard. The murmur is late peaking in severe cases and may even continue past A_2 but stops before P_2. When the degree of stenosis is mild, these findings may be more subtle. The murmur differs from aortic stenosis in its location and radiation but also in its increase with respiration. It is distinguished from atrial septal defect by an ejection click and decreased intensity of P_2. Both atrial septal defect and pulmonic stenosis are reliably diagnosed by Doppler echocardiography.

Holosystolic Murmurs

Differentiation of mitral from tricuspid regurgitation is usually not difficult. The murmur of tricuspid regurgitation will be associated with an abnormal jugular pulse, inspiratory accentuation of the murmur, and

hepatic pulsations. Ventricular septal defect cannot be distinguished from mitral regurgitation by the second heart sound or by response to maneuvers. However, the murmur of ventricular septal defect, usually with a palpable thrill, is best appreciated at the lower left sternal border rather than the apex and axilla.

When mitral regurgitation occurs in a patient with coronary artery disease, papillary muscle ischemia or rupture is suggested. In acute cases, the murmur may end well before S_2. Radiation is to the back, spine, or head if anterior papillary muscle rupture occurs and to the sternal border with posterior papillary muscle rupture.

Mitral Valve Prolapse

The auscultatory findings in mitral prolapse syndrome, like its clinical manifestations, are protean. There may be no abnormal findings, a midsystolic click, a click with a late systolic murmur, or a holosystolic murmur of mitral regurgitation. The prolapse of the valve is dynamic. The click occurs earlier and the murmur is longer (and usually louder) with standing from a squat and with Valsalva strain. Echocardiography is often utilized to diagnose mitral prolapse, but overdiagnosis is frequent if rigid criteria are not applied.[11,12] It appears that many otherwise healthy persons have echocardiographic prolapse without auscultatory or clinical manifestations.

Continuous Murmurs

Patent ductus arteriosus produces a characteristic continuous murmur and thrill at the upper left sternal border, with signs of increased blood flow through both ventricles. Patients with coronary arteriovenous fistulae or ruptured sinus of Valsalva aneurysm have a murmur that is similar but usually not maximal at the same site as in patent ductus. Aortic coarctation produces either a holosystolic or continuous murmur; radiation to the back and a lower extremity pulse deficit are key to its diagnosis.

When both holosystolic and diastolic murmurs are present, the sound may appear to be continuous; careful auscultation will reveal the murmurs to be separate. Another continuous sound, a cervical venous hum, should not be mistaken for a pathologic murmur. It is low-pitched and is abolished by gentle compression or turning of the neck.

REFERENCES

1. American Heart Association, Council on Rheumatic Fever and Congenital Heart Disease. Jones criteria (revised) for guidance in the diagnosis of rheumatic fever. Circulation 1965;32:664–8.
2. Ben-Dov I, Berry E. Acute rheumatic fever in adults over the age of 45 years: an analysis of 23 patients together with a review of the literature. Semin Arthritis Rheum 1980;10:100–10.
3. Braunwald E. The physical examination. In: Braunwald E, ed. Heart disease: a textbook of cardiovascular medicine. Philadelphia: WB Saunders Co, 1988:13–40.
4. Perloff JK. Cardiac auscultation. DM 1980;26:1–47.
5. Lembo NJ, Dell'Italia LJ, Crawford MH, O'Rourke RA. Bedside diagnosis of systolic murmurs. N Engl J Med 1988;318:1572–8.
6. Grewe K, Crawford MH, O'Rourke RA. Differentiation of cardiac murmurs by dynamic auscultation. Curr Probl Cardiol 1988;13:669–721.
7. Nishimura RA, Miller FA Jr, Callahan MJ, Benassi RC, Seward JB, Tajik AJ. Doppler echocardiography: theory, instrumentation, technique, and application. Mayo Clin Proc 1985;60:321–43.
8. Rahko PS. Prevalence of regurgitant murmurs in patients with valvular regurgitation detected by Doppler echocardiography. Ann Intern Med 1989;111:466–72.
9. Braunwald E, Oldham HN Jr, Ross J Jr, Linhart JW, Mason DT, Fort L III. The circulatory response of patients with idiopathic hypertrophic subaortic stenosis to nitroglycerin and to the Valsalva maneuver. Circulation 1964;29:422–32.
10. Stein PD, Sabbah HN. Aortic origin of innocent murmurs. Am J Cardiol 1977;39:665–71.
11. Perloff JK, Child JS. Mitral valve prolapse. Evolution and refinement of diagnostic techniques. Circulation 1989;80:710–1.
12. Krivokapich J, Child JS, Dadourian BJ, Perloff JK. Reassessment of echocardiographic criteria for diagnosis of mitral valve prolapse. Am J Cardiol 1988;61:131–5.

TACHYARRHYTHMIAS

RUEY J. SUNG

SYNONYMS: Fast Heart Rhythm, Rapid Heartbeat

BACKGROUND

Normally, the heart rhythm is generated by an intrinsic pacemaker tissue, that is, the sinoatrial (SA) node, which is located at the junction of the right atrium and the superior vena cava. The activity of the SA node is governed by the autonomic nervous system. At the resting state, the parasympathetic influence predominates, and the SA node delivers electrical impulses at rates between 60 and 90 beats per minute. This resting heart rhythm is called normal sinus rhythm. During exercise, there is withdrawal of parasympathetic tone followed by enhancement of sympathetic tone. Consequently, the sinus rhythm accelerates its rate beyond 100 beats per minute. The fast sinus rhythm is referred to as sinus tachycardia. Sinus tachycardia also occurs as a physiologic response to anemia, fever, hypovolemia, hyperthyroidism, congestive heart failure, and so on, as a result of enhancement of sympathetic tone when oxygen and metabolic demands are increased. On the other hand, the sinus rhythm may decelerate its rate below 60 beats per minute owing to enhanced vagotonia or SA nodal dysfunction (sick sinus syndrome). The slow sinus rhythm is referred to as sinus bradycardia.

This chapter discusses tachyarrhythmias. The prefix *tachy* means "swift," and the suffix *arrhythmias* denotes "abnormal rhythms." Tachyarrhythmias are abnormally fast heart rhythms at a rate greater than 100 beats per minute as documented by the electrocardiogram (ECG). The two most common electrophysiologic mechanisms underlying tachyarrhythmias are re-entry and enhanced automaticity.[1,2] Re-entry occurs when the wavefront of an electrical impulse circulates repetitively within an intracardiac anatomic circuit. Two frequently encountered clinical examples of re-entry are atrioventricular (AV) nodal re-entrant tachycardia and AV reciprocating tachycardia associated with the Wolff-

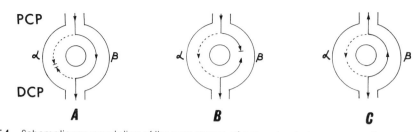

FIGURE 1. Schematic representation of the occurrence of a re-entrant phenomenon. A re-entrant circuit is composed of a proximal common pathway (*PCP*), two conduction pathways (α and β), and a distal common pathway (*DCP*). The β pathway has a faster conduction time (*solid line*), with a longer refractory period, and the α pathway has a slower conduction time (*dashed line*), with a shorter refractory period. *A,* An impulse is conducted over both α and β pathways without initiation of a re-entrant phenomenon. *B,* A premature impulse is blocked in the β pathway but is conducted slowly by way of the α pathway. *C,* The slow conduction in the α pathway is sufficient to allow recovery of excitability of the previously blocked β pathway. The premature impulse can thus be conducted over the β pathway in a retrograde direction, initiating a re-entrant phenomenon. (From Sung RJ, Chang MS, Chiang BN. Clinical electrophysiology of supraventricular tachycardia. Cardiol Clin 1983;1:225–51. Reprinted with permission of WB Saunders Co.)

Parkinson-White syndrome. The anatomic circuit in AV nodal re-entry consists of two AV nodal pathways (fast and slow) and two common pathways (proximal and distal) (Fig. 1), whereas the anatomic circuit in AV reciprocation incorporates the atrium, the AV node-His Purkinje system, the ventricle, and an anomalous AV connection (e.g., Kent bundle). Enhanced automaticity occurs when the speed of normal or abnormal diastolic (phase 4) depolarization of a cardiac tissue is accelerated. Both re-entry and enhanced automaticity may occur spontaneously or in association with a variety of underlying disease processes (e.g., myocardial ischemia or infarction, myocarditis, cardiomyopathy, and degenerative changes) and may be iatrogenic or drug-induced (e.g., electrolyte imbalance, digitalis excess, and proarrhythmic effects of antiarrhythmic agents).

Tachyarrhythmias are generally divided into two types: supraventricular and ventricular. This classification conforms to a simple electrocardiographic distinction: Supraventricular tachyarrhythmias arising at or above the level of the His bundle are characterized by narrow QRS complexes identical to those of normal sinus rhythm, whereas ventricular tachyarrhythmias originating below the level of the His bundle in the ventricle produce wide and bizarre QRS complexes. Although this classification is popular, it is imprecise because (1) supraventricular tachyarrhythmias include AV reciprocating tachycardia, which requires both the atrium and the ventricle to maintain re-entry; and (2) supraventricular tachyarrhythmias may be complicated by ven-

tricular pre-excitation and pre-existing or functional bundle branch block with resultant wide QRS complexes. Based on the ECG characteristics and underlying electrophysiologic mechanisms, both supraventricular and ventricular tachyarrhythmias can further be subdivided into various forms, as listed in Table 1.

The prevalence of tachyarrhythmias increases with advancing age.[3,4] They can complicate a variety of organic heart diseases but may also be observed in apparently healthy subjects.[3,4] In general, ventricular tachyarrhythmias connote a much worse prognosis than supraventricular tachyarrhythmias[1,2,3,4] because of (1) the absence of a protective bar-

TABLE 1.   Classification of Cardiac Tachyarrhythmias

SUPRAVENTRICULAR	VENTRICULAR
Nonparoxysmal SA* node tachycardia	Ventricular tachycardia
Paroxysmal SA node or SA re-entrant tachycardia	Torsades de pointes
Ectopic or re-entrant atrial tachycardia	Ventricular flutter
Chaotic (multifocal) atrial tachycardia	Ventricular fibrillation
Atrial flutter	
Atrial fibrillation	
Accelerated AV† junction rhythm or tachycardia	
Paroxysmal AV nodal re-entrant tachycardia	
Paroxysmal AV reciprocating tachycardia of the orthodromic form	

* SA = sinoatrial.
† AV = atrioventricular.

rier (e.g., the AV node in supraventricular tachyarrhythmias) to limit the rate of ventricular response; (2) the abnormal contractile pattern of the ventricle (wide QRS complex due to electrical asynchrony); and (3) the frequent presence of organic heart disease with compromised left ventricular function. Degeneration of ventricular tachycardia to ventricular fibrillation leading to sudden cardiac arrest and death is not an uncommon occurrence.

Palpitations (heart pounding) and rapid pulses caused by tachyarrhythmias are often felt by the patient. An episode of prolonged tachyarrhythmia may result in incomplete recovery (diastole) time for ventricular filling and may thereby cause a significant drop in blood pressure (hypotension) and/or pulmonary congestion (congestive heart failure), particularly in patients with compromised left ventricular function (ejection fraction equal to or less than 40 per cent). As a consequence, symptoms of dizziness, lightheadedness, fainting (syncope), chest pain (angina pectoris), shortness of breath, and even cardiac arrest (circulatory collapse) may ensue following the onset of a tachyarrhythmia.

HISTORY

History of the Present Illness

If the patient is in a tachyarrhythmia at the time he or she presents, the severity and duration of the presenting symptoms associated with the tachyarrhythmia should be first obtained in order to determine whether or not the tachyarrhythmia should be immediately terminated by an electrical (cardioversion or defibrillation) or pharmacologic means. Hence, in addition to palpitations, symptoms such as dizziness, syncope, chest pain, shortness of breath, and cardiac arrest brought on by the tachyarrhythmia should be elicited and recorded.

The triggering factors should be sought for the onset of the tachyarrhythmia. Is the onset of palpitations initiated by anger, nervousness, exertion, chest pain, or shortness of breath? The experience of chest pain or shortness of breath prior to the onset of palpitations may suggest myocardial ischemia or infarction, pulmonary embolism, or congestive heart failure as the triggering factor rather than resultant symptomatology of the tachyarrhythmia. Substance abuse (e.g., cocaine, heroin, marijuana, amphetamine, etc.) and alco-

hol ingestion (holiday heart syndrome) should also be considered, as either may serve as a triggering factor for the onset of a tachyarrhythmia. This history of recent medication is also important. Is the onset of palpitations related to discontinuation of an antiarrhythmic drug (medical noncompliance) or initiation of a new antiarrhythmic drug (idiosyncratic reaction or proarrhythmic effects of an antiarrhythmic agent)? The possibilities of tachyarrhythmias being caused by diet- or diuretic-induced hypokalemia and drug toxicity such as digitalis intoxication or the excess of antiarrhythmic drugs should also be entertained. Another important question is the history of recent infection such as upper respiratory tract infection, pneumonia, and pleuritis that may also involve the heart (e.g., pericarditis and myocarditis), thereby causing tachyarrhythmias.

Past Medical History

A history of many similar episodes of palpitations dating back to childhood in otherwise apparently healthy subjects favors the diagnosis of re-entrant supraventricular tachycardia such as AV nodal re-entrant tachycardia or AV reciprocating tachycardia.[1] In contrast, the occurrence of a tachyarrhythmia associated with prior myocardial infarction, myocarditis, pericarditis, cardiomyopathy, or congestive heart failure is suggestive of either atrial fibrillation or a ventricular tachyarrhythmia.[1,2,3,4] A previous history of termination of palpitations by vagal maneuvers (e.g., carotid sinus massage, gag reflex, and Valsalva maneuvers) usually identifies a re-entrant supraventricular tachycardia in which the SA or AV node is part of the re-entrant circuit.

Certain tachyarrhythmias are more commonly seen in association with specific organic heart diseases—for example, atrial fibrillation in rheumatic mitral stenosis, hyperthyroidism, pericarditis, and congestive heart failure associated with structural heart diseases; ectopic or re-entrant atrial tachycardia, atrial flutter, and chaotic (multifocal) atrial tachycardia in chronic obstructive lung disease; accelerated AV junction rhythm or tachycardia in hypokalemia, digitalis intoxication, and inferior wall myocardial infarction; ventricular tachyarrhythmias in atherosclerotic coronary heart disease, cardiomyopathy, myocarditis, right ventricular dysplasia, sarcoid heart disease, and mitral valve prolapse syndrome;[3,4,5,6] idiopathic benign ventricular tachycardia in apparently healthy young subjects;[7,8] and torsades de pointes in prolonged QT syndrome which may be congenital or acquired (usually drug-induced), hypokalemia, bradyarrhythmias, and myocardial ischemia with or without coronary arterial spasm.[9]

Focused Queries

1. *Are you having dizziness, chest pain, or breathing difficulty associated with palpitations? Have you ever passed out (fainting or syncope)?* The severity and duration of these symptoms dictate the decision whether or not to terminate the tachyarrhythmia immediately.

2. *How long have you had these episodes of palpitations?* The long duration of recurrent episodes without being associated with an organic heart disease favors the diagnosis of reentrant supraventricular tachycardia.[1]

3. *How do you usually get relief of palpitations?* Tachyarrhythmias that can be terminated by vagal maneuvers are suggestive of a re-entrant supraventricular tachycardia involving the SA or AV node as a part of the re-entrant circuit.[1]

4. *Are the onset and termination of the palpitations abrupt or gradual?* Sudden onset and termination of a tachyarrhythmia suggests the usual paroxysmal nature of a re-entrant mechanism.

5. *Can you think of any provoking factors relative to the onset of palpitations?* Focus on exertion, chest pain, alcohol ingestion, or drug abuse. Identification of these factors is relevant to the future management of the tachyarrhythmias.[2]

6. *What medicines are you currently taking? Have you recently begun or stopped taking any medicine?* Suspect medical noncompliance and entertain the possibility of iatrogenic and drug-induced tachyarrhythmias.

PHYSICAL EXAMINATION

Vital signs (mental status, blood pressure, pulse rate, and respiratory rate) must be immediately obtained. Regardless of the origin of a tachyarrhythmia, the urgency of termination of a tachyarrhythmia is determined by vital signs. In general, patients with ventricular tachyarrhythmias are more likely to have clinically significant organic heart diseases such as atherosclerotic coronary heart disease and

primary or secondary cardiomyopathy and are more likely to be symptomatic with dizziness, syncope, chest pain, congestive heart failure, and even cardiac arrest, compared with those with supraventricular tachyarrhythmias. However, absence of significant clinical symptoms during an episode of palpitations does not exclude a ventricular tachyarrhythmia as the underlying rhythm disturbance.

Arterial Pulses and Jugular Vein

Rapid arterial pulses can usually be felt in carotid, branchial, and radial arteries. If hypotension or congestive heart failure is present, the intensity of arterial pulses is diminished. The presence of irregular arterial pulses with variable pulse intensity is suggestive of atrial fibrillation. Jugular veins may be elevated in the presence of right-sided heart failure. The wave form of venous pulsations should be carefully analyzed. Regular cannon A waves may be seen in atrial tachycardia, AV reciprocating tachycardia, or ventricular tachycardia with 1:1 ventriculoatrial conduction, whereas irregular cannon A waves usually indicate ventricular tachycardia with AV dissociation.

Heart and Lungs

Displacement of the point of the maximal impulse (cardiomegaly) with or without a heart murmur suggests the presence of an organic heart disease. Variation in the intensity of the first heart sound is a sign of AV dissociation suggestive of a ventricular tachyarrhythmia. Atrial fibrillation is noted by irregular heartbeats and a pulse deficit in the carotid or radial artery (the heart rate is greater than the arterial pulse rate). Evidence of congestive heart failure—an S_3 gallop rhythm, moist rales in both lung fields with or without wheezing (cardiac asthma), and decreased breathing sounds with percussion dullness (pleural effusion)—may be found during tachyarrhythmias.

ELECTROCARDIOGRAMS

The 12-lead ECG with a 30-second lead II or aVF rhythm strip is essential for differential diagnoses of tachyarrhythmias. Narrow QRS complex identical to that of sinus rhythm indicates that the tachyarrhythmia is of a supraventricular origin, whereas a broad and bizarre QRS complex (equal to or greater than

FIGURE 2. SA re-entrant tachycardia. *A*, Onset of nonsustained SA re-entry (third and ninth P waves). *B*, Onset of sustained SA re-entrant tachycardia (seventh P wave) at a rate of 105 beats per minute. (From Sung RJ, Chang MS, Chiang BN. Clinical electrophysiology of supraventricular tachycardia. Cardiol Clin 1983;1:225–51. Reprinted with permission of WB Saunders Co.)

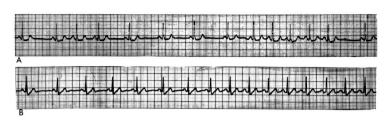

0.12 seconds) implies that the tachyarrhythmia is either a ventricular tachyarrhythmia or a supraventricular tachyarrhythmia with ventricular pre-excitation or bundle branch block (pre-existing or functional).

Nonparoxysmal SA Node Tachycardia and Paroxysmal SA Node or SA Re-entrant Tachycardia

The onset of either tachycardia requires no prolongation of the P-R interval, and the P wave morphology of either tachycardia is identical or similar to that seen in sinus rhythm (Fig. 2). Nonparoxysmal SA node tachycardia is caused by enhanced automaticity presumably due to imbalance of the autonomic nervous system. Vagal maneuvers and intravenous verapamil or adenosine can terminate paroxysmal SA node or SA re-entrant tachycardia but can only slow the rate of nonparoxysmal SA node tachycardia.

Ectopic or Re-entrant Atrial Tachycardia

The P wave morphology during tachycardia is usually different from that seen in sinus rhythm. Both vagal maneuvers and intravenous verapamil or adenosine exert no effects on these two atrial tachyarrhythmias but may transiently slow the ventricular response by depressing AV nodal conduction (Fig. 3). Ectopic atrial tachycardia with AV block in patients taking digitalis should arouse a suspicion of digitalis intoxication (Fig. 4).

Chaotic (Multifocal) Atrial Tachycardia

The ECG features of chaotic atrial tachycardia include (1) the presence of discrete P waves with at least three different configurations; (2) irregular variation of P-P, P-R, and R-R intervals; and (3) an isoelectric line between P waves (Fig. 5).

Atrial Flutter

Typically, the atrial rate during atrial flutter is 300 (280 to 360) per minute. Physiologic block in the AV node frequently limits its ventricular response to 140 to 180 per minute (2:1 AV block). The typical atrial flutter is characterized by a sawtooth appearance of the baseline in standard ECG leads II, III, and aVF and is referred to as type I atrial flutter. Atrial flutter with less distinct atrial flutter waves and with atrial rates of 340 to 430 per minute is referred to as type II atrial flutter. Both vagal maneuvers and intravenous verapamil or

FIGURE 3. Effect of carotid sinus massage on atrial tachycardia. *A*, The rate of ventricular response is 170 beats per minute during tachycardia. *B*, Carotid sinus massage induces AV block and exposes P waves of atrial tachycardia. (From Sung RJ, Chang MS, Chiang BN. Clinical electrophysiology of supraventricular tachycardia. Cardiol Clin 1983;1:225–51. Reprinted with permission of WB Saunders Co.)

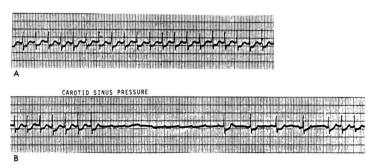

CAROTID SINUS PRESSURE

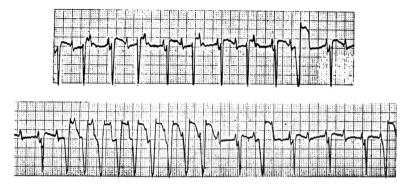

FIGURE 4. Atrial tachycardia with AV block (3:2 AV Wenckebach in the *upper panel* and 2:1 AV block in the *lower panel*) due to digitalis intoxication (serum digoxin level = 4.6 ng/ml). In addition, ventricular premature beats and a short run of ventricular tachycardia presumably caused by digitalis-induced enhanced automaticity are noted. (From Sung RJ, Chang MS, Chiang BN. Clinical electrophysiology of supraventricular tachycardia. Cardiol Clin 1983;1:225–51. Reprinted with permission of WB Saunders Co.)

adenosine can only transiently slow the rate of ventricular responses (thereby allowing better visualization of atrial flutter waves) (Fig. 6*A* and Fig. 6*B*).

Atrial Fibrillation

The ECG hallmarks of atrial fibrillation include irregular baseline oscillation at 400 to 700 per minute and an irregular ventricular response (Fig. 6*C*).

Atrial Flutter and Atrial Fibrillation with Bundle Branch Block or with Ventricular Pre-excitation

The QRS complexes during atrial flutter and atrial fibrillation are usually identical to those of sinus rhythm. However, when there is associated bundle branch block (pre-existing or functional) or ventricular pre-excitation, the QRS complexes are wide, simulating a ventricular tachyarrhythmia (Fig. 7 and Fig. 8). Atrial flutter with 2:1 ventricular pre-excitation is difficult to differentiate from ventricular tachycardia and the antidromic form of AV reciprocating tachycardia. In contrast to ventricular tachycardia and ventricular flut-

ter, atrial fibrillation with ventricular pre-excitation has irregular ventricular responses with different degrees of ventricular fusion (Fig. 8).

Accelerated AV Junctional Rhythm or Tachycardia

The intrinsic AV junctional automatic rhythm originating at the AV node or the His bundle has a rate of 40 to 60 beats per minute. This AV junctional rhythm is normally suppressed by the sinus rhythm. Under pathologic conditions, the AV junctional rhythm may be accelerated to 70 to 100 beats per minute, referred to as accelerated AV junction rhythm, and even to greater than 100 (usually less than 130) beats per minute, referred to as accelerated AV junctional tachycardia. The QRS complex is narrow, similar to that seen in sinus rhythm, and atrial activity is usually not discernible on ECG rhythm strip (Fig. 9).

AV Nodal Re-entrant Tachycardia

The usual (slow-fast) form of AV nodal re-entry uses a slow AV nodal pathway for antegrade conduction and a fast AV nodal path-

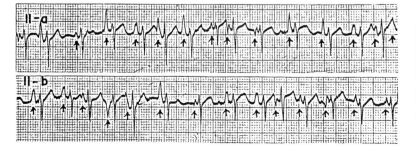

FIGURE 5. Chaotic (multifocal) atrial tachycardia. (From Sung RJ, Chang MS, Chiang BN. Clinical electrophysiology of supraventricular tachycardia. Cardiol Clin 1983;1:225–51. Reprinted with permission of WB Saunders Co.)

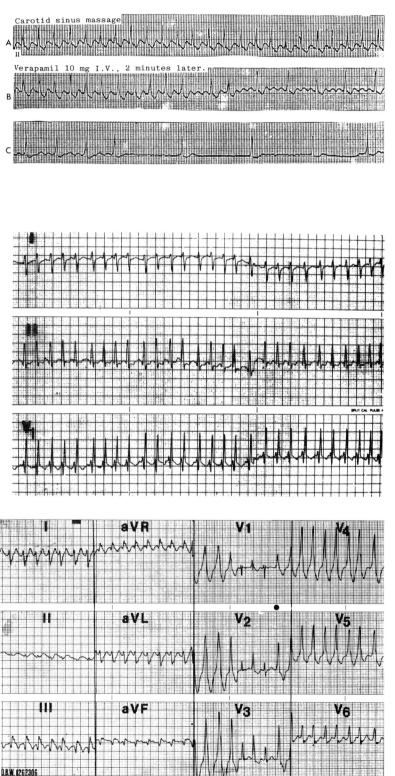

FIGURE 6. Control of the rate of ventricular response during atrial flutter with intravenous verapamil. Tracings of ECG lead II are not continuous. *A,* Carotid sinus massage fails to affect the rate of ventricular response (160 per minute) during atrial flutter with 2:1 AV conduction. *B,* Intravenous verapamil, 10 mg, increases the degree of AV block by its depressive action on the AV node. As a result, the ventricular rate is decreased to 75 to 90 beats per minute. *C,* An incidental finding of conversion of atrial flutter to atrial fibrillation is shown after administration of intravenous verapamil. (From Sung RJ, Chang MS, Chiang BN. Clinical electrophysiology of supraventricular tachycardia. Cardiol Clin 1983;1:225–51. Reprinted with permission of WB Saunders Co.)

Carotid sinus massage

Verapamil 10 mg I.V., 2 minutes later.

FIGURE 7. Atrial fibrillation with complete right bundle branch block.

FIGURE 8. Atrial fibrillation with ventricular pre-excitation (Wolff-Parkinson-White syndrome).

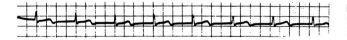

FIGURE 9. Accelerated AV junctional rhythm in acute inferior myocardial infarction. ECG lead II.

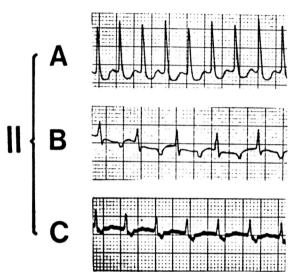

FIGURE 10. *A,* The usual (slow-fast) form of AV nodal re-entrant tachycardia. *B,* The unusual (fast-slow) form of AV nodal re-entrant tachycardia. *C,* The ortho-dromic form of AV reciprocating tachycardia. (From Sung RJ, Chang MS, Chiang BN. Clinical electrophysiology of supraventricular tachycardia. Cardiol Clin 1983;1:225–51. Reprinted with permission of WB Saunders Co.)

WIDE-COMPLEX TACHYCARDIA

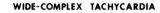

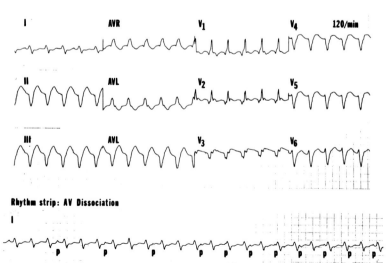

FIGURE 11. Ventricular tachycardia with AV dissociation.

VENTRICULAR TACHYCARDIA

Concordant Precordial Leads

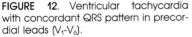

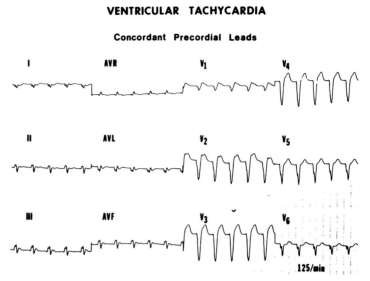

FIGURE 12. Ventricular tachycardia with concordant QRS pattern in precordial leads (V₁-V₆).

way for retrograde conduction. The initiation of tachycardia usually requires prolongation of the P-R interval. Retrograde atrial activation is by way of the retrograde fast AV nodal pathway at a time when the impulse conducts downward to the ventricle. Thus, the retrograde P wave is usually inscribed within the QRS complex, hardly discernible from the surface ECG during the tachycardia (Fig. 10).

In contrast, the unusual form (fast-slow) of AV nodal re-entry has a reverse re-entrant circuit using a fast AV nodal pathway for antegrade conduction and a slow AV nodal pathway for retrograde conduction. Retrograde atrial activation is by way of the slow AV nodal pathway. Thus, the retrograde P wave is inscribed far behind the QRS complex, resulting in an R-P interval longer than the P-R interval during tachycardia (Fig. 10B). Both forms of AV nodal re-entrant tachycardia can be terminated by vagal maneuver and intravenous verapamil or adenosine.[10]

AV Reciprocating Tachycardia

The orthodromic form of AV reciprocation uses the AV node-His Purkinje system for an-

tegrade conduction and an anomalous AV connection for retrograde conduction. The QRS complex during tachycardia is narrow unless there is pre-existing or functional bundle branch block (aberrant conduction). Retrograde atrial activation by way of the anomalous AV connection occurs following the completion of ventricular depolarization. Thus, the retrograde P wave is inscribed immediately after the QRS complex, resulting in an R-P interval shorter than the P-R interval during tachycardia (Fig. 10C).

The antidromic form of AV reciprocation has a reverse re-entrant circuit using the anomalous AV connection for antegrade conduction and the AV node-His Purkinje system for retrograde conduction. The QRS complex during tachycardia represents total ventricular pre-excitation mimicking ventricular tachycardia. Differentiation among antidromic AV reciprocating tachycardia, ventricular tachycardia, and atrial flutter with 2:1 ventricular pre-excitation is extremely difficult. Vagal maneuvers may terminate antidromic AV reciprocating tachycardia by depressing retrograde AV node conduction but usually exert no effects on ventricular tachycardia and atrial flutter with 2:1 ventricular pre-excitation.

FIGURE 13. Torsades de pointes or polymorphic ventricular tachycardia.

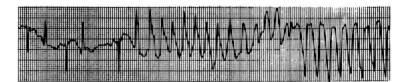

Ventricular Tachycardia and Ventricular Flutter

Ventricular tachyarrhythmias usually produce wide and bizarre QRS complexes. Ventricular tachycardia is usually regular. When its rate reaches 280 to 340 per minute, it is called ventricular flutter. There is no need to distinguish between ventricular flutter and ventricular tachycardia.

Differential diagnosis between ventricular tachycardia and supraventricular tachycardia with bundle branch block (pre-existing or functional) is commonly encountered. Vagal maneuvers usually exert no effects on ventricular tachycardia. The following ECG features are suggestive of ventricular tachycardia:[11]

1. AV dissociation (Fig. 11).
2. QRS duration greater than 0.14 seconds.
3. Captured beat.
4. Fusion beat.
5. Concordance of the QRS complex in precordial leads (V_1-V_6) (Fig. 12).
6. Q waves in lead I and aVL.
7. Rsr or RsR' pattern in V_1.

Torsades de Pointes (Twistings of the Points)

Morphologically, torsades de pointes is a distinct ECG entity. It is often described as a polymorphic ventricular tachycardia characterized by alternating runs of positive and negative wide QRS complexes swinging back and forth above and below the isoelectric baseline

(Fig. 13). Its occurrence is usually associated with prolongation of the Q-T interval.

Ventricular Fibrillation

Ventricular fibrillation is usually a terminal event. On ECG, there is complete absence of properly formed QRS complexes, making the baseline uneven (Fig. 14).

DIAGNOSTIC STUDIES

Which laboratory tests should be ordered depends on clinical suspicion and diagnosis: (1) cardiac enzymes for myocardial infarction or contusion; (2) complete blood counts and virus antibody titers for myocarditis; (3) serum electrolytes for electrolyte imbalance; (4) arterial blood gas for hypoxemia and hypercapnia; (5) digoxin level for digoxin toxicity; (6) serum concentrations of antiarrhythmic drugs for medical noncompliance or drug toxicity; (7) thyroid function test for hyperthyroidism; (8) chest x-ray for congestive heart failure; (9) V/Q lung scan for pulmonary embolism; (10) echocardiograms for cardiac contractility, valvular heart disease, and cardiomyopathy; (11) radionuclide ventriculography for contractile patterns and ejection fraction; (12) treadmill exercise testing with or without [201]thallium imaging for myocardial ischemia and exercise-provocable cardiac tachyarrhythmias; (13) cardiac catheterization with coronary arteriography for atherosclerotic coronary heart disease; and (14)

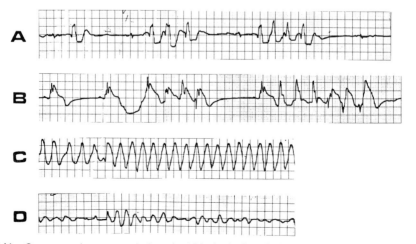

FIGURE 14. Coronary artery spasm–induced ventricular tachyarrhythmias. A chest lead equivalent to V_3 is used for recordings. A, B, Gradual development of intraventricular conduction delay and ST segment elevation followed by short bursts of ventricular tachycardia (polymorphic). C, Rapid ventricular tachycardia. D, Degeneration of ventricular tachycardia to ventricular fibrillation.

invasive cardiac electrophysiology study (programmed electrical stimulation along with intracardiac recordings) for tachyarrhythmias of unknown mechanisms.

MANAGING TACHYARRHYTHMIAS

Differential diagnosis between supraventricular and ventricular tachyarrhythmias is essential for planning immediate diagnostic and therapeutic strategies. In selected cases with difficult ECGs, invasive cardiac electrophysiology study for defining the underlying electrophysiologic mechanisms should be employed. Recognition of acute reversible causes (e.g., hypoxia, myocarditis, myocardial ischemia, electrolyte imbalance, congestive heart failure, toxicity, and proarrhythmic effects of drugs) depends on accurate diagnoses of various types of tachyarrhythmias.

REFERENCES

1. Sung RJ, Chang MS, Chiang BN. Clinical electrophysiology of supraventricular tachycardia. Cardiol Clin 1983;1:225–51.
2. Sung RJ, Shen EN, Morady F, Scheinman MM, Hess D, Botvinik EH. Electrophysiologic mecha-nism of exercise-induced sustained ventricular tachycardia. Am J Cardiol 1983;51:525–30.
3. Barrett PA, Peter CT, Swan HJC, Singh BN, Mandel WJ. The frequency and prognostic significance of electrocardiographic abnormalities in clinically normal individuals. Prog Cardiovasc Dis 1981;23: 299–319.
4. Winkle RA. Ambulatory electrocardiography and the diagnosis, evaluation, and treatment of chronic ventricular arrhythmia. Prog Cardiovasc Dis 1980;23:99–128.
5. Vignola PA, Aonuma K, Swaye PS, et al. Lymphocytic myocarditis presenting as unexplained ventricular arrhythmias: diagnosis with endomyocardial biopsy and response to immunosuppression. J Am Coll Cardiol 1984;4:812–9.
6. Trappe HJ, Brugada P, Talajic M, et al. Prognosis of patients with ventricular tachycardia and ventricular fibrillation; role of the underlying etiology. J Am Coll Cardiol 1988;12:166–74.
7. Adams CW. Functional paroxysmal ventricular tachycardia. Am J Cardiol 1962;9:215–22.
8. Deal BJ, Miller SM, Scagliotti D, Prechel D, Gallastegui JL, Hariman RJ. Ventricular tachycardia in a young population without overt heart disease. Circulation 1986;73:1111–8.
9. Tzivoni D, Keren A, Stern S. Torsades de pointes versus polymorphous ventricular tachycardia. Am J Cardiol 1983;52:639–40.
10. Sung RJ, Elser B, McAllister RG Jr. Intravenous verapamil for termination of reentrant supraventricular tachycardia. Intracardiac studies correlated with plasma verapamil concentrations. Ann Intern Med 1980;93:682–9.
11. Wellens H, Bar F, Lie K. The value of the electrocardiogram in the differential diagnosis of a tachycardia with a wide QRS complex. Am J Med 1978;64:27–33.

TACHYPNEA

CHARLES R. SOWDER, DAVID W. MARSLAND, and STEPHEN M. AYRES

SYNONYMS: Hyperpnea, Hyperventilation, Polypnea, Dyspnea, Rapid Breathing

BACKGROUND

Tachypnea is an excessive rapidity of respiration marked by quick, shallow breathing. Hyperpnea is an abnormal increase in the depth and rate of the respiratory movements. Hyperventilation is an increased amount of air entering the pulmonary alveoli (increased alveolar ventilation), resulting in reduction of carbon dioxide tension and eventually leading to alkalosis. Polypnea is a condition in which the rate of breathing is increased. Dyspnea is difficult or labored breathing.[1]

The normal respiratory rate in adults is between 14 and 20 breaths per minute. Respiratory rates greater than 20 per minute are associated with tachypnea, hyperpnea, hyperventilation, and polypnea, and may or may not be associated with dyspnea, which is a subjective symptom, not a measurable sign.[2]

Neural Control of Breathing

Two separate systems are involved, voluntary and autonomic. The voluntary system is contained in the cerebral cortex and, via the corticobulbar and corticospinal tracts, sends impulses to the respiratory motor neurons. The autonomic system is situated in the pars and medulla, with its efferent system sending impulses to the lower motor neurons via tracts contained in the lateral and ventral portions of the spinal cord.[3]

The sensors for the autonomic system are located peripherally in chemoreceptors, lung, and other receptors and centrally on the ventral surface of the medulla in the vicinity of the ninth and tenth cranial nerves. The following are the responses of these sensors to various stimuli leading to modifications of respiratory rate. For the carotid and aortic bodies, impulses are mediated via the ninth and tenth cranial nerves to the medulla. At a decrease of a P_aO_2 (to 40 torr), ventilation increases by only 17 per cent. With profound hypoxemia, these receptors are suppressed. When blood P_aCO_2 rises, CO_2 diffuses into the cerebrospinal fluid from the cerebral vessels, liberating H^+ (hydrogen) ions that stimulate the central chemoreceptors. These receptors have the most profound effect on ventilation (Table 1).[3,4,5]

In the normal adult, the neural control of breathing maintains finely tuned responses to the metabolic needs of the individual, leading to normal alveolar ventilation. During exercise, in the face of an increased metabolic need, the arterial P_aO_2, P_aCO_2, and pH are maintained within very narrow normal limits. Disease states involving the pulmonary, cardiovascular, or other homeostatic systems can lead to imbalances in this finely tuned system, which in turn produce abnormalities in ventilation. Increased respiratory rate can be associated, as in the example of hyperventilation, with respiratory alkalosis or can be associated when there is rapid inadequate ventilation, as in hypoventilation, with respiratory acidosis. A metabolic acidosis as would occur with diabetes can also be associated with tachypnea owing to the response of central mediators to increased cerebrospinal fluid H^+ ion concentrations.[3,4,5,6]

Blood Gases

Tachypnea is associated with hypoxemia and hypercapnia. Hypoxia pathophysiologically is due to hypoventilation, ventilation-perfusion inequalities, diffusion defects, and shunting. Clinically, these contributing mechanisms often occur in combination. Hypercap-

TABLE 1. Receptors That Influence Ventilation

RECEPTOR	RESPOND TO	EFFECT
Peripheral		
Carotid and aortic bodies	Increase in P_aO_2, decrease in arterial pH, and increase in P_aCO_2	Increase in respiratory rate
Pulmonary stretch receptors	Distension lung	Increase in neural transmission via the sensory vagus nerve, leading to limiting duration and thus depth of inspiration and thus leading to a complementary increase in respiration
Irritant receptors	Noxious gases, inhaled dusts, cold air, cigarette smoke	Same as pulmonary stretch receptors
J receptors	Engorgement of pulmonary capillaries and increases in interstitial fluid volume within the alveolar wall	Same as pulmonary stretch receptors
Nose and airway receptors	Mechanical and chemical stimulation	Sneeze, cough, bronchoconstriction
Joint and muscle receptors	Moving limbs	Stimulate ventilation during exercise
Gamma system	Elongation of muscle units in the intercostal and diaphragm muscles	Sensation of dyspnea
Arterial baroreceptors	Decrease in blood pressure	Hyperventilation
Pain and temperature	Pain	Apnea initially progressing to hyperventilation
	Heat	Hyperventilation
Central		
Chemoreceptors	Increase in hydrogen ion concentration in brain extracellular fluid	Increase in ventilation

nia is due to hypoventilation. At the bedside, it is impossible to sort out these pathophysiologic parameters. When diagnostically imperative, the clinician, by obtaining arterial blood gases on room air and 100 per cent oxygen, pulmonary function studies for carbon monoxide diffusing capacity (DLCO), and ventilation/perfusion (V/Q) scans, can gain great insight into the etiology of the hypoxemia and hypercapnia and then by deduction the tachypnea. Often, however, the history and physical examination alone can provide realistic clues as to the cause.[4,6]

The relationship between the P_aCO_2 and the P_aO_2 may provide important clues to the correct diagnosis. Hyperventilation in the presence of normal lungs leads to a reciprocal increase in P_aO_2 as P_aCO_2 falls. Hyperpnea due to serious pulmonary disease such as pulmonary embolization leads to an inappropriate increase in P_aO_2, and P_aCO_2 falls because of abnormal distribution of ventilation and perfusion. Calculation of the alveolar-arterial oxygen difference becomes a useful differential tool since an increased difference suggests pulmonary abnormalities.

HISTORY

In general, evaluation of tachypnea in the adult requires a systems approach based on age and acuteness of onset. For example, the 60-year-old "pink puffer" with a 30-year pack history is quite different from the acutely tachypnea 18-year-old trumpet player. The understanding of an increased respiratory rate often requires the best of Sherlock Holmes. However, the following represent focused "high-payoff" queries.[7,8,9]

Cardiovascular

1. *Is there chest pain Location? Quality? Timing? Setting? Worse or better with what activity? Associated with?* This is a sequence of query for all symptoms.
2. *Is there breathlessness (dyspnea) with limited exercise? While lying down, relieved by sitting up (orthopnea)? Severe, arousing the patient from sleep and relieved by sitting up (paroxysmal nocturnal dyspnea)? Frank acute dyspnea, as in pulmonary edema?* The severity of dyspnea can be evaluated by assessing cardiovascular functional class (Table 2).[10]

3. *Is there rust- or blood-colored sputum?*
4. *Is there nocturia (early symptom of heart failure)?*
5. *Is there swelling of the ankles?*
6. *Have you had a heart problem since you were a child?*
7. *Has there been any unpleasant awareness of heartbeat (palpitations)? Syncopal episodes?*
8. *Is there a history of cigarette smoking? How many packs for how many years?*

Pulmonary

1. *Is there a cough? Productive? Duration? Blood? Color of sputum? Odor? Consistency?*
2. *Is there a sensation of wheezing or crackling sounds?*
3. *Has there been croup or stridor?*
4. *Is there a sudden onset of breathlessness, or has it been coming on slowly?*

Metabolic

1. *How much alcohol is consumed?*
2. *Is there polyuria, polydypsia, or polyphagia?*
3. *What medications are being used?*
4. *Is there illicit drug use or drug overdose?*
5. *Is there recent weight loss, tremulousness, or prominence of the eyes?*
6. *Have there been tarry stools, excessive menstruation, or blood in bodily secretions?*
7. *Has there been an onset of fever?*
8. *Is there neck or abdominal pain?*

Trauma

1. *Has there been significant injury to the head, thorax, or abdomen?*
2. *Has there been significant injury to the long bones?*
3. *Has there been significant blood loss?*
4. *Has there been loss of consciousness?*

Miscellaneous

1. *Has there been a recent labor and delivery?*
2. *Is the patient stressed or anxious?*
3. *Has the patient been a low-lander coming to the mountains?*
4. *Is the patient a malingerer?*
5. *Has there been exposure to environmental toxins?*

TABLE 2. A Comparison of Three Methods of Assessing Cardiovascular Disability

CLASS	NEW YORK HEART ASSOCIATION FUNCTIONAL CLASSIFICATION	CANADIAN CARDIOVASCULAR SOCIETY FUNCTIONAL CLASSIFICATION	SPECIFIC ACTIVITY SCALE
I	Patients with cardiac disease but without resulting limitations of physical activity. Ordinary physical activity does not cause undue fatigue, palpitation, dyspnea, or anginal pain.	Ordinary physical activity, such as walking and climbing stairs, does not cause angina. Angina with strenuous or rapid or prolonged exertion at work or recreation.	Patients can perform to completion any activity requiring ≥ 7 metabolic equivalents, e.g., can carry 24 lb up eight steps, carry objects that weigh 80 lb; do outdoor work (shovel snow, spade soil); do recreational activities (skiing, basketball, squash, handball, jog/walk 5 mph).
II	Patients with cardiac disease resulting in slight limitation of physical activity. They are comfortable at rest. Ordinary physical activity results in fatigue, palpitation, dyspnea, or anginal pain.	Slight limitation of ordinary activity. Walking or climbing stairs rapidly, walking uphill, walking or stair climbing after meals, in cold, in wind, or when under emotional stress, or only during the few hours after awakening. Walking more than two blocks on the level and climbing more than one flight of ordinary stairs as a normal pace in normal conditions.	Patient can perform to completion any activity requiring ≥ 5 metabolic equivalents but can not and does not perform to completion activities requiring ≥ 7 metabolic equivalents, e.g., have sexual intercourse without stopping, garden, rake, weed, roller skate, dance fox trot, walk at 4 mph on level ground.
III	Patients with cardiac disease resulting in marked limitation of physical activity. They are comfortable at rest. Less-than-ordinary physical activity causes fatigue, palpitation, dyspnea, or anginal pain.	Marked limitation of ordinary physical activity. Walking one to two blocks on the level and climbing more than one flight in normal conditions.	Patient can perform to completion any activity requiring ≥ 2 metabolic equivalents but cannot and does not perform to completion any activities requiring ≥ 5 metabolic equivalents, e.g., shower without stopping, strip and make bed, clean windows, walk 2.5 mph, bowl, play golf, dress without stopping.
IV	Patient with cardiac disease resulting in inability to carry on any physical activity without discomfort. Symptoms of cardiac insufficiency or of the anginal syndrome may be present even at rest. If any physical activity is undertaken, discomfort is increased.	Inability to carry on any physical activity without discomfort—anginal syndrome *may be* present at rest.	Patient cannot or does not perform to completion activities requiring ≥ 2 metabolic equivalents. *Cannot* carry out activities listed above (Specific Activity Scale, Class III).

(From Goldman L, Hashimoto B, Cook EF, Loscalzo A. Comparative reproducibility and validity of systems for assessing cardiovascular functional class advantages of a new specific activity scale. Circulation 1981;64:1227–34. By permission of the American Heart Association, Inc.)

6. *Has there been prolonged immobility?*

7. *Are there joint pains, unusual evanescent rashes, or any unexplained symptom complex?*

PHYSICAL EXAMINATION

To assess tachypnea, it is exceedingly important to count and characterize the respiratory rate for one minute. To avoid higher respiratory rates in the stressed or anxious patient, it is important to have a neutral environment and communication that has a calming effect. In the patient who purposely may be hyperventilating, the respiratory rate can be counted while auscultating the abdomen or taking the pulse.

The rate and rhythm of the breathing should be characterized, as in Table 3. For diagnosis, it is very useful to characterize the respiratory pattern and rate in this manner.[7]

Often, tachypnea is associated with cardiopulmonary failure, especially in the early

TABLE 3.   Abnormalities in Rate and Rhythm of Breathing

When observing respiratory patterns think in terms of *rate, depth,* and *regularity* of the patient's breathing. Describe what you see in these terms. Traditional terms, such as tachypnea, are given below so that you will understand them, but simple descriptions are recommended for use.

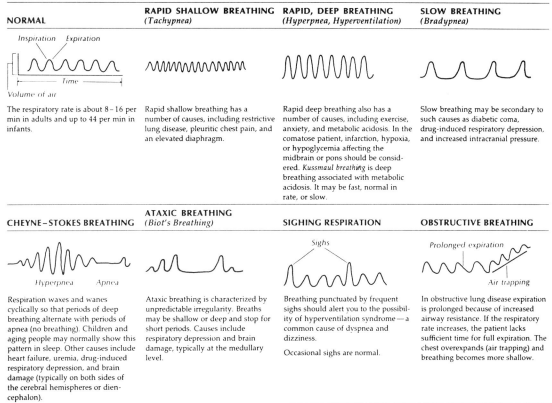

NORMAL	RAPID SHALLOW BREATHING (*Tachypnea*)	RAPID, DEEP BREATHING (*Hyperpnea, Hyperventilation*)	SLOW BREATHING (*Bradypnea*)
The respiratory rate is about 8–16 per min in adults and up to 44 per min in infants.	Rapid shallow breathing has a number of causes, including restrictive lung disease, pleuritic chest pain, and an elevated diaphragm.	Rapid deep breathing also has a number of causes, including exercise, anxiety, and metabolic acidosis. In the comatose patient, infarction, hypoxia, or hypoglycemia affecting the midbrain or pons should be considered. *Kussmaul breathing* is deep breathing associated with metabolic acidosis. It may be fast, normal in rate, or slow.	Slow breathing may be secondary to such causes as diabetic coma, drug-induced respiratory depression, and increased intracranial pressure.
CHEYNE–STOKES BREATHING	ATAXIC BREATHING (*Biot's Breathing*)	SIGHING RESPIRATION	OBSTRUCTIVE BREATHING
Respiration waxes and wanes cyclically so that periods of deep breathing alternate with periods of apnea (no breathing). Children and aging people may normally show this pattern in sleep. Other causes include heart failure, uremia, drug-induced respiratory depression, and brain damage (typically on both sides of the cerebral hemispheres or diencephalon).	Ataxic breathing is characterized by unpredictable irregularity. Breaths may be shallow or deep and stop for short periods. Causes include respiratory depression and brain damage, typically at the medullary level.	Breathing punctuated by frequent sighs should alert you to the possibility of hyperventilation syndrome—a common cause of dyspnea and dizziness. Occasional sighs are normal.	In obstructive lung disease expiration is prolonged because of increased airway resistance. If the respiratory rate increases, the patient lacks sufficient time for full expiration. The chest overexpands (air trapping) and breathing becomes more shallow.

(From Bates B. A guide to physical examination and history taking. Philadelphia: JB Lippincott, Co, 1987:245. Reprinted with permission.)

stages. Thus, in the emergent situation, it is imperative to evaluate impending cardiopulmonary failure, looking for tachypnea, hypertension, hypotension, tachy- or bradycardia, diaphoresis, cyanosis, dyspnea, confusion, panic, obtundation, agitation, use of accessory muscles of respiration, and increased effort in breathing.[11]

Careful evaluation of vital signs (respiration, pulse, blood pressure, weight, height, appearance, and metal status) can help focus the initial evaluation of tachypnea.

The cardiopulmonary examination is also especially important. The following are some of its essential elements that might lead to the elucidation of the cause of tachypnea:[9]

Inspection. Location/intensity of the apical pulse, neck veins distended or not in various positions, anterior-posterior diameter of the chest, inequalities in thoracic cage movement, tracheal deviation, use of accessory muscles of respiration, cyanosis, clubbing, neck or thoracic masses, retraction of intercostal muscles, flaring nasal alae.

Palpation. Intensity of cardiac impulses (precordial, radial, femoral, popliteal, and dorsalis pedis), thrills, heaves, chest wall trigger points, tactile fremitus, and inequalities in respiratory expansion.

Percussion. Heart size, air fluid levels, hyper-resonance, decreased resonance.

Auscultation. First and second sounds (murmurs, gallops, extra sounds, changes by position, regularity), crackles, rubs, rales, rhonchi, wheeze, I:E (inspiratory to expiratory) ratio, egophony, decreased breath sounds.

Other important elements in the examination include assessment of nail beds, color (pale or cyanotic), abdominal distension or pain, presence of visceromegaly, odor of breath, edema (eyes or ankles), and a general trauma review.[12]

TABLE 4.   Differential Diagnosis of Tachypnea*

Pulmonary
  Respiratory distress from infections
  Pleurisy
  Paralysis of respiratory muscles
  Emphysema
  Pneumothorax
  Asthma
  Interstitial fibrosis
  Pulmonary edema
  Thoracic cage deformation
  Inhaled toxins (smoke, chromium)
  Acute and recurrent pulmonary embolism (blood,
    amniotic fluid, fat)
  Primary pulmonary hypertension
  Tumors—lung, pleura, or mediastinum
  Aspiration pneumonitis
  Pulmonary alveolar proteinosis
  Wegener's granulomatosis
  Impending respiratory failure
  Radiation pneumonitis
  Upper airway obstruction
Cardiovascular
  Cardiac insufficiency (decreased cardiac output from
    any cause, right heart failure from any cause)
  Congenital heart defects

  Acquired cardiac defects (mitral or aortic valve insuf-
    ficiency, ruptured interventricular septum)
  Shock (to include septic)
  Peripheral vascular spasm
General
  Exertion
  Fever
  High-altitude pulmonary edema
Metabolic
  Thyrotoxicosis
  Drugs (salicylates, ammonium chloride, etc.)
  Alcohol withdrawal
  Extreme cold, heat
  Anemia, methemoglobinemia, sulfhemoglobinemia
  Metabolic acidosis (diabetic, etc.)
  Drug reactions (heroin, bleomycin, busulfan, nitro-
    furantoin)
Miscellaneous
  Direct pulmonary contusion
  Brain/head trauma
  Abdominal distension with restriction
  Pancreatitis
  Cirrhosis
  Collagen vascular disease
  Transfusion reaction

* See references[2,13,14].

DIAGNOSTIC ASSESSMENT OF TACHYPNEA

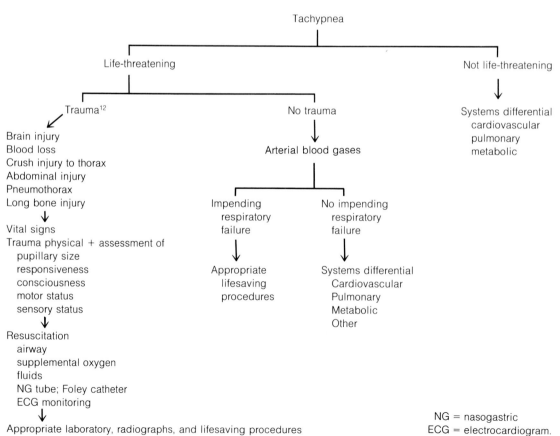

NG = nasogastric
ECG = electrocardiogram.

DIAGNOSTIC STUDIES

The practicing generalist today has at his or her disposal conveniently in the office and hospital the procedural and laboratory studies that would be required to sort out this nonspecific sign, tachypnea. In all situations, it is imperative first to pursue the problem by history and physical examination, thereby selecting those tests needed to arrive, in a cost-effective manner, at the specific correct diagnosis. Sometimes even after exhaustive testing the diagnosis cannot be ascertained with certainty, particularly when the disease process is in its earliest stages.

Laboratory tests that are often helpful include a complete blood count; urinalysis; SMAC; thyroid profile; arterial blood gases; electrocardiogram; echocardiogram; chest radiograph; computed tomography (CT) and magnetic resonance imaging (MRI) scans of the head, thorax, and abdomen; pulmonary function tests (lung volumes, flow rates, carbon monoxide diffusing capacity; ventilation perfusion scans; sputum analysis (cells, bacteria, fungi, etc.); abdominal films; and appropriate bacteriologic studies for urine, sputum, blood, and cerebrospinal fluid. Procedural studies that are helpful include cardiac catheterization, bronchoscopy, mediastinoscopy, and lung biopsy.

ASSESSMENT

The clinician is often faced with the differential that surrounds tachypnea in the acute emergent, hospital ward, and ambulatory environments. The differential is extensive. The common diagnoses contained within the differential are listed in Table 4.

In the algorithm shown, key differential decision points are noted: life-threatening or not life-threatening; trauma or no trauma; and impending or no impending respiratory failure. The complete history and physical examina-

tion for the systems differential with appropriate laboratory tests and studies for confirmation are paramount in importance. Occasionally, even with a complete evaluation, the clinician can be left with a nonspecific diagnosis of tachypnea that then will be followed in time in the ambulatory setting.

REFERENCES

1. Dorland's illustrated medical dictionary. 27th ed. Philadelphia: WB Saunders Co, 1988.
2. Glauser FL. Signs and symptoms in pulmonary medicine. Philadelphia: JB Lippincott Co, 1983:97–106.
3. Ganong WF. 1989 Review of medical physiology. 14th ed. Norwalk, Connecticut: Appleton & Lange, 1989:570–8.
4. West JB. Respiratory physiology—the essentials. 4th ed. Baltimore, Maryland: Williams & Wilkins, 1990:115–29.
5. Weil JV. Dyspnea. In: Horwitz LD, Groves BM, eds. Signs & symptoms in cardiology. Philadelphia: JB Lippincott Co, 1985:28–50.
6. Comroe JH Jr, Forster RE II, Dubois AB, Briscoe WA, Carlsen E. The lung: clinical physiology and pulmonary function tests. 2nd ed. Chicago: Yearbook Medical Publishers, Inc, 1968.
7. Bates DV. Respiratory function in disease. 3rd ed. Philadelphia: WB Saunders Co, 1989:382–6.
8. DeGowin EL, DeGowin RL. Bedside diagnostic examination. 2nd ed. New York: Macmillan Publishing Co, 1969.
9. Bates B. A guide to physical examination and history taking. 4th ed. Philadelphia: JB Lippincott Co, 1987.
10. Goldman L, Hashimoto B, Cook EF, Loscalzo A. Comparative reproducibility and validity of systems for assessing cardiovascular functional class: advantages of a new specific activity scale. Circulation 1981;64:1227–34.
11. Brenner BE. Comprehensive management of respiratory emergencies. Rockville, Maryland: Aspen Publishers, Inc, 1985.
12. Asensio JA, Barton JM, Wonsetler LA, Thomford NR. Trauma: a systematic approach to management. Am Fam Physician 1988;38:97–112.
13. Wyngaarden JB, Smith LH. Cecil textbook of medicine. 18th ed. Philadelphia: WB Saunders Co, 1988:179.
14. Miller WC. Respiratory failure, acute. In: Taylor RB, ed. Difficult diagnosis. Philadelphia: WB Saunders Co, 1985:452–8.

THYROID ENLARGEMENT

KAY F. McFARLAND

SYNONYMS: Goiter, Diffuse Goiter, Multinodular Goiter, Thyroid Nodule

BACKGROUND

Most thyroid disorders involve enlargement of the gland and/or excessive or insufficient thyroid hormone production. The normal gland has a soft, rubbery consistency and is barely palpable. The right lobe is slightly larger than the left; both are less than 2 cm in thickness and 4 cm in length. When the thyroid enlarges, the pyramidal lobe, which is a band of tissue extending upward from the isthmus, sometimes can be felt, often just left of the midline.

Most thyroid disorders affect women more frequently than men. For example, the incidence of hyperthyroidism is 35.5 per 100,000 women and 9.2 per 100,000 men.[1] Up to 7 per cent of the population have a nodular thyroid,[2] and with any lump or nodule, especially ones that can be easily felt and seen, the possibility of cancer is raised. However, the incidence of clinically significant thyroid malignancy is low and accounts for only 1 per cent of all new cancer cases and 0.02 per cent of cancer deaths in the United States.[3] Determining whether or not a thyroid nodule is malignant and evaluating the patient's metabolic status are the principal tasks in evaluating an enlarged thyroid (Table 1).

HISTORY

The risk of thyroid malignancy should be carefully weighed, particularly in patients who present with an enlarging, firm neck mass. Features that suggest malignancy include head or neck irradiation, rapid increase in nodule size, or growth during thyroid hormone suppression. Other clinical characteristics of carcinoma are hoarseness, dysphagia, and a positive family history of thyroid cancer[4] (Table 2). Pain may be associated with a malignancy but is more characteristic of subacute thyroid-itis. A history of an upper respiratory infection or other minor illness followed by fatigue and a sore throat, often thought to be pharyngitis, are other features of subacute thyroiditis.

A history of heat intolerance, weight loss in spite of a good appetite, palpitations, increased sweating, nervousness, fatigue, and dyspnea are all characteristic symptoms of hyperthyroidism. Young patients more often complain of emotional lability than older patients, who are more likely to present with muscle weakness or cardiovascular manifestations such as atrial fibrillation. Many patients will not mention muscle weakness unless they are queried specifically in this regard. This may be done by asking if they have difficulty climbing stairs or arising from a chair without assisting with their hands. Patients with Graves' disease often will give a history of a "gritty" feeling in their eyes, tearing, and periorbital puffiness; proptosis and diplopia are less frequent signs of endocrine eye disease.

In assessing the nonspecific symptoms that so frequently occur in association with hypothyroidism, it is important to determine if there has been a change over time. In the order of their relative diagnostic value, symptoms of hypothyroidism include cold intolerance, hoarseness, decreased sweating, parasthesias, dry skin, constipation, weight gain, and diminished hearing.[5] Parasthesias of the hands and muscle cramps are frequent signs of hypothyroidism and are particularly common after ^{131}I therapy.

Focused Queries

1. *Have you ever had any radiation to the head or neck?* A positive history of head or neck radiation with the presence of a thyroid nodule is an indication for surgical excision, as the incidence of thyroid carcinoma is much higher in these patients.

2. *What medications have you taken within the last three months?* Lithium may cause thyroid enlargement, which is associated most often with hypothyroidism and

TABLE 1.   Evaluation of Goiter

Tests to determine hormonal status
  History
  Physical examination
  Thyroxine
  Tri-iodothyronine uptake
  Free thyroxine index
Other tests to evaluate or determine etiology
  Euthyroid
    Ultrasound
    Radionuclide scan
    Needle aspiration
    Surgery
  Hyperthyroid
    Tri-iodothyronine
    Thyroid stimulating hormone
    Thyroglobulin level
    ^{131}I uptake
  Hypothyroid
    Thyroid stimulating hormone
    Microsomal antibodies

rarely with hyperthyroidism. Iodine excess, particularly the large amounts of iodine contained in expectorants, may precipitate hyperthyroidism or hypothyroidism.

3. *Does anyone in your family have a thyroid disorder?* Most thyroid disorders have a genetic component with the notable exception of goiter secondary to iodine deficiency, a condition that has almost been completely eliminated in developed countries. Medullary carcinoma in particular has a strong familial tendency and may also occur in association with the syndrome of multiple endocrine neoplasia.

4. *When was your last pregnancy?* Women have a much higher incidence of all thyroid conditions, and transient thyroiditis is

TABLE 2.   Clinical Characteristics Increasing Likelihood of Thyroid Cancer

History
  Age <20 or >60 years
  Head or neck irradiation
  Rapid growth
  Family history
  Hoarseness
  Dysphagia
  Growth during thyroid hormone suppression
Physical
  Single nodule
  Stony hard nodule
  Lymphadenopathy
Laboratory
  Normal thyroxine, tri-iodothyronine uptake, free
    thyroxine index
  Cold nodule on iodine scan
  Solid versus cystic
Suspicious/malignant thyroid cells on aspiration

frequently diagnosed in the first three months postpartum.

5. *Do your eyes bother you, for example, burn, itch, or tear?* A positive response suggests Graves' disease.

PHYSICAL EXAMINATION

When the neck is extended, an enlarged thyroid usually can be visualized. However, for palpation, the neck should be partially flexed in order to relax the sternocleidomastoid muscles, allowing the examiner better to define the contour and size of the gland. Medially directed pressure over the larynx and upper portion of one thyroid lobe makes it easier to outline the opposite lobe. Palpation usually can define whether the gland is diffusely enlarged, contains a solitary nodule, or is multinodular. However, at times it is difficult to make an anatomic diagnosis by physical examination alone, and a radionuclide scan or ultrasound may be used to verify the clinical impression.

Physical findings that may be valuable in assessing the metabolic status of the patient include: the heart rate, skin temperature and texture, the relaxation phase of the ankle reflex, and the speed and number of body movements. In relative order of diagnostic value, the physical signs suggestive of hyperthyroidism are: thyroid enlargement; tachycardia; hyperkinesis; hot, moist hands; irregular heart rate; lid retraction; and tremor. Palpation of a vascular thrill is suggestive of hyperthyroidism, and a bruit also indicates that the gland is hyperplastic. Signs that support the diagnosis of hyperthyroidism, listed in order of their discriminant value, include: slow reflex relaxation, coarse skin and hair, slow movements, periorbital puffiness, bradycardia, and cold skin.[5] Usually, more than half of these physical findings are present when the diagnosis is confirmed by thyroid function tests.

Masses in the neck usually can be distinguished easily from thyroid enlargement, as they are in a different position and fail to move with swallowing. The differential diagnosis of neck masses includes thyroid enlargement, bronchial cleft cysts, cystic hygroma, lymphoproliferative disease, and rarely, parathyroid masses. A thyroglossal duct cyst, which is a midline mass, can usually be distinguished from the pyramidal lobe of the thyroid, as the cyst remains attached by the thyroglossal duct to the tongue and moves upward when the tongue is protruded.

There are a number of physical findings that are suggestive of thyroid malignancy. These include hoarseness, which may indicate compression of the recurrent laryngeal nerve; a stoney, hard gland that is fixed to the adjacent tissue and does not move with swallowing; and firm enlargement of the cervical lymph nodes. A single firm nodule is more likely to be malignant than when multiple nodules are present. Tenderness is more suggestive of subacute thyroiditis or hemorrhage into a nodule than carcinoma.

DIAGNOSTIC STUDIES

Thyroid Function Tests

Thyroxine (T_4) and tri-iodothyronine (T_3) levels are increased in hyperthyroidism and decreased in hypothyroidism.[6,7] The T_4 is used for screening and usually is ordered with the T_3 uptake. T_3, sometimes written T_3 RIA (radioimmunoassay), should be distinguished from the T_3 uptake. The T_3 is a particularly valuable test in patients with hyperthyroidism, as T_3 concentrations may be elevated disproportionately to T_4 levels. A number of nonthyroidal conditions and drugs affect T_4 and T_3 levels. For example, oral contraceptives cause an increase in serum thyroxine binding globulin and elevation in T_4 and T_3 levels. As binding protein concentrations increase, more T_4 and T_3 are bound, increasing their serum concentrations. However, the proportion of T_4 or T_3 that is not bound to protein, the free T_4 or T_3 concentration, remains normal and is a better measure of metabolic status than the bound fraction of these hormones. The methods used to determine free T_4 concentrations are cumbersome and expensive, and therefore the free thyroxine index (FTI) has been developed, which utilizes the T_4 and T_3 uptake. This is an indirect measure of thyroxine binding globulin levels and the T_4. The FTI more accurately reflects the metabolically active free hormone concentration than either the T_3 or T_4 concentration.

Thyroid Stimulating Hormone

Thyroid stimulating hormone (TSH) increases when serum thyroxine levels fall. An elevated TSH level indicates primary thyroid gland failure and is the most sensitive method to diagnose primary hypothyroidism. Until recently, the test was not sensitive enough to detect subnormal levels. Now highly sensitive methods for determining TSH have been developed and more accurately distinguish between normal and subnormal TSH levels. TSH levels now aid in the diagnosis of both hyperthyroidism and hypothyroidism.

Serum Thyroglobulin

Serum thyroglobulin levels are decreased in patients who are taking exogenous thyroid hormone and thus are low in patients with thyrotoxicosis factitia.[8] Also, thyroglobulin determinations may be useful in patients who are being followed for thyroid cancer, as levels rise with tumor recurrence. Thyroglobulin levels, however, are not helpful in distinguishing between thyroid enlargement that is benign or malignant, as patients with both conditions may have elevated levels.

Microsomal Antibodies

Microsomal antibodies are found in high titers in 70 per cent of patients with autoimmune thyroiditis and are helpful in confirming this diagnosis.[9] Low titers are also found in patients with other thyroid diseases as well as those with nonthyroidal autoimmune disorders. Thyroglobulin antibody titers may be positive in some patients with autoimmune thyroiditis when the microsomal antibody titers are normal, but these levels are not as specific as microsomal antibodies.

Radioactive Iodine Uptake

^{123}I or ^{131}I uptake usually is not used to measure thyroid function; however, the radioiodine uptake is helpful in calculating the dose of radioactive iodine needed for treatment of hyperthyroidism and when low helps confirm the diagnosis of transient thyroiditis. Scanning with technetium and ^{123}I are more commonly utilized than ^{131}I because a lower radiation dose is delivered to the patient. An ^{123}I scan may be indicated when there is a single nodule, as some solitary malignant nodules will concentrate technetium but not iodine.

Ultrasound

Ultrasound of the thyroid is another way to define thyroid anatomy and is particularly useful in determining whether nodules are solid or cystic. Ultrasound, however, cannot differentiate between malignant and benign nodules.

The major advantage of ultrasound is that one can follow the size of thyroid nodules without exposing the patient to irradiation.

Fine Needle Aspiration

Fine needle aspiration of the thyroid commonly is being used as an initial diagnostic procedure. It is safe, easy to perform, and the most direct method short of surgery in determining whether a thyroid nodule is benign or malignant. The procedure is safe and causes little discomfort, although obtaining an adequate specimen is sometimes difficult. An experienced pathologist is needed to interpret the cytology. Aspiration of a single nodule may eliminate the need for both a scan and surgery if the tissue obtained is benign.

ASSESSMENT

Hyperthyroidism

Thyroid enlargement is present in over 90 per cent of patients who have hyperthyroidism. Thyrotoxicosis and hyperthyroidism are often used synonymously and refer to a clinical syndrome that results from overproduction of thyroid hormone or the ingestion of excessive amounts of thyroid. The diagnosis of hyperthyroidism may be obvious, particularly in those who present with the classical manifestations. Although the severity of symptoms is not linearly related to serum thyroid hormone levels,[10] the T_4, T_3 uptake, and FTI all usually are elevated. However, if the patient appears to be clinically hyperthyroid and these tests are normal, a T_3 and TSH should be done to exclude the diagnosis.

By far the most common cause of hyperthyroidism is Graves' disease, an autoimmune disorder that affects women much more commonly than men. The disease is characterized by hyperthyroidism, diffuse thyroid enlargement, and/or ophthalmopathy. Infiltrative dermopathy and thyroid acropachy are uncommon features.

Thyroiditis, often associated with diffuse goiter, is the second-most common cause of hyperthyroidism. Thyroiditis can be divided into subacute thyroiditis, associated with pain in the thyroid, and autoimmune, or painless, thyroiditis.[11] The hyperthyroidism due to subacute thyroiditis usually lasts a week to a month or so and then subsides but may recur transiently. However, it rarely results in permanent thyroid dysfunction. Painless thyroiditis, which frequently presents postpartum, causes hyperthyroidism for several weeks to months. This may be followed by a transient period of hypothyroidism, although the patient usually recovers normal thyroid function. Thyroid biopsy in this disorder shows evidence of lymphocytic infiltration, indicating that this is likely a variant of chronic autoimmune thyroiditis.

Toxic nodular goiter, another cause of hyperthyroidism, is more common in the fourth and fifth decades of life. The multinodular gland may be enlarged for years before hyperthyroidism develops. A single hyperfunctioning nodule also may cause hyperthyroidism. In these cases, the nodule usually is greater than 3 cm in diameter. T_3 toxicosis is relatively more common in patients with a single thyroid adenoma than in those whose hyperthyroidism is due to other causes. Rare causes of hyperthyroidism include: factitious hyperthyroidism due to exogenous thyroid hormone, struma ovarii, thyroid carcinoma, or TSH excess from a pituitary or trophoblastic tumor.

Hypothyroidism

The most common cause of hypothyroidism is autoimmune thyroiditis. Hypofunction also is frequent following treatment of hyperthyroidism with ^{131}I or thyroidectomy. The latter conditions as well as hypothyroidism due to pituitary failure are rarely associated with thyroid enlargement. Drugs such as lithium as well as the antithyroid drugs may be responsible for hypothyroidism; rarely, the condition is congenital. Often, the diagnosis of hypothyroidism is made on the basis of abnormal thyroid function alone, as many of the symptoms of hypothyroidism are nonspecific.

The T_4, T_3 uptake, and FTI are the primary tests used for diagnosis. The TSH helps to establish whether the condition is primary or secondary. Primary thyroid gland failure causes the TSH to rise; with pituitary failure, the TSH is low or normal. TSH levels may rise prior to the development of overt hypothyroidism, and when elevated without abnormality in thyroxine levels, the condition is called subclinical hypothyroidism.

Painful Thyroid

The thyroid is encapsulated, and so any condition that causes rapid enlargement may result in pain and tenderness of the gland. Hemorrhage into a nodule and irradiation thyroiditis both may cause considerable thyroid tenderness, although the pain usually resolves without treatment. Patients with subacute thyroiditis often present with a sore throat and are exquisitely tender over the thyroid. The pain may radiate to the ear and after a month or so resolve only to recur on the other side of the gland. Treatment may be needed for the pain, although it does not tend to affect the time course of the disorder.

Euthyroid Goiter

Often thyroid gland enlargement is found on a routine examination, although the patient or a family member may be the first to notice an enlargement of the neck or a nodule in the thyroid. Rarely, thyroid enlargement causes symptoms by pressure on the trachea or esophagus. Hoarseness and dysphagia, in fact, are so unusual that when present suggest the possibility of carcinoma. In contrast, complaints of a lump or constriction in the throat are common and more often related to anxiety than to thyroid enlargement.

Thyroid Nodule

The possibility that a mass is cancer, particularly if it is a single nodule in the thyroid, is of concern to both the patient and physician. The problem is really quite frequent, as about half of thyroid glands in adults contain one or more nodules 1 cm or greater in size. When multiple nodules are present and there has not been recent enlargement or a stony hard area in the thyroid, the thyroid enlargement may be considered to be benign. Although levothyroxine therapy is not effective in reducing the size of nodules,[12] enlargement of the thyroid during treatment with thyroxine is an indication for aspiration or excision.

On the other hand, if clinical evaluation or ultrasound indicates that there is only one nodule present, further evaluation is warranted, as a single nodule is more often malignant than when multiple nodules are present. A radionuclide scan may be used to define whether a single nodule is cold or warm. Most thyroid malignancies do not concentrate technetium or radioactive iodine as does normal tissue. When a cold nodule is present on scan, this increases the possibility that the mass is malignant. Actually, more thyroid tumors will concentrate technetium than ^{131}I or ^{123}I, and

therefore an iodine scan may be preferable when a single nodule is being evaluated.

Actually, only a tissue diagnosis can ultimately diagnose or exclude thyroid carcinoma. Fine needle aspiration of the thyroid may be an alternative to surgery in some patients. The sensitivity and specificity of the test vary between series. Sensitivity is reported to be as high as 100 per cent and specificity about 47 per cent.[13] The accuracy of the fine needle aspirate depends both on the sampling and on the experience of the pathologist who interprets the specimen.

In the euthyroid patient, if there is strong clinical evidence of malignancy such as the presence of hoarseness, an enlarging firm nodule, or a history of head or neck irradiation, surgery is usually performed without reliance on any other diagnostic evaluation. On the other hand, if there is some question whether the mass is a single nodule or whether multiple nodules are present, a thyroid ultrasound or scan would be indicated. Surgery is usually recommended for a single cold nodule in a male or child. In women, a course of thyroid hormone suppression may be given for three months. If there is a decrease or no change in the nodule, suppression may be continued. If, however, there is enlargement of the nodule on thyroid suppression, then surgery would be recommended.

Based on data from 5669 patients, of whom 18 per cent had thyroid carcinoma, thyroid aspiration was better than any other diagnostic test in detecting the disease (sensitivity) and correctly identifying those that did not have a malignancy (specificity). Therefore, assuming that there is a single, palpable, or dominant nodule; normal thyroid function tests; no clinical suggestion of a cyst or malignancy; and no history of head or neck irradiation, the most cost-effective method of evaluation to use is fine needle aspiration. This procedure makes a clear diagnosis in 73 per cent of all thyroid nodules.[14] This, of course, assumes that an adequate specimen is obtained and that the pathologist has considerable experience in deciphering the cytologic detail of needle aspirates.

REFERENCES

1. Barker KJP, Phillips DIW. Current incidence of thyrotoxicosis and past prevalence of goitre in 12 British towns. Lancet 1984;2:567–8.
2. Rojeski MT, Gharib H. Nodular thyroid disease:

evaluation and management. N Engl J Med 1985;313:428–36.

3. Cancer statistics 1990. Cancer J Clinicians 1990;40:18–9.

4. Ridgeway EC. Clinical evaluation of solitary thyroid nodules. In: Ingbar SH, Braverman LE, eds. Werner's the thyroid. 5th ed. Philadelphia: JB Lippincott Co, 1986: 1377

5. Utiger RD. The thyroid: physiology, hyperthyroidism, hypothyroidism, and the painful thyroid. In: Felig P, Baxter J, Broodus A, eds. Endocrinology and metabolism. New York: McGraw-Hill Book Co, 1987.

6. De los Santos ET, Mazzaferri EL. Thyroid function tests. Postgrad Med 1989;85:333–50.

7. Gavin LA. The diagnostic dilemmas of hyperthyroxinemia and hypothyroxinemia. Adv Intern Med 1988;33:185–204.

8. Mariotti S, Martino E, Cupini C, et al. Low serum thyroglobulin as a clue to the diagnosis of thyrotoxicosis factitia. N Engl J Med 1982;307:410–2.

9. Hamburger JI. The various presentations of thyroiditis. Ann Intern Med 1986;104:219–24.

10. Trzepacz PT, Klein E, Roberts M, et al. Graves' disease: an analysis of thyroid hormone levels and hyperthyroid signs and symptoms. Am J Med 1989;87:558–61.

11. McGregor AM, Hall R. Thyroiditis. In: Besser GM, Cahill GF, Jr, Marshall JC, et al, eds. Endocrinology. 2nd ed. Philadelphia: WB Saunders Co, 1989:683–701.

12. Gharib H, James EM, Charboneau JW, et al. Suppressive therapy with levothyroxine for solitary thyroid nodules. N Engl J Med 1987;317:70–5.

13. Asp AA, Georgitis W, Waldron EJ, et al. Fine needle aspiration of the thyroid: use in an average health care facility. Am J Med 1987;83:489–93.

14. Van Herle AJ, Rich P, Ljung BE, et al. The thyroid nodule. Ann Intern Med 1982;96:221–32.

TRANSIENT ISCHEMIC ATTACKS

FRANK L. SILVER

SYNONYM: Threatened Stroke

BACKGROUND

Transient ischemic attacks (TIAs) are short episodes of neurologic dysfunction presumed to be on the basis of reversible cerebral ischemia.[1] Many physicians consider TIA a specific diagnosis that should then dictate the appropriate course of management. A TIA is not a distinct disease entity and should be recognized only as a clinical syndrome for which there are many possible causes. To be satisfied with the diagnosis TIA, the physician must first confirm that the patient's symptoms are secondary to cerebral ischemia and then determine the underlying etiology.

Stroke, the broader syndrome, is defined as an acute episode of focal neurologic dysfunction presumed to be on a vascular basis. Arbitrarily, when a patient's deficit completely resolves within 24 hours, the stroke is referred to as a TIA. TIAs, as the name implies, are usually transient. Most last only minutes, and half are less than 30 minutes in duration.[2] When the attack lasts longer than 24 hours but resolves in days (usually within two weeks), the stroke is referred to as a reversible ischemic neurologic deficit (RIND). When the deficit is stable and persistent, the term completed stroke is applied. To round out the definitions, a stroke in evolution refers to a stroke that progresses over time. Therefore, a TIA is simply one end of a continuum of the syndrome stroke. The fact that the symptoms are transient does not make it distinctive, other than indicating the patient's good fortune, at least on that occasion.

Much emphasis has been placed on recognizing TIAs as threatened strokes. Stroke is the third most common cause of death in North America and a major source of disability. Cerebral infarction, the most common pathology underlying stroke, is irreversible, and even early intervention is generally ineffective. The management of acute stroke is primarily aimed at secondary prevention, that is, preventing subsequent strokes. The importance of TIAs is that they identify the stroke-prone patient when, by definition, the patient is still neurologically intact. Therapy is available that can reduce the patient's risk of a future, possibly more devastating, stroke. Unfortunately, according to a population-based study of the first occurrence of cerebral infarction in Rochester, Minnesota, only 9 per cent of patients described preceding TIAs.[3] Other referral-based studies have suggested a much higher percentage of patients with cerebral infarction had preceding TIAs, but this can be attributed to selection bias.

The overall risk of cerebral infarction following a TIA is about 5 per cent per year.[4] The risk is highest in the first month, accounting for 20 per cent of the strokes that occur in the first five years.[5] The long-term survival after TIA is primarily determined by cardiac disease, not stroke,[4] suggesting that a TIA serves as an important marker of coronary artery disease (CAD) in addition to stroke. After the first 30 days following a TIA, there is a 50 per cent chance of surviving seven years.[4]

In making the complete diagnosis of a TIA, there are four questions that need to be addressed:

1. *Is this a stroke syndrome?* Not every sudden episode of neurologic dysfunction is on the basis of cerebral ischemia. Ten per cent of patients with intracranial tumors present in an identical fashion as patients with TIAs.[6] Subdural hematomas have on occasion been incorrectly diagnosed as TIAs.[7] Some patients initially labeled as having TIAs turn out to have focal seizures or migraines. To be considered a TIA, the symptoms must reflect focal neurologic dysfunction, and their onset must be acute. The patient's age and the presence of atherosclerotic risk factors are also

TABLE 1. Nonischemic Causes of TIA-Like Syndromes*

Focal seizures
Migraine
Hyperventilation
Peripheral vestibulopathy (isolated vertigo)
Bell's palsy (isolated facial weakness)
Demyelination (multiple sclerosis)
Hysterical conversion
Cardiac syncope
Intracranial tumors
Subdural hematomas
Hypoglycemia
Other metabolic/toxic disturbance (acute confusional state)

* Listed in order of frequency.

important. In young patients, acute demyelination has to be considered. Attacks in multiple sclerosis (MS) tend to be subacute, progressing over days. Occasionally, they appear rapidly mimicking TIAs. Hysterical conversion should also be considered in the younger age group. In hysteria, the symptoms and signs do not make sense anatomically or physiologically. There is almost always a prior history of functional illness, and the patient is usually getting some "secondary gain" by having the symptoms. Table 1 lists the nonischemic causes of TIA-like events.

2. *Where is the lesion?* This is one of the classical questions of clinical neurology. Localizing the patient's symptoms to a specific area of the brain will also identify the vascular territory involved. Whether the lesion is in the distribution of one of the carotid arteries (anterior circulation) or the vertebrobasilar system (posterior circulation) will help determine management. Table 2 lists the common neurologic symptoms associated with anterior and posterior vascular territories. Note that unilateral weakness (hemiparesis), dysarthria, and hemisensory loss predict only that the lesion is

TABLE 2. Vascular Territory Involved in Common Neurologic Symptoms

CAROTID TERRITORY	VERTEBROBASILAR TERRITORY
Hemiparesis (or a component of face/arm/leg)	Quadraparesis (or a component of bilateral arms or legs)
Hemisensory symptoms (numbness, tingling)	Crossed sensory symptoms (ipsilateral face and contralateral body)
Aphasia (disturbance of speech, reading, writing)	Dysarthria, dysphagia
Monocular visual loss (complete or altitudinal, i.e., upper or lower)	Binocular visual loss (homonymous hemanopia or cortical blindness)
Loss of spatial function	Vertigo, nausea/vomiting, incoordination, ataxia, diplopia, hiccoughs

on the contralateral side of the neural axis. Although a hemispheric localization is statistically more likely, exact localization requires the presence of other accompanying findings.

3. *What is the lesion?* Strokes are classified by their pathology into two main groups: cerebral ischemia/infarction and cerebral hemorrhage. Since TIAs are short-lived, it is often assumed that the ischemia is reversible, leaving no residual infarction. When symptoms persist longer than a few minutes, there is usually some cerebral infarction appropriate to the patient's symptoms. Computed tomography (CT) studies have shown evidence of infarction in 25 per cent of patients after TIAs.[8] The percentage increases when magnetic resonance imaging (MRI) is used. Although patients with intracerebral hemorrhage can present with TIAs, as would be expected, this is rare. This chapter will confine its discussion to ischemic stroke.

TABLE 3.   Causes of Ischemic Stroke

Large artery atherosclerosis
    Artery to artery emboli from carotid bifurcation, siphon, vertebral, basilar arteries
    Hemodynamic from severe stenosis or occlusion of the same arteries
Cardiogenic emboli
    From

        Left atrium—atrial fibrillation, atrial myxoma
        Mitral valve—rheumatic, prosthetic, infected, prolapse
        Left ventricle—mural thrombus, postacute myocardial infarction, left ventricular aneurysm
        Aortic valve—rheumatic, prosthetic, infected, calcific
        Paradoxical—from veins via a right to left shunt (patent foramen ovale, atrial septal defect, anomalous veins)
Lacunar infarction
    Sites—internal capsule, pons, midbrain, medulla
    Classical syndromes—pure motor weakness, pure sensory weakness, clumsy hand dysarthria, ataxic hemiparesis
Nonatherosclerotic arterial disease
    Fibromuscular dysplasia (internal carotid)
    Dissection (extracranial carotid or vertebral, rarely intracranial basilar)
    Arteritis—polyarteritis, meningovascular syphilis, granulomatous angiitis, Takayasu's
    Arterial compression—vertebral artery at osteophytes
    Moyamoya disease—transient ischemic attack precipitated by hyperventilation
Hematologic disorders
    Lupus anticoagulant—"hypercoagulable state" associated with systemic lupus erythematosus
    Hyperviscosity syndromes—polycythemia, thrombocytosis, macroglobulinemia
    Thrombotic thrombocytopenia
    Sickle cell anemia
Complicated migraine

4. *What is the etiology of the stroke?* Any process that leads to inadequate perfusion of a focal area of cerebral tissue can result in a TIA. This includes (a) downstream hypoperfusion (hemodynamic compromise) secondary to stenosis/occlusion of a proximal artery and (b) occlusion of a distal cerebral artery on the basis of embolism or local thrombosis.

Focal ischemia on a hemodynamic basis secondary to atherosclerotic narrowing or occlusion of large proximal cerebral arteries is a relatively rare mechanism for TIAs. Most are embolic, with the embolus originating in the heart (cardiogenic embolism) or proximal large arteries (artery to artery embolism). The important causes of ischemic stroke are summarized in Table 3. The three most common causes to consider are large artery cerebral atherosclerosis (LACA), cardiogenic embolism, and lacunar infarction. LACA results in artery to artery embolism and, less commonly, ischemia on a hemodynamic basis. Cardiogenic embolism occurs most commonly in patients who are in chronic atrial fibrillation, following myocardial infarction, and in presence of valvular disease. Lacunar infarction involves occlusion of small penetrating arteries and has been coined stroke secondary to "small vessel disease."

HISTORY

The diagnosis of TIAs relies almost exclusively on the history provided by the patient. It is often helpful to get an account of the event from an eyewitness, especially when the patient is unable to provide a good description. Usually, by the time the patient is being examined, the symptoms have cleared, and there are no neurologic signs remaining.

History of Present Illness

A detailed description of the onset of the event is essential. It is best to inquire about the patient's condition the day before and the hour leading up to the TIA. Preceding chest pain may suggest an unrecognized myocardial infarction with secondary embolization. Recent trauma may evoke a diagnosis of subdural hematoma. Transient cerebral ischemia results in symptoms that appear suddenly, are generally maximal at onset, and then clear rapidly. There should be no progression of the symptoms at onset as in the rapid march (over seconds) of a jacksonian seizure (e.g., hand, arm, and then leg). Migrainous auras usually evolve slowly, typically over 10 to 30 minutes. Both migrainous auras and focal seizures are associated with positive symptoms such as flashing lights (scintillations), involuntary motor activity, or intense paresthesias ("tingling," "pins and needles"). This is in contrast to the negative symptoms, including visual loss, motor paralysis, and loss of sensation, associated with TIAs.

The symptoms must reflect a focal neurologic lesion. Syncope or presyncope (often described as "lightheadedness"), blurred vision (especially when binocular), and nonvertiginous dizziness ("fullness of the head," "fogginess") should not be considered consistent with TIAs. Episodes of isolated vertigo, diplopia, ataxia, or dysphagia are not usually secondary to cerebral ischemia. When more than one of these symptoms appear together, posterior circulation ischemia is likely.

Transient monocular blindness, amaurosis fugax (AF), deserves special mention. Classically, patients describe a blind or curtain coming down (or up) to obstruct vision in one eye. Vision usually returns to normal within seconds to minutes. AF is usually caused by temporary embolic occlusion of the central retinal artery. The episode is brief since the embolus usually lyses and/or migrates distally. Prolonged occlusion can result in retinal infarction with permanent monocular blindness in the case of a central retina artery occlusion, or a persisting upper or lower altitudinal monocular defect with a central retinal artery branch occlusion. Patients often report a problem with the vision in one eye when there is a binocular hemianopic field defect. Covering each eye in turn will confirm that the disturbance is definitely monocular. AF has been found to result from artery to artery embolism from atherosclerotic disease in the ipsilateral carotid in the majority of cases. Retinal migraine can cause a transient monocular blindness, with or without headache. Evolving scintillating scotomata, without headache, in older patients, are generally benign and have been referred to as "migraine equivalents."[9]

Headache often accompanies TIAs, but rarely is it a predominant feature of the attack. Prospective stroke registries have suggested that 30 per cent of patients with TIAs complain of associated headache.[10] Headache is unusual with AF or when the TIA is found to be secondary to lacunar infarction. Headache is most common with posterior circulation

TIAs. Severe headache, accompanied by nausea, suggests migraine, especially when the focal neurologic symptoms have cleared before the onset of the headache. Progressive headache with nausea, vomiting, and a declining level of consciousness always suggests increased intracranial pressure. A space occupying lesion or subarachnoid bleeding must be considered.

Another intriguing clinical syndrome that should not be regarded as a TIA is transient global amnesia (TGA). The patient is discovered by family or friends to be confused, but on closer examination, the only derangement is a failure of recent memory. The patient will ask the same questions repeatedly, unable to register any new information. Speech, sensation, and motor function are unaffected, and the patient recognizes himself or herself and family members. The attack typically lasts hours, with memory recovering completely except for persisting amnesia of the event. The long duration and the absence of other posterior circulation symptoms insinuate that TGA is unlikely to be secondary to transient cerebral ischemia. The pathogenesis of this syndrome remains a mystery. Fortunately, TGA is usually not recurrent and does not appear to be associated with a higher risk of stroke.[11]

Past Medical History and Family History

It is important to inquire about the presence of risk factors for atherosclerosis including hypertension, diabetes, hyperlipidemia, and family history of CAD or stroke. A history of angina, myocardial infarction, or intermittent claudication suggests atherosclerosis in other vascular beds, raising the likelihood of atherosclerotic cerebrovascular disease. Other cardiac diseases are important to note, especially valvular heart disease, cardiomyopathies, and atrial fibrillation. See Table 3 for a list of cardiac disorders associated with embolic TIAs.

Previous periodic headaches and a family history of headaches suggest a migrainous tendency. Migraine headaches tend to be associated with nausea, are often hemicranial, and, in the classical form, are preceded by an evolving visual aura. Atypical migraine syndromes, including ophthalmoplegic, hemiplegic, and vertebrobasilar migraine, are only distinguished from TIAs by their onset in childhood, recurrent nature, and strong family history. The pathophysiology of migraine is poorly understood, but the current neurogenic theory promotes a primary disturbance of cortical neurons, with lowered cerebral blood flow (demonstrated in classical migraine) a secondary phenomenon. In the case of complicated migraine, the neurologic deficit persists, and cerebral infarction can be demonstrated. In this rare situation, migraine can be considered a valid cause for ischemic stroke.

PHYSICAL EXAMINATION

The general physical examination should not be overlooked in the patient presenting with a TIA. Simply finding an irregular pulse may reveal atrial fibrillation, a probable cause for the TIA. The blood pressure should be recorded since hypertension is the most important risk factor for stroke. If it is excessive and papilledema is present, hypertensive encephalopathy should be considered. A thorough examination of the heart is required to detect valvular disease. Systemic signs such as fever, splinter hemorrhages, digital infarcts, and Roth spots may be indicative of bacterial endocarditis. Arthritis, alopecia, iritis, and skin lesions may provide clues to a diagnosis of systemic vasculitis. The absence of peripheral pulses, femoral bruits, and ischemic skin changes suggest peripheral vascular disease.

The neck should be auscultated for bruits. Their absence is not helpful, since bruits may become inaudible when the stenosis is severe. True carotid bruits are localized (not radiated from the heart) and are heard best just below the angle of the jaw. High pitch and extension into diastole signify severe stenosis. Underlying stenosis of greater than 35 per cent is found by angiography in about 60 per cent of patients with a focal bruit. There is a 30 per cent chance that there is significant disease in the contralateral side.[12] Carotid disease is common in older patients, and the presence of a carotid bruit does not necessarily mean the cause for the TIA has definitely been found.

Funduscopic examination may reveal platelet (white-gray) or cholesterol (refractile) emboli at a bifurcation of the retinal arteries. This is most likely found in the case of amaurosis fugax and is strongly associated with ipsilateral carotid atherosclerosis.

The neurologic examination may unexpectedly uncover residual findings after the patient's symptoms have cleared. Attention should be placed on assessing language function by listening for paraphasic errors (mixed up sounds or words) or word-finding difficulties in spontaneous speech, by asking the patient to repeat sentences (e.g., "No, ifs, ands, or buts"), name objects, read aloud, and write. Subtle spatial deficits (reflecting a right parietal lesion) can be screened for by asking the patient to draw the face of a clock and place the time. On testing the cranial nerves, look for facial weakness detected as asymmetry of facial movement or flattening of one nasolabial fold. Mild pyramidal (upper motor neuron) weakness of the arm can be demonstrated by checking for arm drift with the forearm fully supinated. Weakness, if present, involves the extensors of the upper extremity and the flexors of the lower extremity. Deep tendon reflexes may be increased on the side of the weakness, and the plantar response may be upgoing. Abnormalities of cortical sensation, indicative of a contralateral parietal lesion, can be tested by asking the patient to identify objects placed in the hand (stereognosis), numbers drawn on the palm (graphesthesia), and extinction to simultaneous bilateral stimulation.

DIAGNOSTIC STUDIES

Clinical investigations should be directed at imaging the brain to visualize a lesion, if present, and to determine the etiology of the TIA. The basic laboratory tests done prior to imaging include: a complete blood count (CBC) (to detect polycythemia, anemia, thrombocytosis), sedimentation rate (screening for vasculitis), prothrombin time/partial thromboplastin time (PT/PTT) (to document coagulation status, screen for the lupus anticoagulant), and VDRL (Venereal Disease Research Laboratories) (screen for syphilis, lupus anticoagulant). Baseline electrolytes, blood urea nitrogen (BUN), creatinine, and fasting glucose assess renal status and screen for diabetes. A chest x-ray and electrocardiogram (ECG) are helpful in detecting cardiac disease. Serial electrocardiograms and cardiac enzymes rule out recent myocardial infarction, especially if there is a history of chest pain. Fasting lipid studies should be done six weeks after the TIA so spurious results secondary to the stress of the situation are avoided. A sickle cell screen should be sent on black patients.

The brain can be imaged using x-ray CT or MRI. In the acute setting, CT is generally more readily available and is sufficient to rule out hemorrhage or other structural lesions. MRI is more sensitive than CT for detecting cerebral infarction, especially if the lesion is in the posterior fossa (brain stem or cerebellum). MRI will show the lesion sooner and may give information about the patency of the large cerebral vessels. All patients with TIAs should have a CT or MRI to confirm the exact location and size of the infarct, if present, and to exclude any other pathology. Old infarcts may be found that provide evidence of previous ischemic damage in the same vascular territory as the TIA. If multiple old infarcts are seen in different vascular territories, a cardiac source of emboli is suggested.

The appropriate timing of the CT or MRI is important. The yield of detected infarction is increased if the study is delayed by a few days. A CT scan without contrast should always be done prior to starting anticoagulants. This implies urgent CT scanning when a cardiogenic embolus is suspected or when there are repeated TIAs over a short period ("crescendo TIAs"). Early CT or MRI scanning should also be entertained when the diagnosis of TIA is uncertain. The finding of small, deep infarcts is usually sufficient to make a diagnosis of lacunar infarction.

After the initial workup (described subsequently), if the etiologic diagnosis is certain, no further investigations are necessary. Otherwise the next step, in the case of carotid territory TIAs, is to image the extracranial carotid arteries noninvasively with duplex Doppler studies. This combination of ultrasound imaging and Doppler flow analysis is highly accurate at detecting significant carotid stenosis at the level of the carotid bifurcation. Noninvasive vascular tests should always be considered as a method of screening the carotids, and angiography remains the gold standard. Arterial angiography, which carries about a 1 per cent risk of stroke,[13] should be considered before carotid endarterectomy, a prophylactic operation whose place is now being evaluated by several multicentered clinical trials. Angiography of the posterior circulation is reserved for patients with recurrent vertebrobasilar TIAs, uncontrolled with antiplatelet therapy. Revascularization surgery is only rarely considered, but the presence of occlusive disease of the intracranial vertebral or basilar arteries may dictate the use of anticoagulant therapy. Young patients often deserve angiography when the diagnosis of transient cerebral ischemia is definite, to search for arterial dissection, vasculitis, or evidence of embolic occlusion.

When no arterial disease is detected or cardiogenic embolism is suspected, two-dimensional echocardiography should be considered. The yield of finding a source for emboli is low if there is no clinical evidence of cardiac disease. Transesophogeal echocardiography allows better imaging of the left atrium and mitral valve. Prolonged Holter ECG monitoring may uncover occult paroxysmal atrial fibrillation. Several blood cultures should be drawn if bacterial endocarditis is considered.

ASSESSMENT

After the history, physical examination, and investigations are completed, nonischemic TIAs will be excluded, and both the anatomic and etiologic diagnoses should be known. Mistakes in diagnosis frequently relate to inadequate history taking and jumping to the conclusion of TIA without asking the first question: Is this a stroke? Do not despair if the etiologic diagnosis remains unknown after an extensive evaluation. The recent Stroke Data Bank suggests that the cause of cerebral infarction remains unknown in 40 per cent of cases.[14] Only when the cause is determined can patients be managed in a truly rational way. (Also see chapter on Transient Ischemic Attacks in *Difficult Medical Management*, WB Saunders Co, 1991.)

REFERENCES

1. Ad Hoc Committee of the National Institute of Neurological and Communicative Disorders and Stroke (NINCDS). [Chairman: Millikan C]. A classification and outline of cerebrovascular disease. II. Stroke 1975;6:566–616.
2. Matsumoto NJ, Whisnant JP, Kurland LT, Okazaki H. Natural history of stroke in Rochester, Minnesota, 1955 through 1969: an extension of a previous study, 1945 through 1954. Stroke 1973;4:20–9.
3. Dyken ML, Conneally PM, Haerer AF, et al. Cooperative study of hospital frequency and character of transient ischemic attacks. JAMA 1977;237:882–6.
4. Committee on Health Care Issues, American Neurological Association. Does carotid endarterectomy decrease stroke and death in patients with transient ischemic attacks? Ann Neurol 1987;22:72–6.
5. Sandok BA, Furlan AJ, Whisnant JP, Sundt TM Jr. Guidelines for the management of transient ischemic attacks. Mayo Clin Proc 1978;53:665–74.
6. Loeb C. Clinical evaluation of patients with transient

cerebral ischemia. In: Goldstein ML, Bolis L, Fieschi C, Gorini S, Millikan CH, eds. Advances in neurology, Vol 25: New York: Raven Press, 1979;141–8.

7. Luxon, LM, Harrison MJG. Chronic subdural haematoma. Q J Med 1979;48:43–53.
8. Calandre L, Gomara S, Bermejo F, Millan JM, Del Prozo G. Clinical-CT correlations in TIA, RIND, and strokes with minimum residuum. Stroke 1984;15:663–6.
9. Fisher CM. Late-life migraine accompaniments as a cause of unexplained transient ischemic attacks. Can J Neurol Sci 1980;7:9–17.
10. Gorelick PB, Hier DB, Caplan LR, Langenberg P.

Headache in acute cerebrovascular disease. Neurology 1986;36:1445–50.
11. Shuping JR, Rollinson RD, Toole JF. Transient global amnesia. Ann Neurol 1980;7:281–5.
12. Chambers BR, Norris JW. Clinical significance of asymptomatic neck bruits. Neurology 1985; 35:742–5.
13. Mani RL, Eisenberg RL, McDonald EJ, et al. Complications of catheter cerebral arteriography: analysis of 5000 procedures. I. Criteria and incidence. AJR 1978;131:861–5.
14. Sacco RL, Foulkes MA, Mohr JP, et al. Determinants of early recurrence of cerebral infarction: the Stroke Data Bank. Stroke 1989;20:983–9.

VESICULOBULLOUS DISORDERS

JAMES E. FITZPATRICK and SCOTT D. BENNION

SYNONYMS: Blister, Bulla, Vesicle

BACKGROUND

Numerous cutaneous disorders may produce a vesiculobullous or blistering reaction by a variety of mechanisms. While some vesiculobullous lesions can be diagnosed by their appearance, the human eye often cannot readily distinguish between different blister types. In this chapter, we present a rational approach to the diagnosis of this heterogeneous group of diseases based on patient age, history, location, and distribution of lesions. Special emphasis will be given to diagnostic tests such as cultures, patch testing, and biopsies for routine histology, immunofluorescence, and electron microscopy.

Vesicles are defined as elevated lesions filled with fluid that are less than 5 mm in diameter, whereas bullae are vesicles that exceed 5 mm. Since 5 mm is an arbitrary figure and many diseases have primary lesions that are both vesicles and bullae, the term vesiculobullous is often used to describe this group of diseases. As vesiculobullous lesions mature, several different secondary lesions may be produced. If acute inflammatory cells accumulate in the blister cavity, producing a purulent exudate, the blister may take on the appearance of a pustule. If the blister wall breaks or is denuded by excoriation, an erosion will be produced. As blisters or pustules heal, a crust will be produced. Since certain disorders are more likely to demonstrate particular types of secondary skin lesions, it is important to note which types of secondary skin lesions are present during physical examination.

Vesiculobullous lesions can be produced by splits within one of several different layers of the skin, depending on the disease process. Since vesiculobullous disorders demonstrate characteristic sites at which they split, it is a useful concept both for understanding the disease process and for diagnosis. Blisters can be categorized as subcorneal (beneath the stratum corneum), intraepidermal (through the prickle cell layer), suprabasal (between the basal cell layer and prickle cell layer), intrabasal (through the basal cell layer), subepidermal

The opinions and assertions contained herein are the views of the authors and are not to be considered as reflecting the views of the Department of the Army or the Department of Defense.

(between the epidermis and dermis), or dermal.

Table 1 presents a classification of blisters according to characteristic age of presentation.

HISTORY

Focused Queries

In many instances, the history alone will provide the correct diagnosis or eliminate many possibilities. Focused queries that should be answered include the following:

1. *How long have you had blisters?* This is a crucial question since some blistering disorders such as epidermolysis bullosa are present since birth, whereas others such as allergic contact dermatitis are acquired and have an acute course. It is important to know the exact day the blisters were first noticed, since this will allow the examiner to focus on preceding events that may have triggered the eruption such as new medications, exposure to poison ivy, and so on.

2. *Have you ever had similar blisters?* Many vesiculobullous diseases are recurring

disorders such as bullous erythema multiforme, whereas others such as acute varicella-zoster infection (chickenpox) do not typically recur.

3. *Are you taking any medications?* A vesiculobullous drug eruption should always be considered in the differential diagnosis. While most drug eruptions occur within days or weeks of starting a new drug, the examining physician should always consider the possibility that the patient has had a reaction to one of their chronic medications.

4. *What are you putting on your skin?* Topical medications, especially antibiotic-containing products, are notorious for producing allergic contact dermatitis.

5. *Does anyone else in your family, or do any of your close friends, have blisters?* This will allow the physician to focus in on common exposures such as arthropods, allergic contact dermatitis, infections, and hereditary disorders.

6. *Do your blisters itch?* Some vesiculobullous eruptions such as dermatitis herpetiformis and arthropod bites are characterized by intense pruritus, whereas others such as pemphigus and porphyria cutanea tarda are frequently asymptomatic.

TABLE 1.   Classification of Blisters by Characteristic Age of Presentation

Neonates
   Congenital herpes simplex
   Epidermolysis bullosa (all types except acquired)
   Incontinentia pigmenti
   Staphylococcal scalded skin syndrome
Children and adolescents
   Chickenpox
   Hand-foot-and-mouth disease
Adults
   Bullous lupus erythematosus
   Dermatitis herpetiformis
   Epidermolysis bullosa acquisita
   Erythema multiforme
   Herpes gestationis
   Pemphigus (all types)
   Porphyria cutanea tarda
Elderly
   Bullous lichen sclerosus et atrophicus
   Bullous pemphigoid
   Cicatricial bullous pemphigoid
   Herpes zoster
No age predilection
   Allergic contact dermatitis
   Bullous drug eruptions
   Bullous impetigo
   Bullous dermatophyte infection
   Friction blisters
   Herpes simplex infection
   Linear IgA bullous dermatosis

PHYSICAL EXAMINATION

The physical examination in combination with the history will usually provide the correct diagnosis. The following features should be noted on physical examination:

1.   Size of vesicles and/or bullae.

2.   Type of blister (tense, flaccid, pustular, etc.).

3.   Distribution of primary lesions (i.e., linear, grouped, photodistributed, diffuse, acral, dermatomal, etc.).

4.   Presence or absence of secondary lesions.

5.   Presence or absence of scarring.

6.   Presence or absence of mucosal involvement.

7.   Presence or absence of other types of primary skin lesions (i.e., target lesions, urticarial lesions).

DIAGNOSTIC STUDIES

In general, the most useful laboratory tests are those that are performed on the blister itself or its contents. The most rewarding tests at the time of initial evaluation include bacterial cultures, potassium hydroxide (KOH) examination, Gram stain, Tzanck preparation, and biopsy for hematoxylin and eosin examination. Certain cases also may warrant viral cultures and biopsy for direct immunofluorescence and electron microscopy. Bacterial cultures and Gram stain of the fluid contents are useful in excluding bullous impetigo, whereas a KOH preparation is useful in ruling out a bullous dermatophyte infection. The Tzanck smear is best performed by scraping the blister roof and floor with a #15 scalpel blade and transferring the contents to a glass slide. The slide is then fixed and stained with any one of several different preparations including Papanicolaou's, Wright's, Giemsa, methylene blue, toluidine blue, or polychrome stain. The presence of multinucleated syncytial virocytes indicates infection by either herpes simplex or varicella-zoster virus. Diagnostic virocytes can be demonstrated in approximately two thirds of early vesicles.[1]

Blisters are commonly biopsied since many blistering disorders have a specific or suggestive histology. Early blisters (less than 24 hours old) should be selected for biopsy since they are the most likely to be diagnostic. Vesiculobullous lesions can usually be removed by shave biopsy and should include a portion of surrounding intact epidermis and the superficial dermis. Biopsies also may be taken by the punch or excisional technique, the advantage being that the deeper portion of the dermis and subcutis can be examined. Biopsies for direct immunofluorescence can be either shave or punch biopsies from perilesional skin

that include the blister edge and normal skin (see Table 2).

ASSESSMENT

Neonatal Vesiculobullous Lesions

Neonates with vesiculobullous lesions are a cause for immediate concern since congenital herpes simplex infection is in the differential diagnosis. The lesions often initially involve the location that first contacts the infected maternal site. The primary lesions may be present at birth or develop in the first three weeks. The most common lesions are vesicles measuring 1 to 2 mm in diameter on an erythematous base, but larger bullae also may be seen. Within several days, the lesions become pustular and then crusted. The diagnosis is suggested by a maternal history of cervical herpes simplex infection and a sick neonate with associated vesicular lesions. The diagnosis can be quickly established by a Tzanck preparation. A skin biopsy or viral culture is a more definitive diagnostic procedure, but it takes longer to receive the results.

Epidermolysis bullosa is a constellation of different inherited mechanobullous diseases in which there is an inborn error of attachment of the epidermis or superficial dermis.[2] Clinically, this group of diseases manifests as blisters or sheets of skin that separate from the underlying skin following trauma (Fig. 1). The lesions are typically large and do not demonstrate associated erythema. The diagnosis is established primarily by inheritance pattern, biopsy, electron microscopy, or direct im-

TABLE 2.   Direct Immunofluorescent Patterns in Bullous Diseases

Pemphigus (all types)	IC*—IgG, C3
Bullous pemphigoid	BML†—IgG, C3
Dermatitis herpetiformis	DP‡—IgA
Linear IgA dermatosis	BML—IgA
Bullous lupus erythematosus	BMG§/BML—Ig's$, C's**
Herpes gestationis	BML—IgG, C3
Epidermolysis bullosa acquisita	BML—IgG, C3
Erythema multiforme	DV‖—IgG, C3
Porphyria cutanea tarda	DV—Ig's

* IC = intercellular (between keratinocytes) pattern.
† BML = linear, tubular pattern along basement membrane.
‡ DP = granular pattern in dermal papillae.
§ BMG = linear, granular pattern along basement membrane.
‖ DV = around dermal vessels.
$ Ig's = multiple isotopes of immunoglobulins.
** C's = multiple complement components.

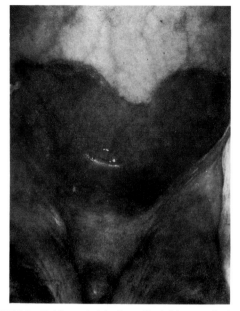

FIGURE 1. Epidermolysis bullosa. The blisters are typically large and leave large denuded areas, as seen here.

munofluorescence. A pediatrician or dermatologist with expertise in this area should be consulted since there are 18 or more different recognized variants.

Incontinentia pigmenti is an uncommon genodermatosis that almost exclusively af-

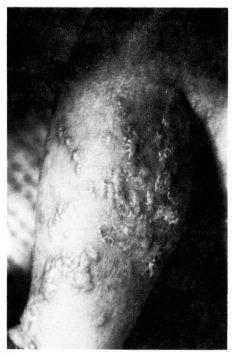

FIGURE 2. Incontinentia pigmenti. Blisters are small and frequently demonstrate linear patterns.

fects females since it is inherited in an X-linked recessive fashion.[3] The primary lesions may be present at birth or develop during the first several weeks. The primary lesions are erythematous plaques with vesicles that may have linear or whorled arrangements (Fig. 2). Verrucous or hyperpigmented lesions also may be present; if present, they represent an important clinical finding. Additional clinical findings include ocular, central nervous system, and bony abnormalities. Peripheral eosinophilia is present in up to 75 per cent of patients and peripheral counts may reach as high as 65 per cent. The diagnosis can be confirmed by biopsy of a blister that will demonstrate intraepidermal blisters filled with eosinophils.

Staphylococcal scalded skin syndrome usually occurs in either newborn infants (Ritter's disease) or young children. It is due to infection by phage group II *Staphylococcus aureus*, which produces an exfoliative toxin. This toxin, which is characteristically hematogenously spread from an asymptomatic focus of infection, is responsible for the subcorneal split that develops in the epidermis. Patients initially present with pharyngitis, rhinorrhea, or conjunctivitis, followed by diffuse tender erythema that is most pronounced around the face and flexural areas. Within 12 to 24 hours, large flaccid bullae develop that quickly rupture. The skin then peels off in large sheets, leaving a moist, erythematous base. The diagnosis is usually suggested by the characteristic clinical presentation. The superficial nature of the split and diagnosis can be quickly established by performing a frozen section on the blister roof and demonstrating a subcorneal split.

Childhood Bullous Eruptions

Acute varicella-zoster infection, or chickenpox, is a highly contagious infection that normally presents in childhood but also may develop in adolescents or adults. The vesicles of chickenpox may begin abruptly or follow a short viral prodrome. The primary lesions are 2 to 3 mm clear vesicles surrounded by erythema ("dewdrops on a rose petal"). The vesicles rapidly become pustular and crust. The lesions occur in crops, with a predominantly central distribution. Mucosal lesions are often present as small erosions. The diagnosis is usually established by the physical examination and confirmed by either a Tzanck prepa-

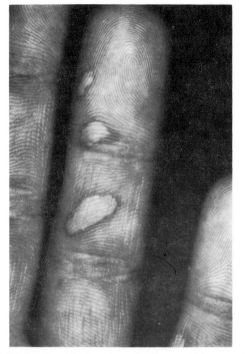

FIGURE 3. Hand-foot-and-mouth disease. Blisters usually demonstrate a characteristic distribution. Individual blisters are oval in shape and opalescent in appearance.

ration, which will demonstrate multinucleated virocytes, or viral culture.

Hand-foot-and-mouth disease is a distinctive viral infection that most commonly affects young children. It is caused by various Coxsackie viruses, most commonly A16. Patients typically demonstrate a mild viral prodrome, followed by oral erosions and oval, opalescent vesicles of the hands and feet (Fig. 3). The number of lesions is usually less than 10, but more may be seen in exceptional cases. The primary lesions are usually vesicles, but bullae up to 1.0 cm or larger may develop. The diagnosis is established by the clinical presentations. However, atypical cases may require viral cultures of blister fluid, pharynx, or stool to prove the diagnosis. Biopsies show an intraepidermal blister that is compatible with, but not diagnostic of, hand-foot-and-mouth disease.

Bullous Eruptions of Adults

Bullous lesions can occur in all forms of lupus erythematosus. The blisters can arise in pre-existing lupus lesions or occur as a widespread generalized eruption on both normal and erythematous skin. The criteria for diagnosis include: (1) a diagnosis of lupus erythe-

matosus based on the American Rheumatism Association criteria; (2) vesicles arising on, but not limited to, sun-exposed skin; (3) histopathologic features consistent with lupus erythematosus or a subepidermal blister containing neutrophils; and (4) direct immunofluorescence studies demonstrating the deposition of immunoreactants in a pattern compatible with lupus erythematosus.[4] The development of blisters in lupus erythematosus is frequently associated with worsening of the systemic symptoms, especially decreased kidney function.

Dermatitis herpetiformis usually presents in the third or fourth decade as an extremely pruritic vesicular eruption symmetrically located on the scalp, elbows, knees, and buttocks.[5] The primary lesions are vesicles that are often grouped (Fig. 4). The vesicles are often destroyed by the incessant scratching of the patient, and frequently only excoriations are present. Almost 100 per cent of these patients have a gluten-sensitive enteropathy, which can be demonstrated by a small bowel biopsy, but the enteropathy is rarely symptomatic. In addition to the enteropathy, 23 to 50 per cent of the patients have been demonstrated to have either antithyroid antibodies or overt thyroid disease. The diagnosis can be made by direct immunofluorescence study of perilesional skin that demonstrates the deposition of IgA in a granular pattern in the papillary dermis (Fig. 5). This finding is present in greater than 90 per cent of the cases and is pathognomonic of dermatitis herpetiformis. Hematoxylin and eosin stained sections of a vesicle reveal a unique histologic pattern of a subepidermal blister associated with neutrophils and, less commonly, eosinophils that fill the dermal papillae.

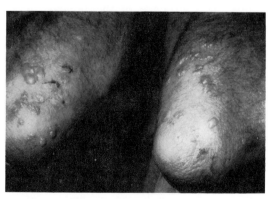

FIGURE 4. Dermatitis herpetiformis. Blisters are usually small, grouped, and frequently involve the elbows, as seen here.

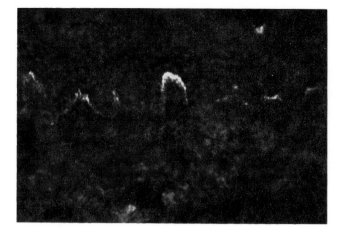

FIGURE 5. Dermatitis herpetiformis. Direct immunofluorescence demonstrating the diagnostic deposition of granular IgA in the dermal papillae.

Epidermolysis bullosa acquisita is a mechanobullous disease that occurs in adults and is associated with deposition of immunoreactants at the basement membrane zone. Clinically, the disease presents as vesicles, bullae, superficial erosions, variable scarring, and milium in areas of trauma including the hands, feet, elbows, and knees. Criteria for the diagnosis include: (1) increased skin fragility that is often evidenced by a positive Nikolsky's sign, (2) adult onset, (3) negative family history of blistering diseases, and (4) exclusion of other bullous diseases. Biopsies demonstrate a subepidermal blister with a sparse mononuclear infiltrate, although occasionally eosinophils and neutrophils may be present. Direct immunofluorescence demonstrates IgG and/or IgM deposition along the basement membrane zone of the floor of a sodium chloride split-skin preparation.

The bullous form of erythema multiforme occurs in an acral distribution usually involving the hands, feet, forearms, genitalia, and mouth, with sparing of the trunk.[6] This disease can occur in childhood but typically occurs in adults. The presence of the typical iris or "bull's eye" lesions and the acral distribution are helpful in differentiating this bullous disease from other vesiculobullous disorders. A history of previous herpes simplex infection or antibiotic ingestion, two of the most common identified etiologic agents of erythema multiforme, can often be elicited. Biopsies of lesional skin demonstrate necrosis of the basal keratinocytes, edema, intrabasal blister formation, and a mononuclear infiltrate. These findings are fairly distinctive and very helpful in diagnosing bullous erythema multiforme. The direct immunofluorescent findings of C3 and IgM in the upper dermal vessels are not specific.

Herpes gestationis is a disease limited to females of childbearing age that usually occurs during middle to late pregnancy or during the postpartum period.[7] The primary lesions consist of urticarial papules and plaques that become vesicular and can be grouped in annular or arcuate patterns. The lesions, which are extremely pruritic, usually begin on the abdomen and umbilicus, then spread to the back, chest, and extremities. Herpes gestationis is not associated with any increased mortality or with any long-term morbidity of the infant or mother. The disease is autoimmune in nature, as manifested by complement-fixing IgG antibodies directed against a herpes gestationis factor present in the basement membrane zone. Direct immunofluorescence reveals C3 and less commonly IgG in a linear pattern along the basement membrane zone. Since herpes gestationis patients have circulating antibodies, indirect immunofluorescent studies also demonstrate C3 staining in the basement membrane zone. Biopsies of blisters are histologically indistinguishable from those of bullous pemphigoid and demonstrate numerous eosinophils and variable numbers of neutrophils associated with subepidermal vesicles.

Pemphigus vulgaris is a blistering disease that typically occurs in the fifth and sixth decades of life.[8] It is the prototype for the pemphigus disease group that includes pemphigus foliaceus, a superficial variant; and pemphigus vegetans, a type characterized by thick crusts. Patients with pemphigus vulgaris present with superficial oral ulcerations in 60 per cent of cases prior to the development of skin lesions. The primary cutaneous skin lesions are flaccid bullae that readily break, leaving an oozing, raw surface (Fig. 6). The flaccid nature of the bullae is a useful clinical finding for excluding

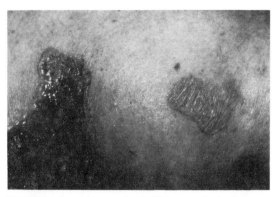

FIGURE 6. Pemphigus vulgaris. Blisters are typically large, flaccid, and easily rupture, leaving denuded areas, as seen here.

subepidermal bullous disorders such as bullous pemphigoid that are characterized by tense bullae. A positive Nikolsky's sign, which is manifest by the lateral sliding of the epidermis with applied finger pressure, is also supportive of pemphigus vulgaris, but it is not specific, as it also may be seen in pemphigus foliaceus, toxic epidermal necrolysis, and some forms of epidermolysis bullosa. The most common cutaneous sites are the groin, scalp, axillae, face, and neck. The disease may remain localized or become generalized; untreated generalized pemphigus vulgaris is associated with a high mortality rate. Although pemphigus vulgaris usually occurs spontaneously, it also may be associated with myasthenia gravis, thymoma, or therapy with captropril, penicillamine, penicillin, or rifampin. The diagnosis is suggested by biopsy of a blister that demonstrates a suprabasal split associated with a blister cavity containing rounded, poorly cohesive keratinocytes. The diagnosis is confirmed by the demonstration of an IgG autoantibody directed against desmosomal proteins; this produces a diagnostic intercellular pattern of fluorescence (Fig. 7). Circulating antibodies to the intercellular substance also can be detected in the serum by indirect immunofluorescence.

Porphyria cutanea tarda is a photosensitive bullous disease characterized by blistering, erosions, crusting, and scarring, especially in areas that are sun-exposed and subject to friction and trauma (Fig. 8).[9] Typical areas where lesions occur are the hands, forearms, and rarely, the face. In addition, there is often facial hypertrichosis around the temples and periorbital areas and hyperpigmentation on the malar areas resembling melasma. The definitive diagnosis and differentiation from rare types of vesiculobullous porphyrias are made by quantitating the increase in uroporphyrins and corproporphyrins in the urine. Their presence in the urine can be qualitatively demonstrated in the office by a pink fluorescence of the urine when exposed to ultraviolet light from a Wood's lamp. Biopsies of lesional skin reveal a noninflammatory subepidermal blister and a deposition of PAS (periodic acid–Schiff)-positive material around the upper dermal vessels. Direct immunofluorescence studies demonstrate a characteristic homogeneous deposition of immunoglobulins and complement around the upper dermal vessels.

Bullous Eruptions of the Elderly

The development of hemorrhagic bullae is an uncommon complication of lichen sclerosus et atrophicus. Lichen sclerosus et atrophicus may occur on almost any site of the body, but bullous lesions most commonly occur on the glans penis. Clinically, the presence of a

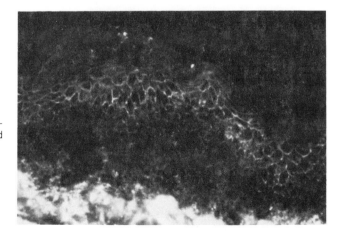

FIGURE 7. Pemphigus vulgaris. Diagnosis is established by demonstrating antibodies directed against the intercellular spaces, as seen here.

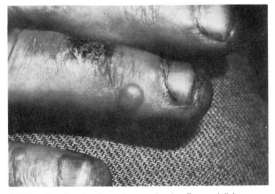

FIGURE 8. Porphyria cutanea tarda. Tense blisters are found on the backs of the hands associated with areas of "fragile" skin that demonstrate scale crust.

hemorrhagic bullae associated with surrounding porcelain white atrophy is virtually diagnostic, although biopsies are occasionally needed in atypical cases. The pathogenesis is presumably due to a mechanical separation of the epidermis from the dermis due to damaged basal keratinocytes.

Bullous pemphigoid is a disease that characteristically occurs in the elderly, but there are reports of patients under the age of 60 years developing bullous pemphigoid.[8] Clinically, the disease presents as nontender, pruritic urticarial plaques associated with variable num-

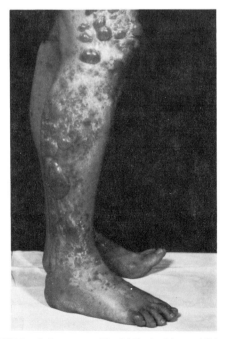

FIGURE 9. Bullous pemphigoid. Typical tense blisters of the lower leg.

bers of tense vesicles and bullae (Fig. 9). The sites of predilection are the flexural areas and lower extremities, with involvement of mucosal surfaces occurring in 10 to 30 per cent of cases. Although the lesions are typically widespread, a localized variant does exist. Previous reports have suggested that bullous pemphigoid is frequently associated with an underlying condition, especially carcinoma; however, more recent controlled studies suggest that this association does not exist. The natural course of this disease is chronic, but it is not life-threatening; bullous pemphigoid usually resolves spontaneously without treatment after several years. The diagnosis is established by a combination of immunofluorescence and light microscopic findings. Direct immunofluorescence demonstrates a linear band of C3 and IgG along the dermal-epidermal junction (Fig. 10). The same findings can be seen with epidermolysis bullosa acquisita; the two can be best differentiated using an indirect immunofluorescent technique on split skin preparations to localize more accurately the deposition of the immunoreactants. The microscopic findings of bullous pemphigoid, while not totally specific, are highly suggestive and consist of a subepidermal blister with the predominant inflammatory cells being eosinophils.

Cicatricial bullous pemphigoid is a bullous disease that mainly affects mucous membranes, especially the mouth, eyes, nose, genitalia, and anus.[10] The majority of patients are 60 years or older, and the most frequent age of onset is in the eighth decade. Typically, these patients present with recurrent bullae and superficial ulcerations of the mouth, eyes, and skin. These lesions are relatively painless and heal with atrophic scarring. Thus, over a period of years, recurring lesions can lead to severe damage in involved areas and produce strictures in the esophagus and larynx and symblepharon, corneal ulceration, and blindness. The skin involvement, although not common, can be widespread and resemble bullous pemphigoid. The diagnosis is established by combining the clinical presentation with a biopsy of a blister that demonstrates a subepidermal blister with a mild mixed inflammatory infiltrate in the upper dermis. The direct immunofluorescence of perilesional skin reveals the deposition of immunoreactants (mainly IgG or C3) in a linear pattern along the dermal-epidermal junction.

Herpes zoster is a recrudescent varicella-zoster infection that demonstrates a predilec-

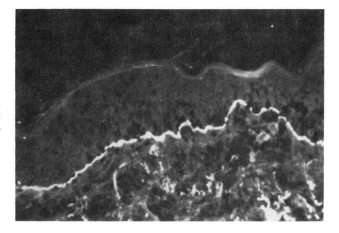

FIGURE 10. Bullous pemphigoid. Direct immunofluorescence demonstrates a linear tubular pattern of reactants (C3, in this case) at the basement membrane zone.

tion for the elderly, but it may develop in any age group.[11] Herpes zoster often initially presents as dermatomal pain or hyperesthesia that may be mistaken for muscular or visceral pain. The cutaneous eruption develops within hours to days and consists of grouped vesicles on an erythematous base that follow a unilateral dermatomal distribution; occasionally, more than one dermatome may be involved. A mild viremia is common, and isolated lesions outside the primary dermatome are not unusual. The most commonly involved dermatomes are in the thoracic area, followed by the cranial, lumbar, and sacral areas. The diagnosis is usually clinically obvious, but atypical cases may require confirmation by Tzanck preparation, biopsy, or viral culture.

Bullous Eruptions Without An Age Predilection

Allergic contact dermatitis is one of the most important vesiculobullous diseases, affecting all age groups. The pathogenesis is due to a cell-mediated immune reaction that produces an intraepidermal blister. Common causes of allergic contact dermatitis include plants (e.g., poison ivy), topical medications, metals (especially nickel), fragrances, and compounds used in production of rubber. Clinically, contact with the offending allergen produces intense pruritus and clinical lesions within 24 to 72 hours after exposure. The primary lesions are erythematous plaques with blisters that are initially distributed in patterns following the points of contact (Fig. 11). New blisters may continue to develop for up to three weeks following a single exposure and may develop at sites distant from contact. The diagnosis is usually readily established by the history and unusual distribution patterns of the blisters. The diagnosis can be confirmed by patch testing to the suspected agent(s) and reproducing clinical disease.

Bullous arthropod reactions occur as solitary or multiple lesions that typically occur on

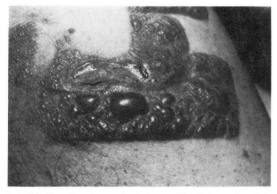

FIGURE 11. Allergic contact dermatitis. Blisters often following the pattern of contact, as demonstrated by this case of allergy to tape.

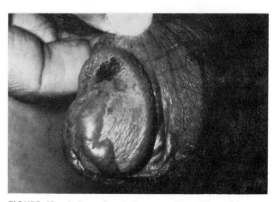

FIGURE 12. Bullous fixed drug reaction. Sites of trauma including the male genitalia are frequent sites of involvement.

the extremities. If more than one lesion is present, the blisters are often grouped. The patient often gives a history of arthropod exposure or actually recalls the bite. The blisters are usually intensely pruritic, but some species of arthropods (especially some beetles and spiders) produce painful blisters. Careful examination of the center of the blister will frequently demonstrate the presence of the diagnostic punctum. The diagnosis of arthropod reactions is made by the history, characteristic distribution and grouping, and presence of a punctum. Unusual cases may require a biopsy that will demonstrate an intraepidermal blister associated with numerous eosinophils.

Bullous drug eruptions occur in two main patterns: a fixed variant that recurs at the same site with each exposure[12] and a generalized variant. The former variant, referred to as a fixed drug eruption, is most commonly associated with certain drugs such as barbiturates, sulfonamides, tetracyclines, and phenolphthalein (laxatives). Fixed drug eruptions most commonly occur on the face, arms, and male genitalia (Fig. 12). Generalized bullous drug eruptions may mimic pemphigus, epidermolysis bullosa, porphyria cutanea tarda, or pemphigoid. The most commonly implicated drugs are cephalosporins, furosemide, sulfonamides, captopril, and piroxicam. The diagnosis is usually established by taking a careful drug history and correlating it with the appearance of the blisters. The diagnosis is usually established by the resolution of the blisters following withdrawal of the offending drug.

Bullous impetigo occurs as a result of infection by certain toxin-producing strains of *Staphylococcus aureus*. The toxin produces a superficial split in the epidermis, resulting in flaccid blisters that quickly crust. A helpful clinical finding is the presence of flaccid blisters that demonstrate a gravity-dependent layer of pus due to the numerous neutrophils (Fig. 13). The diagnosis is strongly suggested by finding gram-positive cocci in the blister fluid and confirmed by a positive culture of the blister contents.

Bullous dermatophyte infections are an uncommon presentation of cutaneous fungal infections.[13] The most frequent site of involvement is the feet, particularly the instep. The primary lesions are tense blisters that are intensely pruritic. Occasionally, the blisters may form annular or arcuate patterns as seen in other forms of dermatophytosis. The diagnosis is established by a KOH preparation that demonstrates abundant hyphae in the blister roof. The diagnosis can be confirmed by fungal cultures.

Friction blisters are easily diagnosed by the history of tense blisters developing at the site of trauma, usually the hands or feet. The patient can usually recall the inciting event, but

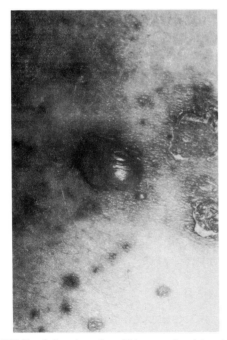

FIGURE 13. Bullous impetigo. Blisters are flaccid and rupture easily. Note the purulent nature of the blister contents.

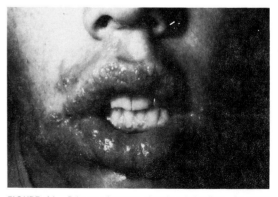

FIGURE 14. Primary herpes simplex infection. As seen here, primary infections usually demonstrate more vesicles than seen in recurrent lesions.

rare patients may require careful questioning to elicit the necessary history. A biopsy is rarely required, but if performed, it demonstrates a characteristic intraepidermal blister without a significant inflammatory cell infiltrate.

Herpes simplex infections occur either as primary, recurrent, or disseminated infections.[14] The primary infections most commonly afflict the oral mucosa and perioral skin, genitalia, or fingers. The primary cutaneous lesions are small 2- to 3-mm vesicles that may or may not be grouped (Fig. 14). The patients often have associated fever, edema, pain, and lymphadenitis. Recurrent herpes simplex infections are commonly instigated by fever, other viral infections, menstruation, stress, or sunburn. Patients typically describe tingling or pain followed by erythema and grouped vesicles. Disseminated herpes simplex infections often occur in immunocompromised hosts or patients with a pre-existing skin disease (eczema herpeticum). The diagnosis is strongly suggested by history and confirmed by either a Tzanck preparation that shows multinucleated virocytes or viral cultures.

Linear IgA dermatosis may occur in childhood (also referred to as "chronic bullous disease of childhood") or in an adult form.[15] The primary lesions are tense blisters that often form arcuate patterns. Clinically and histologically, it may be impossible to differentiate from bullous pemphigoid. The diagnosis is established by demonstrating a linear deposition of IgA along the basement membrane zone using direct immunofluorescence.

REFERENCES

1. Solomon AR. The Tzanck smear: viable and valuable in the diagnosis of herpes simplex, zoster, and varicella. Int J Dermatol 1986;25:169–170.
2. Fine JD. Epidermolysis bullosa: clinical aspects, pathology, and recent advances in research. Int J Dermatol 1986;25:143–57.
3. Carney RG. Incontinentia pigmenti: a world statistical analysis. Arch Dermatol 1976;112:535–42.
4. Camisa C, Sharma HM. Vesiculobullous systemic lupus erythematosus: report of two cases and review of the literature. J Am Acad Dermatol 1983; 9:924–33.
5. Thiers BH. Dermatitis herpetiformis. J Am Acad Dermatol 1981;5:114–7.
6. Huff JC, Weston WL, Tonnesen MG. Erythema multiforme: a critical review of characteristics, diagnostic criteria, and causes. J Am Acad Dermatol 1983;8:763–8.
7. Shornick JF, Bangert JL, Freeman RG, Gilliam JN. Herpes gestationis: clinical and histologic features of twenty-eight cases. J Am Acad Dermatol 1983; 8:214–24.
8. Lever WF. Pemphigus and pemphigoid: a review of the advances made since 1964. J Am Acad Dermatol 1979;1:2–31.
9. Eubanks SW, Patterson JW, May DL, Aeling JL. The porphyrias. Int J Dermatol 1983;22:337–47.
10. Ahmed AR, Hombal SM. Cicatricial pemphigoid. Int J Dermatol 1986;25:90–6.
11. Reuler JB, Chang MK. Herpes zoster: epidemiology, clinical features, and management. South Med J 1984;77:1149–56.
12. Sehgal VN, Gangwani OP. Fixed drug eruption: current concepts. Int J Dermatol 1987;26:67–74.
13. Bennion SD. Annular vesiculation: bullous tinea corporis caused by *Trichophyton rubrum*. Arch Dermatol 1989;125:1569.
14. Raab B, Lorincz AL. Genital herpes simplex—concepts and treatment. J Am Acad Dermatol 1981;5: 249–63.
15. Janninger CK, Wiltz H, Schwartz RA, Kowalewski C, Lambert WC. Adult linear IgA bullous dermatosis: a polymorphic disorder. Cutis 1990;45:37–42.

VISUAL LOSS, UNILATERAL

MITCHELL D. DRUCKER and CURTIS E. MARGO

SYNONYMS: Blindness, Amaurosis (Unilateral)

BACKGROUND

Unilateral visual loss is a manifestation of injury or disease to the anterior visual pathway. This portion of the visual pathway includes the major refracting surfaces of the eye (cornea and lens), the clear ocular media (aqueous and vitreous humor), retina, and optic nerve. At the chiasm, the two separate arms of the pathway merge. From the chiasm to the occipital cortex, the visual pathway is intimately interconnected.

The division of the visual pathway into anterior (prechiasmal) and posterior components has important clinical implications, since lesions occurring at the chiasm or posterior to it will affect vision in both eyes. The hallmark of a posterior visual pathway lesion is the hemianopic field defect, characterized by field loss that respects the vertical meridian at fixation.

In the context of this chapter, the term *visual loss* will refer to either a relative or absolute loss of central or peripheral vision. Although disorders of the anterior branch of the visual pathway commonly affect central visual acuity, there are only three locations in the posterior portion of the pathway that have the potential to cause loss of central acuity: chiasmal lesions, an optic tract lesion, and bilateral occipital lobe disease (usually infarction). Because of the intimate association of nerve axons serving both eyes from the chiasm to occipital cortex, any disease or lesion in this part of the visual pathway will result in bilateral field loss, although at times the loss of peripheral vision in one eye may be subtle.

Unilateral visual loss occurs when the visual system anterior to the optic chiasm is impaired. Visual loss can be insidious, subacute, or acute. Although visual loss may be described by patients as apoplectic, this history is often difficult to substantiate because the

first symptom of visual impairment may be noticed by chance when one eye is covered. Patients may also complain of unilateral vision loss when in fact they have bilateral field loss. A dense left homonymous hemianopia, for example, can be interpreted by some patients as loss of vision in the left eye because objects cannot be seen in the left field of vision. The primary physician who encounters the patient with unilateral visual loss has a crucial role since early diagnosis and treatment of many eye diseases may help hasten the recovery of vision or prevent further deterioration.

HISTORY

Specific questions regarding the circumstances of the visual loss should be asked if patients are not able to describe their symptoms voluntarily. Was the loss of vision painful or painless? Were there any other associated ocular or systemic symptoms? Categorize the time course: Was the event transient, stationary, or progressive? Have the patient be as precise as possible. Transient loss of vision secondary to retinal vascular emboli, for example, will last minutes to hours. In contrast, transient visual obscurations due to elevated intracranial pressure last only a few seconds.

Frequently, obtaining a good history will narrow the differential diagnosis remarkably. Table 1 lists symptoms associated with visual loss and their clinical implications.

PHYSICAL EXAMINATION

There are five basic elements that compose the visual experience: central, peripheral, color, night vision, and stereo acuity. In evaluating a patient with unilateral visual loss, physicians need to assess central acuity, color perception, and peripheral vision.

Visual impairment can result from: (1) interference of light transmission through the cornea, lens, or vitreous; (2) damage to the retina;

TABLE 1. Symptoms Associated with Visual Loss

SYMPTOM	CLINICAL SIGNIFICANCE
Colored halos around lights	Diffraction from corneal edema; angle closure glaucoma
Photophobia, tender eye	Uveitis
Flashes of light in peripheral field of vision	Posterior vitreous detachment; this condition predisposes to retinal detachment
Floaters	Vitreous hemorrhage; may precede retinal detachment
Peripheral monocular visual loss (veil), possibly progressing and affecting central vision	Retinal detachment
Distortion of straight lines	Macular dysfunction
"Spot" in center of visual field	Macular dysfunction
Decrease in peripheral visual field	Retinal detachment, chiasmal disease, advanced glaucoma, bilateral occipital lobe infarcts
Dramatic sudden loss of vision	Vascular obstruction of retinal or optic nerve
Transient obscurations of vision (seconds), usually bilateral	Increased intracranial pressure
Transient visual loss lasting minutes (monocular)	Amaurosis fugax secondary to emboli or giant cell arteritis
Transient visual loss lasting minutes (binocular)	Transient ischemic attacks, migraine
Pain on eye movement	Can be associated with optic neuritis
Headache, temporal tenderness, jaw claudication, myalgias	Giant cell arteritis

(From Drucker MD, Margo CE. Acute visual loss. In: Harwood-Nuss AL, ed. The clinical practice of emergency medicine. Philadelphia: JB Lippincott Co, 1991:42–5. Reprinted with permission.)

(3) injury or dysfunction of the optic nerve; or (4) insult to the intracranial optic pathway—optic chiasm, tract, radiations, or occipital cortex. The cause of visual loss can be addressed by sequentially evaluating each anatomic division. Unilateral visual loss is localized anterior to the chiasm.

The Snellen eye chart is used to measure central acuity. Patients need to wear their glasses when being tested for best corrected acuity. Each eye is tested independently. Viewing the chart through a pinhole often obviates a refractive error. Failure to improve acuity through a pinhole does not preclude a refractive error, as some patients are unable to master its use.

An underlying eye injury may make it difficult to test visual acuity. Swollen eyelids may need to be opened manually. Occasionally, a lid speculum is necessary. Pain may also prohibit a good examination. In such situations a topical anesthetic can be administered to facilitate the examination.

Peripheral visual fields can be tested by the confrontation technique. The examiner sits 1 m in front of the patient with the patient fixating on the examiner's nose. The examiner presents stationary fingers on either side of the vertical and horizontal meridia that divide the center of vision. Each quadrant is tested sequentially, and most important, each eye is tested separately. Carefully performed, the confrontational field test is a reliable way of distinguishing lesions of the retina and optic nerve, which may affect central acuity unilaterally from chiasmal and retrochiasmal processes.

Macular function, corresponding to the central and paracentral visual field, can be tested with an Amsler grid (a square containing a series of vertical and horizontal parallel lines set perpendicular to one another). The grid should be held approximately 30 cm from the eye; each eye is tested separately. Patients that describe wavy or distorted grid lines or amorphous blind spots may have an underlying retinal or optic nerve disorder.

Color vision can be tested in several ways. The evaluation of color vision helps to assess optic nerve function. The loss of color perception can occur early in optic nerve disease when central acuity is still spared. Ishihara's color plates are relatively inexpensive, standardized, and easy to administer.

A penlight or biomicroscope is used to examine the cornea and conjunctiva for foreign bodies, abrasions of the surface epithelium, or edema of the stroma. Corneal abrasions are easier to visualize after the instillation of topical fluorescein; epithelial defects stain green when illuminated by a blue light. Evaluation of the anterior chamber can also be performed with a penlight. Blood in the anterior chamber, referred to as a hyphema, will decrease visual acuity dramatically when interfering with light transmission. Hyphemas are often secondary to trauma but may occur spontaneously owing to juvenile xanthogranuloma, retinoblastoma, or iris neovascularization.

A Schiotz hand-held tonometer or the applanation tonometer on the slit lamp measures intraocular pressure. Glaucoma describes a family of diseases usually involving elevated intraocular pressure. Based on duration of disease and the appearance of the anterior chamber angle, the glaucomas can be classified as acute or chronic and as open or closed angle.

The swinging flashlight test to evaluate pupillary reactions is invaluable in screening for optic nerve dysfunction. A relative afferent papillary defect (RAPD) or Marcus Gunn pupil is a reliable sign of unilateral or asymmetric optic nerve or profound retinal dysfunction. The patient should be evaluated in a dimly lighted room and asked to fixate on a distant target. The light is directed into one eye and then briskly redirected into the other eye. A normal examination will show little, if any, pupillary movement as the light is swung to the second eye because the direct and consensual light responses are equal. Unilateral or asymmetric impairment of impulses along the optic nerves results in a difference between the consensual and direct light reflexes. The pupil on the affected side will appear to dilate when light is directed into it, compared with the normal pupil, which briskly constricts to the light stimulus.

A direct ophthalmoscope can be used to assess the transparency of the vitreous and the appearance of the retina and optic nerve. If the pupil is adequately dilated and the cornea and anterior chamber are clear, then the fundus should be clearly visible. Opacities of the lens or vitreous can obscure this view. The color and topography of the disk (whether it is flat or elevated) and the clarity of the disk margins should be noted.

COMMON CAUSES OF REDUCED VISION

Dry Eye Syndrome

Dry eye syndrome may cause blurred vision, burning, or a foreign body sensation. (Also see chapter on Dry Eye.) The dry eye syndrome results from a lack of an adequate tear film. It is often related to aging, particularly in postmenopausal women; however, various systemic diseases are also associated with dry eyes, including lymphoproliferative

disorders, Sjögren's syndrome, and collagen vascular diseases. Exposure from a seventh cranial nerve paresis can also cause drying. Testing for basic tear secretion is facile; a topical anesthetic, such as proparacaine, is administered to prevent reflex tearing from the filter paper. After the fornices are dried, a piece of Whitman filter paper is placed in the inferior cul-de-sac at the juncture of the middle and lateral third of the inferior lid. Less than 10 mm of wetting after five minutes is consistent with a diagnosis of dry eye. Artificial tears used every three to four hours, with a topical ointment at bedtime, is often all that is needed to ameliorate symptoms.[1]

Other ailments such as Fuch's endothelial dystrophy can cause unilateral visual impairment and pain secondary to corneal edema. It is seen most commonly in postmenopausal women and is inherited as an autosomal dominant trait with variable penetrance.[2]

Glaucoma

Glaucoma is a disease characterized by optic nerve injury usually, but not always, associated with elevated intraocular pressure. Intraocular pressure is measured with a Schiotz or other hand-held tonometer when a slit lamp applanation tonometer is unavailable. Injury to the optic nerve results in typical patterns of visual field loss in the glaucomas. Chronic open angle glaucoma (COAG) is the most common form of glaucoma. Aging, nearsightedness, family history, and black race are all considered risk factors.[3] Visual loss is painless and typically goes unnoticed until very advanced. Initial field loss occurs peripherally, or focally as a small paracentral scotoma. These abnormalities are demonstrated by either manual or automated perimetry. When patients have all the features of COAG with normal elevated intraocular pressure, they have a disorder termed low-tension glaucoma.[4,5]

Closed or narrow angle glaucoma is characterized by obstruction of the anterior chamber angle by the peripheral iris. Angle closure glaucoma is caused by a variety of mechanisms. In each, the trabecular outflow is compromised and intraocular pressure increases. Acute angle closure is characterized by a painful, red eye with cloudy vision. The conjunctiva is injected circumferentially about the corneal lumbus (ciliary flush). The cornea may be cloudy secondary to epithelial and stroma edema. The pupil is often fixed in the mid-dilated position, measuring approximately 5 mm in diameter, with the fixed pupil in contact with the lens behind it; aqueous humor, formed in the posterior chamber by the ciliary body, is trapped, causing the iris to bow forward (iris bombe). Angle closure glaucoma is a medical emergency and requires immediate therapy.

Cataract

Opacification of the crystalline lens is most often related to aging and possibly the result of accumulated exposure to ultraviolet radiation. However, lens opacification can occur from a variety of metabolic or traumatic insults at any time in life. The term *cataract* is clinically used to describe lens opacification that produces some degree of visual impairment.

Age-related cataracts opacify slowly, causing progressive visual loss. Lens fibers become densely packed and sclerotic as the lens increases in size. Urochrome pigment gives the lens nucleus a yellow or brown color. Proliferation of lens epithelium on the inner aspect of the posterior lens capsule results in a posterior subcapsular cataract, a type of cataract also seen in diabetes and with chronic corticosteroid use.

Although the standard clinical test of visual function has been the Snellen acuity chart, Snellen acuity provides limited information regarding functional performance. Contrast sensitivity testing has become an important adjunct in evaluating visual function, particularly in patients with early cataracts.

Surgery to remove cataractous crystalline lenses and insert an artificial posterior chamber lens implant is highly successful. It is an elective procedure, and the decision to operate should be based on the patient's need and desire for better vision.

Age-Related Macular Degeneration

Age-related macular degeneration (ARMD) is a leading cause of unilateral and bilateral central visual loss in patients over the age of 55. It is associated with accumulated exposure to sunlight and occurs more frequently in people with blue, gray, or green irides.[6] Interestingly, hyperopia and cardiovascular disease have been positively correlated with the development of ARMD.[7]

ARMD is divided into two morphologic forms: atrophic (dry) and neovascular/exudative (wet). Drusen are present in both varieties and are deposits of amorphous yellow material found beneath the retinal pigment epithelium (Fig. 1). They are easily seen with the direct ophthalmoscope in the macula that is temporal to the optic disk. The dry form of ARMD shows atrophy of the retinal pigment epithelium. The wet variety has both drusen and a leaky subretinal neovascular membrane.

Visual loss in ARMD may be insidious or abrupt. Subretinal neovascular membranes may leak blood or serous fluid beneath the macula, causing straight lines to appear bent or curved and objects to appear twisted (metamorphopsia). These particular visual symptoms are important to elicit in the history because they are commonly associated with a neovascular membrane that may be amenable to treatment. Therapy for the wet form of ARMD is performed with laser photocoagulation directed at a membrane that must lie 200 μ or more from the center of the fovea.[8]

FIGURE 1. Age-related macular degeneration. Macular drusen.

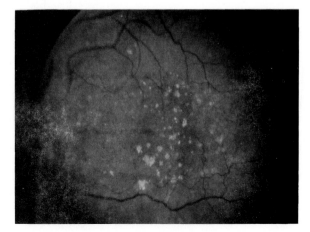

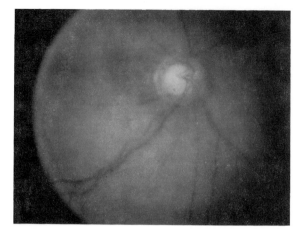

FIGURE 2. Central retinal artery occlusion. Edematous retina.

There is presently no proven effective therapy for dry ARMD. The use of oral zinc to slow its development is presently being studied.[9]

Patients with severe and irreversible visual loss from either atrophic or neovascular ARMD may benefit from consultation with a low vision expert. Optical and nonoptical aids can emotionally, socially, and visually help patients cope with the loss of their vision.

Retinal Detachment

Retinal detachment occurs spontaneously or as a result of trauma. People who are myopic or who have had cataract surgery are at a greater risk than the general population. Symptoms of retinal detachment include flashing lights, floaters, or a visual field defect that is often described as a "shade being drawn." If the macula is not detached, central acuity may be normal. An RAPD suggests that the detachment is chronic and involves a large portion of the retina. Ophthalmoscopy reveals a billowing, elevated pale retina. The treatment is surgical.

Central Retinal Artery Occlusion

A central retinal artery occlusion (CRAO) causes painless, acute, monocular visual loss. Vision may drop to the level of bare light perception and is associated with an RAPD. Men are affected more frequently than women. The condition is found in approximately 1 of 5000 ophthalmology outpatient visits.

When viewed with an ophthalmoscope, the nerve fiber layer of the retina looks white, whereas the fovea, which has no overlying nerve fibers, appears red owing to its underlying choroidal blood. This phenomenon has been termed a "cherry red spot" (Fig. 2). In a branch retinal artery occlusion, retinal edema is limited to the affected area. Visual loss may go unnoticed if central vision is normal. Episodes of amaurosis fugax may precede permanent visual impairment.

CRAO is usually caused by embolic or local thrombotic disease. Emboli from calcified cardiac valves or ulcerated carotid plaques can be visualized with an ophthalmoscope but may have moved "downstream" by the time patients are examined. In such situations, all that is seen is the edematous retina. Cholesterol emboli are yellow, talc or calcium emboli are white, and platelet emboli are fluffy or stringy, according to classic teaching. However, the appearance of a particular embolus is not very reliable. Patients should be evaluated for the source of retinal emboli in the context of their general physical examination.

If no embolus is seen, giant cell arteritis must be considered in the differential diagnosis, and a sedimentation rate should be drawn in patients over the age of 50. Other systemic conditions such as sickle cell hemoglobinopathy and collagen vascular disease are other causes of CRAO.

The treatment of CRAOs (within the first 24 hours) consists of lowering the intraocular pressure and attempting to re-establish retinal blood flow. This can be accomplished by digitally massaging the globe, performing an anterior chamber paracentesis, or using topical or oral medications such as beta blockers or carbonic anhydrase inhibitors. Arterial blood flow can be improved by inhaling a mixture of 95 per cent oxygen and 5 per cent carbon dioxide, which causes dilation of the retinal blood vessels. The sooner therapy is started after the occlusion, the more likely some visual func-

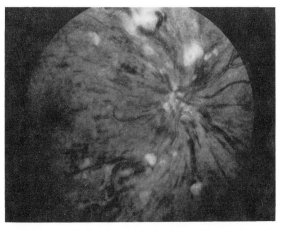

FIGURE 3. Central retinal vein occlusion. Flame-shaped hemorrhages in nerve fiber layer and cotton wool spots.

tion will be recovered. Although these measures are employed within the first 24 hours, the prognosis is poor if more than 12 hours have elapsed.[10,11]

Central Retinal Vein Occlusion

Central retinal vein occlusion (CRVO) causes an acute, painless, often profound loss of vision that is usually, but not always, unilateral. The fundus, when viewed with a direct ophthalmoscope, has flame-shaped hemorrhages throughout the retina with optic nerve head edema and occasionally cotton wool spots (Fig. 3). Other conditions associated with CRVOs include diabetes (15 to 30 per cent), hypertension (60 per cent), open angle glaucoma (6 to 20 per cent), atherosclerosis (25 to 50 per cent), and collagen vascular diseases. Bilateral CRVOs occur in polycythemia vera and dysproteinemias.[12] CRVOs are classified as ischemic or nonischemic by ophthalmologists. Ischemic vein occlusions are more serious. They produce numerous cotton wool spots, cause an RAPD, and often lead to neovascular glaucoma.

Referral to an ophthalmologist is necessary for evaluation and possible treatment with panretinal photocoagulation to prevent neovascular glaucoma.

Anterior Ischemic Optic Neuropathy

Anterior ischemic optic neuropathy (AION) causes an acute, painless, unilateral visual loss due to an infarction of the optic nerve head. The visual acuity may be markedly de-creased. Visual field loss is characteristically an altitudinal defect that does not cross the horizontal midline or an arcuate scotoma. The affected eye shows an RAPD, loss of color vision, and a pale, elevated optic nerve head with splinter hemorrhages[15] (Fig. 4).

AION is classified as arteritic (due to temporal arteritis) or nonarteritic. The nonarteritic variety occurs in people over 50.[13] The optic cup in the contralateral eye is small or absent in many of these patients.[14] Between 20 and 40 per cent of patients may have involvement of the contralateral eye within weeks to months. It is extremely rare for a second event to occur in the same eye—probably less than 1 per cent. There is no therapeutic or prophylactic treatment.

The arteritic form is caused by giant cell (temporal) arteritis, which almost always occurs in people over the age of 60. Systemic symptoms may include temporal tenderness, jaw claudication, headache, proximal muscle weakness, and fever. The erythrocyte sedimentation rate (ESR) is often over 50 mm per hour. However, a normal ESR does not preclude a diagnosis. The contralateral eye is affected in about 80 per cent of patients and may occur within hours of the first eye. It is therefore mandatory that prophylactic treatment with high-dose corticosteroids begin immediately, with intravenous methylprednisolone, 250 mg, every six hours or oral prednisone, 80 mg or more per day. Corticosteroids, with their potential side effects, are needed for months. It is therefore prudent to perform a temporal artery biopsy to obtain a tissue diagnosis to help justify the risk of treatment. Biopsy is usually done within two weeks of initi-

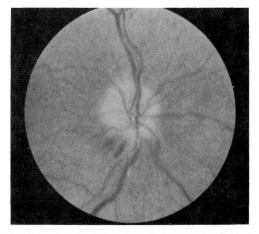

FIGURE 4. Anterior ischemic optic neuropathy. Pale elevated disks with splinter hemorrhages.

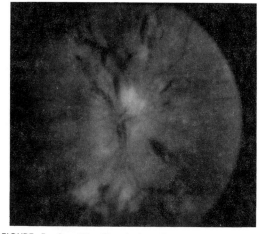

FIGURE 5. Papillitis. Elevated optic disks with blurred margins and peripapillary hemorrhages.

ation of treatment to avoid the chance of a false-negative result.

Optic Neuritis

Optic neuritis is an inflammatory condition of the optic nerve. If inflammation involves the nerve behind the eye, it is termed retrobulbar optic neuritis, and if the optic disk is elevated, it is called papillitis (Fig. 5). Clinically, pain is associated with eye movements in 65 per cent of cases, visual loss ranges from a mild arcuate scotoma with 20/20 acuity to no light perception, color vision is impaired, and there is an RAPD.

Visual acuity decreases over the first week in typical idiopathic optic neuritis and slowly improves over the next 7 to 12 weeks. Optic neuritis is an idiopathic disorder or may be related to multiple sclerosis, sarcoidosis, postviral illness, syphilis, collagen vascular diseases, herpes zoster, or tuberculosis.

The use of corticosteroids for optic neuritis is widespread; however, there is no proof of their clinical efficacy either to shorten the nat-ural course of the disease or to improve the final visual acuity. There is currently a multi-center national clinical study comparing oral or intravenous corticosteroids to placebo.[15]

REFERENCES

1. Moatsopoulos H. Sjögren's syndrome: current issues. Am Int Med 1980;92:212–5.
2. Waring GO, Rodriques MM, Laibson PR. Corneal dystrophies 1. Surv Ophthalmol 1978;23:74–9.
3. Leske MD, Rosenthal J. Epidemiologic aspects of open-angle glaucoma. Am J Epidemiol 1979;109:250–61.
4. Zimmerman TJ, Kooner TS, Kandarakis AS, Ziegler LP. Improving the therapeutic index of topically applied ocular drugs. Arch Ophthalmol 1984;102:551–7.
5. Drance SM, Douglass GR, Airaksinen PJ, Schulzer M, Hitchings RA. Diffuse visual field loss in chronic open-angle and low-tension glaucoma. Am J Ophthalmol 1987;104:577–80.
6. Hyman LG, Lilienfeld AM, Ferris FL III, Fine SL. Senile macular degeneration. A case-control study. Am J Ophthalmol 1983;118:213–9.
7. Sunness JS, Massoff RW, Johnson MA, Bressler NM, Bressler SB, Fine SL. Diminished foveal sensitivity may predict the development of advanced age-related macular degeneration. Ophthalmol 1989;96:375–80.
8. Macular Photocoagulation Study Group. Argon laser photocoagulation for senile macular degeneration: results of a randomized clinical trial. Arch Ophthalmol 1982;100:912–9.
9. Newsome DA, Swartz M, Leone NC, Elston RC. Oral zinc in macular degeneration. Arch Ophthalmol 1988;106:192–8.
10. Brown GC, Margargul LE. Central retinal artery obstruction and visual acuity. Ophthalmol 1982;89:14–9.
11. Gold D. Retinal arterial occlusion. Trans Am Acad Ophthalmol Otolaryngol 1977;83:392–7.
12. Johnston RL, Brucker AJ, Steinmann W, Hoffman ME, Holmes JA. Risk factors of brand retinal vein occlusion. Arch Ophthalmol 1985;103:1831–2.
13. Hayreh SS. Anterior ischemic optic neuropathy. Arch Ophthalmol 1981;99:1030–5.
14. Beck RW, Savino PJ, Repka MX, Schatz NJ, Sergott RC. Optic disc structure in anterior ischemic optic neuropathy. Ophthalmol 1984;91:1334–7.
15. Beck RW. The optic neuritis treatment trial. Arch Ophthalmol 1988;106:1051–2.

WEIGHT GAIN

STEPHEN A. BRUNTON, NANCY CARPENTER, and RALPH R. HALL

SYNONYMS: Overweight, Obesity, Excess Adiposity

BACKGROUND

The terms *overweight* and *obesity* are often used synonymously, but in fact their definitions are quite different. Overweight is defined as excess weight for height as assessed by standards such as actuarial tables (e.g., Metropolitan Life Insurance Company) (see Table 1). Obesity, on the other hand, refers to excess body fat. Overweight is generally accepted as 10 per cent above an ideal or desirable weight, whereas obesity is 20 per cent or more above this point.

The problem of weight gain—and obesity, in particular—is of significant concern in industrialized countries such as the United States. Depending on the definition utilized, between 6 and 15 per cent of children and adolescents can be classified as significantly overweight. It is thought that as many as one half of obese adults had significant weight problems in adolescence. Adolescent obesity rates have been estimated at about 20 to 30 per cent.[1]

The prevalence of obesity is estimated at around 24 per cent for men and 32 per cent for women. The incidence of major weight gain is twice as high in women and highest in persons age 25 to 34 years (3.9 per cent men; 8.4 per cent women). Women between the ages of 25 and 44 who are initially overweight have a 14.2 per cent incidence of weight gain, the highest of any group. Normal-weight individuals have a continuing incidence of developing obesity that is similar in both sexes and highest among the ages 35 to 44 (16.3 per cent in men and 13.5 per cent in women).[2]

There is also an inverse relationship between socioeconomic status and the prevalence of obesity. As many as 30 per cent of economically disadvantaged women are obese, compared with 5 per cent in higher income groups.[3]

Race may also be a factor, with a higher prevalence of obesity in black women compared with white women, whereas white men have a higher prevalence than black men.[4]

One or more parents may pass on a genetic predisposition enabling their children to be overweight and obese, and it appears that family environment by itself is not a major determinant in the development of obesity.[5]

There now exists an emerging body of research and knowledge regarding weight gain leading to weight above ideal standards. Theories of weight gain related to obesity include: genetic influences, the fat cell theory, set point theory, brown versus white fat theory, and the sluggish metabolism theory. These theories are briefly explored.

The fat cell theory is based on the premise that the number of fat cells in the body is fixed during childhood and that although their size may vary, their number does not change despite weight loss. However, it is apparent that the number of fat cells may increase through childhood and into adulthood if a person gains a large amount of weight.[6]

The set point theory proposes that each individual has a natural weight or set point. People who lose and gain 10 to 20 pounds and cannot seem to maintain a lower weight may actually be set biologically at a certain weight possibly regulated by the hypothalamus. Although few research studies have been undertaken in this area, it may help to explain persistent weight maintenance despite rigorous dieting. Exercise may be one mechanism that may change one's set point.

Named because of its pigmentation, brown fat is located between the scapulae, around the heart and aorta, just under the kidneys, and in other localized areas of the chest and abdomen. Brown fat is responsible for thermogenesis, whereas the function of white fat is the storage of excess calories. It has been postulated that lean persons have a larger ratio of brown to white fat, which may be a primary factor in maintaining normal or even lean weight in adults who can eat recklessly and never gain weight.[7]

TABLE 1.   1983 Metropolitan Height and Weight Tables*

MEN					WOMEN				
Height		Small Frame	Medium Frame	Large Frame	Height		Small Frame	Medium Frame	Large Frame
Feet	Inches				Feet	Inches			
5	2	128–134	131–141	138–150	4	10	102–111	109–121	118–131
5	3	130–136	133–143	140–153	4	11	103–113	111–123	120–134
5	4	132–138	135–145	142–156	5	0	104–115	113–126	122–137
5	5	134–140	137–148	144–160	5	1	106–118	115–129	125–140
5	6	136–142	139–151	146–164	5	2	108–121	118–132	128–143
5	7	138–145	142–154	149–168	5	3	111–124	121–135	131–147
5	8	140–148	145–157	152–172	5	4	114–127	124–138	134–151
5	9	142–151	148–160	155–176	5	5	117–130	127–141	137–155
5	10	144–154	151–163	158–180	5	6	120–133	130–144	140–159
5	11	146–157	154–166	161–184	5	7	123–136	133–147	143–163
6	0	149–160	157–170	164–188	5	8	126–139	136–150	146–167
6	1	152–164	160–174	168–192	5	9	129–142	139–153	149–170
6	2	155–168	164–178	172–197	5	10	132–145	142–156	152–173
6	3	158–172	167–182	176–202	5	11	135–148	145–159	155–176
6	4	162–176	171–187	181–207	6	0	138–151	148–162	158–179

* Weights at ages 25 to 59 based on lowest mortality; weight in pounds according to frame (in indoor clothing weighing 5 lbs for men and 3 lbs for women; shoes with 1-in. heels).
(Courtesy of Metropolitan Life Insurance Company.)

It is not clear that a sluggish metabolism causes obesity. However, age, sex, frame size, and nutritional status all contribute to changes in the BMR (basal metabolic rate). Younger people have a higher BMR, whereas women have lower BMRs, as do smaller-framed, less muscular individuals. Poor nutritional status or severe caloric restriction also results in a lowered BMR.

There are many factors involved in the development of obesity. However, the etiology depends predominantly on caloric intake, expenditure, and mechanisms of fat storage, as well as genetic and psychologic influences.

Psychiatric conditions must also be considered. Bulimia nervosa is described as episodes of uncontrollable binge eating alternating with severe dietary restriction. This condition needs to be differentiated from another variant characterized by cycles of binge eating and purging whose sufferers tend to be somewhat underweight. Bulimia nervosa is more common, affecting up to 10 per cent of women in the United States and 1 to 2 per cent of men. The pattern of eating displayed by persons with bulimia nervosa usually leads to obesity. The prevalence of this syndrome increases directly with weight, reaching the prevalence of around 40 per cent with a body mass index (BMI) greater than 35.[8]

The question of an endocrinopathy as the cause of obesity is often raised. The occasional patient with either Cushing's disease or a hypogonadal state as well as the high incidence of obesity at the onset of non–insulin-dependent diabetes necessitates that physicians evaluate the possibility of an endocrine abnormality. However, the likelihood of a hormonal cause of obesity is slight, and the endocrinopathy seen in some obese states is the result rather than the cause of the obesity.[9]

The identification of a hormonal etiology of the obesity such as an adrenal tumor, however, can be important. One may incidentally also identify the patient with alcoholism as a factor in his or her appearing to have an excess of adrenal steroids.

Abnormalities of the hypothalamus, pituitary, thyroid, adrenal glands, pancreas, and gonads need to be considered. Rarely, a hypothalamic lesion affecting the ventromedial hypothalamus resulting from a tumor (most likely a craniopharyngioma), infection, or more rarely, trauma may result in damage to the satiety center, thus giving rise to overfeeding.[10]

A pituitary cause of Cushing's disease or an adrenal cause of Cushing's syndrome is a rare cause of obesity; however, the diagnosis will become apparent with appropriate laboratory testing and evaluation of the patient's signs and symptoms.

The occurrence of obesity in some patients with hypothyroidism has led physicians to consider this as an important factor in weight gain. The weight loss that occurs in patients with hyperthyroidism and the successful weight reduction that results when excess thyroid hormone has been administered further enhance the concept that inadequate thyroid

TABLE 2. Drugs Reported to Cause Weight Gain

Amitriptyline (Elavil, Endep)	Methdilazine (Tacaryl)
Baclofen (Lioresal)	Methenamine mandelate (Mandelamine)
Buspirone (Buspar)	Methyclothiazide (Enduronyl)
Chlorothiazide (Diupres)	Methyldopa (Aldomet)
Chlorpromazine HCL (Thorazine)	Methyldopa/chlorothiazide (Aldoclor)
Chlorthalidone (Demi-Regroton, Regroton)	Methyldopa/hydrochlorothiazide (Aldoril)
Cholestyramine (Questran)	Methysergide maleate (Sansert)
Clofibrate (Atromid)	Nadolol (Corgard)
Clomiphene citrate (Clomid, Serophene)	Nadolol/bendroflumethazide (Corzide)
Clonidine (Catapres)	Norethindprone acetate (Aygestin)
Clonidine/chlorthalidone (Combipres)	Norethindrone/ethinyl estradiol (Brevicon, Micronor,
Conjugated estrogens (Mediatric, Premarin)	Modicon, Norinyl, Nor-QD, Ortho-Novum, Ovcon,
Cortisone acetate (Cortone)	Trinorinyl)
Cryptenamine (Diutensen)	Nortriptyline (Aventyl, Pamelor)
Danazol (Danocrine)	Pargyline (Eutonyl Filmtab)
Dexamethasone (Decadron)	Perphenazine (Etrafon, Trilafon)
Dienestrol (Ortho Dienestrol Crm)	Phenelzine sulfate (Nardil)
Diethylstilbestrol (Stilphostrol)	Pindolol (Visken)
Diltiazem (Cardizem)	Piroxicam (Feldene)
Dimethyl sulfoxide (DMSO)	Polyestradiol (Estradurin)
Disopyramide phosphate (Norpace)	Potassium phosphate (K-Phos)
Doxepin (Adapin, Sinequan)	Prazepam (Centrax)
Estradiol micronized (Estrace)	Prednisdone sodium phosphate (Hydeltrasol)
Estrapipate (Ogen)	Prochlorperazine (Compazine)
Ethinyl estradiol (Estinyl)	Rauwolfia (Raudixin, Rauxide)
Guanadrel sulfate (Hylorel)	Rescinnamine (Moderil)
Hydrochlorothizide (Esidrix, Hydrodiuril, Oretic)	Reserpine hydralazine (Ser-Ap-Es, Serpasil)
Hydrocortisone	Terazosin (Hytrin)
Hydroflumethiazide (Salutensin)	Theophylline
Imipramine (Tofranil)	Thioridizine (Mellaril)
Indomethacin (Indocin)	Tolmetin sodium (Tolectin)
Ketoprofen (Orudis caps)	Trazodone (Desyrel)
Levodopa/carbidopa (Sinemet)	Triethylperazine (Torcan)
Lithium (Cibalith, Eskalith, Lithane, Lithobid)	Trifluoperazine (Stelazine)
Mazindol (Sanorex)	Trimeprazine tartrate (Temaril)
Medroxy progesterone acetate (Amen, Depo-Provera,	Trimipramine maleate (Surmontil)
Provera)	Valproic acid (Depakene, Depakote)
Mesoridazine (Serentil)	

hormone level is a common etiology of obesity.

However, hypothyroidism is not a frequent finding in obesity, and in fact, myxedema patients as a group are not overweight.[11] Weight loss in a hypothyroid patient on a replacement therapy is a result of diuresis since water retention is a feature of myxedema.

Frequently overlooked, but an important consideration in the evaluation of weight gain, is the role of medications (see Table 2).

Antipsychotic agents have frequently been implicated. The mechanism by which this occurs is not well understood, although improvement in well-being together with an increased appetite or carbohydrate craving may contribute. Dose and route of administration may also have an effect on the amount of weight gain. This is seen particularly with oral antipsychotic agents, owing to the larger doses required for therapeutic effects.[12] Drugs with higher sedative properties increase the potential for weight gain (see Table 3.)

Tricyclic compounds used successfully to treat endogenous depression may also be responsible for a patient's reported weight gain. Although the mechanism is unclear, it may be that improved mental status results in better appetite and an increased craving for carbohydrates.[13] Weight gain from tricyclic compounds is a complex issue and involves many interacting pathways, making it difficult to identify one specific mechanism.

Cyproheptadine, an antihistamine with antiseritonergic properties, was first shown to have an effect on weight gain when used on asthmatic children.[14] The exact pathway of

TABLE 3. Highly Sedating Antipsychotic Medications

Chlorpromazine (Chlorzine, Promachlor, Promapar,
   Promaz, Sonazine, Terpium, Thorazine)
Chlorprothixene (Taractan)
Mesoridazine (Lidanil, Serentil)
Thioridazine (Mellaril, Millazine)
Triflupromazine (Vesprin)

this weight gain is unknown. However, it appears largely due to a central effect on the hypothalamus. Similar compounds in structure and antiseritonergic properties such as azatadine most likely cause weight gain by the same mechanism.

Estrogen and estrogen analogues used in birth control pills or for postmenopausal replacement commonly result in weight gain. Danazol, a steroid blocking agent, has also been implicated in weight gain in 3 per cent of the patients receiving various dosages.[15]

Stopping the use of nicotine has been shown to decrease resting metabolic rate and possibly increase caloric intake. In approximately 30 to 50 per cent of individuals, cessation of smoking can result in weight gain that averages 10 pounds.[16] Some individuals, however, have experienced significant weight gain owing to excessive caloric intake.

Less common considerations that present in childhood and carry with them specific stigmata are the rare genetic syndromes of which obesity is a common expression. These include: Prader-Labhart-Willi syndrome, idiopathic adiposogenital dystrophy, Fröhlich's syndrome, Laurence-Moon-Biedl syndrome, Bongiovanni-Eisenmenger syndrome, and Alström's syndrome.

HISTORY

A typical history is that of progressive weight gain through adolescence and early adult life, with several attempts at diet and weight loss but with recurrence of the weight.

The age of onset, rapidity of weight gain, and in particular any specific fat distribution patterns should be asked (e.g., Cushing's syndrome with the typical buffalo hump, moon facies, and truncal obesity).

The dietary history is critical. The patient should be asked about any previous attempts at weight loss. Has the appetite increased or remained the same? Have there been any recent changes? (A diary containing amounts and descriptions of all foods and beverages consumed written contemporaneously by the patient can help to estimate caloric intake. It is not uncommon for an obese patient to markedly understate the quantity of food he or she ingests.)

Focused Queries

Specific questions in the following areas may further aid the diagnostician.

1. *Does the patient exercise? Has this increased or decreased? Has the patient stopped smoking? Is he or she taking any medications?* (see Tables 2 and 3.)

2. *Has there been any change in the menstrual cycle or the development of hirsutism (polycystic ovary or Cushing's syndrome)? Does the patient binge eat or at times feel unable to control his or her appetite (bulimia nervosa)?*

3. *What is the patient's urinary frequency? Is he or she frequently thirsty?* Urinary frequency and thirst may suggest the diagnosis of diabetes mellitus in an obese individual.

4. *Is there decreased libido (due to decreased gonadotrophins)? Intolerance to cold? Visual disturbances (visual field defects or temporal hemianopsia can be seen)? Memory loss? Is there an increase or decrease in hair or change in distribution?* Hypothyroidism secondary to pituitary failure may be implicated by positive responses to these questions.

5. *Any skin changes, such as acne or pigmentation? Weakness in climbing stairs? Mood lability or new emotional problems?* Positive responses to these questions may suggest Cushing's syndrome.

Family History

Are the parents overweight? (Eighty per cent of children of two obese patients will eventually be obese, compared with only 14 per cent of normal-weight parents.) Does the patient have an overweight sibling? (The inheritability of obesity is seen particularly in monozygotic twins.)[17]

PHYSICAL EXAMINATION

As previously mentioned, endocrine causes of weight gain are extremely uncommon. However, exclusion of these conditions is appropriate. During your physical examination, you may determine other findings that may complete the weight gain puzzle.

Pituitary

Findings may include visual field defects such as temporal hemianopsia (seen with chromophobe adenoma). One may also see stigmata of decreased function in pituitary target organs.

Thyroid

Suggestions of hypothyroidism include: sluggish reflexes, enlarged thyroid, possible exophthalmus, nonpitting edema, and dry skin with coarse, dry, brittle hair.

Adrenal

Physical findings in Cushing's syndrome include: hypertension, hirsutism, moon facies, increased fat deposition over the vertebrae in the upper dorsal area (buffalo hump), and truncal obesity. Arms and legs may be thin. There may be purple striae, and the skin is thin, bruising easily in advanced disease.

Ovary

In the polycystic ovary syndrome (Stein-Leventhal syndrome), patients' physical findings vary from mild to moderate hirsutism, and they are often muscular as well as obese. (Clitoral hypertrophy is a manifestation of virilism and occurs in ovarian and adrenal tumors as well as in the adrenogenital syndrome.)

DIAGNOSTIC STUDIES

The initial use of diagnostic procedures needs to be directed toward classifying the patient's weight gain, which may include determining the relative proportion of fat.

Height and weight tables, BMI, underwater weighing, bioelectrical impedance, and measurements of skinfold thickness assess fatness with varying degrees of precision and practicality. It is recommended that a combination of methods be used to ensure validity of the data.

Height and weight tables are convenient to provide initial determination of weight relative to height. These tables reflect data from upper-middle-class Caucasian groups and, although specific for sex and height, are not age specific. Additionally, ranges for a particular height can vary as much as 40 lbs, making this a rather inaccurate tool if used in isolation (see Table 1).

BMI is a more accurate measure and is calculated by dividing a person's nude weight (in kilograms) by the square of the barefoot height (in meters). For ease and convenience, a nomogram may be used instead (see Fig. 1). The index range for normal weights is 20 to 25 for men, and 19 to 24 for women. When BMI exceeds 30, morbidity and mortality rates begin to rise steadily for both men and women. However, a major weakness is that very muscular individuals may be misclassified as obese.

Because over half the body's fat is deposited under the skin and the percentage increases with increasing weight, weight gain can be evaluated with the use of skinfold calipers. Usually, four sites are measured (biceps, triceps, subscapular, and suprailiac skinfolds), and their sum is used to determine fat content as a percentage of body weight.[18] Regression equations have been developed to include variables such as sex and age; however, variations in size of grasp, degree of subject fatness, and level of experience can affect the reliability of the results. Several measures on the same site are recommended to reduce variations in the results. It should be noted that skinfold data are less reliable in children than in adults.

Underwater or hydrostatic weighing, although seldom used in office practice, is considered one of the most accurate means of assessing body composition. A person is submerged in water and weighed after he or she has expended all the air in the lungs. Because muscle is more dense (1.1 gm/cm) and fat less dense (0.9 gm/cu cm), persons with a higher proportion of fat tissue weigh less under water, and so the percentage of body fat can be calculated. This procedure can demonstrate how people who do not exhibit a loss of weight on a conventional scale can lose body fat and increase muscle mass through exercise.

Bioelectric impedance is the newest instrument to measure fatty tissue. The electrical conductivity of nonfatty tissue is far greater than that of fatty tissue.[19] Thus, if a small amount of electrical current is uniformly applied to the body, the conductivity observed should directly relate to the total body water—which theoretically reflects fat-free mass. Unfortunately, these instruments need

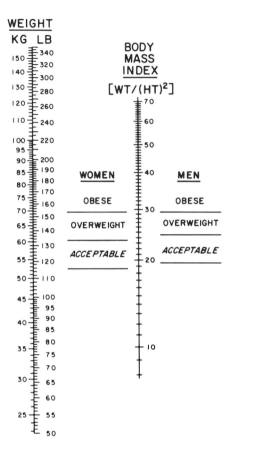

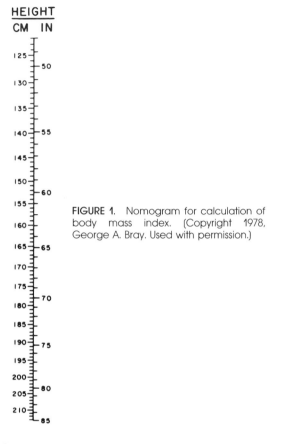

FIGURE 1. Nomogram for calculation of body mass index. (Copyright 1978, George A. Bray. Used with permission.)

further refinements before they can become reliable clinical tools.

Hypothalamus

Impairment of pituitary hormone production such as growth hormone, prolactin, and gonadotropin are frequently found in markedly obese subjects. Cortisol, insulin, and norepinephrine release may also be impaired in response to stimuli such as hypoglycemia and thyrotropin releasing hormone (TRH). The variation in the response to hypoglycemia and TRH raises interesting questions regarding these being the cause or effect of the obesity. An example of this phenomenon is the difference in prolactin response to hypoglycemia and TRH. Those individuals who have a muted response of prolactin to hypoglycemia (about half of those tested) also fail to release norepinephrine in response to hypoglycemia.

Pituitary

A pituitary etiology for Cushing's syndrome is a rare cause of obesity. The diagnosis will become apparent with appropriate laboratory testing and evaluation of the patient's signs and symptoms. Measurement of the plasma cortisol is less expensive and is as accurate as urine testing in establishing the diagnosis of Cushing's syndrome.

The dexamethasone suppression test may help to further establish an etiology. Visualizing the pituitary radiographically is not indicated in the absence of abnormal laboratory findings.[20]

Thyroid

Testing the status of the thyroid has become more precise with the introduction of a new sensitive thyroid stimulating hormone (TSH) determination, such that a normal level of TSH rules out the thyroid as a significant contributor to obesity.

It is important to understand that the serum tri-iodothyronine (T_3) in particular and total and free thyroxine (T_4) and thyroid binding globulin do fluctuate with feeding. T_3 increases with feeding and decreases with fasting; this rise or fall in serum T_3 depends mainly on alteration of carbohydrate intake.

Adrenal

Just as many obese individuals have increased serum levels of T_3 and T_4, many obese subjects have an increased production rate and turnover of cortisol. The observations are reflected by increased urinary excretion of 17-hydroxycorticosteroids. Despite this increase in production of cortisol, plasma levels are normal and respond with a diurnal variation that is within the normal range. In addition, the urinary-free cortisol level is normal and provides a useful measure for ruling out adrenal causes of obesity.

The presence of increased dehydroepiandrosterone (DHA) and DHA sulfate probably result in an increased urine excretion of 17-ketosteroids. This is a measure of adrenal androgen production.

It has been observed that obese subjects fasting for at least 36 hours have a decrease in urinary 17-hydroxycorticosteroid excretion and cortisol secretion rates.[21] However, overfeeding will elevate cortisol production rates.

ASSESSMENT

In the majority of cases, the search for a secondary cause of weight gain will be unrewarding. However, physical stigmata correlated with a laboratory evaluation can provide specific direction.

Certainly if a medication is indicated in the etiology of weight gain, this can be modified and a response evaluated. A detailed family, life-style, and further dietary history can provide additional clues.

Several points need to be considered in the evaluation of endocrine causes. The endocrine response to TRH and hypoglycemia return to normal in those individuals who are able to return to the nonobese state. The length of time required for recovery of organ response after return to the nonobese state varies widely with the individual. This aspect of weight loss also raises the question of whether there are different causes for the weight gain. These features, although intriguing, are not helpful in differentiating the cause of obesity. Therefore, physicians must be aware of these nuances if they are to avoid unnecessary pursuit of an endocrine cause for a patient's obesity.

Subtle variations in the adrenal cortico-trophic hormone (ACTH) secretion due to stress, pulsal secretion, and diurnal variations render ACTH determination misleading unless the change is marked.

Adrenal or pituitary causes of obesity may be ruled out by any of the following: (1) the 24-hour excretion of urinary-free cortisol; (2) the dexamethasone suppression test measuring urinary 17-hydroxycorticosteroid secretion; and (3) the overnight dexamethasone suppression test using the 8:00 A.M. plasma cortisol level. The plasma cortisol, as previously stated, may be the simplest means of establishing that an endocrine abnormality is present.

Indications of normal pituitary-adrenal function include a normal 24-hour urinary-free cortisol excretion, suppression of the urine 17-hydroxycorticosteroids or 17-ketogenic steroids after dexamethasone suppression to less than 3 mg for 24 hours, or a drop in the 8:00 A.M. blood plasma cortisol after 1 mg of dexamethasone the prior evening.

The appearance of patients with Cushing's syndrome and Cushing's disease may be similar to patients with excessive alcohol intake largely owing to their distribution of body fat as well as the plethora that is occasionally present. Both may also have elevated high blood pressure and easy bruising. However, the thin skin frequently seen with excess adrenal steroid production is seldom present in the alcoholic.

Obesity also is associated with changes in gonadotropin secretion as well as disturbances of ovarian function. Both amenorrhea and oligomenorrhea may be associated with obesity. The associated signs of acne, hirsutism, and menstrual irregularities resulting from an increase in adrenal androgens may suggest polycystic ovaries as the cause of weight gain.

MANAGING WEIGHT GAIN

Patients presenting with the problem of weight gain require a detailed history and physical examination and, if indicated, additional laboratory evaluation to investigate the possibility of an endocrine etiology. In the vast majority of cases, secondary causes of obesity are usually eliminated early in the diagnostic evaluation, and so one is left with the conclusion that the origin of the patient's weight gain stems from life-style factors rather than specific pathologic processes.

REFERENCES

1. Pi-Sunyer FX. Obesity. In: Shils ME, Young VR, eds. Modern nutrition in health and disease. 7th ed. Philadelphia: Lea & Febiger, 1988:795–816.
2. Williamson DF, Kahn HS, Remington PL, et al. The 10-year incidence of overweight and major weight gain in U.S. adults. Arch Intern Med 1990;150:665–72.
3. Goldblatt PB, Moore BE, Stunkard AJ. Social factors in obesity. JAMA 1967;192:1039–44.
4. Height and weight of adults ages 18–74 years by socioeconomic status and geographic variables. United States. Hyattsville, Maryland: National Center for Health Statistics, 1981; DHHS Publication no. (PHS) 81–1674.
5. Stunkard AJ, Sorensen TA, Harris C, et al. An adoption study of human obesity. N Engl J Med 1986;314:893–8.
6. Bray GA. Brown tissue and metabolic obesity. Nutr Today 1982;17:23–7.
7. Elliott J. Blame it all on brown fat now. JAMA 1980;243:1983–5.
8. Telch CF, Agras WS, Rossiter EM. Binge eating increases with increasing adiposity. Int J Eating Disorders 1988;7:115–9.
9. Jung R. Endocrinological aspects of obesity. Clin Endocrinol Metab 1984;13:597–612.
10. Bray GF, Gallagher TF Jr. Manifestations of hypothalamic obesity in man: a comprehensive investigation of eight patients and a review of the literature. Medicine 1975;54:301–21.
11. Plummer WA. Body weight in spontaneous myxedema. Trans Am Goiter Assoc Study 1940;88–98.
12. Doss F. The effect of antipsychotic drugs on body weight: a retrospective review. J Clin Psychiatry 1979;54–528–30.
13. Paykel ES. Amitriptyline, weight gain, and carbohydrate craving: a side effect. Br J Psychol 1973;123:123–501.
14. Lavenstein AF, Dacaney EP, Lasagna L, VanMetre TE. Effect of cyproheptadine on asthmatic children. JAMA 1962;180:912–6.
15. Spooner JB. Classification of side effects to danazol therapy. J Int Med Res 1977;5(Suppl 3):15–24.
16. The health consequences of smoking: nicotine addiction. A report of the surgeon general. Rockville, Maryland: US Department of Health and Human Services, Public Health Service, Centers for Disease Control, Center for Health Promotion and Education, Office on Smoking and Health, 1988; DHHS publication no. CDC88–8406.
17. Stunkard AJ, Foch TT, Hrubek Z. A twin study of human obesity. JAMA 1986;256:50–4.
18. Durnin JVGA, Womersley J. Body fat assessed from total body density and its estimation from skinfold thickness: measurements on 481 men and women from 16–72 years. Br J Nutr 1974;31:77–97.
19. Carpenter NS, Brunton SA. Evaluating the severity and causes of adult obesity. Fam Pract Recertification 1988;10(9):59–71.
20. Ashcraft MW, Van Herle AJ, Verner SL, et al. Serum cortisol levels in Cushing's syndrome after low- and high-dose dexamethasone suppression. Ann Intern Med 1982;97:21–6.
21. Simken B. Urinary 17-ketosteroids and 17-ketogenic steroidal excretion in obese patients. N Engl J Med 1961;164:924–27.

XEROSTOMIA

JERRY W. TEMPLER and PETER E. SHAPIRO

SYNONYMS: Dry Mouth, Oral Dryness, Sicca Syndrome, Salivary Dysfunction, Asialorrhea

BACKGROUND

Xerostomia is dryness of the mouth from lack of normal secretion. Hypofunction of the salivary glands results from any process that intrinsically affects the glands or depresses the stimulatory function of the autonomic nervous system. While thought by some patients (and their physicians) to be an annoyance, xerostomia can have profound effects on multiple organ systems. It is, therefore, important to examine the problems with respect to its presentation, etiology, and possible treatments.

The anatomy and physiology of the salivary glands are only recently understood. The ancients thought the glands to have a sievelike role in straining substances such as the "emunctories (evil spirits) of the brain."[1] Later, the saliva was thought to originate from the lymph. It was not until Wharton, in 1656, discovered the duct to the submandibular gland that the concept of salivary secretion was formulated.

Stensen discovered the duct to the parotid and introduced the concept that stimulation of the gland came from the brain via nerves. In the late eighteenth and early nineteenth century, with the discovery of the autonomic nervous system, the connection between brain and glands was found. In the 1850s and 1860s, Ludwig stimulated the lingual nerve, causing secretion in the submandibular gland, and Bernard showed there were medullary centers for control of salivation. Later, Heidenheim discovered the separate functions of the autonomic nervous system by showing that stimulation of the cranial nerves caused watery secretion, whereas sympathetic stimulation caused scant viscid secretion from the submandibular and none from the parotid gland.[1]

The Assyrians, Babylonians, and Egyptians knew that saliva was present in the mouth and that certain conditions and substances could increase or decrease its flow. Belladonna was mentioned in the Assyrian Herbarium of 2000 BCE as useful ''to stop the flow of saliva.''[2] In 1874, Langley showed that jaborandi, a pilocarpine-containing compound, could stimulate the flow of saliva.[1]

The parotid gland is the largest of the salivary glands and is palpable between the ramus of the mandible and the mastoid process.[3] It has a superficial and deep lobe separated by the seventh cranial nerve; however, this designation is probably arbitrary. The duct of the parotid gland (Stensen's) runs across the masseter one finger breadth below the zygomatic arch (along with the buccal branch of the seventh cranial nerve), then turns medially to enter the oral cavity at the level of the second maxillary molar. The gland is surrounded by a capsule that contains numerous lymph nodes as well. The ninth cranial nerve provides secretomotor function to the gland.

The submandibular gland fills the major portion of the submandibular triangle and consists of two lobes: a superficial lobe and a deep lobe that wraps around the mylohyoid. The duct of the submandibular gland (Wharton's) runs from the anterior portion of the gland, between the hyoglossus and the mylohyoid muscles, and terminates as an elevated papilla on the floor of the mouth on either side of the frenulum of the tongue.[3] The sublingual gland occupies the same plane as Wharton's duct, lying in the floor of the mouth and having a series of ductules opening directly into the mouth or into Wharton's duct. The seventh cranial nerve provides secretomotor function to the submandibular and sublingual glands as well as to the numerous minor salivary glands that are present in the mucosa of the lips, gingiva, and pharynx. Sympathetic innervation of all the glands is from the cervical ganglia via the carotid and reaches the glands accompanying the blood vessels.

The central nervous system modulates salivation with efferent information from the salivary center in the medulla. The superior and inferior salivatory nuclei supply the submandibular/sublingual and parotid glands, respectively. Afferent information carried to the salivary center includes unconditioned reflexes (olfaction, taste, mastication, oral stimulation, pharyngeal stimulation, and stimulation of the gastric branch of the vagus nerve), emotional and psychic factors, and conditioned reflexes[4] (see Fig. 1).

With the exception of the vasodilatory action of bradykinin and the stimulation of ductal sodium and potassium ion transport by aldosterone, the autonomic nervous system is almost solely responsible for the physiologic control of the salivary glands.[4] Stimulation of the parasympathetics causes vasodilation and secretion (mostly serous), whereas sympathetic stimuli cause vasoconstriction and the production of only scant amounts of viscid (mucinous) saliva. The parasympathetics have a direct stimulatory effect, whereas the sympathetic effect is due either to weak stimulation or to contraction of myoepithelial cells, or both.[4]

There may be a mechanical component to salivary flow as well. The anatomic position of the salivary glands is such that they lie within pockets of the muscles of mastication. With chewing, these muscles massage the glands and promote flow.

Saliva plays many important physiologic roles: Lubrication aids in swallowing, mechanical cleaning, and immunologic defense; digestion is aided by emulsification of food and enzymatic cleavage of some starches by alpha-amylase; some hormones are produced; antibodies, blood group–reacting substances, iodine, and viruses are actively secreted; and taste is mediated by delivery of chemicals to the taste buds.[5] Therefore, the patient with xerostomia is subject to stresses on the tissues in the oral cavity and oral pharynx, leading to dysfunction of speech, chewing, swallowing, taste, and digestion, as well as possible systemic processes.

Saliva contains inorganic electrolytes, organic compounds (urea, ammonia, uric acid, glucose, cholesterol, fatty acids, amino acids, and proteins), and polypeptides (nerve growth factor, epidermal growth factor, kallikrein, renin, and possibly erythropoietin, glucagon, angiotensin II, mesodermal growth factor,

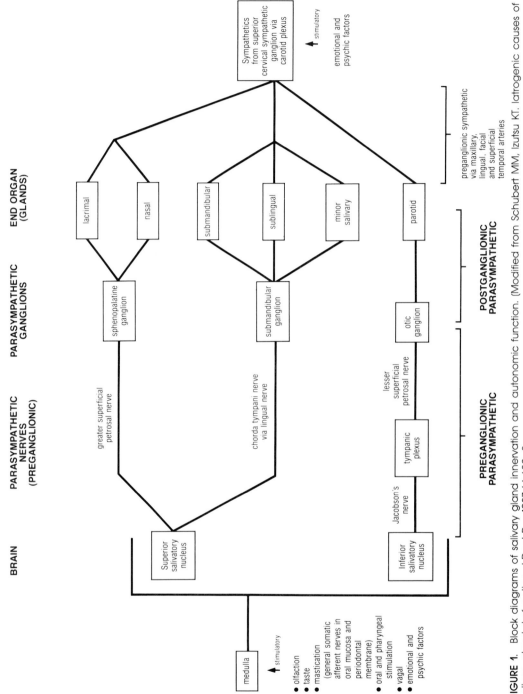

FIGURE 1. Block diagrams of salivary gland innervation and autonomic function. (Modified from Schubert MM, Izutsu KT. Iatrogenic causes of salivary gland dysfunction. J Dent Res 1987;66:680–8.

lymphoid factors, somatostatin, and gastrin, as well as others).[5] Some of these probably serve undiscovered functions; others may be an ultrafiltrate of serum.

There is some controversy as to factors that affect salivary flow in normal healthy subjects. Dawes[6] compiled information from many authors and concluded that the following factors affect normal salivary flow:

1. *Hydration.* When body water content was reduced by 8 per cent, salivary flow decreased virtually to zero.

2. *Body position.* Flow was higher and lower with standing and lying, respectively.

3. *Exposure to light.* There was greater flow in light.

4. *Smoking.* There was increased flow in smokers.

5. *Olfaction.* Flow increased with subjection to stimulation.

6. *Circadian rhythm.* There was greater flow in the afternoon and virtually none during sleep.

7. *Circannual rhythm.* There was greater flow in the winter months.

8. *Drugs.*

Factors that did not affect flow were: gender, age, body weight, gland size, and strangely, psychic factors.

Because xerostomia is not a recognized illness per se but rather a sign or symptom, its prevalence may be underestimated. Xerostomia is found primarily in the elderly. Osterberg et al. studied 1148 individuals over the age of 70 years and found that up to 16 per cent of men and 25 per cent of women had a dry mouth. Gilliland et al. surmised that because half of patients with rheumatoid arthritis suffer from xerostomia and that 0.15 to 3.8 per cent of the population of the United States carries the diagnosis of rheumatoid arthritis, between 0.5 and 4 million people suffer from dry mouth.[7] In a study of a normal population presenting to a family health clinic, Sreebny and Valdini found that 29 per cent had a dry mouth.[8]

It is difficult to set physiologic parameters that define xerostomia because it is the subjective feeling of oral dryness. This feeling, however, is almost always accompanied by a severe reduction in the secretion of unstimulated saliva. In the study of dental students given atropine and other anticholinergic drugs, Dawes found that the perception of dryness was reported when unstimulated salivary flow

had fallen to 40 to 50 per cent of the value after placebo consumption.[6] Because the perception of moisture in the mouth is dependent on the neural mechanisms of secretion including higher cortical function, mucosal and glandular integrity, and the quality as well as quantity of saliva, xerostomia could be the initial complaint of a patient with a variety of local or systemic disorders.[9]

The most common causes of xerostomia are drugs that inhibit the flow of saliva, systemic or local autoimmune processes, and irradiation damage to the salivary glandular tissue.

There are over 400 drugs that possess the ability to inhibit salivary flow (see Tables 1 and 2). In 1983, the National Center for Health Statistics reported on the frequency of drugs prescribed, and 4 of the top 20 were xerogenic. Furthermore, of the most frequently taken drugs with a xerogenic side effect, half of them are mood altering.[12] In a study by Sreebny et al., 60 per cent of patients who reported a dry mouth were taking xerogenic drugs.[13] In a study of the geriatric population in a nursing home, Handelman et al. found that there was a statistical significance in the use of hyposalivatory drugs by level of health care and age: Patients in a health-related facility rather than a skilled-care facility and older patients received more. This might indicate that xerostomia attributed to age may in fact be from medication.[12]

Systemic or local autoimmune diseases can cause xerostomia, the most common of which is Sjögren's syndrome.[14] The primary form, or sicca syndrome, is characterized by xerosto-

TABLE 1. The 15 Most Frequently Prescribed Drugs with a Xerogenic Effect*

Amitriptyline (Elavil)
Ibuprofen (Motrin, Advil, Rufen, Nuprin, and others)
Thioridazine (Mellaril)
Diphenhydramine (Benadryl)
Trifluoperazine (Stelazine)
Doxepin (Sinequan, Adapin)
Methyldopa (Aldomet)
Diazepam (Valium)
Sulindac (Clinoril)
Oxazepam (Serax)
Flurazepam (Dalmane)
Carbidopa-levodopa (Sinemet)
Propoxyphene napsylate with aspirin or acetaminophen (Darvon-N, 100; Darvocet-N, 50, 100)
Chlordiazepoxide (Librium)
Temazepam (Restoril)

* (Data from Handelman SL, Baric JM, Espeland MA, Berglund KL. Prevalence of drugs causing hyposalivation in an institutionalized geriatric population. Oral Surg 1986;62:26–31.)

TABLE 2. Xerogenic Drugs*

General, by mode of action
 Parasympatholytics
  Examples—atropine, scopolamine, propantheline,
   dicyclomine, phenothiazines, belladonna, amitrip-
   tyline, maprotiline, chlorpromazine, clonidine,
   biperiden, disopyramide, clidinium
 Sympathomimetics
  Examples—norepinephrine, synephrine, epineph-
   rine, ephedrine, amphetamine, isoproterenol,
   terbutaline
 Central nervous system inhibitors
  Examples—general anesthetics, benzodiazepines,
   diphenhydramine, levodopa
Specific, by therapeutic indication
 Analgesics
 Anticonvulsants
 Antiemetics
 Antihistamines
 Antihypertensives
 Antinauseants
 Anti-parkinson's agents
 Antipruritics
 Antineoplastic agents
 Antispasmodics
 Anxiolitics
 Appetite suppressants
 Cardiac antiarrhythmics
 Cold medicines
 Diuretics
 Decongestants
 Expectorants
 Muscle relaxants
 Psychotropic drugs
  Central nervous system depressants
  Dibenzazepine derivatives
  Phenothiazine derivatives
  Monoamine oxidase inhibitors
  Tranquilizers
  Sedatives

* Compiled from references 4, 10, 11.

TABLE 3. Systemic Factors and Illnesses Causing Xerostomia

In normals
 Hydration
 Body position
 Olfaction
 Light exposure
 Circadian rhythm
 Circannual rhythm
 Age (?)
Central
 Psychiatric disorders/psychogenic factors
 Increased sympathetic tone
 Brain tumor
 Encephalitis
 Status postneurosurgical operation
 Diabetes insipidus
 Drugs
Peripheral
 Collagen vascular disease
  Rheumatoid arthritis
  Sarcoidosis
  Autoimmune hemolytic anemia
  Systemic lupus erythematosus
  Scleroderma
  Raynaud's disease
  Polymyositis/dermatomyositis
  Sjögren's syndrome
  Sicca syndrome
 Drugs
 Irradiation
 Chemotherapy
 Trauma/physical damage
 Salivary gland aplasia
 Salivary gland duct calculi
 Salivary gland inflammation
 Salivary gland tumors
 Systemic inflammatory
  Tuberculosis
  Syphilis
  Sarcoid
  Heerfordt's disease (uveoparotid fever)
 Graft versus host disease
 Primary biliary cirrhosis
 Hyposecretory states
  Atrophic gastritis
  Pancreatic insufficiency
  Sicca syndrome
  Cystic fibrosis
 Type V hyperlipoproteinemia
 Vitamin deficiency
 Nasal obstruction/mouth breathing
 Pernicious anemia
 Plummer-Vinson syndrome
 Electrolyte problems
  Dehydration
  Uremia
  Diabetes insipidus
  Cardiac failure

mia and xerophthalmia. The secondary form is the sicca syndrome along with a systemic autoimmune process, most commonly rheumatoid arthritis (but can include systemic lupus erythematosus, scleroderma, Raynaud's disease, polymyositis/dermatomyositis, sarcoidosis). The salivary gland histopathology in Sjögren's syndrome is referred to as the lymphoepithelial lesion and is characterized by reticular cell proliferation, ductal hyperplasia, and replacement of acini by lymphoid tissue.[7]

It has been shown that the patient with Sjögren's syndrome is more likely to develop a lymphoproliferative malignancy. This progression, however, usually takes years to develop. The patient with Sjögren's should be carefully monitored for parotid swelling, lymphadenopathy, and splenomegaly because these symptoms carry with them a greater risk of progression to lymphoma.[15]

A systemic autoimmune process is thought to affect the salivary glands as it might other exocrine glands in the body by tissue destruction from the chronic inflammatory cells. Therefore, xerostomia may be associated with other hyposecretory states such as atrophic gastritis and pancreatic insufficiency. This is also the basis for the supposition that systemic treatment with anti-inflammatory agents may effect a cure.

Xerostomia during irradiation therapy is seen early in the course, owing to local inflammation. The permanent hyposalivatory effect is caused by disorganization and destruction of acinar cells, with preservation of the ductal cells, the mechanism of which is thought to be due to the action of free radicals on cellular metabolism. The glands' radiation sensitivity decreases, in order, from parotid to submandibular/sublingual to minor, with serous cells being affected more than mucous cells. Studies have shown a 76 per cent decrease in stimulated flow and a 95 per cent decrease in unstimulated flow, which indicates the ability of the irradiated gland to respond, at least partially, to strong stimuli.[4,7]

There are other, less common causes of xerostomia. Studies have shown that chemotherapeutic agents cause ductal dilation and acinar degeneration in up to 50 per cent of patients.[4] Psychogenic factors such as threat and fear, hypnotism, transcendental meditation, mental stress, various personality traits, and depression can cause xerostomia. Decreased mastication with loss of general somatic afferent nerve stimulation (from nerves located in the periodontal membrane and oral mucosa) produces salivary gland atrophy. This problem occurs in patients fed a liquid or powdered diet. Anatomic factors such as salivary gland aplasia, ductal blockage by calculi, infection, and tumors all can cause xerostomia.[14] A more extensive list of causes of xerostomia is found in Table 3.

HISTORY

The patient may or may not present with xerostomia as the chief complaint. Therefore, in the general medical history, a question about dry mouth should be asked. The time course, degree of disability, associated symptoms, exacerbating factors, and modes of treatment are ascertained to better understand the problem. A list of the patient's current medications, both prescription and over-the-counter, is obtained. Prior surgery or irradiation therapy and habits such as smoking and coffee and alcohol consumption are important factors.

Pointed questions to focus on xerostomia should include degree of dryness and associated disability such as difficulty eating, swallowing, or even speaking. A decrease in food enjoyment with ageusia or even dysgeusia is common. Mastication is made difficult, especially with dry foods such as crackers. Swallowing is a problem, and the patient might note increased fluid consumption at meals or "washing one's food down." An increase in fluid intake at night is often manifested by the patient's keeping a glass of water at the bedside.

The patient's subjective feeling of oral dryness may manifest itself as smarting, burning, or soreness, especially on the tongue. There may be painful ulceration in the oral cavity and signs of increased dental caries. The patient may complain of difficulty with dental appliances, such as trouble getting dentures to secure properly or irritation or frank ulceration beneath a seemingly well-fitting appliance.

In a study by Sreebny and Valdini, the most common symptoms associated with oral dryness (seen in 48 per cent of the patients) were: the need to do something to keep the mouth moist, the need to get out of bed at night to drink water, and difficulty with speech articulation. Less common (seen in 13 to 30 per cent of patients) were: the need to keep fluids at the bedside, problems with taste, difficulties with chewing dry foods, burning and tingling sensations on the tongue, the presence of cracks or fissures at the angle of the lips, and difficulty in swallowing.[8]

Fox et al. studied the correlation of subjective symptoms with objective measurements of salivary flow and found that the following symptoms did not correlate with decreased flow: dryness at night or on awakening, daytime dryness, keeping a glass of water at the bedside, and chewing gum or candy. Symptoms that did correlate with decreased salivary flow included: dryness while eating a meal, difficulty swallowing, and the need to sip while swallowing. They concluded that these findings revealed that the greatest disability was present when there was a loss of salivary flow at times of maximal stimulation. This is indicative of extensive glandular dysfunction and is more serious than an alteration in unstimulated output.[15]

Xerostomia is often associated with dryness in other areas of the body, revealing dysfunction of the lacrimal, respiratory, alimentary, or vaginal mucous glands. Sreebny et al. showed that ocular dryness, blurred vision, throat and nasal dryness, and vaginal itching

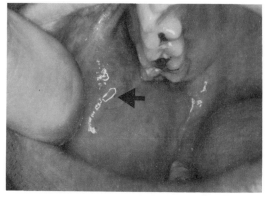

FIGURE 2. The papilla and opening to the parotid (Stensen's) duct are demonstrated by the *arrow*. Clear saliva may be expressed from the duct by massaging the gland. The duct may be cannulated to inject contrast media for sialography.

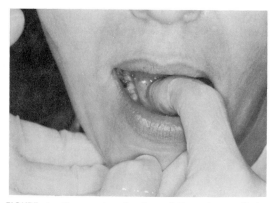

FIGURE 4. Bimanual palpation of the submandibular gland. The submandibular glands and ducts are best palpated by placing one hand under the chin and a finger in the mouth. Structures are rolled between the palpating fingers for the most sensitive evaluation.

were more prevalent in xerostomic individuals.[13] (Also see chapter on Dry Eye.)

PHYSICAL EXAMINATION

As with any new patient, a complete physical examination is warranted. This is especially true with the xerostomic patient because the cause of the problem can be any number of systemic disease processes, and these need to be ruled out.

Obviously, the oral examination will be the most revealing, and one should always be systematic in examination to avoid overlooking subtle signs. Begin in one anatomic area—for instance, the lips—and systematically move through the remainder of the examination.

The lips may show fissuring with angular cheilitis. Evert the lips and dry the buccal mucosa, watching for the normal production of mucinous saliva. The mucosa may be pale and dry owing to epithelial atrophy and the loss of mucous coating. A wooden tongue depressor tends to stick to mucosa with scant viscid saliva. The mucous membrane may be erythematous from local irritation and inflammation.

Stensen's duct, adjacent to the second maxillary molar, may be erythematous and swollen. One can dry the orifice and watch for serous salivary flow (Fig. 2). Also look for flow from Wharton's duct, which lies on the floor of the mouth on either side of the frenulum of the tongue (Fig. 3). Express saliva by posterior to anterior massage across the parotid or submandibular gland. A voluntary yawn frequently expresses submandibular saliva. Crystal-clear saliva is expressed from normal glands. The glands themselves may feel swollen, firm, or tender. Pain on palpation indicates acute or chronic inflammation (Fig. 4).

The tongue may have fissuring and coating on its dorsum. There is an absence of keratin at the edges owing to wear from lack of protection. The filiform papillae along the dorsum may be atrophied.

Xerostomia causes an unusual pattern of dental caries, which develop at the zone of gingiva-tooth contact. In fact, root surface caries and cavities forming around the necks of teeth may be pathognomonic. This is due to alterations in the oral microbial ecology: Absence of saliva in turn means a decrease in dissolved oxygen to the tooth surface, with a concomitant increase in the proportion of anaerobes.[14]

Tests for the ability to taste are difficult because taste is a subjective sign, and it is inti-

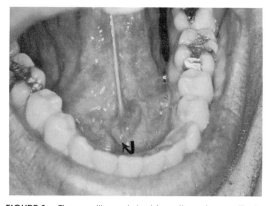

FIGURE 3. The papilla and duct from the submandibular gland. Stones may be palpated within the duct. The duct may be cannulated for sialography.

mately associated with olfaction. Altered taste is due to loss of the dissolution and presentation of food by the saliva as well as from damage to the taste buds themselves, but it is not specific for decreased salivation.

Associated signs include dryness of other exocrine glands such as the lacrimal, alimentary, and respiratory tracts and the mucous glands of the vagina.[7] Ophthalmologic examination of the patient with Sjögren's syndrome reveals keratoconjunctivitis sicca.

DIAGNOSTIC STUDIES

The symptoms of xerostomia are subjective; therefore, salivary gland hypofunction should be confirmed with objective measurement of decreased salivary flow. There are many laboratory and office tests that may be of help—the availability and feasibility of performing the test will depend on the type and location of the practice. The diagnostic test of primary importance is the physical examination; all other tests should be a confirmation of that information.

Sialometry

Sialometry is the measure of salivary flow and can be performed in the office. In one modification of the test, the patient is asked to collect and expectorate accumulated secretions for six minutes. However, one must remember that whole saliva also includes food debris, bacterial products, and desquamated cells. To obtain a more accurate appraisal of gland secretion, parotid saliva can be collected with a modified Carlson-Crittenden cup and submandibular/sublingual saliva with a 100-μL pipette.[9] Alternatively, cannulation of the ducts is an excellent method of obtaining saliva, and it is easily quantitated. Following passive collection (unstimulated flow), the glands are stimulated with paraffin or citric acid, and saliva is collected (stimulated flow).

Unstimulated salivary flow is normally 0.3 to 0.5 ml per minute. Stimulated flow rate is normally 1 to 2 ml per minute. In a study by Sreebny and Valdini,[8] mean flow rates for unstimulated and stimulated secretion in xerostomic patients were, respectively, one third and one half of the flow rates in normals. They concluded that the subjective feeling of oral dryness is associated with a marked decrease in the rate of flow. Others have surmised that

low flow rates are rare unless there is massive (60 to 70 per cent) salivary gland impairment.[7]

Salivary Scintigraphy

Salivary scintigraphy is an indicator of salivary function and is generally available in any radiology department. Technetium pertechnetate is a radioactive, gamma-emitting, nonallergenic salt with a six-hour half-life. After intravenous injection, it is actively taken up by the salivary glands, concentrated, and then excreted into the saliva. There are two phases seen in the test—the uptake, or vascular phase, and the excretory phase—which allows differentiation in abnormalities of uptake and secretion. Fox et al.[9] found, in patients undergoing irradiation therapy, that after 4000 to 6000 rads there is decreased uptake due to destruction and fibrosis of the vasculature. In contrast, after 1000 to 3000 rads, there is increased uptake secondary to acute inflammation.

Sialography

Sialography is the radiographic imaging of the salivary gland duct system. It involves the intraoral cannulation of the ducts and retrograde injection of radiopaque material. Mechanical blockage is readily revealed. In the Sjögren's syndrome patient, one may see punctate sialectasis. Because sialography is difficult to perform and invasive in nature, it is of little benefit in the xerostomic patient.

Labial Biopsy of Minor Salivary Glands

Labial biopsy of minor salivary glands is the single most useful diagnostic test for the clinician. Histopathologic findings in the minor salivary glands correlate well with those seen in the major glands because they suffer from the same infiltration of inflammatory cells. The minor salivary glands of the lower lip are readily accessible beneath the mucous membrane and a thin layer of connective tissue but above the muscle layer (Fig. 5). The lower lip is everted and local anesthetic infiltrated. An ellipse of mucosa with the underlying tissue down to the muscle layer is removed and sent to the pathologist. The mucosa is then closed primarily with an absorbable suture.

On histologic section, there is marked infiltration with lymphocytes and histiocytes. There may be periductal or acinar invasion or

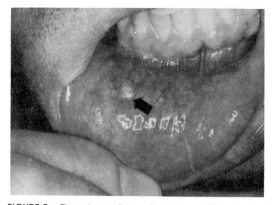

FIGURE 5. The minor salivary glands are easily palpated just under the mucosa of the lower lip. Glands are removed for biopsy by making an incision over a gland and excising it with scissors and grasping forceps.

replacement. There also may be formation of "epimyothelial islands," which are conglomerates of hyperplastic ductal epithelial cells surrounded by lymphocytes.[15]

Sialochemistry

Sialochemistry is the analysis of the components of saliva. It is not generally available. Salivary IgA is elevated in xerostomic patients. It has also been shown that there is an elevated sodium and potassium concentration in whole unstimulated saliva of patients with Sjögren's syndrome.[15]

Xerostomia may be seen alone but is often associated with either the sicca syndrome or a generalized autoimmune disorder. Therefore, tests for associated signs and symptoms should be performed.

The Schirmer test is a simple office evaluation of lacrimal secretion. It involves the placement of a strip of filter paper in the lower fornix of the conjunctival sac and measuring the extent of wetting. The sum of the lengths of wetted filter paper for both eyes of less than 25 mm is considered pathologic. A slit lamp examination after application of a rose bengal or fluoroscein stain that shows filamentary keratitis is diagnostic of keratoconjunctivitis sicca.[16]

Systemic autoimmune disease should be evaluated with hematologic testing. There are several serologic markers of autoimmune disease including: rheumatoid factor (positive), antinuclear antibodies (positive), erythrocyte sedimentation rate (elevated), serum immunoglobulins (polyclonal hyperglobulinemia), and specific extractable nuclear anti-

gens, such as SS-A [Ro] and SS-B [La] (present in the majority of patients with primary Sjögren's). If these are positive, further studies include serum and urine immunoelectrophoresis, serum anti-DNA (deoxyribonucleic acid) binding, and HLA haplotyping.[9,15] In patients with Sjögren's syndrome, a decrease in serum IgM usually heralds progression to malignant disease.[16]

ASSESSMENT

Xerostomia is a symptom complex that the patient may or may not present as the chief complaint. It is most frequently an iatrogenic problem, caused by the prescription of xerogenic medication for nonassociated medical problems. It may also be seen frequently as a postirradiation complication. Less common, but nonetheless very important, xerostomia may be the initial presentation of a patient with a serious systemic autoimmune process and should be investigated until the cause is found. Labeling xerostomia as idiopathic should be condemned and reserved only for that situation in which the cause has meticulously been sought but remains elusive.

Xerostomia may be underdiagnosed because of lack of physician (or patient) concern, but it is a problem that significantly affects the patient's quality of life, causing

TABLE 4. Treatment of Xerostomia

Gland stimulable
  Seek to stimulate remaining gland activity
    Gustatory stimulants (e.g., citric acid, sour candy)
    Mechanical stimulants (e.g., frequent chewing/meals)
    Drugs (e.g., pilocarpine [cholinergic])
Gland not stimulable
  Topical/symptomatic treatment
    Saliva substitutes (e.g., carboxymethylcellulose, hydroxymethylcellulose, water, glycerin, mineral oil, mucin)
Alter drug therapy
  Stop the drug
  Change the drug
  Alter the dosing schedule
Treat the autoimmune disorder
  Anti-inflammatory drugs
Correct the anatomic abnormality
  Remove the stone
  Treat the inflammation
  Treat the nasal obstruction
Oral hygiene
  Sodium fluoride/stannous fluoride
  Dentist
Palliative
  Avoid dry foods, alcohol, coffee, tobacco

problems of speech, taste, swallowing, digestion of food, and loss of teeth. While not thought of as a life-threatening problem, xerostomia may be the initial complaint of a patient with Sjögren's syndrome, a disease known to impart a greater risk of lymphoproliferative malignancy.

The diagnosis is clinical and can be inferred from the history. The subjective feeling of oral dryness is present, with a severe reduction in salivary flow, and indicates a significant injury to the glands themselves. The physical examination is important in verifying the patient's symptoms, and the diagnostic tests are used mainly as an adjunct. The laboratory tests of consequence are those used to rule out a serious systemic autoimmune process.

The treatment of xerostomia can be categorized into two groupings: (1) topical or symptomatic treatment and (2) systemic. The systemic treatment can be further broken down into those methods that seek to stimulate remaining gland activity and those that attempt to treat an underlying systemic illness (see Table 4). Xerostomia is a difficult problem to treat because of the poor correlation between the subjective complaint and objective measure of actual gland function.[17]

REFERENCES

1. Garrett JR. Changing attitudes on salivary secretion—a short history on spit. Proc R Soc Med 1975;68:553–60.
2. Rankow R, Polayes I. Diseases of the salivary glands. Philadelphia: WB Saunders Co, 1976:1.
3. Graney DO. Anatomy. In: Cummings CW, Frederickson JM, Harker LA, Krause CJ, Schuller DE, eds. Otolaryngology—head and neck surgery. St. Louis: CV Mosby Co, 1986:961–8.
4. Schubert MM, Izutsu KT. Iatrogenic causes of salivary gland dysfunction. J Dent Res 1987;66:680–8.
5. Batsakis JG. Physiology. In: Cummings CW, Fredrickson JM, Harker LA, Krause CJ, Schuller DE, eds. Otolaryngology—head and neck surgery. St. Louis: CV Mosby Co, 1986:969–79.
6. Dawes C. Physiological factors affecting salivary flow rate, oral sugar clearance, and sensation of dry mouth in man. J Dent Res 1987;66:648–53.
7. Sreebny LM, Valdini A. Xerostomia—a neglected symptom. Arch Intern Med 1987;147:1333–7.
8. Sreebny LM, Valdini A. Xerostomia. Part I: relationship to other oral symptoms and salivary gland hypofunction. Oral Surg 1988;66:451–8.
9. Fox PC, Weiffenbach JM, van der Ven PF, Baum BJ, Sonies BC. Xerostomia: evaluation of a symptom with increasing significance. J Am Dent Assoc 1985;110:519–25.
10. Rice DH. Salivary gland physiology. In: Work WP, Johns ME, eds. Salivary gland diseases. The Otolaryngologic Clinics of North America. Philadelphia: WB Saunders Co, 1977;10(2):273–85.
11. Treatment of xerostomia. Med Lett Drugs Ther 1988;30:74–6.
12. Handelman SL, Baric JM, Espeland MA, Berglund KL. Prevalence of drugs causing hyposalivation in an institutionalized geriatric population. Oral Surg 1986;62:26–31.
13. Sreebny LM, Valdini A, Yu A. Xerostomia. Part II: relationship to nonoral symptoms, drugs, and diseases. Oral Surg 1989;68:419–27.
14. Navazesh M, Ship II. Xerostomia: diagnosis and treatment. Am J Otolaryngol 1983;4:283–92.
15. Fox PC, Busch KA, Baum BJ. Subjective reports of xerostomia and objective reports of salivary gland performance. Am Dent Assoc 1987;115:581–4.
16. Glass BJ, Van Dis ML, Langlais RP, Miles DA. Xerostomia: diagnosis and treatment planning considerations. Oral Surg 1984;58:248–52.
17. Fox PC. Systemic therapy of salivary gland hypofunction. J Dent Res 1987;66:689–92.

INDEX

Page numbers in *italics* refer to illustrations; page numbers followed by t refer to tables.

Abscess formation, in upper airway obstruction, 437–438
Abdominal pain, chylomicronemia and, 227
    ectopic pregnancy and, 145, 146
    fever associated with, 163
    ovarian cysts and, 334
Abdominal pain, chronic, 1–6
    assessment of, 5–6
    causes of, 2t
    definition of, 1
    diagnostic studies in, 4–5
    diverticulitis and, 6
    epigastric pain and, 5–6
    fiber endoscopy in diagnosis of, 5
    history in, 1–3
    implications of, 6
    irritable bowel syndrome (IBS) and, 6
    lower, 6
    physical examination and, 3–4
    in right upper quadrant (RUQ), 6
Abdominal ultrasound, cholestasis assessment using, 89
Abetalipoproteinemia, ataxia associated with, 39
    steatorrhea in, 435
Abortion, β-hCG levels in, 340
Absence seizures, 412, 417
    evaluation of, 414
Abstinence syndrome, hallucinations in drug withdrawal, 174, 177
Abuse, substance, tachyarrhythmia associated with, 455
Acanthocytosis, ataxia associated with, 39
Acanthosis nigricans, 236, 312
    abdominal pain associated with, 3
Acidosis, azotemia associated with, 49
    renal tubular, hyperuricemia associated with, 245
    tachypnea associated with, 464
    uric acid underexcretion associated with, 243
Acoustic neuroma, 182, 184
Acquired immune deficiency syndrome (AIDS). See also *Human immunodeficiency virus (HIV) infection.*
    anorexia associated with, 17
    anxiety associated with, 33
    cough associated with, 113
    diarrhea associated with, 120
    intracranial infection associated with, 284
    PGL as sign of progression of HIV infection in, 299
    referral to NIH AIDS Clinical Trial Group, 222
    risk of progression to, in HIV-positive males, 219t
Acrocyanosis, Raynaud's phenomenon versus, 390
Acromegaly, acanthosis nigricans and, 236
    hyperpigmentation in, 237t

Acro-osteolysis, pseudoclubbing associated with, 95
Acuity, central, evaluation of, 493
Acute necrotizing ulcerative gingivitis (ANUG), oral ulcers associated with, 321
Acute tubular necrosis (ATN), 46
Addison's disease, acanthosis nigricans and, 236
    anorexia associated with, 17
    hyperpigmentation in, 237t
Adenoma, adrenal, secondary hypertension and, 410
Adenopathy, liver disease associated with, 119–200
Adenosine diphosphate (ADP), metabolism of, 243
Adenosine triphosphatase (ATP), activity of, cholestasis and, 87
Adiposogenital dystrophy, idiopathic, weight gain in, 502
Adjustment disorder, anxious mood associated with, 35–36
    insomnia associated with, 266
Adnexal mass, pelvic, 337–338
Adolescents, anorexia in, 20
    causes of, 17t
Adrenal adenoma, secondary hypertension and, 410
Adrenal cortical carcinoma, secondary hypertension and, 410
Adrenal gland, anxiety, and pathology of, 32
    hyperplasia of, and secondary hypertension, 410
    obesity and, 503, 505
Adrenergic response, in hypoglycemia, 249, 253
Adrenocorticotropic hormone (ACTH), androgen secretion and, 312
    ectopic production of, 303
    West's syndrome treatment with, 417
Adults, anorexia in, causes of, 17t
    blisters in, causes of, 482t
    urinary protein values in, 380t
Aerophagia, 276–277, 279
Affective disturbance, hypersomnia and, 429
Afferent papillary defect (RAPD), relative, 494, 498
Agammaglobulinemia, mediastinal mass associated with, 303
Age-related macular degeneration (ARMD), 495
Aging process, ANA positive titer and, 23
    and androgen levels, 313
    and bone pain, changing causes of, 53t
    and breast mass, assessment of, 69–70
    and cataract development, 495
    and dysuria, 140
    and IPF incidence, 268
    and oral ulcers, 321
    and pelvic mass
    changing causes of, 355
        etiology of, 334
    and phantogeusia, 353
    and scrotal pain, changing causes of, 396
    and seizures, 412t
    and tachyarrhythmia prevalence, 454

Aging process (*continued*)
    and thyroid cancer likelihood, 471
    and uric acid level, 239
    and xerostomia, 509
    dyslipidemia evaluation in older adults, 231
    polyps and cancer increase during, 193
Agoraphobia, 29
    anxiety associated with, 35
AIDS. See *Acquired immune deficiency syndrome*
    (AIDS); Human immunodeficiency virus (HIV)
    infection.
Air Force School of Aerospace Medicine study (coronary artery disease), 421
Airway obstruction, upper, causes of, 437t
Airway wall, normal and obstructed, *439*
Alanine aminotransferase (ALT), hepatomegaly evaluation and, 201
Albumin, 379
Albuminuria. See also *Proteinuria.*
  in diabetic nephropathy, 382
Alcohol consumption, abdominal pain and, 3
    ataxia associated with, 39
    blackout following, 14
    breast cancer risk and, 68
    diarrhea and, 119
    hallucinations associated with, 174
    hepatitis and, hepatomegaly associated with, 199
    hepatomegaly associated with, 199, 202
    hypertriglyceridemia exacerbated by, 230
    hyperuricemia associated with, 243
    hypomagnesemia caused by, 258, 259
    insomnia and, 264
    polycythemia and, 373
    sleep disturbance and, 427
    tachyarrhythmia associated with, 455
    thiamine deficiency and, 12
Aldosteronism, primary, diagnostic assessment of, *409*
    secondary hypertension and, 410
Aliageusia, 354
    versus phantogeusia, 349
Alkaline phosphatase, cholestasis and, 86
    elevated levels of, drug-induced, 88t
        evaluation of, 89t
    hepatomegaly and, 201
    hyperuricemia associated with, 245
    polyarticular arthritis and, 367
    polycythemia and, 374
Alkalosis, primary aldosteronism and, 410
    tachypnea associated with, 464
Allergens, dyspareunia caused by, 132
Allergic conjunctivitis, 127
Allergic contact dermatitis, 489, *489*
Allergic keratoconjunctivitis, symptoms, 124t
Alpha-1-antitrypsin, hepatomegaly associated with deficiency of, 198, 200
    intestinal clearance of, and protein-losing enteropathy, 435
Alpha-fetoprotein (AFP), and scrotal pain, evaluation of, 397
    tumor marker, 338
Alström's syndrome, weight gain in, 502
Alveolar cell carcinoma, cough in, 112
Alveolitis, 268. See also *Interstitial pulmonary disease.*
Alzheimer's disease, amnesia in, 15
Amaurosis fugax (AF), 478
Amazia, 68
Amenorrhea, 309, 340
    anorexia-related, 18
    obesity associated with, 505
    secondary, pelvic mass and, 335

Aminotransferase, cholestasis and, 88
Amiodarone, hyperpigmentation induced by, 238t
Amnesia, 7–15
    alcoholic blackout and, 14
    anterograde, 11
        Korsakoff psychosis and, 13
    assessment of, 8
    cerebral concussion and, 10–11
    cerebrovascular disease and, 14–15
    chylomicronemia and, 227
    definition of, 8
    dementia and, 7, 15
    electroconvulsive therapy and, 14
    infection and, 15
    memory and, 7
    mental status examination and, 7–8
    post-traumatic, 11
    psychogenic, 15
    retrograde, 9, 10–11
        Korsakoff psychosis and, 13
    recovery after infection, 15
    seizure-related, 413
    situational, 15
    thiamine deficiency and, 13
    transient global (TGA), 8–10, 478
    vertebrobasilar insufficiency and, 9
    Wernicke-Korsakoff syndrome and, 11–14
Amphetaminelike drugs, athetosis caused by, 43
Amphetamines, hallucinations associated with, 174
Ampullary ectopic pregnancy, *149*
Amylase serum levels, and azotemia, 49
    and cholestasis, 88
Amyloidosis, larynx and trachea involvement, 214
    steatorrhea with, 435
Anabolic steroids, liver disease risk and, 198
Anaerobic fermentation, hydrogen and methane produced by, 274
Anaphylaxis, food-allergy related, 168t
    on oral challenge, 170
Androgen insensitivity, amenorrhea associated with, 313
Androgenic disorders, 311–313
Anemia, aplastic, mediastinal mass associated with, 303
    azotemia associated with, 49
    bone pain associated with, 56
    fatigue associated with, 157
    intestinal bloating associated with, 278
    iron deficiency, interstitial pulmonary disease and, 273
    lecithin:cholesterol acyltransferase deficiency and, 227
    Sjögren's syndrome and, 127
    systolic murmurs associated with, 446
Aneurysms, aortic, 401
    mediastinal mass in, 303
    mediastinal mass caused by, 301
    polyarteritis and, 362
Angina, Prinzmetal's, 73, 83
    stable, 421
        evaluation of, 423
    unstable, 76–77, 421
        evaluation of, 423
    walk-through, 76
Angina pectoris, 75–77
    and systolic murmurs, 445–446
    functional classification of, 76t
Angiofollicular lymph node hyperplasia, 301
Angiography, 407
    ataxia for evaluation of, 39
    chest pain evaluation using, 83
    coronary, chest pain assessment with, 85

Angiography (*continued*)
  hematochezia evaluation using, 192
  polyarteritis study using, 362
  pulmonary, chest pain assessment with, 85
  thoracic, for mediastinal mass evaluation, 303–304
Angiotensin-converting enzyme (ACE) inhibitors, cough associated with, 112
Anhedonia, 153
Ankylosing spondylitis (AS), 363
  anorexia associated with, 17
  bone pain associated with, 59
  myofascial pain versus, 318–319
Anorectal manometry, constipation assessment and, 108
Anorexia, 16–21
  assessment of, 20–21
  causes of, by age group, 17t
  diagnostic studies in, 19–20
  history in, 17–18
  liver disease and, 197
  physical examination and, 19
  prognostic implications of, 21
Anorexia nervosa, 17
  amenorrhea and, 310
Anosmia, 355
Anterior ischemic optical neuropathy (AION), 497, *497*
Anthrax, 294
Antiarrhythmics, anorexia as side effect, 18
Antibiotic therapy, empirical, for fever, 165–166, 165(t)
  erythema multiforme associated with, 486
Antibody assay(s), ANA, 22–28
  ELISA, 217–218, 220
  IgE, and diagnosis of food allergies, 169–179
  radioimmunoassay for C-peptide measurement, 255
  RAST, 169–170
  RIPA, 218
Antibody(ies), anticentromere (ACA), 4, 390
  antineutrophil cytoplasmic, polyarteritis and, 361
  antitopoismerase, scleroderma and, 390
  in cardiolipin syndrome, 24, 26–27
    FANA, percentage positive , 23
  thyroglobulin, Sjögren's syndrome and, 127
Anticentromere antibody (ACA), CREST syndrome and, 4
  scleroderma and, 390
Anticholergenic agents, renal clearance of uric acid by, 240
Anticoagulants, TIA evaluation with, 480
Anticonvulsants, athetosis caused by, 43
Antidepressants, hallucinations caused by, 174
Antifungal drugs, anorexia as a major side effect, 18
Antigen tests, intracranial infection evaluation and, 283, 285
  markers for narcolepsy and hypersomnia identified with, 429
Antigen, carcinoembryonic (CEA), as a tumor marker, 338
Antihypertensive drugs, anorexia as a side effect, 18
Antineutrophil cytoplasmic antibody, polyarteritis indicated by, 361
Antinuclear antibody (ANA), arthritis juvenile rheumatoid, and, 27–28
  rheumatoid, and, 27
  assessment of significance of, 28
  cardiolipin antibody syndrome and, 26–27
  diagnostic studies in, 25–28
  diseases associated with, nonrheumatic, 24t
  drugs inducing, 24t, 27
  FANA test for, 22–34
  history in, 23–25
  joint examination in, 25

Antinuclear antibody (ANA) (*continued*)
  physical examination and, 25
  polyarticular arthritis evaluation and, 367
  positive titer, 22–28
  rheumatic diseases associated with, 23t
  serologic tests for evaluation of, 26t
  systemic lupus erythematosus and, 26
Antipsychotic medications, highly sedating, 501t
  weight gain and, 501
Antitopoisomerase antibody, scleroderma and, 390
Antituberculin drugs, anorexia and, 18
Anxiety, 29–36
  adjustment disorder and, 35–36
  AIDS and HIV associated with, 33
  anorexia and, 20
  assessment of, 32–36
  definition of, 29–30
  diagnostic studies in, 32
  differential diagnosis of, 32t
  endocrine disorders and, 32
  existential, 30
  history in, 30–31
  insomnia associated with, 266
  intestinal bloating associated with, 278
  myofascial pain associated with, 316
  neoplastic disease and, 33
  obsessive-compulsive disorder and, 35
  phobias and, 34–35
  physical examination and, 31–32
  post-traumatic stress disorder and, 31–32, 35
  psychologic theories of, 30
  separation, 30
  somatic ailments associated with, 33t
  specific syndromes of, 34–36
Aorta, coarctation of, and systolic murmurs, 450
  hypertension and, 405
Aortic aneurysm, mediastinal mass in, 303
  rupture of, and scrotal pain, 401
Aortic dissection, chest pain associated with, 74–75, 77–78, 79
  excluding in thrombolytic therapy, 85
Aortic ejection murmurs, 450–451
Aortic stenosis, hemodynamically significant, 451
Aortitis, syphilitic, chest pain associated with, 75
Aortography, for chest pain evaluation, 83
Aphasia, post-traumatic amnesia associated with, 11
Aphthous ulcers, 321, 326
Aplastic anemia, mediastinal mass associated with, 303
Apolipoprotein deficiency, A-I and C-III, 227
  C-II, 230
Apoproteins, 224
  defective E, and hypercholesterolemia, 231
Apparitions. See *Hallucinations.*
Appendix epididymis, 393
  torsion of, with scrotal pain, 398
Appendix testis, 393
  torsion of, with scrotal pain, 398
Apraxia, post-traumatic amnesia associated with, 11
Argyria, hyperpigmentation in, 237t
Arnold-Chiari malformation, ataxia associated with, 37
Arrhythmia(s), hypomagnesemia-related, 259–260, 261
Arterial blood gases (ABGs), stridor evaluation with, 442
Arterial embolus, 389
Arterial pulse, systolic murmur evaluation, 447
Arterial stenosis, renal, progression of, 4
Arteriography, hepatic, hepatomegaly evaluation with, 201
  renal, 407
Arteriosclerosis, Raynaud's phenomenon and, 387

Arteritis, Takayasu's, 389
Artery disease, premature coronary, silent myocardial ischemia associated with, 422
Arthralgia, cardiolipin antibody syndrome and, 26
    connective tissue diseases and, 24
    versus arthritis, 363
Arthritis, axial psoriatic, diagnostic imaging for evaluation of, 368
    bone pain associated with, 58, 59
    connective tissue diseases and, 24
    gonococcal, 365, 369
    gouty, 246, 368
    infectious, 246
    juvenile rheumatoid arthritis (JRA), 23, 23(t), 27–28, 290
    limb pain associated with, 287, 289–290
    Lyme disease and, 369
    lymphadenopathy and, 296
    night pain in, 55
    oligoarticular reactive, HIV-related, 365
    osteoarthritis (OA), 319, 363
        diagnostic imaging to evaluate, 368
        polyarthritis in, 369
    polyarticular, 363–371
        diagnostic assessment of, *370*
    psoriatic, 368
    pyogenic, 369
    rheumatoid (RA), 214, 363
        ANA positive test in, 27
        diagnostic imaging to evaluate, 368
        FANA and, percent positives with, 23t
        lymphadenopathy in, 294
        polyarthritis in, 369
        proteinuria associated with, 383
        psoriatic arthritis versus, 368
        Sjögren's syndrome associated with, 124
    septic, bone pain associated with, 58
Arthrocentesis, 246
Arthropathy, crystal-induced, 371
Arthroscopy, 368
Asbestos/asbestosis, environmental exposure, and pulmonary fibrosis, 268
    interstitial pulmonary disease associated with, 272
Ascites, cardiac failure and, 101
Asherman's syndrome, and amenorrhea, 313
Aspartate aminotransferase (AST), and hepatomegaly, evaluation of, 201
Asphyxia, athetosis due to, 42
Aspirin, hematochezia caused by, 189
    inhibition of uric acid transport by, 241
Asthma, cardiac, 100, 112
    cough associated with, 111
    occupational, 115
Ataxia, 36–40
    and Wernicke encephalopathy characterized by, 12
        recovery time in, 13–14
    assessment of, 40
    definition of, 36
    diagnostic studies in, 39–40
    hemispheric lesions and, 40
    history in, 37
    hypomagnesemia and, 259
    midline lesions and, 40
    neurologic examination and, 38–39
    optic, 36–37
        atrophy associated with, 38
    physical examination and, 37–39
    sensory, 36
Ataxiatelangiectasia, 39

Atherosclerosis, dyslipidemias and, 231
    high-density lipoprotein (HDL) and, 223
    hypertension and, 405
    premature, 228
Athetosis, 41–45
    assessment of, 45
    characteristics of, 42t
    definition of, 41–42
    diagnostic studies in, 44–45
    drug-caused, 43
    history in, 43–44
    metabolic disorders as causes of, 43
    movement disorders compared with, 42t
    movement-induced reflex epilepsy (MIRE) and, 45
    neurometabolic disorders and, 42–43
    paroxysmal dyskinesias, genetically caused, 43
    physical examination and, 44
Atrial fibrillation, 455–456, 458
    TIA caused by, 479
Atrial flutter, 457–458
    ventricular response during, *459*
Atrial tachycardia, carotid sinus massage effect on, *457*
    with AV block, *458*
Atrioventricular (AV) nodal re-entrant tachycardia, 453
Atrioventricular block, *64*
Atrioventricular reciprocating tachycardia, and Wolff-Parkinson-White syndrome, 453–454
Atrophy, dyspareunia, superficial, caused by, 133
    olivopontocerebellar (OPCA), ataxia associated with, 38
    testicular, mumps and, 399
Attention span deficits, in amnesia, 8
Audiologic evaluation, 182
Auditory brain stem response (ABR), 182
Auras, 413
    migraine, 416
Auscultation, cardiac, 448, 449t
    dynamic, 449, 449t
Autoimmune chronic active hepatitis, 198, 199
Autoimmune disorders, hearing loss in, steroid responsive, 184
    herpes gestationis, 486
    oophoritis, 311
    post-myocardial injury pericarditis and, 346–347
    systemic, xerostomia and, 510–511
    thyroiditis, 473
        microsomal antibodies in, 472
    thyrotoxicosis, 472
Automatic behavior, narcolepsy as, 428
Autonomic denervation in myocardial ischemia, 420
Autonomic nervous system, salivary gland control by, 507
Autonomic neuropathy, diabetes and, 252
Autonomous erythrocytosis, 375–376
    erythropoietin in, 374
Avascular necrosis, bone pain associated with, 54
    of the femoral head, 57
Axillary nodes, 298
Azidothymidine (AZT), 221, 222
Azotemia, acute, 46–51. See also *Renal failure.*
    assessment of, 50
    biochemical changes in, 48t
    causes of, 47t
    definition of, 46
    diagnostic studies in, 48–50, *50*
    extracellular fluid (ECF) and, 48
    history in, 46–47
    mortality rate in, 51
    neurologic disturbances associated with, 47–48
    physical examination and, 47–48

Azotemia (*continued*)
  postpartum, mortality rate in, 51
  prerenal, differentiation from renal azotemia, 49,
    49t
  urine diagnostic indices in, 49t
  urine sediment findings in, 49t

Babcock sentence, 8
Bacteremia, age-related risk of, 159
Bacterial epiglottitis, 437
Bacteriologic localization, in urethritis and prostatitis,
  141
Bacteriuria, 140
Ballism, characteristics of, 42t
Barium enema, constipation evaluation using, 108
  hematochezia evaluation using, 191
Barium x-rays, abdominal pain evaluation using, 4
Bartholin's gland inflammation, dyspareunia associated
  with, 131
Bartter's syndrome, hyperuricemia in, 243, 245
Bassen-Kornzweig syndrome, ataxia associated with, 39
Battle's sign, middle-ear deafness associated with, 183
Behçet's disease, pain with, 365
Belching, 276–277
Bell's palsy, proteinuria associated with, 383–384
Belladonna, and saliva flow, 507
Bence Jones protein, 379, 380
Benzodiazepines, anxiolytic effects of, 30
Beryllium disease, chronic, uric acid clearance in, 244
Beta-endorphin, serum levels in PMS, 155
Beta-hCG. See *β-Human chorionic gonadotropin.*
Beta-sympathomimetics, anorexia as a side effect of, 18
Beta-2-microglobulin levels, HIV infection and, 220
Bicarbonate, and acute renal failure, levels in, 48t
Bile duct stone, 87
Biliary cirrhosis, acanthosis nigricans and, 236
  hyperpigmentation in, 237t
Biliary scintigraphy, abdominal pain evaluation using, 4
Bilirubin, cholestasis, elevated levels in, 88
Bioelectric impedance, fatty tissue measurement with,
  503–504
Biopsy, assessment of pelvic masses and, 340
  blister, 483
  bone marrow, for polycythemia evaluation, 374
  brain, 285–286
  cervix, 330
  dyspareunia evaluation and, 131–132
  labial, of minor salivary glands, 513–514
  lung, 271–272
  lymph node, 297
  muscle, for polyarteritis identification, 360, 362
  nerve, for polyarteritis identification, 360, 362
  of mediastinal masses, 304–306
  renal, 50, 384
    for polyarteritis identification, 362
  small bowel, 435
Bipolar (manic-depressive) disorder, hallucinations in,
  153, 154, 173, 177
Birth, premature, pyelonephritis associated with, 140
  trauma at, athetosis due to, 42
Birth control pills, liver disease risk and, 198
Bleomycin, hyperpigmentation induced by, 238t
  infiltrative lung disease caused by, 268
Blepharitis, 127
  dry eye syndrome associated with, 123
  incidence of, 124
  symptoms of, 124t
Blepharospasm, bilateral, phantogeusia associated with,
  354

Blisters, 481–491
  biopsy of, 483
  classification of, 482t
Blood glucose, constipation and, 107
Blood Pressure Control in Children, Second Task Force
  on, 383
Blood products, HIV risk from use of, 216
Blood urea nitrogen (BUN), and azotemia, 46
  and renal failure, acute, 48t
Body mass index, and hyperuricemia, 239
  nomogram for calculation of, *504*
Bone, categories of disease in, 58t
  hyperuricemia and deposits in, 246
  lesions, differential diagnosis of, *59*
  marrow biopsy, polycythemia evaluation using, 374
  pain in, 52–60
  tumors of, primary, 59t
Bone pain, 52–60
  assessment of, 57–60
  categories of disease causing, 58t
  clubbing and, 94
  diagnostic studies in, 56–57
  history in, 53–56
  in adults, causes of, 53t
  lesions, and differential diagnosis of, *59*
    bone tumors simulated by, 59t
  musculoskeletal, evaluation of, 57t
  physical examination and, 56
Bongiovanni-Eisenmenger syndrome, weight gain in,
  502
Bradycardia, 60–66. See also *Bradytachycardia.*
  AV block and, electrocardiogram, *64*
  causes of, 61–62
  conditions associated with, 62t
  definition of, 60–61
  depolarization repolarization phases and, *61*
  diagnostic studies in, *66*
  heart failure and, 101
  history in, *65–66*
  junctional, 63, *64*, 65
  myocardial infarction and, 66
  physical examination and, *66*
  pseudobradycardia and, *65*
  sinoatrial exit block and, 63
  sinus, 62, *62*, *64*
  types of, 62–65
  ventricular ectopy induced by, 65
  ventricular escape rhythm and, *64*
  ventricular rhythm and, 65
Bradycardia-tachycardia syndrome, *63*, 430
Bradykinin, and bone pain, 53
Bradytachycardia, nocturnal, and sleep apnea, 430
Brain biopsy, 285
  herpes simplex encephalitis evaluation with, 285–286
Brain stem, lesions of, and auditory hallucinations,
  173
  response (ABR), auditory, 182
Breast lump, 67–72
  diagnostic studies in, 69–72
  history in, 68
  in children, 69
  in gravid women, 71–72
  in males, 72
  in nongravid women, 69–71
  incidence of, 68
  physical examination and, 68–69
Breath holding, seizure simulated by, 415
Breathing, abnormalities in rate and rhythm of, 467t
  neural control of, 464
  shortness of, tachyarrhythmias with, 455

Bromocriptine, hyperprolactinemia treated with, 313
  prolactinoma treated with, 310
Bronchiolitis obliterans interstitial pneumonitis (BIP), 267
Bronchitis, cough and, 115
Bronchoalveolar lavage (BAL), 271
Bronchogenic carcinoma, clubbing associated with, 96
Bronchoscopy, fiberoptic (FOB), 115
  mediastinal mass evaluation with, 305
  stridor evaluation with, 442–443
Bronchospasm, paroxysmal nocturnal dyspnea (PND) and, 445
Brown fat, 499
Budd-Chiari syndrome, polycythemia vera and, 376
Buerger's disease, 390
Bulimia, 17, 20
  nervosa, 500
Bullae, defined, 481
Bullosa, epidermolysis, 483, 484
Bullous disorder(s), arthropod reaction as, 489–490
  dermatophyte infection, 490
  fixed drug reaction in, 489
  immunofluorescent patterns in, 483t
  impetigo as, 490, 490
  pemphigoid as, 488, 488, 489
Bundle branch block, atrial fibrillation with complete right, 459
  atrial flutter and atrial fibrillation with, 458
Bundle of His, AV block site relative to, and bradycardia, 61
Burnout. See Fatigue, chronic.
Bursitis, differentiating from myofascial pain, 319–320
Busulfan, hyperpigmentation induced by, 238t

Cachexia, cancer, 17
  hepatomegaly and, 199
Cacogeusic taste sensation, 349, 354
Caffeine consumption, anxiety associated with, 34
  hoarseness and, 208
Calcium, constipation, and serum level of, 107
  homeostasis, maintenance by Mg, 261
Calcium pyrophosphate dihydrate (CPPD) deposition disease, 368
Cancer. See also Malignancy; Tumors.
  anxiety or depression with, 33
  colon, incidence, 194
Cancer cachexia, 17
Candidiasis, oral, HIV and, 217
Cannon waves, bradycardia associated with, 66
Captopril, cough caused by, 112
Carbamazepine, ataxia caused by, 40
Carbohydrate malabsorption, osmotic diarrhea and, 118
Carbon dioxide, panic induced by, 29
Carbon dioxide laser, for treating cervical dysplasia, 332–333
Carboxyhemoglobin determination, 374
Carcinoembryonal antigen (CEA), tumor marker, 338
Carcinoid syndrome, screening for, 4
  secretory diarrhea associated with, 118
Carcinoma, adrenal cortical, secondary hypertension and, 410
  alveolar cell, cough in, 112
  bronchogenic
    clubbing in, 96
    small cell, mediastinal mass in, 303
  hepatocellular, polycythemia associated with, 378
  renal cell, polycythemia associated with, 378

Carcinoma (continued)
  squamous cell, 323
    hoarseness associated with, 214
    pelvic mass associated with, 336
    ulcerated, 327
Cardiac arrhythmias, classification of tachyarrhythmias, 454t
  seizures simulated by, 416
Cardiac asthma, 112
  congestive heart failure and, 100
Cardiac catheterization, indications for, 423, 450
  pericarditis evaluation using, 345–346
Cardiac disorder(s), congenital, 445t
  pericarditis caused by trauma as, 343
  polyarteritis, juvenile form of, 360
Cardiac disorders, subsequent to TIA, 476
Cardiac glycosides, anorexia as a side effect of, 18
Cardiac palpation, systolic murmur evaluation and, 447–448
Cardiac tamponade, 343
  diagnosis with echocardiography, 345
Cardiolipin antibody syndrome, 24, 26–27
  percentage positive FANA with, 23t
Cardiomegaly, hepatomegaly associated with, 200
  tachyarrhythmias associated with, 456
Cardiomyopathy, hypertrophic obstructive, 451
  peripartum, 100
Cardiopulmonary failure, tachypnea associated with, 466
Cardiovascular disorder(s), anxiety associated with, 33t
  clubbing associated with, 97
  evaluation of systolic murmur in, 446t
  methods of assessing, 466t
Carotid sinus hypersensitivity, and bradycardia, 66
Carvallo's sign, 449
Castleman's disease, mediastinal mass associated with, 301
Castration anxiety, 30
Cataplexy, narcolepsy and, 428
Cataract, 495
Catecholamines, fatigue and depression with low levels of, 153–154
Catheterization, Swan-Ganz, 102–103
Cat-scratch fever, 294
Cauda equina syndrome, 55
CD4 (helper) cell, immune deficiency caused by loss of, 219
Celiac disease, anorexia associated with, 17
Central nervous system (CNS), depressants for, causing sleep apnea, 427
  dysfunction of, disorientation due to, 8
  intracranial infection and, 283
  polyarteritis and, 359
  polyarticular arthritis and, 366
  salivation modulation by, 507
  thiamine deficiency and, 11
  uric acid levels and, 240
Cerebellar hemangioblastoma, polycythemia associated with, 378
Cerebellopontine angle tumors, 182
Cerebral blood flow, regional (rCBF) changes in, 10
Cerebral infarction, 475–476
Cerebral injury, amnesia following concussion, 10–11
  seizures and, 414
Cerebral ischemia, TIAs and, 475
Cerebrospinal fluid (CSF), intracranial infection and, 282
Cerebrovascular disease, 14–15

Ceroid lipofuscinosis, athetosis associated with, 44
Ceruloderma, 235
Cervical biopsy, 330
Cervical intraepithelial neoplasia (CIN), 329
Cervix, anatomy of, 328
  conization of, 330–331
  cytology of, diagnostic terminology, 332
  dysplasia of, 328–329
  lesions of, premalignant, 329
  lymphadenopathy of, 297–298
    and mediastinal lymphadenopathy, 303
  pelvic mass originating from, 336
Charles-Bonnet syndrome, hallucinations associated
    with, 174
Chemicals. See also *Environmental exposure; Occupa-*
    tional exposure.
  dry eye syndrome caused by, 128
  dyspareunia caused by, 132
  dysuria caused by, 139
Chemotherapy, anorexia as a side effect of, 18
  ovarian failure caused by, 311
"Cherry red spot" in CRAO, 496
Chest pain, 73–85, 445–446
  mediastinal mass and, 302
  pericarditis and, 342
  tachyarrhythmias with, 455
Chest pain, acute, angina pectoris and, 75–77
    functional classifications of, 76t
  causes of, 74t
  diagnostic studies in, 80–84, 84t
  exercise-thallium imaging, indications for, 84t
  gastrointestinal causes of, 78–79
  history in, 76–79
  myocardial infarction and, 77, 85
  neuromusculoskeletal causes of, 78
  physical examination and, 79–80
  pulmonary angiography for diagnosis of, 85
  pulmonary embolism and, 85
Chest x-ray, 344
  for chest pain evaluation, 80
  for congestive heart failure evaluation, 102
  for cough evaluation, 114
  for hypoglycemia evaluation, 255
  for mediastinal mass evaluation, 306
  for pericarditis evaluation, 344
Chicken pox (varicella-zoster infection), 484–485
Chilblains, versus Raynaud's phenomenon, 390
Children, absence seizures in, 417–418
  anorexia in, 20
    causes of, 17t
  athetotic movements in, 42
  azotemia in, causes of, 46
  blisters in, causes of, 482t
  bone pain evaluation in, 54
  breast masses in, 69
  bullous eruptions in, 484–485
  dysuria assessment in, 139
  epididymitis in, 396
  fever in, 159–166
  generalized lymphadenopathy in, 298–299
  hematochezia in, 186
    causes of, 188t
  Henoch-Schönlein purpura in, 401
  hoarseness in, 212
  hypercholesterolemia assessment in, 231
  hypertension in, 383
  idiopathic nephrotic syndrome in, 385
  IgA dermatosis in, 491

Children (*continued*)
  limb pain in, 287–291
  linear IgA dermatosis in, 491
  pheochromocytoma in, 407
  proteinuria in, 381–382
  scrotal pain in, 396
  seizures in, 411–418
    etiology of, 412, 412t
  systolic murmurs in, 445
  upper airway obstruction in, 437
  uric acid levels in, 239
  urinary protein values in, 380t
Chlamydia trachomatis, dysuria, and infection by, 136
Chloasma, 233
Chlorpromazine, hyperpigmentation induced by, 238t
Cholangiopancreatography endoscopic retrograde
    (ERCP), 5
Cholangitis, liver disease and, 197
  sclerosing, 88
Cholecystitis, chest pain associated with, 78–79
Cholecystokinin, 17
Choledocholithiasis, abdominal pain in, 2
Cholestasis, 86–90
  alkaline phosphatase elevation in, 88(t), 89t
  assessment of, 89–90
  biochemical definition of, 86–87
  definition of, 86
  diagnostic studies in, 88–89
  extrahepatic, 89–90
  hepatocellular
    differentiation from extrahepatic, 88t
  history in, 87–88
  liver disease and, 89, 197
  pathophysiology of, 87
  physical examination and, 88
  syndromes associated with, 87t
Cholesterol. See also *Lipoproteins.*
  blood levels of, 227
  metabolism of, 229–230
  transport of, 224–225
Cholesterol Education Program (NCEP), National,
    Expert Panel, 228
Cholesterol ester transfer protein (CETP), 225
Cholesterol Lowering Atherosclerosis Study, 223
Cholestyramine, treatment of LDL with, 223
Chondrocalcinosis, 371
  diagnostic imaging to evaluate, 368
  polyarthritis and, 371
Chondromalacia patellae, limb pain associated with, 287
Chorea, characteristics of, 42t
  muscular atrophy and ataxia in, 39
Choreoacanthocytosis, 43
Choreoathetosis, 41
  paroxysmal, 416
Chorioretinitis, 414
Chromium isotope test, for hematochezia evaluation,
    186–187
Chronic fatigue syndrome (CFS), 152–158
Churg-Strauss syndrome, 269, 360
  interstitial pulmonary disease associated with, 272
Chvostek's sign, 31
Cicatricial pemphigoid, bullous, 488t
  ocular, 123, 127–128
Cigarette smoking. See *Smoking.*
Cilazapril, cough associated with, 112
Circadian rhythm(s), anginal events in, 76
  narcolepsy and, 425
Circulatory failure. See *Congestive heart failure.*

Cirrhosis, biliary, and acanthosis nigricans, 236
    hyperpigmentation in, 237
    hepatomegaly associated with, 199
Clitoral hypertrophy, 503
Clonazepam, for paroxysmal dyskinesias, 43
    for seizures, 418
Clonidine, for challenge testing, in PMS, 156
Clubbing, 91–97, 446–447
    assessment in, 95–97
    bone pain and, 94
    cardiovascular disorders and, 97
    cough and, 113
    definition of, 91
    diagnostic studies in, 95
    differential diagnosis in, 96–97
    history in, 94
    hormonal theories of, 93
    hypertrophic osteoarthropathy and, 93t
    identification and measurement, 92
    IPF and asbestosis associated with, 269
    neural mechanism explaining, 92–93
    physical examination and, 94–95
    pseudoclubbing, 95t, 96
    respiratory disorders and, 96
    unilateral, 94t
    vasodilation and, 92
Cocaine, chest pain associated with, 77
    cough associated with, 113
    hallucinations associated with, 174
Cognitive impairment, hallucination and, 176
    sleep apnea and, 429
Collagen diseases, hallucinations associated with, 174
    vascular, 268
Colon cancer, incidence of, 194, 194
Colonoscopy, abdominal pain evaluation with, 4
    compared with sigmoidoscopy, 194
    hematochezia evaluation with, 191
Color vision, evaluation of, 493
Colorectal constipation, 106t
    assessment of, 109
Colposcopy, cervical evaluation with, 331
    dyspareunia evaluation with, 131
    dysuria evaluation with, 138
Combined hyperlipidemia (FCHL), 230
Complex partial seizures, 412
    hallucinations associated with, 178
Computed tomography (CT), 345
    abdominal pain evaluation with, 4–5
    adrenal scan, 407, 410
    ataxia evaluation with, 39
    breast mass assessment with, 70
    cholestasis assessment using, 89
    cough assessment with, 114
    fever assessment with, 164
    head trauma evaluation with, 11
    hearing loss evaluation with, 182
    hepatic, 196
    hepatomegaly evaluation with, 201
    hoarseness evaluation using, 211
    hypoglycemia evaluation and, 255
    infarction identification in TIA, 477
    interstitial pulmonary disease evaluation with, 270
    intracranial infection evaluation with, 284
    lymphadenopathy evaluation, 296–297
    mediastinal mass evaluation with, 300, 304, 306–307
    correlation of image with etiology, 305t
    menstrual dysfunction evaluation with, 310
    pelvic mass evaluation with, 338
    pericarditis assessment with, 345
    polyarticular arthritis evaluation with, 368–369

Computed tomography (CT) (continued)
    scrotal pain evaluation with, 397
    seizure evaluation with, 415
    TGA evaluation with, 10
    TIA evaluation with, 480
Conception rate, and oligomenorrhea, 314
    following ectopic pregnancy, 151
Conduction disturbances, polyarteritis associated with, 360
Condyloma acuminata, pelvic mass associated with, 336
Confabulation, cerebrovascular disease and, 14
    Korsakoff psychosis and, 13
Congenital disorders. See also Hereditary disorders; Neonates.
    chloridorrhea, secretory diarrhea and, 118
    Down's syndrome, hyperuricemia in, 244
    Turner's syndrome, 311
Congestive heart failure, 98–104
    acute myocardial infarction and, 103
    assessment of, 103–104
    cardiac asthma and, 100
    classic causes of, 99t
    definition of, 98
    diagnostic studies in, 102–103
    evaluation of, 99t
    history in, 99–100
    normal ejection fraction and, 103–104
    pathophysiology of, 98–99
    pericarditis versus, 342–343
    physical examination and, 100–102
    polyarteritis associated with, 360
    proteinuria caused by, 379–380
    signs and symptoms of, 99t
    systolic versus diastolic dysfunction, 99
Conjunctivitis, allergic, 127
Conn's disease, secondary hypertension and, 410
Connective tissue disease (CTD), ANA diagnostic test for, 23
    pericarditis associated with, 347
    polyarteritis and, 361, 371
    Raynaud's phenomenon, associated with, 387, 388, 389
    progressing to, 390–391
Constipation, chronic, 105–109
    assessment of, 108–109
    classification of, 106(t)
    diagnostic studies in, 107–109
    environmental, 108
    hematochezia associated with, 189
    history in, 105–107
    implications of, 109
    medications causing, 107t, 108
    metabolic, 109
    neurologic, 109
    pharmacologic, 106t
    physical examination and, 107
    risks associated with, 105
Coombs test, positive, and SLE, 26
Cooper's ligaments, 67
Copper, zinc antagonist role of, 157
Corditis, polypoid, 213
Coronary angiography, 85
Coronary artery spasm, 462
Coronary Artery Surgery Study (CASS) Registry, 421
Coronary Drug Project, 223
Corpus luteum cyst, pregnancy and, 337
Corticosteroids. See also Adrenocorticotropic hormone (ACTH).
    anterior ischemic optic neuropathy, treatment with, 497–498

Corticotropin releasing factor, appetite and, 16–17
Cortisol, hypoglycemia and, 252
    levels in chronic fatigue, 156
    plasma glucose level maintenance by, 250
    production rate and turnover in obesity, 505
Cost-effectiveness, sigmoidoscopy compared with col-
        onoscopy, 194
Cough, epiglottitis and, 441
    hoarseness with, 206, 211
    interstitial pulmonary disease and, 269
    mediastinal mass and, 302
    paroxysmal nocturnal dyspnea (PND) and, 445
Cough, chronic, 110–116
    assessment in, 115–116
    causes by receptor location, 111t
    causes in nonsmoking patients, 111
    clubbing associated with, 113
    complications of, 116, 116t
    diagnostic studies in, 114–115
    drugs associated with, 112t
    history in, 112–113
    occupation-related causes of, 113
    physical examination and, 113–114
    skin disorders associated with, 113
    smoking and, 110–111
Courvoisier's law, 90
Coxsackie virus, 485
    herpangina caused by, 325
C-peptide, hypoglycemia evaluation and, 255
Cranial neuropathies, polyarteritis associated with, 359
C-reactive protein, polyarticular arthritis evaluation, 367
Creatine phosphokinase (CPK), serum levels, and azote-
        mia, 49
Creatinine, changes in acute renal failure, 48t
Creatinine kinase, levels in EBV infection, 154
Cremasteric reflex, 397
CREST syndrome, 3
    abdominal pain and, 4
    Raynaud's phenomenon preceding, 391
Creutzfeldt-Jakob disease, amnesia in, 15
Crigler-Najjar syndrome, 86
Crohn's disease, 434
    intestinal bloating associated with, 279
    pain and, 3
    steatorrhea and, 435
Croup, 437
Cryoglobulinemia, associated with Sjögren's syndrome,
        127
Cryoglobulins, false positive ELISA tests associated
        with, 218
Cryotherapy, for treating cervical dysplasia, 332–333
Cryptogenic fibrosing alveolitis. See Interstitial pulmo-
        nary disease.
Culdocentesis, for ectopic pregnancy evaluation, 148–
        149
Cushing's syndrome, 500
    obesity and, 503, 504, 505
Cyanosis, 446–447
    cough and, 113
Cyclic adenosine monophosphate (AMP), secretory
        diarrhea and, 118
Cyclothymia, fatigue related to, 154
Cyproheptadine, weight gain associated with, 501–502
Cystic fibrosis, clubbing and, 92
    cough and, 112, 115
Cystoscopy, dysuria evaluation with, 138
Cysts, Gartner's duct, 336
    hydatid, 338
    theca lutein, pregnancy and, 337
    thyroglossal duct, 471

Cytomegalovirus (CMV) infection, 296
    lymphadenopathy associated with, 299
    polyarteritis associated with, 358
    retinitis in, and HIV infection, 217

Deafness. See Hearing loss.
Defecography, constipation assessment and, 108
Dehydroepiandrosterone (DHA), 505
Dehydroepiandrosterone sulfate (DHEA-S), 313
Delusions. See Hallucinations.
Dementia, amnesia in, 15
    ataxia associated with, 38
    differentiating from amnesia, 7
    multi-infarct, 15
Demyelination, ataxia associated with, 37
Dental problems, caries, xerostomia associated with,
        512
    plaque, bacteria in, 325
Depression. See also Manic-depressive disorder.
    anorexia associated with, 20
    anxiety associated with, 31, 33–34
    cancer and, 33
    chronic fatigue associated with, 153–154
    fugue state associated with, 15
    hallucinations in, 177
    myofascial pain associated with, 316
    phantogeusia associated with, 354
Dermatitis herpetiformis, gluten-sensitive enteropathy
        and, 485
Dermatologic dysfunction. See also Skin.
    allergic contact dermatitis, 489
    dermatitis herpetiformis, 485, 485, 486
    dermatitis, immune complexes in, 491
    dermato/polymyositis
        ANA positive test in, 27
        FANA positive test in, 23t
    dermatomyositis, and limb pain, 290
    food allergy and, 168t
Deruloderma, 233
Desipramine, scrotal pain associated with, 395
Desquamative interstitial pneumonitis (DIP), 267
Dexamethasone suppression test (DST), for depression,
        154
Diabetes insipidus, hyperuricemia associated with, 244
Diabetes mellitus, 311
    anorexia associated with, 17
    diabetic nephropathy and, 382
    hyperlipidemias secondary to, 231
    hyperpigmentation associated with, 236
    hyperuricemia associated with, 244
    hypoglycemia in insulin-treated, 251–252
    silent myocardial ischemia associated with, 422
Diabetes, brittle, hypoglycemia associated with, 252
Diagnostic Assessment of Premenopausal Patients, 71,
        71
Diagnostic imaging. See also Computed tomography
        (CT); Magnetic resonance imaging (MRI).
    for abdominal pain, chronic, evaluation, 4–5
    for azotemia evaluation, 49–50
    for biliary tract evaluation, 89
    for constipation evaluation, 107–108
    for hepatomegaly evaluation, 201–203
    for hoarseness evaluation, 211
    for intracranial structural evaluation, 283–284
    for polyarticular arthritis evaluation, 368–369
Diaphanography, for breast mass assessment, 70
Diarrhea, acute, 117–122
    assessment of, 121–122
    causes of, 120t

Diarrhea (*continued*)
  clinical features of, 118t
  definition of, 117
  diagnostic studies in, 120–121
  drugs causing, 120t
  hematochezia associated with, 189
  history in, 119–120
  intestinal motility in, 118–119
  laboratory studies in, 121t
  osmotic, 118
    versus secretory diarrhea, 118t, 121
  pathophysiology of, 117–118
  physical examination and, 120
  secretory, 118
    versus osmotic diarrhea, 118t
Diastolic dysfunction, diagnosis of, 104
Diet. See also *Nutrition.*
  and breast cancer risk, 68
Dietary stress, uric acid levels and, 240
Diethylstilbestrol (DES), ectopic pregnancy and exposure to, 143
Digital subtraction angiography (DSA), renal evaluation using, 407
Digitalis, ectopic atrial tachycardia and, 457
  hypokalemia and hypomagnesemia associated with, 261
Digoxin, diastolic ventricular dysfunction and, 103–104
Dilantin. See *Phenytoin (Dilantin).*
Diphtheria, stridor associated with, 438
Disaccharidase deficiencies, 434
Disorder of excessive somnolence (DOES), 263
Disorder of initiating or maintaining sleep (DIMS), 263–266
Disorder(s), neurologic, constipation and, 106t
Distal interphalangeal (DIP) joints, 371
Diuretics, diastolic ventricular dysfunction and, 103–104
  hyperuricemia caused by, 244
  hypomagnesemia caused by, 259
Diverticula, incidence of, 192–193
  Zenker's diverticulum, 352
    cough and, 112
Diverticulitis, pain associated with, 6
Doppler echocardiography, 450, 451
  for chest pain evaluation, 83
  for congestive heart failure evaluation, 102
  for TIA evaluation, 480
Down's syndrome, hyperuricemia in, 244
Drugs. See also *Medications,* and specific drug.
  ANA-inducing, 24t
  anorexia as a side effect of, 18
  anxiety associated with abuse of, 31
  bradycardia caused by, 62t
  bullous eruptions caused by, 490
  chemotherapeutic, and anorexia, 18
  clubbing and, 97
  cough and, 112, 112t
  diarrhea caused by, 120, 120t
  gynecomastia caused by, 72
  hallucinations induced by, 174
  hyperuricemia caused by, 243, 244
  hypomagnesemia caused by, 258
  interstitial pulmonary disease caused by, 272–273
  lupus associated with, 364
  osmotic diarrhea caused by, 118
  pericarditis induced by, 347
  phantogeusia and, 351
  scrotal pain and, 395
  tachyarrhythmia associated with, 455
  voice quality and, 207t
  weight gain caused by, 501–502, 501t

Drugs (*continued*)
  xerogenic effect of, 509t, 510t
  xerostomia caused by, 509
Dry eye, 122–128, 494. See also *Sjögren's syndrome.*
  allergic conjunctivitis and, 127
  assessment of, 127–128
  blepharitis and, 127
  chemical burns causing, 128
  classification of, 123t
  diagnostic studies in, 126–127
  epidemiology of, 123–124
  history in, 124–126
  liver disease associated with, 199
  physical examination and, 126
  polyarticular arthritis associated with, 366
  symptoms, comparison of different disorders, 124t
Dubin-Johnson syndrome, 86
Dynorphin, appetite and, 16–17
Dysarthria, ataxia with, 38
Dysbetalipoproteinemia, 224, 231
Dysgeusia, anorexia related to, 19
Dysgeusia, anorexia related to, 19
Dyskinesia, athetosis and, 41–45
  paroxysmal, versus movement-induced reflex epilepsy (MIRE), 45
Dyslipidemias. See *Hypercholesterolemia; Lipoproteins.*
Dysmenorrhea, endometriosis and, 335
Dyspareunia, 128–134
  assessment of, 132–134
  causes of, 129, 130t
  chemicals and allergens associated with, 132
  developmental anomalies and, 133
  diagnostic studies in, 131–132
  endometriosis and, 335
  history in, 129–130
  physical examination and, 130
  surgical causes of, 133–134
Dysphagia, thyroid enlargement with, 470
Dysphonia. See also *Hoarseness.*
  functional, 207
  muscle tension and, 213
  plica ventricularis and, 213–214
  spastic, 214
Dyspnea, defined, 463
  interstitial pulmonary disease and, 269
  systolic murmurs associated with, 445
Dysthymia, fatigue related to, 153, 154
Dystonia, characteristics of, 42t
  dystonic choreoathetosis (PDC), paroxysmal, 43
Dysuria, 135–141
  assessment of, 139–141
  bacteriologic localization of, *141*
  definition of, 135
  diagnostic studies in, 136–139, *138*
  genitourinary system and, 137t
  history in, definition of, 136
  management of, 141
  physical examination and, 136

Ear, anatomy of, *180*
  external, hearing loss and, 182
  inner, hearing loss and, 183
Echocardiography, for chest pain evaluation, 83
  for congestive heart failure assessment, 102
  for fever assessment, 164
  for hypoglycemia evaluation, 255
  for pericardial effusion diagnosis, 344–345

Echocardiography (*continued*)
    for systolic murmur evaluation, 449–450
    for TIA evaluation, 480
    M-mode, 450
Ectopic pregnancy, 142–151, 309, 335, 337
    β-hCG levels in, 340
    abdominal examination in, 146t
    ampullary, *149*
    anatomic locations of, *144*
    assessment of, 149–151, *150*
    diagnostic studies in, 148–149
    history in, 144–146
    human chorionic gonadotropin levels and, 146–147,
        147
    laboratory studies in, 146–148, *148*
    mortality rate in, 142–143
        by race and age group, *143*
    physical examination and, 146–148
    progesterone levels and, 147, *148*
    rates of, *143*
Ectopy, ventricular, bradycardia-induced, 65
Eczema herpeticum, 491
Edema, 446
    cardiac failure and, 101
    systolic murmurs and, 447
Eisenmenger reaction, 445, 446
Ejection fraction (EF), CAD evaluation and, 82
    congestive heart failure and, 99, 102, 103–104
    normal, in congestive heart failure, 103–104
Ejection murmurs, pulmonic, 452
Elderly, anorexia in, 20–21
    causes of, 17t
    blisters in, causes of, 482t
    bullous eruptions of, 487–488
Electrocardiography (ECG), acute pericarditis stages
        seen in, 344t
    for chest pain assessment, 80, 85
    for congestive heart failure assessment, 102
    for hypoglycemia evaluation, 255
    for myocardial ischemia evaluation, 421
        silent, 422
    for pericarditis evaluation, 344
    for systolic murmur evaluation, 449
    for tachyarrhythmia evaluation, 453, 456–457
    P wave in, 457, 461
    Q wave in, 422
Electroconvulsive therapy (ECT), amnesia following, 14
Electroencephalography (EEG), for hypoglycemia
        evaluation, 255
    for intracranial infection evaluation, 284
    for seizure evaluation, 415
    for TGA evaluation, 10
    narcolepsy and patterns of, 425
Electrolytes, serum, constipation and, 107
Electromyography, for constipation assessment, 108
Electronystamography, for fibrositis evaluation, 155
Elimination diets, for allergy testing, 168–169
Embolism, CRAO caused by, 496
    TIAs and, 477
Embolus, arterial, 389
Emphysema, cough and, 115
    mediastinal, 300
    subcutaneous, and pneumomediastinum, 302
Enalapril, cough associated with, 112
Encephalopathy, and herpes encephalitis, amnesia
        associated with, 15
    encephalomyelitis syndrome
        causes of, 285t
    hepatic, 197, 200
        diarrhea induced by treatment for, 118

Encephalopathy (*continued*)
    seizures associated with, 413
    Wernicke's, 11–12, 40
Endocarditis, polyarticular arthritis associated with, 366
    subacute bacterial, 369
Endocrine disorders, acanthosis nigricans associated
        with, 236
    anxiety and, 32, 33t
    insomnia associated with, 266
    obesity-related, 500
Endometriosis, abdominal pain in, 2, 6
    cystic masses produced in, 335
    dyspareunia during treatment for, 133
    ectopic pregnancy and, 145
Endoscopic retrograde cholangiopancreatography
        (ERCP), 5
    hepatomegaly evaluation with, 201
Endoscopy, 5
    for constipation assessment, 108
    for hematochezia evaluation, 191
Endothelial dystrophy, unilateral visual impairment in,
        494
Enterokinase deficiency, 434
Enteropathy, dermatitis herpetiformis and gluten-sensi-
        tivity, 485
    eosinophilic enteritis, steatorrhea with, 435
    protein-losing, 434, 435
Enuresis, constipation-related, 105
Environmental constipation, 106t
    assessment of, 108
Environmental exposure, farmer's lung and, 268
    to aflatoxin, and liver disease, 198
    to asbestos, and pulmonary fibrosis, 268
    to oxygen, and pulmonary fibrosis, 268
Enzyme-linked immunosorbent assay (ELISA), for HIV
        diagnosis, 217–218
    for staging HIV infection, 220
Eosinophilic enteritis, steatorrhea with, 435
Eosinophilic pneumonia, interstitial pulmonary disease
        associated with, 272
Epidermolysis bullosa, 483, *484*
    acquisita, 486
    versus bullous pemphigoid, 488
Epididymitis, 396
    dysuria associated with, 141
    scrotal pain and, 398–399
Epididymo-orchitis, 396
Epigastric pain, 5–6
Epiglottis, "cherry red", 443
Epiglottitis, 441, 443
    bacterial, 437
    stridor associated with, 441
Epilepsy, 411. See also *Seizures*.
    classification of seizures in, 412t
    grand mal seizures and hypomagnesemia, 260
    movement-induced reflex epilepsy (MIRE), 45
    syndromes, 417–418
Epilepsy, International League Against, 412
Epileptiform discharge, cyclic phantogeusia and, 350
Epinephrine, dry eye syndrome caused by, 123
    hypoglycemia and, 252
    plasma glucose level maintenance by, 250
    starvation and, 250
Epithelial cell abnormalities, cervical, 332
Epitrochlear nodes, 298
Epstein-Barr virus (EBV) infection, 438
    fatigue associated with, 154
    liver disease associated with, 199
    lymphadenopathy associated with infection, 296,
        298–299

Erythroid colony growth, endogenous, in polycythemia, 374
Erythema, multiforme, 486
  cough and, 113
  nodosum, abdominal pain and, 3
  oral lesions in, 326
  palmar, abdominal pain and, 3
Erythematosus. See *Lupus erythematosus (LE); Systemic lupus erythematosus (SLE).*
Erythremia. See *Erythrocytosis, primary.*
Erythrocyte sedimentation rate (ESR), hearing loss and, 184
Erythrocytosis. See also *Polycythemia.*
  absolute, 375–377
  primary, 377
  relative, 375
  secondary, 375t
    appropriate, 377
    inappropriate, 378
Erythropoietin (epo), 372
  in autonomous erythrocytosis, 374
Escape rhythm, cardiac, 61, *63*
  junctional, *64*
  ventricular, *64*
Escherichia coli, dysuria and infection by, 136
Esophageal disorders, anorexia associated with dysmotility, 17
  chest pain associated with dysmotility, 78
  chronic cough and, 112
Essential hypererythropoietinemia, 378
Essential hypertension, asymptomatic proteinuria in, 381
Estrogen, dependence of the bladder epithelium on, 140
  dyspareunia and, 133
  hyperpigmentation and, 236
  hypertension and, 410
  levels during lactation, 134
  supplementation of, 310
Ethanol. See *Alcohol.*
Ethosuximide, treating seizures with, 418
Ethyl alcohol. See *Alcohol.*
Ethylenediamine tetraacetic acid (EDTA), insulin interaction with, 255
Euthyroid goiter, 474
Ewing's tumor, 54
Exercise, allergic reactions induced by, 167
  amenorrhea and, 310
  angina induced by, 76
  diarrhea following, 120
  silent myocardial ischemia, and level of, 422
Exercise test, abnormal, evaluation of, 420
  chest pain evaluation with, 81
  recommendations for, 423–424
  silent myocardial ischemia evaluation with, 422–423
  thallium imaging with, indications for, 84t
Existential anxiety, 30
Extracellular fluid (ECF), prerenal azotemia caused by reduction in, 48
Extrahepatic cholestasis, 89–90
Extramedullary hematopoiesis, mediastinal mass associated with, 301
Extrathoracic obstruction, airway dynamics associated with, *439*
  flow-volume loop in, *443*
Eye disorders. See also *Dry eye; Sjögren's syndrome.*
  ataxia, optic, 36–37, 38
  blepharitis, 123, 124, 124t
  cataract, 495
  chorioretinitis, 414
  cicatricial pemphigoid, 127–128

Eye disorders (*continued*)
  comparison of symptoms of, 124t
  endothelial dystrophy, unilateral impairment in, 494
  glaucoma, 494–495
  hemianopsia, temporal, 503
  iritis, 28
  and juvenile rheumatoid arthritis, 28
  nystagmus, and hypomagnesemia, 259–260
  ocular cicatricial pemphigoid, 123, 127–128
  ocular motility, 38
  ocular surface pathology
    dry eye syndrome and, 123
  optic neuritis, 498
  retinal detachment, 496
  retinal infarction, 478
  retinal migraine, 478
  retinitis, cytomegalovirus (CMV) infection and, 217
  retinitis pigmentosa, 38

Familial disorders. See also *Hereditary disorders.*
  cancer syndrome, 189
  dysautonomia, 162
  Mediterranean fever, 162
  myocardial infarction and FCHL, 230
Farmer's lung, environmental exposure and, 268
Fat cell theory, 499
Fatigue, chronic, 152–158
  epidemic of, 156
  etiology of, 152–153
  interactive disease states with, *153*
  liver disease and, 197
Fear, 29
  bradycardia associated with, 61
Febrile seizure, 413, 417
Felty's syndrome, ANA positive test in, 27
Females. See also *Gender differences.*
  dysuria in, 140
  masses in the gastrointestinal system of, 335–336
Femoral head, avascular necrosis of, 57
Fermentation, anaerobic, hydrogen and methane produced by, 274
Fertility, and oligomenorrhea, 314
  conception rate following ectopic pregnancy, 151
Fever, rheumatic, limb pain associated with, 287
  polyarthritis in, 369
  seizures associated with, 413, 417
  systolic murmurs associated with, 445
Fever in childhood, 159–166
  antibiotic therapy for, 165t
  assessment of, 164–166
  causes of, in fever of unknown origin, *161*
  diagnostic studies of, 163–164
  evaluation of fever of unknown origin, 164t
  history and, 160, 162
  physical examination and, 162–163
  risk factors for occult bacteremia in, 160t
Fever of unknown origin, 162–163
  causes of, *161*
  diagnostic studies of, 163–164
  laboratory evaluation of, 164t
Fiberoptic bronchoscopy (FOB), for cough evaluation, 115
Fiberoptic laryngoscopy, and hoarseness, diagnosis of, 209–210
Fibrillation, atrial, 455–456, 458
  magnesium deficiency and, 261
  tachyarrhythmias associated with, 456
  TIA caused by, 479
  ventricular, 462

Fibroadenoma, breast mass associated with, 69
Fibrocystic changes, breast mass associated with, 69
Fibromuscular dysplasia, renal artery stenosis secondary to, 403
Fibromyalgia. See *Fibrositis*.
Fibrosis, replacement congestive heart failure and, 98
Fibrositis, fatigue associated with, 155
  myofascial pain versus, 320, 320t
  Symthe criteria for, 155
Fine needle aspiration of the thyroid, 474
Fisheye disease, 227
Flatulence, 274–280
Fluorescein staining, dry eye evaluation with, 126
Fluorouracil, hyperpigmentation induced by, 238t
Fluorescent antinuclear antibody test (FANA), 22–23, 384
Flutter, atrial, 457–458
  ventricular response during, 459
Food allergy, 167–171
  common manifestations of, 168t
  diagnostic studies of, 168–171, 168t
  food/symptom diary evaluation, 169
  history in, 167
  physical examination and, 167–168
Food intolerance, 167–171
  milk-induced chronic pulmonary disease due to, 170
Foreign body aspiration, stridor and, 437
Framingham Study, 419
Frederickson-Levy classification of dyslipidemias, 229
Friction blisters, 490–491
Friedrich's ataxia, 38, 39–40
Frontal lobe, amnesia as a symptom of dysfunction in, 8
Fructose, hyperuricemia caused by, 243
  intestinal bloating caused by malabsorption of, 277
Fröhlich's syndrome, weight gain in, 502
Fuch's endothelial dystrophy, unilateral visual impairment in, 494
Fugue state, 15
Functional cyst, pelvic mass and, 340
Functional dysphonia, 207
Functional murmurs, 444–453
Funduscopy, 414
  TIA evaluation with, 479

Gaisböck's syndrome, 375
Gait ataxia, and Wernicke encephalopathy, recovery time in, 13–14
  characterized by, 12
Gamma-aminobutyric acid (GABA) receptor, 30
Gamma-glutamyl transferase (GGT), levels in cholestasis, 86
Gartner's duct cysts, pelvic mass associated with, 336
Gas-bloat syndrome, 277
Gaseousness, 274–280
Gastric outlet obstruction, anorexia associated with, 17
Gastroenteritis, acute. See *Diarrhea, acute*.
Gastroesophageal reflux (GER), cough associated with, 111, 115
Gastrointestinal disorders, and resorption of liquid, 117
  chest pain and, 78–79
  clubbing associated with, 97
  food allergy and, 168t
  inflammatory bowel disease and, 290
  masses in, in females, 335–336
  mediastinal mass associated with, 302
  polyarteritis associated with, 359–360
  polycythemia vera and, 376

Gaucher's disease, bone pain associated with, 58
Gender differences. See also *Females; Males*.
  in aphthous ulcer occurrence, 326
  in arthritis type, 364
  in breast development and breast cancer risks, 68
  in chronic fatigue incidence, 153
  in colorectal cancer, 194
  in constipation incidence, 105
  in croup incidence, 437
  in dysuria incidence, 135
  in hereditary clubbing and, 94
  in hypersomnia incidence, 426
  in hyperthyroid incidence, 470
  in IPF incidence, 268
  in pachydermoperiostosis incidence, 94
  in phantogeusia incidence, 353
  in Raynaud's phenomenon incidence, 386
  in risk factors for CAD, 225, 232
  in secondary hypertension incidence, 403
  in serum uric acid levels, 239
  in ulcer causes, 321–322
  male inheritance of Lesch-Nyhan syndrome, 43
Generalized anxiety disorder, 34
Generalized lymphadenopathy, 292 persistent (PGL), 299
Genetic disorders. See *Hereditary disorders*.
Genitourinary system, cancer of, incidence and age correlation, 140
  dysuria, and causes of, 137t
  laboratory tests for infection of, 139t
Gestational age, pregnanediol-3-glucuronide (PDG) values and, *148*
Giant cell arteritis, 364, 496, 497
Giant cell interstitial pneumonitis (GIP), 267
Gilbert's disease, 86
Gingivitis, acute necrotizing ulcerative, 321
Glands, submandibular, 507, *512*
Glaucoma, 494–495
  open angle, chronic (COAG), 494
Global amnesia, transient (TGA), 8–10, 478
Global confusional state, Wernicke encephalopathy and, 12
Glomerulonephritis, proteinuria in, 382
Glossopyrosis, phantogeusia associated with, 351
Glucagon, hypoglycemia and, 252
  plasma glucose level maintenance by, 250
  starvation and, 250
Gluconeogenesis, 250
Glucose metabolism, azotemia and, 49
  dependence on thiamine, 13
  homeostasis in, *251*
  hypoglycemia evaluation and, 255
  pathways of, *250*
Glucose tolerance test, androgenic disorder evaluation with, 312
  oral (OGTT), 256
Glucose-6-phosphate dehydrogenase deficiency, 199
Glucose-6-phosphatase deficiency, 243
Glutathione reductase mutation, 243
Gluten-sensitive enteropathy, 485
Glycogenolysis, 250
Goiter. See also *Thyroid enlargement*.
  euthyroid, 474
  evaluation of, 471t
Gonadotropins, elevated, in neonates, 334
  obesity associated with, 505
Gonococcal arthritis, 365, 369
Goodpasture's syndrome, 271, 273

Gout, 363–364, 365. See also *Pseudogout*.
 and hyperuricemia, 249
 myofascial pain distinguished from, 318
 polyarthritis in, 369
Grand mal seizures, hypomagnesemia-associated, 260
Granulomas, intubation, 213
Granulomatosis, Wegener's, 271, 360
 interstitial pulmonary disease and, 272
Graves' disease, 32, 470, 473
 acanthosis nigricans in, 236
 hyperpigmentation in, 237t
Grief, hallucinations associated with, 174, 177
Growing pains, 291
Growth factor, platelet-derived (PDGF), 93
Growth hormone, hypoglycemia and, 252
 plasma glucose level maintenance by, 250
Growth retardation, seizures and, 414
Guillain-Barré syndrome, bradycardia associated with,
 62t
Gynecomastia, 72
 abdominal pain associated with, 3
 clubbing associated with, 96
 germ cell tumors associated with, 303
 hepatomegaly associated with, 200

Hairy leukoplakia, HIV and, 217
Halban's syndrome, 335
Hallervorden-Spatz disease, 42
Hallucinations, 172–178
 assessment of, 177–178
 biologic theories of, 172
 causes of, 173t
 clinical aspects of, 173–174
 definition of, 172
 diagnostic studies of, 176–177
 functional psychoses and, 177t
 history in, 174–175
 hypnagogic, 428
 laboratory studies and results in, 176t
 mental status examination and, 175–176
 optic tract damage and, 173
 organic mental syndromes and, 178t
 physical examination and, 175
 responses to, 175t
 types of, 173t
Hammond's Disease. See *Athetosis*.
Hand-foot-and-mouth disease, 485, *485*
Hartnup's disease, 42
Hashimoto's thyroiditis, 311
Head and neck, sagittal view of, *204*
Head trauma, seizures associated with, 413
Hearing, Weber test of, 181–182
Hearing loss, hereditary nephritis and, 383
 idiopathic sudden, 184–185
 otosyphilis and, 183
 sudden, 179–185
  assessment of, 183–185
  diagnostic studies in, 182
  etiology of, 181t
  history in, 179–181
  idiopathic, 184–185
  physical examination and, 181–182
 Waldenström's macroglobulinemia and, 184
Heart failure, congestive, 98–104
 classic causes of, 99
 evaluation of, 99
 polyarteritis associated with, 360
 proteinuria caused by, 379–380
 signs and symptoms of, 99
 versus pericarditis, 342–343

Height and weight tables, 500t
Heiner syndrome, 170
Helsinki Heart Trial, 223
Hemangioblastoma, cerebellar, polycythemia associated
 with, 378
Hemangiomas, subglottic, 212
Hematocele, scrotal pain associated with, 400
Hematochezia, 186–194
 assessment of, 192–193
 causes of, emergent and nonemergent, 187t
  rare, 188(t)
 colorectal cancer and, 194, *194*
 definition of, 186
 diagnostic studies in, 190–192
 emergent, 192–193
  causes of, 187(t)
 history in, 189
 in children, 188(t)
 nonemergent, 193–194
 physical examination in, 189–190
Hematologic diseases, hemochromatosis congestive
  heart failure in, 103
 hemoglobinopathies, 377
 hepatomegaly associated with, 198
 hyperpigmentation in, 236, 237
 hyperuricemia associated with, 243
Hematopoiesis, extramedullary, mediastinal mass associated with, 301
Hematuria, polycystic kidney disease in, 385
Hemianopia, homonymous, 492
Hemianopsia, temporal, obesity associated with, 503
Hemispheric lesions, ataxia associated with, 40
Hemochromatosis, congestive heart failure in, 103
 hepatomegaly associated with, 198
 hyperpigmentation in, 236, 237t
Hemoglobin P_{50} measurement, 374
Hemoglobinopathies, 377
Hemoptysis, interstitial pulmonary disease with, 269
Hennebert's sign, 183
Henoch-Schönlein purpura, 401
 azotemia associated with, 48
 limb pain and, 287, 289, 396
Heparin, hematochezia caused by, 189
 insulin interaction with, 255
Hepatic encephalopathy, 197, 200
 diarrhea induced by treatment for, 118
Hepatitis, abdominal pain and, 4
 alcoholic, hepatomegaly associated with, 199
 autoimmune chronic active, 198, 199
Hepatitis B virus (HBV) infection, joint involvement
  associated with, 369
 polyarteritis associated with, 358
Hepatocellular carcinoma, polycythemia associated
 with, 378
Hepatocellular cholestasis, and extrahepatic cholestasis,
 88t
Hepatomegaly, 195–203
 abdominal pain in, 2
 arteriography for evaluating, 201
 assessment of, 202–203
 causes of, 202t
 diagnostic studies in, 200–202
 history in, 196–199
 physical examination and, 199–200
 right heart failure and, 101
Hepatosplenomegaly, HDL deficiency and, 227
Hereditary disorders, 17-alpha-hydroxylase deficiency,
 311
  ANA positive titer and SLE, 23, 25
  apolipoprotein C-II deficiency, 230

Hereditary disorders (*continued*)
  ataxia in, 37, 38, 39
  bilirubin transport defects, 86–87
  clubbing, 91, 95–96
  combined familial hyperlipidemia (FCHL), 230
  congenital chloridorrhea, 118
  erythrocytosis syndromes, 373
  familial cancer syndrome, 189
  familial defective apo B-100, 230
  familial dysautonomia, 162
  familial Mediterranean fever, 162
  Fuch's endothelial dystrophy, 494
  galactosemia, 311
  glucose-6-phosphatase deficiency, 243
  glutathione reductase mutation, 243
  HDL deficiencies, 227
  HGPRT deficiency, 242–243
  Hirschsprung's disease, 105
  hypercholesterolemia, 224, 230
  hypersomnia, 426
  hypoalphalipoproteinemia, 231
  incontinentia pigmenti, 484
  increased PRPP-S activity, 242
  Lesch-Nyhan syndrome, 43, 243
  lipoprotein levels and, 226–227, 226t
  lipoprotein lipase deficiency, 230
  lipoprotein lipase inhibitor deficiency, 230
  liver dysfunction associated with, 198
  multiple endocrine adenomatosis, 403
  nephritis, 383
  obesity caused by, 502
  pachydermoperiostosis, 94
  paroxysmal dyskinesias, 43
  polyarticular arthritides, 365
  polycystic kidney disease, 403
  polycythemia, 377
  rheumatoid arthritis, 288
  rolandic epilepsy, 418
  secondary hypertension and, 404t
  Sjögren's syndrome, 125
  sleep apnea, 427
  spondyloarthropathy, 288
  systemic lupus erythematosus, 288
  vesiculobullous, 483–484
  von Recklinghausen's disease, 180
Herniorrhaphy, scrotal pain following, 396
Heroin, beta-endorphin similarity to, 156
Herpangina, 325
Herpes gestationis, 486
Herpes simplex infection, 324, *490*, *491*
  congenital, 483
  encephalitis in, 284
    amnesia associated with, 15
    brain biopsy to confirm, 285–286
  erythema multiforme associated with, 486
  intraoral lesions, *324*
  oral ulcers associated with, 321
Herpes zoster infection (shingles), 488–489
  chest pain associated with, 78
  intraoral, 324
Hiccups, persistent, 277
High-density lipoprotein (HDL), hypercholesterolemia
    and, 229, 231
  atherosclerosis and, 231
Hippocampal formation, amnesia as a symptom of
    dysfunction in, 8
Hirschsprung's disease, 105, 107, 108, 109
Histamine, food-allergy related levels of, 170
HIV infection. See *Human immunodeficiency virus
    (HIV) infection.*

HLA antigens, 429
  spondyloarthropathies and, 365
Hoarseness, 203–214
  assessment of, 212–214
  definition of, 203
  diagnostic studies in, 211–212
  direct laryngoscopy in diagnosis of, 211, *211*
  drugs causing, 207t
  fiberoptic laryngoscopy in diagnosis of, 209–210, *210*
  history in, 206–208
  mediastinal mass and, 302
  physical examination and, 208–211
  stridor and, 441
  thyroid dysfunction and, 470, 472
  videostroboscopy in diagnosis of, 210–211, *210*
Hodgkin's lymphoma, 293
  breast cancer risk in, 68
  chest pain associated with, 78
Holosystolic murmur, 450, 452
  genesis of, *451*
Homonymous hemianopia, 492
Homosexuality, anorexia associated with, 18
Hormones. See also *Estrogen.*
  glucose-regulating, *251*
  hypoglycemia and, counter-regulatory responses in,
    252
  influence on taste and smell function, 356
  luteinizing hormone-releasing hormone (LHRH), 133
  progesterone, in pathologic pregnancies, 147
    pain from effect on smooth muscle and, 2
  testosterone, levels in chronic fatigue, 156
  thyroid stimulating (TSH), primary hypothyroidism
    levels, 472
    thyrotropin releasing (TRH), 504
Horner's syndrome, chest pain associated with, 79
β-Human chorionic gonadotropin (β-hCG), diagnosis of
    problem pregnancies by following, 146–147, *147*
  identification of normal pregnancy, 340
  pregnancy evaluation using levels of, 144
  testicular tumor and, 397
Human immunodeficiency virus (HIV) infection, 215–
    222. See also *Acquired immune deficiency syn-
    drome (AIDS).*
  assessment of, 221–222
  diagnostic studies in, 217–221
  history in, 216–217
  lymphadenopathy in, 294, 296
  necrotizing vasculitis in individuals with, 358
  oligoarticular reactive arthritis and, 365
  physical examination and, 217
  pneumocystics carinii pneumonia and, 221, 221(t)
  relative risks of, 216(t)
  stages of, 221(t)
  staging of patients with, 219–221
Human papilloma virus (HPV), and cervical neoplasia,
    328
    dyspareunia-associated infection, 131
Huntington's disease, 42
Hydatid cysts, 338
Hydrocele, scrotal pain associated with, 400
Hydrocephalus, amenorrhea associated with, 309
Hydrostatic weighing, 503
17-Hydroxycorticosteroids, urinary excretion of, 505
Hyperapobetalipoproteinemia, 230–231
Hypercalcemia, hyperuricemia associated with, 245
    multiple myeloma or bone metastases associated
    with, 54
Hypercapnia, tachypnea associated with, 464–465
Hypercatecholaminemia, hypomagnesemia associated
    with, 260

Hypercholesterolemia, 79, 223–232, 423. See also
    Cholesterol; Lipoproteins.
  apoprotein E and, 231
  assessment of, 228–232
    in children, 231–232
  definition of, 223
  diagnostic studies in, 227–228
  history in, 225–226
  lipoprotein disorders, classifications of, 229–230, 229(t)
  lipoprotein testing for adults, criteria for, 228(t)
  management of, 232
  physical examination and, 226–228, 226(t)
  secondary causes of, 229
  silent myocardial ischemia and, 422
Hyperchylomicronemia, 230
Hyperemesis gravidarum, thiamine deficiency in, 12
Hypererythropoietinemia, essential, 378
Hypergammaglobulinemia, Sjögren's syndrome associated with, 127
Hyperkalemia, azotemia, acute and, 48
    bradycardia associated with, 62t
Hyperlipidemia, combined familial (FCHL), 230
    myocardial ischemia, silent associated with, 422
Hyperlipoproteinemia, hyperuricemia associated with, 244
Hypermagnesemia, 49
    fatigue associated with, 157
Hypermobility syndrome, limb pain associated with, 287
    in children, 291
Hypernatremia, primary aldosteronism and, 410
Hyperparathyroidism, 403
  bone pain associated with, 58
  hyperuricemia associated with, 244
Hyperpigmentation, generalized, 233–238
    assessment of, 233
      studies in, 237
    drug-induced, 238t
    etiology of, 235t, 237(t)
    hepatomegaly associated with, 199
    history in, 235–236
    liver disease associated with, 197
    physical examination and, 236–237
    process of skin pigmentation and, 234–235, *234*
Hyperplasia, angiofollicular lymph node, 301
    atypical lymphoid, 293
Hyper-reflexia, secondary seizure disorder and, 414
Hypersensitivity pneumonitis, 115
    interstitial pulmonary disease associated with, 272
Hypersomnia, 425, 426
    differentiating from other sleep disorders, 430–431, 430t
    idiopathic, 430t
    symptoms of, 428
Hypersplenism, hepatomegaly associated with, 199
    hepatosplenomegaly, HDL deficiency and, 227
Hypertension, 423, 479
    causes of secondary, 404t
    essential, asymptomatic proteinuria in, 381
    estrogen-induced, 410
    genetic conditions associated with, 404(t)
    nonessential, 403–410
    proteinuria in, 385
    relative erythrocytosis associated with, 375
    renovascular, 405–407, 405t
      diagnostic assessment of, 406
      symptoms raising suspicion of, 405
    risk factor for aortic dissection, 74–75
    secondary, 403–410. See also *Secondary hypertension.*
    silent myocardial ischemia associated with, 422

Hyperthyroidism, 473
  anorexia associated with, 17
  incidence of, 470
  screening for, in anxiety, 32
  signs of, 471
  systolic murmurs associated with, 446
Hypertonicity, secondary seizure disorder and, 414
Hypertriglyceridemias, 230–231
Hypertrophic obstructive cardiomyopathy, 451
Hypertrophic osteoarthropathy (HOA), clubbing and, 91, 93t
Hypertrophy, cellular, congestive heart failure and, 98
    clitoral, 503
    ventricular, chest pain with, 73
Hyperuricemia, 49, 239–248
  approach to patient with, 244–247
  definition of, 239
  etiology of, 242–244, 242t
  history in, 245
  laboratory studies in, 245
  management of, 247–248
  pathophysiology of, 242
  physical examination and, 245
  prevalence of, 240
  purine synthesis and degradation cycle, *241*
  renal control of uric acid and, *241*
Hyperventilation, 416
  defined, 463
  panic induced by, 29
  seizures associated with, 413
Hyphemas, 493–494
Hypoalphalipoproteinemia, CAD and, 231
Hypocalcemia, azotemia associated with, 49
    hypomagnesemia coexisting with, 260
Hypocomplementemia, 26
Hypogammaglobulinemia, mediastinal mass associated with, 303
Hypoglycemia, 249–257, 504
  anxiety associated with, 32
  assessment of, 256–257
  definition of, 249–250
  diagnostic studies of, *254*, 255–256
  etiologies of, 252(t)
  glucose homeostasis and, *251*
  glucose metabolic pathways and, *250*
  history in, 253
  iatrogenic, 250
  physical examination and, 253–255
  types of, 250–252
Hypoglycemic agents (OHAS), oral, 252
Hypokalemia, fatigue associated with, 157
    hypomagnesemia and, 261–262
      coexisting with, 260
    primary aldosteronism and, 410
    tachyarrhythmia associated with, 455
Hypomagnesemia, 258–262
  aldosteronism, primary, and, 410
  and cisplatin, 261
  assessment of, 261–262
  causes of, 259t
  diagnostic studies in, 260
  false positive tests for, 260
  frequency of, in hospitalized patients, 258
  history and, 258–259
  physical examination and, 259–260
Hyponatremia, acute azotemia and, 48
    hypomagnesemia coexisting with, 260
Hypophosphatemia, hypomagnesemia coexisting with, 260

Hypoprothrombinemia, cholestasis associated with, 87
Hyposmia, 354–355
Hypothalamic-pituitary disorders, menstrual dysfunction associated with, 309–310
Hypothalamus, appetite and, 16
Hypothermia, bradycardia associated with, 62t
Hypothyroidism, 473
    bradycardia associated with, 62t
    breast cancer risk in, 68
    fatigue associated with, 157–158
    hyperlipidemia secondary to, 229, 231
    hyperuricemia associated with, 244
    obesity associated with, 500–501, 503
Hypoxanthine guanine phosphoribosyl transferase (HGPRT) deficiency, 242–243
Hypoxemia, 81
    erythrocytosis due to, 377
        secondary, 374
    hyperuricemia associated with, 243
    tachypnea associated with, 464–465
Hypoxia, excessive sleepiness and, 426
        perinatal, and seizures, 412
Hysterical conversion, TIAs similar to, 476

Iatrogenic hypoglycemia, 250
Idiopathic hypersomnia, 430t
Idiopathic hyperuricemia, 242
Idiopathic sudden hearing loss, 184–185
Illusions. See *Hallucinations.*
Imaging studies. See *Computed tomography (CT); Diagnostic imaging; Magnetic resonance imaging (MRI).*
Immune complexes, food-allergy studies of, 170
        linear IgA dermatitis and, 491
        vasculitis and, 358
Immune deficiencies, cell-mediated, 217
        chronic fatigue and, 152
        helper cells and, 219
        ulcers secondary to, 325–326
Immunity. See also *Autoimmune disorders.*
    markers associated with interstitial pulmonary disease, 271
    mechanisms of, and aphthous ulcers, 321
Immunofluorescence technique, direct, IgA detection with, 491
        IgG detection with, 488
Immunofluorescent technique, indirect (FANA), 22–23, 384
Impulse anxiety, 30
Incontinentia pigmenti, *484*
Infant death syndrome, sudden, bradycardia associated with, 62t
Infants. See also *Neonates.*
    anorexia in, 20
        causes of, 17t
    athetosis in, 43–44
    bradycardia associated with SIDS, 62t
    breath holding in, 415
    hoarseness in, 212
    infantile spasms in, 417–418
    pallid infantile syncope in, 415–416
    seizure etiology in, 412, 412(t)
Infarct-avid imaging, chest pain evaluation with, 82
Infarction. See also *Myocardial infarction.*
    retinal, 478
    watershed, amnesia in, 14–15
Infection, amnesia associated with, 15
    anxiety associated with, 33t
    arthritis and, evaluation of, 368

Infection (*continued*)
    deafness following, 183
    mononucleosis, stridor associated with, 438
    pericarditis and, 347
Infertility, varicocele associated with, 400
Infiltrative disorders, hepatomegaly associated with, 292–293
Inflammatory diseases, arthropathies, 318–319
    bowel, clubbing and, 92, 97
    diarrhea and, 121
    dyspareunia caused by, 132–133
    limb pain associated with, 290
Inguinal canal, anatomy of, 392–394, 394t
    boundaries of, *393*
    nodes, 298
    scrotal pain and, 395, 395t
    in hernia of, 399–400
Insomnia, 263–266
    assessment of, 265–266
    conditions associated with long-term, 264(t)
    diagnostic studies in, 265
    history in, 263–264
    management of, 266
    medical conditions associated with, 266
    physical examination and, 264–265
    psychophysiologic, 264, 265
Insulin, hypoglycemia evaluation and, 255
Insulinoma, hypoglycemia associated with, 256, 257
Interstitial lung disease, 266–273
    assessment of, 272–273
    causes of, 267(t)
    diagnosis of, 273
    diagnostic studies of, 270–272
    history in, 268–269
    pathogenesis of, 268
    physical examination and, 269–279
    pulmonary function tests (PFTs) for diagnosis of, 270–271
    radiologic patterns in, 270t
Interstitial pulmonary disease, Churg-Strauss syndrome associated with, 272
Intestinal bloating and gas, assessment of, 278–280
    diagnostic studies in, 278
    foods and flatus, 280t
    functional gas syndromes, 276–278
    gas composition and, 274–275
    history in, 275–278
    physical examination and, 278
Intestinal dysfunction, abnormal motility, and diarrhea, 118–119
    thiamine deficiency and obstruction, 12
Intoxication. See *Alcohol; Drugs; Environmental exposure; Medications; Occupational exposure.*
Intracranial disorder(s), amenorrhea associated with tumors, 309–310
    infection as, acute, 280–286
        assessment of, 284–286
        categories of, 281(t)
        diagnostic studies of, 283–284, 283t
        history in, 281–282
        meningitic syndrome and, 285t
        meningitis syndrome and, 285t
        physical examination and, 282–283
Intrahepatic cholestasis, 89
Intrathoracic obstruction, airway dynamics associated with, *440*
Intrauterine device (IUD), ectopic pregnancy and, 145
Intravenous (IV) drugs, abdominal pain source and, 3
Intravenous pyelography, 406

Intravenous urography (IVU), dysuria evaluation with, 138
Inverted nipple, 67
Iritis, and juvenile rheumatoid arthritis, 28
Iron deficiency anemia, 273
Irradiation therapy, xerostomia during, 511
Irritable bowel syndrome (IBS), 275, 277 pain in, 2, 6
Ischemia. See also *Myocardial ischemia; Silent myocardial ischemia.*
   abdominal pain, chronic, and, 1
   and AION, 497
   bradycardia associated with, 62t
   cerebral
     and TGA, 9
     and TIAs, 475
   marker of residual, 424
   myocardial, silent, 419–424
   polyarteritis associated with, 360
   reversible ischemic neurologic deficit (RIND), 475
   stroke, and causes of, 477t
Isoproterenol, anxiety precipitated by, 29

Jaborandi, and saliva flow, 507
Jakob-Creutzfeldt syndrome, 39
Jaundice, bradycardia associated with, 62t
   cholestasis versus, 86–87
   hepatomegaly and, 199
Joints, ANA positive tests and condition of, 25
   and HBV infection, 369
   distal interphalangeal (DIP), 371
   examination of, in limb pain evaluation, 288–289
   in myofascial pain evaluation, 317
   pain of, in polyarticular arthritis, 363–371
Jugular vein, and heart failure, 101
   pulsations of, systolic murmur evaluation and, 447
Junctional bradycardia, 64
Junctional rhythm, AV, 458, 460
   bradycardia associated with, 63–65

Kaposi's sarcoma, cough and, 113
   HIV infection and, 217
   polyarticular arthritis and, 366
Kawasaki's disease, 360
   limb pain and, 289
Kayser-Fleischer rings, liver disease associated with, 199
Kearns-Sayre syndrome, 426
Keratoconjunctivitis, allergic, symptoms of, 124
   incidence of, 124
   medicamentosa, 127
   toxic, symptoms of, 124t
Keratoconjunctivitis sicca (KCS). See also *Dry eye.*
   incidence of, 124
   symptoms of, 124t
   systemic conditions associated with, 125t
Kidney disease. See also *Azotemia, acute; Renal disease/dysfunction; Renal failure.*
   polycystic
     hematuria in, 385
     hypertension and, 405
     hyperuricemia in, 243
     secondary hypertension and, 403
Kinase, creatinine, levels in EBV infection, 154
Kinesigenic choreoathetosis (PKC), paroxysmal, 43
Kleine-Levin syndrome, 428
Korsakoff psychosis, 11–14
Krebs cycle, 13
Kussmaul's sign, 343, 345

Laboratory studies, in abdominal pain, 3
   in acute diarrhea, 121t
   in differential diagnosis of anxiety, 32t
   in hallucination evaluation, 176t
   in hematochezia evaluation, 190–191
   in hepatomegaly evaluation, 200–201
   in hyperuricemia, 245
   in hypomagnesemia, 260
   in intracranial infection evaluation, 283t
Lactase deficiency, 279
   diarrhea associated with, 119
   fecal hydrogen production in, 274
   intestinal gas associated with, 276
Lactate, ataxia and serum levels of, 40
   panic induced by high levels of, 29
Lactose intolerance, 168
   osmotic diarrhea and, 118
Laparoscopy, for abdominal pain evaluation, 5
   for dyspareunia evaluation, 132
   for dysuria evaluation, 138
   for ectopic pregnancy, diagnosis of, 149
     management of, 144
     treatment of, 151
Laparotomy, hematochezia evaluation with, 192
   pelvic mass evaluation with, 340
Laryngitis. See also *Hoarseness.*
   acute, 212
   chronic, 212–213
Laryngocele, hoarseness in, 214
Laryngomalacia, 212
Laryngoscopy, fiberoptic, 209–210, *210*
   stridor evaluation in, 442–443
Laryngotracheobronchitis, viral (croup), 437
Larynx, coronal view of, *205*
   malignant tumors of, 214
   mirror examination of, 209–211, *209*
   papillomas of, 212
   phonation activity of, 204
   webs of, 212
Late luteal phase dysphoric disorder. See *Premenstrual syndrome (PMS).*
Laurence-Moon-Biedl syndrome, weight gain in, 502
Learning theory, anxiety defined in, 30
Lecithin:cholesterol acyltransferase (LCAT), 225
   deficiency of, 227
Left ventricular dysfunction, cough and, 115
   diastolic, 103
   systolic versus diastolic, 99
Leiomyoma, uterine, polycythemia associated with, 378
Leiomyomata, uterine, 335
Lenegre's diffuse conduction system disease, bradycardia associated with, 62(t)
Lennox-Gastaut syndrome, 417
Lesch-Nyhan syndrome, 43, 240, 243
Leucine aminopeptidase, levels in cholestasis, 86
Leukemia, limb pain associated with in children, 290
   lymphocytic, chronic, lymphadenopathy in, 294
Leukoencephalopathy, progressive multifocal, MRI evaluation of, 284
Leukoplakia, hairy, HIV and, 217
Levodopa, athetosis caused by, 43
Liability risk, in failure to identify HIV infection, 215
Lichen planus, oral ulcers associated with, 326, *326*
Limb pain in childhood, 287–291
   assessment of, 291
   diagnostic studies in, 289–291
   grading of muscle strength in, 288(t)
   growing pains as, 291
   history in, 287–288

Limb pain in childhood (*continued*)
  joint examination in, 288–289
  physical examination and, 288–289
Linear IgA dermatosis, 491
Lipids, dry eye syndrome and, 123
  transport system, 224
Lipids Research Clinics (LRC) Primary Prevention
      Trial, 223
Lipoprotein lipase, deficiency of, 230
  inhibitor deficiency, 230
Lipoproteins, atherosclerosis and, 223
  classifying disorders of, 229t
  genetic disorders and, 226
  high-density (HDL), 223
  low-density lipoprotein (LDL) receptor gene, 223,
      229–230
  Lp(a), 225
  metabolism of, 224–225
  testing for, in adults, 228(t)
  very low-density (VLDL), and athero-sclerosis, 223
Lithium, athetosis caused by, 43
  hypothyroidism associated with, 473
Livedo reticularis, and cardiolipin antibody syndrome,
      26
Liver, biopsy of, 89
  cholestasis arising from disorders of, 87
  EBV-related dysfunction of, 154
  enlarged. See *Hepatomegaly.*
Lonidamine, scrotal pain associated with, 395
Lovibond's angle, 94–95
Low blood sugar level. See *Hypoglycemia.*
Low-density lipoprotein (LDL), assessment of hyper-
      cholesterolemia and, 228–231
  atherosclerosis, 223
  in hyperapobetalipoproteinemia, 230–231
  receptor gene for, 229–230
Lumbar puncture, 285
  for fever assessment, 165
  for intracranial infection, 283
Lung, abscessed, cough and, 112
  biopsy of, 271–272
  interstitial disease of, 266–273. See also *Interstitial
      lung disease.*
Lupus erythematosus (LE), 485. See also *Systemic
      lupus erythematosus (SLE).*
  cell test for, 23
  FANA for identification of, 22
Luteinizing hormone-releasing hormone (LHRH), 133
Lyme disease, 294
  arthritis in, 364, 369
  bone pain in, 59
  limb pain in, 287, 289
  polyarticular arthritis and carditis in, 366
Lymphadenopathy, 292–299
  anatomic location of lymph nodes, *295*
      head and neck, 297–298
  assessment in, 297–299
  causes of, 293t
  definition of, 292
  diagnostic studies in, 296–297
  generalized, 298–299
  history in, 293–294
  HIV and AIDS associated with, 299
  mediastinal mass and, 301
  mediastinal, CT detection of, 307
  oral ulcers associated with, 325
  persistent generalized (PGL), 299
  physical examination and, 294–296
  postauricular, 297

Lymphadenopathy (*continued*)
  submandibular, 297
  ulcers associated with, 323
Lymphangiectasia, steatorrhea with, 435
Lymphatic drainage, breast, 67
Lymphocyte stimulation, food-allergy studies, 170
Lymphocytic interstitial pneumonitis (LIP), 267
Lymphocytic leukemia, chronic, lymphadenopathy in,
      294
Lymphomas, 293
Lymphoproliferative malignancy, 510
Lymphoreticular malignancy, nephropathy following
      treatment for, 248
Lysergic acid diethylamide (LSD), 174

Macular function, evaluating, 493
  degeneration of, 495–496, *495*
Magenblase syndrome, 277
Magnesium deficiency. See *Hypomagnesemia.*
Magnetic resonance imaging (MRI), for abdominal pain
      evaluation, 5
  for ataxia evaluation, 39
  for bone pain evaluation, 57
  for differentiating benign and malignant breast
      neoplasms, 71
  for fever assessment, 164
  for hearing loss evaluation, 182
  for hepatomegaly evaluation, 201
  for hoarseness evaluation, 212
  for infarction identification in TIA, 477
  for intracranial infection evaluation, 284
  for intracranial tumor evaluation, 310
  for limb pain evaluation, 290
  for mediastinal and hilar blood vessel study, 304
  for pelvic mass evaluation, 338
  for pericarditis evaluation, 345
  for polyarticular arthritis evaluation, 369
  for scrotal pain evaluation, 397
  for seizure evaluation, 415
  for TGA evaluation, 10
  for TIA evaluation, 480
  hepatic, 196
Major histocompatibility complex (MHC), rheumatoid
      arthritis and, 365
Malabsorption, carbohydrates and, 118
  diagnostic assessment of, *434*
  diarrhea and, 117, 121
  intestinal gas associated with, 276
  physical findings and signs associated with, 433t
  steatorrhea associated with, 432
Maldigestion, intestinal gas associated with, 276
Males. See also *Gender differences.*
  breast mass in, 72
  dysuria in, 140–141
Malignancy. See also *Cancer; Tumors*, and specific
      neoplasm.
  acanthosis nigricans associated with, 236
  bone pain associated with, 55
  lymphoproliferative, Sjögren's syndrome as risk
      factor in, 510
  lymphoreticular, nephropathy following treatment for,
      248
  pericarditis associated with, 346
Mammography, for breast mass assessment, 70
Manic-depressive disorder, 154
  fatigue related to, 153
  hallucinations in, 173, 177
Marcus Gunn pupil, 494

Marfan's syndrome, aortic dissection associated with, 74–75
  systolic murmurs associated with, 446
Marinesco-Sjögren's syndrome, ataxia associated with, 38
Markers, antigen, narcolepsy and hypersomnia identified with, 429
  tumor, 338
Maternal deaths. See *Mortality rate, in ectopic pregnancy*.
Mazindol, scrotal pain associated with use of, 395
MEA III syndrome, hypertension and, 405
Mediastinal mass, 300–307
  assessment of, 306–307, *306*
  biopsy of, 304–305
  diagnostic studies in, 303–304, *306*
  etiology of, 301–302, 302t, 305t
  occult, 303t
  physical signs in, 302–303
  symptoms of, 302
Mediastinoscopy, for mediastinal mass evaluation, 305
Mediastinum, anatomy of, 300
    diagram of compartments of, *301*
    disease(s) of, CT for evaluating, 304t
      emphysema (pneumomediastinum), 300
      infection, 438
      mediastinitis, 300–301
Medications, unintended effects of. See also *Drugs; Oral contraceptives*.
  ANA induced by, 24–25t
  anorexia as a side effect of, 18
  anticonvulsant toxicity and ataxia, 40
  anxiety associated with, 31
  athetosis due to, 43
  constipation assessment and, 108
  constipation caused by, 107t
  diarrhea and, 119
  dry eye syndrome and, 123
  ectopic pregnancy and oral contraceptives, 143
  excessive sleepiness and, 426
  fibrositis from interleukin-2-therapy, 155
  hallucinations associated with, 178
  hallucinations caused by, 174
  heart failure precipitated by, 101
  hematochezia associated with, 189
  hoarseness caused by, 206
  hyperpigmentation induced by, 238t
  hypertriglyceridemia exacerbated by, 230
  hypomagnesemia caused by, 258
  interstitial pulmonary disease caused by, 268
  keratoconjunctivitis medicamentosa, 127
  lupus induced by, 27
  lymphadenopathy caused by, 294
  Raynaud's phenomenon induced by, 387
  secondary hypertension associated with, 403
  sleep patterns and, 427
  xerostomia caused by, 514
Melanin, 233
  synthesis of, *234*
Melanoderma, 233
Melanoma, malignant, breast cancer risk in, 68
Melanosis, 233
Memory, 7. See also *Amnesia*.
  damage to, in Korsakoff psychosis, 14
Menarche, normal progression of, 309
Meniere's syndrome, 183
Meningitic syndrome (neutrophil predominant CSF), etiologies of, 285t
Meningitis, tuberculous, amnesia associated with, 15

Meningitis syndrome (lymphocyte predominant CSF), etiologies of, 285t
Menopause, premature, 310–311
Menstrual dysfunction, 308–314
  androgenic disorders and, 311–313
  hypothalamic-pituitary disorders associated with, 309–310
  oligomenorrhea and, obesity associated with, 505
  outflow obstruction to menses, 335
  ovarian cyst and, 334–335
  ovaries
    polycystic, weight gain and, 505
    premature failure of, 310–311
  treatment of, 313–314
Mental disorders, organic syndromes, 178t
    sleepiness, excessive, secondary to, 428
    Wernicke encephalopathy, confusion in, 12
Mental retardation, secondary seizure disorder and, 414
Mental status examination (MSE), 282
  in anxiety evaluation, 31–32
  in hallucination assessment, 175–176
  in memory deficit identification, 414
Metabolic disorders, athetosis due to, 43
    constipation in, 106t
      chronic, 109
    hallucinations associated with, 174, 177
    phantogeusia and, 349
Metabolism, of purines, 240
  synthesis and degradation of, *241*
Metaplasia, 328
  squamous, 123
Metastases, pelvic masses in, 336
  to bone, 54
Methane excretion, intestinal gas associated with, 275
Methemoglobinemia, 377–378
3-Methoxy-4-hydroxy phenethyleneglycol (MHPG), 154
N-Methyl-D-aspartate receptors, zinc relationship to, 156–157
Methylxanthines, anorexia as a side effect of, 18
Microcephaly, seizures and, 414
Microvascular angina, chest pain with, 73
Middle age, anorexia in, 20–21
Middle ear, hearing loss and, 182
Midline lesions, ataxia associated with, 40
Midsystolic murmur, 450
Migraines, equivalents of, 478
    headaches versus TIAs, 478–479
    retinal, 478
    seizures versus, 416
    TGA and, 9–10
Milk line, aberrant, 67
Minocycline, hyperpigmentation induced by, 238t
Mitral regurgitation, systolic murmurs with, 451
Mitral valve prolapse (MVP), 452
  anxiety associated with, 32–33
  chest pain associated with, 74, 77
Mixed connective tissue disease (MCTD), 27
M-mode echocardiography, 450
"Mono syndrome," 298–299
Mononeuritis syndrome, polyarteritis associated with, 359
Mononucleosis, infectious, stridor associated with, 438
Monosodium urate (MSU), deposition in gouty arthritis, 246
Montgomery glands, 67
Mood disorders, insomnia associated with, 266
Mortality rate, in acute renal failure, 51
  in azotemia, postpartum, 51
  in ectopic pregnancy, 142–143, *143*

Mortality rate (*continued*)
  in emergent GI bleeding, 192
  in epiglottitis, 437
  in upper airway obstruction, 436
Motility, ocular, 38
Movement disorders, 42t. See also *Ataxia; Athetosis;*
    Dyskinesia; Paroxysmal disorders.
  paroxysmal dyskinesias versus MIRE, 45
Mucin deficiency, dry eye syndrome and, 123t
Multiple endocrine adenomatosis (MEA), secondary
    hypertension and, 403
Multiple myeloma, 54
  alkaline phosphatase levels in, 86
  bone pain associated with, 56
  hypercalcemia associated with, 245
Multiple sclerosis (MS), ataxia associated with, 40
  hearing loss associated with, 184
  TIAs and, 476
Multiple sleep latency tests (MSLTs), 265, 431
Mumps, orchitis in, 399
Munchausen's syndrome, by proxy, and fever, 160
  electronic, 65
Murmurs, continuous, 452–453
  crescendo-decrescendo, 450
  holosystolic, 450, *451*, 452
  systolic, 79–80, 444–453
    ejection, *451*
    etiology of, 448t
Murphy's sign, 80
Muscle biopsy, for polyarteritis identification, 360, 362
Muscle strength, grading of, 288t
Musculoskeletal pain, radiographic evaluation of, 57t
Myasthenia gravis, hoarseness and, 214
  mediastinal mass in, 303
Mycobacterium tuberculosis, oral ulcers associated
    with, 325
Myocardial cells, 61
  depolarization of, *61*
Myocardial infarction, acute, diagnosis of, 85
  bradycardia due to, 66
  chest pain associated with, 77
  congestive heart failure and, 103
  FCHL incidence associated with, 230
  polyarteritis associated with, 360
Myocardial ischemia. See also *Hypoxemia; Silent*
    myocardial ischemia.
  autonomic denervation in, 420
  causes of, 74
  chest pain with, 73
  pericarditis versus, 342–343
  silent, 76, 419–424
Myocardium, congestive heart failure and, 98–99. See
    also *Myocardial infarction; Myocardial ischemia.*
Myoclonus, characteristics of, 42t
Myofascial pain, 315–320
  assessment of, 318–320
  diagnostic studies in, 318
  differential diagnosis of regional pain in, 319t
  history in, 316–317
  physical examination and, 317–318
  trigger points in, 317–318
Myomatous uterus, 337
Myopathy, chemotherapy-induced, 103
  hoarseness and, 208
Müllerian agenesis, amenorrhea associated with, 313

Narcolepsy, 425–426, 429
  sleep disorders versus, 430–431, 430t
  symptoms of, 427–428

Narcotics. See also *Drugs; Medications.*
  bone pain relief with, 55
National Center for Health Statistics, 509
Necrosis, congestive heart failure and, 98
  in testicular vasculitis, 361
Neonates. See also *Infants.*
  blisters in, causes of, 482t
  cyanosis in, 446
  fever in, 162, 163, 164, 165–166
  pelvic mass in, 334
  pyelonephritis associated with premature birth,
    140
  seizure etiology in, 412, 412t
  steatorrhea in, 433
  vesiculobullous lesions in, 483–484
Neoplasia, See also *Cancer; Malignancy; Tumors.*
  abdominal pain and, 1, 3
  anxiety associated with, 33t
  ataxia associated with, 37, 40
  bone pain associated with, 54, 59
  cervical, 328
    intraepithelial (CIN), 329
  cholestasis associated with, 87
  hyperuricemia associated with, 243
  ulcers secondary to, 327
  vasculitis associated with, 358–359
Nephropathy, diabetic, 382
  hyperuricemia and, 246–247
  lead, hyperuricemia in, 243
  lymphoreticular malignancy and, 248
  nephrotic syndrome, 385
Nerves, biopsy of, for polyarteritis identification, 360,
    362
  scrotal, 393–394, 394t
Neurologic disorders, anxiety associated with, 33t
  azotemia-related, 47–48
  constipation, 106t
    chronic, caused by, 109
  hallucinations in, 173, 177
  neuroacanthocytosis, 43
  neuroblastoma, and limb pain in children, 290
  neuroglycopenic response to hypoglycemia, 249–
    250
  neuropathy, hoarseness and, 208
    scrotal pain associated with, 401
  neurovascular compression syndrome, 387–388
  optic neuritis, 498
  polyarteritis and, 359
  vascular territory involved in symptoms, 476t
Neuroma, acoustic, 184
Neurometabolic disorders, athetosis due to, 42
Neuromuscular system, chest pain and, 78
Neuropathy, anterior ischemic optic (AION), 497
Neutrophil chemotaxis, food-allergy studies, 170
Nicotine, anxiety associated with, 34
Nicotinic acid, hyperuricemia caused by, 243
Nikolsky's sign, 326
Nitrofurantoin, pneumonitis caused by, 268
Nitroglycerin, for pain relief in angina, 76
Nocturnal dyspnea, paroxysmal (PND), 445
Nocturnal myoclonus, 265
Non-islet cell tumor, hypoglycemia associated with,
    257
Nonessential hypertension, 403–410
Non-Hodgkin's lymphoma, 293
Nonrheumatic disease-ANA associations, 24, 24t
Nonsteroidal anti-inflammatory drugs (NSAIDs), bone
    pain and, 54, 55
  hematochezia caused by, 189
  renal impairment caused by, 247

Norepinephrine, anxiety and, 29, 30
    appetite and, 16–17
    PMS symptoms caused by, 156
Nucleic acids, hyperuricemia, and turnover rates of, 243
5-Nucleotidase, levels in cholestasis, 86
Nutrition, assessment of, in foods, and flatus, 280
    deficient, ataxia in, 39
    in anorexia, tests for, 20
    in hypercholesterolemia, 226
    in hypomagnesemia, 258
    in steatorrhea, 432
    management of, for hypercholesterolemia, 232
        for hyperuricemia, 248
Nystagmus, and hypomagnesemia, 259–260

Obesity. See also *Weight gain.*
    hepatomegaly and, 203
    in hypoglycemia, 253–254, 255
    serum uric acid levels and, 239
    silent myocardial ischemia associated with, 422
    sleep apnea and, 265
Obsessive-compulsive disorders, anxiety associated with, 31, 35
Obstruction, chronic abdominal pain associated with, 3
    extrathoracic, airway dynamics associated with, *439*
        flow-volume loop in, *443*
    in sleep apnea, 430t
Occupational exposure, asthma from, 115
    cough and, 113
    interstitial pulmonary disease and, 269
    liver disease and, 198
    lymphadenopathy related to, 294
    Raynaud's phenomenon and, risk of, 387
    to chemicals causing hypersomnia, 426
    to stress, anorexia due to, 18
Ocular disorders. See also *Optic disorders; Visual loss.*
    cicatricial pemphigoid, 123, 127–128
    motility and, ataxia associated with, 38
    surface pathology, dry eye syndrome and, 123t
Olfactory hallucinations, olfactory pathway pathology and, 173–174
Oligoarticular reactive arthritis, HIV-related, 365
Oligomenorrhea, obesity associated with, 505
    treatment of, 313–314
Olivopontocerebellar atrophy (OPCA), ataxia associated with, 38
Open angle glaucoma (COAG), chronic, 494
Ophthalmoplegia, Wernicke encephalopathy characterized by, 12
Optic disorders. See also *Ocular disorders; Visual loss.*
    and hallucinations, 173
    ataxia, 36–37
        atrophy associated with, 38
    neuritis, 498
    neuropathy (AION), anterior ischemic, 497
Oral challenge, food-allergy identification, 170
Oral contraceptives, liver disease risk and, 198
    zinc deficiency caused by, 157
Oral glucose tolerance test (OGTT), 256
Oral hypoglycemic agents (OHAs), 252
Oral pain, phantogeusia as an atypical form of, 349
Oral ulcers, 321–327
    assessment of, 324–327
    diagnostic studies of, 323–324
    history in, 321–322
    physical examination and, 322–323
Orchialgia. See *Scrotal pain.*
Orchitis, scrotal pain associated with, 399

Organic mental syndromes, differential diagnosis of, 178t
Orientation/disorientation, with respect to time, 8
Oropyrosis, phantogeusia associated with, 351
Orthostatic (postural) proteinuria, 380, 385
Osmotic diarrhea, 118
    versus secretory diarrhea, 118t, 121
Osmotic gap, in secretory diarrhea and osmotic diarrhea, 121
Osteoarthritis (OA), 319, 363
    diagnostic imaging to evaluate, 368
    polyarthritis in, 369
Osteoarthropathy, hypertrophic (HOA), clubbing and, 91, 93t
Osteogenic sarcoma, 54
Osteoid osteoma, limb pain associated with in children, 291
Osteomalacia, 53
Osteomyelitis, bone pain associated with, 58
    limb pain associated with, 290
Otorhinolaryngology, and sleep apnea evaluation, 429
Otosyphilis, inner-ear deafness associated with, 183
Ovary, cancer of, 335
    cyst in, 334–335
    neoplasms of, 337
    obesity, and functioning of, 503
    ovarian pregnancy, incidence of, 143
    polycystic syndrome (Stein-Leventhal syndrome), 503
    premature failure of, 310–311
Oxygen, environmental exposure to, and pulmonary fibrosis, 268
    erythrocytosis due to defective transport of, 377

P wave, 461
    morphology during tachycardia, 457
Pacemaker cells, 61
    depolarization in, *61*
Pachydermoperiostosis, 91, 94
Paget's disease, 86
    hyperuricemia associated with, 245
Pain, abdominal, chronic, causes of, 2t
    anxiety, and control of, 33
    bone, 52–60
        referred, 52
    bradycardia associated with, 61
    epigastric, 5–6
    factors that alter, 3
    in polyarticular arthritis, 363–371
    musculoskeletal, radiographic evaluation of, 57t
    myofascial, referred, 317
    oral ulcers and, 322
    parietal, 1
    pelvic, in endometriosis, 335
    perception of, 1
    phantogeusia as atypical, 349, 356
    polyarticular arthritis and, 364
    referred, 1, 317, 394, 401–402
        trigger points and, 315
    regional, 319t
        differential diagnosis of, 319
    scrotal, 392–402
        causes of, 395t, *398*
        inguinal causes of, 395, 395t
        pathology and, 395, 395t
        referred, 401–402
    substernal. See *Chest pain.*
    threshold, and silent myocardial ischemia, 420

Pain (*continued*)
   thyroid, 473–474
      enlargement accompanied by, 470
      visceral disease, and referred, 318
Pallid infantile syncope, seizure simulated by, 415–416
Palmar erythema, abdominal pain associated with, 3
Panarteritis, *358*
Pancreatic insufficiency, diarrhea and, 121
Pancreatitis, characterizing, 435
   chronic, serum trypsinogen
      radioimmunoassay (RIA) for
      diagnosis, 434
Panic disorder, anxiety associated with, 35
   experimentally induced, 29
Pap smear, abnormal, 328–333
   assessment of, 332–333, *332*
   diagnostic assessment of, 330–332, *333*
   history in, 329–330
   physical examination and, 330
Papilledema, funduscopy to identify, 414
Papillitis, *498*
Papillomas, 213
Paragangliomas, 307
Paraneoplastic syndrome, 39
Parasitic infestation, anorexia associated with, 17
Parasomnias, 416
Parasympathetic system, uric acid regulation by, 240
Parietal pain, 1
Parkinson's disease, insomnia associated with, 266
   muscular atrophy and ataxia in, 39
   voice quality in, 205
Parotid duct, 507, *512*
Paroxysmal disorders, dyskinesias versus MIRE, 45
   dystonic choreoathetosis (PDC), 43
   kinesigenic choreoathetosis (PKC), 43
   nocturnal dyspnea (PND), 445
Partial thromboplastin time (PTT), for polyarticular
      arthritis evaluation, 367
Parvovirus, polyarteritis associated with, 358
Patellofemoral syndrome, limb pain associated with, in
      children, 291
Pavor nocturnus, 416
Pelizaeus-Merzbacher disease, 42–43
Pelvic congestion syndrome, 134
Pelvic mass in female patient, assessment of, 338–
      340, *339*
   diagnostic studies of, 338
   history in, 334–336
   physical examination and, 336–338
Pelvic pain, endometriosis and, 335
Pelvic surgery, deep dyspareunia and, 133–134
Pemphigoid, cicatricial bullous, 488
Pemphigus vulgaris, 486–487, *487*
   oral ulcers in, 326
Penicillamine, zinc deficiency caused by, 157
Peptic ulcer disease, 275
   chest pain associated with, 78
Percutaneous transhepatic cholangiography (PTC), 5
   for cholestasis evaluation, 89
   for hepatomegaly evaluation, 201
Pericardial tamponade, 344
Pericardiocentesis, 346
Pericarditis, 341–348
   acute, electrocardiographic stages of, 344t
   assessment of, 346
   causes of, 342t
   chest pain associated with, 77
   definition of, 341–342
   diagnostic studies in, 344–346
   drugs causing, 347t

Pericarditis (*continued*)
   history in, 342–343
   physical examination and, 343–344
   polyarteritis associated with, 360
   precordial pain with, 74
Peripartum cardiomyopathy, 100
Peritoneoscopy, hepatomegaly evaluation with, 202
Persistence, of asymptomatic viral infections, 220
Persistent generalized lymphadenopathy (PGL), 299
Petit mal seizure, 417–418
Ph, vaginal, 132
Phantogeusia, 348–356
   characteristics of, 349–352
   definition of, 348
   etiology of, 351–352, 352t
   management of, 356
   patient diagnosis and, 354, 354t
   phantosmia associated with, 355, 355t
   quality of taste in, descriptive, 353t
   taste and smell changes associated with, 355t
   taste distortions in, *349*
   types of, 350t
Phantosmia, phantogeusia and, 355t
Pharmacologic constipation, 106t
Phencyclidine (PCP), hallucinations and, 174
Phenytoin (Dilantin), ataxia caused by, 38, 40
   athetosis caused by, 43
Pheochromocytoma, 304, 403, 407–408, 410
   diagnostic assessment of, *408*
   hypertension and, 405
   laboratory findings in, 408t
Phobias, defined, 29
   simple, 34
   social, 34–35
Phosphokinase, creatine, (CPK) serum levels, and
      azotemia, 49
5-Phosphoribosyl-1-pyrophosphate synthetase (PRPP-S)
      increase, in purine metabolism, 242
Photic stimulation, seizures associated with, 413
Physical exertion, angina induced by, 76
   diarrhea following, 120
Phytanic acid, ataxia associated with elevated levels, 39
Phytase, zinc deficiency caused by, 157
Pilocarpine, dry eye syndrome caused by, 123
Pituitary, damage to, and amenorrhea, 310
   hormone impairment in obese subjects, 504
   obesity and, 503, 504
Pituitary-adrenal function, obesity associated with, 505
Plasma creatinine levels (Pcr), azotemia defined by, 46
Plasma glucose levels, hypoglycemia evaluation and,
      255
Platelet-derived growth factor (PDGF), clubbing and, 93
Platybasia, ataxia associated with, 37
Pleuritis, polyarticular arthritis associated with, 366
Pneumoconioses, 113
Pneumocystis carinii pneumonia (PCP), diagnosis with
      BAL, 271
   prophylaxis against, 221, 221t
Pneumomediastinum (mediastinal emphysema), 300
Pneumonia, *Pneumocystis carinii* (PCP), diagnosis with
      BAL, 271
   eosinophilic, interstitial pulmonary disease associ-
      ated with, 272
   prophylaxis against, 221, 221t
Pneumonitis, bronchiolitis obliterans interstitial (BIP),
      267
   desquamative interstitial (DIP), 267
   hypersensitivity, 115
   interstitial lymphocytic (LIP), 267
   nitrofurantoin and, 268

Pneumoscrotum, 397, 401–402

Pneumothorax, interstitial pulmonary disease with, 269

Poisoning, hallucinations associated with, 174

Polyarteritis, 357–362

  assessment of, 361–362

  clinical features of, 359–360, 359t

  diagnostic criteria for the classification of, 361, 361t

  diagnostic studies in, 360–361, 361t

  nodosa, azotemia associated with, 48

  vasculitides, classification of, 358t

Polyarticular arthritis, 363–371

  assessment of, 369–371, *370*

  definition of, 363

  diagnostic assessment of, *370*

  diagnostic studies in, 367–369, 367t

  history in, 364–365

  physical examination and, 366

Polycythemia, primary erythrocytosis and, 377

Polycystic kidney disease, hematuria in, 385

  hypertension and, 405

  hyperuricemia in, 243

  secondary hypertension and, 403

Polycystic ovary syndrome (Stein-Leventhal syndrome), obesity associated with, 503

Polycythemia, 372–378, 446–447

  assessment of, 375–378

  definition of, 372

  diagnostic criteria in polycythemia vera, 376t

  diagnostic studies in, 373–375, 375t

  evaluation of, and vitamin B_{12}-binding capacity, 374

  history in, 373

  physical examination and, 373

  serum uric acid levels in, 239

  smokers', 377

Polycythemia vera, 376

  hearing loss associated with, 184

  laboratory findings in, 375t

Polycythemia Vera Study Group (PVSG), diagnostic criteria suggested by, 376, 376t

Polymerase chain reaction (PCR) assay, HIV diagnosis with, 217, 219

  HIV infection staging with, 220–221

Polymyalgia rheumatica, 369

Polymyositis, Raynaud's phenomenon associated with, 391

Polypnea, defined, 463

Polypoid corditis, 213

Polyps, hematochezia associated with, 193

Polysomnographic study of sleep patterns, 265

Porphyria cutanea tarda, 487, *488*

  hyperpigmentation in, 237t

Positron emission tomography (PET), 172

Postauricular lymph nodes, lymphadenopathy of, 297

Postnasal drip, cough associated with, 111

Postpartum azotemia, mortality rate in, 51

Postprandial hypoglycemia, 256

Post-traumatic stress disorder, anxiety associated with, 31, 35

  insomnia associated with, 266

Post-traumatic amnesia, 11

Potassium. See also *Hyperkalemia; Hypokalemia.*

  changes in acute renal failure, 48t

  hypomagnesemia associated with deficiency, 261

Prader-Labhart-Willi syndrome, weight gain in, 502

Precocious puberty, endocrinologically active tumor and, 334

Precordial discomfort, gastrointestinal disorders associated with, 78–79

Preeclampsia, hyperuricemia in, 243

Pregnancy, 309. See also *Ectopic pregnancy.*

  abnormal pap smear during, 332

  alkaline phosphatase levels in, 86

  breast lump assessment during, 71–72

  cardiomyopathy associated with, 100

  clubbing in, 97

  dyspareunia related to, 134

  dysuria associated with, 139–140

  ELISA tests during, false positives, 218

  enlarged uterus caused by, 337

  hyperemesis gravidarum, thiamine deficiency in, 12

  hyperpigmentation in, 236

  miscarriages and cardiolipin antibody syndrome, 26

  outcomes of, and positive ANA, 24

  pelvic mass associated with, 335

  peripartum cardiomyopathy and, 100

  pheochromocytoma in, 407

  postpartum azotemia in, 51

  postpartum painless thyroiditis in, 473

  preeclampsia in, 243

  testing for, 338

  thiamine deficiency in, 12

  ultrasonography, and diagnosis of abnormal, 148

Pregnanediol-3-glucuronide (PDG), ectopic pregnancy and levels of, *148*

Prehn's sign, 396–397

Premature births, pyelonephritis associated with, 140

Premature coronary artery disease, silent myocardial ischemia associated with, 422

Premature menopause, 310–311

Premature ovarian failure, 310–311

Premenopausal patients, assessment of breast mass in, *70*

Premenstrual syndrome (PMS), fatigue associated with, 155–156

  late luteal phase dysphoric disorder, 152–153

Prerenal azotemia, renal azotemia versus, 49, 49t

Primary bone tumors, lesions that simulate, 59t

Prinzmetal's angina, 83

  chest pain with, 73

Progesterone, levels in pathologic pregnancies, 147

  pain from effect on smooth muscle and, 2

Progressive multifocal leukoencephalopathy, MRI evaluation of, 284

Proinsulin, hypoglycemia evaluation and, 256

Prolactin level, for seizure diagnosis, 417

  response, to hypoglycemia and TRH, 504

  seizure-related, 415

Prolactinoma, 309

  amenorrhea associated with, 310

Prostaglandins, and bone pain, 53

  fever and, 159

Prostatitis, dysuria associated with, 141, *141*

Protein values, urinary, 380t

Protein-losing enteropathy, 434, 435

Proteinuria, 379–385

  assessment of, 384–385

  causes of, 381t

  definition of, 380

  diagnostic studies in, 384

  history in, 382–383

  laboratory evaluation of, 384t

  physical examination and, 383–384

  urinary protein values in, 380t

Prune-belly syndrome, 383

Pruritus, cholestasis and, 87, 197

  polycythemia vera and, 376

Pseudobradycardia, 65

Pseudocholinesterase levels, PMS and, 155

Pseudoclubbing, 95t, 96–97
Pseudogout, 364, 371. See also *Gout.*
　diagnostic imaging to evaluate, 368
　myofascial pain versus, 318
　polyarthritis in, 369
Pseudomyasthenia, mediastinal mass in, 303
Pseudoseizures, 415, 416–417
Psoriatic arthritis, 368
Psychiatric disorders. See also *Mental disorders.*
　anxiety associated with, 31
　hallucinations associated with, 173, 177
　hypersomnia, secondary, associated with, 426
　insomnia and, 264
Psychogenic factors, in amnesia, 15
　in chest pain, 79
　in hypersomnia, 430t
　in seizures, 416–417
　in xerostomia, 511
Psychophysiologic insomnia, 264, 265
Psychoses, differential diagnosis of, 177t
Puberty, precocious, and endocrinologically active
　　tumors, 334
Puerperal sepsis, thiamine deficiency in, 12
Pulmonary angiography, for chest pain assessment, 85
Pulmonary dysfunctions, chest pain associated with, 78
　edema and congestive heart failure and, 100
　embolism as, 85
　fibrosis as, 266–273
　liver disease and, 198
　mediastinal mass simulated by lesions and, 302
　neoplasms as, clubbing associated with, 96
　polyarteritis associated with, 360
　systolic murmurs and artery stenosis and, 450
　thromboembolism as, chest pain associated with, 75
Pulmonary function tests (PFTs), 270–271
　cough assessment with, 114–115
　stridor evaluation with, 442
Pulmonic ejection murmurs, 452
Pulse, arterial, and systolic murmur evaluation, 447
Purine metabolism, 240
　synthesis and degradation in, *241*
Purkinje system, 461
Pyelography, intravenous, 406
　retrograde, 49–50
Pyelonephritis, premature births associated with, 140
Pyogenic arthritis, 369
Pyrexia. See *Fever.*
Pyrogens, 159
Pyrosine, levels in chronic fatigue, 156
Pyruvate metabolism, in Friedrich's ataxia, 39–40

Q waves, in silent myocardial ischemia, 422

Racoon eyes, middle-ear deafness associated with, 183
Radiation dose, and iodine isotopes, choice of, 472
Radiation-induced pericarditis, 347
Radiculopathy, hypoglycemia and, 253
Radioactive iodine uptake, thyroid enlargement evalua-
　　tion using, 472
Radioallergosorbent test (RAST), 169
Radiocontrast media, nephrotoxicity of, 47
Radiographs, limb pain evaluation with, 290
Radioimmunoassay, C-peptide measurement, 255
Radioimmunoprecipitation assay (RIPA), HIV infection
　　identified with, 218
Radioisotope scans, 304
　for interstitial pulmonary disease evaluation, 270

Radioisotope scans (*continued*)
　for intracranial infection evaluation, 283t
　for polycythemia evaluation, 373–374
　for scrotal pain evaluation, 397
　for testicular torsion evaluation, 397
　technetium, for bone assessment, 56–57
Radionuclide imaging, 290
　angiograms, congestive heart failure assessment with,
　　103
　auditory evaluation with, 182
　chest pain assessment with, 81–82, 85
　exercise testing measurement with ventriculography,
　　422
　fever assessment with, 164
　hematochezia evaluation with, 186, 191–192
　renal function evaluation with, 49
　thyroid evaluation with, 474
Radiotherapy, ovarian failure caused by, 311
Ramsay Hunt syndrome, 297
　inner-ear deafness associated with, 125t, 183
Rapid eye movement (REM) sleep, fibrositis and,
　　155
　　hallucinations associated with disturbance in,
　　　172
　　narcolepsy and, 425, 430
Rat-bite fever, 294
Raynaud's phenomenon, 155, 386–391
　and associated diseases, 388t
　　assessment of, 390–391
　azotemia associated with, 48
　chest pain associated with, 77
　connective tissue disease and, 390–391
　　definition of, 386
　　diagnostic studies in, 389–390
　　history in, 387–388
　　incidence of, 386–387
　　physical examination and, 388–389
　　primary, 390–391
　scleroderma and, 391
　　secondary, 390
　underlying condition in, 389t
Receptors, chronic cough causes and, 111
　ventilation and, 464t
Reciprocating tachycardia, AV, 461
Rectal bleeding. See *Hematochezia.*
Red cell mass, determination of, 373–374
　hyperuricemia and, 239
Re-entrant tachyarrhythmias, 454
Re-entrant tachycardia, 458–459, 460, 461
Referred pain, 1, 394
　bone, 52
　myofascial, 317
　scrotal, 401–402
　trigger points and, 315
　visceral disease and, 318
Reflex, cremasteric, 397
Refsum's disease, 39
　ataxia associated with, 38
Regional lymphadenopathy, 292
Regional pain, differential diagnosis of, 319
Reiter's syndrome, 363, 365, 371
　diagnostic imaging to evaluate, 368
Relative afferent papillary defect (RAPD), 494, 498
Relative erythrocytosis, laboratory findings in, 375
Renal biopsy, 50, 384
　for polyarteritis identification, 362
Renal cell carcinoma, polycythemia associated with,
　　378
Renal control, of uric acid, 240–242, *241*

Renal disease(s)/dysfunction(s), arterial lesion as, hypertension and, 405
  arterial stenosis as, progression of, 4
  contrast-dye induced, 360
  erythrocytosis due to, 378
  polyarteritis and, 359
  transplantation in, and erythrocytosis, 378
  tubular acidosis as, hyperuricemia associated with, 245
  uric acid underexcretion associated with, 243
Renal failure. See also *Azotemia.*
  and hyperuricemia, incidence in, 247
  biochemical changes in acute, 48t
  hyperpigmentation in, 237t
  insomnia associated with, 266
  lecithin:cholesterol acyltransferase deficiency and, 227
Renin-angiotensin system, congestive heart failure and, 98
Renovascular hypertension, 405–407, 405t
  diagnostic assessment of, 406
  symptoms raising suspicion of, 405
Replacement fibrosis, congestive heart failure and, 98
Respiratory dysfunction, anxiety and, 32, 33t
  clubbing associated with, 96
  food allergy and, 168t
Retinal disorders, central artery occlusion (CRAO), 496, *496*
  central vein occlusion, 497, *497*
  detachment, 496
  infarction, 478
  migraine and, 478
  retinitis pigmentosa, ataxia associated with, 38
Retinoids, dry eye syndrome caused by, 123
Retrograde amnesia, 9, 10–11
  Korsakoff psychosis and, 13
  recovery after infection, 15
Retrograde cholangiopancreatography (ERCP), hepatomegaly evaluation with, 201
Retrograde pyelography, 49–50
Retroperitoneal causes for referred scrotal pain, 394, 395t
Retrovir. See *Azidothymidine (AZT).*
Reversible ischemic neurologic deficit (RIND), 475
Reye's syndrome, 197, 202
Rheumatic fever, limb pain associated with, 287
  polyarthritis in, 369
  systolic murmurs associated with, 445
Rheumatoid arthritis (RA), 214, 363
  ANA positive test in, 27
  diagnostic imaging to evaluate, 368
  differentiating from psoriatic arthritis, 368
  lymphadenopathy in, 294
  percentage positive FANA with, 23t
  polyarthritis in, 369
  proteinuria associated with, 383
  Sjögren's syndrome associated with, 124
Rheumatoid factor, associated with Sjögren's syndrome, 127
  ELISA tests, false positive associated with, 218
  gouty arthritis and, 246
  polyarteritis and, 360
Rhythm, ventricular, bradycardia associated with, 65
Right upper quadrant (RUQ) pain, 6
Rinne test of hearing, 182
Risk factors, for acute azotemia, 51
  for atherosclerosis, 223, 478
  for avascular necrosis of the femoral head, 54
  for breast cancer, 68
  for cervical neoplasias, 329

Risk factors (*continued*)
  for colorectal cancer, 193
  for congestive heart failure, 100
  for coronary artery disease (CAD), 77, 79, 223, 225, 248, 422
    by gender, 232
  for dysplasia with polyps and bleeding, 193
  for ectopic pregnancy, 143, 145, 145t
  for HIV infection, 216, 216t
  for occult bacteremia, 160t
  for ovarian tumors, 311
  for Raynaud's phenomenon, 387
  in lymphadenopathy, for diseases associated with, 298
Ritter's disease, 484
Rokitansky-Kuster-Hauser syndrome, amenorrhea associated with, 313
Rolandic epilepsy, 418
Romberg test, 182
Rose bengal staining, for dry eye evaluation, 126
Rotator cuff tendinitis, 55
Rotor's syndrome, 86–87

Salicylates, hyperuricemia caused by, 244
Salivary gland(s), 506
  biopsy of, 513–514
  innervation and autonomic function, *508*
  labial biopsy of minor, 513–514
  minor, *514*
Salivary scintigraphy, xerostomia evaluation with, 513
Salpingitis, 335
  ectopic pregnancy associated with, 143
Sarcoidosis, cough and, 115
  interstitial pulmonary disease associated with, 267, 272
  mediastinal mass associated with, 301
Sarcoma, osteogenic, 54
Sarcoma botryoides, pelvic mass associated with, 336
Savage's syndrome, 311
Schamroth's sign, 95
Schirmer test, dry eye evaluation with, 126
Schizophrenia, hallucinations in, 173, 177
  insomnia associated with, 266
Scintigraphy, biliary, abdominal pain evaluation with, 4
  hepatic, 196
  hepatomegaly evaluation with, 201
  pheochromocytoma evaluation with, 407–408
  renal, 407
  salivary, xerostomia evaluation with, 513
Scleroderma, acanthosis nigricans, 236
  ANA positive test in, 27
  azotemia associated with, 48
  hyperpigmentation in, 237t
  myofascial pain distinguished from, 318
  percentage positive FANA with, 23t
  polyarticular arthritis associated with, 366
  Raynaud's phenomenon associated with, 389–390
  systemic lupus erythematosus (SLE) associated with, 391
Sclerosing cholangitis, 88
Scrotal pain, 392–402
  causes of, 395t, 397–402, *398*
  diagnostic studies in, 397
  differential diagnosis of, 394–395, 395t
  history in, 395–396
  inguinal causes of, 395, 395t

Scrotal pain (*continued*)
  management of, 402
  pathology and, 395, 395t
  physical examination and, 396–397
Scrotum, anatomy of, 392–394, 394t
Seattle Heart Watch study, 420
Secondary hypertension, 403–410
  assessment of, 405–410
  causes of, 404t
  definition of, 403
  diagnostic studies in, 405
  estrogen-induced, 410
  genetic conditions associated with, 404t
  history in, 403–404
  pheochromocytoma and, *408*
    laboratory findings in, 408t
  physical examination and, 404–405
  primary aldosteronism and, 409–410, *409*
  renovascular hypertension and, 405–407, 405t
    diagnosis of, 406, *406*
Secretory diarrhea, 118
  osmotic diarrhea versus, 118t
Sedative withdrawal, anxiety associated with, 34
Seizures. See also *Epilepsy.*
  complex partial, 412
  etiologies of, 412t
  grand mal, 260
  head trauma and, 413
  hypersomnia and, 426
  hypertonicity, and secondary disorder, 414
  partial complex, hallucinations associated with, 178
  petit mal, 417–418
  TGA differentiated from, 10
Seizures in childhood, assessment of, 415–418
  classification of, 412t
  definition of, 411
  diagnostic studies in, 414–415
  differential diagnosis of, 415–417
  etiologies of, by age, 412t
  history in, 412–413
  management of, 418
  physical examination and, 413–414
Sensory ataxia, 36–37
Separation anxiety, 30
Septic arthritis, bone pain associated with, 58
Seroconversion syndrome, in HIV infection, 221
Serologic tests, evaluating the significance of a positive ANA, 26t
Serum calcium, constipation and, 107
Serum electrolytes, constipation and, 107
Serum trypsinogen radioimmunoassay (RIA), 434
Set point theory, 499
Sexual response, functional interference with, 129
Sexually transmitted diseases, 335
  HPV infection, 328
Shortness of breath, tachyarrhythmias with, 455
Shuddering attacks, seizures simulated by, 416
Shy-Drager syndrome, 39
Sialochemistry, xerostomia evaluation and, 514
Sialography, xerostomia evaluation with, 513
Sicca syndrome, 27, 509–510
Sigmoidoscopy, compared with colonoscopy, 194
Silent myocardial ischemia, 76, 419–424
  assessment of, 423–424
  classification of patients in, 419
  diagnostic studies in, 422–424
  history in, 421–422
  mechanism of, 419–420

Silent myocardial ischemia (*continued*)
  physical examination and, 422
  prognosis in, 420–421
Single photon emission computed tomography (SPECT), chest pain evaluation with, 81
  hallucination evaluation with, 172
Sinoatrial (SA) exit block, bradycardia associated with, 63
Sinoatrial (SA) node, 453
Sinus bradycardia, 62, *62*, *64*
Sinus x-rays, cough assessment with, 114
Sinusitis, cough associated with, 111
Sitophobia, anorexia and, 17–18
Situational-related amnesias, 15
Sjögren's syndrome, 25, 26, 509–510, 515. See also *Dry eye.*
  ANA positive test in, 27
  defined, 124
  FANA positive test in, 23t
  hoarseness in, 209, 214
  phantogeusia associated with, 354
  polyarticular arthritis associated with, 366
  Raynaud's phenomenon associated with, 388
  rheumatoid factor and, 127
Skeletal disorders, mediastinal mass caused by, 302
Skeletal survey, in bone pain assessment, 57
Skin. See also *Dermatologic dysfunction.*
  abnormality in, and abdominal pain, 3
  ANA positive tests and condition of, 25
  conductance of, during hallucinations, 172
  lesions, polyarteritis associated with, 360
  lipoprotein disorders and, 226t
  pachydermoperiostosis and, 95
  pigmentation, *234*
Skin testing, allergic response evaluation, 169
Skinfold calipers, for obesity measurement, 503
SLE. See *Systemic lupus erythematosus (SLE).*
Sleep disorders. See also *Sleepiness, excessive.*
  apnea, 264–265, 425, 426–427, 426t, 429, 430
    differentiating from other sleep disorders, 430–431, 430t
    obstructive, 430t
    REM sleep in, 430
    symptoms of, 428–429
  DIMS, 263–266
  DOES, 263
  myofascial pain associated with, 316
  nocturnal myoclonus, 265
  paralysis during sleep, 428
  paroxysmal nocturnal dyspnea (PND), 445
Sleep Disorders Association, American, 265
Sleep patterns, polysomnographic study of, 265
Sleepiness, excessive, 425–431. See also *Sleep disorders.*
  assessment of, 430–431
  clinical characteristics of sleep apnea, 426t
  definitions of disorders associated with, 425
  diagnostic studies in, 429–430
  differentiation among disorders causing, 430t
  history in, 427–429
  physical examination and, 429
Sleep-onset REM periods. See *Rapid eye movement (REM) sleep.*
Smell, changes associated with phantogeusia, 355t
Smoking, 269, 373
  breast cancer risk associated with, 68
  cervical cancer associated with, 329
  chronic cough and, 110–111
  hoarseness and, 208

Smoking (*continued*)
  ischemia associated with, 420
  laryngitis caused by, 213
  polycythemia associated with, 374, 377
  relative erythrocytosis associated with, 375
  silent myocardial ischemia associated with, 422
  sleep disturbance and, 427
  squamous cell carcinoma and, 327
  weight gain following cessation of, 502
Socioeconomic class, cervical cancer associated with, 329
Solute gap in osmotic diarrhea, 118
Somnambulism, 416
Somnolence, disorder of excessive (DOES), 263
Somogyi effect, 252
Sonography, for kidney size assessment, 49
    for mediastinal mass evaluation, 304
Sorbitol, diarrhea and, 118, 119
Spasms, characteristics of, 42t
Spermatic cord, *393*
Spermatic granuloma, 401
Sphincter of Oddi pressures, 5, 6
Splenomegaly, lymphadenopathy associated with, 296
    polycythemia vera associated with, 376
Spondyloarthropathies, seronegative, 371
Spondylolysis, 54
Sprue, diagnosing, 435
Sputum, cytologic examination, 114
Squamous cell carcinoma, 323
  hoarseness associated with, 214
  pelvic mass associated with, 336
  ulcerated, *327*
Squamous metaplasia, 123
ST depression, exercise testing measurement, 422
    ischemia marker, 424
    morbidity and mortality associated with, 421
Stable angina, 421
  evaluation of, 423
Starvation, insulinoma verification with, 257
Status marmoratus, 42
Steatocrit, steatorrhea evaluation with, 433
Steatorrhea, 432–435
  assessment of, 433–435, *434*
  associated with cholestasis, 87
  diagnostic studies in, 433
  history in, 432–433
  intestinal gas associated with, 276
  malabsorption and, physical findings, 433t
Stein-Leventhal syndrome, 312–313
Sterilization, tubal, reversal of, and ectopic pregnancy, 145
Steroids, anabolic, liver disease risk and, 198
  17-hydroxy, and chronic fatigue, 158
Stevens-Johnson syndrome, 123, 127–128, 326
Stool examination, in diarrhea evaluation, 120, 121
Storage disorder, seizures and, 414
Stress, abdominal pain associated with, 3
    amenorrhea and, 310
    anxiety and, 32
    dietary, uric acid levels and, 240
    fatigue associated with, 156
    fugue state precipitated by, 15
    hypersomnia, secondary, associated with, 426
    insomnia and, 264
    ischemia associated with, 420
    mechanical, and myofascial pain, 315–316
    myocardial ischemia, silent, associated with, 422
    occupational, and anorexia, 18
    oral ulcers and, 322, 325

Stress (*continued*)
    post-traumatic
      anxiety associated with, 31, 35
      insomnia associated with, 266
      postural, and myofascial pain, 316
      TGA precipitated by, 10
Stress fractures, 53, 56
  bone pain in, 54
Stridor, 436–443
  assessment of, 442–443
  definition of, 436
  history in, 440–441
  management of, 443
  mechanisms of, 438–439, *438, 440, 443*
  physical examination and, 441
  upper airway obstruction in, causes of, 437–438, 437t
Stroke, differentiating from TIAs, 475
  incidence among TGA patients, 9
Stroke Data Bank, 480
Subglottic hemangiomas, 212
Submandibular gland, 507, *512*
Submandibular lymph nodes, lymphadenopathy of, 297
Substance abuse. See also *Alcohol consumption; Drugs.*
  anxiety associated with, 34
  cocaine, 77, 113, 174
  heroin, 156
  tachyarrhythmia associated with, 455
Substance P, and bone pain, 53
Substernal pain. See *Chest pain.*
Sudan stain, steatorrhea evaluation with, 433
Sudden infant death syndrome, bradycardia associated with, 62t
Suicide, fugue state associated with, 15
Superego anxiety, 30
Supraventricular tachyarrhythmias, 454, 456
  differentiating from ventricular tachyarrhythmias, 463
Swan-Ganz catheterization, 102–103
Sympathoadrenal system, congestive heart failure and, 98
Sympathomimetic compounds, anxiety associated with, 34
Symthe criteria for fibrositis, 155
Syncope, pallid infantile, seizure simulated by, 415–416
    seizures simulated by, 416
Syndrome of Wallenberg, ataxia associated with, 40
Syndrome X. See *Microvascular angina.*
Synovial fluid analysis, 367t
Syphilis, false-positive tests for, 26
    inner-ear deafness associated with, 183
    oral chancre, tongue, *325*
    oral ulcers associated with, 321, 325
    secondary, and lymphadenopathy, 296
Syphilitic aortitis, chest pain associated with, 75
Systemic diseases, associated with KCS, 126
    autoimmune, xerostomia and, 510–511, 514
Systemic lupus erythematosus (SLE), 363. See also
    Lupus erythematosus (LE).
  ANA positive tests in, 26
  anorexia associated with, 17
  azotemia associated with, 48
  false positive ELISA tests associated with, 218
  FANA positive tests in, percentage of, 23t
  interstitial lung disease accompanying, 268
  limb pain associated with, 290
  lymphadenopathy in, 294
  proteinuria and, 383
  Raynaud's phenomenon and, 388, 391
  Sjögren's syndrome associated with, 127

Systemic vasculitis. See also *Polyarteritis*.
  necrotizing, radiographic studies in, 360
  polyarteritis group features, 359t
Systolic murmurs, 79–80, 444–453
  assessment of, 450–453
  cardiovascular examination in, 446t
  congenital cardiac disorders and, 445t
  diagnostic studies in, 449–450
  ejection, genesis of, *451*
  etiology of, 448t
  functional, 451–452
  history in, 445–446
  mitral valve prolapse and, 452
  physical examination and, 446–449
    cardiac auscultation, 448–449, 449t
  second heart sound and, 448t

Tachyarrhythmias, 453–463
  atrial, chaotic, electrocardiogram in, *458*
    electrocardiogram in, *457*
    fibrillation and RBBB, *459*
    fibrillation in WPW syndrome, *459*
    flutter and, electrocardiogram, *459*
    with AV block, electrocardiogram in, *458*
  AV junctional rhythm, electrocardiogram, *460*
  classifications of, 454t
  definition of, 453
  electrocardiograms in, 456–462
  history in, 455–456
  management of, 463
  physical examination and, 456
  prevalence of, 454
  re-entrant, 454
    electrocardiogram, *454, 457, 457, 460*
  supraventricular, 454, 456, 463
    torsades de pointes, electrocardiogram, *461*
  ventricular, 454, 456, 462
    electrocardiogram, *461, 462*
    with AV dissociation,
      electrocardiogram, *460*
Tachycardia, atrial, *458*
  carotid sinus massage effect on, 457
  P wave in, 457
  with AV block, 458
    atrioventricular (AV) nodal re-entrant, 453
    P wave morphology during, 457
    re-entrant, 458–459, 460, 461
      SA, 457, *457*
    reciprocating AV, 453, 461
    re-entrant, 453
    stress-associated, 156
    ventricular, 261, 456, *460, 461*
    Wolff-Parkinson-White syndrome and, 453–454

Tachypnea, 463–469
  assessment of, *468*, 469
  definition of, 463
  diagnostic studies in, *468*, 469
  differential diagnosis of, 468t
  emergent, 467t
  history in, 465–466
  physical examination and, 466–468
  rate and rhythm of breathing and, 467t
  receptors that control ventilation, 464t
Takayasu's arteritis, 389
Tamm-Horsfall mucoprotein, 379
Tamponade, cardiac, 343
  diagnosis of, 345

Tangier disease, 226t
Taste, cacogeusic sensation in, 349, 354
  distortions of, *349*, 355t
  torqueguesic sensation in, 349, 354
Taste and Smell Clinic, Washington, D.C., 353
Tay-Sachs disease, athetosis associated with, 44
Tears, 123
  deficiency, dry eye syndrome and, 123t
Telangiectasias, abdominal pain associated with, 3
Temporal hemianopsia, obesity associated with, 503
Temporal lobe dysfunction, amnesia as a symptom of, 8
Tendinitis, myofascial pain versus, 319–320 rotator cuff,
  55
Testicular disorders, mumps and atrophy of, 399
  torsion, 396
    scrotal pain associated with, 397–398
  vasculitis, necrotizing, 361
Testicular pain. See *Scrotal pain.*
Testosterone, levels in chronic fatigue, 156
Theca lutein cyst, pregnancy and, 337
Thelarche, normal progression of, 309
Thermography, for breast mass assessment, 70
Thiamine, deficiency, and amnesia, 11
  glucose metabolism, dependence on, 13
  Wernicke encephalopathy and, treatment with, 12
Thoracic angiography, for mediastinal mass evaluation,
  303–304
Thoracotomy, 307
  and mediastinal mass evaluation, 305–306
Thromboangiitis obliterans, Raynaud's phenomenon
  versus, 390
Thromboembolism, pulmonary, chest pain associated
  with, 75
Thromboplastin time (PTT), partial, 367
Thrombosis, spermatic vein, 396
Thymoma, 307
Thyroglobulin antibody, Sjögren's syndrome and, 127
Thyroglobulin levels, 472
Thyroglossal duct cyst, 471
Thyroid. See also *Hyperthyroidism; Hypothyroidism;
  Thyroid enlargement; Thyroid stimulating hormone (TSH).*
  acropachy, clubbing associated with, 97
  and constipation, 107
  and depression, 154
  and likelihood of cancer, 471t
  and obesity, 503
  cancer of, hoarseness and, 472
Thyroid enlargement, assessment of, 473–474
  autoimmune thyrotoxicosis and, 472
  diagnostic studies in, 472–473
  goiter
    euthyroid and, 474
    evaluation and, 471, 471t
  history in, 470–471
  hyperthyroidism and, 473
  hypothyroidism and, 473
  incidence of, 470
  malignancy and, 474
  physical examination and, 471–472
  primary hypothyroidism, diagnosis of, 472
  radioiodine uptake in, 472
  thyroid cancer and, 471t
Thyroid stimulating hormone (TSH), for thyroid function evaluation, 504
Thyroiditis, 473
  associated with connective tissue diseases, 24
  Hashimoto's, 311
Thyrotoxicosis, congestive heart failure in, 103

Thyrotropin releasing hormone (TRH), 504
Thyroxine (T₄) test, 472
TIA-like syndromes, causes of, 476t
Tics, characteristics of, 42t
Tietze's syndrome, chest pain associated with, 78
Todd's paralysis, 413
Tolbutamide test, 257
Tophi, hyperuricemia and, 246
Torqueguesic taste sensation, 349, 354
Torsades de pointes, 456, *461*, 462
   magnesium deficiency associated with, 261
Toxic keratoconjunctivitis, symptoms of, 124t
Toxic reactions, hallucinations in, 177–178
Toxoplasmosis, lymphadenopathy associated with, 294, 299
   MRI evaluation of, 284
Transhepatic cholangiography (PTC), percutaneous, 5
   for cholestasis assessment, 89
   for hepatomegaly evaluation, 201
Transient global amnesia (TGA), 8–10, 478
Transient ischemic attacks (TIAs), 475–480
   assessment of, 480
   diagnostic studies and, 479–480
   history in, 477–479t
   ischemic stroke and, causes of, 477t
   neurologic symptoms and vascular territory in, 476t
   nonischemic causes of, 476t
   physical examination and, 479
Transillumination, for cough assessment, 114
Trauma, dyspareunia caused by, 133
   dysuria associated with, 139
   pericarditis caused by, 347
   scrotal pain associated with, 399
   stridor associated with, 438
   ulcers caused by, 324, *324*
Tremors, characteristics of, 42t
Trench mouth, 325
Tricuspid insufficiency, 447
Trigger points, 317–318
   latent and active, 315
Triglycerides (TG), hypercholesterolemia and, 228, 230–231
Tri-iodothyronine (T₃) test, 472
Trypsinogen radioimmunoassay (RIA), serum, 434
Tryptophan, and chronic fatigue, 156
Tubal pregnancy. See *Ectopic pregnancy*.
Tubal sterilization, and ectopic pregnancy, 145
Tuberculosis, anorexia associated with, 17
   hoarseness and, 213
   oral ulcers associated with, 321
Tuberculous meningitis, amnesia associated with, 15
Tularemia, 294
Tumors. See also *Cancer; Malignancy*.
   cerebellopontine angle, 182
   erythrocytosis associated with, 378
   insulin-producing, and hypoglycemia, 256–257
   larynx, 214
   markers of, 338
   primary bone, lesions that simulate, 59t
   stridor associated with, 438
   testicular, scrotal pain associated with, 399
Tympanometry, 182
Typhoid fever, thiamine deficiency in, 12
Tyrosinase, melanin and, 233

Ulcerative gingivitis, acute necrotizing, 321
Ulcers, 324
   aphthous, 321, 326

Ulcers (*continued*)
   oral, 321–327
   peptic, 275
      chest pain associated with, 78
   traumatic, *324*
Ultrasonography, for abnormal pregnancy diagnosis, 148
   for hepatomegaly evaluation, 201
   for scrotal pain evaluation, 397
   hepatic, 196
Ultrasound, abdominal, for cholestasis assessment, 89
   for abdominal pain evaluation, 4
   for dysuria evaluation, 138
   for limb pain evaluation, 290
   for pelvic mass evaluation, 338
   for thyroid enlargement evaluation, 472–473
   for TIA evaluation, 480
   vaginal probe, 132
Unilateral clubbing, 94t
Unstable angina, 76–77, 421
   evaluation of, 423
Upper airway obstruction, causes of, 437t
Urea nitrogen, blood (BUN), renal failure, acute, and, 48
Uremic pericarditis, 347
Uric acid, acute renal failure and, 48t
   biosynthesis of, 240
   elevated level of, 239–248
   renal handling of, *241*
   underexcretion of, 243–244
Uricase, purine metabolism and, 240
Urinary protein values, 380t
Urinary tract infection, constipation-related, 105
Urine, azotemia diagnostic indices, 49t
   in azotemia, 48
   sediment findings and azotemia-related disorders, 49t
Urolithiasis, hyperuricemia and, 247
Urologic masses, 336
Usual interstitial pneumonitis (UIP), 267
   interstitial pulmonary disease and, 267
Uterine curettage, ectopic pregnancy and, 149
Uterus, 336–337

Vagina, masses in, 336
Valproate, treating seizures with, 418
Varicella-zoster infection (chicken pox), 484–485
Varicocele, scrotal pain associated with, 400
Vascular insufficiency, bone pain associated with, 58–59
Vasculitides, classification of, 358t
Vasculitis, systemic, necrotizing, radiographic studies in, 360
   polyarteritis group features, 359t
Vasectomy, scrotal pain following, 396, 401
Vasodilation, in clubbing, 92
Vasopressin, scrotal pain associated with use of, 395
Venography, hepatic, hepatomegaly evaluation with, 201
Ventilation-perfusion imaging (V/Q scan), chest pain evaluation using, 83–84
Ventricular disorders, 456
   ectopy, bradycardia-induced, 65
   fibrillation, 462
      magnesium deficiency and, 261
   hypertrophy, chest pain with, 73
   pre-excitation, atrial fibrillation with, *459*
   rhythm and, and bradycardia associated with, 65
   tachyarrhythmias, 454, 462

Ventricular disorders (*continued*)
  tachycardia, 456, *460*, *461*
    hypomagnesemia associated with, 261
Vertebrobasilar insufficiency, amnesia in, 9
Very low-density lipoprotein (VLDL), atherosclerosis,
    and levels of, 223
Vesicles, defined, 481
Vesicoureteral reflex, constipation-related, 105
Vesiculobullous disorders, 481–491
  allergic contact dermatitis, *489*
  assessment of, 483–491
  blisters, classification by age of presentation, 482t
  bullous arthropod reactions, 489–490
  bullous drug eruptions, *489*, *490*
  bullous impetigo, 490, *490*
  bullous pemphigoid, 488, *488*, *489*
  definitions of, 481
  dermatitis herpetiformis, *485*, *486*
  diagnostic studies in, 482–483
  empidermolysis bullosa, *484*
  hand-foot-and-mouth disease, *485*
  herpes gestationis and, 486
  herpes simplex infection, primary, *490*
  history in, 482
  immunofluorescent patterns in, 483t
  incontinentia pigmenti and, *484*
  pemphigus vulgaris, 486–487, *487*
  physical examination and, 482
  porphyria cutanea tarda, 487, *488*
Vestibulitis, 131
Viral laryngotracheobronchitis (croup), 437
Viral pericarditis, 346
Viral ulcers, oral, 324–325
Visceral pain, 1
Visions. See *Hallucinations.*
Visual loss, bilateral versus unilateral vision loss, 492
    polyarteritis associated with, 360
    unilateral, 492–498
      age-related macular degeneration and, 495–496,
        495
      anterior ischemic optical neuropathy and, 497–
        498, *497*
      cataract and, 495
      causes of, 494–498
      definition of, 492
      dry eye and, 494
      glaucoma and, 494–495
      history in, 492
      optic neuritis and, 498, *498*
      physical examination and, 492–494
      retinal artery occlusion, central, 496–497, *496*
      retinal detachment and, 496, *496*
      retinal vein occlusion, central, and, 497, *497*
      symptoms associated with, 493, 493t
Vitamin B$_{12}$-binding capacity, polycythemia evaluation
    and, 374
Vitamin deficiency(ies), cholestasis and, 87
  dry eye syndrome and, 123
  steatorrhea and, 432
  vitamin E, ataxia associated with, 40
  vitamin K, cholestasis associated with, 88
Vocal abuse and misuse, 206
Vocal cord, bowing of, 214
  hoarseness
    and granulomas, 213
    and nodules or polyps on, 213
  nodules on, 212
  paralysis of, 212, 213
Vogt's disease, 42

Voice production, 204–205. See also *Dysphonia;*
    Hoarseness; Vocal cord.
Von Recklinghausen's disease, 180
  hypertension and, 405
Vulvar masses, 336
Vulvitis, 131
Vulvovaginitis, dysuria associated with, 139

Waldenström's macroglobulinemia, hearing loss associ-
    ated with, 184
Walk-through angina, 76
Warfarin, hematochezia caused by, 189
    hyperuricemia caused by, 243
Watershed infarction, amnesia in, 14–15
Weber test of hearing, 181–182
Wegener's granulomatosis, 271, 360
  interstitial pulmonary disease associated with, 272
Weight gain, 499–505
  assessment of, 505
  body mass index for measuring, 503, *504*
  diagnostic studies in, 502–505
  drugs reported to cause, 501–502, 501t
  history in, 502
  management of, 505
  medications and, 501–502, 501t
  Metropolitan height and weight tables, 500t
  obesity and, 499
    theories, 499–500
  physical examination and, 502–503
  prevalence of, 499
  psychiatric conditions and, 500
  smoking cessation and, 502
Weight loss, abdominal pain and, 3
Wernicke's encephalopathy, 11–12, 40
Wernicke-Korsakoff syndrome, hallucinations associ-
    ated with, 11–14, 174
West's syndrome, 417–418
Western blot test, HIV diagnosis with, 218
Wheezing, differentiating from stridor, 439–440
Whipple's disease, 250
  steatorrhea with, 435
Wilms' tumor, polycythemia associated with, 378
Wilson's disease, 200
  athetosis associated with, 44
  hepatomegaly associated with, 198, 199
Window period phenomenon, in HIV infection, 218
Wolff-Parkinson-White syndrome, AV reciprocating
    tachycardia and, 453–454
    Q waves in, 80
    atrial fibrillation with, *459*

Xanthine oxidase inhibitor (allopurinol), hyperuricemia
    treated with, 248
Xanthoderma, 233
Xanthomas, abdominal pain associated with, 3
    and familial hypercholesterolemias, 227
Xerostomia, 506–515
  assessment in, 514–515
  definition of, 506
  diagnostic studies in, 513–514
  drugs causing, 509t, 540t
  glands involved in, *512*
  history in, 511–512
  illnesses caused by, 510t
  minor salivary glands and, *514*
  phantogeusia associated with, 354
  physical examination and, 512–513

Xerostomia (*continued*)
  salivary gland and, *508*
  systemic factors and illnesses causing, 510t
  treatment of, 514t
X-rays, chest. See *Chest X-ray.*
  interstitial pulmonary disease evaluation with, 270
  lymphadenopathy evaluation with, 296–297
  mediastinal mass evaluation with, 303
  sinus, cough assessment with, 114
  stridor evaluation with, 442
  D-Xylose test, 434–435

Yohimbine, anxiety precipitated by, 29
Young adults, anorexia in, 20

Zenker's diverticulum, 352
  cough and, 112
Zidovudine. See *Azidothymidine (AZT).*
Zinc deficiency, chronic fatigue and, 156–157
Zollinger-Ellison syndrome, secretory diarrhea associated with, 118
  screening for, 4